Tumors of the Adrenal Gland and Extra-Adrenal Paraganglia

Atlas of Tumor Pathology

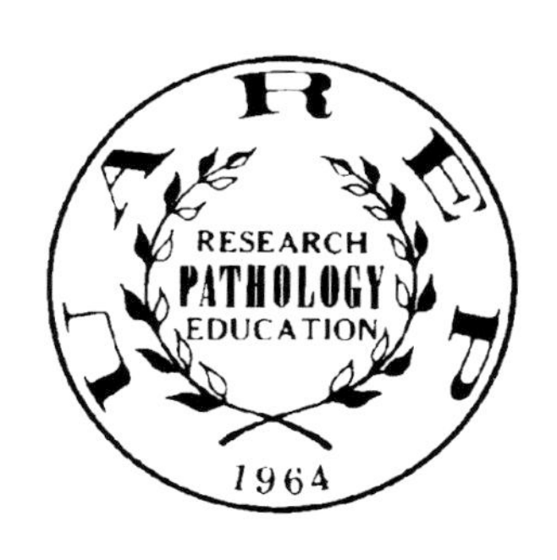

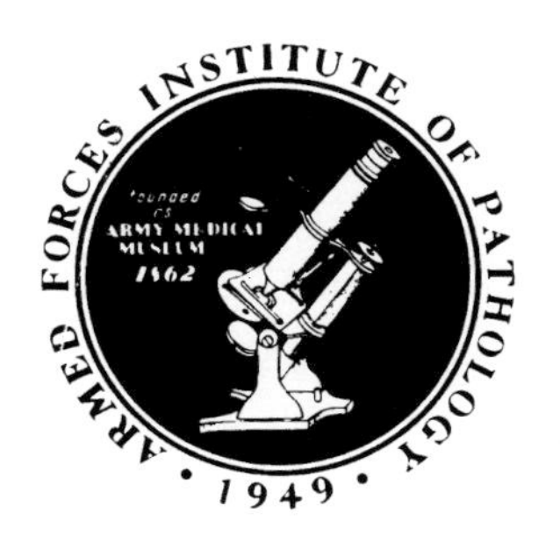

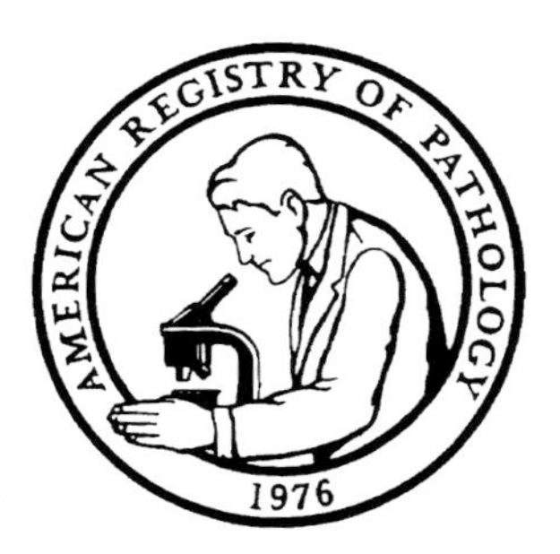

D1127452

ATLAS OF TUMOR PATHOLOGY

Third Series
Fascicle 19

TUMORS OF THE ADRENAL GLAND AND EXTRA-ADRENAL PARAGANGLIA

by

ERNEST E. LACK, M.D.
Director of Anatomic Pathology and
Professor of Pathology
Georgetown University School of Medicine
Washington, D.C. 20007

Published by the
ARMED FORCES INSTITUTE OF PATHOLOGY
Washington, D.C.

Under the Auspices of
UNIVERSITIES ASSOCIATED FOR RESEARCH AND EDUCATION IN PATHOLOGY, INC.
Bethesda, Maryland
1997

Accepted for Publication
1995

Available from the American Registry of Pathology
Armed Forces Institute of Pathology
Washington, D.C. 20306-6000
ISSN 0160-6344
ISBN 1-881041-28-X

ATLAS OF TUMOR PATHOLOGY

EDITOR
JUAN ROSAI, M.D.
Department of Pathology
Memorial Sloan-Kettering Cancer Center
New York, New York 10021-6007

ASSOCIATE EDITOR
LESLIE H. SOBIN, M.D.
Armed Forces Institute of Pathology
Washington, D.C. 20306-6000

EDITORIAL ADVISORY BOARD

Jeffrey Cossman, M.D.	Georgetown University School of Medicine Washington, D.C. 20007
Ronald A. DeLellis, M.D.	Tufts University School of Medicine Boston, Massachusetts 02111
Glauco Frizzera, M.D.	New York University Medical Center New York, New York 10016
Leonard B. Kahn, M.D.	Long Island Jewish Hospital New Hyde Park, New York 11042
Richard L. Kempson, M.D.	Stanford University Medical School Stanford, California 94305
Paul Peter Rosen, M.D.	Memorial Sloan-Kettering Cancer Center New York, New York 10021
Robert E. Scully, M.D.	Harvard Medical School and Massachusetts General Hospital Boston, Massachusetts 02114
Steven G. Silverberg, M.D.	University of Maryland School of Medicine Baltimore, Maryland 21201
Sharon Weiss, M.D.	University of Michigan School of Medicine Ann Arbor, Michigan 48109-0602

EDITORS' NOTE

The Atlas of Tumor Pathology has a long and distinguished history. It was first conceived at a Cancer Research Meeting held in St. Louis in September 1947 as an attempt to standardize the nomenclature of neoplastic diseases. The first series was sponsored by the National Academy of Sciences-National Research Council. The organization of this Sisyphean effort was entrusted to the Subcommittee on Oncology of the Committee on Pathology, and Dr. Arthur Purdy Stout was the first editor-in-chief. Many of the illustrations were provided by the Medical Illustration Service of the Armed Forces Institute of Pathology, the type was set by the Government Printing Office, and the final printing was done at the Armed Forces Institute of Pathology (hence the colloquial appellation "AFIP Fascicles"). The American Registry of Pathology purchased the Fascicles from the Government Printing Office and sold them virtually at cost. Over a period of 20 years, approximately 15,000 copies each of nearly 40 Fascicles were produced. The worldwide impact that these publications have had over the years has largely surpassed the original goal. They quickly became among the most influential publications on tumor pathology ever written, primarily because of their overall high quality but also because their low cost made them easily accessible to pathologists and other students of oncology the world over.

Upon completion of the first series, the National Academy of Sciences-National Research Council handed further pursuit of the project over to the newly created Universities Associated for Research and Education in Pathology (UAREP). A second series was started, generously supported by grants from the AFIP, the National Cancer Institute, and the American Cancer Society. Dr. Harlan I. Firminger became the editor-in-chief and was succeeded by Dr. William H. Hartmann. The second series Fascicles were produced as bound volumes instead of loose leaflets. They featured a more comprehensive coverage of the subjects, to the extent that the Fascicles could no longer be regarded as "atlases" but rather as monographs describing and illustrating in detail the tumors and tumor-like conditions of the various organs and systems.

Once the second series was completed, with a success that matched that of the first, UAREP and AFIP decided to embark on a third series. A new editor-in-chief and an associate editor were selected, and a distinguished editorial board was appointed. The mandate for the third series remains the same as for the previous ones, i.e., to oversee the production of an eminently practical publication with surgical pathologists as its primary audience, but also aimed at other workers in oncology. The main purposes of this series are to promote a consistent, unified, and biologically sound nomenclature; to guide the surgical pathologist in the diagnosis of the various tumors and tumor-like lesions; and to provide relevant histogenetic, pathogenetic, and clinicopathologic information on these entities. Just as the second series included data obtained from ultrastructural (and, in the more recent Fascicles, immunohistochemical) examination, the third series will, in addition, incorporate pertinent information obtained with the newer molecular biology techniques. As in the past, a continuous attempt will be made to correlate, whenever possible, the nomenclature used in the Fascicles with that proposed by the World Health Organization's International Histological Classification of Tumors. The format of the third series has been changed in order to incorporate additional items and to ensure a consistency of style throughout. Close cooperation between the various authors and their respective liaisons from the editorial board will be emphasized to minimize unnecessary repetition and discrepancies in the text and illustrations.

To its everlasting credit, the participation and commitment of the AFIP to this venture is even more substantial and encompassing than in previous series. It now extends to virtually all scientific, technical, and financial aspects of the production.

The task confronting the organizations and individuals involved in the third series is even more daunting than in the preceding efforts because of the ever-increasing complexity of the matter at hand. It is hoped that this combined effort—of which, needless to say, that represented by the authors is first and foremost—will result in a series worthy of its two illustrious predecessors and will be a suitable introduction to the tumor pathology of the twenty-first century.

Juan Rosai, M.D.
Leslie H. Sobin, M.D.

ACKNOWLEDGMENTS

This third series Fascicle, Tumors of the Adrenal Gland and Extra-Adrenal Paraganglia, includes topics covered in two previous second series Fascicles - Tumors of the Extra-Adrenal Paraganglion System (Including Chemoreceptors) by Drs. George G. Glenner and Philip M. Grimley and Tumors of the Adrenal by Drs. David L. Page, Ronald A. DeLellis, and Aubrey J. Hough, Jr. Both of these Fascicles provide a sound, basic framework upon which to expand existing concepts, focus on specific neoplasms and tumor-like lesions, and highlight newly recognized or evolving entities. A broad array of topics are covered herein, and to achieve a better understanding of the various neoplasms of the adrenal cortex, medulla, and extra-adrenal paraganglia, morphologic aspects of normal anatomy and hyperplasia are illustrated in some detail.

The contributions of cytology and fine needle aspiration to diagnosis are emphasized particularly with respect to adrenal tumors. Some of the benign adrenal (and occasionally extra-adrenal) tumors can be diagnosed by cytologic evaluation, thus avoiding unnecessary surgery, and therefore some of these lesions may not become surgical pathology specimens. The imaging characteristics of the lesions on computed tomographic (CT) scan or magnetic resonance imaging (MRI) are very important in correlation with the cytologic findings, and in essence they become the gross pathology in some cases. Appropriate emphasis is given, therefore, to imaging studies. The author wishes to thank Dr. Richard Patt for kindly providing succinct information on the imaging characteristics of a number of different entities of the adrenal glands.

Several physicians have contributed photographic material for this Fascicle, and they are acknowledged in the corresponding figure legends or text. I thank Ms. Eileen Rusnock for the technical assistance, Ms. Kiran Verma for the preparation of electron micrographs, the Educational Media at Georgetown University for their skillful services, and Mr. Oscar Rodbell for his photographic assistance. The author also acknowledges the skillful typing of the manuscript by Mr. Harold Brayman and, as a final note, the thoughtful comments and suggestions of the reviewers and in particular the guidance, patience, and support of Dr. Juan Rosai.

A large token of appreciation is also expressed to the editorial staff, Ms. Dian Thomas, Mr. Andrew Male, and Ms. Audrey Kahn for their assistance in the preparation of this Fascicle. I would also like to thank Mr. Ken Stringfellow for his skillful color separation and preparation of the many figures used in this Fascicle.

Ernest E. Lack, M.D.

Permission to use copyrighted illustrations has been granted by:

American Medical Association:
Arch Pathol 1962;335:345–55. For figure 7-20.
Arch Pathol Lab Med 1980;104:46–51. For figure 12-15.

American Society for Investigative Pathology:
Am J Pathol 1985;119:301–14. For figure 15-5.

Appleton & Lange:
Pathol Annu 1992;27:1–53. For figures 6-1, 6-4, 6-5, 6-7, and 6-23.

Blackwell Scientific:
Endocr Pathol 1992;3:116–128. For figure 6-2, tables 6-1 and 6-2.
Acta Physiol Scand 1951;22:14–43. For figure 14-4.

Churchill Livingstone:
Pathology of the Adrenal Glands, 1990. For figures 1-1, 1-9, 1-10, 1-19, 1-44, 2-2, 2-8, 2-12, 2-20, 3-22, 5-3, 5-25, 7-12, 8-13, 8-15, 10-41, 10-49, 11-3, 12-2, 12-10, 23-16, 23-32, 23-50, 23-56, 23-59, 23-60, and Table 5-1.

Humana Press:
J Urol Pathol 1994;2:265–72. For figure 7-30.

John Wiley and Sons:
Cancer 1961;14:421–5. For figure 23-70B.
Cancer 1979;43:269–78. For figure 20-5.
Cancer 1992;69:2197–211. For figure 23-52.

Lippincott-Raven:
J Computr Assist Tomogr 1991;15:773–779. For figure 3-21.
Am J Surg Pathol 1979;3:85–92. For figure 19-3.
Am J Surg Pathol 1980;4:109–120. For figure 12-15.
Am J Surg Pathol 1983;7:699–705. For figure 23-70A.
Diagnostic Surgical Pathology, 1994. For figure 15-1.

Radiology Society of America:
Radiology 1979;132:99–105. For figure 17-7.

Springer-Verlag:
Anat Embryol 1983;166:439–451. For figure 1-2.

Taylor and Francis:
Ultrastruct Pathol 1985;8:333–343. For table 22-1.

WB Saunders:
Hum Pathol 1979;10:191–218. For figures 16-26 and 19-4.
J Clin Oncol 1984;2:719–32. For figures 23-1, 23-3, 23-41 and 23-54.
Pathology of the Adrenal and Extra-adrenal Paraganglia. Major Problems in Pathology, Vol. 29, 1994. For figures 1-32, 1-34, 1-37, 1-39, 1-47, 9-2, 10-16, 10-18, 11-7, 12-16, 13-6, 15-10, 16-3, 16-5–16-7, 17-2, 17-4, 17-6, 17-16, 18-2, 18-11, 20-9, 21-4, 22-3–22-8, 22-16, 23-4, 23-5, 23-12, and 23-33.

Contents

TUMORS OF THE ADRENAL GLAND AND EXTRA-ADRENAL PARAGANGLIA

1
DEVELOPMENTAL, PHYSIOLOGIC, AND ANATOMIC ASPECTS OF ADRENAL CORTEX AND MEDULLA

The adrenal cortex plays a vital role in the regulation of water and electrolyte balance, mainly by secretion of mineralocorticoids, and it also mediates important changes in intermediary metabolism affecting proteins, carbohydrates, and fat. Glucocorticoids modulate a variety of processes including wound healing, growth, and inflammation, and affect the immune system. The adrenal glands are also involved in reacting to stress and changes in the environment which mandate rapid adaptations. This homeostatic role is mediated largely by the adrenal medullae which secrete catecholamines, mainly epinephrine (7); the physiologic changes are rapid and the effects are short term. The adrenal cortex is also involved in reacting to stress through activation of the hypothalamic-pituitary axis and trophic stimulation of the glands by adrenocorticotropic hormone (ACTH). The physiology and endocrinology of the adrenal cortex and medulla are far too complex to be adequately addressed here. It is essential, however, to have a fundamental knowledge of the physiology, structure, and function of the adrenal cortex and medulla in the investigation of endocrinologic abnormalities of the adrenal glands.

EMBRYOLOGY AND BIOSYNTHETIC PATHWAYS

Embryologic Development of the Adrenal Cortex

Crowder (4) detailed the early events in the embryonic development of the adrenal cortex and medulla in staged human embryos; the important Carnegie stages in embryogenesis of the adrenal glands are shown in Table 1-1 (9). The adrenal cortical primordia first appear during Carnegie stage 14 just lateral to the dorsal mesentery near the cephalic end of the mesonephros; at this time there is a change in the characteristics of the cells of the coelomic epithelium, which are of mesodermal origin. At stage 15 there is a cellular proliferation continuous with overlying epithelium in an area designated as the adrenal ridge (fig. 1-1). From stages 15 to 18 the adrenal primordia are cigar shaped and extend from vertebral segments T6 to L1 lateral to aorta and mesogastrium (9). The first group of cells, called C1 cells (fig. 1-2), migrate to the area of the adrenal ridge, enlarge, and become polyhedral with eosinophilic cytoplasm. According to Crowder, a new group of cells (C2) appears in the medial wall of the mesonephric glomeruli and migrates into the adrenal primordium at stage 15; these appear to give rise to the connective tissue framework and capsule of the developing adrenal gland. A second wave of cells (C3) from coelomic epithelium appears at Carnegie stage 16, and both C1 and C3 cells enter the adrenal primordia.

The developing adrenal gland grows as new cells accumulate in the subcapsular zone, also

Table 1-1

IMPORTANT CARNEGIE DEVELOPMENTAL STAGES IN EARLY EMBRYOGENESIS OF HUMAN ADRENAL GLANDS*

Carnegie Stage	Size (mm)	Age (days)
15	7–9	33
16	8–11	37
17	11–14	41
19	16–18	47.5
23	27–31	56.5

*From reference 9.

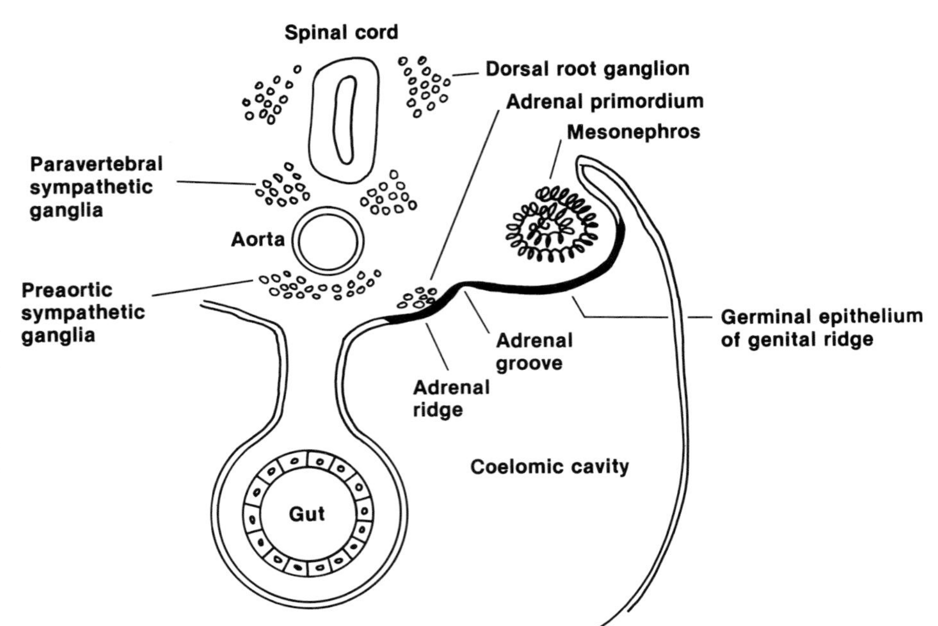

Figure 1-1
PRIMORDIA OF ADRENAL GLANDS

Schematic cross section of a human embryo shows primordia of adrenal glands located lateral to the base of the dorsal mesentery, close to the urogenital ridge. (Fig. 1-3 from Lack EE, Kozakewich HP. Embryology, developmental anatomy and selected aspects of non-neoplastic pathology. In: Lack EE, ed. Pathology of the adrenal glands. New York: Churchill Livingstone, 1990:1–74.)

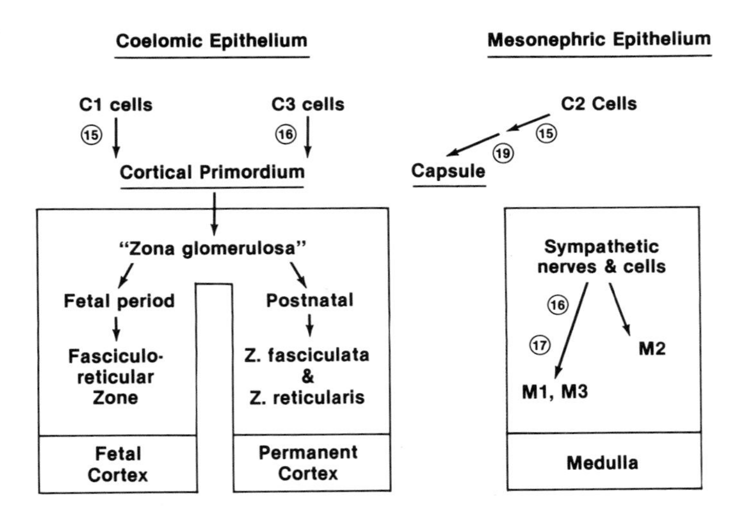

Figure 1-2
CROWDER'S INTERPRETATION OF DEVELOPMENTAL STAGES IN EMBRYOGENESIS OF THE ADRENAL GLANDS

Important stages appear as numerals within circles. C1, C2, C3: cell types in cortex; M1, M2, M3: cell types in medulla. (Modified from fig. 1 from O'Rahilly R. The timing and sequence of events in the development of the human endocrine system during the embryonic period proper. Anat Embryol 1983;166:439–51.)

referred to as the zona glomerulosa. Mitotic figures can be identified in this area. New cells seem to migrate or are forced vis a tergo by replicating cells in a centripetal direction thus forming the inner part of the gland, with irregular cords of cortical cells and intervening sinusoids. The portion of the developing cortex which becomes most prominent is referred to as the fetal or provisional zone. At about 4 months' gestation the adrenal glands are slightly larger than the kidney and most of the glands are composed of fetal cortical cells (fig. 1-3).

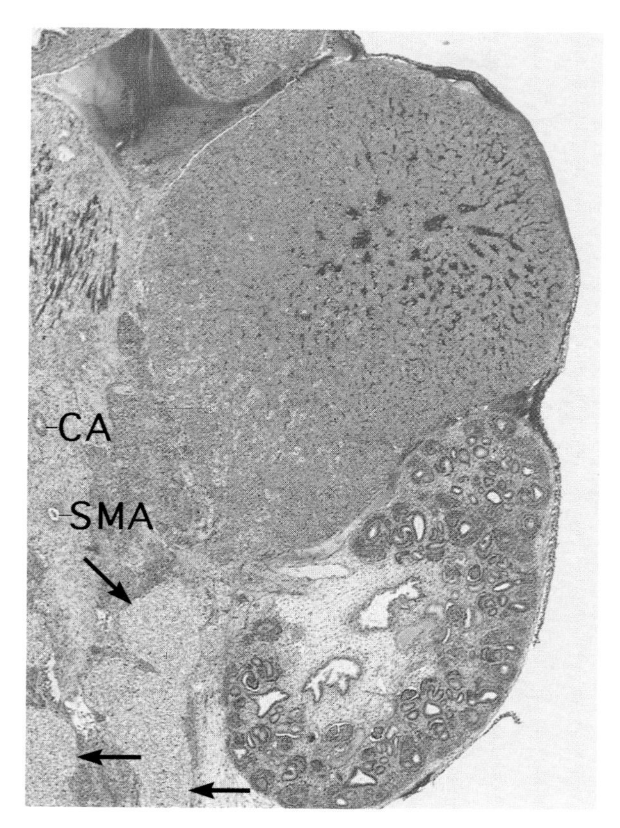

Figure 1-3
CORONAL SECTION OF FETAL KIDNEY AND ADRENAL GLAND AT ABOUT 11 WEEKS' GESTATIONAL AGE

Note the close relation of developing para-aortic sympathetic plexus with medial and inferior aspects of the adrenal gland. Small pale-staining clusters of cells separate cords of provisional or fetal cortical cells in the inferomedial aspect of the gland. Note large collections of extramedullary chromaffin tissue (arrows) representing organs of Zuckerkandl. Celiac (CA) and superior mesenteric (SMA) arteries are also present.

There are two polar theories explaining cell turnover and replacement of adrenal cortical cells. The "cell migration" theory of Gottschau (6) proposes that cortical cells in the zona glomerulosa migrate centripetally, suggesting that a cell is sequentially capable of secreting all of the major classes of cortical steroids. The "zonation" theory of Chester Jones (2) suggests that each zone of the adrenal cortex replaces cells independently. A recent study using cellular kinetics in the experimental animal provided evidence supporting the cell migration theory with the displaced adrenocytes producing all three classes of steroids in sequence through their migration. In this experimental model the "streaming" adrenal cortex is replenished by a subcapsular stem cell (capsular blastema) (14).

Biosynthetic Pathway of Adrenal Corticosteroids

There are three major classes of steroids that are synthesized in the adrenal cortex: mineralocorticoids, glucocorticoids, and sex steroids; their respective biosynthetic pathways are illustrated in figure 1-4. The precursor of steroid hormones is cholesterol, which is stored in an esterified form in the lipid droplets of cortical cells. Aldosterone is produced by cells of the zona glomerulosa, while cortisol is synthesized mainly in the zona fasciculata, with a smaller contribution from the zona reticularis. Sex steroids, mainly dehydroepiandrosterone sulfate, are synthesized in the zona reticularis, although the zona fasciculata is also capable of sex steroid production (10). The secretion of cortisol is regulated by trophic stimulation by ACTH. Aldosterone secretion is stimulated by altered fluid and electrolyte status or decrease in volume of extracellular fluid. The renin-angiotensin system is particularly important in physiologic stimulation of the zona glomerulosa, with angiotensin II acting on these cells to cause synthesis and secretion of aldosterone (12). Other stimulating factors that regulate aldosterone secretion include potassium, atrial natriuretic peptide, and ACTH. Adrenal androgen secretion rises throughout childhood reaching a peak at puberty (adrenarche), and begins to decline at 40 to 50 years of age (adrenopause) (12). The mechanism(s) regulating secretion of adrenal androgens is not entirely clear, but ACTH is a potent stimulant.

Embryologic Development of Adrenal Medulla

At Carnegie stages 16 and 17 (see Table 1-1), a large para-aortic neural complex forms from paravertebral sympathetic ganglia T6 through T12, and usually including L1; included are primordia of adrenal medullae, as well as celiac, superior mesenteric, and renal plexuses. The paravertebral sympathetic ganglia increase in size due to cell division and addition of nerve fibers from the rami communicantes. The ganglia contain three types of cells, M1, M2, and M3,

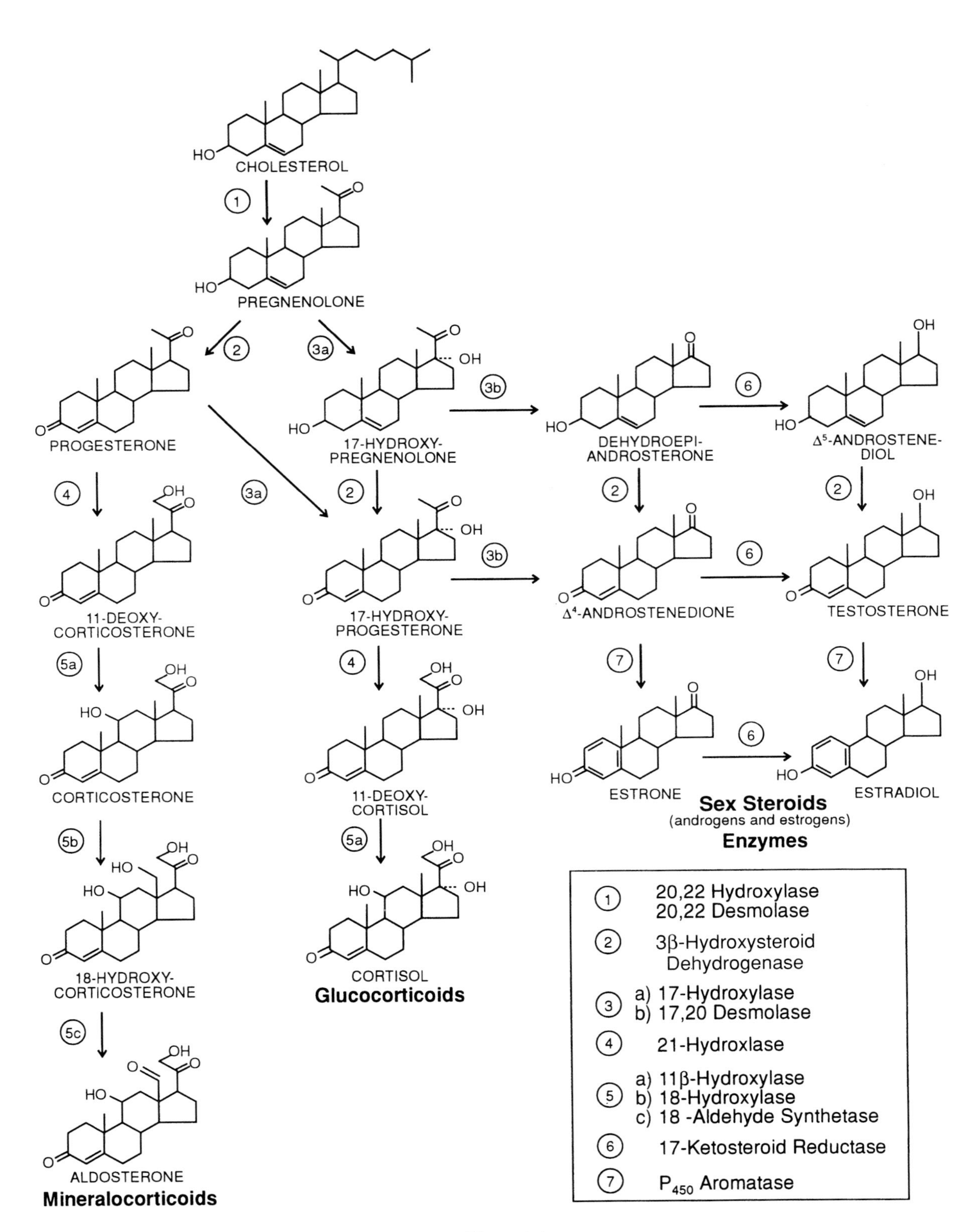

Figure 1-4
ADRENAL CORTICAL STEROIDS
Biosynthetic pathway of the three major classes of adrenal cortical steroids.

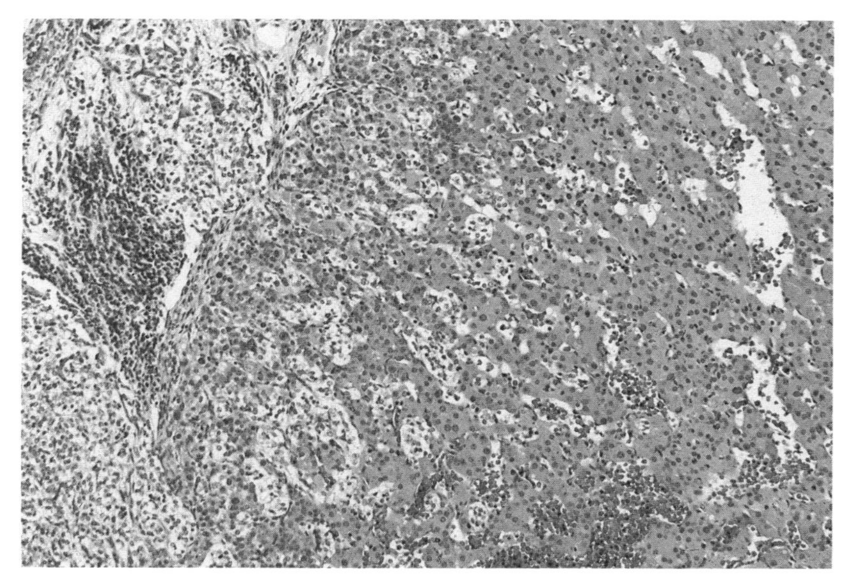

Figure 1-5
MEDIAL ASPECT OF
DEVELOPING ADRENAL GLAND
IN HUMAN FETUS

Note the close association between the developing sympathetic plexus and small nests of pale-staining cells (mostly future chromaffin cells) separating cords of provisional or fetal cortical cells. Primitive cells of the sympathetic plexus (left) contrast with pale-staining cells and those located between cords of cortical cells. Definitive (or adult) cortex is difficult to recognize in this area of developing adrenal gland.

which can be distinguished by size and shape (4). Bundles of nerve fibers and small primitive cells (sympathicoblasts) pass laterally, and enter the dorsal and medial aspect of the adrenal glands, with small collections of cells separating cords of cortical cells (figs. 1-3, 1-5). This separation and disruption of preexisting structures is referred to as "invasion" by Crowder (4), and involves mainly the medial and dorsal aspects of the gland; the ventrolateral part remains relatively intact. Nerve fibers from paravertebral ganglia accompany M1 and M3 cells; M2 cells remain within the ganglia to become sympathetic ganglion cells (fig. 1-2) (9). The M3 (or paraganglion) cells are scattered like seeds along the course of the nerve fibers; these immature cells have sometimes been referred to as pheochromoblasts. The nerve fibers entering the gland before formation of the adrenal capsule maintain their place of entry indefinitely (4).

At stage 19 there are small nests of immature cells scattered throughout most of the cortex, and at stage 23, paraganglion (M3) cells begin to multiply rapidly with some evidence of maturation into chromaffin cells. At the 50-mm size or later a positive chromaffin reaction can be observed (4). Compared to the primitive sympathicoblasts, developing chromaffin cells have slightly enlarged nuclei with dispersed chromatin and pale staining cytoplasm. With postnatal regression of the fetal cortex there is some loss of support for neural elements, which migrate to the area of the central vein.

Clusters of primitive sympathicoblasts (neuroblastic nodules) are an integral histologic component in the normal development of the adrenal glands (fig. 1-6, left), and may linger until birth or early infancy (11). Some neuroblastic nodules may be superficial near the adrenal capsule (fig. 1-6, right), but in the older fetus are located towards the central aspect of the gland due to inward migration, attrition, or relatively greater growth of cortex. There is an increase in number and maximum size of neuroblastic nodules with age, with a peak at 17 to 20 weeks' gestational age, and there is a tendency to regress in older fetuses. Some nodules may be cystic, but usually not until the 16th week of gestation (fig. 1-7). In all age groups combined nodules range from 60 by 60 μm to a maximum of 200 by 400 μm (11). The neuroblastic nodules become significant in the differential diagnosis of in situ neuroblastoma (1).

Biosynthesis of Catecholamines

The biosynthetic pathway for catecholamines is shown in figure 1-8. The substrate for the cytosolic enzyme L-aromatic amino acid decarboxylase is 3,4 dihydroxyphenylalanine (DOPA) which is converted to dopamine. This substance is transported into the storage vesicle where the membrane-bound enzyme dopamine beta-hydroxylase forms norepinephrine (5). The terminal

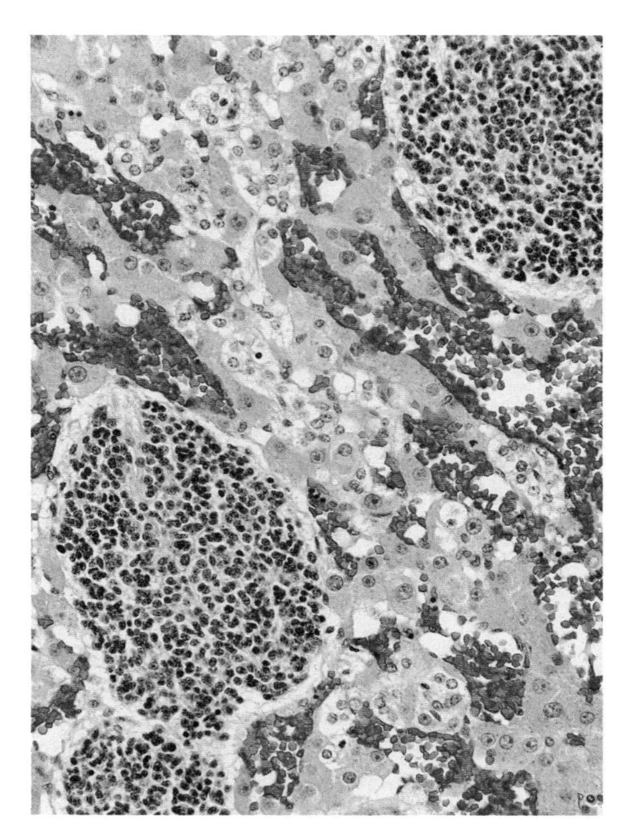

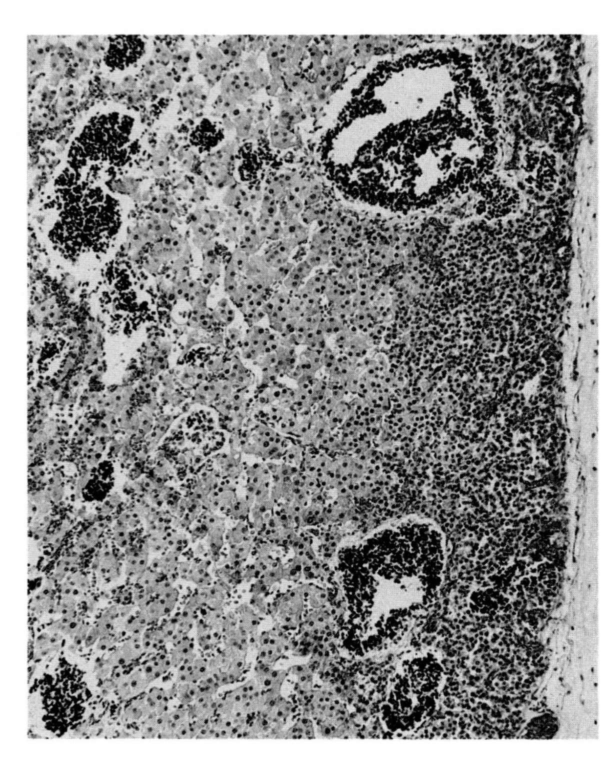

Figure 1-6
DEVELOPING FETAL ADRENAL GLAND

Left: Small nodules of primitive neuroblastic cells are present within the inner aspect of provisional or fetal cortex. A small amount of pale fibrillary matrix is evident in some neuroblastic nodules. Some cells with pale-staining cytoplasm and slightly larger nuclei show early chromaffin cell differentiation.

Right: In an earlier fetus nodules of primitive neuroblastic cells separate columns and cords of provisional or fetal cortical cells. Some are near the adrenal capsule.

Figure 1-7
FETAL ADRENAL GLAND
AT 16 WEEKS' GESTATION

There is prominent cystic change in the neuroblastic nodules, with formation of pale, stringy, proteinaceous contents.

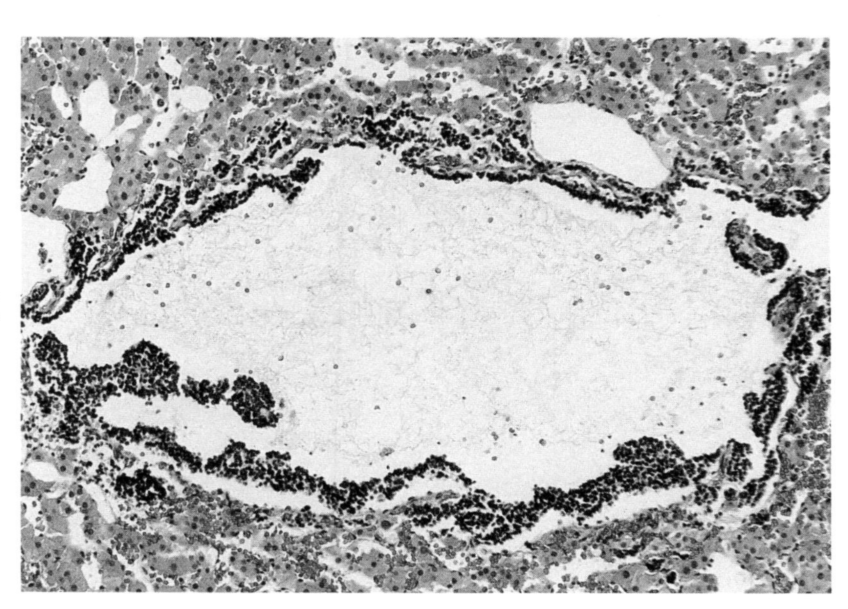

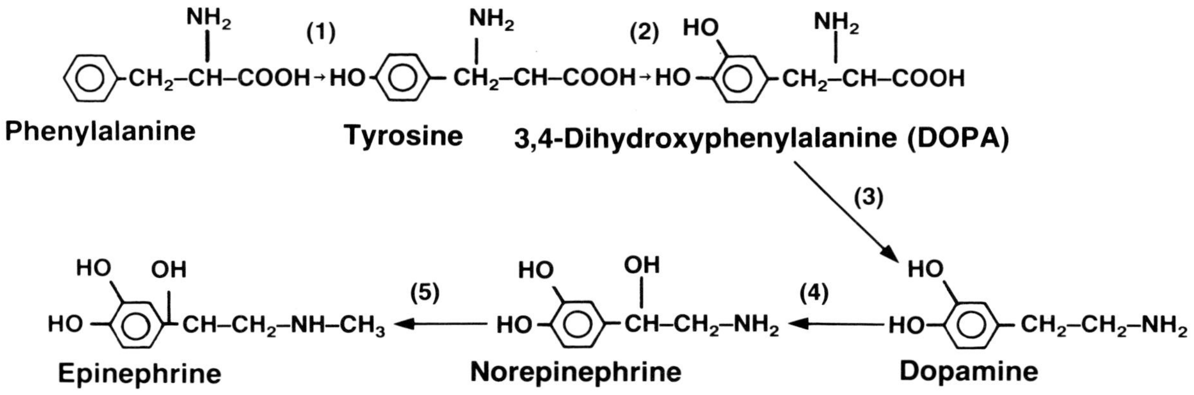

Phenylalanine (1) → Tyrosine (2) → 3,4-Dihydroxyphenylalanine (DOPA) (3) → Dopamine (4) → Norepinephrine (5) → Epinephrine

(1) Phenylalanine hydroxylase, (2) tyrosine hydroxylase, (3) L-aromatic amino acid decarboxylase, (4) dopamine β-hydroxylase, (5) phenylethanolamine N-methyltransferase.

Figure 1-8
BIOSYNTHETIC PATHWAY OF CATECHOLAMINES AND VARIOUS INVOLVED ENZYMES

enzyme in catecholamine synthesis is phenylethanolamine-N-methyltransferase (13), and it is present in the cytosol. This enzyme methylates norepinephrine to form epinephrine which is then taken up again into the vesicle for storage. The chromaffin cell is in essence a postganglionic sympathetic neuron. Following depolarization with influx of calcium, the secretory vesicles move toward the plasma membrane, and through a process of exocytosis the granule contents are expelled into the extracellular space (3). The clearance of catecholamines within the blood is rapid, and epinephrine and norepinephrine have a half life of only 1 to 2 minutes (5). The ratio of epinephrine to norepinephrine in the normal adrenal medulla in adults is about 4 to 1 (8).

FUNCTION OF FETAL ADRENAL GLANDS

The adrenal glands are essentially two endocrine glands in one: in humans, the medulla is completely enveloped by cortex, thus ensuring a microenvironment rich in corticosteroids. The fetal adrenal gland exhibits functional zonation of fetal versus adult cortex. The corticosteroid produced in largest quantity by cells of the fetal zone is dehydroepiandrosterone sulfate (DHAS) while cells of the adult or definitive cortex produce mainly cortisol. Glucocorticoids have an important role in initiation of parturition in some animals, but such a function has not been established in humans (16). Cortisol in particular may have an important role in the induction and maturation of different enzyme systems that are involved in lung maturation, deposition of glycogen in the liver, and induction of several enzymes in fetal brain, retina, pancreas, and gastrointestinal tract (17). Corticosteroids also facilitate synthesis of epinephrine by stimulation or induction of phenylethanolamine-N-methyltransferase (19). DHAS is metabolized in the fetal liver to 16-hydroxy DHAS, and both of these steroids can be hydrolyzed in the placenta with subsequent aromatization to form estrone, estradiol, and estriol; estriol is the major estrogen in the pregnant female (16). This underscores the interdependence of fetus, placenta, and mother in the formation of estrogens. It has been shown that chronic stimulation of fetal cortical cells by ACTH in vitro can give rise to a functional phenotype similar to cells of the adult cortex with increased production of cortisol (18).

Most of the chromaffin tissue in fetal life resides in extra-adrenal sites, particularly the organs of Zuckerkandl where norepinephrine is the predominant catecholamine. It is generally assumed that a high proportion of norepinephrine in the fetal adrenal medulla is indicative of functional immaturity (15). There is some suggestion that fetal chromaffin tissue might be involved in the

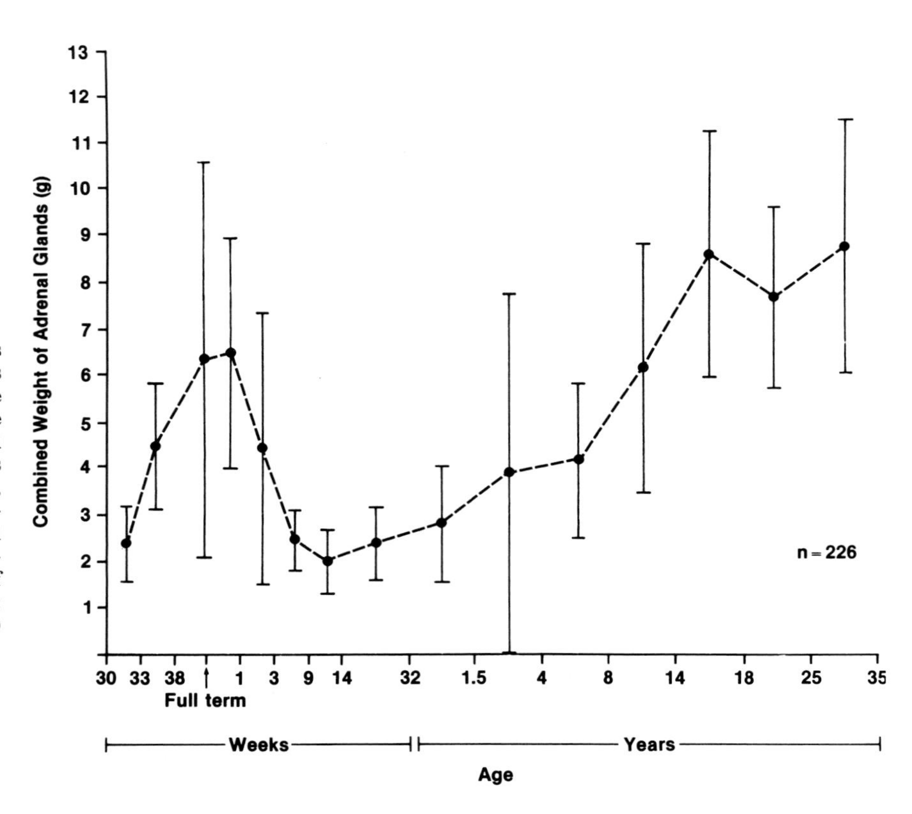

Figure 1-9
AVERAGE COMBINED WEIGHT OF ADRENAL GLANDS FROM 226 PATIENTS AT AUTOPSY

The patients in these autopsies ranged from 30 weeks to 35 years in age. Vertical bars represent one standard deviation. Note the marked decrease in combined weight during the first few weeks of life. (Fig. 1-11 from Lack EE, Kozakewich HP. Embryology, developmental anatomy and selected aspects of non-neoplastic pathology. In: Lack EE, ed. Pathology of the adrenal glands. New York: Churchill Livingstone, 1990:1–74.)

homeostatic maintenance of vascular tone and blood pressure in utero. By 10 to 15 weeks' gestation, epinephrine (soon to be the major catecholamine in the medulla) and norepinephrine are detectable in medullary chromaffin cells (16).

ANATOMY OF ADRENAL GLANDS

Adrenal Weight

The individual or combined weight of the adrenal glands depends upon a number of factors such as age, abnormalities in development, presence and chronicity of diseases of various types, and most importantly, the effort taken to carefully remove adherent connective tissue and fat for accurate specimen weight. Data regarding adrenal weights in infancy and childhood are based per force upon postmortem studies (38). Figure 1-9 shows the average combined weights of meticulously dissected adrenal glands from 226 individuals ranging in age from 30 weeks' gestation to 35 years; the adrenal glands grow considerably towards the end of pregnancy (27). Tähkä (39) studied the average combined weight of adrenals from infants at various postnatal periods: 6.50 g at 0 to 7 days, 6.11 g at 8 to 14 days, and 4.52 g at 15 to 30 days. In another study involving adrenals from 84 children, the average combined weight at birth was 10 g (range, 2 to 17 g), by 7 days had decreased to 6 g (range, 3 to 12 g), and at 2 weeks it was 5 g (range, 2 to 8 g) (35). The rather marked decrease in adrenal weights in the first few weeks of life (fig. 1-9) is attributed almost entirely to regression of the fetal cortex.

In a study of adrenal glands obtained surgically from adult females undergoing staged bilateral adrenalectomy for advanced breast cancer, the average weight of individual glands was 4.0 g (1 SD = 0.80 g); adrenals obtained at autopsy were heavier (average, 6.0 g), probably due to trophic stimulation by ACTH (36). Adrenal glands from patients given a crude extract of ACTH prior to surgery underwent a nearly twofold enlargement (average weight, 8.1 g), and showed conversion of pale, lipid-rich cells of zona fasciculata to cells with compact eosinophilic cytoplasm (36). In children and adults there are no significant differences in adrenal weights with regard to sex or laterality. Since 98 percent of apparently normal glands removed surgically weigh less than 6.0 g, adrenals heavier than this

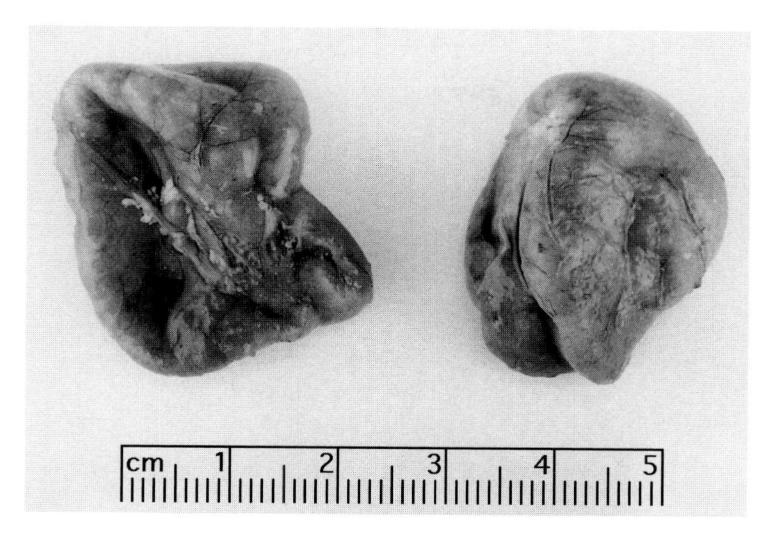

Figure 1-10
DORSAL ASPECT OF FETAL ADRENAL GLANDS
The dorsal aspect of both adrenal glands from a premature fetus shows a longitudinal ridge (or crista) and a relatively smooth cortical surface.

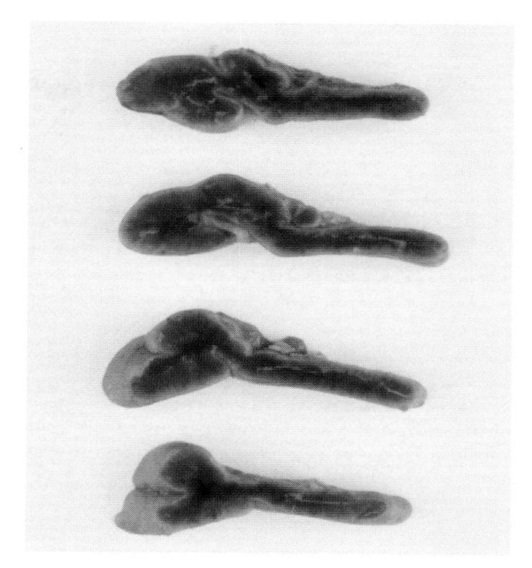

Figure 1-11
TRANSVERSE SECTION OF ADRENAL GLAND FROM A PREMATURE FETUS
Note the dark appearance of much of the provisional or fetal cortex.

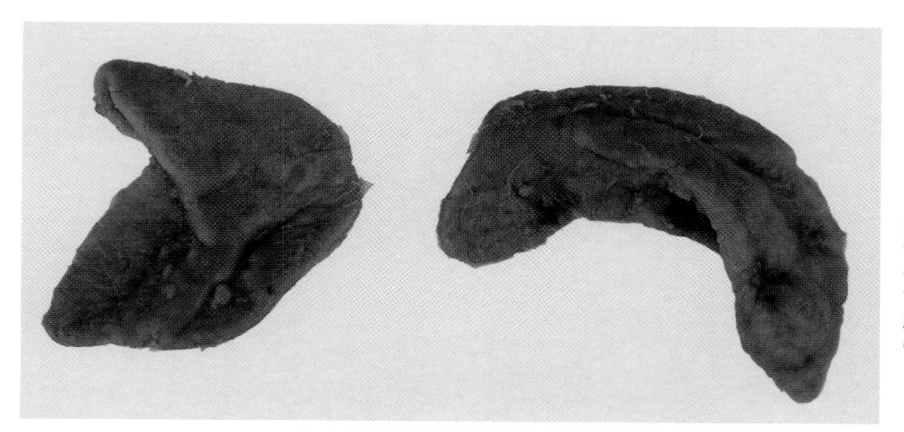

Figure 1-12
DORSAL ASPECT OF ADULT ADRENAL GLANDS
The dorsal aspect of both adrenal glands from an adult shows the pyramidal shape of the gland on the right (left side of photo), while the left adrenal is more elongate. A few small capsular extrusions are seen.

may be abnormal (36), but this assessment must be based upon weights of meticulously dissected glands and correlation with clinical and endocrinologic data. Gross dissection and weighing of adrenal medulla has shown that this component accounts for about 10 percent of the weight of the entire gland (0.431 g left, 0.448 g right) (33).

Gross Anatomy

In newborns the adrenal glands have a relatively smooth capsular surface (fig. 1-10); in transverse sections they may appear dark reddish brown due to a combination of regressed fetal cortex, congestion, and increased density of vascular sinusoids (fig. 1-11). On gross inspection this appearance may give the erroneous impression of adrenal hemorrhage or apoplexy; in addition the glands may be quite soft. Medullary tissue is not grossly identifiable in the newborn gland under normal circumstances since it constitutes less than 1 percent of the total gland volume (37).

In adults the right adrenal gland is roughly pyramidal in shape while the left is more elongate or crescentic (fig. 1-12). The anterior surface is relatively smooth or flattened, and there may be a shallow groove, usually on the left side, which contains a segment of the central adrenal

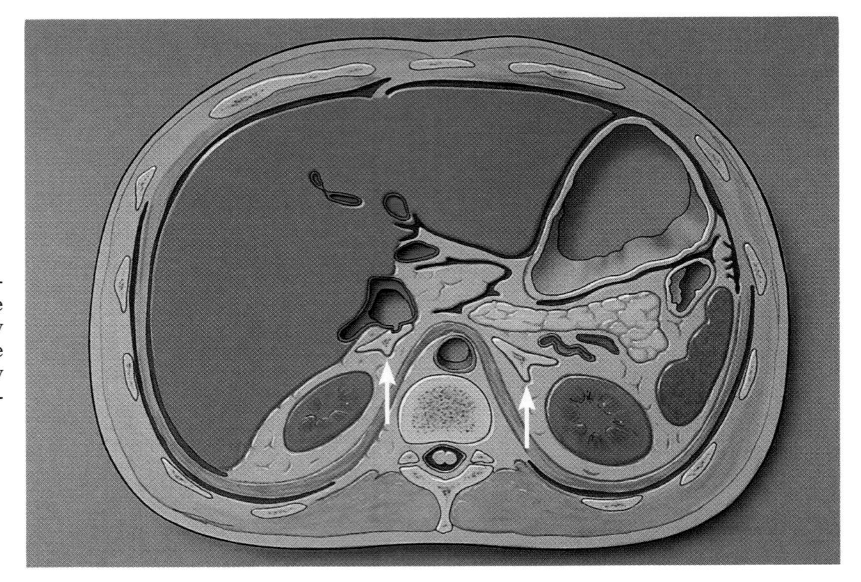

Figure 1-13
CONFIGURATION OF ADRENAL GLANDS IN SITU IN TRANSVERSE PLANE THROUGH ABDOMEN

In this schematic diagram the adrenal ridge (or crista) is located on the dorsal aspect (arrows) and is flanked by medial and lateral limbs (or alae). The right adrenal gland has a relatively short adrenal vein which drains directly into the inferior vena cava.

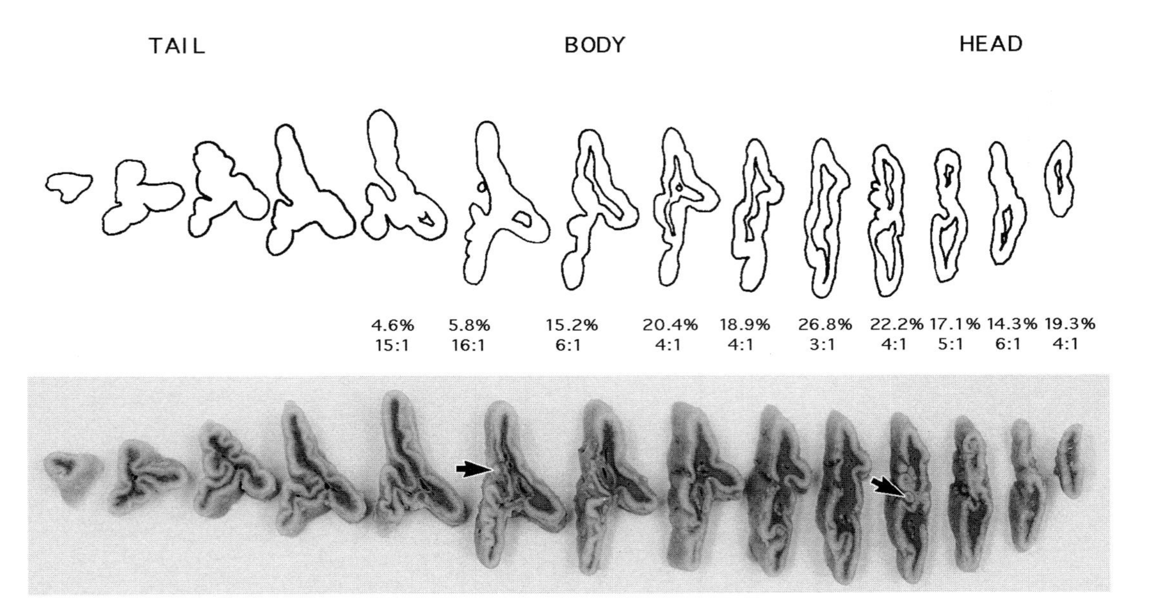

Figure 1-14
SERIAL TRANSVERSE SECTIONS OF ADULT ADRENAL GLAND

Three regions of the gland are seen, including the head (medial and inferior in situ), body, and tail (superior and lateral in situ). Most of the chromaffin tissue is concentrated in the body and head of gland with none present in the tail. The percentage of cross sectional area occupied by medulla is indicated along with the ratio of area occupied by cortex versus medulla (overall ratio about 10:1). Note the few cortical extrusions (arrows).

vein. This vein is much longer on the left and normally drains into the renal vein, while the right adrenal vein is short and empties into the inferior vena cava (fig. 1-13). The arterial supply to the adrenal gland is three-fold: from the inferior phrenic artery, the aorta, and the renal artery. The posterior or dorsal surface of the gland is convex with a ridge (or crista) that is often more prominent in the tail of the gland on the superior and lateral aspects (fig. 1-14). The crista is flanked by flattened projections or alae (wings); these medial and lateral limbs are evident with

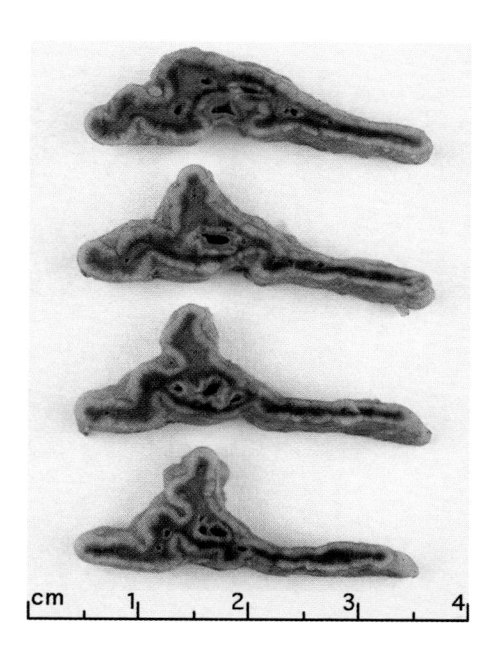

Figure 1-15
TRANSVERSE SECTIONS THROUGH BODY OF NORMAL ADRENAL GLAND FROM AN ADULT PATIENT AT AUTOPSY

The medullary compartment appears dull gray in contrast to the bright yellow cortex. Partial to complete cuffs of cortex are present around tributaries of the central adrenal vein. Note also the brown zona reticularis at the inner cortex.

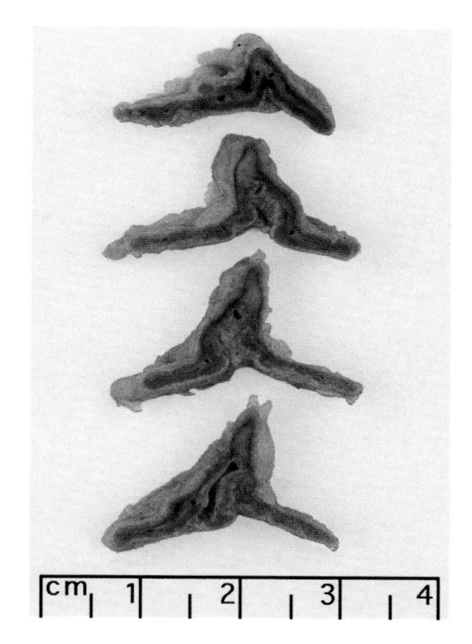

Figure 1-16
ADULT ADRENAL GLAND AFTER CORTICOSTEROID THERAPY

Transverse sections of adrenal glands at autopsy from an adult patient who had received suppressive doses of corticosteroids. The cortex is atrophic while the medullary compartment appears relatively prominent. Accurate morphometric evaluation for adrenal medullary hyperplasia (e.g., relative surface areas of cortex versus medulla) may be affected by alterations in cortex such as atrophy or nodularity/hyperplasia.

computed tomography or magnetic resonance imaging (fig. 1-13) (21,22,25,30,31). When sectioned in the transverse plane perpendicular to the long axis, the gland can arbitrarily be divided into three regions: the head (inferomedial one third), the body (middle one third), and the tail (superolateral one third). Chromaffin tissue is concentrated in the head and body of the gland with little extension into one or the other ala (figs. 1-14, 1-15) (26,27).

The medulla has an ellipsoid shape near the extremity of the head and an omega or sickle shape in sections near the body. It appears as a gray-white zone concentrated in the head and body of the gland (fig. 1-14). Using planimetry or other quantitative techniques, the ratio of the area occupied by cortex to that of the medulla is about 10 to 1 overall, but in making this assessment it is necessary to exclude areas occupied by structures such as blood vessels and collections of cortical cells associated with vascular structures. Atrophy of adrenal cortex may make the medulla appear relatively prominent (fig. 1-16), while the reverse may occur with cortical nodularity or hyperplasia. In areas of the gland there may be no intervening medulla, and where cortex abuts upon cortex there is a raphé (cristal or interalar).

The normal adrenal cortex in children and adults has a radiant, yellow-gold hue due to lipid accumulation within cortical cells, but this may not be uniform throughout. The thin zona reticularis is darker, and may contrast sharply with the gray-white medulla. Frequently, a partial or complete cuff of lipidized cortical cells is seen about the intraglandular portion of the central vein or its tributaries, and it is very common to see small (usually 1 to 2 mm), round extrusions of cortex (figs. 1-12, 1-15). These may appear partially or entirely encapsulated, with or without connection to underlying cortex, or they may lie free in periadrenal connective tissue.

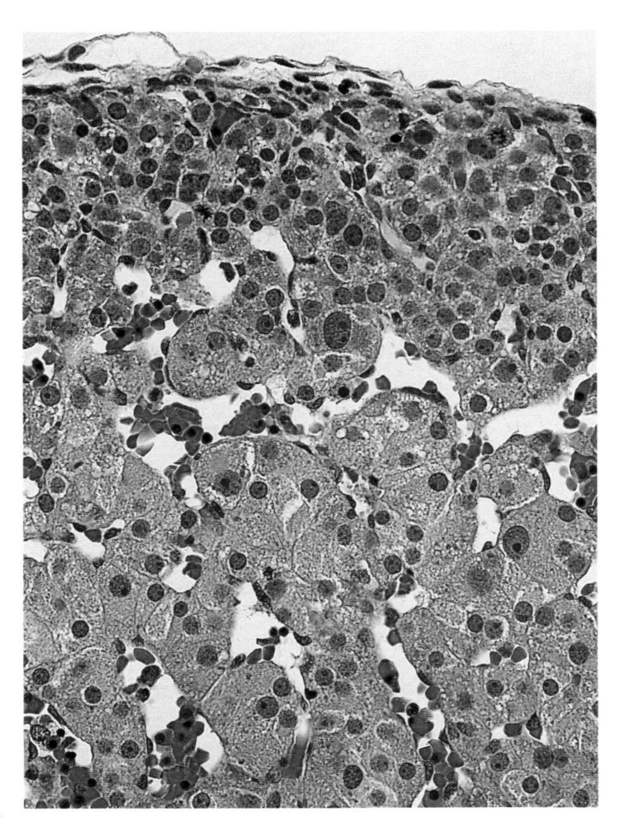

Figure 1-17
ADRENAL GLAND FROM A PREMATURE INFANT
Definitive or adult cortex forms a thin rim of subcapsular cells with a high nuclear/cytoplasmic ratio. Most of the cortex is composed of provisional or fetal cortical cells.

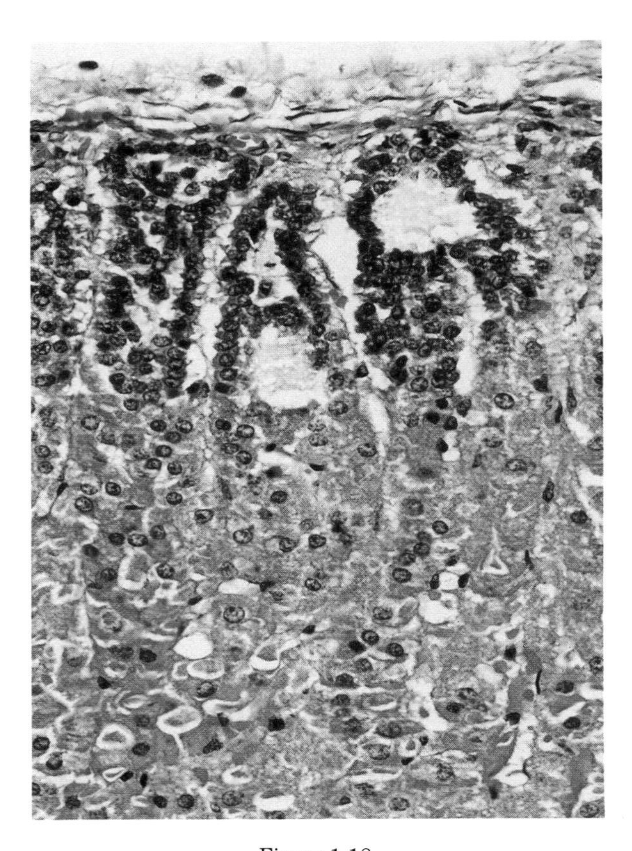

Figure 1-18
ADRENAL GLAND FROM A PREMATURE STILLBORN
Microcystic change is present in the definitive or adult cortex.

Microscopic Anatomy

Microscopic Anatomy of Newborn Adrenal Cortex. The adrenal cortex of the fetus and newborn has a biphasic structure: a thin subcapsular adult or definitive zone and a wide inner zone composed of fetal or provisional cortical cells (fig. 1-17). At birth the adult or definitive cortex is 0.1 to 0.2 mm thick, and by 9 days it is about 0.5 mm thick. The adult cortex is 0.8 to 1.0 mm thick by the end of the 12th year (35). It is only in the 2nd to 4th weeks of life that some differentiation of zona glomerulosa and zona fasciculata can be seen (35). Cells of the adult cortex are small with dark staining nuclei and scant cytoplasm, whereas the fetal cortical cells have larger, more vesicular nuclei, often with a small nucleolus and more voluminous compact cytoplasm that is granular and eosinophilic. About 70 to 85 percent of the cortex in the normal newborn adrenal gland is composed of fetal or provisional cells: it is this prominent zone (much thicker than the adult cortex) that undergoes marked regression in the first few weeks of life. In anencephaly the fetal cortex is markedly thin, although it is often normal in size and structure until approximately 20 weeks' gestation (28).

Microcysts have been reported in the adult or definitive cortex in premature stillborns and newborn infants (fig. 1-18), and have been attributed to a degenerative change associated with in utero stress (32), although some believe they may be a manifestation of the normal developmental process. Microcysts have been correlated with a shorter gestational period and shorter survival time following birth (34). Vacuolar change of cells in the outer fetal cortex has been noted in infants with erythroblastosis fetalis (20), and nearly identical changes have been observed in thalassemia

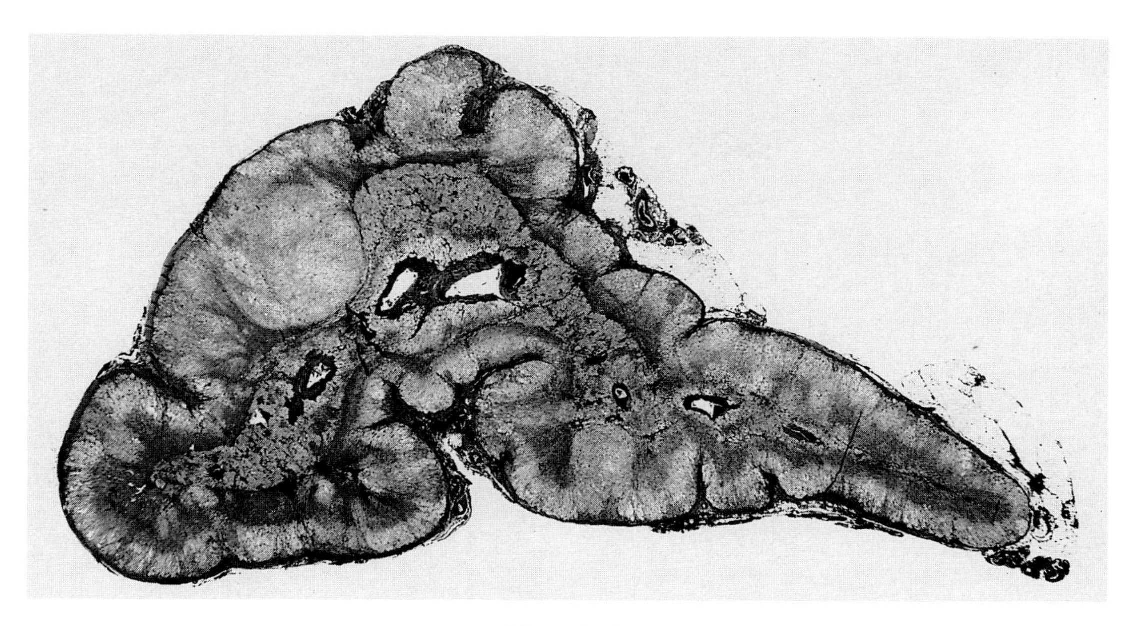

Figure 1-19
EUCORTICAL ADRENAL GLAND

This is a transverse section through the body of an adrenal gland from an adult woman who underwent bilateral adrenalectomy for metastatic breast carcinoma. The patient was eucortical. Note the irregular cortical nodularity, with the darker zone next to the medulla being the zona reticularis. Tributaries of the central adrenal vein are partially surrounded by small cuffs of cortical cells. (Fig. 1-18A from Lack EE, Kozakewich HP. Embryology, developmental anatomy and selected aspects of non-neoplastic pathology. In: Lack EE, ed. Pathology of the adrenal glands. New York: Churchill Livingstone, 1990:1–74.)

major (28). A connection with intrauterine stress and hypoxia has been proposed (20).

Microscopic Anatomy of Adult Adrenal Cortex. The normal adrenal cortex in adults is almost 2 mm thick, but there may be variation from gland to gland, or thicker areas in different areas of the same gland (fig. 1-19). This variation is particularly evident in elderly individuals and those with hypertension or diabetes mellitus, due to an increased incidence of cortical nodularity. Distinct zonation can be found in the normal gland. The zona glomerulosa is a thin, usually discontinuous layer beneath the capsule, with a ball-like arrangement of cells; it comprises 5 to 10 percent of the cortex in some areas of the gland. Cells of the zona glomerulosa have less abundant cytoplasm compared with cells of the zona fasciculata. The zona fasciculata comprises about 70 percent of the thickness of the cortex and has radial columns or cords of cells with ample, lipid-rich cytoplasm (fig. 1-20, left). Close scrutiny of these cells reveals a lattice-like partitioning or fine vacuolization of cytoplasm that is pale staining due to lipid accumulation. There may be small clear spaces due to confluent lipid, which in some instances may be recognizable as lipomatous foci (fig. 1-20, right). The inner zona fasciculata often merges imperceptibly with the zona reticularis; the latter is composed of cells with compact eosinophilic cytoplasm and there may be prominent lipochrome pigment. The radial cord-like and reticular arrangement of cells can be accentuated by staining for reticulin (fig. 1-21). The corticomedullary interface is often smooth or delicately undulating, but can be irregular with intermingled cortical and chromaffin cells (fig. 1-22). Depending upon the plane of section, some of the cortical extrusions may be connected with the underlying cortex (fig. 1-23, left) or lie free in adjacent fat (fig. 1-23, right). Postmortem autolysis may result in "fissure" formation with cavitation, particularly after physical manipulation of the gland (fig. 1-24), and in the extreme example there may be a cavity filled with detritus and blood and almost complete separation of medulla from cortex. Autolysis may be preceded by a toxic or infectious process, but the association is not constant. This postmortem

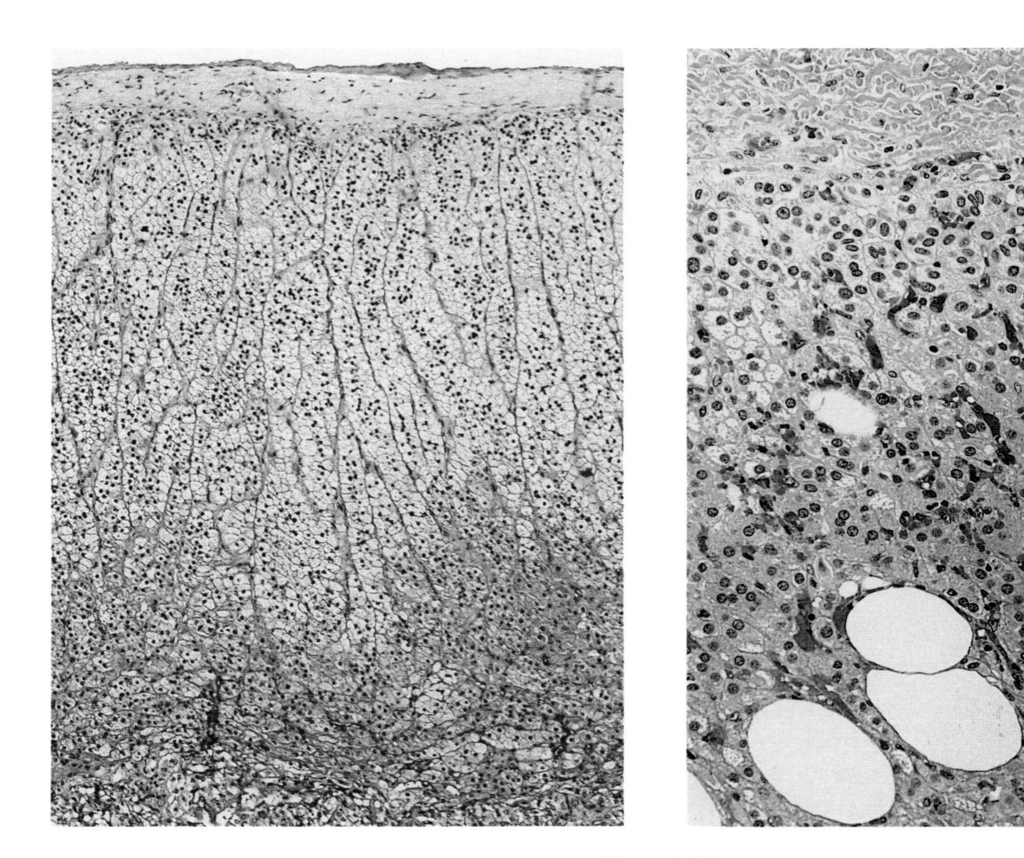

Figure 1-20
NORMAL ADRENAL GLAND

Left: Normal adrenal cortex in an adult shows radial cords of lipid-rich cells of the zona fasciculata and an indistinct, discontinuous zona glomerulosa.

Right: Normal adrenal gland from an adult with a few areas of lipomatous change.

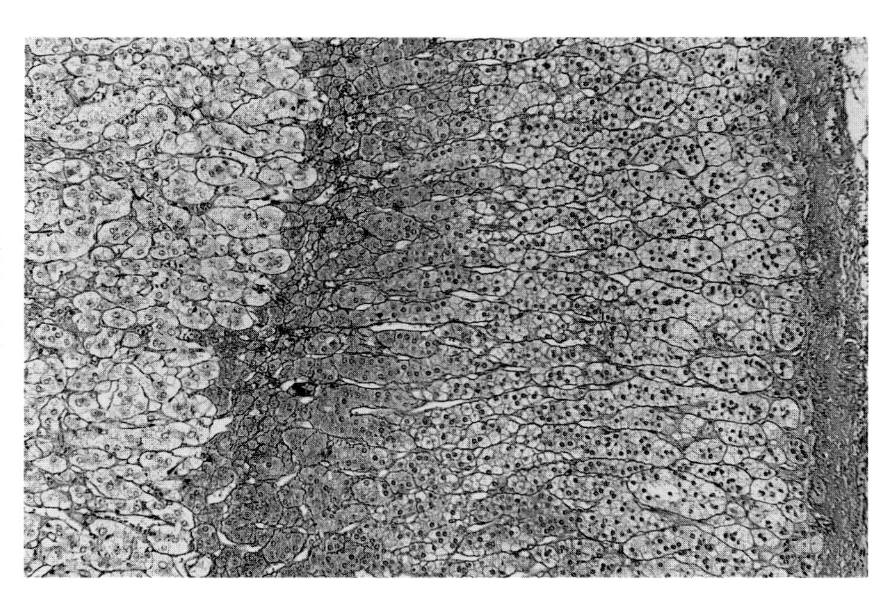

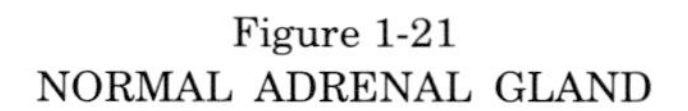

Figure 1-21
NORMAL ADRENAL GLAND

Radial cords of zona fasciculata contrast with the smaller nesting pattern of zona reticularis. The left side of the field shows the organoid nesting pattern of the chromaffin cells of the adrenal medulla. (X100, Reticulum stain)

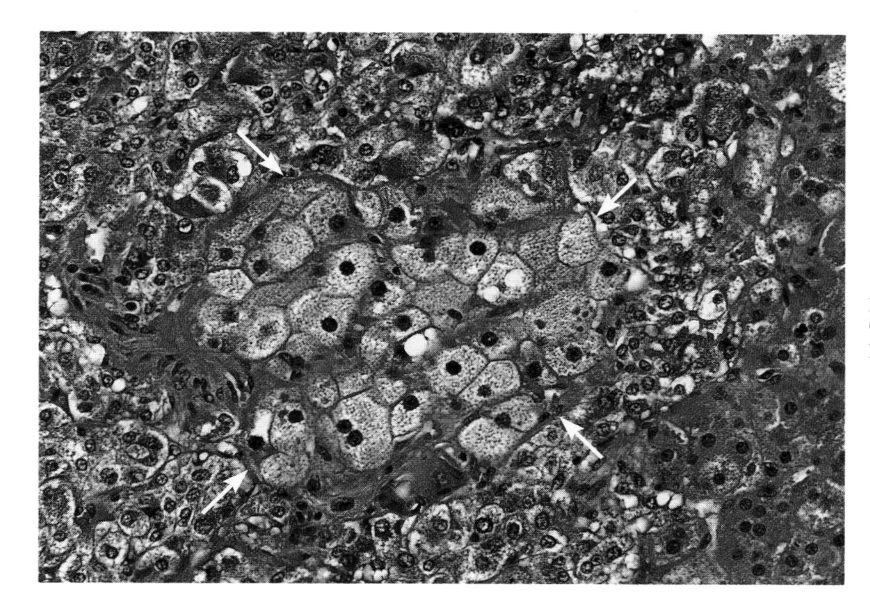

Figure 1-22
NORMAL ADRENAL GLAND
Intermingling of partially lipid-depleted cortical cells (arrows) among chromaffin cells. Zona reticularis is present on the right.

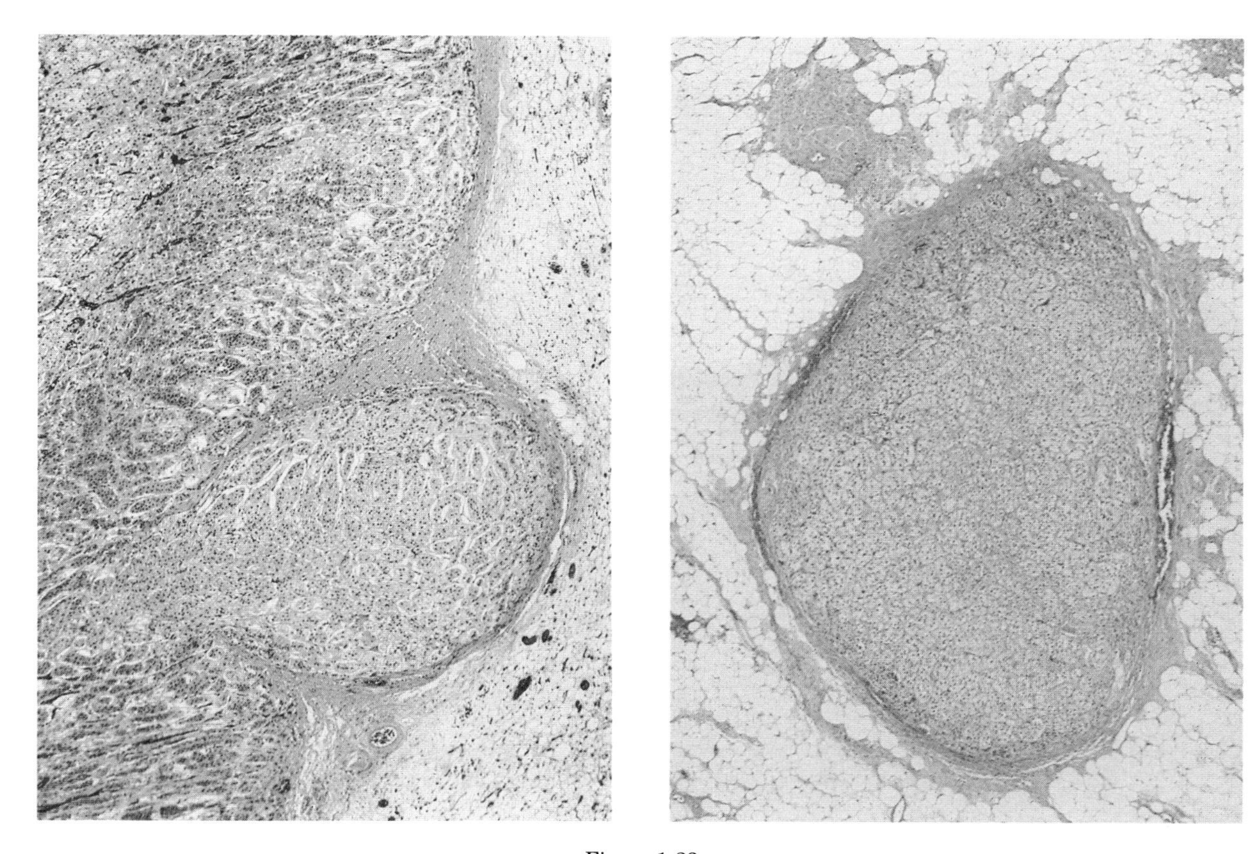

Figure 1-23
NORMAL ADRENAL GLAND
Left: Partially encapsulated cortical extrusion in a normal adrenal gland has a "mushroom"-like configuration with a narrow connection to the underlying cortex.
Right: Encapsulated nodule of adrenal cortex was located free in the periadrenal adipose tissue of an adult patient.

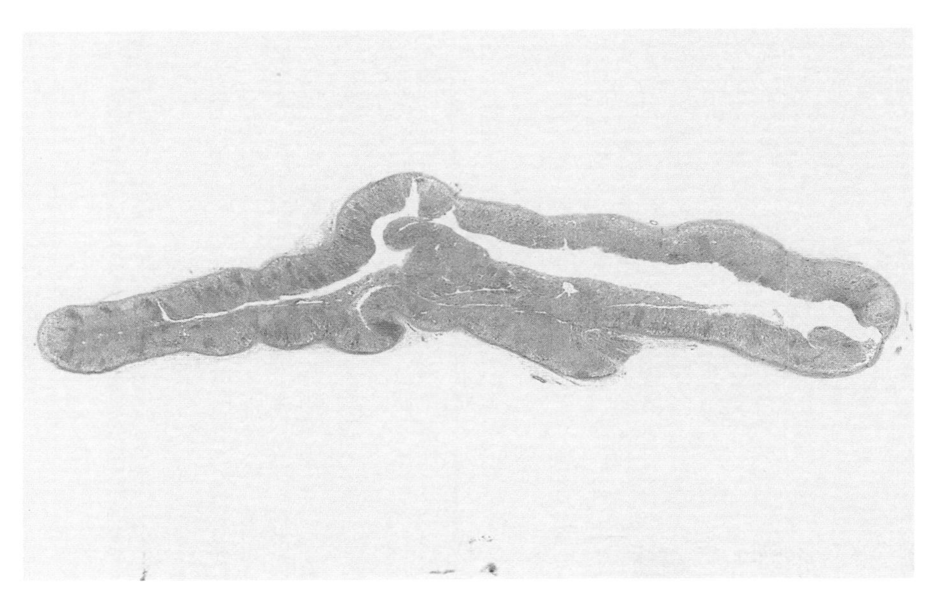

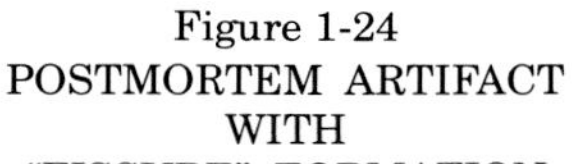

Figure 1-24
POSTMORTEM ARTIFACT WITH "FISSURE" FORMATION

Tissue separation or "fissure" formation is largely through the interalar raphé or region of the corticomedullary junction, but does not indicate a clear demarcation between cortex and medulla. There is no inflammatory reaction.

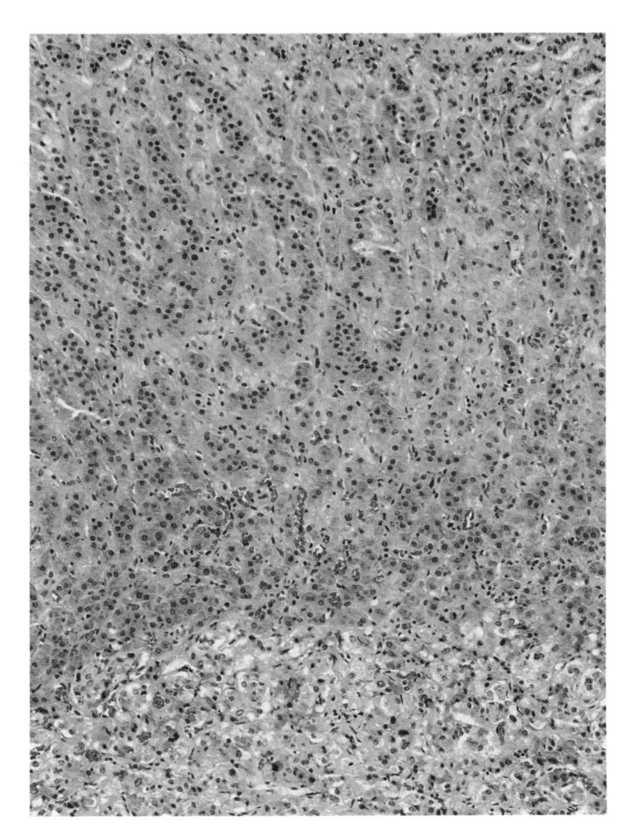

Figure 1-25
ADRENAL GLAND IN AIDS

Adrenal gland from a patient who died of infectious complications of acquired immunodeficiency syndrome (AIDS). The entire cortex shows marked lipid depletion with cells having compact, eosinophilic cytoplasm. Medulla is present at the bottom of the field.

change undoubtedly contributed to the misconception of the adrenal glands as hollow organs (hence the term "suprarenal capsules") and the early belief that they were involved in purifying or altering "black bile" (or "atrabilia").

The most common stress-related change in the adrenal is lipid depletion in which there is conversion of pale-staining, lipid-rich cells of the zona fasciculata to cells with compact, eosinophilic cytoplasm; the zona reticularis may appear widened or the entire thickness of cortex may be involved (fig. 1-25). There is a pattern of patchy lipid depletion referred to as lipid reversion (fig. 1-26) in which lipid is absent in the outer cortex, usually scanty in the zona reticularis, but prominent in the intervening zona fasciculata; this appearance suggests recovery from stress with replenishment of lipid in cells of the inner zona fasciculata (38). Tubular degeneration is evidenced by conversion of normally solid cords of cells in the outer cortex to tubular structures (fig. 1-27) lined by flattened cells that may contain proteinaceous material or occasional degenerated cells (40). Intracytoplasmic globules are sometimes noted within cells of the zona fasciculata in humans dying of streptococcal meningitis, chronic renal failure, pneumonia, and overexposure to cold. Since these globules can be induced in the experimental animal by ACTH administration, it is assumed that they are the result of overstimulation of the adrenal cortex (40).

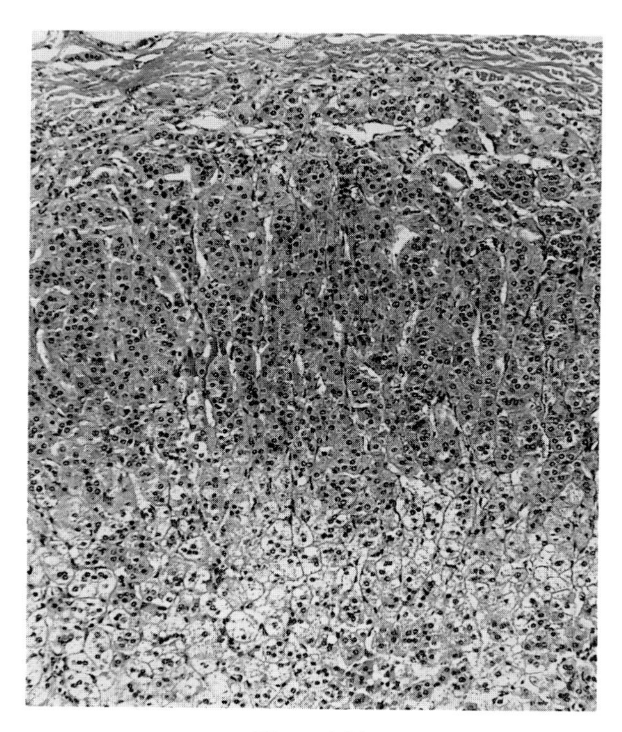

Figure 1-26
LIPID REVERSION PATTERN
Lipid reversion pattern in which the outer aspect of zona fasciculata is composed of cells with lipid-depleted, eosinophilic cytoplasm and the inner zone is composed of pale-staining, lipid-rich cells. Features suggest recovery from stress.

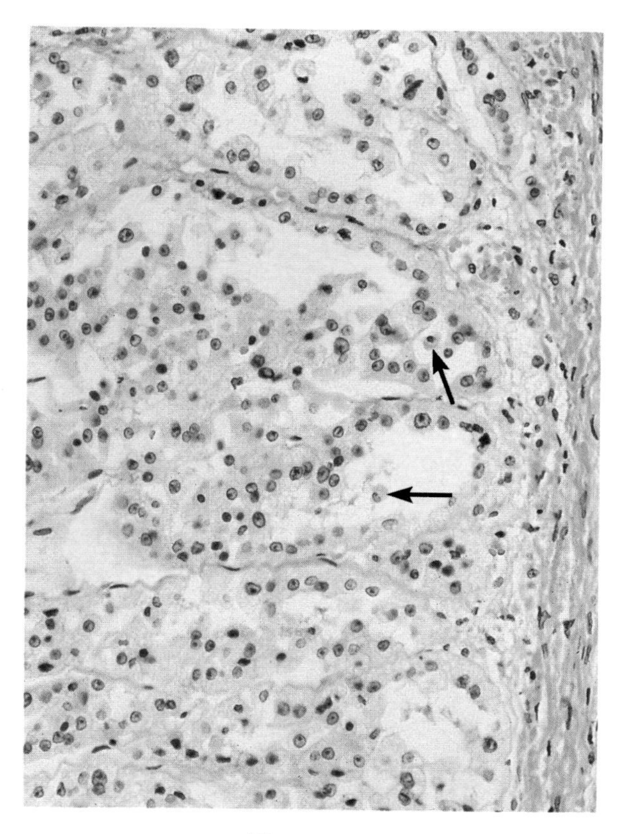

Figure 1-27
TUBULAR DEGENERATION OF OUTER ZONA FASCICULATA
Solid columns and cords of lipid-depleted cells are converted into hollow tubules which contain rare necrobiotic cortical cells (arrows).

Microscopic Anatomy of Adrenal Medulla. Chromaffin cells of the adrenal medulla are arranged in discrete nests or short anastomosing cords (fig. 1-28), a more diffuse or solid arrangement, or an admixture of different architectural patterns within the same gland. Staining for reticulin highlights the organoid arrangement of the cells (see fig. 1-21). Chromaffin cells have amphophilic to basophilic cytoplasm, indistinct borders, and usually a single nucleus that is often slightly eccentric in location. The nuclear contour and size may be normal, but in some glands there is considerable nuclear variation, with enlargement and hyperchromasia. Mitotic figures are virtually absent in the normal medulla, but can be found in diffuse or nodular adrenal medullary hyperplasia as seen in the multiple endocrine neoplasia (MEN) syndrome types IIa and IIb. Pinpoint basophilic granules, which are barely identifiable with the light microscope, are seen on close examination of cell cytoplasm; most of these correspond to dense-core neurosecretory granules. Scattered ganglion cells can be found in the medulla either singly (fig. 1-29, left), or in association with small myelinated nerve bundles (fig. 1-29, right). Depending upon the delay in or method of fixation, the cytologic details of chromaffin cells may be altered with cytoplasmic vacuolization or apparent disruption of cell membranes.

Intracytoplasmic hyaline globules have been reported in 79 percent of adrenal glands from adults, although they may be difficult to find on casual inspection (fig. 1-30). In 86 percent of cases in one study the globules were scored as "minimal" in number, requiring extensive search with the high dry microscope objective while in only 3 percent were the globules "numerous" being present in nearly every high-power field (23). The

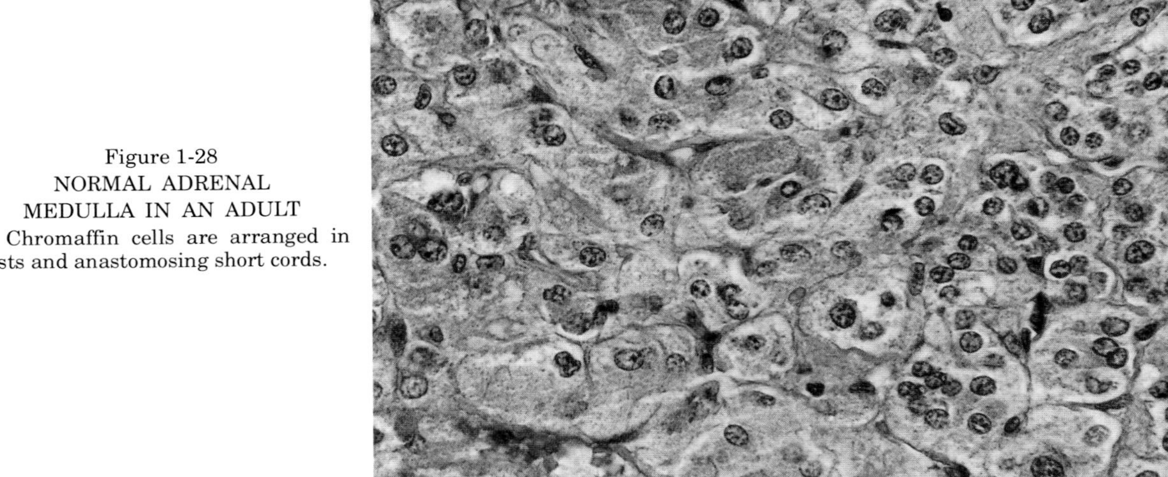

Figure 1-28
NORMAL ADRENAL MEDULLA IN AN ADULT
Chromaffin cells are arranged in nests and anastomosing short cords.

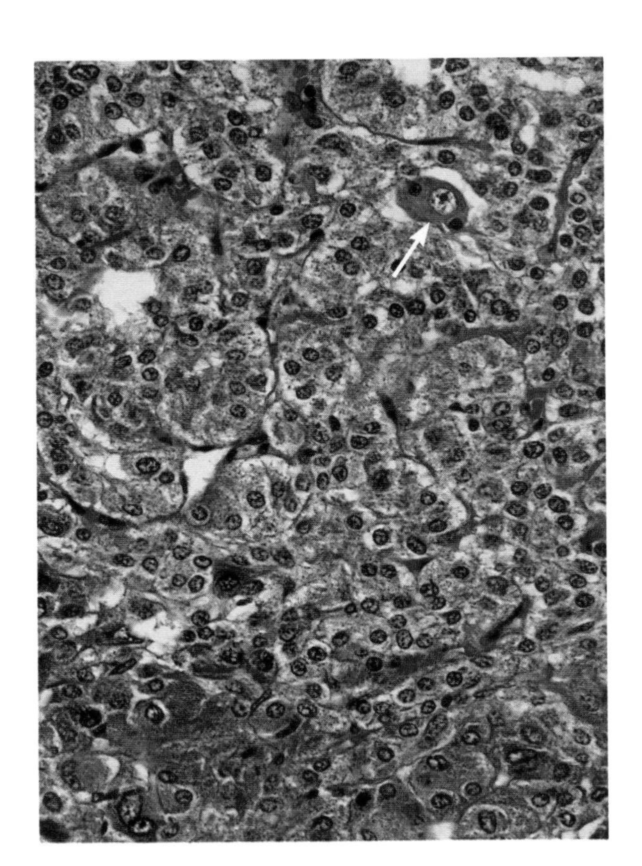

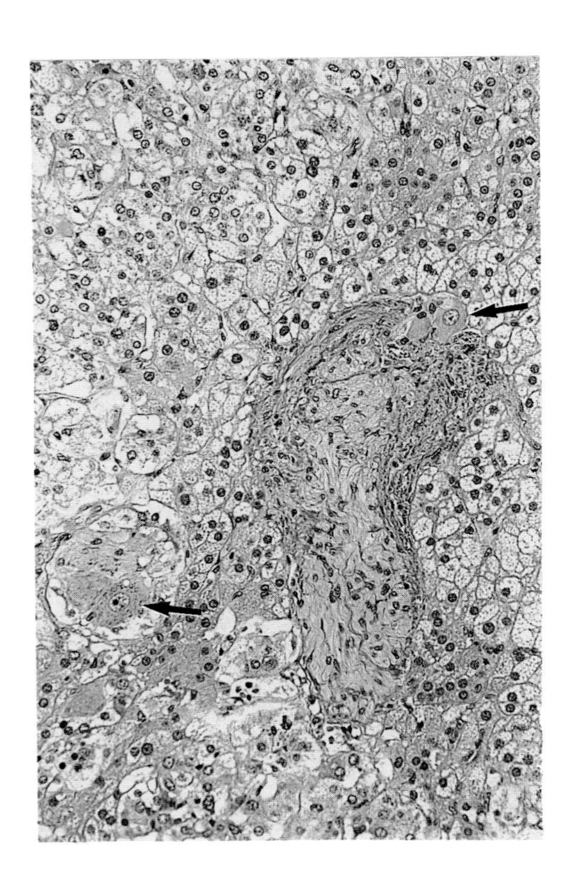

Figure 1-29
NORMAL ADRENAL GLAND FROM AN ADULT PATIENT
Left: Chromaffin cells contain a myriad of pinpoint cytoplasmic granules. A mature ganglion cell is also apparent (arrow).
Right: Myelinated nerve bundles are present near the corticomedullary junction along with several ganglion cells (arrows). Chromaffin cells are present in the lower part of the field.

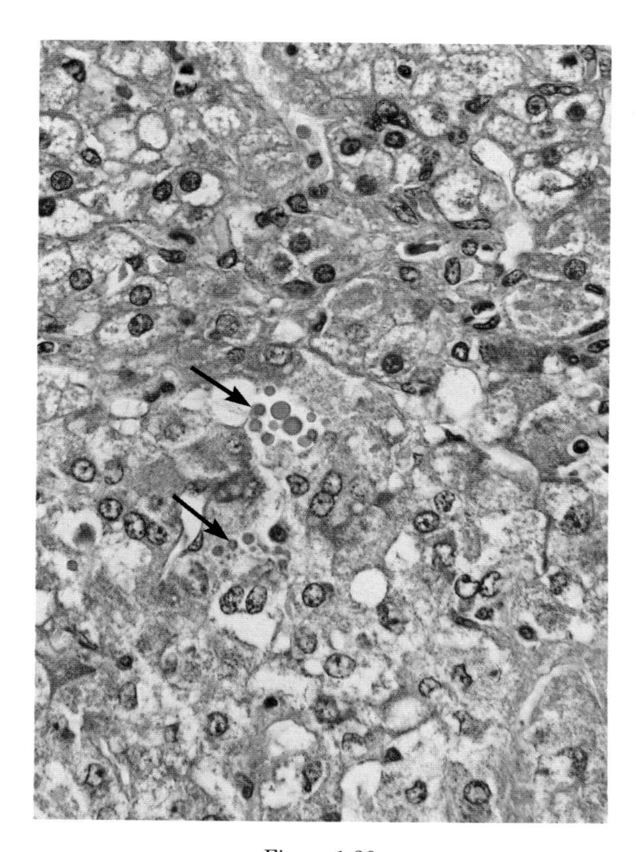

Figure 1-30
INTRACYTOPLASMIC HYALINE GLOBULES
Intracytoplasmic hyaline globules are present in several chromaffin cells near the corticomedullary junction (arrows). Cortical cells with finely vacuolated to eosinophilic cytoplasm are present in the upper portion of the field.

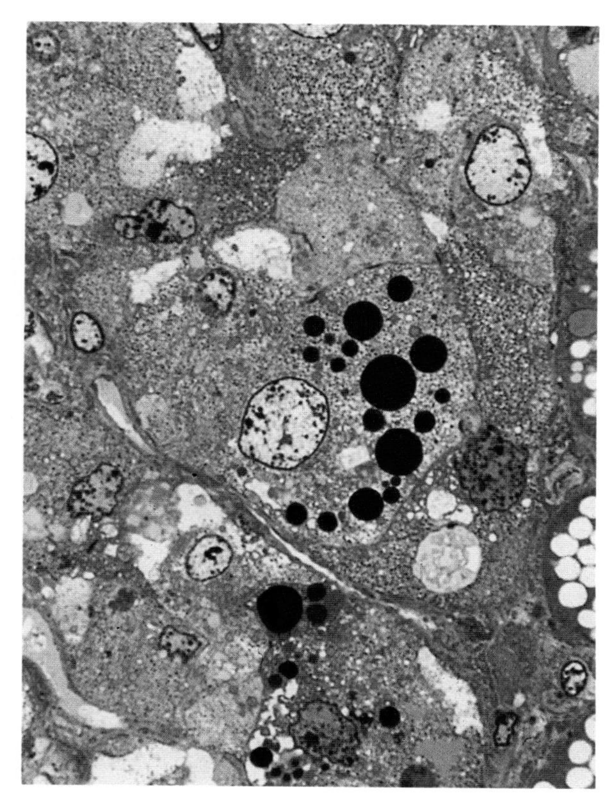

Figure 1-31
INTRACYTOPLASMIC HYALINE GLOBULES
Intracytoplasmic hyaline globules are numerous in this field and are blue-black with toluidine blue stain. Note the delicate microvasculature which winds between nests and short cords of chromaffin cells. (X1,000, Toluidine blue stain)

globules are eosinophilic, ranging in size from 1 to 25 μm, and are periodic acid–Schiff (PAS) positive and resistant to diastase predigestion. There appears to be no correlation with sex, race, or age, but in the author's experience they are uncommon in the pediatric age group. The globules have been described with increased frequency in patients with chronic neurologic disorders such as Parkinson's disease (28). In 1-μm-thick sections stained with toluidine blue the globules are readily detected as blue-black structures which vary considerably in size (fig. 1-31); some give the impression of having small budding projections, but this is probably due to superimposition of adjacent globules in most cases. Ultrastructurally, the globules may be partially or completely membrane bound, and have small curvilinear or circular profiles at the periphery with size, shape, and electron density similar to adjacent dense-core neurosecretory granules (fig. 1-32) (23). This feature suggests a relationship with the secretory activity of the chromaffin cells (29).

Anatomy of Adrenal Vasculature. The three arteries supplying the adrenal glands divide repeatedly into as many as 50 branches which, as the capsular arterioles, partially supply the capsule (24). There is a single central or main adrenal vein; typically, an invaginated cuff of cortical tissue envelopes it throughout its length in much of the gland. It merges imperceptibly with the cortex in the tail of the gland; only in the head are there small venous radicles lying freely in the medulla (24). The microscopic anatomy of the central adrenal vein and its tributaries is remarkable for the seemingly dysmorphic array of medial musculature organized into discontinuous pillars of longitudinal bundles (fig. 1-33).

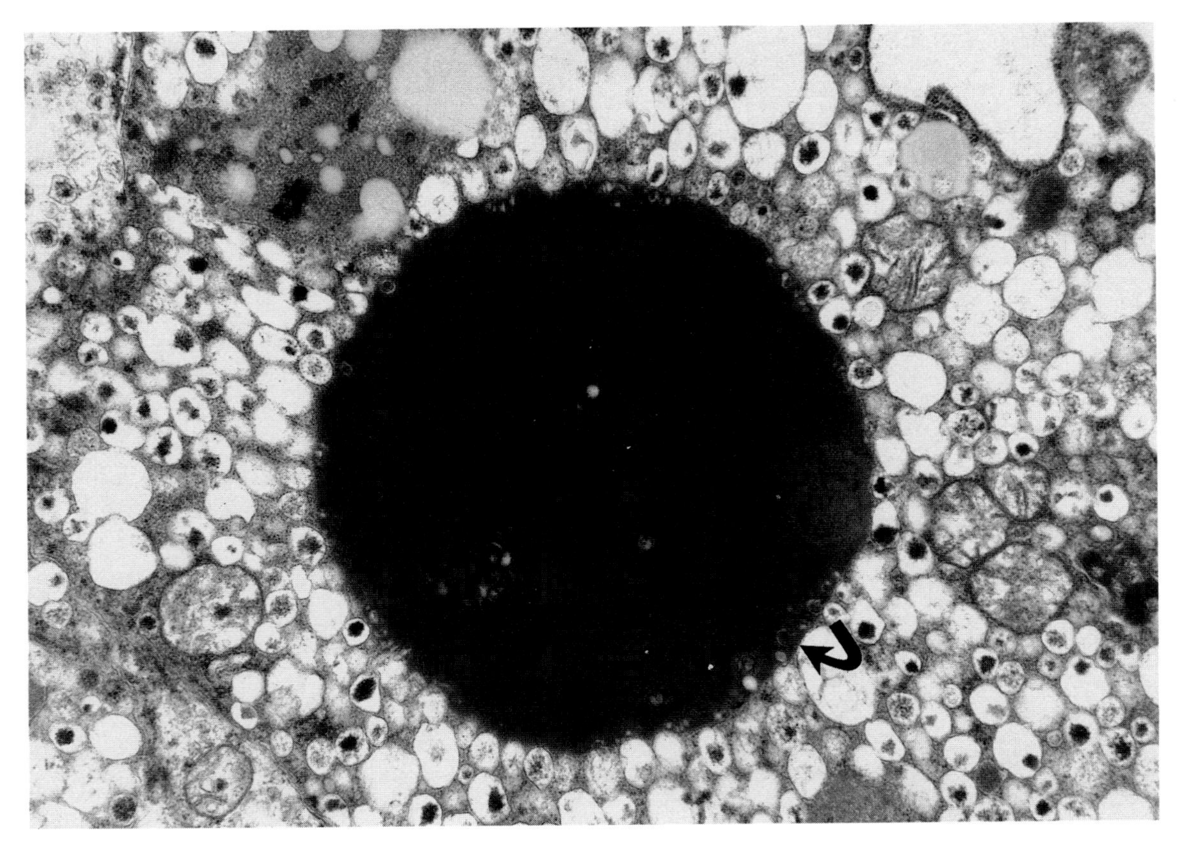

Figure 1-32
INTRACYTOPLASMIC HYALINE GLOBULES

The ultrastructure of normal chromaffin cells of the adult adrenal medulla is shown. The electron-dense structure represents an intracytoplasmic hyaline globule. Note the circular structures at the periphery of the globule: some have the same electron density (curved arrow) as the cores of neurosecretory granules. Some partially empty secretory vesicles slightly indent the matrix of the globule. (X17,000) (Fig. 10-22 from Lack EE. Pathology of adrenal and extra-adrenal paraganglia. Major problems in pathology, Vol. 29. Philadelphia: WB Saunders, 1994:202.)

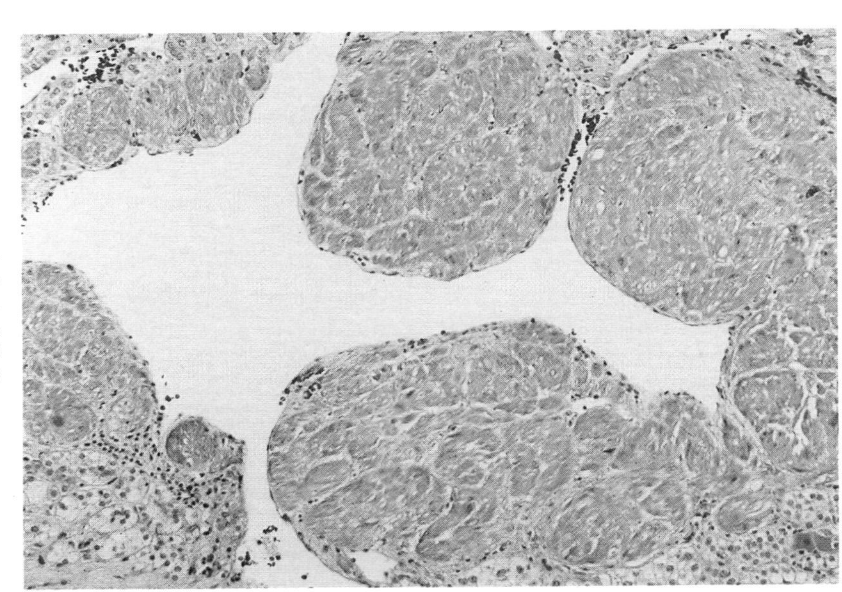

Figure 1-33
NORMAL ADRENAL GLAND

This figure shows dysmorphic arcades of smooth muscle around a tributary of the central adrenal vein. Where smooth muscle is deficient, medullary (chromaffin) or cortical cells may come into close proximity with the vascular space.

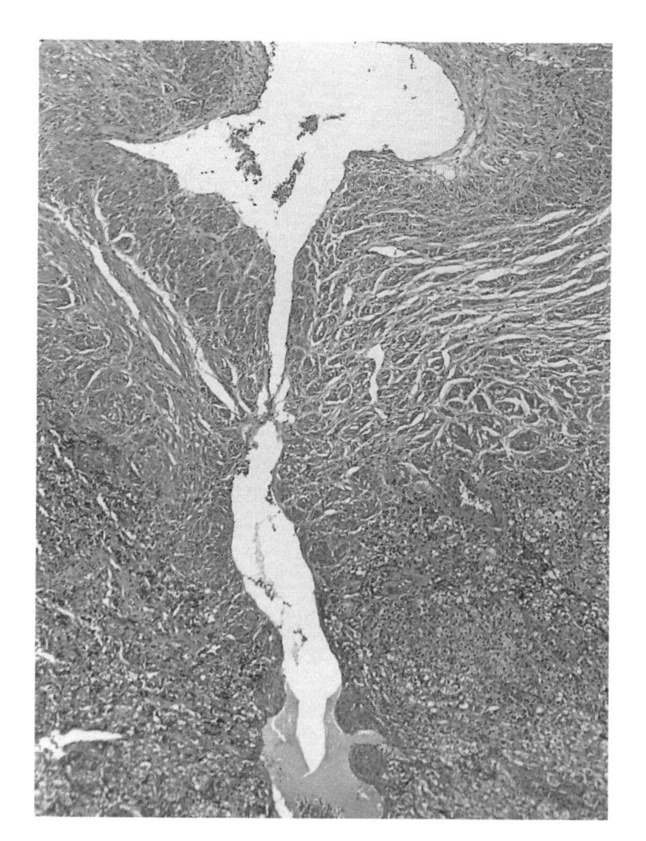

Figure 1-34
NORMAL ADRENAL GLAND
Venous sinusoids within the medullary compartment of the adrenal gland drain into a larger venous channel, which has stout bundles of smooth muscle. Contraction of smooth muscle may cause congestion of venous tributaries.

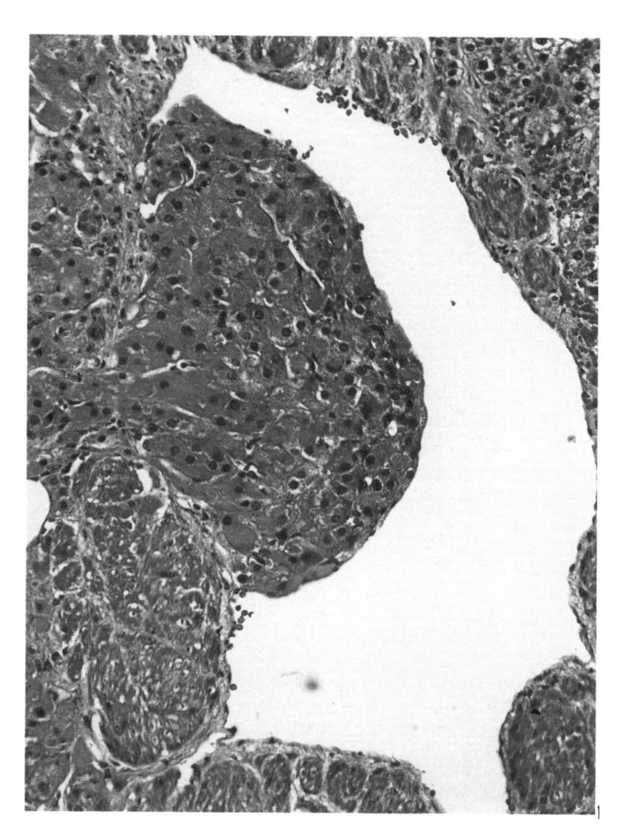

Figure 1-35
NORMAL ADRENAL GLAND
Normal adrenal gland showing extension of cuff of cortical cells through the wall of the tributary of the central adrenal vein where there is discontinuity of smooth muscle bundles.

There is a selective gathering of muscle bundles in the medulla facing segments of veins in certain regions (medullary tropism).

Once the arterioles penetrate the cortex they enter a thin subcapsular plexus that gives rise to capillary channels. These channels course centrally through the zona fasciculata to reach the zona reticularis and then join a rich vascular plexus. Blood courses into venous sinuses in the medulla to enter tributaries of the central adrenal vein. In areas of the gland with no medulla, the blood from the reticular plexus courses directly into tributaries of the central adrenal vein. Contraction of the longitudinal muscle bundles aids in the damming up of blood in the venous sinuses and reticular plexus (fig. 1-34); in this way the muscles act as "sluice gates" regulating the degree of congestion of the zona reticularis and inner zona fasciculata. With relaxation of muscle bundles and elastic recoil of venous sinuses there may be rapid, intermittent release of hormones into the central vein (24). One of the remarkable aspects of the venous structures is the close proximity of cortical or medullary cells to the vascular lumen (fig. 1-35), a feature that is significant when interpreting vascular intrusions in hyperplastic and neoplastic conditions.

Immunohistochemistry and Distribution of Steroidogenic Enzymes

Immunofluorescent studies on frozen sections of fresh tissue and immunoperoxidase staining of formalin-fixed paraffin-embedded tissue have shown cytokeratin localized within the cytoplasm of normal adrenal cortical cells and lack of

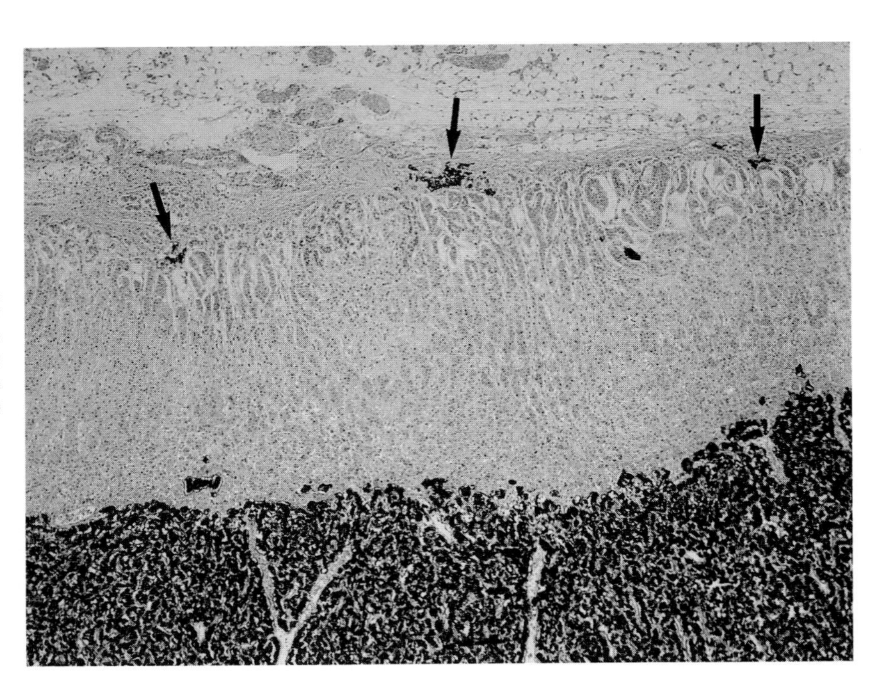

Figure 1-36
NORMAL ADRENAL GLAND
Immunostain for chromogranin in the normal adrenal gland intensely decorates the cytoplasm of chromaffin cells, and also demonstrates small nests of chromaffin cells in the outer zona fasciculata or adjacent to the capsule of the gland (arrows).

vimentin reactivity except for stromal elements (41–43). Negative immunoreactivity has been reported for epithelial membrane antigen (EMA) (42) and neurofilament protein (43). Lectin binding of wheat germ agglutinin (WGA) and concanavalin (Con A) has been reported in most adrenal cortical cells of all zones (44).

Immunostaining for neuroendocrine markers such as chromogranin A (CGA) can highlight chromaffin cells to a remarkable degree, demonstrate intermingling with cortical cells, and even highlight small nests of chromaffin cells near the capsule of the gland (fig. 1-36). Rarely, there may be "extrusion" or "unmasking" of medullary tissue that is continuous with chromaffin cells deeper in the gland (fig. 1-37). Cells that typically escape detection with routine light microscopy, and even electron microscopy, are sustentacular cells, located at the periphery of small clusters and cords of chromaffin cells. These cells are most vividly demonstrated by immunostaining for S-100 protein (fig. 1-38). Neurofilament protein immunostains demonstrate fine neuritic processes which largely correspond to the rich splanchnic innervation by sympathetic fibers (fig. 1-39).

The intracortical distribution of P-450 cytochromes, which are important in corticosteroidogenesis, has been investigated using immunohistochemistry and results underscore the functional zonation of the adrenal cortex. P-$450_{17\alpha}$ is not present in the zona glomerulosa, thus confirming the exclusive localization of glucocorticoid and androgen biosynthesis in the zona fasciculata and zona reticularis; P-450_{C21} (C21-hydroxylation) is present in all three zones of adrenal cortex, reflecting its enzymatic importance in biosynthesis of both mineralocorticoids and glucocorticoids (45). Some data suggest that the outer zona fasciculata is the most active area of corticosteroid biosynthesis (45).

MISCELLANEOUS MICROSCOPIC FEATURES

Adrenal Cytomegaly

Adrenal cytomegaly has been reported in about 3 percent of newborns and 6.5 percent of premature stillborns (47); it is usually an incidental finding in glands that are otherwise grossly normal. It occurs in infants up to 2 months of age (47), and occasionally in older children and even adults (48,55). Affected cells are limited to the fetal cortex and may be focal or diffuse (fig. 1-40). Cells may be as large as 120 μm in diameter (47), and show marked nucleomegaly with pleomorphism and hyperchromasia. These cells were once thought to be precursors of virilizing adrenal cortical tumors in childhood (47), but are almost

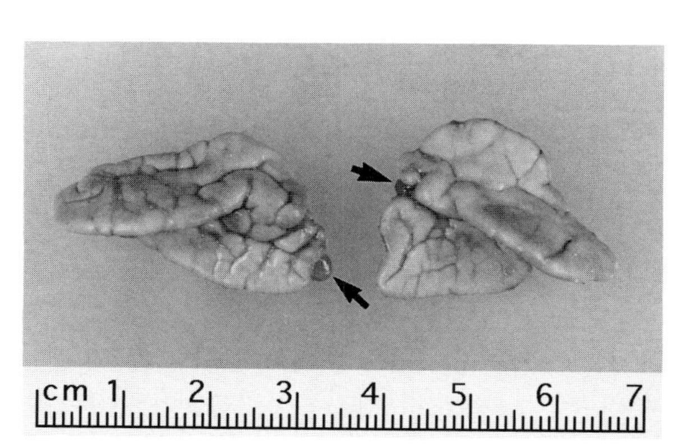

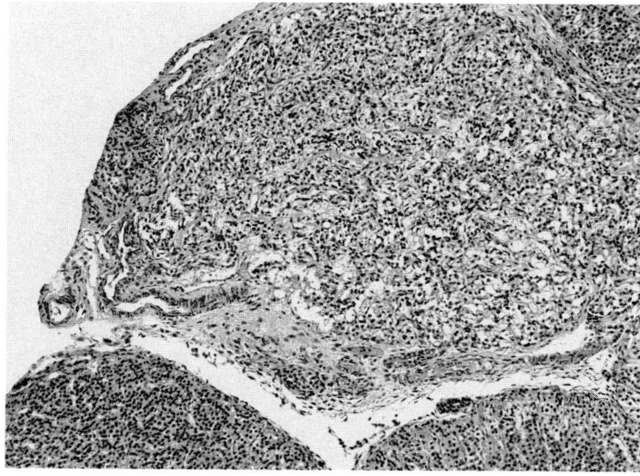

Figure 1-37

ADRENAL GLAND FROM A CHILD WITH "EXTRUDED" OR "UNMASKED" MEDULLARY TISSUE

Left: On the medial, inferior aspect of each adrenal gland from a young infant is a small nodule of "extruded" or "unmasked" medullary tissue (arrows) which was continuous with the adrenal medulla in the head of the gland. A longitudinal ridge or crista is on the dorsal surface of each gland and terminates in the outer (superolateral in situ) aspect of each gland. (Fig. 10-16B from Lack EE, Kozakewich, HP. Embryology, developmental anatomy and selected aspects of non-neoplastic pathology. In: Lack EE, ed. Pathology of the adrenal glands. New York: Churchill Livingstone, 1990:1–74.)

Right: Nodule of "extruded" or "unmasked" medullary tissue. (Fig. 10-16C from Lack EE. Pathology of adrenal and extra-adrenal paraganglia. Major problems in pathology, vol. 29. Philadelphia: WB Saunders Co, 1994:200.)

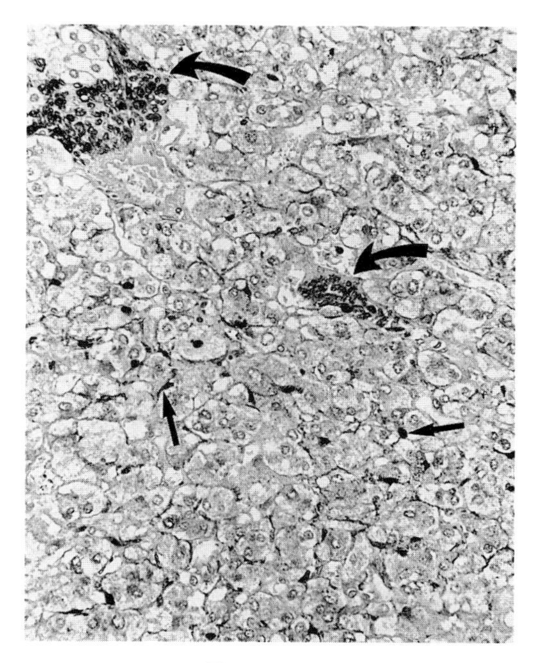

Figure 1-38

NORMAL ADRENAL MEDULLA

Sustentacular cells in the normal adrenal medulla appear as slender, dendritic cells at the periphery of nests and cords of chromaffin cells (straight arrows). Many show strong staining of cytoplasm as well as nuclear staining. Small components of myelinated nerve bundles are also present (curved arrows). (X200, Peroxidase-antiperoxidase stain)

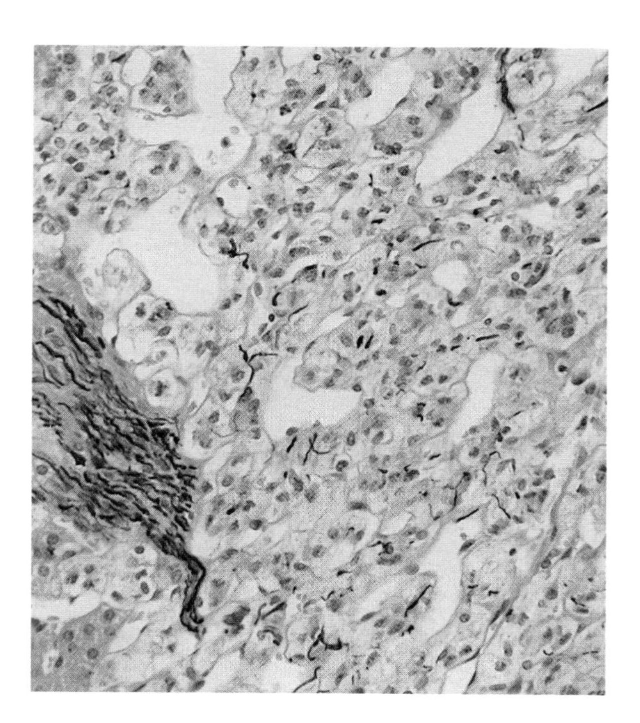

Figure 1-39

NORMAL ADRENAL MEDULLA

Immunostain for neurofilament protein highlights the thin neuritic processes between nests of chromaffin cells as well as the filaments of the nerve bundle.

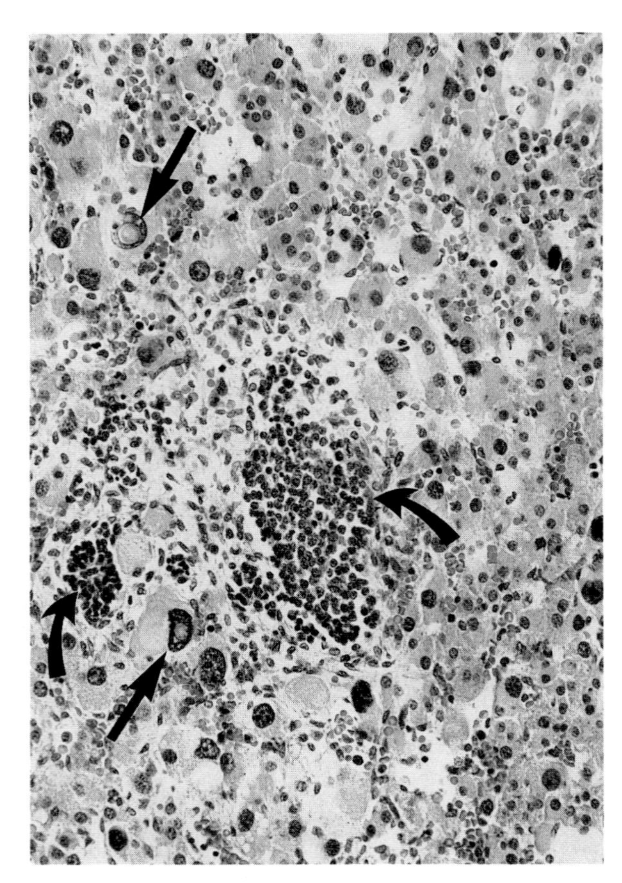

Figure 1-40
ADRENAL CYTOMEGALY IN A STILLBORN INFANT
Note the nuclear "pseudoinclusions" (straight arrows) as well as the small nests of neuroblastic cells (curved arrows).

always an incidental finding. Cytomegalic cells may contain over 25 times the normal amount of nuclear DNA, underscoring the fact that polyploidy/aneuploidy per se is not an entirely specific marker of neoplasia (48). Characteristically, there are no identifiable mitotic figures. The occasional nuclear "pseudoinclusions," which in the past caused some concern about a viral etiology, have been shown ultrastructurally to have no viral inclusions; instead there is nuclear indentation or folding with intranuclear protrusion of cell cytoplasm (51,52,55).

Focal "Adrenalitis"

Focal "adrenalitis" has been reported in 48 percent of patients at autopsy and is most frequent in elderly patients of both sexes (50). Rather than being an intrinsic adrenal disease, small foci of lymphocytes and plasma cells, mainly in a perivenous location (fig. 1-41), are thought to accompany retroperitoneal chronic inflammatory processes, such as chronic pyelonephritis. The significance of these cellular infiltrates is not known.

Ovarian Thecal Metaplasia

Occasionally, small, partially hyalinized, fibroblastic nodules, which are often wedge shaped and attached to the adrenal capsule, are identified (fig. 1-42). Groups of spindle cells often extend between or surround small nests of cortical cells. This mesenchymal proliferation, which is most common in postmenopausal females, has been referred to as nodular hyperplasia of adrenal cortical blastema (53), but morphologically resembles mesenchymal cells of ovarian stroma, thus prompting the designation ovarian thecal metaplasia (54). This lesion is noted in 4.3 percent of females, but has also been documented in men on rare occasion (53). The maximum size of the nodules is about 2 mm, and the lesions are multiple in about half of the cases and bilateral in roughly a third (49). Rarely, macroscopic spindle cell lesions occur which also resemble ovarian cortical stroma, but in one case there was a suggestion of origin from Schwann cells (46).

ELECTRON MICROSCOPY

Electron Microscopy of Adrenal Cortex

The normal ultrastructure of the adrenal cortex in humans has been addressed in a number of selected studies (58–61,63), and optimal results depend upon examination of glands obtained surgically without significant derangement in factors that would impact upon physiologic function by induction of "stress." In a study of glands surgically resected from three women for palliative treatment of breast cancer, the three traditional zones of the cortex could be distinguished on the basis of size, shape, and internal architecture of mitochondria (58). All three zones of the adult cortex have a basement membrane surrounding clusters of several cells (63).

The zona glomerulosa is distinguished by cells with relatively little lipid and lower cytoplasmic volume compared with cells of the zona

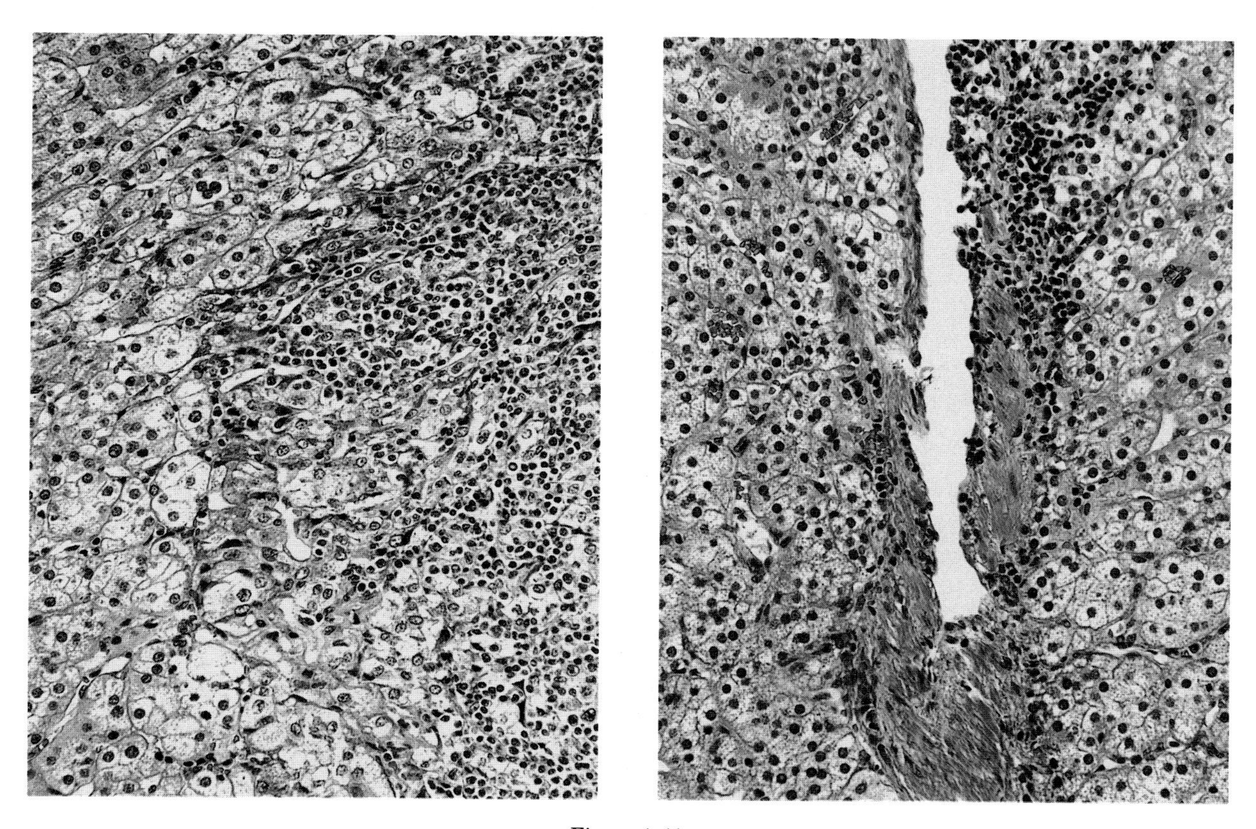

Figure 1-41
CHRONIC INFLAMMATION OF ADRENAL GLAND

Left: A prominent chronic inflammatory infiltrate is present near the corticomedullary junction and consists of mainly lymphocytes.

Right: Mild chronic inflammation is present around a small venous channel near the corticomedullary junction.

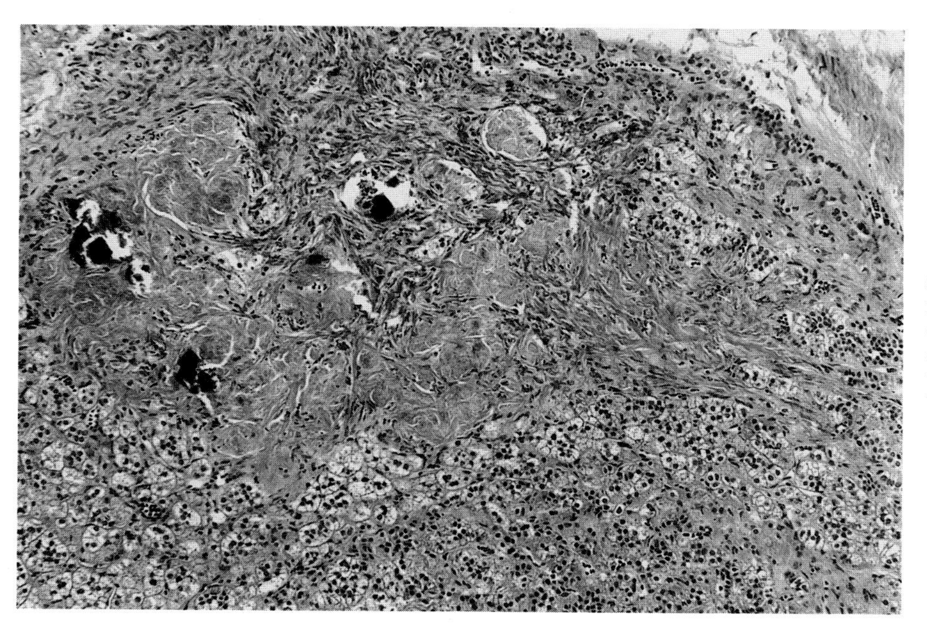

Figure 1-42
OVARIAN THECAL METAPLASIA

A focus of ovarian thecal metaplasia with dystrophic calcification is attached to the adrenal capsule. Small nests of cortical cells are present between some of the bands of hyalinized connective tissue.

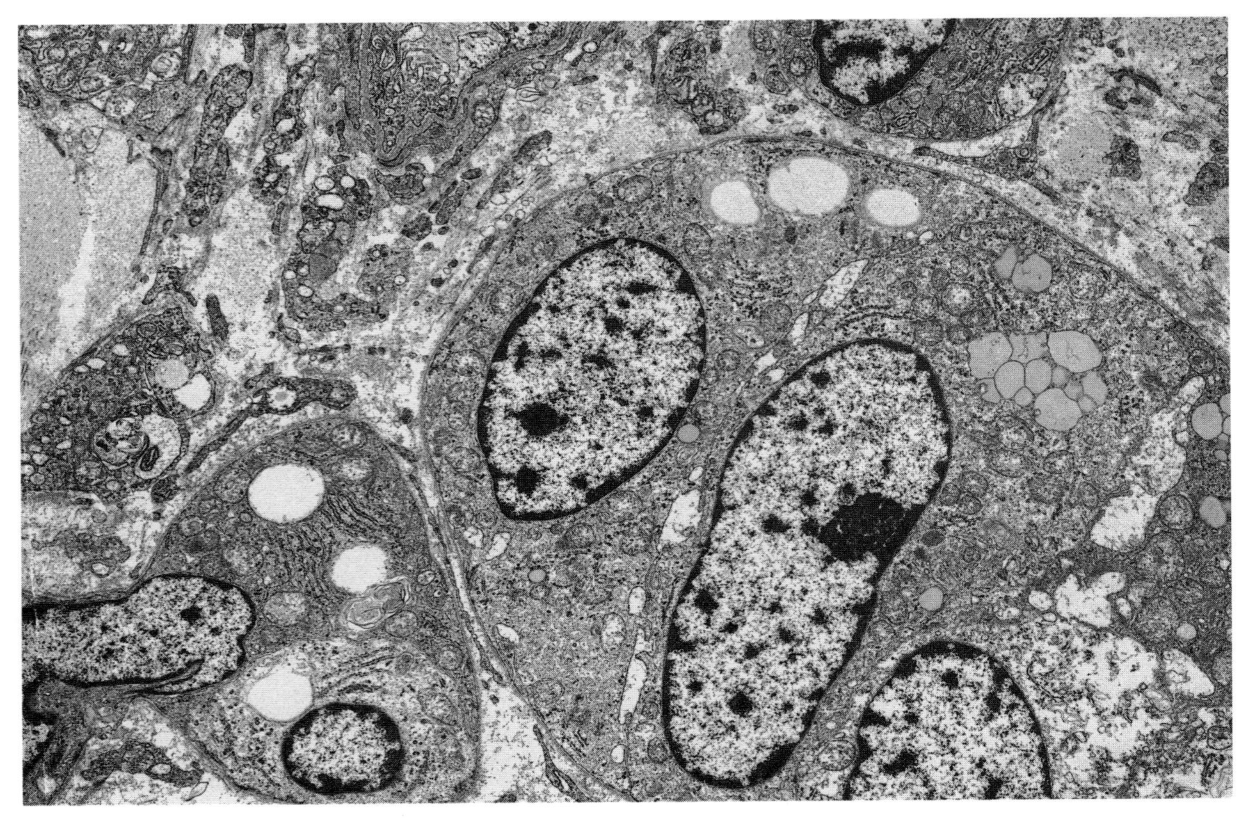

Figure 1-43
ZONA GLOMERULOSA OF NORMAL ADRENAL CORTEX
Cells of the zona glomerulosa contain relatively sparse lipid and have mitochondria that are round or ovoid. On closer view, the mitochondria had lamellar cristae. A clusteb of cells is surrounded by a continuous basement membrane. Both smooth and rough endoplasmic reticulum are present. (X5,000)

fasciculata (59,61), and mitochondria that are elongate to round with lamellar or plate-like cristae (fig. 1-43) (58). Lipofuscin granules and lysosomes are sparse. The surface of cortical cells may have short microvillous projections which are most prominent in the inner zona fasciculata (58,60).

Cells of the zona fasciculata have mitochondria that are usually round to ovoid, and possess short and long tubular cristae (fig. 1-44) (58). Lipid droplets are a prominent feature and may be quite large; some droplets may appear as empty vacuoles depending upon the method of fixation and processing for electron microscopic study. Cells often contain an abundant smooth endoplasmic reticulum which may form a complex network of anastomosing tubules. Profiles of rough endoplasmic reticulum may also be present, but in small amount. The cytoplasmic volume in this zone tends to be large relative to the other zones. Microvillous cytoplasmic projections can also be prominent. Junctional complexes are scanty, with close apposition of the plasmalemma of adjacent cordical cells resembling tight junctions (58).

The zona reticularis is distinguished by cells with sparse lipid and often numerous lipofuscin granules and lysosomes. Mitochondria are usually spherical to ovoid, and have cristae with a mixture of short and long tubular invaginations of the inner membrane (58).

Ultrastructural study of early fetal cortical cells shows an abundant smooth endoplasmic reticulum which accounts in large part for the granular eosinophilic appearance by light microscopy; mitochondria are spherical to ovoid with tubular cristae, and contain sparse lipid at about 8 weeks' gestation (60). The cell surface is covered with short microvilli which project both into the intercellular space and toward the sinusoidal

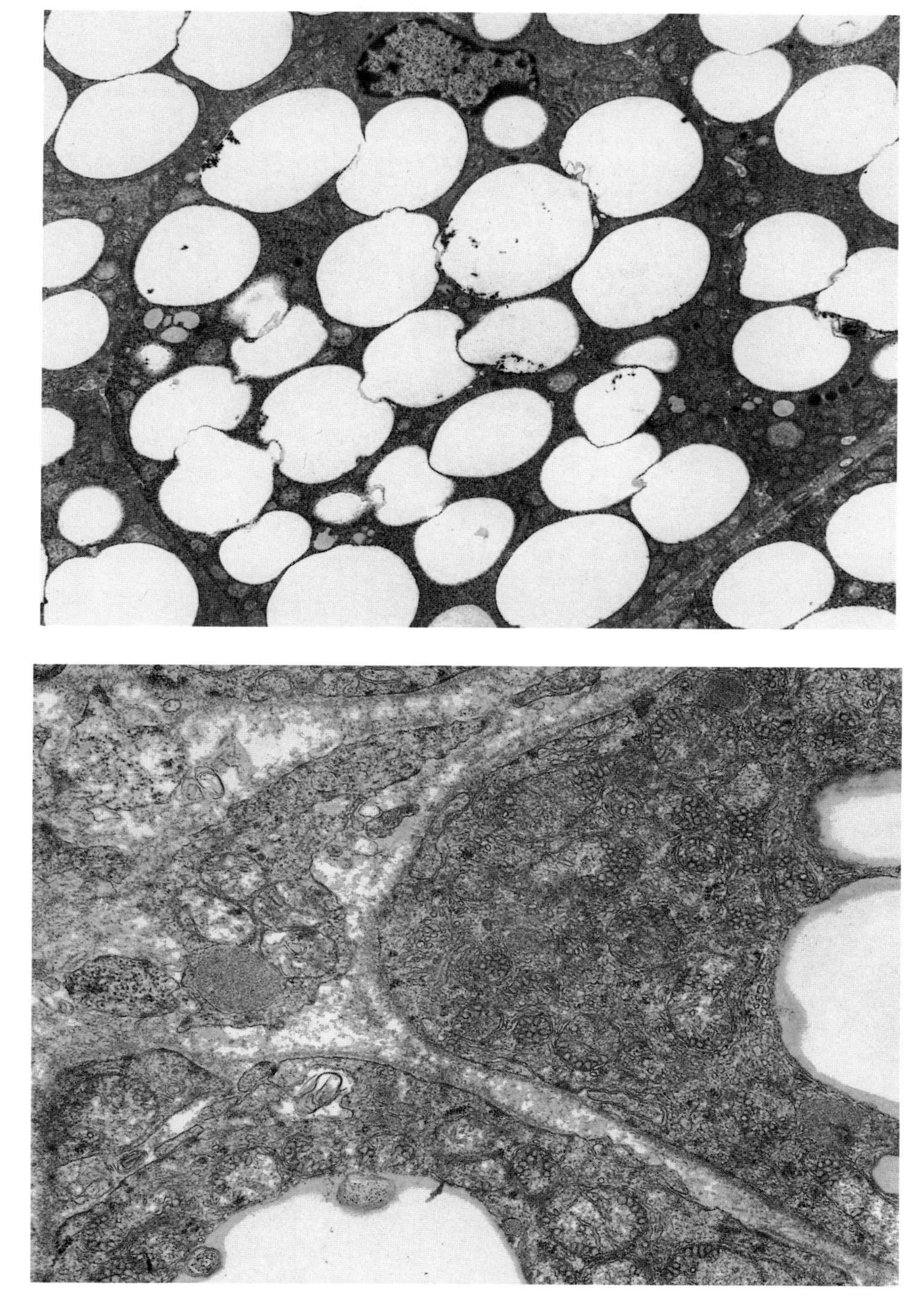

Figure 1-44

ZONA FASCICULATA OF NORMAL ADRENAL CORTEX

Top: Cells of the zona fasciculata contain abundant, large lipid droplets. Focally, lipid droplets distort the nuclear contour. (X5,250)

Bottom: Cells of the zona fasciculata contain mitochondria which are roughly circular, with short tubular or vesicular cristae. Smooth endoplasmic reticulum is also prominent. (X21,250) (Fig. 1-24 from Lack EE, Kozakewich HP. Embryology, developmental anatomy and selected aspects of non-neoplastic pathology. In: Lack EE, ed. Pathology of the adrenal glands. New York: Churchill Livingstone, 1990:1–74.)

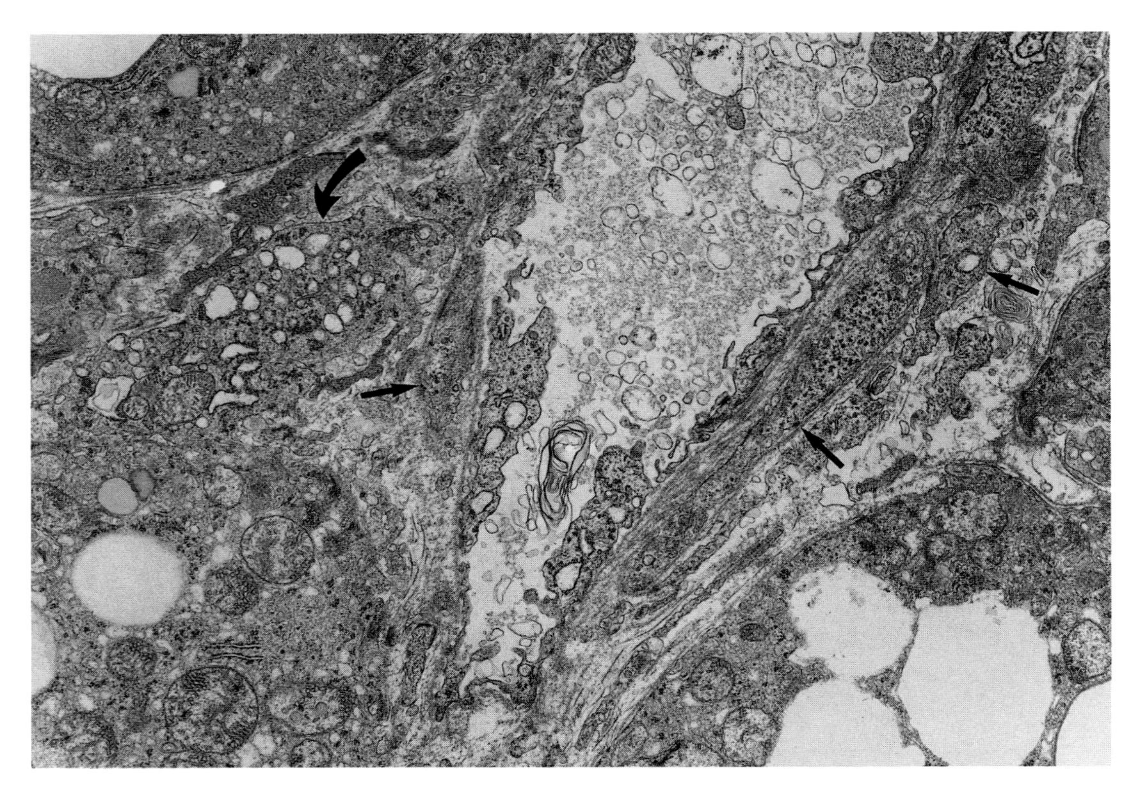

Figure 1-45
ZONA FASCICULATA OF NORMAL ADRENAL CORTEX
The capillary is lined by endothelial cells with cytoplasmic fenestrations. The cytoplasmic processes of the pericytes partially encircle the vascular channel (straight arrows), and have closely apposed basement membrane material. Occasional cells resemble fibroblasts (curved arrow). (X8,500)

endothelium. Cells often contain a large Golgi complex with numerous associated dense bodies which are described as lysosome-like and are perhaps involved in the fetal pattern of steroid metabolism (60).

Almost all of the cortical cells are in close proximity to capillary channels. Capillary spaces are lined by an attenuated endothelium with fenestrations, and in most areas there is a continuous well-developed basal lamina with scattered pericytes (fig. 1-45). The perivascular spaces within the adrenal cortex have been considered similar to the space of Dissé in the liver, and occasional macrophages have been noted in this area (63).

Electron Microscopy of Adrenal Medulla

Chromaffin cells in the adult adrenal gland show some interdigitation of blunt to elongate cytoplasmic processes with few small, rudimentary intercellular attachments (not true desmosomes). The density of cellular organelles may vary from cell to cell, contributing to the impression of a dichotomous or dual cell population with both "dark" and "light" cells. The dominant ultrastructural feature is the presence of dense-core neurosecretory-type granules that also vary in density from one cell to another, and even in the same cell (fig. 1-46) (56). The granules range in morphology from small, uniform dense cores having a tight limiting membrane and symmetric halo to granules with a wide asymmetric halo (fig. 1-47); the former granules have been associated with epinephrine storage and the latter with norepinephrine (62). Granule morphology can vary considerably, with pleomorphic, elongate, crescentic, or "dumbbell" shaped granules (fig. 1-46), and association of granule morphology by itself with storage of any particular regulatory peptide or hormone is not reliable. Neurosecretory granules usually range in size from 150 to 250 nm (62).

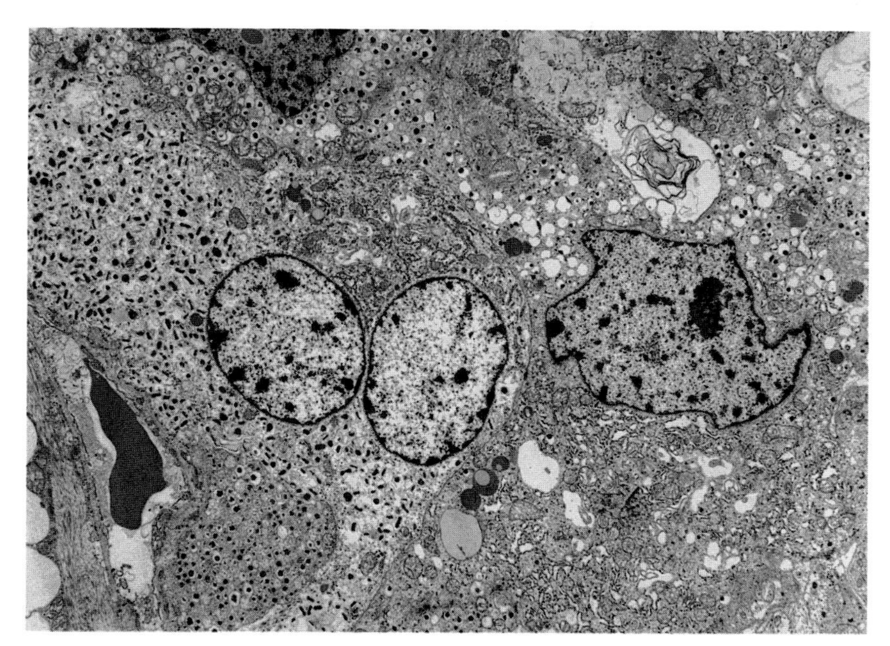

Figure 1-46
NORMAL ADRENAL
CHROMAFFIN CELLS

The density of the dense-core neurosecretory granules varies from cell to cell. Some neurosecretory granules are pleomorphic (cells on left) with many having an elongate, indented, or "dumbbell" configuration. Some chromaffin cells have prominent rough endoplasmic reticulum. Lipofuscin can also be identified. (X4,000)

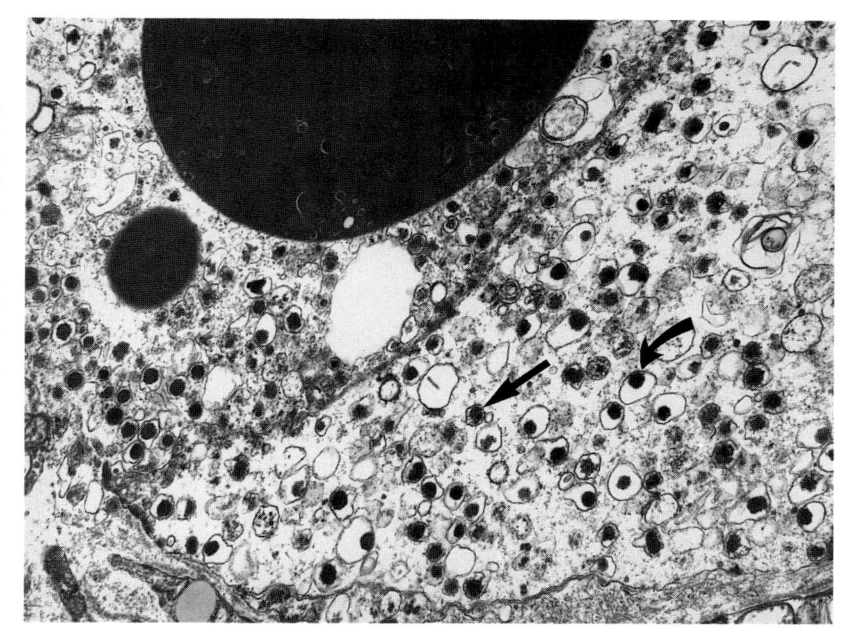

Figure 1-47
MAFFIN CELLS
IN NORMAL MEDULLA

Two adjacent chromaffin cells contain numerous neurosecretory granules. Some granules have a wide, asymmetric halo between the electron-dense core and limiting membrane (curved arrow), a morphologic feature associated with norepinephrine storage. Other granules have a more uniform morphology with a narrow, symmetric halo (straight arrow) which has been associated with storage of epinephrine. These ultrastructural features by themselves may not be reliable in predicting the granule content of any particular hormone or neuropeptide. Note also the large intracytoplasmic hyaline globule with small round to oval structures at the periphery. (X17,000) (Fig. 10-37 from Lack EE. Pathology of adrenal and extra-adrenal paraganglia. Major problems in pathology. vol 29. Philadelphia: WB Saunders, 1994:215.)

A small to moderate amount of rough endoplasmic reticulum is seen in some chromaffin cells (fig. 1-46), but overall, smooth endoplasmic reticulum is sparse. Lipochrome pigment is present in some cells in association with sparse lipid, and is typically not as electron dense as in the structures corresponding to the hyaline globules. Nuclei often show peripheral aggregation of chromatin, and the nuclear membrane is usually smooth and regular in contour, but may show some indentation or folding. Occasionally, there are simple intercellular attachments between chromaffin cells, and rarely even with an adjacent cortical cell (57). The vascular network is delicate, lined by endothelial cells with some cytoplasmic fenestrations, similar to that present in the cortex.

REFERENCES

Embryology and Biosynthetic Pathways

1. Beckwith JB, Perrin EV. In situ neuroblastomas: a contribution to the natural history of neural crest tumors. Am J Pathol 1963;43:1089–104.
2. Chester Jones I. Variation in the mouse adrenal cortex with special reference to the zona reticularis and to brown degeneration, together with a discussion of the "cell migration" theory. Qtr J Micros Sci 1948;89:53–74.
3. Coupland RE. The natural history of the chromaffin cell—twenty-five years on the beginning. Arch Histol Cytol 1989;52:331–41.
4. Crowder RE. The development of the adrenal gland in man, with special reference to origin and ultimate location of cell types and evidence in favor of the "cell migration" theory. Contributions to embryology. Vol 36, publication no. 611, Carnegie Institute of Washington, 1957:242–51.
5. Gilles Bouloux PM. Phaeochromocytomas and related tumours. In: Grossman A, ed. Clinical endocrinology. London: Blackwell Scientific, 1992;459–85.
6. Gottschau M. Struktur und embryonale entwickelung der nebennieren bei säugetieren. Arch fur Anat und Endwicklungsgeschichte. Anatomischer Abteilung 1883;9:412–58.
7. Lack EE, Kozakewich HP. Embryology, developmental anatomy, and selected aspects of non-neoplastic pathology. In: Lack EE, ed. Pathology of the adrenal glands. New York: Churchill Livingstone, 1990:1–74.
8. Neville AM. The adrenal medulla. In: Symington T, ed. Functional pathology of the adrenal gland. Baltimore: Williams & Wilkins, 1969:219–324.
9. O'Rahilly R. The timing and sequence of events in the development of the human endocrine system during the embryonic period proper. Anat Embryol 1983;166:439–51.
10. Pescovitz OH, Cutler GB Jr, Loriaux DL. Synthesis and secretion of corticosteroids. In: Becker KL, ed. Principles and practice of endocrinology and metabolism. Philadelphia: JB Lippincott, 1990:579–91.
11. Turkel SB, Itabashi HH. The natural history of neuroblastic cells in the fetal adrenal gland. Am J Pathol 1974;76:225–36.
12. Vinson GP, Whitehouse BJ, Hinson JP. Structure and function of the adrenal cortex. In: Grossman A, ed. Clinical endocrinology. London: Blackwell Scientific, 1992:373–92.
13. Wurtman RJ. Catecholamines. N Engl J Med 1965; 273:637–46, 693–700, 748–53.
14. Zajicek G, Ariel I, Arber N. The streaming adrenal cortex: direct evidence of centripetal migration of adrenocytes by estimation of cell turnover rate. J Endocr 1986;111:477–82.

Function of Fetal Adrenal Glands

15. Artul R. Fetal adrenal medulla. Clin Obstet Gynecol 1980;23:825–36.
16. Challis JR, Mitchell BF, Lye SJ. Activation of fetal adrenal function. J Dev Physiol 1984;6:93–105.
17. Pepe GJ, Albrecht ED. Regulation of the primate fetal adrenal cortex. Endocr Rev 1990;11:151–76.
18. Simonian MH, Capp MW. Characterization of steroidogenesis in cell cultures of the human fetal adrenal cortex: comparison of definitive zone and fetal zone cells. J Clin Endocrinol Metab 1984;59:643–51.
19. Wurtman RJ, Axelrod J. Control of enzymatic synthesis of adrenaline in the adrenal medulla by adrenal cortical steroids. J Biol Chem 1966;241:2301–5.

Anatomy of Adrenal Glands

20. Bartman J, Driscoll SG. Fetal adrenal cortex in erythroblastosis fetalis. Arch Pathol 1969;87:343–6.
21. Bretan PN Jr, Lorig R. Adrenal imaging. Computed tomographic scanning and magnetic resonance imaging. Urol Clin North Am 1989;16:505–13.
22. Consensus conference. Magnetic resonance imaging. JAMA 1988;259:2132–8.
23. Dekker A, Oehrle JS. Hyaline globules of the adrenal medulla of man. A product of lipid peroxidation? Arch Pathol 1971;91:353–64.
24. Dobbie JW, Symington T. The human adrenal gland with special reference to the vasculature. J Endocrinol 1966;34:479–89.
25. El-Sherief MA, Hemmingsson A. Computed tomography of the normal adrenal gland. Pathologic implications. Acta Radiol 1982;23:433–42.
26. Lack EE. Adrenal medullary hyperplasia and pheochromocytoma. In: Lack EE ed. Pathology of the adrenal glands. New York: Churchill Livingstone, 1990:173–235.
27. Lack EE. Pathology of adrenal and extra-adrenal paraganglia. Major problems in pathology, Vol 29. Philadelphia: WB Saunders, 1994.
28. Lack EE, Kozakewich HP. Embryology, developmental anatomy, and selected aspects of non-neoplastic pathology. In: Lack EE, ed. Pathology of the adrenal glands. New York: Churchill Livingstone, 1990:1–74.
29. Mendelsohn G, Olson JL. Pheochromocytomas [Letter]. Hum Pathol 1978;9:607–8.
30. Mezrich R, Banner MP, Pollack HM. Magnetic resonance imaging of the adrenal glands. Urol Radiol 1986;8:127–38.
31. Mitty HA, Cohen BA. Adrenal imaging. Urol Clin N Am 1985;12:771–85.
32. Oppenheimer EH. Cyst formation in the outer adrenal cortex. Studies in the human fetus and newborn. Arch Pathol 1969;87:653–9.
33. Quinan C, Berger AA. Observations on human adrenals with especial reference to the relative weight of the normal medulla. Ann Int Med 1933;6:1180–92.
34. Rodin AE, Hsu FL, Whorton EB. Microcysts of the permanent adrenal cortex in perinates and infants. Arch Pathol Lab Med 1976;100:499–502.
35. Stoner HB, Whiteley HJ, Emery JL. The effect of systemic disease on the adrenal cortex of the child. J Path Bact 1953;66:171–83.

36. Studzinski GP, Hay DC, Symington T. Observations on the weight of the human adrenal gland and the effect of preparations of corticotropin of different purity on the weight and morphology of the human adrenal gland. J Clin Endocrinol Metab 1963;23:248–54.
37. Swinyard CA. Growth of the human suprarenal glands. Anat Rec 1943;87:141–50.
38. Symington T. Functional pathology of the human adrenal gland. Baltimore: Williams & Wilkins, 1969.
39. Tähkä H. On the weight and structure of the adrenal glands and the factors affecting them in children of 0-2 years. Acta Pediatrica 1951;40 (Suppl 81):4–95.
40. Wilbur OM Jr, Rich AR. A study of the role of adrenocorticotropic hormone (ACTH) in the pathogenesis of tubular degeneration of the adrenals. Bull Johns Hopkins Hosp 1954;93:321–47.

Immunohistochemistry and Distribution of Steroidogenic Enzymes

41. Cote J, Cordon-Cardo C, Reuter VE, Rosen PP. Immunopathology of adrenal and renal cortical tumors. Coordinated change in antigen expression is associated with neoplastic conversion in the adrenal cortex. Am J Pathol 1990;136:1077–84.
42. Gaffey MJ, Traweek ST, Mills SE, et al. Cytokeratin expression in adrenocortical neoplasia: an immunohistochemical and biochemical study with implications for the differential diagnosis of adrenocortical, hepatocellular, and renal cell carcinoma. Hum Pathol 1992;23:144–53.
43. Miettinen M, Lehto VP, Virtanen I. Immunofluorescence microscopic evaluation of the intermediate filament expression of the adrenal cortex and medulla and their tumors. Am J Pathol 1985;118:360–6.
44. Sasano H, Nose M, Sasano N. Lectin histochemistry in adrenocortical hyperplasia and neoplasms with emphasis on carcinoma. Arch Pathol Lab Med 1989;113:68–72.
45. Sasano N, Sasano H. The adrenal cortex. In: Kovacs K, Asa SL, eds. Functional endocrine pathology. London: Blackwell Scientific, 1991:546–84.

Miscellaneous Microscopic Features

46. Carney JA. Unusual tumefactive spindle-cell lesions in the adrenal glands. Hum Pathol 1987;18:980–5.
47. Craig JM, Landing BH. Anaplastic cells of fetal adrenal cortex. Am J Clin Pathol 1951;21:940–9.
48. Favara BE, Steele A, Grant JH, Steele P. Adrenal cytomegaly: quantitative assessment by image analysis. Pediatr Pathol 1991;11:521–36.
49. Fidler WJ. Ovarian thecal metaplasia in adrenal glands. Am J Clin Pathol 1977;67:318–23.
50. Griffel B. Focal adrenalitis. Its frequency and correlation with similar lesions in the thyroid and kidney. Virchows Arch [A] 1974;364:191–8.
51. Nakamura Y, Yano H, Nakashima T. False intranuclear inclusions in adrenal cytomegaly. Arch Pathol Lab Med 1981;105:358–60.
52. Oppenheimer EH. Adrenal cytomegaly: studies by light and electron microscopy. Comparison with the adrenal in Beckwith's and virilism syndromes. Arch Pathol 1970;90:57–64.
53. Reed RJ, Patrick JT. Nodular hyperplasia of the adrenal cortical blastema. Bull Tulane Univ Med Fac 1967;26:151–7.
54. Wong TW, Warner NE. Ovarian thecal metaplasia in the adrenal gland. Arch Pathol 1971;92:319–28.
55. Yamashima M. Focal adrenocortical cytomegaly observed in two adult cases. Arch Pathol Lab Med 1986;110:1072–5.

Electron Microscopy

56. Brown WJ, Barajas L, Latta H. The ultrastructure of the human adrenal medulla: with comparative studies of white rat. Anat Rec 1971;169:173–83.
57. Lack EE. Pathology of adrenal and extra-adrenal paraganglia. Major problems in pathology, Vol 29. Philadelphia: WB Saunders, 1994.
58. Long JA, Jones AL. Observations on the fine structure of the adrenal cortex of man. Lab Invest 1967;17:355–70.
59. Mackay A. Atlas of human adrenal cortex ultrastructure. In: Syminton T, ed. Functional pathology of the human adrenal gland. Baltimore: Williams & Wilkins, 1969:346–489.
60. McNutt NS, Jones AL. Observations on the ultrastructure of cytodifferentiation in the human fetal adrenal cortex. Lab Invest 1970;22:513–27.
61. Neville AM, O'Hare MJ. Aspects of structure, function, and pathology. In: James VH, ed. The adrenal gland. New York: Raven Press, 1979:1–65.
62. Tannenbaum M. Ultrastructural pathology of adrenal medullary tumors. Pathol Annu 1970;5:145–71.
63. Tannenbaum M. Ultrastructural pathology of the adrenal cortex. Pathol Annu 1973;8:109–56.

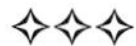

2
CONGENITAL ADRENAL HETEROTOPIA, HYPERPLASIA, AND BECKWITH-WIEDEMANN SYNDROME

ADRENAL ADHESION, UNION, AND FUSION

Adrenal union and adrenal adhesion are distinguished by the presence or absence of a continuous connective tissue capsule (1): in adrenal adhesion there is an intervening capsule, while with adrenal union there is intermingling of respective parenchymal cells (fig. 2-1). The term fusion has been used synonymously with union (2). The morphologic features are probably identical to adrenal-renal heterotopia. Both have involved the liver and kidney. Adrenal fusion is a rare anomaly in which the adrenal glands are united in the midline with some medial deviation of kidneys in most cases (fig. 2-2). This abnormality is sometimes associated with midline congenital defects such as spinal dysraphism, indeterminate visceral situs, and occasionally the Cornelia de Lange syndrome (mental and growth retardation, synophrys, anteverted nostrils, low-set ears, and spade-like hands with short tapering fingers) (3). Renal agenesis is sometimes associated with abnormally shaped adrenal glands, which may be oval with a smooth contour (3). Complete absence or aplasia of adrenal glands has been barely described, and may be familial (4).

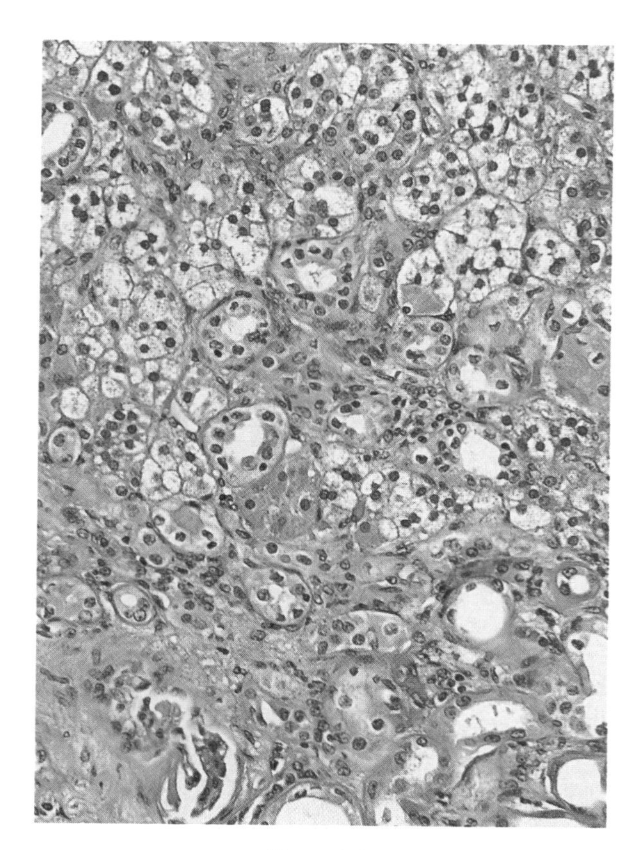

Figure 2-1
ADRENAL-RENAL UNION
There is union of adrenal and renal parenchyma without an intervening capsule.

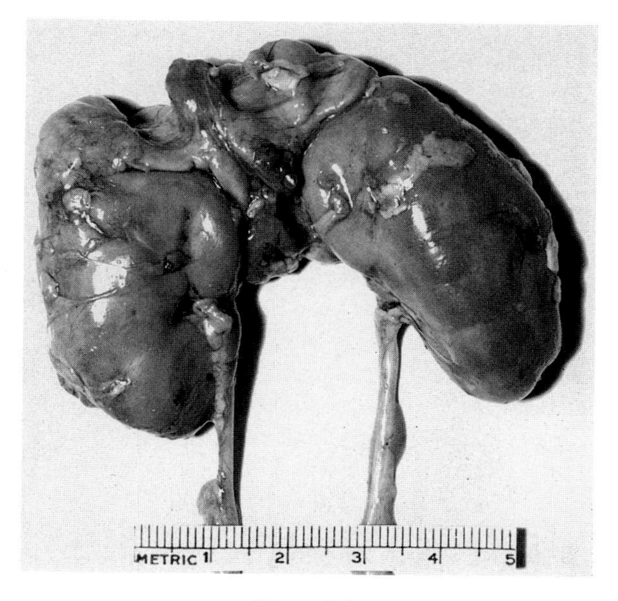

Figure 2-2
MULTIPLE CONGENITAL ANOMALIES
This 1-month-old child had multiple congenital anomalies including spinal dysraphism. At autopsy the kidneys were more medially situated and the adrenal glands were fused in the midline. (Fig. 1-29 from Lack EE, Kozakewich HP. Embryology, developmental anatomy, and selected aspects of nonneoplastic pathology. In: Lack EE, ed. Pathology of the adrenal glands. New York: Churchill Livingstone, 1990:1–74.)

Table 2-1

LOCATION OF ACCESSORY AND HETEROTOPIC ADRENAL TISSUE

Area of celiac axis	32 %
Kidney, usually subcapsular upper pole	<0.1–6 %
Broad ligament	23%
Adnexa of testes	7.5%
Spermatic cord	3.8 –9.3%
Rare sites: placenta, liver, lung, intracranial	

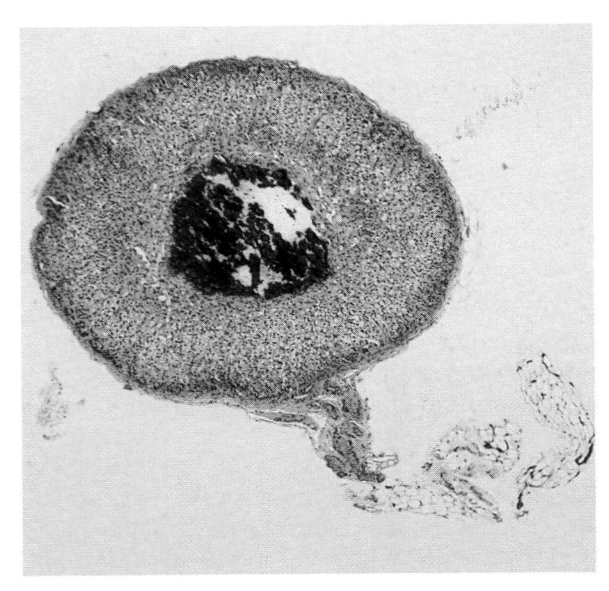

Figure 2-3
HETEROTOPIC ADRENAL CORTICAL TISSUE
A small nodule of heterotopic adrenal cortical tissue was located along the spermatic cord and was removed during inguinal hernia repair in a child. Dystrophic calcification is present centrally.

HETEROTOPIC AND ACCESSORY ADRENAL TISSUES

Heterotopic and accessory adrenal tissues are found in the upper abdomen or anywhere along the path of descent of the gonads. This anatomic location can be explained on an embryologic basis given the close spatial relationship between the developing kidneys and adrenal glands. In rare cases, adrenal heterotopia occurs in bizarre anatomic sites which defy logical embryologic explanation: in placenta (16), lung (7,8), and the intracranial cavity (26). An unusual example of intra-adrenal hepatic heterotopia has also been reported (14). One of the most frequent sites for accessory adrenal tissue is the area of the celiac axis: in a study of 100 consecutive autopsies, accessory adrenal cortical tissue was identified in the area of the celiac plexus in 32 percent of cases, and in half of these (16 percent) the accessory tissue consisted of both cortex and medulla (13). Accessory or heterotopic adrenal cortical tissue has been noted in the kidney, usually in a subcapsular location in the upper pole, in 0.1 to 6.0 percent of individuals at autopsy (6,19,21). Complete removal of the renal capsule with exposure of the entire cortical surface may facilitate recognition of accessory adrenal tissue, which is usually less than 3 to 4 mm in size. The resemblance of adrenal cortex to cells of renal cell carcinoma led Grawitz in 1883 to postulate that hypernephromas arise from misplaced adrenal tissue (22). Ectopic cortical tissue has also been noted within the wall of the gallbladder (9). Small adrenal cortical rests (fig. 2-1) should be distinguished from adrenal-renal (or adrenal-hepatic) heterotopia. Adrenal-renal heterotopia can be complete or incomplete: in the complete form, the entire adrenal gland is located beneath the renal capsule over the superior pole or anterior surface of the kidney; in the incomplete form, the subcapsular portion of the gland is firmly attached to the surface of the kidney while a part of the gland may be contained in peculiar folds of the capsule or outside the capsule. The latter form is rare (10), and was seen in only 0.16 percent of autopsies in one study (22).

Accessory adrenal tissue in sites further removed from the upper abdomen consists almost solely of cortex without a medullary component. Marchand (17) identified accessory adrenal tissue in the broad ligament near the ovary in infants. In 23.3 percent of cases of one study (Table 2-1), accessory cortical tissue was identified in the broad ligament anywhere from the junction with the mesosalpinx to its lateral attachment; it was bilateral in 6.7 percent of cases (12). Accessory adrenal cortical tissue was found along the spermatic cord in 3.8 percent of children, undergoing inguinoscrotal surgery and in 9.3 percent who were operated on for an undescended testis (fig. 2-3) (18). Using

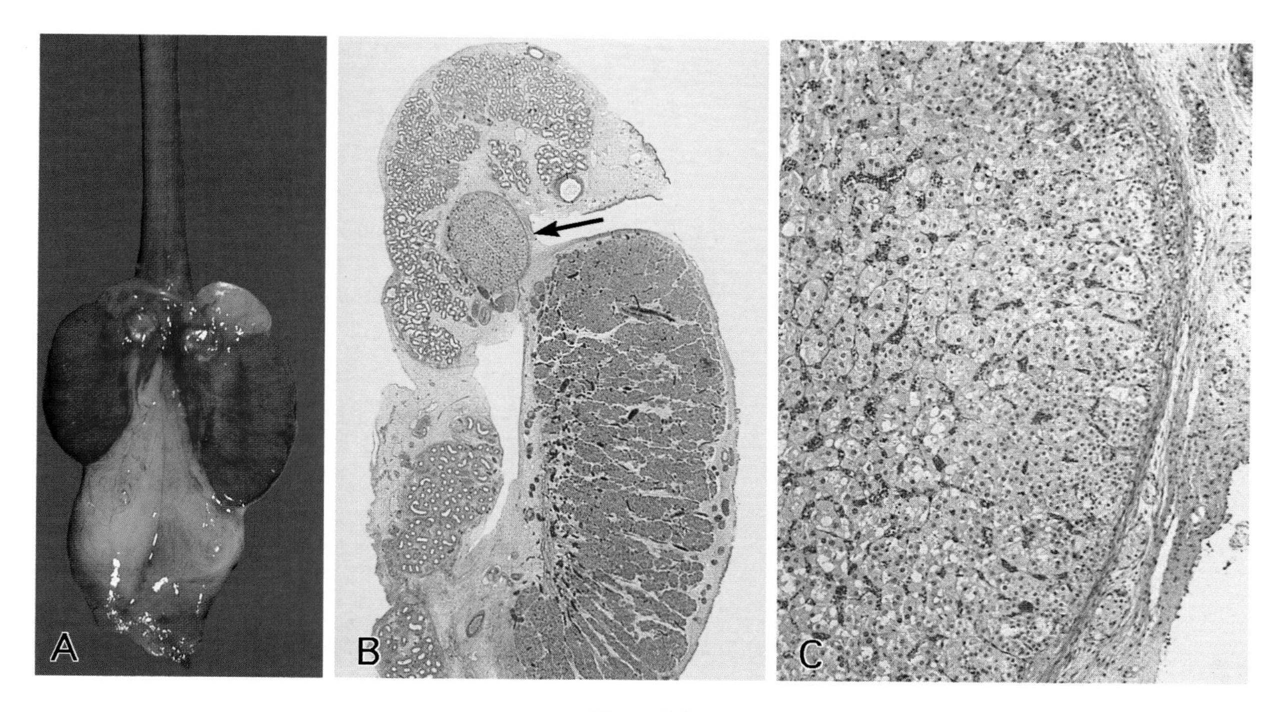

Figure 2-4
ACCESSORY ADRENAL TISSUE

A: Bisected testis from a newborn infant who died of disseminated herpes simplex infection. A small nodule of accessory or heterotopic adrenal cortex is present in the hilum of the testis near the junction with the head of the epididymis and microscopically showed herpetic necrosis similar to necrosis seen in orthotopic adrenal glands. Attached pale connective tissue was markedly edematous.

B: Longitudinal section of a newborn testis shows a nodule of accessory/ heterotopic adrenal cortical tissue in the hilum of the testis adjacent to the head of the epididymis (arrow).

C: The adrenal cortical tissue from case seen in B is composed of only cortical cells, without a medullary component.

a serial blocking technique, accessory adrenal cortical tissue was found in 15 of 200 testes from 100 male infants less than 1 year of age (7.5 percent); it was bilateral in 4 percent (11). The nodules were circumscribed, round to ovoid, measured 0.5 to 7 mm in diameter, and were located in connective tissue of the distal spermatic cord or the area of the hilum of the testis (fig. 2-4). It is rare to see an adrenal cortical rest actually located within testicular parenchyma (23) or in the substance of the ovary (24). The occurrence of adrenal tissue in ectopic locations helps explain adrenal cortical neoplasms that arise in unusual sites such as scrotum (20) and liver (25), although some examples defy ready embryologic explanation (15). Hyperplastic adrenal cortical nodules have been reported within the pancreas, and can be confused with metastatic renal cell carcinoma or a primary pancreatic endocrine neoplasm (5).

CONGENITAL ADRENAL HYPERPLASIA

The first unmistakable and thorough account of congenital adrenal hyperplasia (CAH), or the *adrenogenital syndrome*, was given by the Italian anatomist de Crecchio in 1865 (29). CAH results from a defect in any one of the five enzymatic steps involved in steroid synthesis (fig. 2-5). This disorder is an inborn error of metabolism which has an autosomal recessive mode of inheritance and is the most common cause of ambiguous genitalia in infants (36). About 90 to 95 percent of all cases of CAH are due to 21-hydroxylase deficiency, a disorder of cortisol and aldosterone biosynthesis resulting from mutations in the *CYP*21 gene encoding adrenal 21-hydroxylase P-450c21 (30,35). There are several forms of CAH: 1) a “classic” form, with an incidence between 1:5,000 and 1:15,000 live births in most

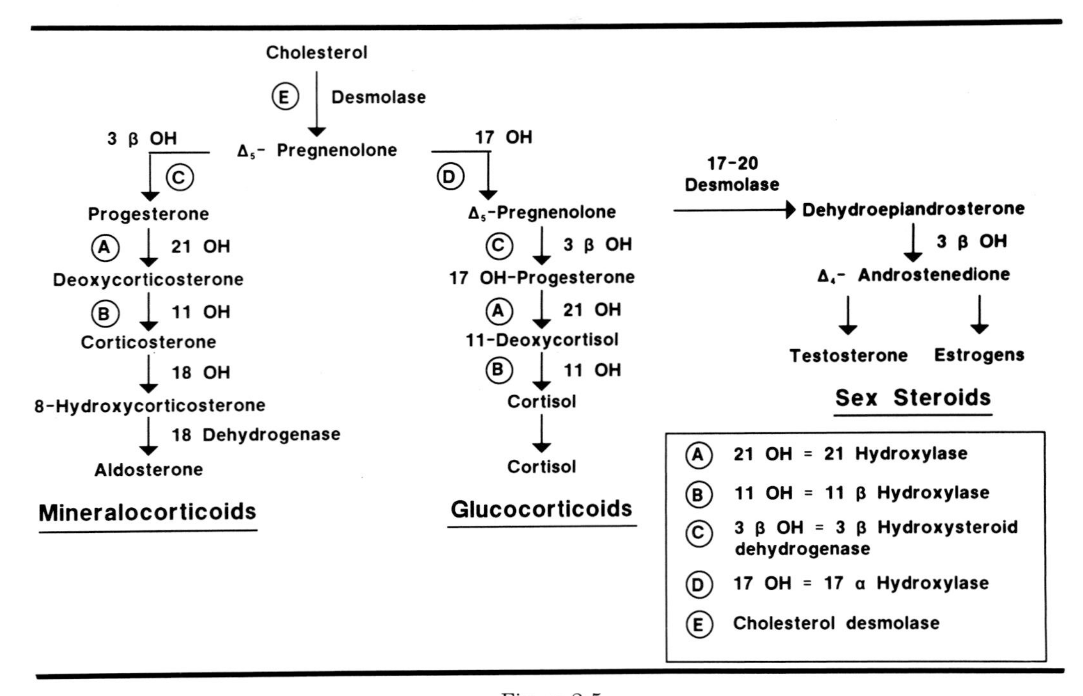

Figure 2-5
BIOSYNTHETIC PATHWAYS OF MINERALOCORTICOIDS, GLUCOCORTICOIDS, AND SEX STEROIDS
Sites of enzymatic block in congenital adrenal hyperplasia (CAH) are indicated by letters with the corresponding enzymes.

white populations; 2) a "nonclassic" form, one of the most frequent autosomal recessive disorders in the general white population; and 3) a "cryptic" form in which biochemical abnormalities may exist but the patients are asymptomatic. In two thirds of patients with the classic form of CAH, biosynthesis of aldosterone is blocked, resulting in "salt-wasting"; the remaining one third have a simple virilizing form of the disease. There are several recent reviews of this topic (28,32,33). Other enzymatic deficiencies causing CAH include: 1) 11-beta-hydroxylase deficiency which causes virilization and often hypertension due to accumulation of deoxycorticosterone; 2) 3-beta-hydroxysteroid dehydrogenase deficiency which results in intersexuality, and salt-wasting in severe cases; 3) 17-hydroxylase deficiency which is associated with hypertension, hypokalemia, and incomplete masculinization (27); and 4) cholesterol desmolase deficiency which affects the earliest step in the steroid biosynthetic pathway, and is usually fatal despite replacement therapy.

Clinical manifestations of CAH are the result of a deficiency of a particular steroid such as cortisol or the effects of steroids that accumulate proximal to the site of enzymatic deficiency and may be shunted into alternate biosynthetic pathways, particularly androgen synthesis. Males with the salt-losing form of 21-hydroxylase deficiency are at particular risk for salt-wasting, with symptoms (vomiting, dehydration, and hypotension) that resemble an Addisonian crisis within a few weeks of birth (fig. 2-6). If the female fetus is exposed to increased androgens in utero, there is a variable degree of virilization of external genitalia, while the internal female organs are relatively normal. The typically ambiguous genitalia in these female infants include clitoromegaly and fusion of labioscrotal folds which may be bulbous and rugated, thus simulating a scrotum (fig. 2-7). The clitoris may be bound somewhat by a "chordee." In a small number of infants the degree of virilization may be so marked that there is a fully masculinized penile urethra. The masculinized female may be incorrectly classified as a male (fig. 2-7), but the error is usually recognized when a salt-losing crisis develops at 1 to 4 weeks of age (28). Prenatal

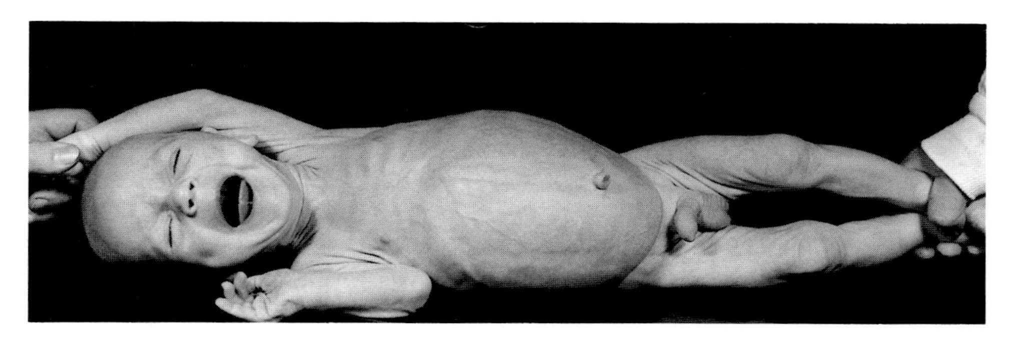

Figure 2-6
CONGENITAL ADRENAL HYPERPLASIA
Infant with the severe salt-losing form of CAH which was fatal due to dehydration, hypotension, and electrolyte imbalance.

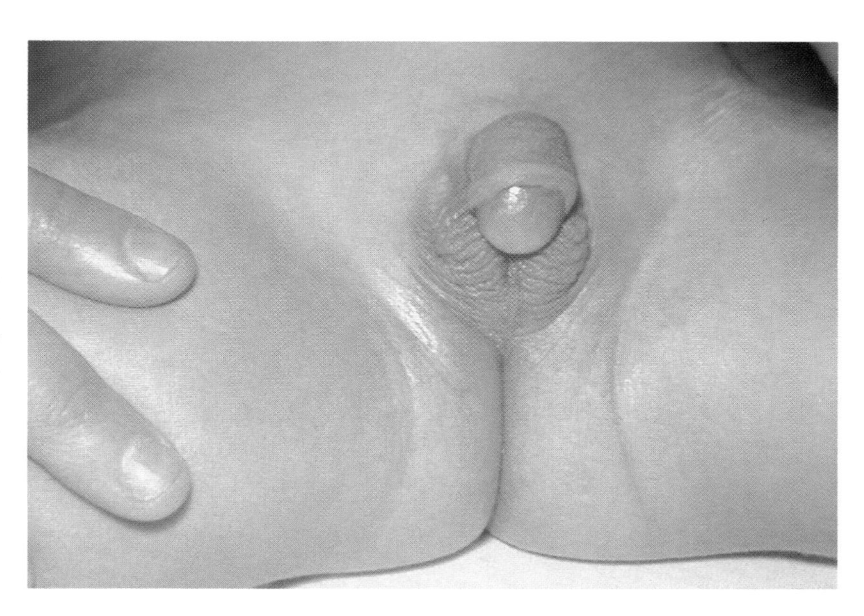

Figure 2-7
CONGENITAL ADRENAL HYPERPLASIA
This 18-month-old female was mistakenly assigned a male gender. Marked clitoromegaly resembles a penis. The hypertrophied clitoris had a urethral opening near the base. Note the rugosity of the partially fused labioscrotal folds which simulates a scrotum. (Photograph courtesy of Dr. Wellington Hung, Washington, DC.)

diagnosis is possible, and successful treatment may prevent virilization of the female fetus thus obviating the need for corrective genital surgery after birth (34).

Pathology of Adrenal Glands in CAH

CAH may be fatal if unrecognized or untreated. At autopsy the adrenal glands are enlarged, often tan or brown, with a convoluted or cerebriform surface due to cortical hyperplasia with redundant folds (fig. 2-8). Individual adrenal glands in children may weigh 10 to 15 g, while in older patients they may be 30 to 35 g (31). In most untreated cases of CAH the adrenal glands are darker than normal (fig. 2-9). In cholesterol desmolase deficiency, accumulation of cholesterol and cholesterol esters gives rise to a nodular cortex that is bright yellow or whitish, and microscopically there may be cholesterol clefts with a foreign body giant cell reaction and dystrophic calcification. In CAH, persistent and intense trophic stimulation by adrenocorticotropic hormone (ACTH) results in marked hyperplasia of the zona fasciculata with conversion of pale-staining, lipid-rich cells into lipid-depleted cells with compact, eosinophilic cytoplasm, similar to those of the zona reticularis (fig. 2-10, top); these morphologic findings, however, may be varied if the patient is partially treated with exogenous corticosteroids (fig. 2-10, bottom). This contributes, in large measure, to the dark color of the glands. With partial

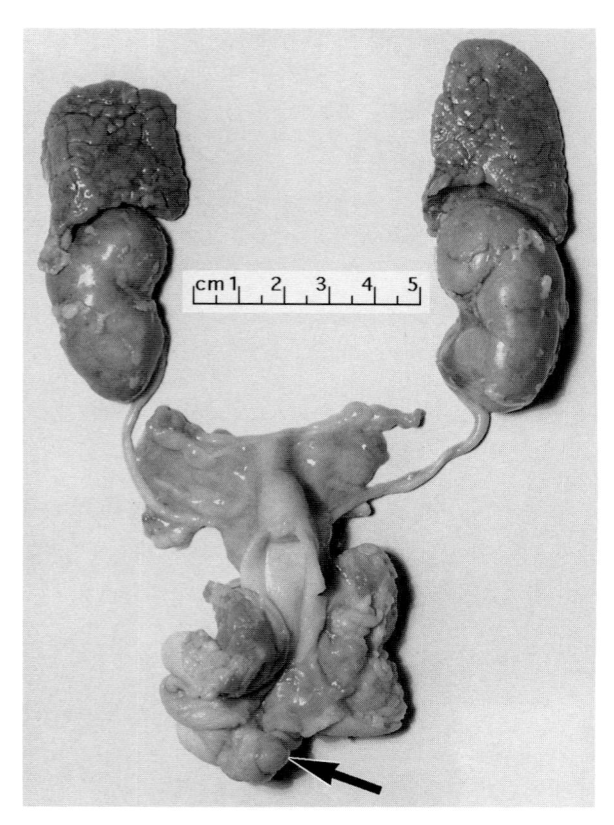

Figure 2-8
CONGENITAL ADRENAL HYPERPLASIA

Autopsy of an infant with CAH shows normal development of female reproductive tract including vagina, uterus, fallopian tubes, and ovaries. Both adrenal glands are markedly enlarged and hyperplastic with excessive cerebriform folds of cortex. Greatly enlarged clitoris is present near the bottom (arrow). (Fig. 1-45 from Lack EE, Kozakewich HP. Embryology, developmental anatomy, and selected aspects of non-neoplastic pathology. In: Lack EE, ed. Pathology of the adrenal glands. New York: Churchill Livingstone, 1990:1–74.)

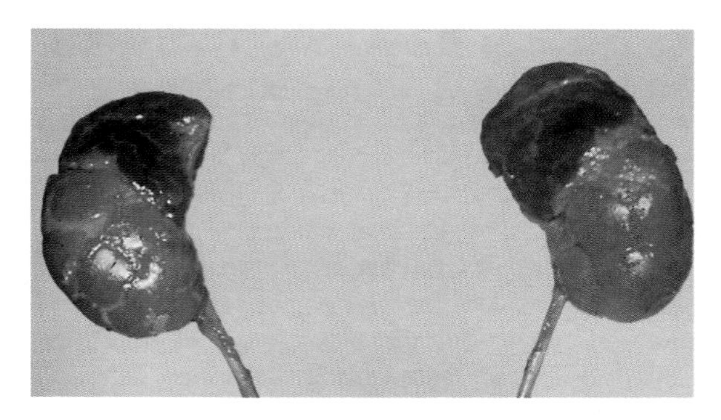

Figure 2-9
CONGENITAL ADRENAL HYPERPLASIA

Adrenal glands in congenital adrenal hyperplasia are enlarged and appear dark brown due to conversion of cortical cells into cells with compact, lipid-depleted cytoplasm.

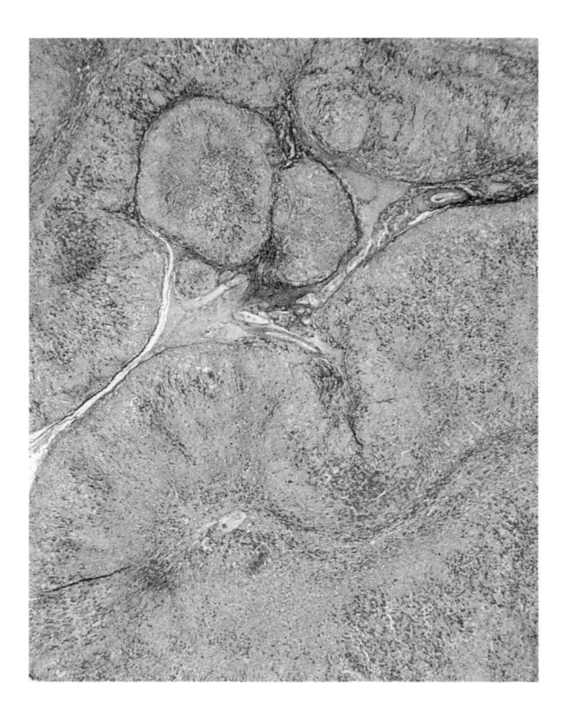

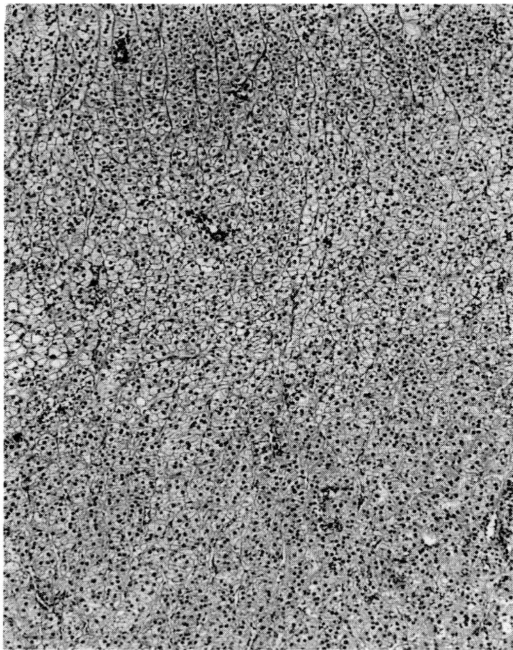

Figure 2-10
ADRENAL CORTICAL HYPERPLASIA

Top: Adrenal cortical hyperplasia with marked expansion of the zona fasciculata in a child with CAH. Many cells have lipid-depleted cytoplasm due to sustained ACTH stimulation. Note enlarged hyperplastic accessory cortical nodules or extrusions. (X100, Toluidine blue eosin stain)

Bottom: Hyperplastic adrenal cortex in a different case of CAH that had been partially treated. Expanded zona fasciculata contains cells with pale-staining, lipid-rich cytoplasm.

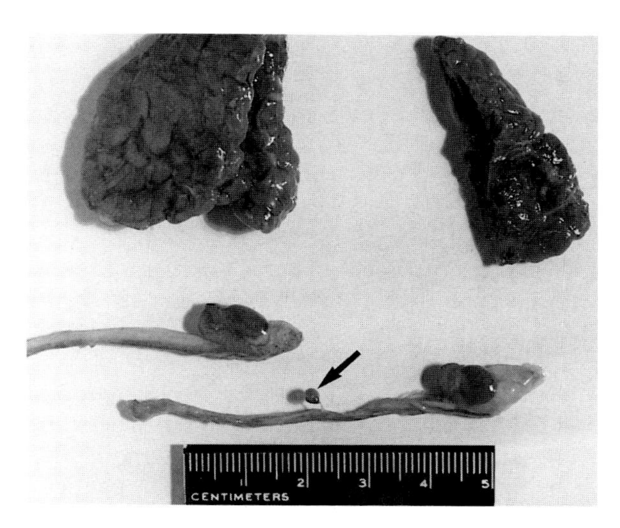

Figure 2-11
ENLARGED HYPERPLASTIC ADRENAL GLANDS IN A FATAL CASE OF CAH
Note enlarged accessory (heterotopic) nodule of adrenal cortex along spermatic cord (arrow).

or incomplete steroid replacement, the histologic picture may become altered, with columns and cords of lipid-rich cells admixed with some cells having lipid-depleted cytoplasm. Heterotopic or accessory adrenal cortical tissue can also become enlarged and hyperplastic (fig. 2-11).

OCCURRENCE OF TUMORS IN THE SETTING OF CAH

Adrenal Cortical Neoplasms

Persistent trophic stimulation of adrenal cortical tissue by ACTH gives rise to a diffuse, and at times, slightly nodular hyperplasia, and there have been rare cases of adrenal cortical neoplasia occurring in the setting of CAH (42). Involved neoplasms include both adrenal cortical adenomas (38,44) and carcinomas (37,41). In two cases, adrenal cortical carcinomas developed in patients with a longstanding (30 years and 36 years) history of virilization with onset in childhood, suggesting untreated CAH (39,43). Activation of virilizing adrenal rest tumors has been reported in a patient with Nelson's syndrome (45) in the areas of accessory adrenal cortical tissue, originally described by Marchand. An increased incidence of incidental adrenal nodule(s) has been noted in patients with homozygous (82 percent of patients; 2 cases were bilateral) and heterozygous (45 percent of patients) traits for CAH; the lesions were assumed to be adrenal cortical adenomas without evidence of excess steroid secretion (40). In the group of patients with the homozygous trait, tumors were 5 to 9 mm (9 patients), 1 to 2 cm (7 patients), and over 5 cm (2 patients); the tumors in the heterozygous group showed a similar size distribution (40). It is uncertain whether these lesions represent a true cortical neoplasm that is nonhyperfunctional or a dominant macronodule arising in a background of cortical hyperplasia.

Testicular Tumors in CAH

Definition. This is a tumefactive lesion of uncertain histogenesis in the setting of CAH which histologically resembles a Leydig or interstitial cell tumor, but may have features in common with hyperplastic adrenal cortical cells under the trophic influence of ACTH. Endocrinologic evaluation of the testicular lesions may reveal ACTH dependency with ability to produce glucocorticoids.

General Considerations. Testicular hilar nodules have been identified in a large proportion of cases of CAH when the testicular hilus was adequately studied (61), and while most of these collections of cells morphologically resemble Leydig cells (fig. 2-12) (55) some consider them to be a primordial rest (61). Extratesticular Leydig-like cells have been noted in the tunica albuginea, rete testis, epididymis, and spermatic cord (56,57): in a recent prospective study, extratesticular Leydig cells were detected in 87 percent of surgical specimens that included paratesticular connective tissue as compared with a detection rate of 30 percent in a retrospective analysis (50). These cells are usually seen in association with nerves or, occasionally, small vascular channels. Curiously, they do not stain immunohistochemically for testosterone while all intratesticular Leydig cells do (50).

Ultrasonography is more sensitive for detecting testicular nodules than manual palpation (60); using this modality, testicular abnormalities were noted in 27 (63) to 47 percent (64) of male patients with CAH. Many of these testicular nodules were clinically undetectable. In one study, the nodules were hypoechoic, ranged in size from 0.2 to 2.8 cm (average, 1.6 cm), were bilateral in 6 of 8 patients (75 percent), and multifocal in each case

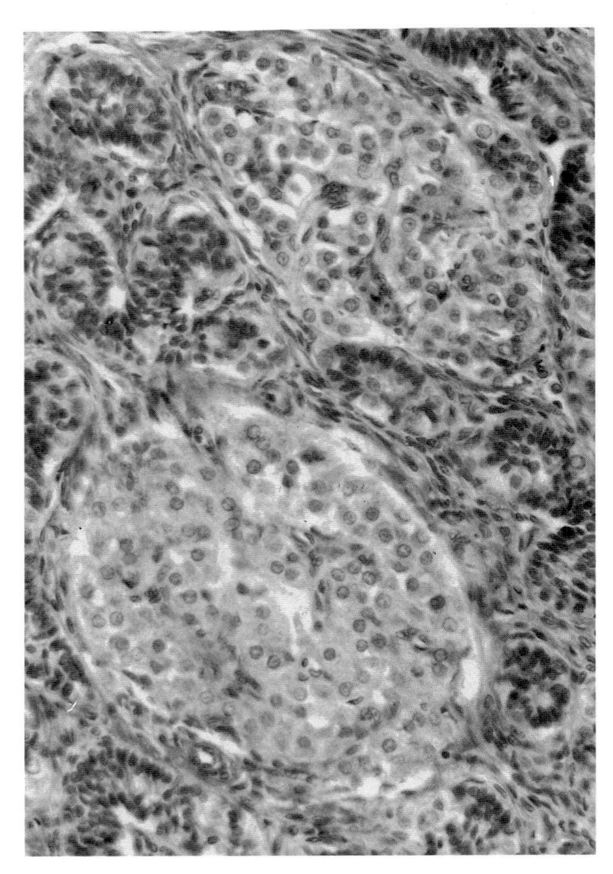

Figure 2-12
TESTIS FROM A CHILD WHO DIED OF SEVERE SALT-LOSING FORM OF 21-HYDROXYLASE DEFICIENCY

A few microscopic nodules of steroid-secreting cells were present within the testicular parenchyma near the hilum. (Fig. 1-47 from Lack EE, Kozakewich HP. Embryology, developmental anatomy, and selected aspects of non-neoplastic pathology. In: Lack EE, ed. Pathology of the adrenal glands. New York: Churchill Livingstone, 1990:1-74.)

(63). In another study, 3 of 36 males with CAH (8.2 percent) followed over a 30-year period developed a testicular mass 1 to 2 cm in size; the nodules were bilateral in 2 patients, and typically occupied the upper half of the testicle near the hilum (Note the location of the adrenal cortical rest in fig. 2-4A and B.) (62). Poor patient compliance with replacement steroid therapy has in some cases led to excess ACTH stimulation in CAH (54,62). "Adrenal rest" tumors or hyperplasia have also been noted in patients with Nelson's syndrome (51) and primary Addison's disease (60).

Pathology. A review of testicular tumors in CAH showed that two thirds of the masses were palpable (up to 10 cm), occurrence was usually in early adult life (average age, 22.5 years), smaller tumors (less than 2 cm) were usually seen in children, and 86 percent were located in the hilum of the testis (59). The tumors were bilateral in 83 percent of cases (59) compared to only 2.5 percent for Leydig cell tumors (52). On cross section the larger tumors are unencapsulated, bulging, multinodular masses separated by prominent bands of fibrous connective tissue (fig. 2-13). They are often light tan-brown due in part to lipochrome pigment and probably diminished cytoplasmic lipid, particularly in cases with inadequate suppression of ACTH. In several cases there have been multiple extratesticular nodules as large as 1.5 cm along the spermatic cord or adjacent to the epididymis (59). Microscopically, there are interconnecting sheets and nests of cells with granular pink cytoplasm and relatively distinct cell borders (fig. 2-14, left). The tumor also has an intimate pattern of reticulum with isolation of individual or small nests of cells (fig. 2-14, right). This is in contrast to the broad radial cords of cells usually seen in hyperplasia of entopic or heterotopic adrenal cortex. Occasionally, there are interstitial adipocytes (fig. 2-15). Sections taken through the testicular hilum and rete testis may show involvement by tumor (fig. 2-16).

Most tumor cells contain prominent lipochrome pigment (lipofuscin). Nuclei are fairly uniform, round to oval, with one or two small, central to eccentric nucleoli; occasionally there may be some nuclear enlargement. Mitotic figures are uncommon (fig. 2-17). There is a great resemblance to Leydig cells, and indeed the diagnosis usually made is Leydig or interstitial cell tumor. The cells also resemble the lipid-depleted cells of adrenal myelolipoma which arise in the setting of CAH. Reinke crystalloids, a pathognomonic marker for Leydig cells, can be found in about 35 percent of Leydig cell tumors (52), but are not a feature of testicular tumors of CAH. Adjacent testicular parenchyma may appear almost normal, or atrophic with sclerosis and decreased spermatogenesis. Ultrastructurally, the cells have features of steroid-producing cells: abundant smooth endoplasmic reticulum, numerous mitochondria, and accumulation of

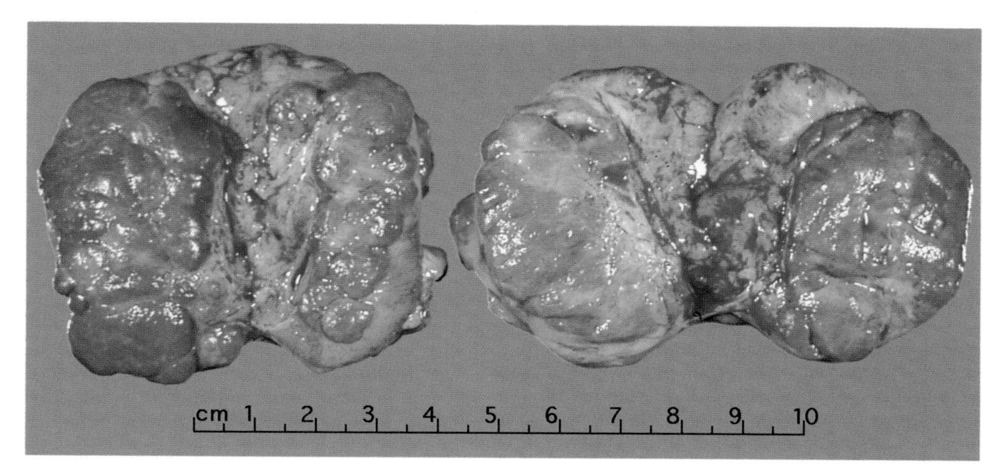

Figure 2-13
BILATERAL ORCHIECTOMY SPECIMENS FROM A 25-YEAR-OLD WHITE MALE WITH SALT-LOSING FORM OF 21-HYDROXYLASE DEFICIENCY

On cross section both testes are almost completely replaced by bulging nodules of tan tumor. Surgery was done to alleviate severe pain and swelling which was not adequately controlled with suppressive doses of dexamethasone. The testicular tumor was shown to be ACTH dependent.

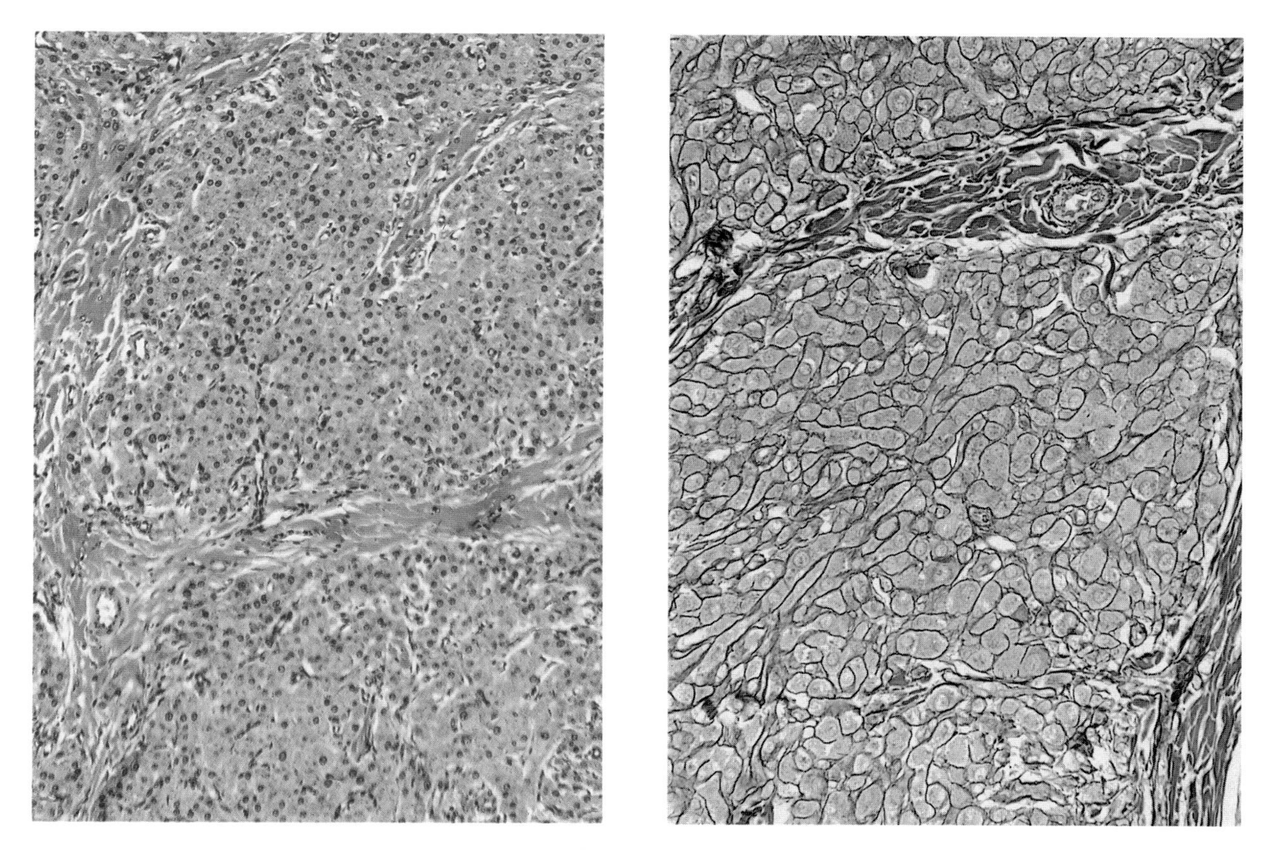

Figure 2-14
TESTICULAR TUMOR IN PATIENT WITH SALT-LOSING FORM OF 21-HYDROXYLASE DEFICIENCY

Left: Tumor cells grow in lobules and solid sheets with some intervening fibrous stroma.
Right: Reticulum pattern isolates individual and small groups of cells. (X175, Reticulum stain)

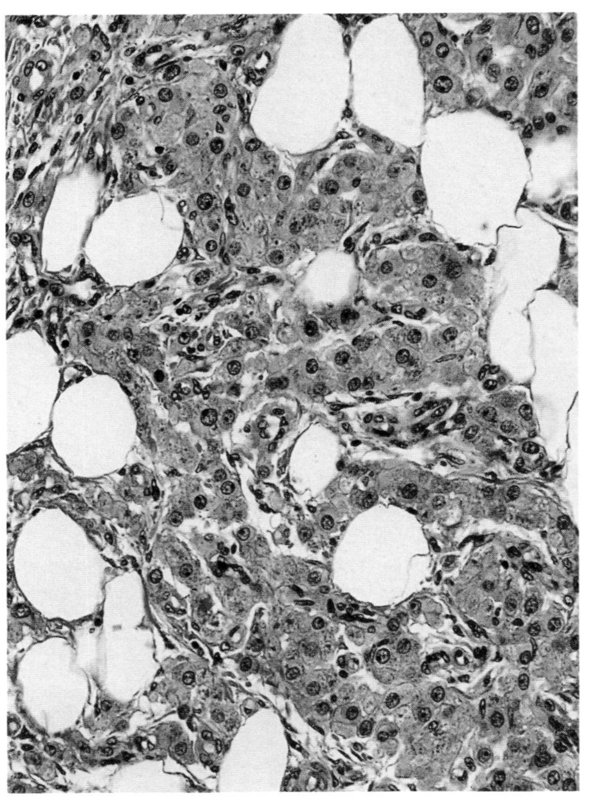

Figure 2-15
TESTICULAR TUMOR IN CAH
This testicular tumor shows small clusters of mature, adipose tissue representing lipomatous metaplasia.

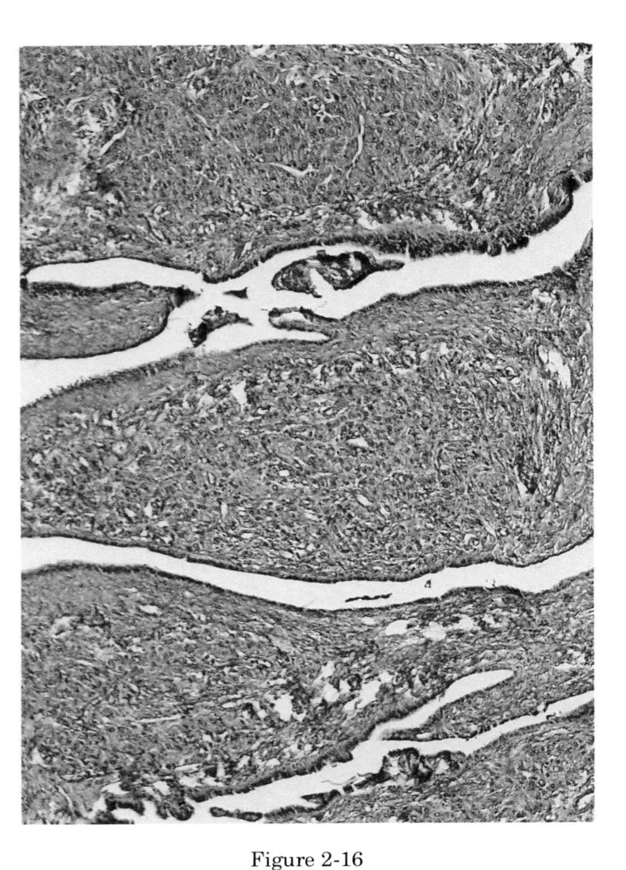

Figure 2-16
TESTICULAR TUMOR IN CAH
Rete testis is involved by testicular tumor in CAH. One may find accessory/heterotopic adrenal cortical tissue under normal conditions in this area (see fig. 2-4A and B).

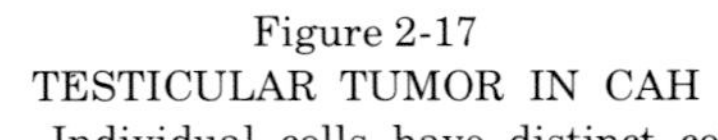

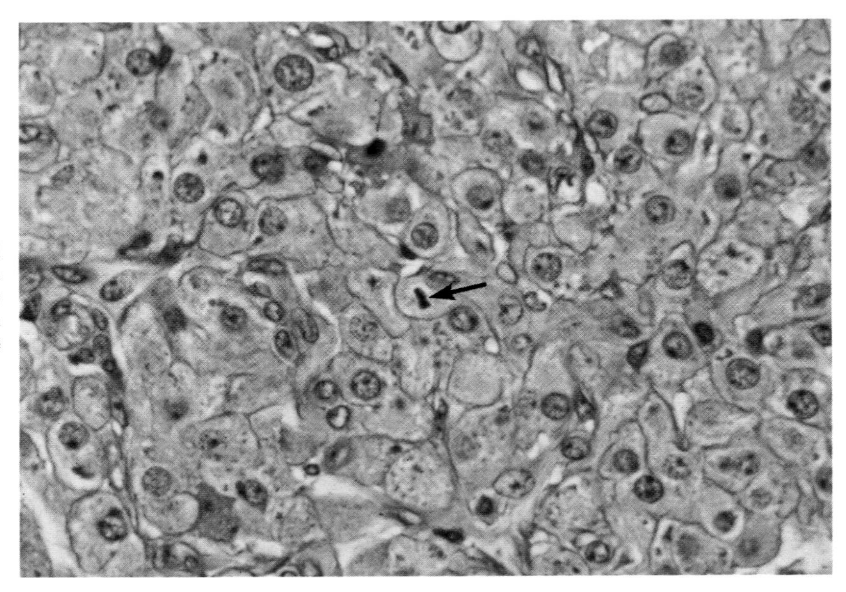

Figure 2-17
TESTICULAR TUMOR IN CAH
Individual cells have distinct cell borders and rounded nuclei, often with one or two eccentric nucleoli. Many cells contain coarse, granular pigment which is lipofuscin. Note the mitotic figure near the center of the field (arrow).

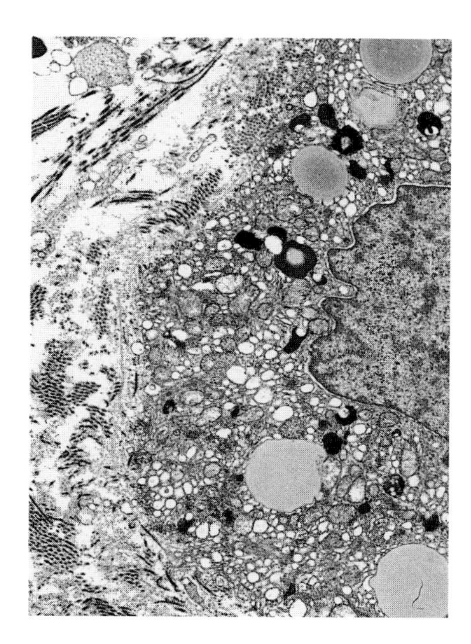
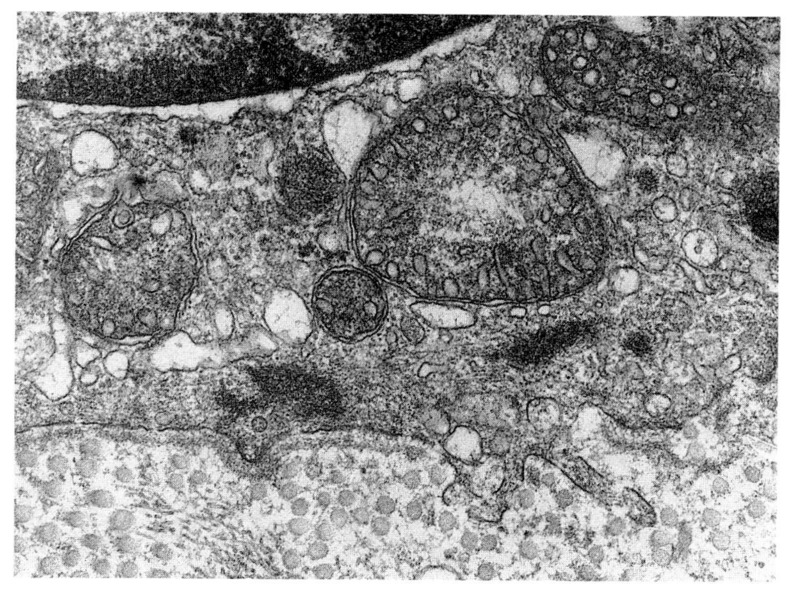

Figure 2-18
TESTICULAR TUMOR IN CAH
Left: The tumor cell contains electron-dense granular material associated with lipid (lipofuscin) as well as some free lipid droplets. The cell also contains abundant mitochondria. (X13,000)
Right: Similar to left, some cells show distinct basal lamina. Mitochondria have vesicular or tubular cristae with intervening granular matrix. (X22,000)

lipofuscin (fig. 2-18, left). The mitochondrial cristae may be lamellar or vesicular (fig. 2-18, right).

Histogenesis and Biologic Behavior. The cell of origin for these tumors is uncertain, but they can be distinguished from Leydig cell tumors by their distinctive clinical, biochemical, and pathologic features. Several studies have documented a dependence on ACTH, with increased levels of steroids (17-hydroxyprogesterone, cortisol, and 11-beta-hydroxylated steroids) in the testicular venous effluent (46,53,58). Suppression of ACTH with dexamethasone can greatly decrease testicular size to near normal, while trophic stimulation can cause testicular enlargement with recurrence of pain and tenderness (fig. 2-13). Orchiectomy may not be necessary since the tumor may not be truly neoplastic in view of its dependence on ACTH and the lack of malignant behavior in cases reported to date (54,59). Conflicting opinions exist as to whether the tumor arises from Leydig cells, adrenal cortical rests, or multipotent testicular stromal cells that are capable of multidirectional differentiation depending upon the microenvironment and hormonal milieu.

Other Tumors. Adrenal myelolipoma has been reported in the setting of CAH in a patient with 21-hydroxylase deficiency (47), and in another with deficiency of 17-hydroxylase (48); in these cases there was marked hyperplasia of adrenal cortical cells admixed with the myelolipoma (fig. 2-19). Several extra-adrenal, seemingly unrelated neoplasms have been reported such as osteosarcoma, Ewing's sarcoma, and astrocytoma (49).

BECKWITH-WIEDEMANN SYNDROME

The estimated frequency of the Beckwith-Wiedemann syndrome (BWS) is 1 in 13,000 births. Of reported cases, 85 percent are sporadic; some form of Mendelian inheritance is responsible for familial cases, with one study reporting an autosomal dominant pattern with incomplete penetrance (71). The infant death rate is about 20 percent; failure to recognize the associated hypoglycemia may lead to permanent brain damage, mental deficiency, or death (71). In a review by Wiedemann (74), 7.5 percent of children with

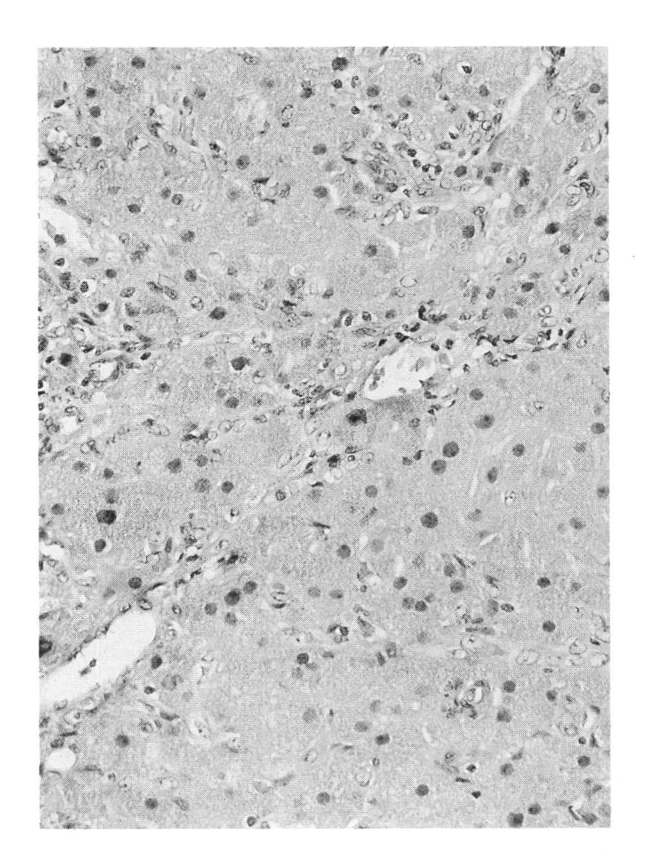

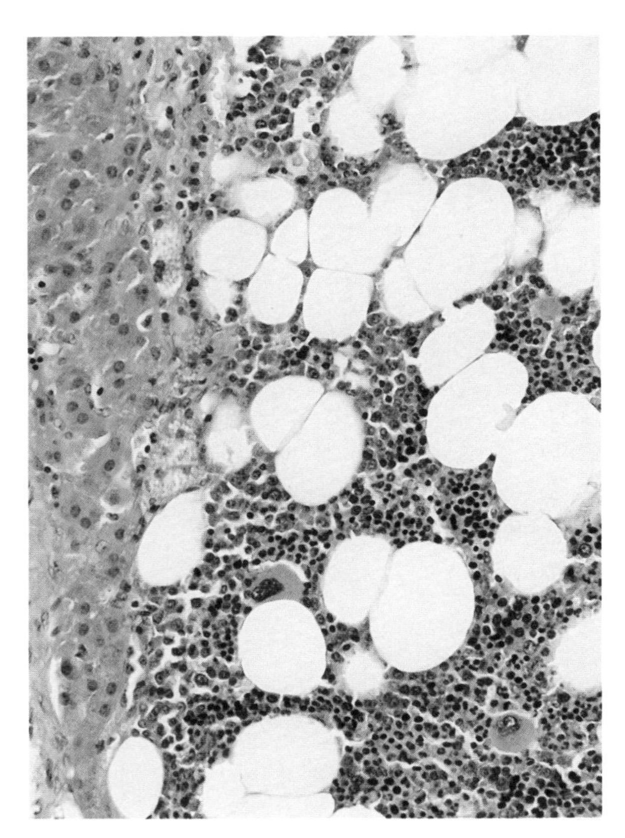

Figure 2-19
MYELOLIPOMA AND CAH

Left: Huge bilateral adrenal myelolipomas in an adult male with CAH. The hyperplastic adrenal cortical tissue is remarkably similar to that of the testicular tumor of CAH illustrated previously. Note granular pigment within some cells which represents lipofuscin.

Right: Most of the bilateral adrenal tumors were composed of myelolipoma (same case as left).

BWS developed a malignant tumor, usually nephroblastoma (Wilms' tumor) or adrenal cortical carcinoma; other reported neoplasms are neuroblastoma, pancreatoblastoma (69), and pheochromocytoma (72). Cytogenetic abnormalities are reported with BWS as well as loss of somatic heterozygosity for a locus on chromosome 11 in adrenal cortical neoplasms in this disorder; the gene involved in predisposition to adrenal cortical neoplasms has been mapped to region 11p15.5 (66,67).

BWS is sometimes referred to by the acronym *EMG (exomphalos, macroglossia, gigantism) syndrome.* The disorder was described by Beckwith in 1963 (65) and by Wiedemann the following year (73), and includes a variety of abnormalities: craniofacial features such as ear creases or pits, nevus flammeus, midfacial hypoplasia, abdominal wall defects, visceromegaly, gigantism, and macroglossia (71). The adrenal glands are enlarged with a combined weight often up to 16 g, and due to cortical hyperplasia may show redundant cortical folds and nodularity which may have a cerebriform configuration (fig. 2-20) (69). Marked adrenal cytomegaly is a characteristic feature and is bilateral, usually affecting most cells in the fetal cortex (fig. 2-21, left). In addition to enlarged, pleomorphic nuclei, pseudoinclusions can be seen (fig. 2-21, right). Chromaffin cells have been reported to be strikingly hyperplastic within adrenal and extra-adrenal sites (65,68) and one may find cortical microcysts in the adult cortex on histologic examination (fig. 2-22). Rarely, hemorrhagic macrocysts of the adrenal cortex may be the cause of an abdominal mass in the fetus and neonate with BWS (70).

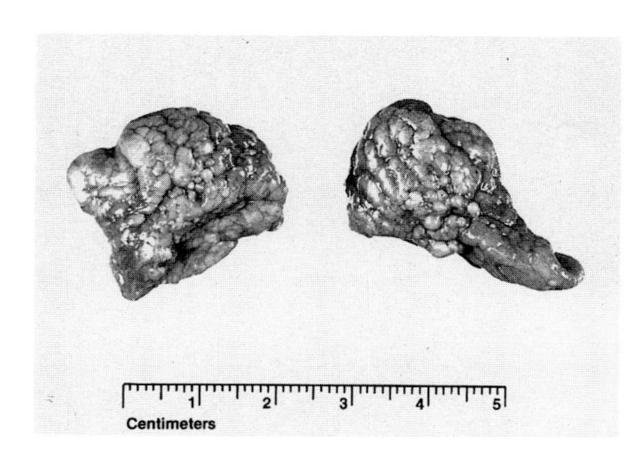

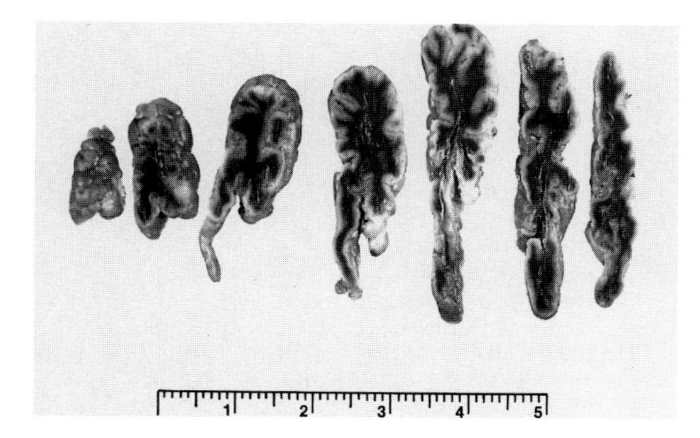

Figure 2-20
BECKWITH-WIEDEMANN SYNDROME

Left: Adrenal glands from a 3-week-old infant with Beckwith-Wiedemann syndrome are enlarged and show excessive cortical nodularity and redundant folds on the external aspect.

Right: In transverse section, much of the fetal cortex is deeply congested. Bilateral cytomegaly affected the fetal or provisional zone. (Figs. 1-36A,B modified from Lack EE, Kozakewich HP: Embryology, developmental anatomy, and selected aspects of non-neoplastic pathology. In: Lack EE, ed. Pathology of the adrenal glands. New York: Churchill Livingstone, 1990:1–74.)

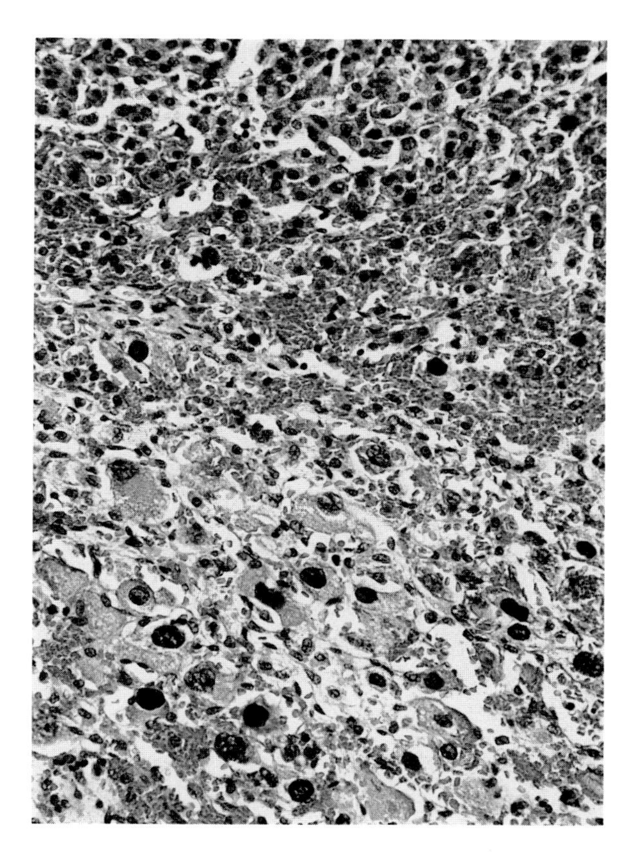

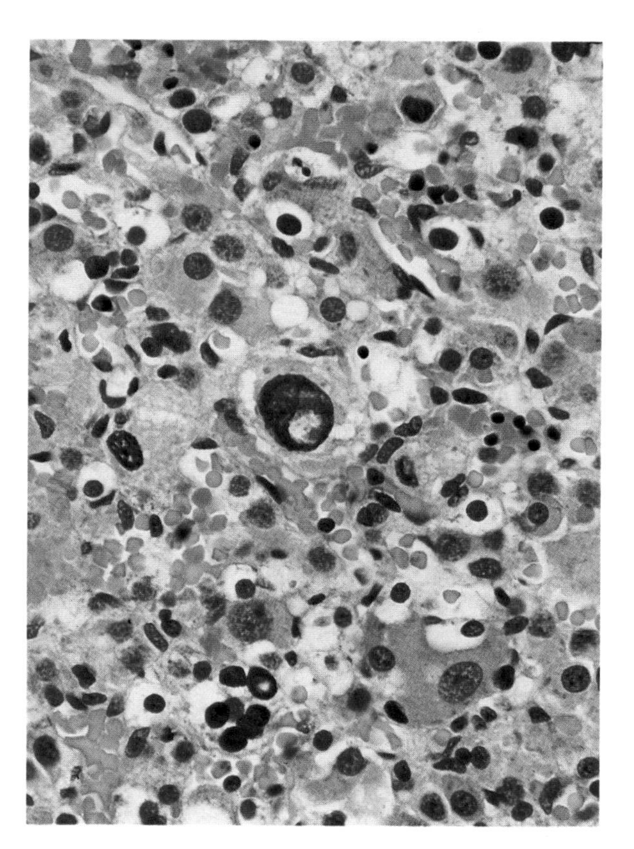

Figure 2-21
BECKWITH-WIEDEMANN SYNDROME

Left: Marked adrenal cytomegaly involves cells of the fetal or provisional cortex. Note the nucleomegaly and hyperchromasia.

Right: Nuclear enlargement and hyperchromasia with nuclear "pseudoinclusion" near the center of field. Mitotic figures were not identified.

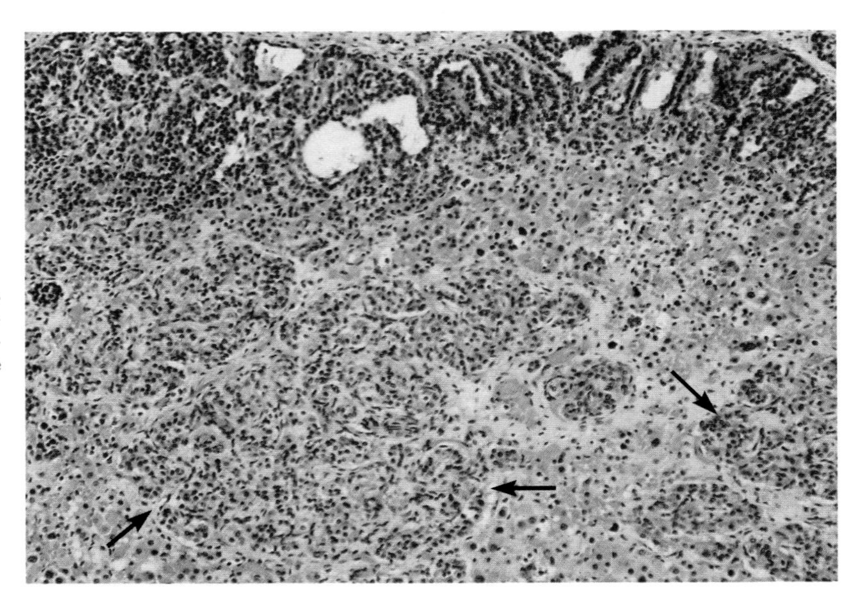

Figure 2-22
NEWBORN WITH BECKWITH-WIEDEMANN SYNDROME

Nests of adrenal chromaffin cells (arrows) are hyperplastic and inappropriately mature for this stage of development. Note also the microcysts in the adult cortex.

REFERENCES

Adrenal Adhesion, Union, and Fusion

1. Dolan MF, Janovski NA. Adreno-hepatic union. (Adrenal dystopia). Arch Pathol 1968;86:22–4.
2. Honma K. Adreno-hepatic fusion. An autopsy study. Zentralbl Pathol 1991;137:117–22.
3. Lack EE, Kozakewich HP. Embryology, developmental anatomy, and selected aspects of non-neoplastic pathology In: Lack EE, ed. Pathology of the adrenal glands. New York: Churchill Livingstone, 1990:1–74.
4. Pakravan P, Kenny FM, Depp R, Allen AC. Familial congenital absence of adrenal glands: evaluation of glucocorticoid, mineralocorticoid, and estrogen metabolism in the perinatal period. J Pediatr 1974;84:74–8.

Heterotopic and Accessory Adrenal Tissue

5. Albores-Saavedra J. The pseudometastasis. Patologia 1994;32:63–71.
6. Apitz K. Die geschwülste und gewebsmissbildungen der nierenrinde. I. Die intrarenalen nebenniereninseln. Virchows Arch Pathol Anat 1944;311:285–305.
7. Armin A, Castelli M. Congenital adrenal tissue in the lung with adrenal cytomegaly. Case report and review of the literature. Am J Clin Pathol 1984;82:225–8.
8. Bozic C. Ectopic fetal adrenal cortex in the lung of a newborn. Virchows Arch [A] 1974;363:371–4.
9. Busuttil A. Ectopic adrenal within the gall-bladder wall. J Pathol 1974;113:231–3.
10. Culp OS. Adrenal heterotopia. A survey of the literature and report of a case. J Urol 1939;41:303–9.
11. Dahl EV, Bahn RC. Aberrant adrenal cortical tissue near the testis in human infants. Am J Pathol 1962;40:587–98.
12. Falls JL. Accessory adrenal cortex in the broad ligament. Incidence and functional significance. Cancer 1955;8:143–50.
13. Graham LS. Celiac accessory adrenal glands. Cancer 1953;6:149–52.
14. Honoré LH. Intra-adrenal hepatic heterotopia. J Urol 1985;133:652–4.
15. Kepes JJ, O'Boynick P, Jones S, Baum D, McMillan J, Adams ME. Adrenal cortical adenoma in the spinal canal of an 8-year-old girl. Am J Surg Pathol 1990;14:481–4.
16. Labarrere CA, Caccamo D, Telenta M, Althabe O, Gutman R. A nodule of adrenocortical tissue within a human placenta: light microscopic and immunocytochemical findings. Placenta 1984;5:139–44.
17. Marchand F. Ueber accessorische nebennieren im ligamentum latum. Virchows Arch 1883;92:11–9.
18. Mares AJ, Shkolnik A, Sacks M, Feuchtwanger MM. Aberrant (ectopic) adrenocortical tissue along the spermatic cord. J Ped Surg 1980;15:289–92.
19. Mitchell N, Angrist A. Adrenal rests in the kidney. Arch Pathol 1943;35:46–52.
20. Morimoto Y, Hiwada K, Nanahoshi M, et al. Cushing's syndrome caused by malignant tumor in the scrotum: clinical, pathologic and biochemical studies. J Clin Endocr Metab 1971;32:201–10.

21. Nelson AA. Accessory adrenal cortical tissue. Arch Pathol 1939;27:955–65.
22. O'Crowley CR, Martland HS. Adrenal heterotopia, rests and the so-called Grawitz tumor. J Urol 1943;50:756–68.
23. Roosen-Runge EC, Lund J. Abnormal sex cord formation and an intratesticular adrenal cortical nodule in a human fetus. Anat Rec 1972;173:57–68.
24. Symonds DA, Driscoll SG. An adrenal cortical rest within the fetal ovary. Report of a case. Am J Clin Pathol 1973;60:562–4.
25. Wallace EZ, Leonidas JR, Stanek AE, Avramides A. Endocrine studies in a patient with functioning adrenal rest tumor of the liver. Am J Med 1981;70:1122–6.
26. Wiener MF, Dallgaard SA. Intracranial adrenal gland. A case report. Arch Pathol 1959;67:120–5.

Congenital Adrenal Hyperplasia

27. Biglieri EG, Kater CE. 17-α-hydroxylation deficiency. Endocrinol Metab Clin N Am 1991;20:257–68.
28. Cutler GB Jr, Laue L. Congenital adrenal hyperplasia due to 21-hydroxylase deficiency. N Engl J Med 1990;323:1806–13.
29. de Crecchio L. Sopra un caso di apparenzi virili in una donna. Morgagni 1865;7:154–88.
30. Kalaitzoglou G, New MI. Congenital adrenal hyperplasia. Molecular insights learned from patients. Receptor 1993;3:211–22.
31. Lack EE, Kozakewich HP. Embryology, developmental anatomy, and selected aspects of non-neoplastic pathology. In: Lack EE, ed. Pathology of the adrenal glands. New York: Churchill Livingstone, 1990:1–74.
32. Migeon, CJ, Donohoue PA. Congenital adrenal hyperplasia caused by 21-hydroxylase deficiency. Its molecular basis and its remaining therapeutic problems. Endocrinol Metab Clin N Am 1991;20:277-96.
33. Miller WL. Congenital adrenal hyperplasia. Endocrinol Metab Clin N Am 1991;20:721-49.
34. Pang S, Pollack MS, Marshall RN, Immken L. Prenatal treatment of congenital adrenal hyperplasia due to 21-hydroxylase deficiency. N Engl J Med 1990;322:111-5.
35. Spieser PW, Agdere L, Ueshiba H, White PC, New MI. Aldosterone synthesis in salt-wasting congenital adrenal hyperplasia with complete absence of adrenal 21-hydroxylase. N Engl J Med 1991;324:145–9.
36. White PC, New MI, Dupont B. Congenital adrenal hyperplasia. N Engl J Med 1987;316:1519–24, 1580–6.

Adrenal Cortical Neoplasms

37. Bauman A, Bauman CG. Virilizing adrenocortical carcinoma. Development in a patient with salt-losing congenital adrenal hyperplasia. JAMA 1982;248:3140–1.
38. Daeschner GL. Adrenal cortical adenoma arising in a girl with congenital adrenogenital syndrome. Pediatrics 1965;36:140–2.
39. Hamwi GJ, Serbin RA, Kruger FA. Does adrenocortical hyperplasia result in adrenocortical carcinoma? N Engl J Med 1957;257:1153–7.
40. Jaresch S, Kornely E, Kley HK, Schlaghecke R. Adrenal incidentaloma and patients with homozygous or heterozygous congenital adrenal hyperplasia. J Clin Endocrinol Metab 1992;74:685–9.
41. Jaursch-Hancke C, Allolio B, Metzler U, Bidlingmaier F, Winkelmann W. Adrenocortical carcinoma in patients with untreated congenital adrenal hyperplasia (CAH). Acta Endocrinol 1988;117:146–7.
42. Lack EE, Kozakewich HP. Embryology, developmental anatomy, and selected aspects of non-neoplastic pathology. In: Lack EE, ed. Pathology of the adrenal glands. New York: Churchill Livingstone, 1990:1–74.
43. Nogeire C, Fukushima DK, Hellman L, Boyar RM. Virilizing adrenal cortical carcinoma. Cancer 1977;40:307–13.
44. Pang S, Becker D, Cotelingam J, Foley TP Jr, Drash AL. Adrenocortical tumor in a patient with congenital adrenal hyperplasia due to 21-hydroxylase deficiency. Pediatrics 1981;68:242–6.
45. Verdonk C, Guerin C, Lufkin E, Hodgson SF. Activation of virilizing adrenal rest tissues by excessive ACTH production. An unusual presentation of Nelson's syndrome. Am J Med 1982;73:455–9.

Testicular and Other Tumors in Congenital Adrenal Hyperplasia

46. Blumberg-Tick J, Boudou P, Nahoul K, Schaison G. Testicular tumors in congenital adrenal hyperplasia: steroid measurements from adrenal and spermatic veins. J Clin Endocrinol Metab 1991;73:1129–33.
47. Boudreaux D, Waisman J, Skinner DG, Low R. Giant adrenal myelolipoma and testicular interstitial cell tumor in a man with congenital 21-hydroxylase deficiency. Am J Surg Pathol 1979;3:109–23.
48. Condom E, Villabona CM, Gómez JM, Carrera, M. Adrenal myelolipoma in a woman with congenital 17-hydroxylase deficiency. Arch Pathol Lab Med 1985;109:1116–8.
49. Duck SC. Malignancy associated with congenital adrenal hyperplasia. J Pediatr 1981;99:423–4.
50. Grignon DJ, Ro JY, Ordonez NG, Ayala AG. Extratesticular interstitial cells [Letter]. Am J Surg Pathol 1988;12:735–6.
51. Johnson RE, Scheithauer B. Massive hyperplasia of testicular adrenal rests in a patient with Nelson's syndrome. Am J Clin Pathol 1982;77:501–7.
52. Kim I, Young RH, Scully RE. Leydig cell tumors of the testis. A clinicopathological analysis of 40 cases and review of the literature. Am J Surg Pathol 1985;9:177–92.
53. Kirkland RT, Kirkland JL, Keenan BS, Bongiovanni AM, Rosenberg HS, Clayton GW. Bilateral testicular tumors in congenital adrenal hyperplasia. J Clin Endocrinol Metab 1977;44:369–78.
54. Knudsen JL, Savage A, Mobb GE. The testicular tumor of adrenogenital syndrome—a persistent diagnostic pitfall. Histopathology 1991;19:468–70.
55. Lack EE, Kozakewich HP. Embryology, developmental anatomy, and selected aspects of non-neoplastic pathology. In: Lack EE. Pathology of the adrenal glands. New York: Churchill Livingstone, 1990:1–74.

56 McDonald JH, Calams JA. A histological study of extraparenchymal Leydig-like cells. J Urol 1958;79:850–8.
57. Nistal M, Paniagua R. Histogenesis of human extraparenchymal Leydig cells. Acta Anat 1979;105:188–97.
58. Radfar N, Bartter FC, Easley R, Kolins J, Javadpour N, Sherins RJ. Evidence for endogenous LH suppression in a man with bilateral testicular tumors and congenital adrenal hyperplasia. J Clin Endocrinol Metab 1977;45:1194–204.
59. Rutgers JL, Young RH, Scully RE. The testicular tumor of the adrenogenital syndrome. A report of six cases and review of the literature on testicular masses in patients with adrenocortical disorders. Am J Surg Pathol 1988;12:503–13.
60. Seidenwurm D, Smathers RL, Kan P, Hoffman A. Intratesticular adrenal rests diagnosed by ultrasound. Radiology 1985;155:479–81.
61. Shanklin DR, Richardson AP Jr, Rothstein G. Testicular hilar nodules in adrenogenital syndrome. Am J Dis Child 1963;106:43–50.
62. Srikanth MS, West BR, Ishitani M, Isaacs H Jr, Applebaum H, Costin G. Benign testicular tumors in children with congenital adrenal hyperplasia. J Ped Surg 1992;27:639–41.
63. Vanzulli A, DelMaschio A, Paesano P, et al. Testicular masses in association with adrenogenital syndrome: US findings. Radiology 1992;183:425–9.
64. Willi U, Atares M, Prader A, Zachmann M. Testicular adrenal-like tissue (TALT) in congenital adrenal hyperplasia: detection by ultrasonography. Pediatr Radiol 1991;21:284–7.

Beckwith-Wiedemann Syndrome

65. Beckwith JB. Macroglossia, omphalocele, adrenal cytomegaly, gigantism, and hyperplastic visceromegaly. Birth Defects: Original Article Series 1969;5:188–96.
66. Hayward NK, Little MH, Mortimer RH, Clouston WM, Smith PL. Generation of homozygosity of the c-Ha-ras-1 locus on chromosome 11p in an adrenal adenoma from an adult with Wiedemann-Beckwith syndrome. Cancer Genet Cytogenet 1988;30:127–32.
67. Henry I, Jeanpierre M, Couillin P, et al. Molecular definition of 11p 15.5 region involved in Beckwith-Wiedemann syndrome and probably in predisposition to adrenocortical carcinoma. Hum Genet 1989;81:273–7.
68. Lack EE. Pathology of adrenal and extra-adrenal paraganglia. Major problems in pathology, vol 29. Philadelphia: WB Saunders, 1994.
69. Lack EE, Kozakewich HP. Embryology, developmental anatomy, and selected aspects of non-neoplastic pathology. In: Lack EE, ed. Pathology of the adrenal glands. New York: Churchill Livingstone, 1990:1–74.
70. McCauley RG, Beckwith JB, Elias ER, Faerber EN, Prewitt LH Jr, Berdon WE. Benign hemorrhagic adrenocortical macrocysts in Beckwith-Wiedemann syndrome. Am J Roentgenol 1991;157:549–59.
71. Pettenati MJ, Haines JL, Higgins RR, Wappner RS, Palmer CG, Weaver DD. Wiedemann-Beckwith syndrome: presentation of clinical and cytogenetic data on 22 new cases and review of the literature. Hum Genet 1986;74:143–54.
72. Schnakenburg K, Müller M, Dörner K, et al. Congenital hemihypertrophy and malignant giant pheochromocytoma—a previously undescribed coincidence. Europ J Pediatr 1976;122:263–73.
73. Wiedemann HR. Complexe malformatif familial avec hernie ombilicale et macroglossie—un "syndrome nouveau"? J Genet Hum 1964;13:223–32.
74. Wiedemann HR. Tumours and hemihypertrophy associated with Wiedemann-Beckwith syndrome. Eur J Pediatr 1983;141:129.

3
ADRENAL CORTICAL NODULES AND TUMOR-LIKE LESIONS

ADRENAL CORTICAL HYPERPLASIA

Definition. Adrenal cortical hyperplasia is a non-neoplastic condition characterized by an increase in the number of cortical cells; this may be diffuse or nodular. There is usually an increase in size or weight of the adrenal glands which may be symmetric or asymmetric. Nodular hyperplasia with one or more dominant nodules may simulate an adrenal cortical neoplasm.

General Remarks. Hyperplasia of the adrenal cortex can be diffuse, localized with formation of one or more nodules, or a mixture of both patterns. It is virtually always bilateral, although rare cases of putative unilateral hyperplasia have been reported (1). Diffuse hyperplasia appears as a generalized thickening of the adrenal cortex, usually without any well-defined nodularity, although occasional small nodules may be detected with a magnifying glass or a microscope. Nodular hyperplasia is divided into micronodular and macronodular types based upon the size of the nodules. Some classify micronodules as less than 0.5 cm in diameter, while others designate nodules of 1.0 cm or more as macronodules (1). Diffuse, micronodular, and macronodular forms of adrenal cortical hyperplasia appear to be a continuum of morphologic alteration making their distinction in some cases somewhat arbitrary. With the sensitive imaging of computed tomography (CT) and magnetic resonance imaging (MRI), adrenal cortical nodules less than 1 cm in size can be detected. Correct pathologic identification of adrenal cortical hyperplasia can be difficult, particularly if the gross and microscopic morphology show only subtle changes. For this reason careful gross dissection of the adrenal glands, with removal of all periadrenal connective tissue and fat, may be necessary for accurate determination of size and weight (1). Some of the smaller nodules may not be apparent on external examination of the intact gland, therefore, transverse sectioning at 3-mm intervals is recommended.

The gross morphologic classification of adrenal cortical hyperplasia is shown in Table 3-1; a functional classification based upon the presence or absence of a particular endocrine syndrome is

Table 3-1

MORPHOLOGIC CLASSIFICATION OF ADRENAL CORTICAL HYPERPLASIA

Bilateral Adrenal Cortical Hyperplasia
Diffuse hyperplasia
Nodular hyperplasia
Micronodular (less than 1 cm in diameter)
Macronodular (greater than 1 cm)
Combined micronodular and macronodular
Combined diffuse and nodular hyperplasia
Dominant cortical nodule with diffuse hyperplasia
Multiple nodules with diffuse hyperplasia
Macronodular hyperplasia with marked adrenal enlargement
Primary pigmented nodular adrenocortical disease
Incidental pigmented nodules
Unilateral Adrenal Cortical Hyperplasia
Diffuse and/or nodular hyperplasia
Incidental pigmented nodule(s)

Table 3-2

CLINICAL ENDOCRINE SYNDROMES ASSOCIATED WITH DIFFUSE OR NODULAR HYPERPLASIA

Endocrine Syndrome	Adrenal Cortical Hyperplasia
Hypercortisolism	
Cushing's syndrome	
Pituitary-dependent (Cushing's disease)	Diffuse and/or nodular
Ectopic ACTH production	Predominantly diffuse
Primary pigmented nodular adrenocortical disease	Predominantly micronodular
Macronodular hyperplasia with marked adrenal enlargement	Macronodular
Ectopic secretion of CRF	Predominantly diffuse
Hyperaldosteronism	Diffuse and/or micronodular
Virilization (congenital adrenal hyperplasia)	Predominantly diffuse
Eucorticalism	Diffuse and/or nodular

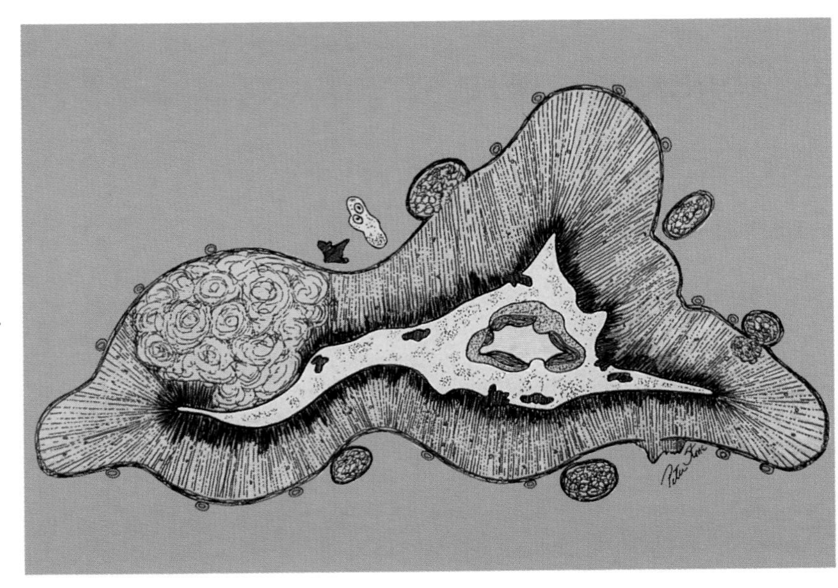

Figure 3-1
SCHEMATIC VIEW OF NODULAR ADRENAL GLAND IN TRANSVERSE SECTION

Cortical extrusions with various configurations are shown, with some lying free in the periadrenal area. A larger dominant intracortical nodule is present on the left. Note also intermingling of nests of cortical cells with chromaffin cells and the close anatomic relationship that both cortex and medulla can have with the vascular space due to discontinuity of smooth muscle in vessel walls.

shown in Table 3-2. The most common presentation of cortical hyperplasia (or neoplasia) with adrenomegaly is an asymptomatic patient who is eucortical. Adrenal cortical hyperplasia associated with noniatrogenic hypercortisolism can be pituitary dependent (Cushing's disease); associated with ectopic production of adrenocorticotrophic hormone (ACTH) (or rarely corticotropin-releasing factor [CRF]); or due to primary pigmented nodular adrenocortical disease (PPNAD) or macronodular hyperplasia with marked adrenal enlargement. The functional approach to classification usually requires careful correlation of morphologic findings with clinical and endocrinologic data. Virilization is typically associated with congenital adrenal hyperplasia while feminization is either poorly characterized or exists only with cortical neoplasia (1).

ADRENAL CORTICAL NODULE (OR ADENOMA) WITH EUCORTICALISM

Adrenal Cortical Nodule at Autopsy

Incidence. The nodular adrenal gland from autopsy material, and even in tissue obtained at surgery from individuals without evidence of hypercorticalism, is a diagnostic challenge for the pathologist (fig. 3-1). Much of the confusion about the nodular adrenal gland results from a combination of factors: vague terminology; continuing difficulty in distinguishing an adrenal cortical neoplasm from a dominant macronodule; overlap in morphology of adrenal cortical lesions in patients with different endocrine syndromes; absence of correlation between pathology and clinical/endocrinologic data; and incomplete understanding of the etiology and pathogenesis of the nodular gland in patients who have no evidence of cortical hyperfunction (8,9). Prior to the availability of CT scanning and other sensitive imaging techniques, the "nonfunctioning" nodular adrenal gland was usually an incidental finding at autopsy. Currently, it often presents as an incidental finding on high resolution CT scan during examination for an unrelated problem or during staging work-up of a patient with a known malignancy elsewhere. The incidence of cortical nodules at autopsy is difficult to estimate since there are no universally accepted morphologic criteria to define a cortical "nodule" in terms of size, number, and other distinguishing characteristics. Early studies considered any solitary adrenal cortical nodule of 3 to 5 mm in diameter to be a "nonfunctioning adenoma." In several large studies, cortical adenomas were detected in 1.4 to 2.9 percent of autopsies (3,7,11).

Several autopsy series report a higher incidence of cortical nodules or adenomas in elderly individuals (4,13) and in patients with hypertension (4,12). Spain and Weinsaft (13) identified solitary adenomas in 29 percent of 100 consecutive autopsies on elderly females (average, 81 years)

(13). Other autopsy studies report adenomas of 1.5 cm or more in as many as 20 percent of patients with systemic hypertension (12). Adenomas 2 mm to 4 cm in size were identified in 8.7 percent of 739 consecutive autopsies, but roughly twice as many occurred in patients with diabetes mellitus (6).

Functional Considerations and Classification. A dominant macronodule might be regarded as an adenoma even though there is no evidence of autonomous hyperfunction or even if close inspection of multiple transverse sections of the ipsilateral or contralateral gland shows coexisting diffuse or micronodular hyperplasia. It can be very difficult or impossible to prove that the macronodule is indeed a neoplasm (i.e., an adenoma), and final classification can be quite arbitrary. A solitary lesion with evidence of autonomous growth favors a diagnosis of neoplasia. Because some of these cortical nodules could be related to vascular sclerosis and aging, it may not always be appropriate to use the designation adenoma, which means a true neoplasm; furthermore, since these lesions are nonfunctional (or nonhyperfunctional), use of the term adrenal "nodule" or "nodular adrenal" seems preferable to hyperplasia in spite of the undoubted increase in mass of cortical cells.

By definition, hyperplasia denotes an increase in number of cells in a tissue or organ, and is usually associated with hypertrophy. When the adrenal cortex becomes hyperplastic (diffuse or nodular hyperplasia) it may cause adrenal hyperfunction or hypercorticalism; this is uncommon, however, based upon the prevalence of nodular adrenal glands in large autopsy studies or the frequency of serendipitous nodular adrenal glands discovered in vivo. Scintigraphic studies using radioiodinated cholesterol, a precursor in steroid biosynthesis, provide insight into the functional status of these silent adrenal nodules (or adenomas) detected in living patients (5,10). The adrenal nodule (or adenoma) is visualized using this technique, and quantitation of cortisol levels in the adrenal vein shows the largest concentration on the side of the mass (unilateral cases), or on the side of the largest nodule in patients with bilateral adrenal masses (5). The nodule or adenoma, therefore, appears to be nonhyperfunctional. The findings suggest a condition analogous to nodular euthyroid (nontoxic) goiter with partial suppression of normal tissue characterized scintigraphically by heterogeneous foci of increased tracer accumulation compared to overall normal hormone secretion (5). Prolonged follow-up of some of these incidentally discovered adrenal nodules (or adenomas) would be of interest to see if an endocrine syndrome does develop. In one report a patient had an adrenal nodule that did not change in size over a 5-year period, and no clinical evidence of Cushing's syndrome, yet preoperative endocrine tests were abnormal, indicating autonomous secretion of cortisol (2). A variety of enzymes involved in steroid biosynthesis have been detected immunohistochemically in small adrenal cortical adenomas found incidentally in asymptomatic patients, indicating a capacity to produce biologically active steroids including cortisol (14).

Even in some cases with atrophy of the attached cortex, the secretion of cortisol may be insufficient to cause detectable clinical or laboratory abnormalities. A recent study of 15 small adrenal cortical nodules or adenomas without apparent endocrinologic hyperfunction indicated a capability for producing biologically active steroids, including cortisol, although this was not associated with obvious hypercorticalism (14). This study used immunohistochemical analysis of various steroidogenic enzymes (P-450 side-chain cleavage enzyme, 3-beta-hydroxysteroid dehydrogenase, P-450 C21-hydroxylase, P-450 17-alpha-hydroxylase, and P-450 11-beta-hydroxylase). Results indicated that autonomous neoplastic production and secretion of cortisol was present, but insufficient to cause clinical or routine laboratory abnormalities. This nonhyperfunction may be sufficient to subtly alter the hypothalamic-pituitary-adrenal axis by suppressing ACTH secretion, CRF secretion, or both which can lead to atrophy of the attached ipsilateral adrenal cortex in some cases (14).

Pathologic Findings. A detailed study of the nodular adrenal gland was provided by Dobbie (4) who identified mild to distinct nodularity in 65 percent of adrenal glands obtained from 113 consecutive autopsies on adult patients. When large nodules (or adenomas) were encountered (fig. 3-2, top), careful examination of the glands revealed that they were not in fact solitary; in each case smaller nodules and capsular extrusions were identified in other parts of the ipsilateral or contralateral gland, suggesting that the

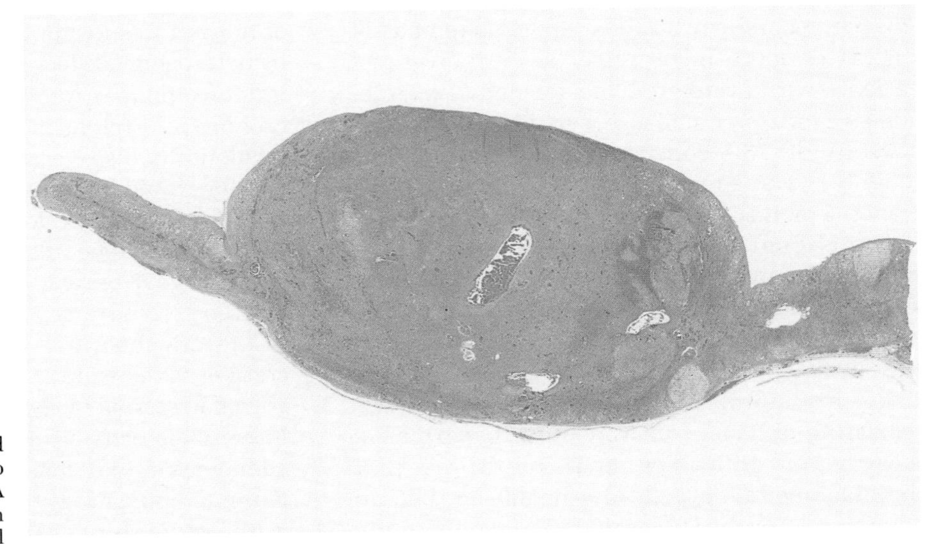

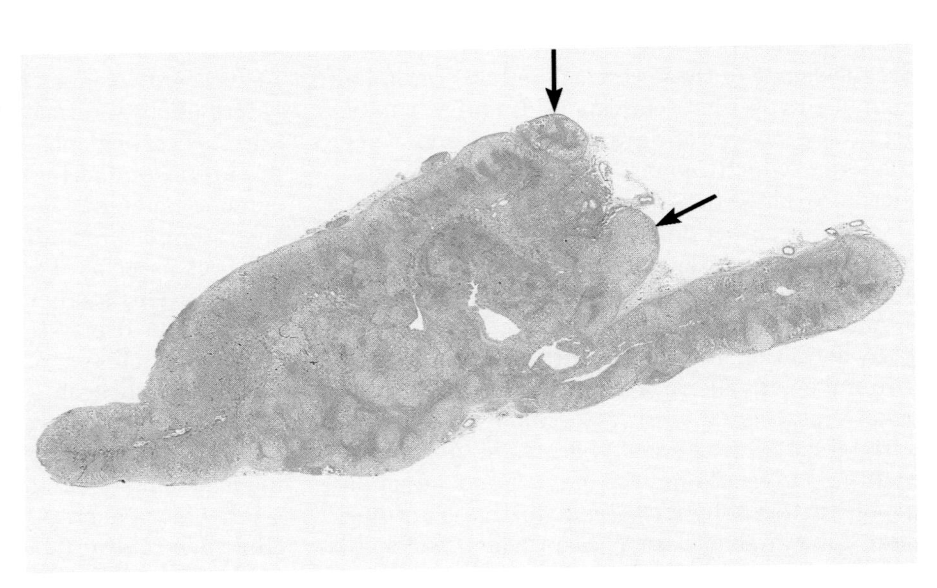

Figure 3-2
NODULAR
ADRENAL GLAND

Top: Nodular adrenal gland at autopsy of a patient with no evidence of hypercorticalism. A dominant macronodule can simulate an adrenal cortical adenoma. Other smaller nodules were also present.

Bottom: The opposite adrenal gland has discrete and confluent nodularity. Note also cortical extrusions (arrows).

larger nodules were an extension of the hyperplastic process (fig. 3-2, bottom). The range of cortical nodularity illustrated schematically in figure 3-1 underscores the fact that nodules are frequently multiple and bilateral. The most common nodules are extrusions of cortex which may project in a hemispheric or roughly "hourglass" configuration (fig. 3-2, bottom), often with continuous extension of the adrenal capsule. Sometimes the nodule may appear to reside on the surface of the gland, with complete encapsulation or connection with the adrenal capsule, but depending upon the plane of section, there is usually a point of continuity with underlying cortex (see fig. 3-1), a configuration likened to a "mushroom" or "door handle" (4,8). At times the cortical cells are unencapsulated and stream into periadrenal fat (fig. 3-3), or form a discrete cortical nodule on the surface of the gland or in adjacent connective tissue without any attachment to the adrenal gland. With hyperplasia, these cortical extrusions and juxta-adrenal nodules may become accentuated (fig. 3-4), as can the cuff of cortical cells in association with the central adrenal vein or its tributaries. Nodules can be seen in every region of the cortex, and the degree of nodularity can vary widely from gland

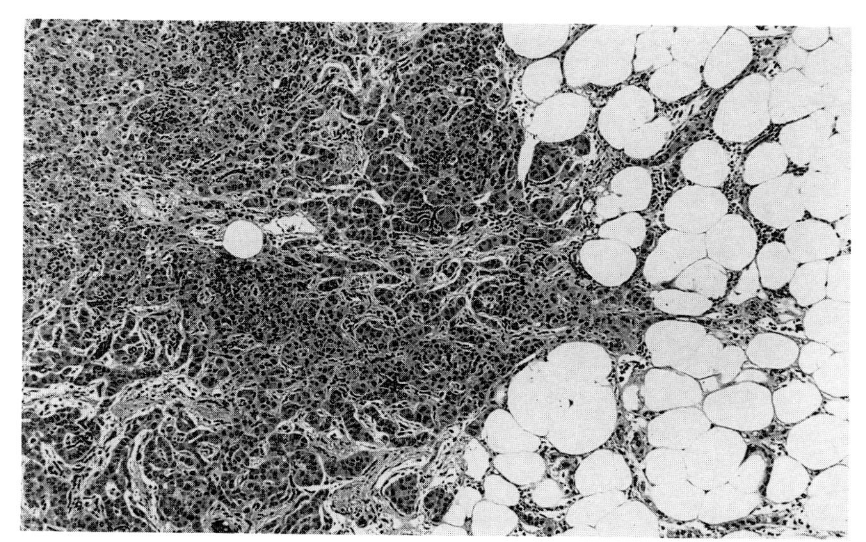

Figure 3-3
UNENCAPSULATED
EXTENSION OF
CORTICAL CELLS
INTO PERIADRENAL FAT

Irregular cortical extrusion extends into periadrenal fat without any encapsulation.

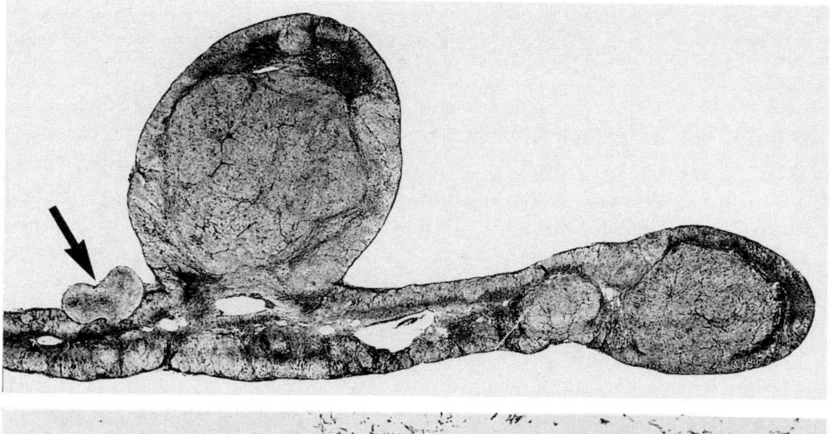

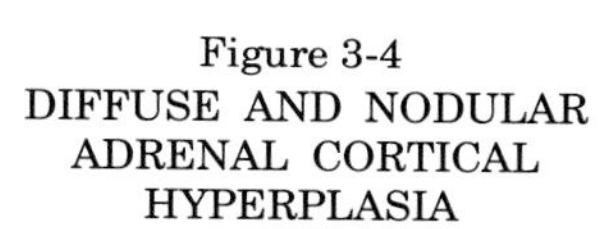

Figure 3-4
DIFFUSE AND NODULAR
ADRENAL CORTICAL
HYPERPLASIA

Top: Macronodular adrenal cortical hyperplasia in a patient with pituitary-dependent Cushing's disease. Several smaller nodules are present including a cortical extrusion (arrow).

Bottom: Higher magnification of cortical extrusion above. Hyperplastic lesion has configuration of a "doorhandle" or "mushroom."

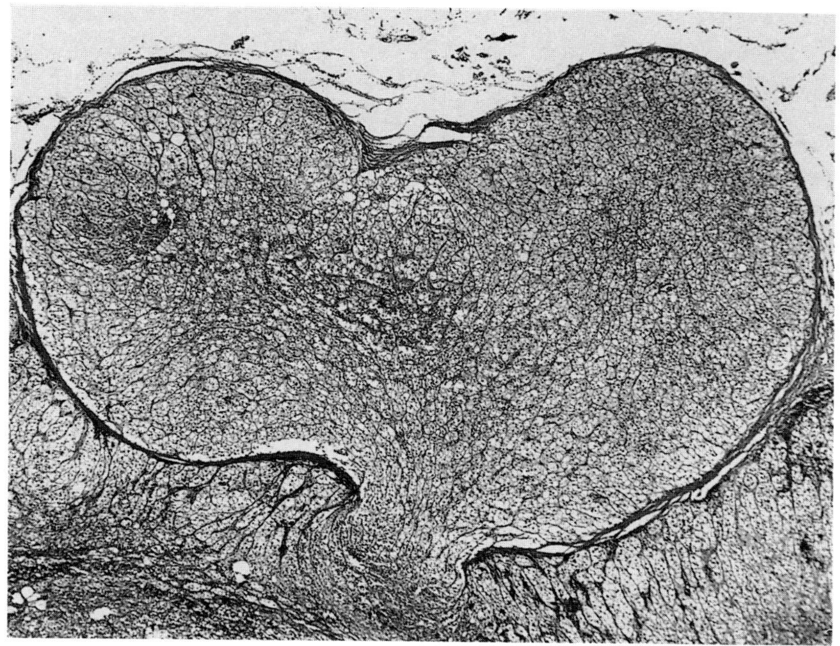

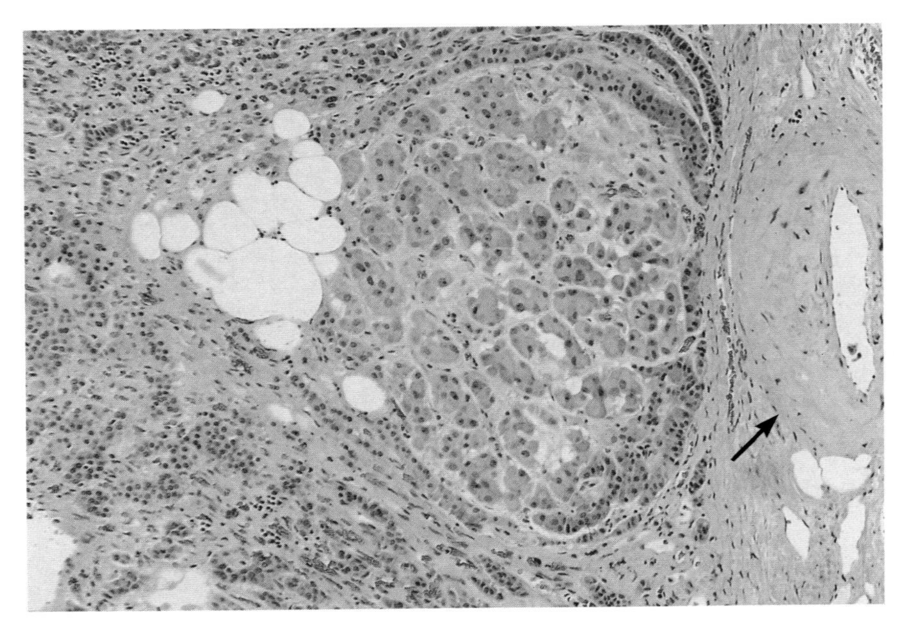

Figure 3-5
INCIDENTAL NODULAR ADRENAL GLAND

Incidental nodular adrenal gland obtained surgically from a patient without any evidence of cortical hyperfunction. A small focus of lipomatous metaplasia is present beneath the micronodule. Medial sclerosis of the capsular arteriole (arrow) is seen.

to gland. The larger nodules may be greater than 2 cm in diameter, and may have areas of myelolipomatous, or even osseous, metaplasia (4). An association between cortical nodularity and degenerative change in capsular arteries and arterioles (capsular arteriopathy) has been reported, suggesting that focal hyperplasia may be a response to localized ischemia (fig. 3-5) (4).

There are many architectural patterns associated with the nodular adrenal gland (fig. 3-6): alveolar, trabecular, gyriform ribbon-like, and "pseudoglandular." It may be difficult or impossible to distinguish an individual dominant macronodule from a cortical neoplasm on purely morphologic grounds since one or more of these varied patterns is also seen in the latter (see chapter 4). Pseudoglandular areas are rare but may have well-defined luminal borders and contents which consist of stringy amorphous or basophilic material (see figs. 3-6D, 4-39) or a few degenerated cortical cells. The adrenal medulla may be deformed due to compression by nodules or penetration of the medulla by cortical cells (4). The functional status of a dominant nodule may be determined by examination of the remaining ipsilateral or contralateral cortex. The presence of cortical atrophy may indicate hypercortisolism; hyperplasia of zona glomerulosa might be an indication of hyperaldosteronism. The large nonhyperfunctional cortical nodule or adenoma may show some advanced degenerative features such as cystic change, hyalinization, or old hemorrhage. Sclerosis may be patchy or involve much of the nodule and may be accompanied by dystrophic calcification. Rarely, there are areas resembling amyloid (figs. 3-7, 3-8).

Incidental Pigmented Cortical Nodules

Small brown or black pigmented nodules of the adrenal cortex are common findings at autopsy or in surgical material. These nodules usually range from 1 mm to 1.5 cm or more in diameter. When the nodule is large it can grossly distort the gland and be seen beneath the capsular surface (fig. 3-9, left); in transverse sections it may present as a tumefactive lesion (fig. 3-9, right). Retrospective autopsy studies have revealed pigmented nodules in 2.2 to 10.4 percent of cases (15,16); when these lesions were prospectively searched for in 3-mm sections from both adrenal glands, they were found in 37 percent of patients (16). As many as five separate pigmented nodules have been found in a single gland, and in 11 percent of cases the lesions were bilateral. In some reports the small pigmented nodules have been referred to as adenomas although there was no known functional significance attached to them. Distinction from a true neoplasm may be impossible, but when the lesions are multiple and bilateral a hyperplastic process is favored.

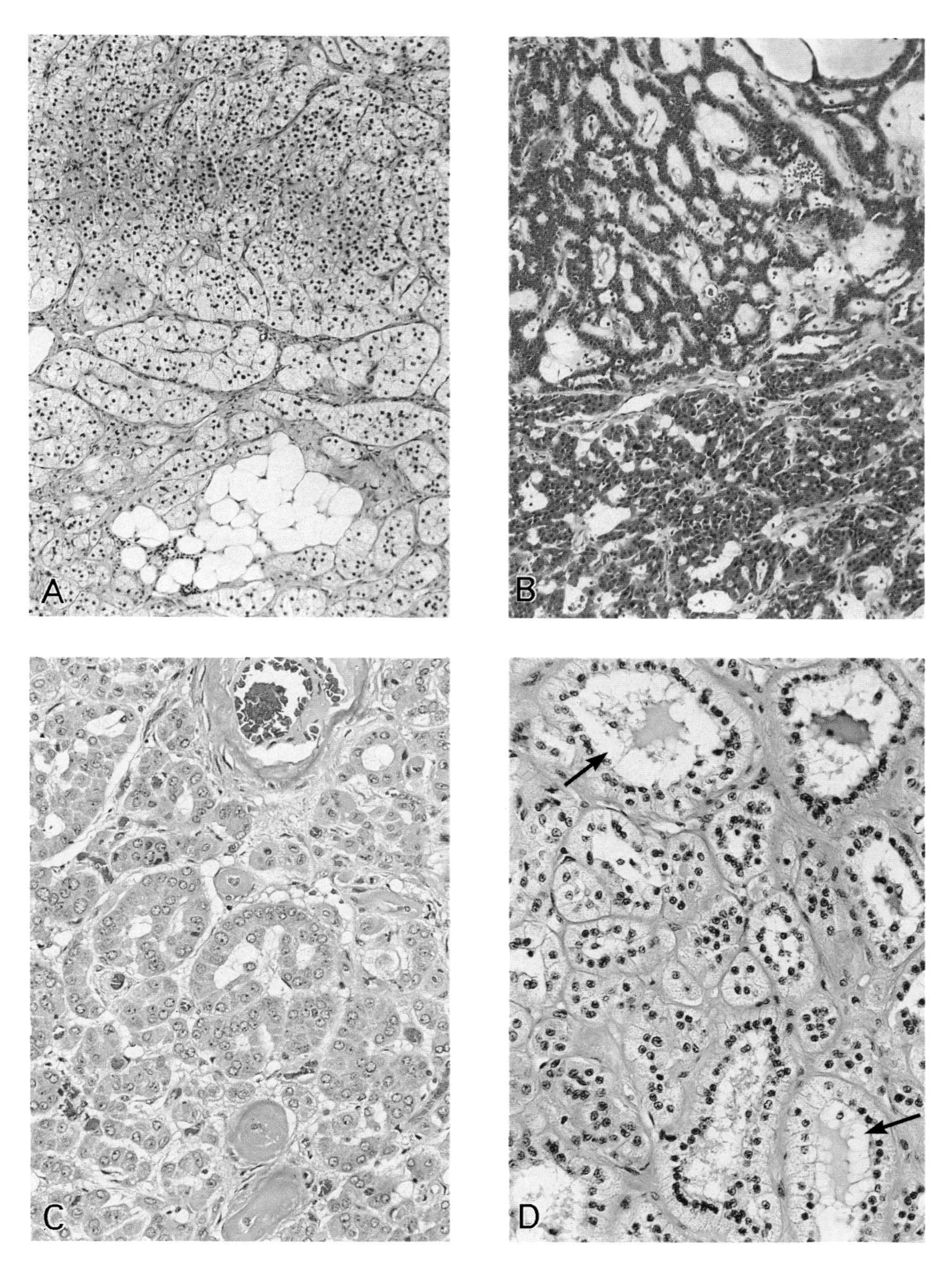

Figure 3-6

DIFFERENT FIELDS IN AN INCIDENTAL NODULAR ADRENAL GLAND FROM AN ADULT WHO HAD NO EVIDENCE OF HYPERCORTICALISM

A: Nodules with lipid-rich cells and smaller cells with compact eosinophilic cytoplasm. Small lipomatous component is at the bottom of the field. The cell cytoplasm is "clear" but contains small vacuolar spaces.

B: Two poorly demarcated nodules are composed of blunt cords and trabeculae as well as thin serpentine columns of cells (top).

C: Irregular cords and clusters of cells with compact eosinophilic cytoplasm. A few hyalinized vessels are also present.

D: Alveolar (or nesting) arrangement of cells, with some showing gland-like spaces (arrows).

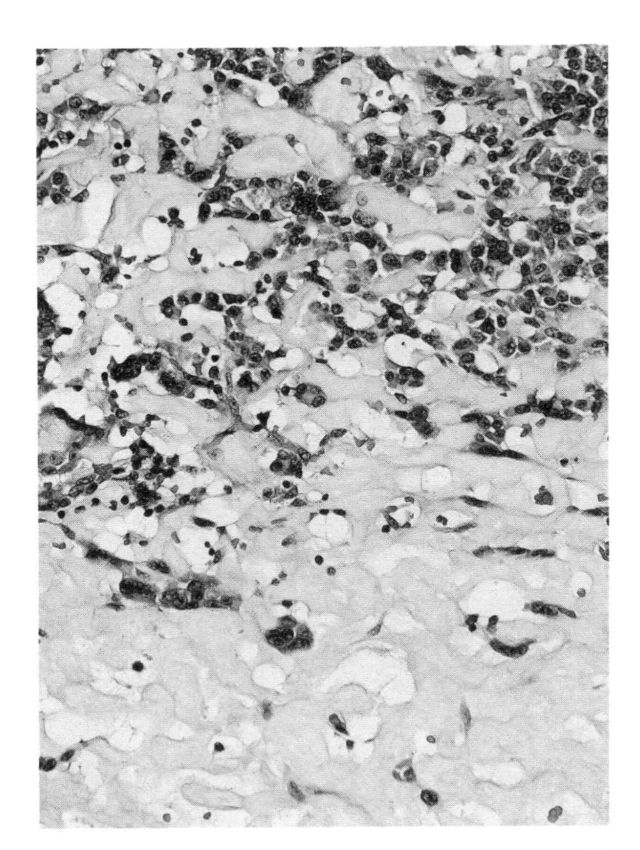

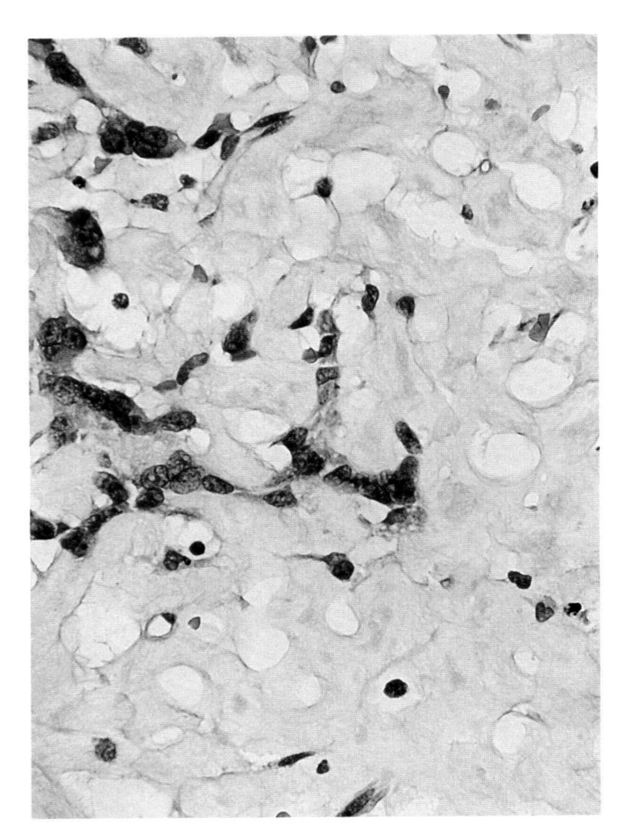

Figure 3-7
HYALINIZED AND PARTIALLY CALCIFIED LEFT ADRENAL MASS

This mass was discovered incidentally on a chest roentgenogram in an 11-year-old girl. The biochemical work-up for increased adrenal function was completely negative.

Left: Nonhyperfunctional adrenal cortical nodule or adenoma shows extensive stromal sclerosis.

Right: Portions of same cortical nodule or adenoma as on the left are extensively hyalinized, with areas resembling amyloid, but Congo red stain was reported to be negative.

The microscopic nature of the lesion at low magnification may not be as distinctive as that seen on gross examination (fig. 3-10). When the pigmented nodule is small it is characteristically centered on the zona reticularis (fig. 3-11, left), and there may be some indentation or distortion of the adrenal medulla. The pigmented lesions are unencapsulated, and are composed largely of cells with compact, eosinophilic cytoplasm, although there may be an admixture of cells with lipid-rich, vacuolated cytoplasm. The dark color of the lesion is imparted to a minor degree by the lipid-depleted cells, but a more conspicuous component is the intracytoplasmic coarse granular pigment representing lipofuscin (fig. 3-11, right). Nuclei are usually uniform, round to oval, with a single, small, dot-like nucleolus, although occasionally there may be some nuclear irregularity. The cells strongly resemble cells of the zona reticularis although greatly expanded in cell density and volume. A recent study suggested the presence of a component of neuromelanin (15).

Serendipitous Cortical Nodule Discovered In Vivo

An unsuspected nonhyperfunctioning adrenal mass has been reported in 0.6 to 1.3 percent of patients examined by CT scan of the upper abdomen (17,25,31); this incidence could be even higher depending upon the patient population (patients with hypertension, diabetes mellitus, and elderly patients may theoretically show an increased frequency). In one study, all of the patients with known malignancy were excluded

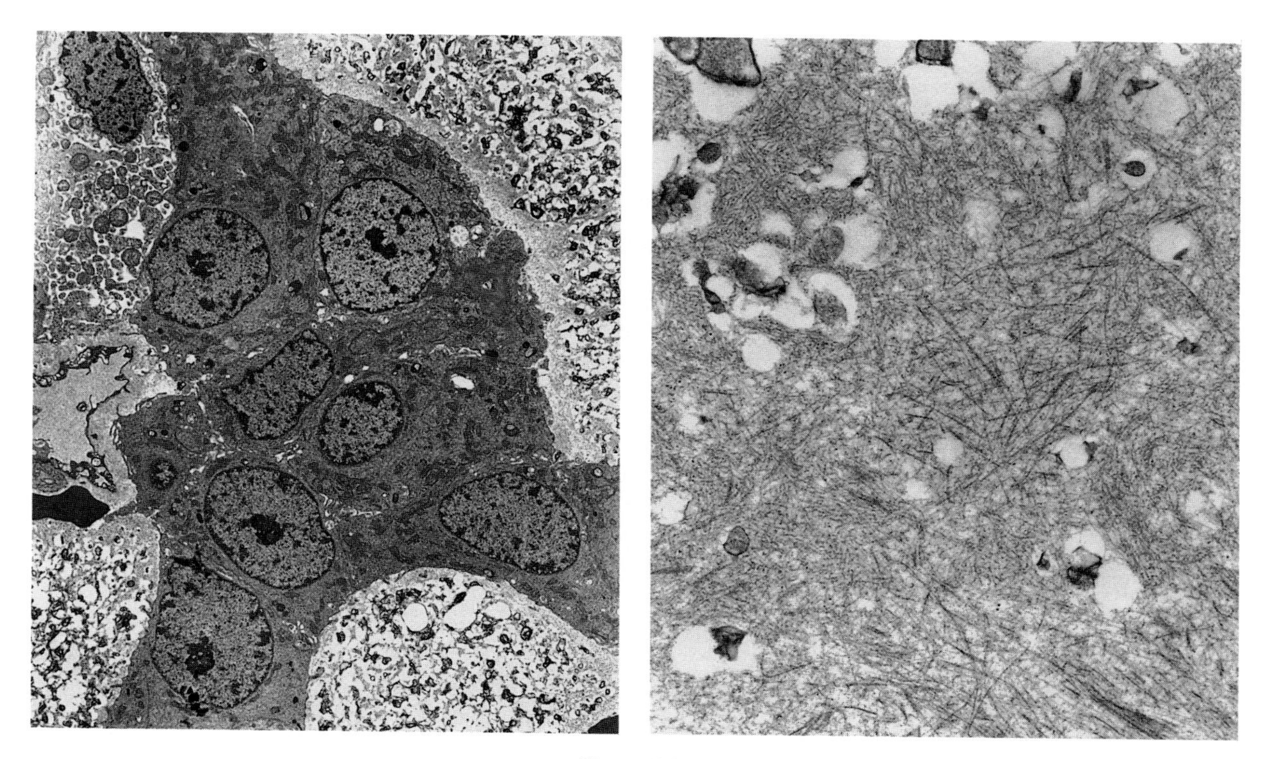

Figure 3-8

HYALINIZED AND PARTIALLY CALCIFIED LEFT ADRENAL MASS

This mass was discovered incidentally on a chest roentgenogram in an 11-year-old girl. It is the same adrenal cortical nodule or adenoma as in figure 3-7.

Left: Cells of cortical adenoma have lipid-depleted cytoplasm and a moderate number of mitochondria with slight pleomorphism. Amorphous matter and fibrillar material separate cells. (X2,200)

Right: Ultrastructure of intensely hyalinized stroma. Some of the rigid, nonbranching filaments resemble amyloid. (X15,500) (Electron microscopic photographs courtesy of Ms. Lynne Farr, Providence, RI.)

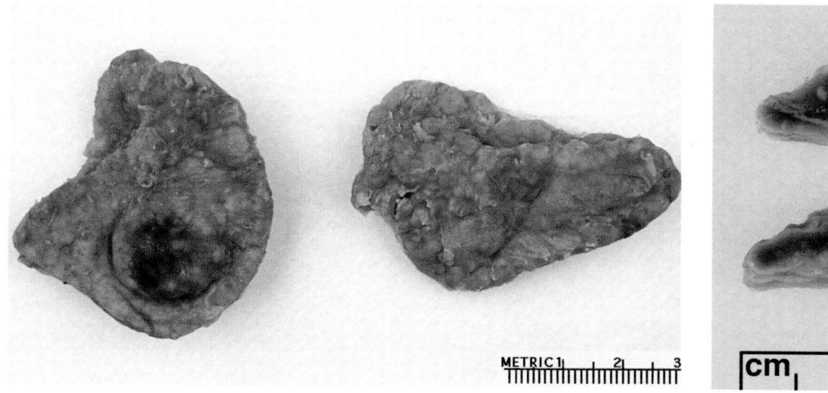

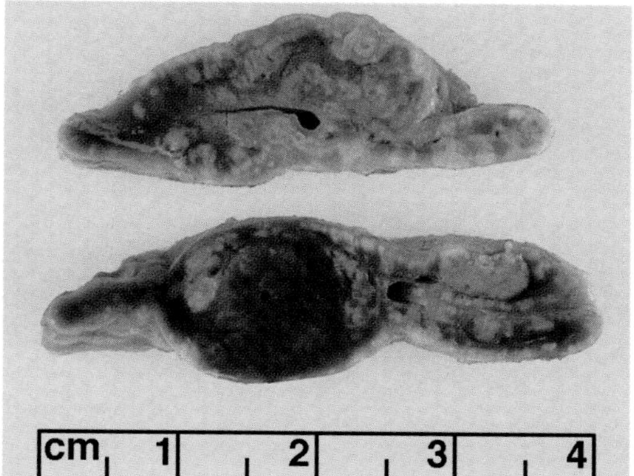

Figure 3-9

NODULAR ADRENAL GLAND WITH INCIDENTAL PIGMENTED MACRONODULE

Left: Dorsal surface of nodular adrenal glands obtained at autopsy of an adult. Note the darkly pigmented nodule projecting beneath the capsule.

Right: Incidental pigmented nodule in transverse section of gland. Numerous micronodules are present in the adjacent cortex.

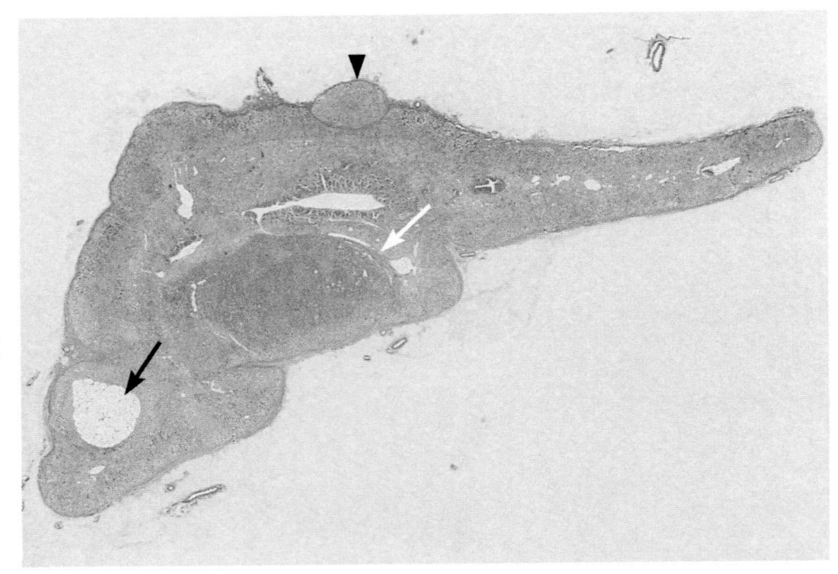

Figure 3-10
INCIDENTAL
PIGMENTED NODULE

Incidental pigmented nodule (white arrow) has expansile borders but lacks encapsulation. A small focus of lipomatous metaplasia (black arrow) as well as capsular extrusion (black arrowhead) are shown.

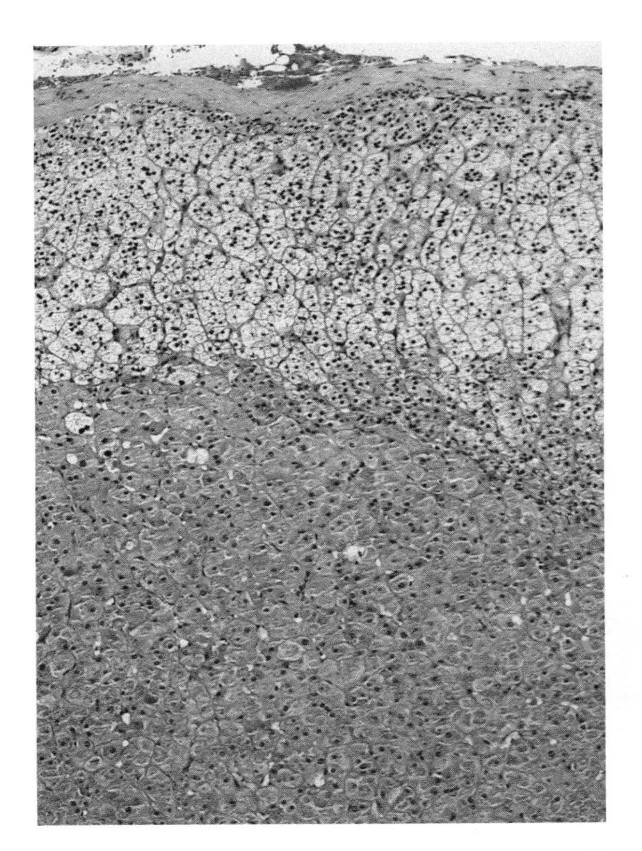

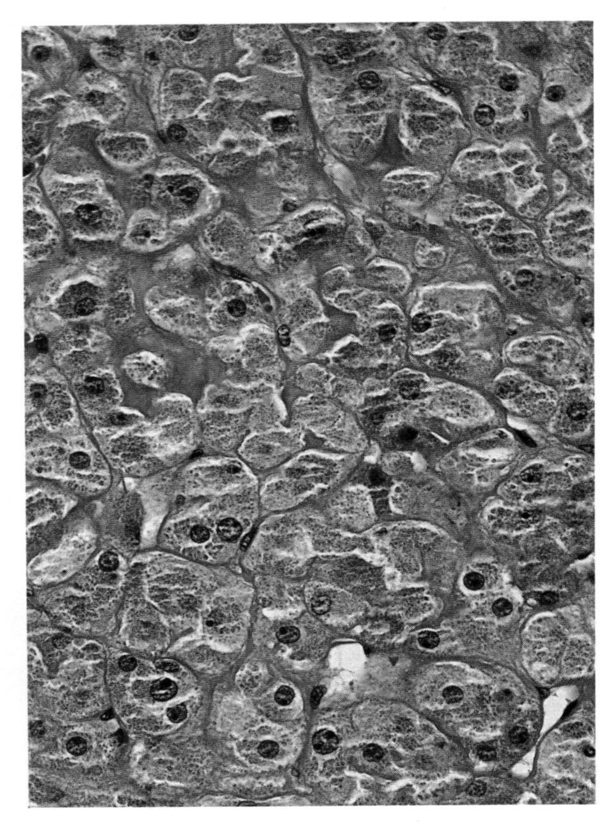

Figure 3-11
INCIDENTAL PIGMENTED NODULE

Left: Incidental pigmented nodule has epicenter in the zona reticularis and expansile borders impinging slightly on the outer cortex.

Right: Cortical cells contain variable amount of granular dark brown pigment. Nuclei tend to be round to oval and vary only slightly in size.

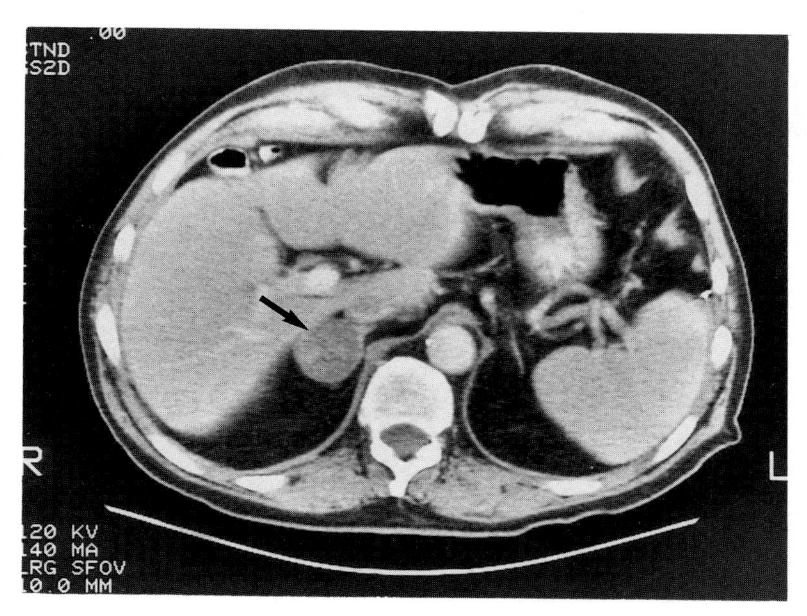

Figure 3-12
INCIDENTAL BENIGN
ADRENAL CORTICAL NODULE

The benign adrenal cortical nodule or "nonhyperfunctioning" adenoma on the right side (arrow) was discovered incidentally in an elderly patient with a history of bladder carcinoma. On CT scan the lesion was round, well circumscribed, and showed low attenuation with intravenous contrast.

(17), while in the other all lesions with classic CT characteristics of cysts or myelolipoma were eliminated (26). An incidental nonhyperfunctional adrenal cortical nodule (or adenoma), as seen on CT scan, is usually round to oval with smooth contour, has a well-delineated margin clearly separate from adjacent structures (fig. 3-12), and typically shows no detectable growth on serial scanning of the abdomen. A smaller nodule may distort the medial or lateral limb of the gland. The average age in one series was 62 years and nearly 60 percent of patients were female (27). The average size in several studies is 2.4 to 2.8 cm (17,26,27,31); the largest lesions are usually 5 to 6 cm. Preclinical Cushing's syndrome (autonomous cortisol production without signs or symptoms of hypercortisolism) has been reported in 1 percent (27) to 12 percent (32) of patients with incidentally discovered adrenal tumors who have been studied biochemically. A major risk of adrenalectomy in some patients is adrenal cortical insufficiency (32).

With the availability of high resolution CT scan, an adrenal mass less than 1 cm may be visualized, and with wider application of this imaging modality an increasing number of asymptomatic patients with an adrenal mass will likely be detected. The benign nonhyperfunctioning adrenal cortical macronodule (or adenoma) is the most common type of incidentally discovered adrenal mass, followed by a metastasis from a known primary tumor elsewhere, especially lung and breast (30). It may not be possible to reliably distinguish a metastasis from an adrenal cortical nodule or neoplasm on CT scan (24), and fine-needle aspiration under CT or ultrasound guidance (fig. 3-13) can provide valuable information which must be correlated with imaging characteristics of the lesion as well as any available clinical or endocrinologic data. Cell block preparations may also provide valuable information (fig. 3-14).

For the large group of adrenal lesions that appear unexpectedly on CT scan in the nononcologic patient, size becomes an important criterion in determining the future course of action, i.e., observation with repeat scan several months later or surgical resection. MRI can separate nonhyperfunctional adenomas (low signal intensity) and pheochromocytomas (high signal intensity) (23,25,28), but many lesions have overlapping patterns (21). The size of the adrenal mass is important since adrenal cortical carcinoma (ACC) is usually over 6 cm in diameter, whereas adenomas are typically smaller in size. Assuming that the prevalence of biochemically silent ACC is about 1 per 250,000 population, it has been estimated that over 60 operations have to be done on patients with an adrenal mass 6 cm or greater to remove one ACC (22). In a large series from the Mayo Clinic, 4 of 342 patients with an incidentally discovered adrenal tumor (55 underwent

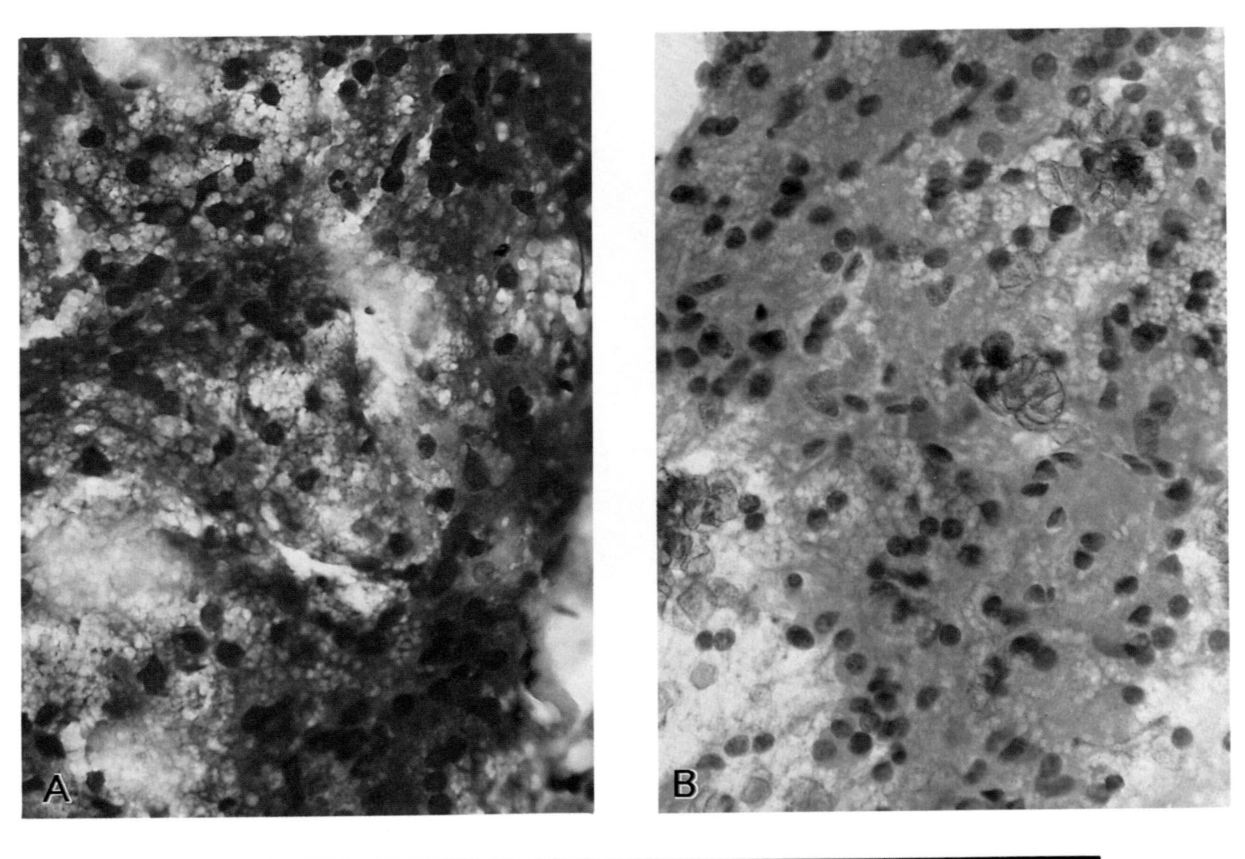

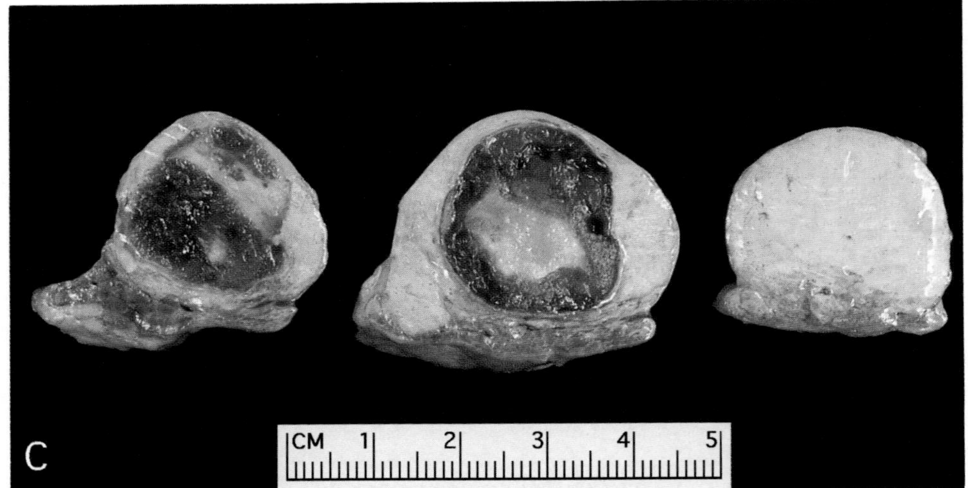

Figure 3-13

INCIDENTAL BENIGN ADRENAL CORTICAL NODULE

A: Fine-needle aspiration of a serendipitous adrenal nodule. The cluster of cells shows relatively uniform nuclei and small vacuolar spaces within the cytoplasm. (X400, Diff Quik stain) (A and B are from the same case as figure 3-12.)

B: Greater nuclear detail is shown. Cells contain numerous cytoplasmic vacuoles representing lipid droplets. (X400, Papanicolaou stain)

C: Incidentally discovered nonfunctional adrenal cortical adenoma in a 73-year-old man who had gallstones. Fine-needle aspirate did not yield sufficient material for diagnosis. Right adrenalectomy was also performed during elective cholecystectomy. The adrenal adenoma weighed 28 g and measured nearly 3.5 cm in diameter. Note the central organizing hematoma following attempt at needle aspiration. Different case than A and B.

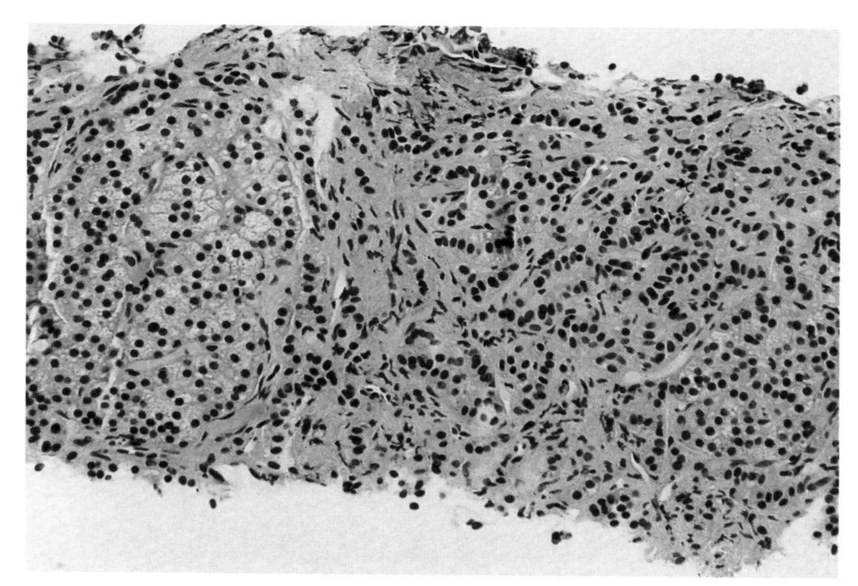

Figure 3-14
INCIDENTAL ADRENAL CORTICAL NODULE

The cell block preparation of fine-needle aspiration biopsy of an incidentally discovered adrenal nodule. "Nonhyperfunctional" cortical nodule or adenoma has vague alveolar and trabecular architecture and most cells have compact, granular eosinophilic cytoplasm.

adrenalectomy) had an ACC (tumor diameters 5.5 cm, 8.5 cm, 8.7 cm, and 17.0 cm); 3 of the 4 died, while the patient with the smallest tumor had no evidence of tumor at 5 years follow up (27). An approach for the evaluation of the asymptomatic adrenal adenoma identified by CT scan or MRI is shown in Table 3-3 using 6 cm as a size criterion; parameters used to make a therapeutic decision included 1) extent and size on CT, 2) hormonal assessment, and 3) MRI (18,22,33). It should be remembered, however, that the threshold of size as a distinguishing feature varies from 3 cm (19) to 4 cm (20,27) to 5 cm (29,34), or slightly larger, depending upon the source.

Table 3-3

EVALUATION OF THE "INCIDENTAL," NONFUNCTIONAL ADRENAL ADENOMA DISCOVERED IN VIVO BASED ON SIZE AND MRI*

Tumor should be resected if larger than 6 cm, if functional or even if less than 6 cm and nonfunctional but has an MRI-T_2-weighted signal intensity of greater than 3 (adrenal vs. liver)
Fine-needle aspiration (before deciding on resection) for nonfunctional tumor less than 6 cm with MRI-T_2 signal intensity of more than 1.4 but less than 3
Nonfunctional tumors less than 6 cm with MRI-T_2 signal intensity less than or equal to 1.4 should have studies yearly and should be resected if growth is greater than 1.0 cm per year.

*Data from reference 18.

ADRENAL CORTICAL HYPERPLASIA WITH HYPERCORTISOLISM

There are several major causes of noniatrogenic Cushing's syndrome (fig. 3-15) (43,49), and the incidence depends in large part on age at diagnosis. In adults, noniatrogenic hypercortisolism can be due to: pituitary-dependent ACTH overproduction (Cushing's disease) which accounts for about 59 percent of cases (50); an autonomously secreting adrenal cortical neoplasm (or rare forms of pituitary or ACTH-independent adrenal cortical hyperplasia), accounting for 17 percent (39), 20 percent (53), and 25 percent (50) of cases in various studies; ectopic production of ACTH, seen in 15 percent (39,53) or 16 percent (50) of cases; or rarely, hypercortisolism due to ectopic production of corticotropin-releasing factor (CRF) (35, 37). Ectopic production of both ACTH and CRF has also been reported, and the biochemical pattern may be that of pituitary ACTH-dependent hypercortisolism (52,57). The age and sex of the patient may have some influence on the relative incidence of these different forms of hypercortisolism. The adrenal form of Cushing's syndrome, for example, predominates in children, particularly those in the first decade of life (47);

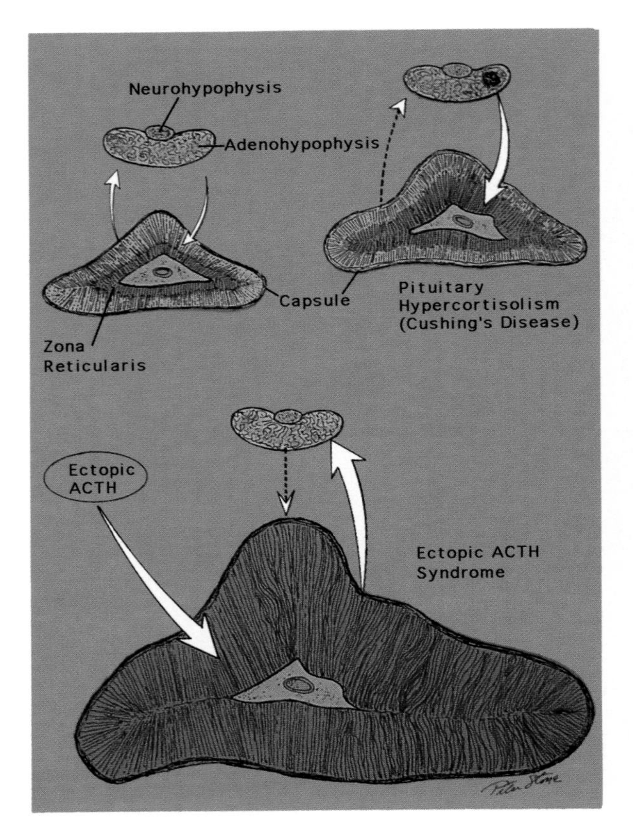

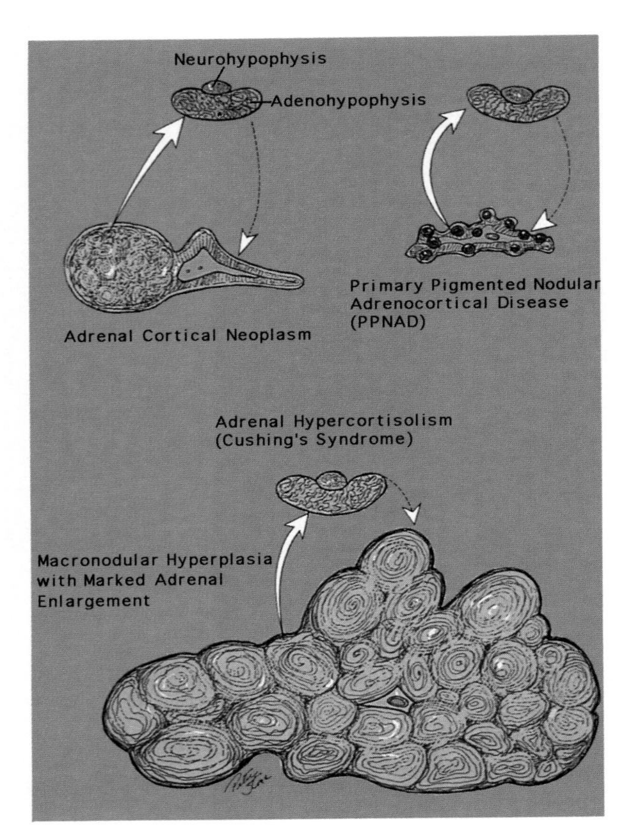

Figure 3-15

ETIOLOGY OF NONIATROGENIC CUSHING'S SYNDROME

Left: Schematic diagram of normal hypothalamic-pituitary-adrenal axis (upper left), pituitary-dependent Cushing's disease (upper right), and ectopic ACTH syndrome.

Right: Adrenal Cushing's syndrome due to either an adrenal cortical adenoma or carcinoma (upper left), primary pigmented nodular adrenocortical disease (PPNAD) (upper right), a rare form of pituitary (or ACTH)-independent Cushing's syndrome,and macronodular hyperplasia with marked adrenal enlargement (lower half).

Cushing's syndrome due to ectopic ACTH production is largely a disease of men, and most patients with Cushing's disease are women of reproductive age (44).

In children under the age of 7 years an adrenal cortical neoplasm (either adrenal cortical adenoma or carcinoma) appears to be the most common cause of Cushing's syndrome (42,47,48). When there is a pituitary source for ACTH overproduction (i.e., Cushing's disease) in childhood, Nelson's syndrome can develop following adrenalectomy (55), and some studies indicate a higher risk of this complication in children compared with adults (54).

There are other causes of Cushing's syndrome that are rare, but provide insight into the regulatory mechanisms at the molecular level (36). The McCune-Albright syndrome consists of a triad of polyostotic fibrous dysplasia, skin pigmentation with café au lait spots, and sexual precocity, but there may be associated endocrine disorders, including Cushing's syndrome (38). The McCune-Albright syndrome is due to somatic mutation within exon 8 of the lambda subunit of stimulatory G protein, a protein that activates adenylate cyclase, which in turn causes authentic autonomous overproduction of cortisol in multiple adrenal cortical nodules in which this mutation is expressed (56). Food-dependent Cushing's syndrome has also been reported secondary to inappropriate sensitivity of the adrenal glands to normal postprandial increase in secretion of gastric inhibitory polypeptide (GIP) (41,51). The primary cause does not appear to be GIP, but more likely "illicit" or "ectopic" expression of GIP receptors on the plasma membrane of adrenal cortical cells. There are also atypical

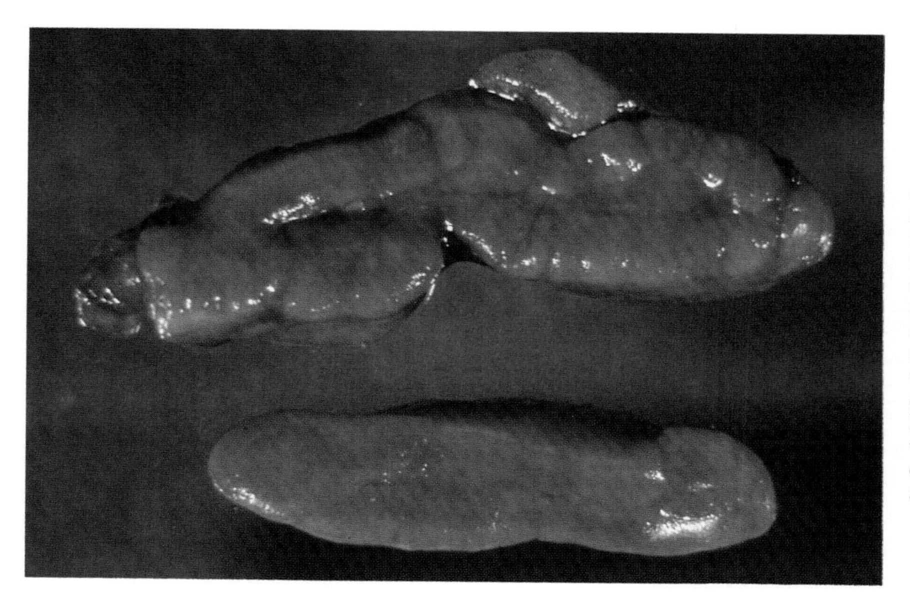

Figure 3-16
CUSHING'S DISEASE

Transverse sections of a 3.5 g adrenal gland surgically resected from an 8-year-old boy with Cushing's disease in 1974. Patient underwent several attempts at transsphenoidal pituitary resection as well as radiation therapy (4800 rads), but the tumor recurred on several occasions. Initially there was no abnormality on tomograms of the sella turcica, but the patient later developed Nelson's syndrome with radiologically detectable changes in the sella. (Figures 3-16 and 3-17 are from the same case.)

forms of Cushing's syndrome which may be difficult to diagnosis, as for example the pseudo-Cushing's syndrome, a reversible form of hypercortisolism related to alcohol abuse (40), or cyclic Cushing's disease with intermittent hypersecretion of ACTH (46).

Pituitary-Dependent Hypercortisolism

Cushing provided a detailed description in 1932 of the disease which came to bear his name (61). (An interesting biography of Cushing was written by Fulton in 1946 [64].) Most cases of Cushing's disease are due to an ACTH-producing pituitary adenoma, usually a microadenoma (less than 10 mm in diameter), which may be difficult to identify with even the most contemporary imaging techniques (63,66,71,74). Advances in dynamic laboratory testing, such as bilateral petrosal venous sinus sampling (71), and improvements in pituitary microsurgical techniques have increased the success rate for resection of microadenomas to over 90 percent in the past decade (66). Plasma ACTH levels are usually within the normal range or only moderately elevated in ACTH (or pituitary)-dependent Cushing's disease. The microadenoma can be very small and located deep in the central wedge of the pituitary gland near the neurohypophysis, making surgical (or pathologic) detection difficult; nonetheless, transsphenoidal adenomectomy remains the treatment of choice for most patients with Cushing's disease. A small proportion of patients with pituitary-dependent Cushing's syndrome appear to have underlying hyperplasia of ACTH-producing corticotroph cells, either as a primary abnormality (76), or one due to entopic (hypothalamic) or ectopic excess production of CRF (58).

Diffuse and Micronodular Hyperplasia. Currently, the pathologist seldom has the opportunity to examine adrenalectomy specimens from patients with Cushing's disease. Because excess corticosteroid secretion may be detected at an earlier phase today, some of the resected adrenal glands may be only mildly stimulated, with very subtle changes, and thus the gland may be regarded as "normal." Careful correlation of morphology with clinical and hormonal data is crucial (67). The adrenal gland usually shows diffuse (fig. 3-16) or diffuse and micronodular hyperplasia. Gland enlargement is usually minimal, with individual weights of 6 to 12 g (67). On transverse sections the gland may appear expanded with rounded edges, and careful inspection may reveal a faint, somewhat irregular junction between the pale yellow outer aspect of the cortex and the inner third to half; this portion is darker, often tan to brown, due to conversion of vacuolated, lipid-rich cells to lipid-depleted cells with more compact, eosinophilic cytoplasm (fig. 3-17). Micronodular hyperplasia may be evident as small irregular nests of cortical cells with

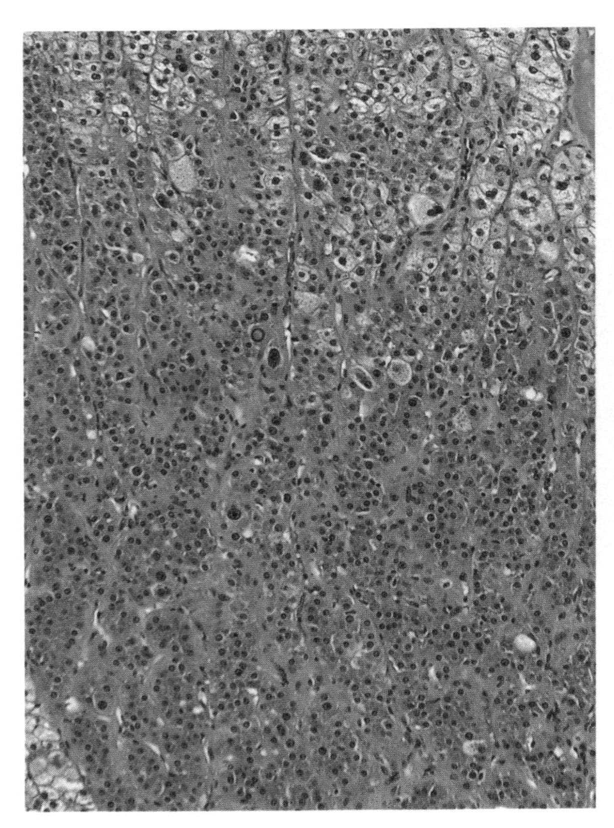

Figure 3-17
CUSHING'S DISEASE
Much of zona fasciculata is converted to cells with compact, eosinophilic cytoplasm under the trophic influence of ACTH.

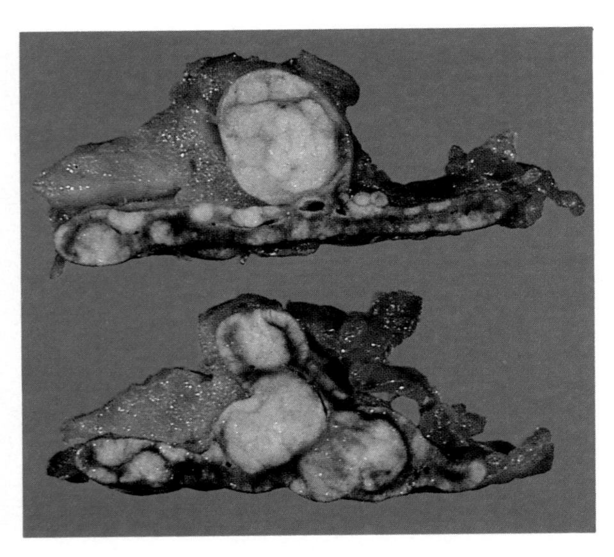

Figure 3-18
MACRONODULAR ADRENAL CORTICAL HYPERPLASIA IN CUSHING'S DISEASE
The patient was a 36-year-old man with multiple endocrine neoplasia (MEN) syndrome type I who underwent right radical nephrectomy for an angiomyolipoma which simulated a renal cell carcinoma. Pale yellow cortical nodules range in size from 0.5 cm to over 1.0 cm. Note the few areas of capsular extrusion. (Figures 3-18 and 3-19 are from the same case.)

expansile pushing borders, occasionally with compression of the adjacent cortex. The extent to which lipid-rich cells of the zona fasciculata are converted to compact lipid-poor cells is variable, and physiologic factors may have some bearing on the overall morphology (67). There may be irregular extension of zona fasciculata cells into periadrenal fat and a conspicuous mantle of cortical cells may be present around tributaries of the central adrenal vein. The adrenal medulla appears normal, although there may be intermingling of cortical and chromaffin cells. Ultrastructural changes have been reported in cortical cells (73), but there may be dynamic endocrinologic and physiologic changes as well.

Macronodular Hyperplasia. Macronodular hyperplasia (MNH), often used synonymously with nodular hyperplasia, has been reported in 10 percent (62) to 20 percent (69,70) of patients with pituitary-dependent Cushing's disease. A relatively high incidence of 40 percent was recorded by Smals et al. (75), but the definition of macronodular is entirely arbitrary. A macronodule is defined by Doppman et al. (62) as any nodule visible on CT scan; when they used 5-mm thick sections the smallest nodule was 6 mm in diameter. MNH is considered to be a distinct form of ACTH-dependent hypercortisolism with rather confusing biochemical and radiologic findings (75). When it is characterized by a single dominant nodule there is a risk of confusing this lesion with a unilateral autonomous adrenal cortical adenoma, and performing an inappropriate unilateral adrenalectomy (62). The term multinodular adrenal was used by Page et al. (72) to emphasize that the nodules are rarely, if ever, solitary (72). MNH is defined by others as the presence of one or more prominent yellow nodules visible to the naked eye in glands in which the remaining cortex is hyperplastic (69).

In MNH the adrenal glands are enlarged and often show a multinodular configuration on transverse sections (fig. 3-18). One or more dominant nodules may distort the intact gland and

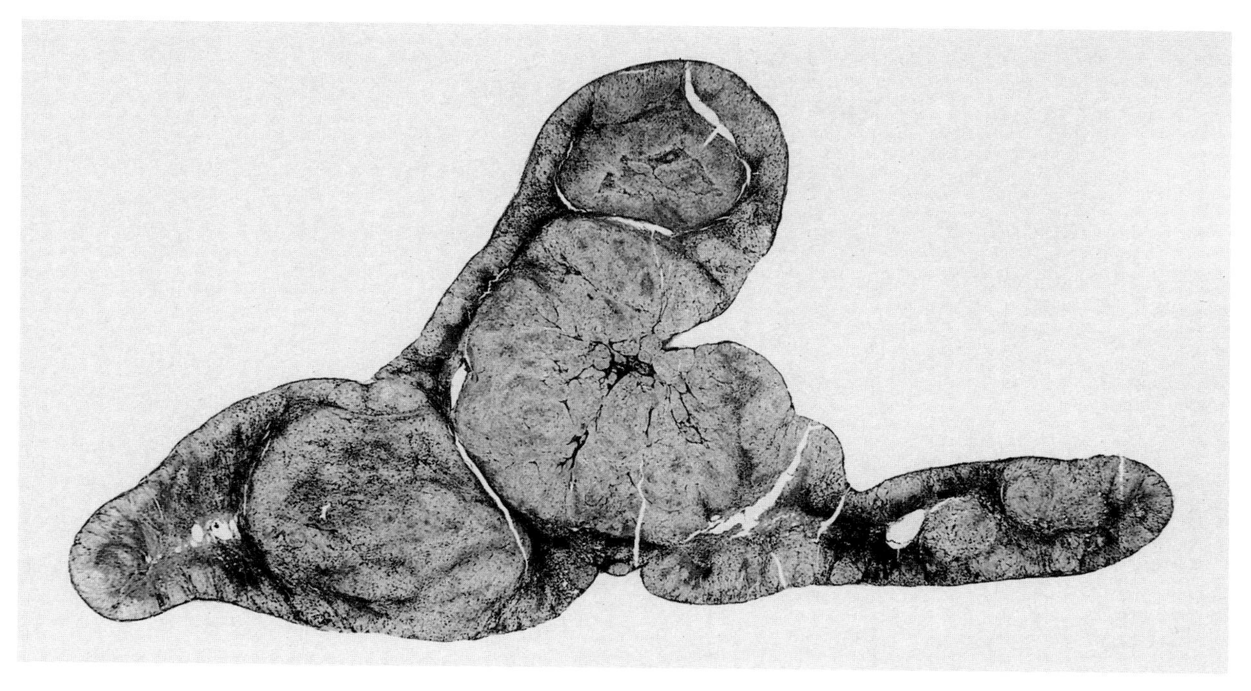

Figure 3-19
PITUITARY (ACTH)-DEPENDENT CUSHING'S SYNDROME
Macronodular hyperplasia with irregular expansile cortical nodules which merge with adjacent hyperplastic cortex.

form a round projection from virtually any region. In one study, the average individual weight of the adrenal gland in MNH was about 16 g, and in one case both adrenal glands weighed 87.5 g (75). In an earlier series of patients with Cushing's disease undergoing subtotal (about 90 percent) adrenalectomy, most glands had a combined weight of 14 to 26 g (60). Some patients undergoing subtotal bilateral adrenalectomy developed "adenoma-like" recurrences (59), thus underscoring the possibility of confusing MNH with an adrenal cortical neoplasm. Nodules vary in size from 0.5 to over 5 cm (62,75), but most are less than 2 cm in diameter. There may be a disparity between size and weight of individual glands.

Grossly, the nodules appear discrete and sharply demarcated, and some dominant macronodules may give the impression of encapsulation; on microscopic study, however, the nodules are less well defined, and blend almost imperceptibly with the adjacent hyperplastic cortex (fig. 3-19). There is a variable mixture of pale-staining, lipid-rich cells and lipid-depleted cells with compact, eosinophilic cytoplasm (fig. 3-20). Some nodules are composed almost exclusively of lipid-rich cells, and correspond to the yellow nodules seen on gross inspection. Prominent cortical nodules may compress and distort the adrenal medulla, and it may be difficult to recognize the medullary compartment in histologic sections (60). There may be foci of lipomatous or myelolipomatous metaplasia.

There are data suggesting that MNH may be the result of longstanding Cushing's disease with varying degrees of pituitary dependency and adrenal cortical autonomy (75). In one study there was a good correlation between the weight of the adrenal gland and the duration of disease (Table 3-4). Some data suggest that cortical cells of MNH may require lower circulating levels of ACTH to sustain the hypercortisolism compared with diffuse hyperplasia (68). The plasma levels of ACTH in some cases may be lower than in classic Cushing's disease, or even undetectable, and there may be absence of suppression with low-dose and high-dose dexamethasone. Some advocate bilateral adrenalectomy as the treatment of choice for some cases of MNH in this setting (75).

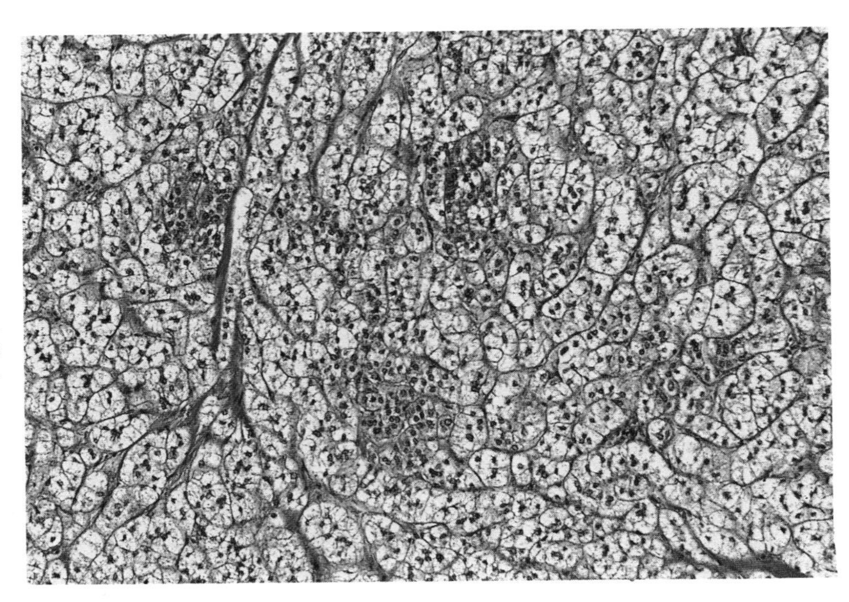

Figure 3-20
MACRONODULAR ADRENAL CORTICAL HYPERPLASIA IN CUSHING'S DISEASE

Nodules are composed of predominantly pale-staining, lipid-rich cells with scattered collections of lipid-depleted cells.

Table 3-4

COMPARISON OF DIFFUSE AND MICRONODULAR HYPERPLASIA WITH MACRONODULAR HYPERPLASIA IN CUSHING'S DISEASE*

	Diffuse and Micronodular Hyperplasia	Macronodular Hyperplasia
Female/male	5 to 1	5 to 1
Age (average)	31 yrs	44 yrs
Duration of disease (avg.)	2 yrs	8 yrs
Adrenal weight (avg.)	8 g each (less disparity in weight)	16 g each (may be some disparity in weight)
Nodule size	less than 0.5 cm	0.5 to 5.3 cm

*Data from reference 75.

It is difficult to determine whether these dominant macronodules are truly neoplastic, or represent autonomous hyperplasia that requires no ACTH or only very low levels to maintain the hypercortisolism. A recent report showed evidence of transition from a pituitary-dependent to adrenal-dependent Cushing's syndrome (65); the situation may be similar to nodular goiter in which one or more thyroid nodules become "toxic" with autonomous hyperfunction (67).

Macronodular Hyperplasia with Marked Adrenal Enlargement

Definition. Macronodular hyperplasia of the adrenal cortex with marked adrenal enlargement (MHMAE), as defined by sensitive imaging and endocrinologic study, is a putative primary (autonomous) adrenal cause of Cushing's syndrome. It may simulate an adrenal cortical neoplasm.

General Considerations. The few cases of MHMAE reported in the literature suggest that it is a very rare cause of primary autonomous adrenal hypercortisolism in which there is tumefactive enlargement of both adrenal glands (fig. 3-21) (77,79). Endocrine studies, including dynamic testing, show elevated plasma cortisol levels with loss of diurnal rhythmicity and undetectable plasma ACTH levels; there is no suppression of adrenal cortisol secretion with dexamethasone, but some studies indicate a response to ACTH stimulation (77,79,82). There is no abnormality of the sella turcica or pituitary fossa on imaging studies, even in one patient who was reinvestigated almost 26 years later (79,82). Results of petrosal venous sinus sampling are also negative for a low-level pituitary source of ACTH (79). In one report, plasma ACTH rose slightly above the normal range following bilateral adrenalectomy (total combined adrenal gland weight of 161 g), suggesting a primary abnormality of the hypothalamic-pituitary axis before the development of autonomous adrenal hyperfunction

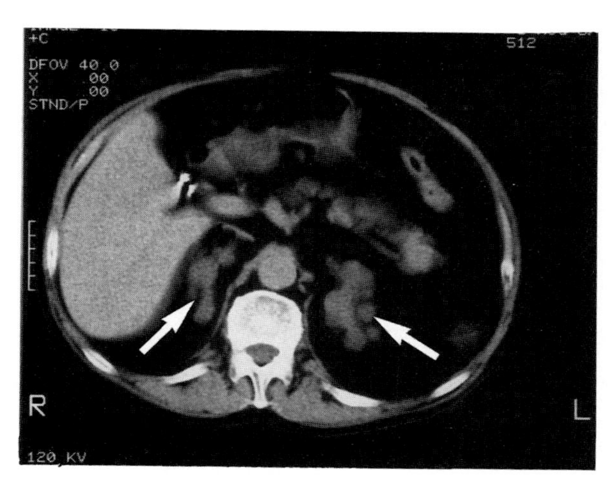

Figure 3-21
MACRONODULAR HYPERPLASIA
WITH MARKED ADRENAL ENLARGEMENT

Extensive endocrine evaluation and imaging studies of sella and pituitary fossa indicated a primary adrenal form of Cushing's syndrome. Normal configuration of adrenal glands (arrows) is obscured by multiple macronodules up to 3.8 cm in diameter. This marked enlargement can simulate a neoplasm. Combined weight of adrenal glands was 94 g. (Fig. 2 from Doppman JL, Nieman LK, Travis WD, et al. CT and MR imaging of massive macronodular adrenocortical disease: a rare cause of autonomous primary adrenal hypercortisolism. J Computr Assist Tomogr 1991;15:773–9.)

(81). An increased plasma cortisol response to insulin-induced hypoglycemia suggests a hyperreaction of adrenal glands to small changes in plasma ACTH, which may not be detected by radioimmunoassay, or stimulation by "unknown factors" which might be increased by hypoglycemia (80,83). An unusual case of ACTH-independent MHMAE has been reported in which the patient presented with feminization in addition to Cushing's syndrome; the combined adrenal weight was 86 g (84).

In the few cases reported to date there has been a slight predilection for male patients (77,79); other types of Cushing's syndrome affect females more often. The average age at diagnosis is about 50 years, with the duration of Cushing's syndrome ranging from 1 1/2 to 10 years in one study (79). Patients are typically older than those with diffuse or micronodular hyperplasia or MNH associated with Cushing's disease (87). Some of the features of MHMAE are summarized in Table 3-5.

Gross Findings. The adrenal glands in MHMAE can be markedly enlarged, with a combined weight of 60 to 180 g (fig. 3-22) (77,79).

Table 3-5

CUSHING'S SYNDROME DUE TO MACRONODULAR ADRENAL CORTICAL HYPERPLASIA WITH MARKED ADRENAL ENLARGEMENT

Average age about 50 years with slight male predominance
Bilateral macronodular hyperplasia; combined adrenal weights usually 60 to 180 g
Bilateral adrenalectomy considered treatment of choice in most cases
Elevated plasma cortisol with loss of diurnal variation
No suppression of adrenal cortisol secretion by dexamethasone
Variable response to ACTH stimulation
No abnormality on petrosal venous sinus sampling
Lack of abnormality of sella or pituitary fossa

There is an extraordinary degree of nodular cortical hyperplasia, which is macronodular, and gross distortion of the glands is seen on external examination (fig. 3-23). In one study the nodules ranged in size from 0.2 to 3.8 cm (79). On gross examination, the external aspect of the intact adrenal gland is often coarsely bosselated, with discrete to closely aggregated nodules that are either round or distorted due to close apposition. On cross section the nodules have a yellow to golden-yellow hue, sometimes with small irregular light brown foci. The nodules are unencapsulated, and may give the impression of coalescence or fusion (fig. 3-24). The medullary compartment may be distorted and difficult to recognize, and random sections of the gland may fail to reveal this. A gland that is grossly distorted by macronodules may be difficult to orient for good transverse sections. It is easy to see why MHMAE can simulate a tumor.

Microscopic Findings. Cortical cells have a variable amount of lipid-rich, pale, vacuolated cytoplasm (fig. 3-25), and there may be some cells, random in distribution, with compact, eosinophilic cytoplasm. Rarely, cells with "ballooned" vacuolated cytoplasm are present (fig. 3-26, left). Nuclear pleomorphism is usually inconspicuous and mitotic figures are rare. An unusual feature is the presence of pseudoglandular foci with stringy,

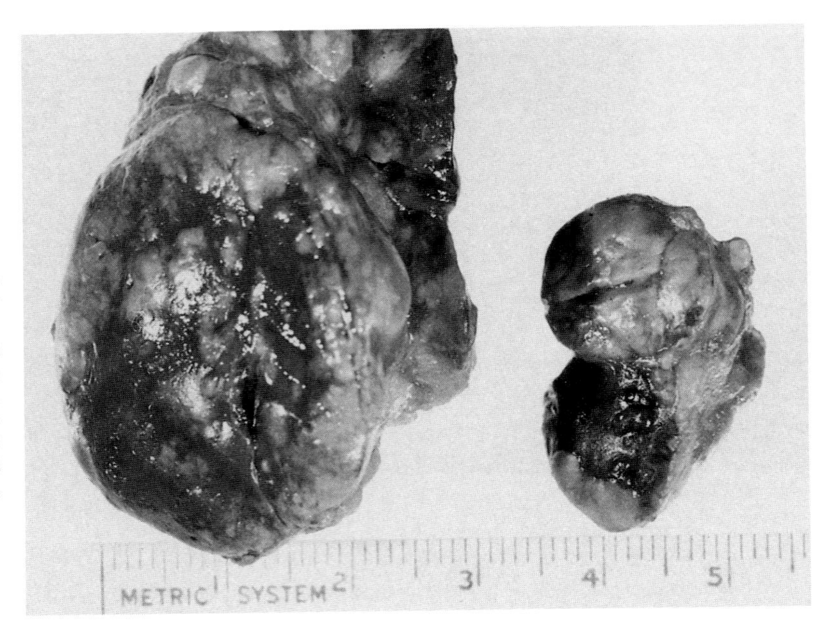

Figure 3-22
BILATERAL MACRONODULAR HYPERPLASIA WITH MARKED ADRENAL ENLARGEMENT

Bilateral adrenalectomy was performed on a 40-year-old woman who had longstanding Cushing's syndrome for about 9 years. Both glands together weighed 84 g, and were greatly distorted by multiple bright yellow nodules ranging in size from 0.2 to 3.5 cm. Patient was reevaluated nearly 26 years later and found to have no evidence of a pituitary tumor. (Fig. 2-12 from Lack EE, Travis WD, Oertel JE. Adrenal cortical nodules, hyperplasia and hyperfunction. In: Lack EE, ed. Pathology of the adrenal glands, New York: Churchill Livingstone, 1990:75–113.)

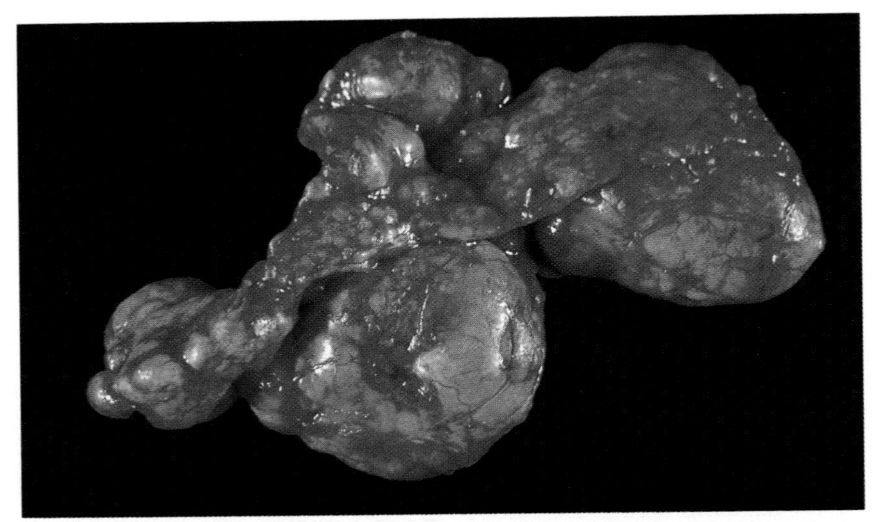

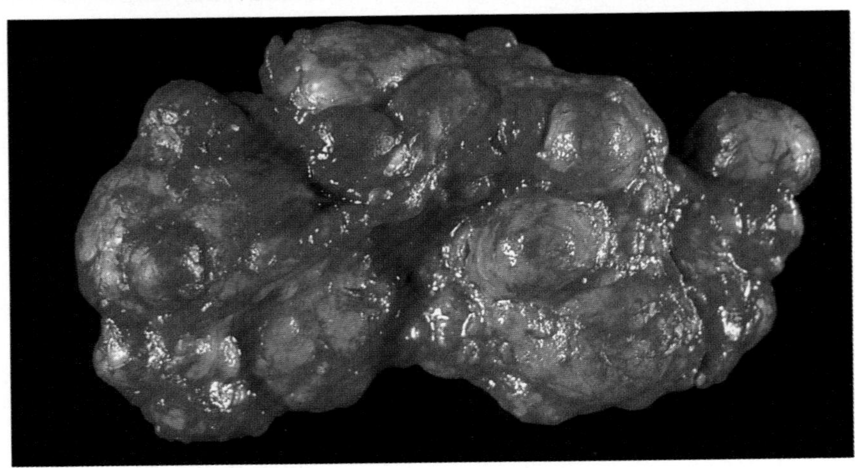

Figure 3-23
MACRONODULAR ADRENAL CORTICAL HYPERPLASIA WITH MARKED ADRENAL ENLARGEMENT

Top, bottom: Combined weight of both glands was about 85 g. External contour of both adrenal glands is greatly distorted by large cortical nodules. Endocrinologic work-up and sensitive imaging studies indicated a primary adrenal form of Cushing's syndrome. (Courtesy of Dr. William D. Travis, Bethesda, MD.)

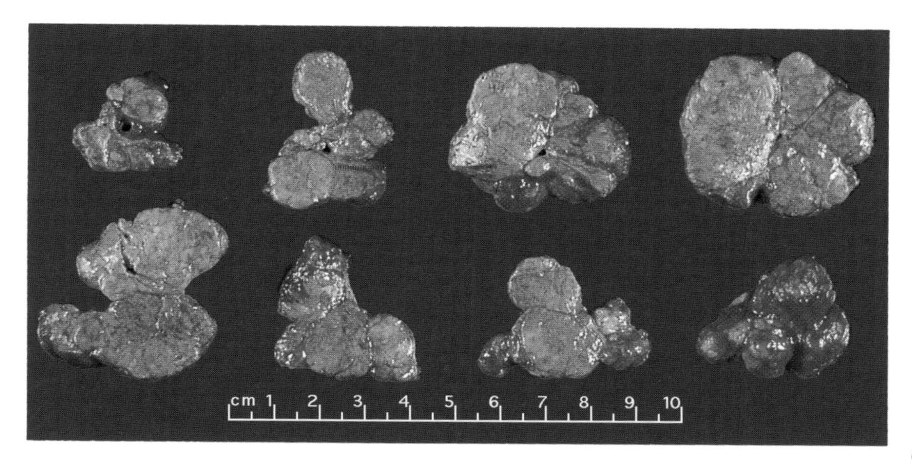

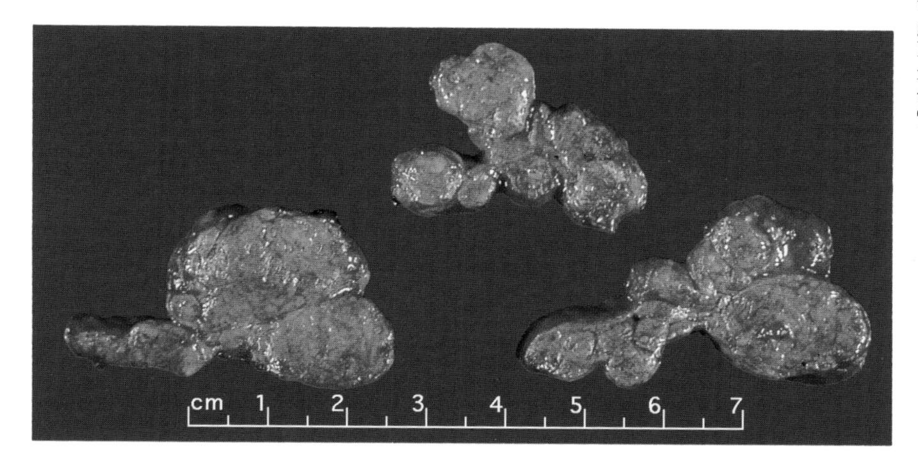

Figure 3-24
MACRONODULAR ADRENAL CORTICAL HYPERPLASIA WITH MARKED ADRENAL ENLARGEMENT

Top, bottom: Transverse sections of both adrenal glands show marked thickening and nodularity of the golden-yellow cortex. The nodules have ill-defined borders. Medulla is not evident in these transverse sections. (Courtesy of Dr. William D. Travis, Bethesda, MD.)

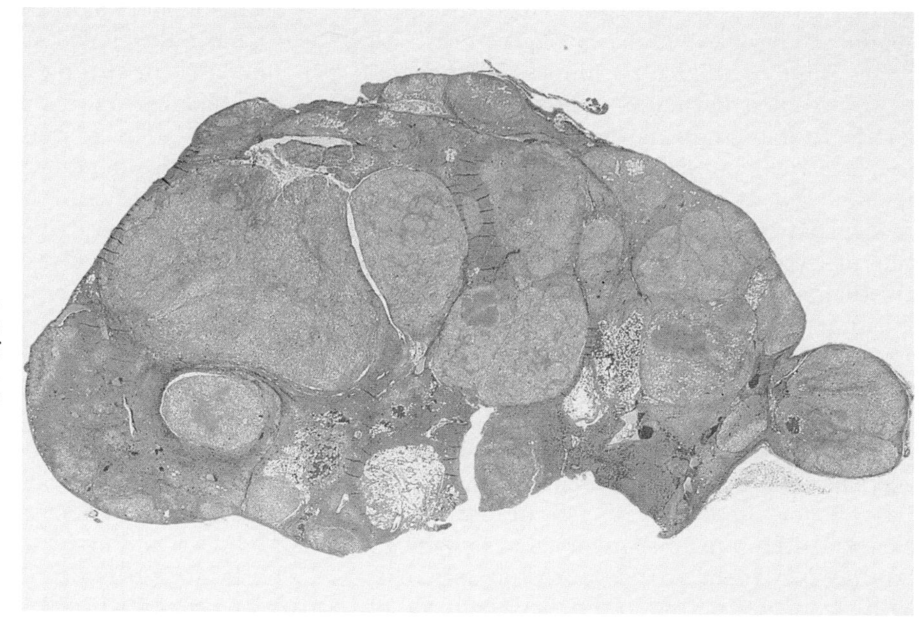

Figure 3-25
MACRONODULAR HYPERPLASIA WITH MARKED ADRENAL ENLARGEMENT

The gland is greatly distorted by large cortical nodules composed predominantly of pale-staining, lipid-rich cells. Some hyperplastic cortical cells extended into periadrenal fat.

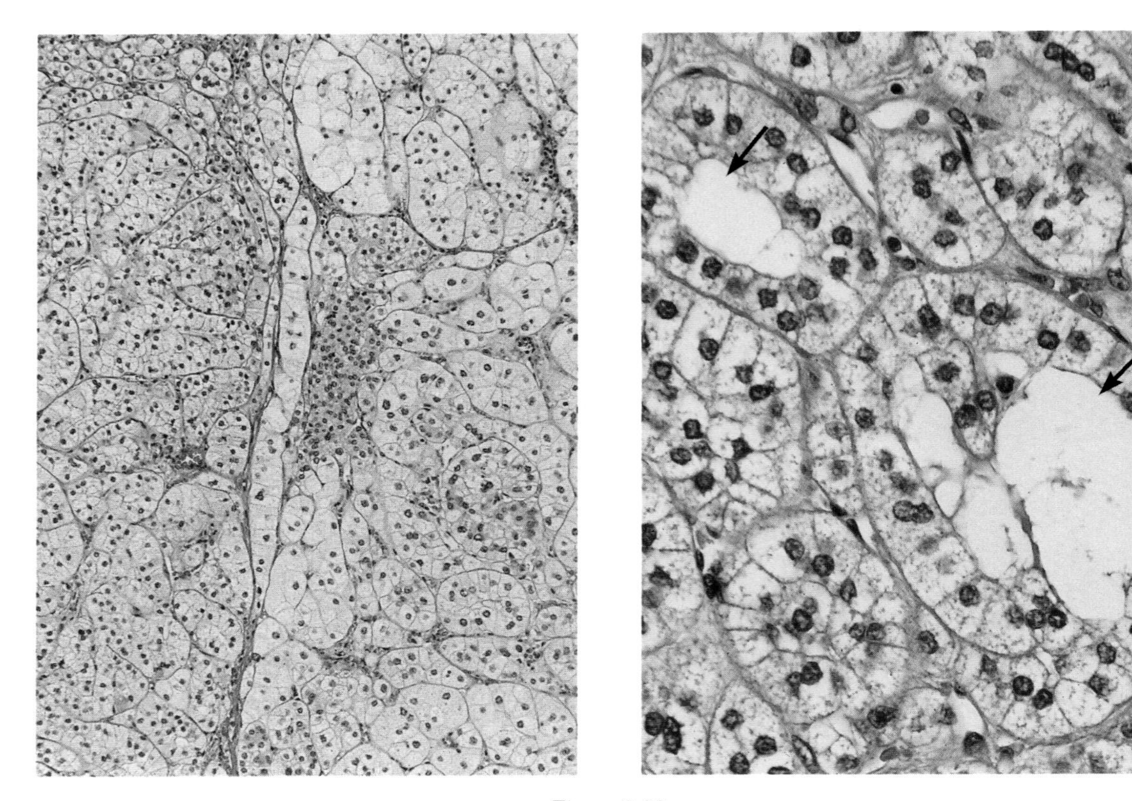

Figure 3-26
MACRONODULAR HYPERPLASIA WITH MARKED ADRENAL ENLARGEMENT

Left: Cells have prominent pale-staining cytoplasm which is finely vacuolated due to abundant lipid. Some cells have a "ballooned" appearance.

Right: Most hyperplastic cortical cells resemble those of the zona fasciculata. Note several pseudoglandular spaces (arrows).

lightly basophilic material, but staining for mucin or glycogen has been negative (fig. 3-26, right). It may be difficult or impossible to identify an intervening normal or diffusely hyperplastic cortex. In one study the non-nodular cortex appeared atrophic in some areas, consistent with a disorder that is ACTH-independent (77). Irregular capsular extensions of cortical cells are common in sections from the periphery of the hyperplastic gland (fig. 3-27, left), and circumscribed capsular extrusions may appear more prominent than usual. Occasionally, there may be lipomatous or myelolipomatous foci, with rare bony metaplasia (fig. 3-27, right). The author has seen one case in which there was focal ischemic necrosis with dystrophic calcification. Weak reactivity for 3-beta-hydroxysteroid dehydrogenase and other enzymes involved in steroidogenesis has been reported in MHMAE in comparison with stronger staining in the usual adrenal cortical adenoma. Ultrastructural study has shown a poorly developed smooth endoplasmic reticulum (77). In situ hybridization of P-450c17 has also been used to localize the site of steroidogenesis (86). These studies suggest that effective corticosteroidogenesis by individual cortical cells is limited, and that a significant increase in cell number (i.e., hyperplasia) is necessary before excess cortisol production occurs, with resultant Cushing's syndrome. By contrast, cortical cells within nodules of primary pigmented nodular adrenocortical disease (PPNAD) have been shown to have intense activity for steroidogenic enzymes (78,85); the nodules consist largely of cells with compact, eosinophilic cytoplasm and have a significantly developed smooth endoplasmic reticulum. A possible relationship between MHMAE and MNH of Cushing's disease cannot be established with certainty in most cases reported to date (fig. 3-28).

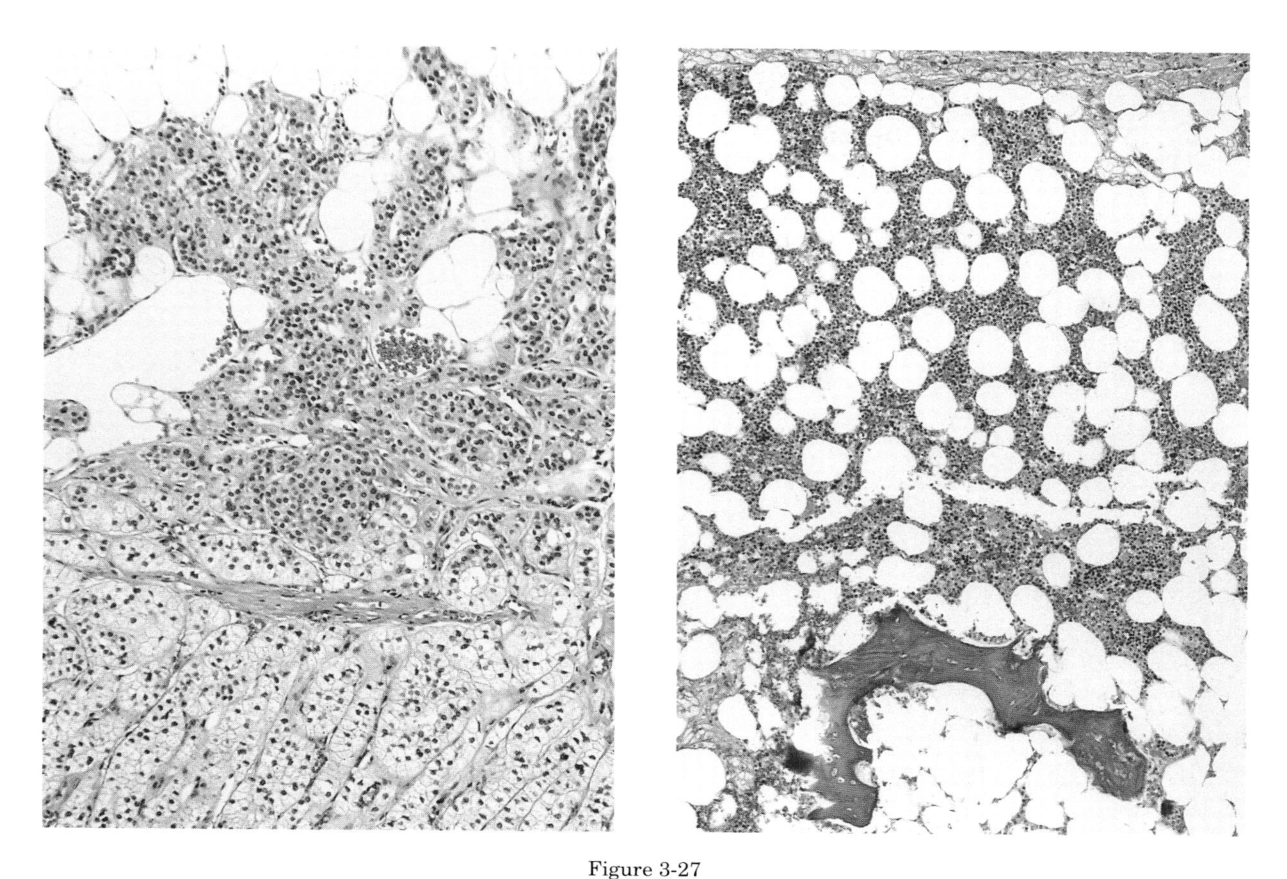

Figure 3-27
MACRONODULAR HYPERPLASIA WITH MARKED ADRENAL ENLARGEMENT
Left: Hyperplastic cortical cells stream out into periadrenal adipose tissue. Some cells have compact, lipid-depleted cytoplasm. Right: Myelolipomatous metaplasia with bone formation.

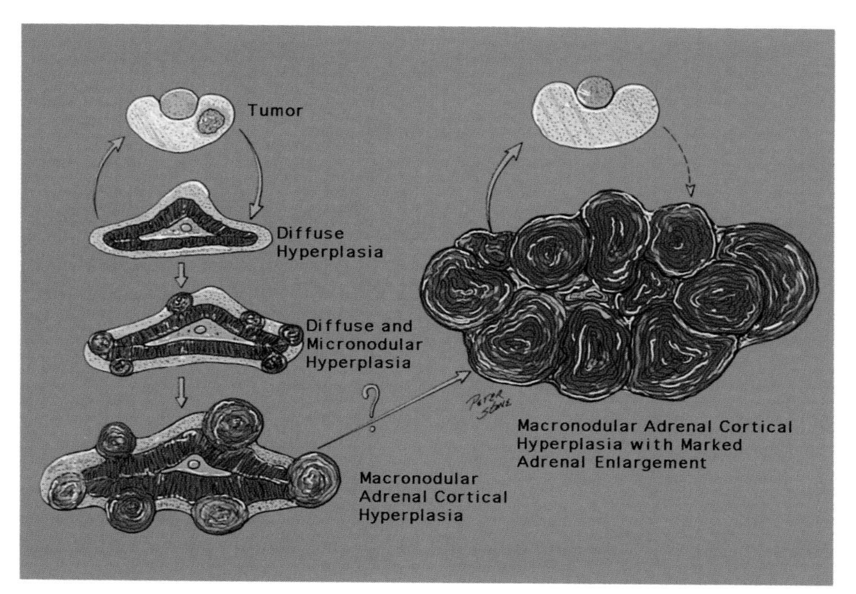

Figure 3-28
MACRONODULAR HYPERPLASIA WITH MARKED ADRENAL ENLARGEMENT

Sensitive endocrinologic testing and imaging studies indicate a rare primary form of ACTH-independent Cushing's syndrome. Some have wondered whether macronodular hyperplasia in Cushing's disease (left) can progress to bilateral autonomous Cushing's syndrome (right).

Table 3-6

CLINICAL FEATURES OF PRIMARY PIGMENTED NODULAR ADRENOCORTICAL DISEASE (PPNAD)*

Slight female predominance: 60%

Young age at diagnosis: average, 18 years; range, 4 to 32 years

Signs or symptoms of hypercortisolism: 82%; overt PPNAD

Associated conditions as main manifestation: 18%; subclinical or latent PPNAD

Average duration of hypercortisolism: 4.3 years (range, 0.3 to 18 years)

Osteoporosis, often severe: 39%

Cyclic hypersecretion of glucocorticoids: 4%

Treatment of choice: bilateral adrenalectomy; 35% of patients with unilateral or subtotal adrenalectomy required completion of total adrenalectomy

Spontaneous regression of Cushing's syndrome: rare

50% of cases familial and associated with unusual conditions

*Data from reference 90.

Table 3-7

SIGNS AND SYMPTOMS OF CUSHING'S SYNDROME IN 72 PATIENTS WITH PRIMARY PIGMENTED NODULAR ADRENOCORTICAL DISEASE*

Sign or Symptom	Frequency (%)
Central obesity	62
Weight gain	61
Hirsutism	44
Hypertension	42
Osteoporosis	39
Abdominal striae	35
Menstrual cycle changes	33
Short stature	29
Muscular weakness	24
Acne	23
Easy bruising	20
Back pain	11
Depression	11
Precocious puberty	9
Renal lithiasis	9
Hypokalemia	8

*Data from reference 90.

Treatment. Bilateral adrenalectomy is the treatment of choice for this rare form of primary (autonomous) Cushing's syndrome.

Primary Pigmented Nodular Adrenocortical Disease (PPNAD)

Definition. Primary pigmented nodular adrenocortical disease (PPNAD) is a descriptive term for a distinctive but rare form of ACTH- or pituitary-independent Cushing's syndrome; there is bilateral nodular (usually micronodular) hyperplasia with a variable degree of pigmentation within the nodules due to accumulation of lipofuscin (see fig. 3-15, right) (95,98). The adrenal glands in this disorder may be small, normal in size, or mildly enlarged.

Clinical and Endocrinologic Features. This disorder has been referred to by a wide variety of terms which reflect an incomplete understanding of etiology and pathogenesis. PPNAD typical affects young individuals, with a predilection for females, and the associated Cushing's syndrome may be severe (Tables 3-6, 3-7) (96). This disorder can be overt, subclinical, or latent with no clinical or laboratory evidence of Cushing's syndrome; cyclic or intermittent hypersecretion of glucocorticoids can occur (90). Endocrinologic studies, including dynamic testing, indicate a primary adrenal source for the hypercortisolism (Table 3-8). Sensitive imaging of the sella and pituitary fossa shows no abnormalities, and selective venous sampling of the inferior petrosal sinus has not indicated a pituitary source of ACTH. Some patients have undergone unsuccessful pituitary ablation because the correct nature of the condition was not recognized. In several reports the adrenal glands in PPNAD have been described as normal on CT scan, but unilateral or bilateral nodularity has also been reported, and in older patients macronodules (larger than 1 cm) have been detected (92).

Table 3-8

ENDOCRINOLOGIC FEATURES IN PRIMARY PIGMENTED NODULAR ADRENOCORTICAL DISEASE (PPNAD)*

Autonomous Hypersecretion of Glucocorticoids	
Plasma ACTH	Low or undetectable, 92% Normal, 8%
Plasma cortisol	High, 94% Normal, 6%
24-hour urine levels	
Cortisol	High, 95% Normal, 5%
17-OHCS/KGS**	High, 97% Normal, 3%
17-Ketosteroids	High, 49% Normal, 46% Low or undetectable, 5%
Results of Dynamic Testing	
Lack of dexamethasone suppression, low and high dose	
Occasional paradoxical increase in glucocorticoids with high-dose dexamethasone	
Failure of stimulation of glucocorticoid secretion with metyrapone	
Uptake of [6β^{131}I] Iodomethyl-19-Norcholesterol on Adrenal Scintigraphy	

*Data from reference 90.
**OHCS: hydroxycorticosteroids, KGS: ketogenic steroids.

Gross Findings. In a recent review, the weight of individual adrenal glands varied from 0.9 to 13.4 g (average, 4 g), with an average combined weight of 9.6 g (range, 4.3 to 17.0 g); the glands were usually normal in size (90). Gross examination of the external surface of the intact gland may reveal scattered pigmented nodules, usually 1 to 3 mm in size, beneath the capsule or bulging into periadrenal connective tissue (fig. 3-29). The "lumpy bumpy" contour of some glands may interfere with complete removal of adherent fat and connective tissue, which makes some recorded weights artificially high. In transverse sections, there may be a spectacular array of small pigmented nodules studding the cortex, ranging from light gray, gray-brown, dark brown, to jet black (figs. 3-30, 3-31). A few nodules may be yellow. Some glands contain pigmented or nonpigmented macronodules measuring 1.8 to 3 cm in diameter; in some cases these result from a confluence of smaller micronodules. The term micronodular is entirely arbitrary since many of the intensely pigmented nodules can be detected on gross examination even when they are smaller than 1 mm.

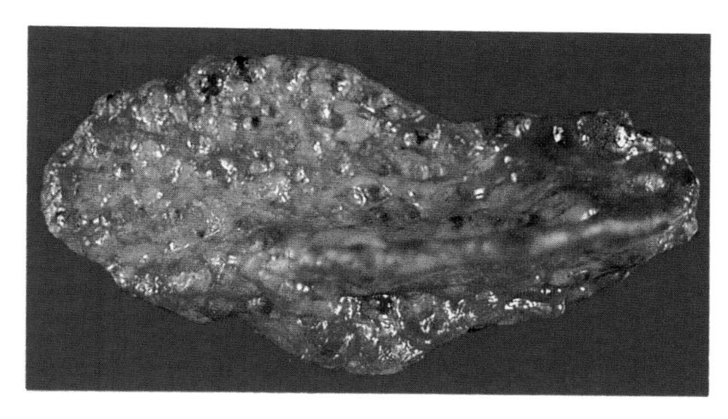

Figure 3-29
PRIMARY PIGMENTED NODULAR ADRENOCORTICAL DISEASE (PPNAD)
Numerous jet black nodules are visible through the capsule on the dorsal surface of the intact gland. Both adrenal glands were small in size and weight, and the internodular cortex showed marked atrophy. (Courtesy of Dr. William D. Travis, Bethesda, MD.)

Microscopic Findings. The conspicuous nature of PPNAD on gross examination may be less obvious once the gland is evaluated histologically (fig. 3-32). The pigmented nodules are round to oval or have an irregular contour; some may have a silhouette which is reminiscent of an "hourglass," "string of beads," or "links of sausage." The nodules are unencapsulated, and are often deep within the cortex centered on the zona reticularis or straddle the corticomedullary junction with expansile borders (fig. 3-33). Some nodules occupy nearly the entire thickness of cortex, and occasionally there is extension into periadrenal fat without any encapsulation (fig. 3-34). Occasionally, there is intraluminal projection of a nodule into tributaries of the central adrenal vein in association with discontinuities in bundles of smooth muscle (fig. 3-35).

Most cells within the nodules have lipid-depleted, compact, eosinophilic cytoplasm, although there may be an admixture of cells with more lipid-rich, vacuolated cytoplasm. Cellular enzymes, which are markers for steroidogenesis, are intensely active in almost all of the cells,

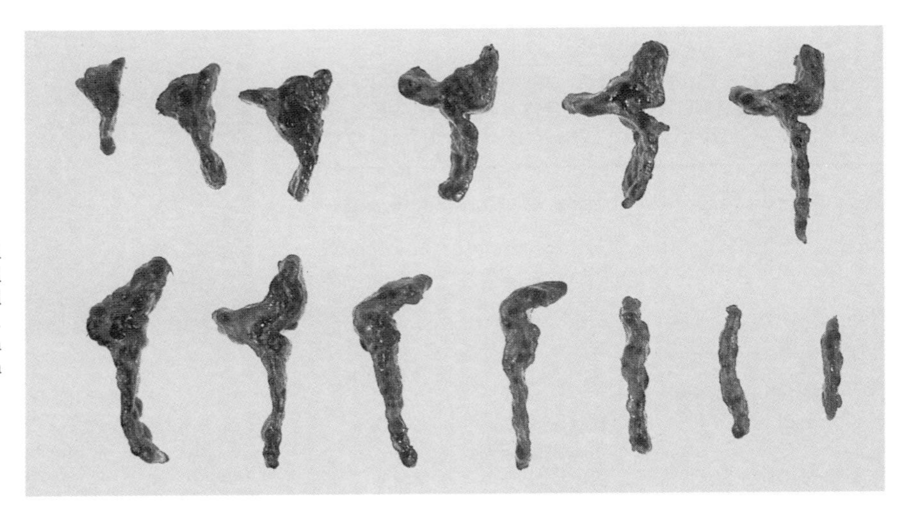

Figure 3-30
PRIMARY PIGMENTED NODULAR ADRENOCORTICAL DISEASE (PPNAD)

Transverse sections of adrenal gland are studded by pigmented micronodules. Many are located along the inner aspect of cortex. Note atrophy of cortex between nodules. (Courtesy of Dr. William D. Travis, Bethesda, MD.)

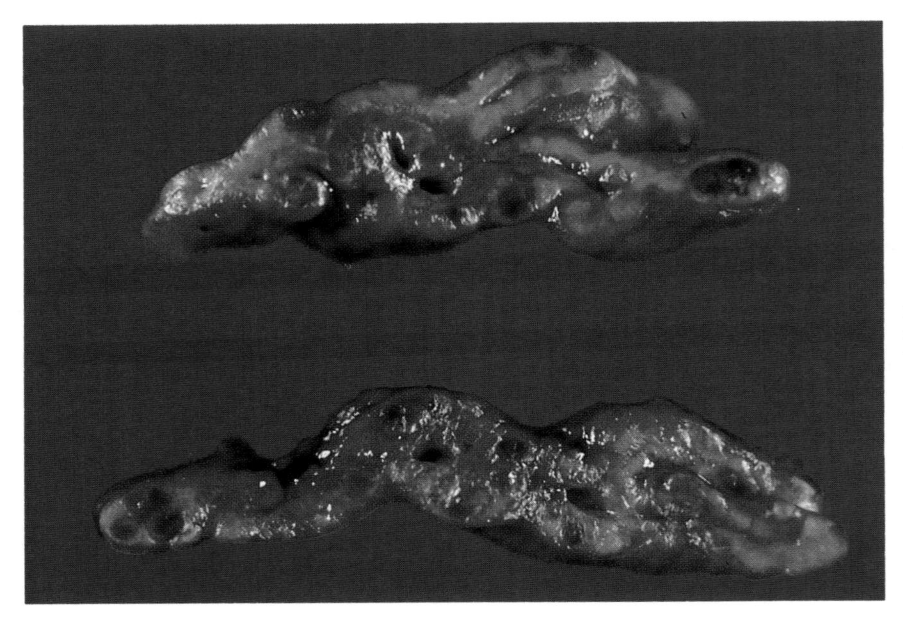

Figure 3-31
PRIMARY PIGMENTED NODULAR ADRENOCORTICAL DISEASE (PPNAD)

There is no atrophy of internodular cortex and pigmented nodules are not as jet black. (Courtesy of Dr. William D. Travis, Bethesda, MD.)

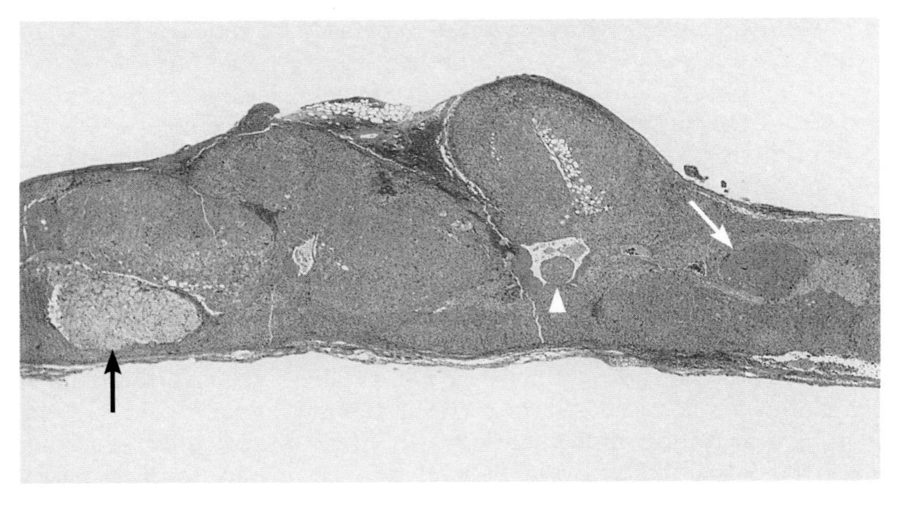

Figure 3-32
PRIMARY PIGMENTED NODULAR ADRENOCORTICAL DISEASE (PPNAD)

Transverse section through body of gland. Micronodules are less well-defined compared with the gross appearance. Some nodules straddle the corticomedullary junction and impinge on chromaffin cells (white arrow). Note the nodule composed of lipid-rich cells (black arrow) and the small hyperplastic nodule protruding into the vascular lumen between discontinuous bundles of smooth muscle (white arrowhead).

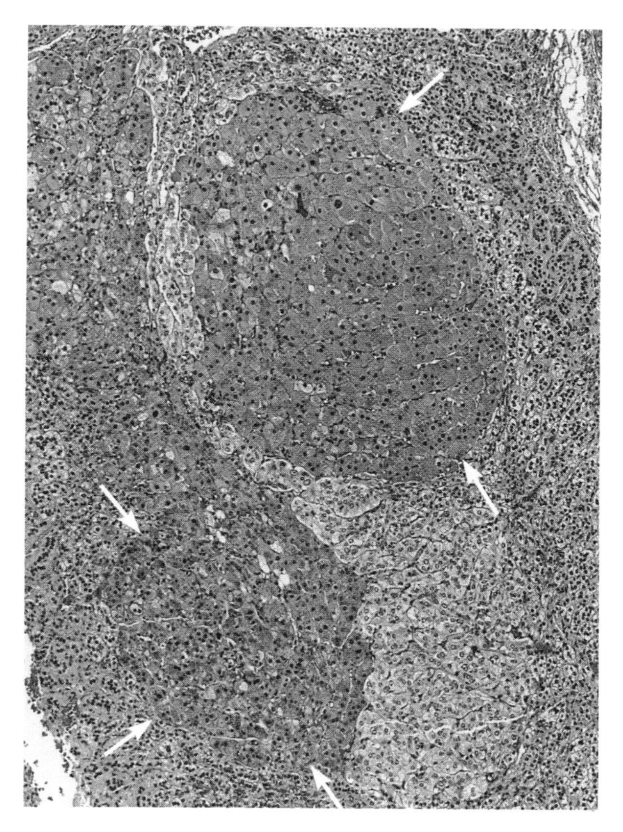

Figure 3-33
PRIMARY PIGMENTED NODULAR ADRENOCORTICAL DISEASE (PPNAD)

Micronodules (arrows) are present at the corticomedullary junction on either side of the medulla. The nodules contain cells with compact, eosinophilic cytoplasm and focally prominent pigment.

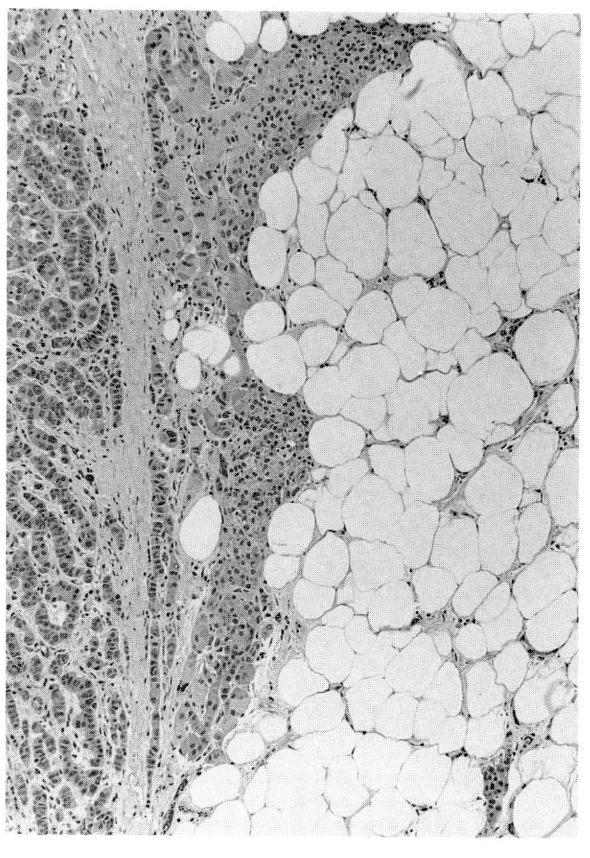

Figure 3-34
PRIMARY PIGMENTED NODULAR ADRENOCORTICAL DISEASE (PPNAD)

Cortical cells with compact and variably pigmented cytoplasm extend in irregular fashion into periadrenal adipose tissue.

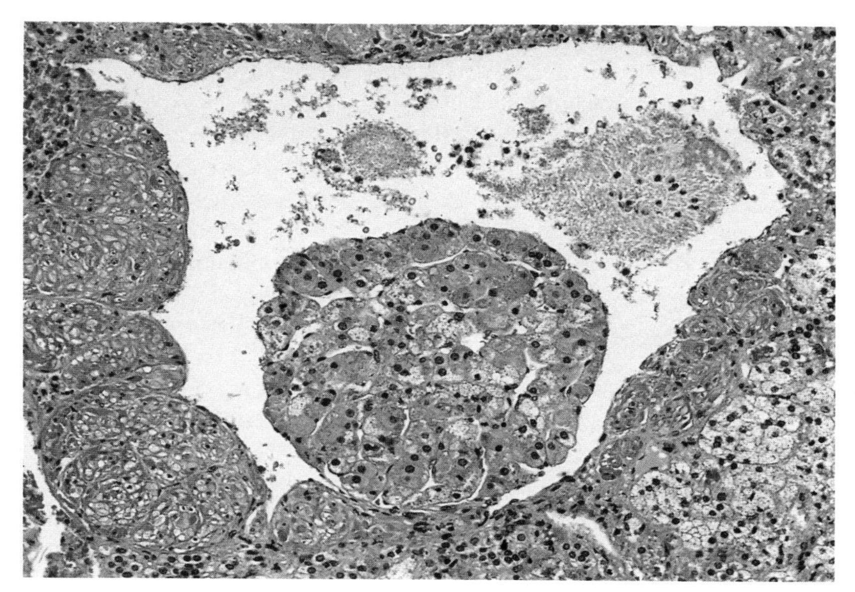

Figure 3-35
PRIMARY PIGMENTED NODULAR ADRENOCORTICAL DISEASE (PPNAD)

A hyperplastic micronodule extends into the tributary of the central adrenal vein. There is a deficiency of smooth muscle in the vessel wall and intact endothelium over the surface of the micronodule projecting into the lumen.

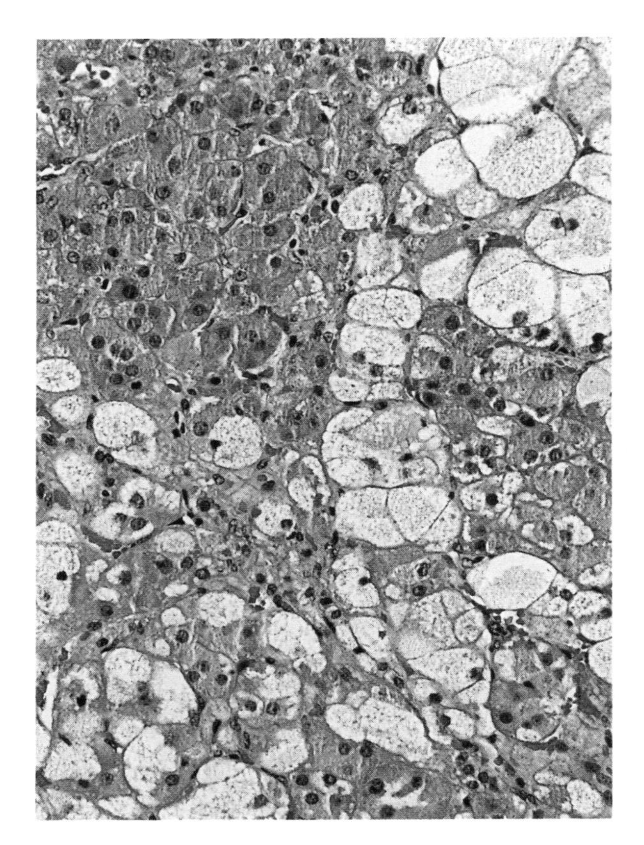

Figure 3-36
PRIMARY PIGMENTED NODULAR ADRENOCORTICAL DISEASE (PPNAD)
This nodule is composed of cells with vacuolated, lipid-rich cytoplasm along with compact, lipid-depleted cells, both of which contain a variable amount of finely granular pigment representing lipofuscin. There is a mild degree of nuclear pleomorphism.

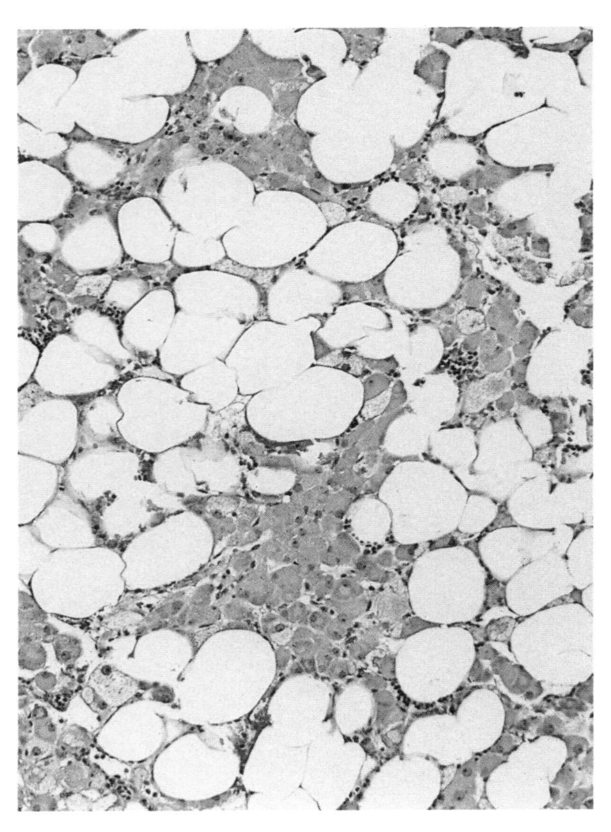

Figure 3-37
PRIMARY PIGMENTED NODULAR ADRENOCORTICAL DISEASE (PPNAD)
This nodule has prominent lipomatous metaplasia with a small component of lymphocytes. Myeloid metaplasia can also be found in some cases.

especially those with abundant eosinophilic cytoplasm (88,97); this enzymatic profile may explain the paradox that adrenal glands that are normal in size or small can cause Cushing's syndrome (88). In one study there was strong reactivity of enzymes in cells located in the zona reticularis, but not elsewhere in the adjacent internodular cortex, suggesting an abnormality of the zona reticularis in the pathogenesis of PPNAD (97). Some nodules contain abundant lipid-rich cells which may show some "ballooning" (fig. 3-36). Occasionally, there is a lipomatous (fig. 3-37) or even myelolipomatous component which represents a metaplastic phenomenon. This is often apparent in adrenal cortical lesions (hyperplastic and neoplastic) characterized by hyperfunction. Sparse lymphocytic infiltrates have occasionally been noted, mainly around vessels but also within the nodules (99,100). These cells have been characterized as suppressor cytotoxic T cells or T-helper cells (100).

Cytologically, the cell features are uniform, although occasionally, cells are binucleated or multinucleated, or have enlarged hyperchromatic nuclei with prominent nucleoli (99). Mitotic figures are rare. The intracytoplasmic pigment has the staining reaction (fig. 3-38) and ultrastructural morphology of lipofuscin. Occasionally, treatment of sections with $KMN0_4$ abolishes this reaction, which suggests a neuromelanin component (95).

Etiology and Pathogenesis. The etiology and pathogenesis of PPNAD are unknown, but the following have been proposed: 1) hamartomatous malformation or dysplasia of the adrenal cortex, a view supported in part by the varying amount of mature fat cells within the nodules

(89); 2) a primary abnormality of the zona reticularis (97); 3) an occult ACTH-secreting pituitary tumor with cortical nodules that become functionally autonomous; 4) an embryonic developmental error in the adrenal cortex at the adrenarche (90); 5) a block in the evolution of zona fasciculata–type cells to cells of the zona reticularis, with accumulation of cells at the interface, and formation of hyperfunctioning nodules that eventually become autonomous or ACTH-independent (90); and 6) a form of autoimmune hypercortisolism (Table 3-9). The last theory is based upon reports of a circulating adrenal-stimulating immunoglobulin (ASI) which has a stimulatory effect on segments of guinea pig adrenal gland in vitro as indicated by quantitation of nuclear DNA (100–103). These observations support the hypothesis that PPNAD may represent an organ-specific autoimmune form of Cushing's syndrome (93) with the ASI directed against the ACTH receptor or domains of this receptor (102). Atrophy of the internodular cortex may be due to heterogeneous responsiveness of cortical cells to autoimmune stimulation or some paracrine effect (103). Further investigation is needed to determine whether PPNAD is truly an autoimmune disorder or one in which the circulating ASI is merely an epiphenomenon. Kindreds have been reported with circulating ASI, yet there is no clinical or biochemical evidence of hypercortisolism (103); an analogous situation may exist with patients who have circulating thyroid-stimulating antibodies, but are euthyroid on clinical evaluation and laboratory testing.

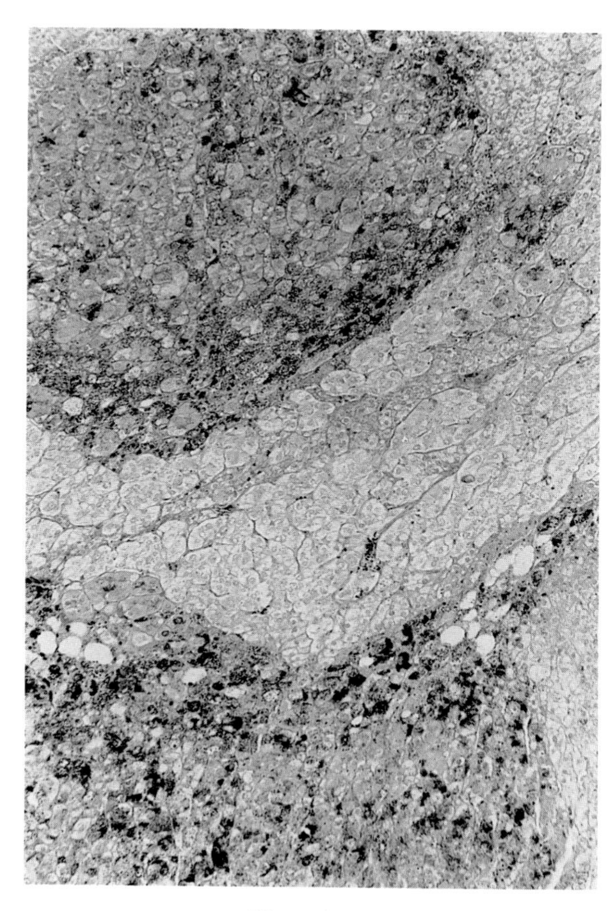

Figure 3-38
PRIMARY PIGMENTED NODULAR ADRENOCORTICAL DISEASE (PPNAD)
Many of the cells of the micronodules are strongly argentaffin positive. (X250, Fontana-Masson stain)

Table 3-9

VARIOUS THEORIES FOR THE ETIOLOGY AND PATHOGENESIS OF PRIMARY PIGMENTED NODULAR ADRENOCORTICAL DISEASE

Hamartomatous malformation or dysplasia of adrenal cortex
Primary abnormality of zona reticularis
Occult ACTH-producing pituitary adenoma with adrenal cortical nodules becoming functionally autonomous
Embryonic developmental error in adrenal cortex at the adrenarche
Block in evolution of zona fasciculata–type cells into cells of zona reticularis with accumulation of autonomous cells at interface
Organ-specific form of autoimmune hypercortisolism (Cushing's syndrome)

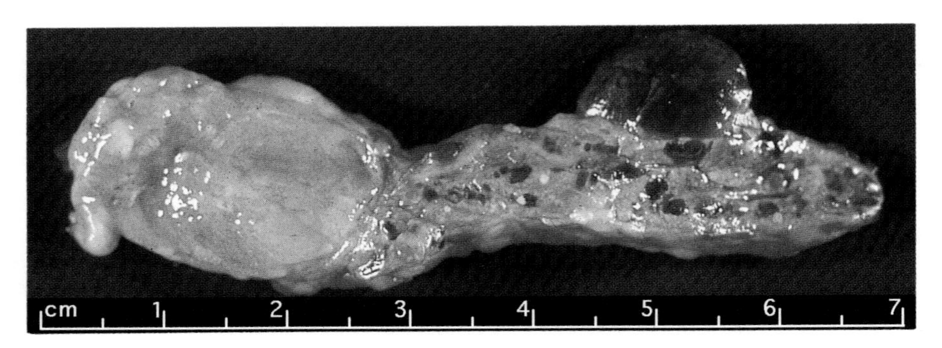

Figure 3-39

PRIMARY PIGMENTED NODULAR ADRENOCORTICAL DISEASE (PPNAD)

The adrenal gland from a young female with PPNAD. Note the large pigmented macronodule. A larger pale yellow nodule had small areas of necrosis as well as occasional mitotic figures. The patient was part of a family pedigree with the complex of myxomas, spotty pigmentation, and endocrine overactivity (Carney's complex). There was a complex history of a retrogastric melanotic schwannoma, fibrolamellar hepatoma, hyperpigmentation of the inner canthus of both eyes, and most recently an ovarian serous cystadenoma. She developed multiple pulmonary nodules which histologically were consistent with adrenal cortical origin (? metastases), but paradoxically has been in good health for the last several years. (Courtesy of Dr. William D. Travis, Bethesda, MD.)

Table 3-10

COMPLEX OF MYXOMAS, SPOTTY PIGMENTATION, AND ENDOCRINE OVERACTIVITY*
(n=40: 16 males, 24 females)

Cardiac myxoma: 72% (n=29)
  Average age, 24.4 years
  Multiple myxomas: 45%

Cutaneous abnormalities: 80% (n=32)
  Pigmented lesions: 44% (n=14); lentigines, ephelides, blue nevi
  Cutaneous myxoma: 19% (n=6)
  Pigmented lesions and cutaneous myxoma: 38% (n=12)

Primary pigmented nodular adrenocortical disease (PPNAD): 45% (n=18)

Testicular tumors: 56% of males (n=9); frequently bilateral, multicentric
  Large cell calcifying Sertoli cell tumor
  Leydig cell tumor
  Adrenal cortical rest tumor

Mammary myxoid fibroadenoma: 42% of females; gynecomastia in 2 males

Pituitary macroadenoma: 10% (n=4)
  Gigantism: 2 patients
  Acromegaly: 2 patients

Uterine myxoma: 8% of females (n=2)

Oral cavity myxoma: 8% of patients (n=3)

Psammomatous melanotic schwannoma: 5% (n=2)**

*Data from reference 90
**Originally classified as a calcifying pigmented neuroectodermal tumor.

Treatment. Bilateral adrenalectomy is the treatment of choice for PPNAD (94), although some cases may permit less than total resection (90). The surgeon must be prepared to remove both adrenal glands, which may appear normal or even small in size. About one third of the patients initially treated by unilateral or subtotal adrenalectomy required consequent total adrenalectomy due to persistence or recurrence of signs or symptoms of Cushing's syndrome (90). Nelson's syndrome has not been reported following bilateral adrenalectomy in patients with PPNAD. Rarely, Cushing's syndrome has been reported to regress spontaneously although dynamic endocrine testing showed persistent autonomous adrenal cortical function (103). It is of interest that one of the patients originally described by Cushing in 1932 (Minnie G) experienced gradual resolution of Cushing's syndrome (91).

THE COMPLEX OF MYXOMAS, SPOTTY PIGMENTATION, AND ENDOCRINE OVERACTIVITY

This is a complex array of diverse abnormalities which is reported to have a Mendelian autosomal dominant mode of inheritance (108). In a recent review of PPNAD, about half of the cases occurred in a nonfamilial or sporadic setting, while the rest were familial (fig. 3-39), and often associated with unusual conditions (Table 3-10) (106,107,109). Some examples of this complex have been published with acronyms such as the

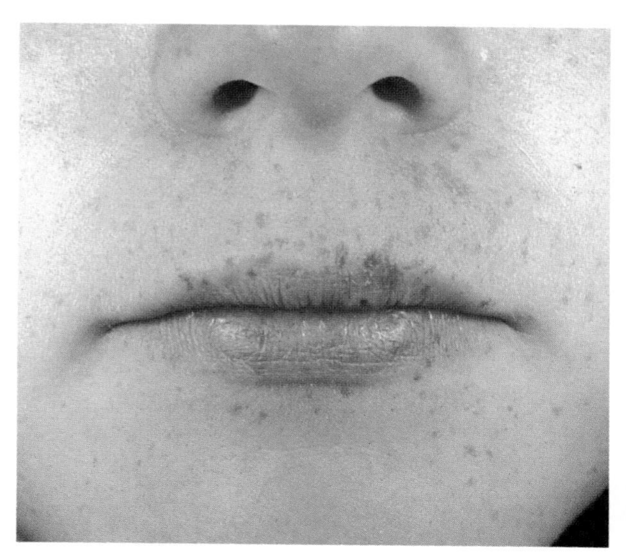

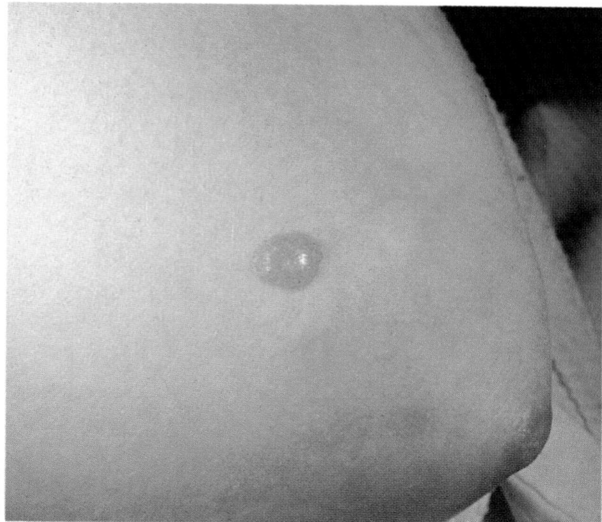

Figure 3-40
COMPLEX OF MYXOMA AND SPOTTY PIGMENTATION

Left: Young girl with multiple pigmented lesions about the mouth. The patient also had a darkly pigmented lesion on the vulva, probably a blue nevus.

Right: Cutaneous myxoma on the breast of the same patient who also had a cardiac myxoma. There was no evidence of adrenal abnormality and no Cushing's syndrome. (Courtesy of Dr. Arthur Rhodes, Pittsburgh, PA.)

LAMB syndrome (lentigines, atrial myxoma, mucocutaneous myxomas, blue nevi) (111) and the *NAME syndrome* (nevi, atrial myxoma, myxoid neurofibroma, ephelides) (104). Hedinger (110) suggested that the entity be referred as the Swiss syndrome, but the detailed collation of cases by Carney has led to the designation *Carney's complex* (105), which has been adopted by others (109).

If patients are identified with two or more elements of this complex, particularly PPNAD, bilateral large cell calcifying Sertoli cell tumors of testis, or mucocutaneous pigmentation of the type described by Carney et al. (fig. 3-40) (107), investigation for possible cardiac myxoma is recommended to permit early detection and treatment (107,109). The cardiac tumors present at a relatively early age (average, 24 years) and are frequently multiple (107).

ECTOPIC ACTH SYNDROME WITH HYPERCORTISOLISM

About 15 percent of Cushing's syndrome in adults is due to ectopic production of ACTH (123, 124,128); the source is usually a neoplasm, but there have been isolated reports of unusual non-neoplastic conditions associated with the syndrome (119,120,122). Some have pointed out that virtually all normal tissues produce small amounts of a biologically inactive precursor of the ACTH molecule, probably pro-opiomelanocortin (POMC). Cancers produce this same substance in increased quantities, although only a select number convert POMC into biologically active ACTH to produce the "ectopic" ACTH syndrome; in this context ectopic ACTH production is not necessarily ectopic (127). It may be possible to detect mRNA expression of POMC with molecular probes such as in situ hybridization. Since pituitary microsurgery is the treatment of choice for Cushing's disease, correct identification of the source of ACTH secretion becomes essential, and unfortunately, failure to recognize it may occasionally result in unnecessary pituitary surgery. Cushing was correct in assuming that secretions from pituitary basophilic adenomas were responsible for the pluriglandular syndrome, but two of his original nine patients who were autopsied had no evidence of a pituitary lesion (116,121).

The neoplastic sources of ectopic ACTH production include bronchial carcinoid tumor, pulmonary and extrapulmonary small cell carcinoma

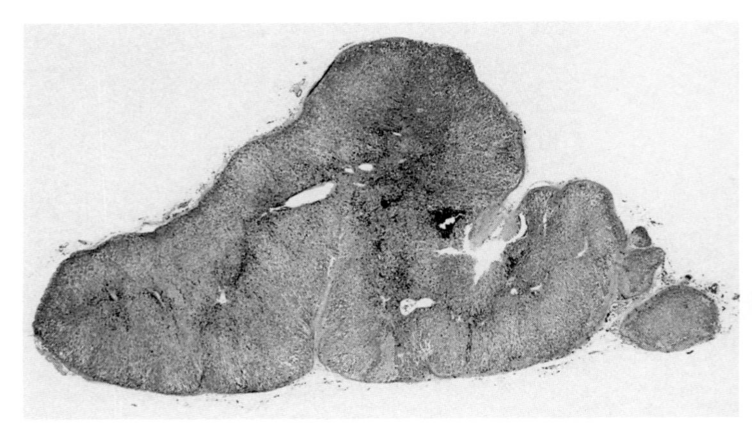

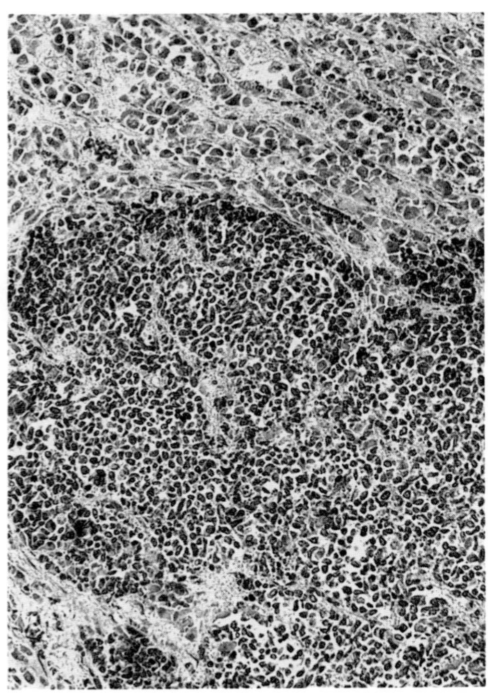

Figure 3-41
ECTOPIC ACTH SYNDROME

Above: Adrenal gland at autopsy of an elderly man who had disseminated small (oat) cell carcinoma of lung. There was no clinical evidence of Cushing's syndrome, but both adrenal glands were markedly enlarged, weighing about 20 g each. The cortex is diffusely hyperplastic with suggestion of vague nodularity in some areas.

Right: Same case as above, showing area of hyperplastic adrenal gland with metastatic small cell carcinoma from lung.

(fig. 3-41), pancreatic islet cell carcinoma (fig. 3-42), medullary thyroid carcinoma, thymic carcinoid, pheochromocytoma (fig. 3-43), and a variety of other tumors (118,125). There are also cases of ectopic CRF production (113,114) which may be accompanied by ectopic ACTH secretion as well (129,130). In some instances the ectopic ACTH production is clinically and biochemically indistinguishable from pituitary-dependent Cushing's disease (126); in the ectopic ACTH syndrome, however, ACTH levels are usually quite elevated (127), sometimes over 250 pg/ml (126), whereas in Cushing's disease ACTH levels are often "normal" (upper range of normal) or only slightly elevated (127), and rarely over 200 pg/ml (123). Occasionally, ovarian neoplasms of various type are associated with Cushing's syndrome (115). A remarkable case of severe Cushing's syndrome has been reported due to a corticotroph cell pituitary adenoma arising in a benign cystic teratoma of the ovary (112).

The clinical features of Cushing's syndrome may be absent in patients with aggressive neoplasms such as bronchogenic small cell carcinoma, and instead the clinical picture may be dominated by cachexia or electrolyte disturbances with hypokalemia and metabolic acidosis (125). Other neoplasms, such as bronchial carcinoid tumor, may be associated with florid Cushing's syndrome, while the primary tumor remains indolent and occult, sometimes for several years. The "occult" ectopic ACTH syndrome has been defined as ACTH-dependent hypercortisolism of greater than 6 months' duration without emergence of an obvious cause or source (117).

The adrenal glands are symmetrically enlarged with rounded contours, and usually weigh 10 to 15 g each (fig. 3-44); sometimes the individual weight may exceed 20 g and rarely 30 g (125). Under conditions of rather intense and constant stimulation by ACTH, there is diffuse hyperplasia, sometimes accompanied by vague nodularity. On transverse sections, the glands are usually tan to brown due to conversion of pale-staining, lipid-rich cells to cortical cells with compact, eosinophilic cytoplasm (fig. 3-45, left). The cortex is often 0.3 to 0.4 cm thick, but may be even wider. The hyperplastic cortex may thus resemble a greatly expanded zona reticularis. Some cortical cells may be hypertrophied, with abundant eosinophilic cytoplasm and moderately enlarged nuclei (fig. 3-45, right), an appearance similar to the enlarged

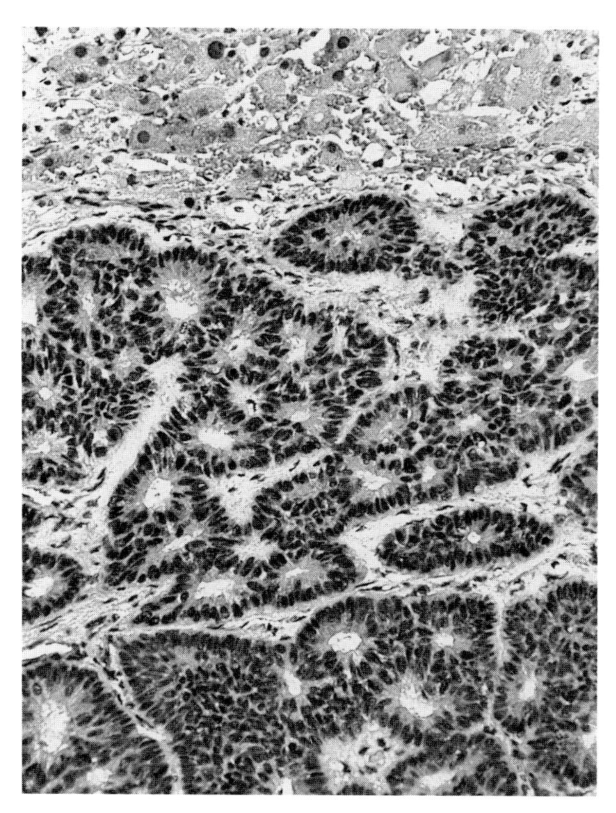

Figure 3-42
ECTOPIC ACTH SYNDROME

Ectopic ACTH syndrome in a patient with islet cell carcinoma, which here has metastasized to hyperplastic adrenal gland. Hyperplastic cortical cells are evident at top of field.

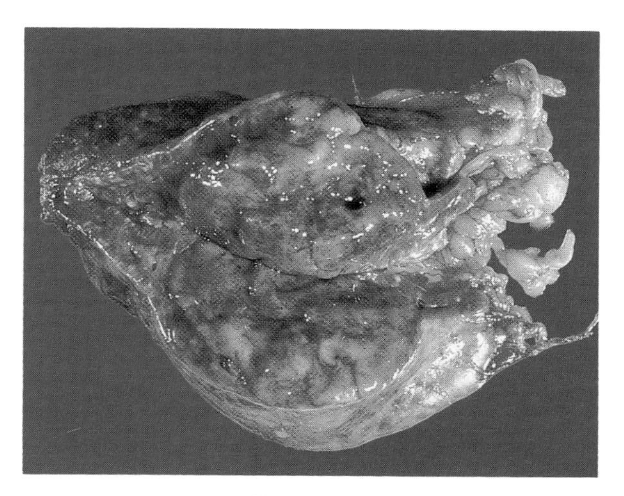

Figure 3-43
ECTOPIC ACTH SYNDROME
DUE TO PHEOCHROMOCYTOMA

A 51-year-old white female presented with hypertension, facial swelling, and hirsutism. There were elevated steroid metabolites in the urine which could not be suppressed with high-dose dexamethasone. Skull X rays showed no abnormalities of the sella. Following surgical removal of a 3-cm pheochromocytoma hirsutism regressed and steroid levels normalized. Surgery was complicated by hypotensive episode(s). The hyperplastic adrenal cortex was largely lipid depleted. Biopsy of opposite hyperplastic adrenal gland was identical.

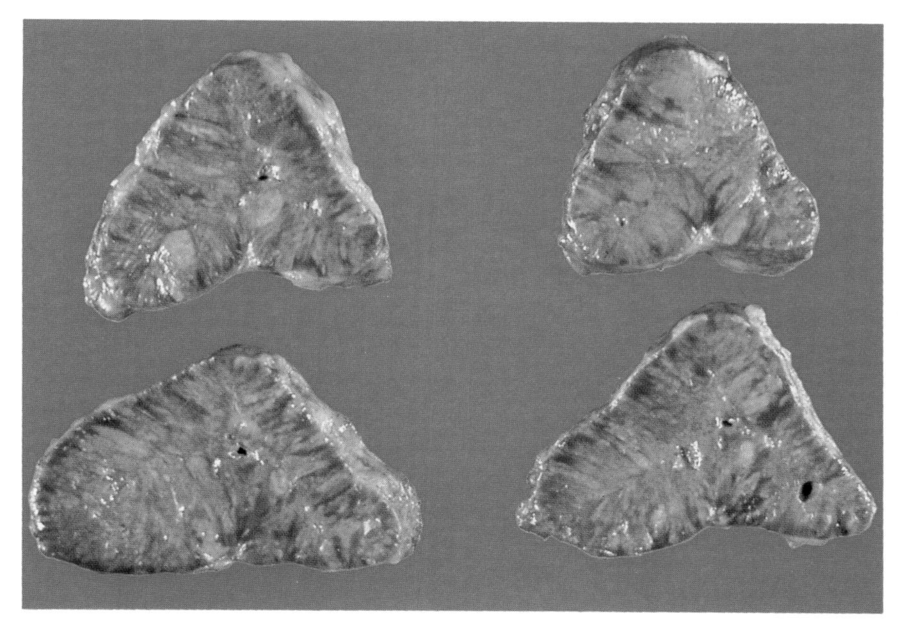

Figure 3-44
ECTOPIC ACTH SYNDROME

Transverse sections of adrenal glands surgically resected from a patient with ectopic ACTH syndrome due to a bronchial carcinoid tumor. The tumor had remained occult for several years. The right adrenal gland weighed 12 g and the left 11 g. The dark appearance is due to intense stimulation by ACTH. Vague nodularity is seen in some areas. (Courtesy of Dr. William D. Travis, Bethesda, MD.)

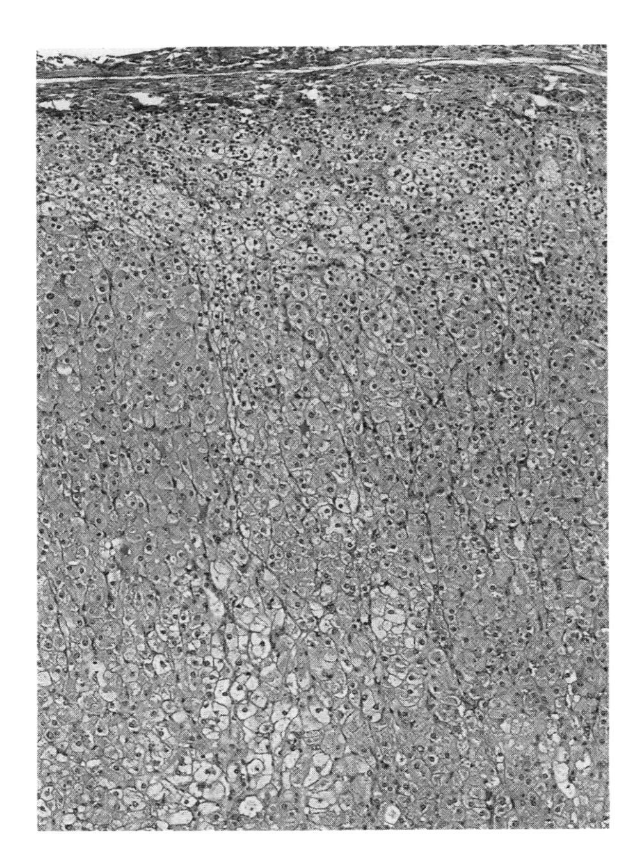

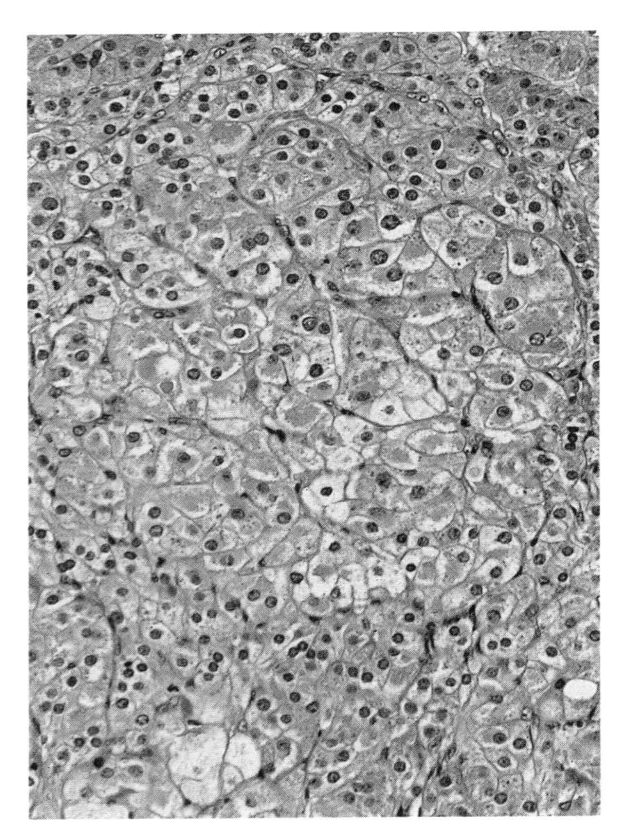

Figure 3-45

ECTOPIC ACTH SYNDROME DUE TO OCCULT BRONCHIAL CARCINOID TUMOR

Left: The cortex shows diffuse hyperplasia with lipid depletion of most of the zona fasciculata.

Right: Same case with area of vague nodularity and hypertrophy of cortical cells. Some cells contained sparse granular pigment representing lipofuscin.

cortical cells in advanced idiopathic or autoimmune Addison's disease. There may also be small clusters of lipid-rich cortical cells randomly distributed in the zona fasciculata. Occasionally, there is lipomatous metaplasia.

MULTIPLE ENDOCRINE NEOPLASIA SYNDROME TYPE I

Multiple endocrine neoplasia (MEN) syndrome type I, also referred to as *Wermer's syndrome,* is inherited as an autosomal dominant trait. Expression is variable and it may appear in sporadic form or affect family members in whom manifestations are detectable only after close scrutiny. Factors other than heredity may be important in MEN type I as evidenced by nonidentical expression of the syndrome in identical twins (131). The genetic defect responsible for the syndrome has been mapped to chromosome 11 (11q13) (135). In a review by Ballard et al. (132) of cases of MEN I, the most common abnormalities were hyperparathyroidism (87 percent), pancreatic islet cell tumors (81 percent), and pituitary adenomas (65 percent) (Table 3-11). Autopsy protocols of 31 patients described adrenal pathology consisting of cortical adenomas, "miliary" adenomas, hyperplasia, multiple adenomas, and nodular hyperplasia, but only one patient had clinical hypercorticalism with increased aldosterone secretion. The pituitary-independent adrenal cortical proliferation does not appear to be the primary lesion in MEN type I, and some postulate that it may be a secondary phenomenon, perhaps related to growth factors produced by a pancreatic endocrine neoplasm (135). Surprisingly, there is little clinical significance ascribed to these adrenal

Table 3-11

MULTIPLE ENDOCRINE NEOPLASIA (MEN) SYNDROME, TYPE I

Endocrine Glands Involved	Percent of Cases	Associated Endocrine Syndrome
Parathyroid	87	Hyperparathyroidism
Pancreatic islets	81	Zollinger-Ellison syndrome or diarrheal syndromes; insulin-induced hypoglycemia
Pituitary tumors	65	Acromegaly, amenorrhea/galactorrhea, nonfunctional
Adrenal cortical nodules/adenomas	36	Nonfunctioning
Thyroid nodules/adenomas	19	Nonfunctioning
Carcinoid tumors including thymic carcinoids	<10	Cushing's syndrome

*Data from reference 132.

cortical alterations, even though they occur in about 40 percent of patients with MEN type I. In a recent review of 33 patients from 20 different families, 37 percent had adrenal cortical pathology, with one case reported as adrenal cortical carcinoma, but there were no biochemical disturbances in the hypothalamic-pituitary-adrenal axis (135). Cushing's disease has been reported in MEN type I (see figs. 3-18, 3-19), but it is uncommon (133). In a series of 1,500 pituitary adenomas surgically resected at the Mayo Clinic, 41 (2.7 percent) arose in patients with MEN type I; these included three corticotroph adenomas, two of which occurred in the setting of Nelson's syndrome and one classified as a "silent corticotrophic adenoma" (134). One of two monozygotic twins had Cushing's disease due to corticotroph cell hyperplasia, which raises the possibility of abnormal CRF secretion either from the hypothalamus or an ectopic source.

ADRENAL HYPERFUNCTION WITH PRIMARY HYPERALDOSTERONISM

Primary hyperaldosteronism is due to excessive secretion of aldosterone by the adrenal glands. Under normal conditions the most important regulators of aldosterone secretion are the renin-angiotensin system and potassium, but ACTH can also stimulate secretion of this mineralocorticoid (150). The clinical spectrum of primary hyperaldosteronism is complex and several unusual forms are recognized. The glucocorticoid-remediable (or dexamethasone-suppressible) form of primary hyperaldosteronism is a rare disorder with an autosomal dominant inheritance pattern (139). There are high levels of abnormal adrenal steroids (18-hydroxycortisol and 18-oxocortisol) which are under the control of ACTH and suppressible with glucocorticoids (149). A genetic abnormality has recently been discovered in this disorder in which the coding sequence for aldosterone synthetase fuses with the 5′-regulatory region of the 11-beta-hydroxylase gene, thus permitting illicit production of aldosterone by the zona fasciculata (146). A syndrome of mineralocorticoid excess has also been reported in children and young adults in which the levels of aldosterone and all known mineralocorticoids are either very low or absent; it seems likely that the functioning "mineralocorticoid" in this disorder is cortisol which circulates in normal amounts, but exerts a mineralocorticoid effect because of incomplete metabolism at target tissues (149). This syndrome has an autosomal recessive pattern of inheritance. Rare cases of hyperaldosteronism have been ascribed to autonomous production of aldosterone by ovarian tumors (137,144,148).

It has been estimated that 15 to 35 percent of cases of primary hyperaldosteronism are idiopathic, with bilateral hyperplasia of the zona glomerulosa (147), although with increased awareness of milder forms of primary hyperaldosteronism, an incidence of 45 percent (151) or even greater (140) has been reported. In the idiopathic form, clinical features such as hypertension, headache, easy fatigability, and weakness are often less pronounced compared with cases of primary hyperaldosteronism due to an adrenal cortical neoplasm. Pathologists rarely have the opportunity to study the nontumorous adrenal glands in these patients since adrenalectomy is reserved almost exclusively for patients with an aldosterone-producing adenoma because of the much more predictable response in terms of amelioration or normalization of systemic hypertension (140,145,151); patients with idiopathic hyperaldosteronism due to hyperplasia are usually managed medically (140). Two unusual subsets of primary hyperaldosteronism have been described in which cure or amelioration of the effects of aldosterone excess can be achieved by subtotal or total adrenalectomy: one was designated primary adrenal hyperplasia and the other an aldosterone-producing renin-responsive adenoma (143).

On gross inspection the adrenal glands in idiopathic primary hyperaldosteronism may not demonstrate distinguishing features, or they may be slightly enlarged with grossly visible micronodules or macronodules. The hyperplastic zona glomerulosa may form a continuous band of cells, or the hyperplasia may be focal and vary from one part of the gland to another, thus necessitating multiple sections to detect the abnormality (145,147). In a study involving patients with primary hyperaldosteronism and no evidence of a neoplasm, 50 percent of cases showed hyperplasia of the zona glomerulosa with micronodules, and the remainder were divided into three groups: 1) hyperplasia of zona glomerulosa with micronodules and macronodules; 2) hyperplasia of zona glomerulosa without nodules; and 3) normal appearing zona glomerulosa with micronodules (147). The etiology of this disorder is unclear, but some investigators have implicated an aldosterone-stimulating factor of anterior pituitary origin (136,140).

There are a variety of conditions that can cause activation of the renin-angiotensin system with resultant secondary hyperaldosteronism (142). Hyperplasia of the zona glomerulosa has been reported in patients with cystic fibrosis and may be related to chronic loss of salt (141). An unusual cause of secondary hypermineralocorticoidism is excess ingestion of licorice which can cause sodium and water retention with systemic hypertension, but renin levels are low; a recent study suggests that licorice probably inhibits an enzyme system in the cortical cells resulting in a state analogous to children with 11-beta-hydroxysteroid dehydrogenase deficiency (138).

UNILATERAL ADRENAL CORTICAL HYPERPLASIA

A few cases of putative unilateral adrenal cortical hyperplasia have been reported in association with Cushing's syndrome (152,154), hyperaldosteronism (153,155), and the ectopic ACTH syndrome (156). In the latter case it was speculated that local ACTH stimulation by metastatic tumor in one gland caused unilateral hyperplasia, and the resulting hypercortisolemia caused feedback inhibition of endogenous ACTH production resulting in atrophy of the contralateral gland.

REFERENCES

Adrenal Cortical Hyperplasia

1. Lack EE, Travis WD, Oertel JE. Adrenal cortical nodules, hyperplasia, and hyperfunction In: Lack EE, ed. Pathology of the adrenal glands. New York: Churchill Livingstone, 1990:75–113.

Adrenal Cortical Nodules with Eucorticalism

2. Charbonnel B, Chatal JF, Ozanne P. Does the corticoadrenal adenoma with "pre-Cushing's syndrome" exist? J Nucl Med 1981;22:1059–61.
3. Commons RR, Callaway CP. Adenomas of the adrenal cortex. Arch Intern Med 1948;81:37–41.
4. Dobbie JW. Adrenocortical nodular hyperplasia: the ageing adrenal. J Pathol 1969;99:1–18.
5. Gross MD, Wilton GP, Shapiro B, et al. Functional and scintigraphic evaluation of the silent adrenal mass. J Nucl Med 1987;28:1401–7.
6. Hedeland H, Östberg G, Hökfelt B. On the prevalence of adrenocortical adenomas in an autopsy material in relation to hypertension and diabetes. Acta Med Scand 1968;184:211–4.
7. Kokko JP, Brown TC, Berman MM. Adrenal adenoma and hypertension. Lancet 1967;1:468–70.
8. Lack EE, Travis WD, Oertel JE. Adrenal cortical nodules, hyperplasia, and hyperfunction In: Lack EE, ed. Pathology of the adrenal glands. New York: Churchill Livingstone, 1990:75–113.
9. Neville AM. The nodular adrenal. Invest Cell Pathol 1978;1:99–111.
10. Rizza RA, Wahner HW, Spelsberg TC, Northcutt RC, Moses HL. Visualization of nonfunctioning adrenal adenomas with iodocholesterol: possible relationship to subcellular distribution of tracer. J Nucl Med 1978;19:458–63.
11. Russi S, Blumenthal HT, Gray SH. Small adenomas of the adrenal cortex in hypertension and diabetes. Arch Intern Med 1945;76:284–91.
12. Shamma AH, Goddard JW, Sommers SC. A study of the adrenal status in hypertension. J Chronic Dis 1958;8:587–95.
13. Spain DM, Weinsaft P. Solitary adrenal cortical adenoma in elderly female. Frequency. Arch Pathol 1964;78:231–3.
14. Suzuki, T, Sasano, H, Sawai, T, et al. Small adrenocortical tumors without apparent clinical endocrine abnormalities: immunolocalization of steroidogenic enzymes. Path Res Pract 1992;188:883–9.

Incidental Pigmented Cortical Nodules

15. Damron TA, Schelper RL, Sorensen L. Cytochemical demonstration of neuromelanin in black pigmented adrenal nodules. Am J Clin Pathol 1987;87:334–41.
16. Robinson MJ, Pardo V, Rywlin AM. Pigmented nodules (black adenomas) of the adrenal. An autopsy study of incidence, morphology, and function. Hum Pathol 1972;3:317–25.

Incidental Cortical Nodule In Vivo

17. Abecassis M, McLoughlin MJ, Langer B, Kudlow JE. Serendipitous adrenal masses: prevalence, significance, and management. Am J Surg 1985;149:783–8.
18. Bravo EL. Pheochromocytoma: new concepts and future trends [clinical conference]. Kidney Internat 1991;40:544–56.
19. Carpenter PC. Cushing's syndrome: update of diagnosis and management. Mayo Clin Proc 1986;61:49–58.
20. Case records of the Massachusetts General Hospital. Case 46-1988. N Engl J Med 1988;319:1336–43.
21. Case records of the Massachusetts General Hospital. Case 6-1991. N Engl J Med 1991;324:400–8.
22. Copeland PM. The incidentally discovered adrenal mass. Ann Intern Med 1983;98:940–5.
23. Doppman JL, Reinig JW, Dywer AJ, et al. Differentiation of adrenal masses by magnetic resonance imaging. Surgery 1987;102:1018–26.
24. Francis IR, Smid A, Gross MD, Shapiro B, Naylor B, Glazer GM. Adrenal masses in oncologic patients: functional and morphologic evaluation. Radiology 1988;166:353–6.
25. Glazer GM, Woolsey EJ, Borrello J, et al. Adrenal tissue characterization using MR imaging. Radiology 1986;158:73–9.
26. Glazer HS, Weyman PJ, Sagel SS, Levitt RG, McClennan BL. Nonfunctioning adrenal masses: incidental discovery on computed tomography. AJR Am J Roentgenol 1982;139:81–5.
27. Herrera MF, Grant CS, van Heerden JA, Sheedy PF II, Ilstrup DM. Incidentally discovered adrenal tumors: an institutional perspective. Surgery 1991;110:1014–21.
28. Krestin GP, Friedmann G, Fishbach R, Neufang KF, Allolio B. Evaluation of adrenal masses in oncologic patients: dynamic contrast-enhanced MR vs. CT. J Comput Assist Tomogr 1991;15:104–10.
29. Nadler JL, Radin R. Evaluation and management of the incidentally discovered adrenal mass. Endocrinologist 1991;1:5–9.
30. O'Leary TJ, Ooi TC. The adrenal incidentaloma. Can J Surg 1986;29:6–8.
31. Prinz RA, Brooks MH, Churchill R, et al. Incidental asymptomatic adrenal masses detected by computed tomographic scanning. Is operation required? JAMA 1982;248:701–4.
32. Reincke M, Nieke J, Krestin GP, Saeger W, Allolio B, Winkleman W. Preclinical Cushing's syndrome in adrenal incidentalomas. Comparison with adrenal Cushing's syndrome. J Clin Endocrinol Metab 1992;75:826–32.
33. Ross NS, Aron DC. Hormonal evaluation of the patient with an incidentally discovered adrenal mass. N Engl J Med 1990;323:1401–5.
34. Roubidoux M, Dunnick NR. Adrenal cortical tumors. Bull NY Acad Med 1991;67:119–30.

Adrenal Cortical Hyperplasia with Hypercortisolism

35. Belsky JL, Cuello B, Swanson LW, Simmons DM, Jarrett RM, Braza F. Cushing's syndrome due to ectopic production of corticotropin-releasing factor. J Clin Endocrinol Metab 1985;60:496–500.
36. Bertagna X. New causes of Cushing's syndrome. N Engl J Med 1992;327:1024–5.
37. Carey RM, Varma S, Drake CR Jr, et al. Ectopic secretion of corticotropin-releasing factor as a cause of Cushing's syndrome. A clinical, morphologic, and biochemical study. N Engl J Med 1984;311:13–20.
38. Danon M, Robboy SJ, Kim S, Scully R, Crawford JD. Cushing syndrome, sexual precocity, and polyostotic fibrous dysplasia (Albright syndrome) in infancy. J Pediatr 1975;87:917–21.
39. Gold EM. The Cushing syndromes: changing views of diagnosis and treatment. Ann Int Med 1979;90:829–44.
40. Grizzle WE, Dunlap N. Cushing's syndrome. Diagnosis of the atypical patient [Editorial]. Arch Pathol Lab Med 1989;113:727–8.
41. Hamet P, Larochelle P, Franks DJ, Cartier P, Bolte E. Cushing's syndrome with food-dependent periodic hormonogenesis. Clin Invest Med 1987;10:530–3.
42. Kaplan SA. Disorders of the adrenal cortex I. Ped Clin N Amer 1979;26:65–76.
43. Kuhn JM, Proeschel MF, Sevrin DJ, Bertagna XY, Luton JP, Girard FL. Comparative assessment of ACTH and lipotropin plasma levels in the diagnosis and follow-up of patients with Cushing's syndrome: a study of 210 cases. Am J Med 1989;86:678–84.
44. Lack EE, Travis WD, Oertel JE. Adrenal cortical nodules, hyperplasia, and hyperfunction. In: Lack EE, ed. Pathology of the adrenal glands. New York: Churchill Livingstone, 1990:75–113.
45. Lacroix A, Bolté E, Tremblay J, et al. Gastric inhibitory polypeptide-dependent cortisol hypersecretion—a new cause of Cushing's syndrome. N Engl J Med 1992;327:974–80.
46. Liddle GW. Cushing's syndrome. Ann New York Acad Sci 1977;297:594–602.
47. Mandel S. Cushing's syndrome in infancy. Endocrinologist 1994;4:28–32.
48. McArthur RG, Hayles AB, Salassa RM. Childhood Cushing disease: results of bilateral adrenalectomy. J Pediatr 1979;95:214–9.
49. Miller J, Crapo L. The biochemical diagnosis of hypercortisolism. Endocrinologist 1994;4:7–16.
50. Orth DN, Liddle GW. Results of treatment in 108 patients with Cushing's syndrome. N Engl J Med 1971;285:243–7.
51. Reznik Y, Allali-Zerah V, Chayvialle JA, et al. Food-dependent Cushing's syndrome mediated by aberrant adrenal sensitivity to gastric inhibitory polypeptide. N Engl J Med 1992;327:981–6.
52. Schteingart DE, Lloyd RV, Akil H, et al. Cushing's syndrome secondary to ectopic corticotropin-releasing hormone—adrenocorticotropin secretion. J Clin Endocrinol Metab 1986;63:770–5.
53. Scott HW Jr, Abumrad NN, Orth DN. Tumors of the adrenal cortex and Cushing's syndrome. Ann Surg 1985;20:586–94.
54. Thomas CG Jr, Smith AT, Benson M, Griffith J. Nelson's syndrome after Cushing's disease in childhood: a continuing problem. Surgery 1984;96:1067–77.
55. Thomas CG Jr, Smith AT, Griffith JM, Askin FB. Hyperadrenalism in childhood and adolescence. Ann Surg 1984;199:538–48.
56. Weinstein LS, Shenker A, Gejman PV, Merino MJ, Friedman E, Spiegel AM. Activating mutations of the stimulatory G protein in McCune-Albright syndrome. N Engl J Med 1991;325:1688–95.
57. Zárate A, Kovacs K, Flores M, Morán C, Félix I. ACTH and CRF-producing bronchial carcinoid associated with Cushing's syndrome. Clin Endocrinol 1986;24:523–9.

Pituitary-Dependent Hypercortisolism

58. Asa SL, Kovacs K, Tindall GT, Barrow DL, Horvath E, Vecsei P. Cushing's disease associated with intrasellar gangliocytoma producing corticotrophin-releasing factor. Ann Int Med 1984;101:789–93.
59. Cohen RB. Observations on cortical nodules in human adrenal glands. Their relationship to neoplasia. Cancer 1966;19:552–6.
60. Cohen RB, Chapman WB, Castleman B. Hyperadrenocorticism (Cushing's disease): a study of surgically resected adrenal glands. Am J Pathol 1959;35:537–61.
61. Cushing H. The basophil adenomas of the pituitary body and their clinical manifestations (pituitary basophilism). Bull Johns H Hosp 1932;50:137–95.
62. Doppman JL, Miller DL, Dwyer AJ, et al. Macronodular adrenal hyperplasia in Cushing's disease. Radiology 1988;166:347–52.
63. Friedberg SR. Transsphenoidal pituitary surgery in the treatment of patients with Cushing's disease. Urol Clin North Am 1989;16:589–95.
64. Fulton JF. Harvey Cushing. A Biography. Springfield, IL: Charles C. Thomas, 1946:505–6.
65. Hermus AR, Pieters GF, Smals AG, et al. Transition from pituitary-dependent to adrenal-dependent Cushing's syndrome. N Engl J Med 1988;318:966–70.
66. Klibanski A, Zervas NT. Diagnosis and management of hormone-secreting pituitary adenomas. N Engl J Med 1991;324:822-831.
67. Lack EE, Travis WD, Oertel JE. Adrenal cortical nodules, hyperplasia, and hyperfunction. In: Lack EE, ed. Pathology of the adrenal glands. New York: Churchill Livingstone, 1990:75–113.
68. Lamberts SW, Bons EG, Bruining HA. Different sensitivity to adrenocorticotropin of dispersed adrenocortical cells from patients with Cushing's disease with macronodular and diffuse adrenal hyperplasia. J Clin Endocrinol Metab 1984;58:1106–10.
69. Neville AM, O'Hare MJ. Histopathology of the human adrenal cortex. Clin Endocrinol Metab 1985;14:791–820.
70. Neville AM, Symington T. The pathology of the adrenal gland in Cushing's syndrome. J Pathol Bacteriol 1967;93:19–35.

71. Oldfield EH, Doppman JL, Nieman LK, et al. Petrosal sinus sampling with and without corticotropin-releasing hormone for the differential diagnosis of Cushing's syndrome. N Engl J Med 1991;325:897–905.
72. Page DL, DeLellis RA, Hough AJ Jr. Tumors of the adrenal gland. Atlas of Tumor Pathology, 2nd Series. Fascicle 23. Washington, D.C.: Armed Forces Institute of Pathology, 1986.
73. Reidbord H, Fisher ER. Electron microscopic study of adrenal cortical hyperplasia in Cushing's syndrome. Arch Path 1968;86:419–26.
74. Sheeler LR. Cushing's syndrome—1988. Cleve Clin J Med 1988;55:329–37.
75. Smals AG, Pieters GF, van Haelst UJ, Kloppenborg PW. Macronodular adrenocortical hyperplasia in long-standing Cushing's disease. J Clin Endocrinol Metab 1984;58:25–31.
76. Young WF Jr, Scheithauer BW, Gharib H, Laws ER Jr, Carpenter PC. Cushing's syndrome due to primary multinodular corticotropic hyperplasia. Mayo Clinic Proc 1988;63:256–62.

Macronodular Hyperplasia with Marked Adrenal Enlargement

77. Aiba M, Hirayama A, Iri H, et al. Adrenocorticotropic hormone-independent bilateral adrenocortical macronodular hyperplasia as a distinct subtype of Cushing's syndrome. Enzyme histochemical and ultrastructural study of four cases with a review of the literature. Am J Clin Pathol 1991;96:334–40.
78. Aiba M, Hirayama A, Iri H, et al. Primary adrenocortical micronodular dysplasia: enzyme histochemical and ultrastructural studies of two cases with a review of the literature. Hum Pathol 1990;21:503–11.
79. Doppman JL, Nieman LK, Travis WD, et al. CT and MR imaging of massive macronodular adrenocortical disease: a rare cause of autonomous primary adrenal hypercortisolism. J Computr Assist Tomogr 1991;15:773–9.
80. Hashimoto K, Kawada Y, Murakami K, et al. Cortisol responsiveness to insulin-induced hypoglycemia in Cushing's syndrome with huge nodular adrenocortical hyperplasia. Endocrinol Jpn 1986;33:479–87.
81. Hidai H, Fujii H, Otsuka K, Abe K, Shimizu N. Cushing's syndrome due to huge adrenocortical multinodular hyperplasia. Endocrinol Jpn 1975;22:555–60.
82. Kirschner MA, Powell RD Jr, Lipsett MB. Cushing's syndrome: nodular cortical hyperplasia of adrenal glands with clinical and pathological features suggesting adrenocortical tumor. J Clin Endocr 1964;24:947–55.
83. Makino S, Hashimoto K, Sugiyama M, et al. Cushing's syndrome due to huge nodular adrenocortical hyperplasia with fluctuation of urinary 17 OHCS excretion. Endocrinol Jpn 1989;36:655–63.
84. Malchoff DC, Rosa J, DeBold CR. Adrenocorticotropin-independent bilateral macronodular adrenal hyperplasia: an unusual cause of Cushing's syndrome. J Clin Endocrinol Metab 1989;68:855–60.
85. Sasano H, Miyazaki S, Sawai T, et al. Primary pigmented nodular adrenocortical disease (PPNAD): immunohistochemical and in situ hybridization analysis of steroidogenic enzymes in eight cases. Mod Pathol 1992;5:23-9.
86. Sasano H, Suzuki T, Nagura H. ACTH-independent macronodular adrenocortical hyperplasia: immunohistochemical and in situ hybridization studies of steroidogenic enzymes. Mod Pathol 1994;7:215–9.
87. Smals AG, Pieters GF, van Haelst UJ, Kloppenborg PW. Macronodular adrenocortical hyperplasia in long-standing Cushing's disease. J Clin Endocrinol Metab 1984;58:25–31.

Primary Pigmented Nodular Adrenocortical Disease

88. Aiba M, Hirayama A, Iri H, et al. Primary adrenocortical micronodular dysplasia: enzyme histochemical and ultrastructural studies of two cases with a review of the literature. Hum Pathol 1990;21:503–11.
89. Böhm N, Lippmann-Grob B, Petrykowski W. Familial Cushing's syndrome due to pigmented multinodular adrenocortical dysplasia. Acta Endocrinol 1983;102:428–35.
90. Carney JA, Young WF Jr. Primary pigmented nodular adrenocortical disease and its associated conditions. Endocrinologist 1992;2:6–21.
91. Cushing H. The basophil adenomas of the pituitary body and their clinical manifestations (pituitary basophilism). Bull Johns H Hosp 1932;50:137–95.
92. Doppman JL, Travis WD, Nieman L, et al. Cushing syndrome due to primary pigmented nodular adrenocortical disease: findings at CT and MR imaging. Radiology 1989;172:415–20.
93. Findling JW. The Cushing syndromes: an enlarging clinical spectrum. N Engl J Med 1989;321:1677–8.
94. Grant CS, Carney JA, Carpenter PC, van Heerden JA. Primary pigmented nodular adrenocortical disease: diagnosis and management. Surgery 1986;100:1178–84.
95. Lack EE, Travis WD, Oertel JE. Adrenal cortical nodules, hyperplasia, and hyperfunction. In: Lack EE, ed. Pathology of the adrenal glands. New York: Churchill Livingstone, 1990:75–113.
96. Larsen JL, Cathey WJ, Odell WD. Primary adrenocortical nodular dysplasia, a distinct subtype of Cushing's syndrome. Case report and review of the literature. Am J Med 1986;80:976–84.
97. Sasano H, Miyazaki S, Sawai T, et al. Primary pigmented nodular adrenocortical disease (PPNAD): immunohistochemical and in situ hybridization analysis of steroidogenic enzymes in eight cases. Mod Pathol 1992;5:23–9.
98. Shenoy BV, Carpenter PC, Carney JA. Bilateral primary pigmented nodular adrenocortical disease. Rare cause of the Cushing syndrome. Am J Surg Pathol 1984;8:335–44.
99. Travis WD, Tsokos M, Doppman JL, et al. Primary pigmented nodular adrenocortical disease. A light and electron microscopic study of eight cases. Am J Surg Pathol 1989;13:921–30.
100. van Berkhout TF, Croughs RJ, Kater L, et al. Familial Cushing's syndrome due to nodular adrenocortical dysplasia. A putative receptor-antibody disease? Clin Endocrinol 1986;24:299–310.

101. Wulffraat NM, Drexhage HA, Jeucken P, van der Gaag RD, Wiersinga WM. Effects of ACTH and ACTH fragment on DNA synthecis in guinea-pig adrenal segments kept in organ culture. J Endocrinol 1987;115:505–10.
102. Wulffraat NM, Drexhage HA, Wiersinga WM, van der Gaag RD, Jeucken P, Mol JA. Immunoglobulins of patients with Cushing's syndrome due to pigmented adrenocortical micronodular dysplasia stimulate in vitro steroidogenesis. J Clin Endocrinol Metab 1988;66:301–7.
103. Young WF Jr, Carney JA, Musa BU, Wulffraat NM, Lens JW, Drexhage HA. Familial Cushing's syndrome due to primary pigmented nodular adrenocortical disease. Reinvestigation 50 years later. N Engl J Med 1989;321:1659–64.

Complex of Myxomas, Spotty Pigmentation and Endocrine Overactivity

104. Atherton DJ, Pitcher DW, Wells RS, MacDonald DM. A syndrome of various cutaneous pigmented lesions, myxoid neurofibromata and atrial myxoma: the NAME syndrome. Br J Dermatol 1980;103:421–9.
105. Bain J. Carney's complex [Letter]. Mayo Clin Proc 1986;61:508.
106. Carney JA. Psammomatous melanotic Schwannoma. A distinctive, heritable tumor with special associations, including cardiac myxoma and the Cushing syndrome. Am J Surg Pathol 1990;14:206–22.
107. Carney JA, Gordon H, Carpenter PC, Shenoy BV, Go VL. The complex of myxomas, spotty pigmentation, and endocrine overactivity. Medicine 1985;64:270–83.
108. Carney JA, Hruska LS, Beauchamp GD, Gordon H. Dominant inheritance of the complex of myxomas, spotty pigmentation and endocrine overactivity. Mayo Clin Proc 1986;61:165–72.
109. Carney JA, Young WF Jr. Primary pigmented nodular adrenocortical disease and its associated conditions. Endocrinologist 1992;2:6–21.
110. Hedinger C. Kombination von herzmyxomen mit primärer nodulärer dysplasie der nebennierenrinde, fleckförmigen haut pigmentierung und myxomartigen tumoren anderer lokalisation-ein eigenartiger familiärer symptomenkomplex ("Swiss-syndrome"). Schweiz Med Wschr 1987;117:591–4.
111. Rhodes AR, Silverman RA, Harrist TJ, Perez-Atayde AR. Mucocutaneous lentigines, cardiomucocutaneous myxomas and multiple blue nevi: the LAMB syndrome. J Am Acad Dermatol 1984;10:72–82.

Ectopic ACTH Syndrome

112. Axiotis CA, Lippes HA, Merino MJ, de Lanerolle NC, Stewart AF, Kinder B. Corticotroph cell pituitary adenoma within an ovarian teratoma. A new cause of Cushing's syndrome. Am J Surg Pathol 1987;11:218–24.
113. Belsky JL, Cuello B, Swanson LW, Simmons DM, Jarrett RM, Braza F. Cushing's syndrome due to ectopic production of corticotropin-releasing factor. J Clin Endocrinol Metab 1985;60:496–500.
114. Carey RM, Varma SK, Drake CR Jr, et al. Ectopic secretion of corticotropin-releasing factor as a cause of Cushing's syndrome. A clinical morphologic and biochemical study. N Engl J Med 1984;311:13–20.
115. Clement PB, Young RH, Scully RE. Clinical syndromes associated with tumors of the female genital tract. Semin Diagn Pathol 1991;8:204–33.
116. Cushing H. The basophil adenomas of the pituitary body and their clinical manifestations (pituitary basophilism). Bull Johns H Hosp 1932;50:137–95.
117. Doppman JL. The search for occult ectopic ACTH-producing tumors. Endocrinologist 1992;2:41–6.
118. Doppman JL, Nieman L, Miller DL. Ectopic adrenocorticotrophic hormone syndrome: localization studies in 28 patients. Radiology 1989;172:115–24.
119. Drasin GF, Lynch T, Temes GP. Ectopic ACTH production and mediastinal lipomatosis. Radiology 1978;127:610.
120. Dupont AG, Somers G, van Steirteghem AC, Warson F, Vanhaelst L. Ectopic adrenocorticotropin production: disappearance after removal of inflammatory tissue. J Clin Endocrinol Metab 1984;58:654–8.
121. Findling JW. Eutopic or ectopic adrenocorticotropic hormone-dependent Cushing's syndrome? A diagnostic dilemma [Editorial]. Mayo Clin Proc 1990;65:1377–80.
122. Georgitis WJ. Clinically silent congenital adrenal hyperplasia masquerading as ectopic adrenocorticotropin syndrome. Am J Med 1986;80:703–8.
123. Gold EM. The Cushing syndromes. Changing views of diagnosis and treatment. Ann Int Med 1979;90:829–44.
124. Grua JR, Nelson DH. ACTH-producing tumors. Endocrinol Metab Clin N Am 1991;20:319–62.
125. Lack EE, Travis WD, Oertel JE. Adrenal cortical nodules, hyperplasia, and hyperfunction. In: Lack EE, ed. Pathology of the adrenal glands. New York: Churchill Livingstone, 1990:75–113.
126. Leinung MC, Young WF Jr, Whitaker MD, Scheithauer BW, Trastek VF, Kvols LK. Diagnosis of corticotropin-producing bronchial carcinoid tumors causing Cushing's syndrome. Mayo Clin Proc 1990;65:1314–21.
127. Odell WD. Ectopic ACTH secretion. A misnomer. Endocrinol Metab Clin N Am 1991;20:371–9.
128. Orth DN, Liddle GW. Results of treatment in 108 patients with Cushing's syndrome. N Engl J Med 1971; 285:243–7.
129. Schteingart DE, Lloyd RV, Akil H, et al. Cushing's syndrome secondary to ectopic corticotropin-releasing hormone—adrenocorticotropin secretion. J Clin Endocrinol Metab 1986;63:770–5.
130. Zárate A, Kovacs K, Flores M, Morán C, Félix I. ACTH and CRF-producing bronchial carcinoid associated with Cushing's syndrome. Clin Endocrinol 1986; 24:523–9.

Multiple Endocrine Neoplasia Syndrome Type I

131. Bahn RS, Scheithauer BW, van Heerden JA, Laws ER Jr, Horvath E, Gharib H. Nonidentical expressions of multiple endocrine neoplasia, type I, in identical twins. Mayo Clin Proc 1986;61:689–96.
132. Ballard HS, Frame B, Hartsock RJ. Familial multiple endocrine adenoma—peptic ulcer complex. Medicine 1964;43:481–516.
133. Miyagawa K, Ishibashi M, Kasuga M, Kanazawa Y, Yamaji T, Takaku F. Multiple endocrine neoplasia type I with Cushing's disease, primary hyperparathyroidism, and insulin-glucagonoma. Cancer 1988;61:1232–6.
134. Scheithauer BW, Laws ER Jr, Kovacs K, Horvath E, Randall RV, Carney JA. Pituitary adenomas of the multiple endocrine neoplasia type I syndrome. Sem Diagn Pathol 1987;4:205–11.
135. Skogseid B, Larsson C, Lindgren PG, et al. Clinical and genetic features of adrenocortical lesions in multiple endocrine neoplasia type 1. J Clin Endocrinol Metab 1992;75:76–81.

Adrenal Hyperfunction with Hyperaldosteronism

136. Carey RM, Sen S, Doland LM, Malchoff CD, Bumpus FM. Idiopathic hyperaldosteronism. A possible role for aldosterone-stimulating factor. N Engl J Med 1984;311:94–100.
137. Ehrlich EN, Dominguez OV, Samuels LT, Lynch D, Oberhelman H Jr, Warner NE. Aldosteronism and precocious puberty due to an ovarian androblastoma (sertoli cell tumor). J Clin Endocrinol Metab 1963;23:358–67.
138. Farese RV Jr, Biglieri EG, Shackleton CH, Irony I, Gomez-Foutes R. Licorice-induced hypermineralocorticoidism. N Engl J Med 1991;325;1223–7.
139. Giebink GS, Gotlin RW, Biglieri EG, Katz FH. A kindred with familial glucocorticoid suppressible aldosteronism. J Clin Endocrinol Metab 1973;36:715–23.
140. Gill JR Jr. Hyperaldosteronism. In: Becker KL, ed. Principles and practice of endocrinology and metabolism. JB Lippincott, 1990:631–43.
141. Hawkins E, Singer DB. The adrenal cortex in cystic fibrosis of the pancreas. Am J Clin Pathol 1976;66:710–41.
142. Hsuch WA, Tuck ML. Aldosterone and the renin-angiotensin system. In: Becker KL, ed. Principles and practice of endocrinology and metabolism. Philadelphia: JB Lippincott, 1990:623–31.
143. Irony I, Kater CE, Biglieri EG, Shackleton CH. Correctable subsets of primary aldosteronism. Primary adrenal hyperplasia and renin responsive adenoma. Am J Hypertens 1990;3:576–82.
144. Kulkarni JN, Mistry RC, Kamat MR, Chinoy R, Lotlikar RG. Autonomous aldosterone-secreting ovarian tumor. Gynecol Oncol 1990;37:284–9.
145. Lack EE, Travis WD, Oertel JE. Adrenal cortical nodules, hyperplasia, and hyperfunction. In: Lack EE, ed. Pathology of the adrenal glands. New York: Churchill Livingstone, 1990:75–113.
146. Lifton RP, Dluhy RG, Powers M, et al. A chimaeric 11-beta-hydroxylase/aldosterone synthase gene causes glucocorticoid-remediable aldosteronism and human hypertension. Nature 1992;355:262–5.
147. Neville AM, O'Hare MJ. Histopathology of the human adrenal cortex. Clin Endocrinol Metab 1985;14:791–820.
148. Todesco S, Terribile V, Borsatti A, Mantero F. Primary aldosteronism due to a malignant ovarian tumor. J Clin Endocrinol Metab 1975;41:809–19.
149. Ulick S. Two uncommon causes of mineralocorticoid excess. Syndrome of apparent mineralocorticoid excess and glucocorticoid-remediable. Endocrinol Metab Clin North Am 1991;20:269–76.
150. White PC. Disorders of aldosterone biosynthesis and action. N Engl J Med 1994;331:250–8.
151. Young WF Jr, Hogan MJ, Klee GG, Grant CS, van Heerden JA. Primary aldosteronism: diagnosis and treatment. Mayo Clin Proc 1990;65:96–110

Unilateral Adrenal Cortical Hyperplasia

152. Catania A, Reschini E, Orsatti A, Motta P, Airaghi L, Cantalamessa L. Cushing's syndrome due to unilateral adrenal nodular hyperplasia with incomplete inhibition of one adrenal gland. Hormone Res 1986;23:9–15.
153. Ganguly A, Zager PG, Luetscher JA. Primary aldosteronism due to unilateral adrenal hyperplasia. J Clin Endocrinol Metab 1980;51:1190–4.
154. Josse RG, Bear R, Kovacs K, Higgins HP. Cushing's syndrome due to unilateral nodular adrenal hyperplasia. A new pathophysiological entity? Acta Endocrinol 1980;93:495–504.
155. Oberfield SE, Levine LS, Firpo A, et al. Primary hyperaldosteronism in childhood due to unilateral macronodular hyperplasia. Case Report. Hypertension 1984;6:75–84
156. Sigman LM, Wallach L. Unilateral adrenal hypertrophy in ectopic ACTH syndrome. Arch Intern Med 1984;144:1869–70.

4
ADRENAL CORTICAL ADENOMA

Definition. Adrenal cortical adenoma (ACA) is a benign neoplasm arising from adrenal cortical cells which may or may not have functional activity as evidenced by a recognizable syndrome or biochemical evidence of hypercorticalism.

General Features. ACAs are typically unilateral, solitary, benign neoplasms which are often associated with an endocrine syndrome because of excess secretion of one or more of the three major classes of adrenal steroids. The incidence of ACAs is relatively low if the incidentally discovered adrenal nodule (or adenoma) that is typically nonhyperfunctional is excluded. The most frequent endocrine abnormality associated with ACA is primary hyperaldosteronism, followed by Cushing's syndrome, virilization, and occasionally feminization (3). In one series of 26 ACAs, in which patients with primary hyperaldosteronism were excluded, 21 were associated with Cushing's syndrome (81 percent), 2 caused virilization, and 3 tumors were "nonfunctional" (1). As previously noted, many nonfunctional tumors are capable of taking up radio-labeled steroid precursor, but are unable to secrete sufficient steroids to cause signs or symptoms of hypercorticalism (hence the term nonhyperfunctional).

Hypersecretion of adrenal steroids may manifest as a fully developed endocrine syndrome that is often "pure," i.e., primary hyperaldosteronism or Cushing's syndrome; by abnormal laboratory data; or by cortical atrophy of the ipsilateral or contralateral adrenal cortex. The presence of virilization, either as part of a pure or mixed endocrine syndrome (Cushing's syndrome and virilization), may indicate malignancy, particularly in large neoplasms weighing over 100 g (4). The presence of feminization is a particularly ominous endocrine feature: in the review by Gabrilove et al. (2) most tumors causing feminization were malignant. In general, ACAs have a predilection for female patients, and are equally distributed on either side. Although there are some gross and microscopic features that are more likely to be associated with tumors producing a particular endocrine syndrome, it may be very difficult (or impossible) to predict the associated endocrine syndrome based upon morphologic features alone without correlation with clinical or endocrinologic data. This chapter deals with ACAs associated with a particular endocrine syndrome. In some cases there may be significant overlap in morphology; indeed, the range in morphology of even a dominant macronodule (nonhyperfunctional nodule or adenoma) can mimic almost any ACA associated with known endocrine syndromes of various types.

On computed tomographic (CT) scan, adrenal cortical adenoma (and nonhyperfunctional adenoma or nodule) is usually well-defined, has a smooth contour, and is homogeneous, with attenuation values less than those of normal adrenal tissue depending upon the amount of lipid present. The tumor may enhance mildly after contrast administration. On magnetic resonance imaging (MRI), ACAs tend to be homogeneous, with signal intensity less than fat but greater than muscle on all pulse sequences; the intensity is similar to that of liver on T1- and T2-weighted sequences. The tumor may enhance mildly; it may also be darker than the rest of the gland, when out-of-phase imaging, which is highly sensitive to the presence and amount of lipid, is used.

ADRENAL CORTICAL ADENOMA WITH CUSHING'S SYNDROME

Gross Findings. ACAs associated with Cushing's syndrome are usually solitary, unilateral, and unicentric neoplasms which often weigh less than 50 g. Only rarely have bilateral ACAs been reported in association with Cushing's syndrome (5). Occasionally, very unusual cases of macronodular hyperplasia with marked adrenal enlargement may appear to be a primary autonomous cause of Cushing's syndrome and may simulate a neoplasm. On cross section, ACAs appear sharply circumscribed or even encapsulated (fig. 4-1). In one study the average diameter of ACAs causing Cushing's syndrome was 3.6 cm (range, 1.5 to 6 cm) (10). Many tumors weigh between 10 and 40 g (17). The largest ACA reported by Bertagna and Orth (6) was 126 g, and on occasion the tumor can

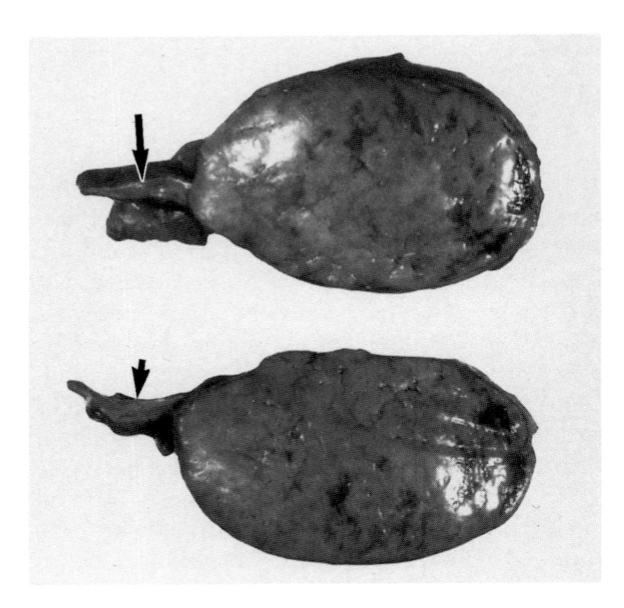

Figure 4-1
ADRENAL CORTICAL ADENOMA
On cross section, this adrenal cortical adenoma from a 22-year-old female with Cushing's syndrome has a slightly bulging surface and is yellow-orange. Note atrophy of the attached adrenal cortex (arrows), which measured less than 1 mm in thickness throughout.

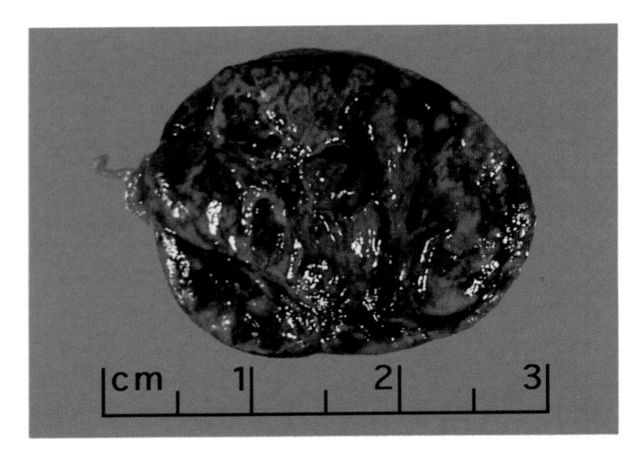

Figure 4-2
ADRENAL CORTICAL ADENOMA
This adrenal cortical adenoma from a 32-year-old woman with Cushing's syndrome measured 2.1 cm in diameter. On cross section there are geographic to mottled zones of dark pigmentation. This was due to lipid depletion of neoplastic cortical cells as well as accumulation of lipofuscin.

weigh several hundred grams. The contralateral adenoma is sometimes nonhyperfunctional (12). There is some suggestion in the literature that an adrenal cortical neoplasm weighing over 100 g (actually 95 g in the study by Tang and Gray [21]) is probably a carcinoma until proven otherwise. Tumor weight alone, however, is insufficient to categorically type an adrenal cortical tumor as benign or malignant. While it is true that adrenal cortical carcinomas tend to be quite large, often 400 g or more, some very large tumors associated with Cushing's syndrome fail to metastasize, and rare tumors less than 50 g prove to be malignant (14). Clearly, criteria other than weight alone are necessary to predict biologic behavior.

On cross section, ACAs may appear homogenous yellow or golden-yellow throughout, or there may be irregular foci of dark discoloration. The latter can be attributed to recent or old hemorrhage, areas of lipid depletion within the tumor, or the presence of increased lipofuscin (fig. 4-2). In the study by O'Leary et al. (18), microscopic examination revealed lipofuscin in each adrenal cortical lesion (including ACAs) associated with Cushing's syndrome. When the tumor is diffusely dark brown (fig. 4-3) or black, the term *black adenoma* has been used (14). Occasionally, areas of degeneration with fibrosis and cystic change are seen, but areas of confluent or geographic tumor necrosis are uncommon (14). Some tumors have vague nodularity on cross section (fig. 4-4), but typically without the coarse lobulations with broad fibrous bands associated with adrenal cortical carcinoma. If these qualities are present in larger tumors, malignancy should be suspected. Use of all available histologic and nonhistologic parameters may be necessary for a correct diagnosis (14).

Microscopic Findings. While an ACA may appear encapsulated on gross examination, on histologic study the tumor may have a relatively smooth "pushing" border without a well-defined fibrous capsule. In some tumors the compressed fibrous connective tissue at the periphery is, in essence, a fibrous pseudocapsule, whereas some tumors may acquire a fibrous capsule from the adrenal capsule itself. A "classic" ACA is easy to define in many instances, particularly in adults, but the tumor may reside in a nodular cortex making a straightforward definition difficult (14).

Most tumors have broad fields of pale-staining, lipid-rich cells with relatively uniform nuclei, and cytoplasm that appears optically "clear" at low magnification (fig. 4-5). The most common architectural patterns are cells in a nesting or

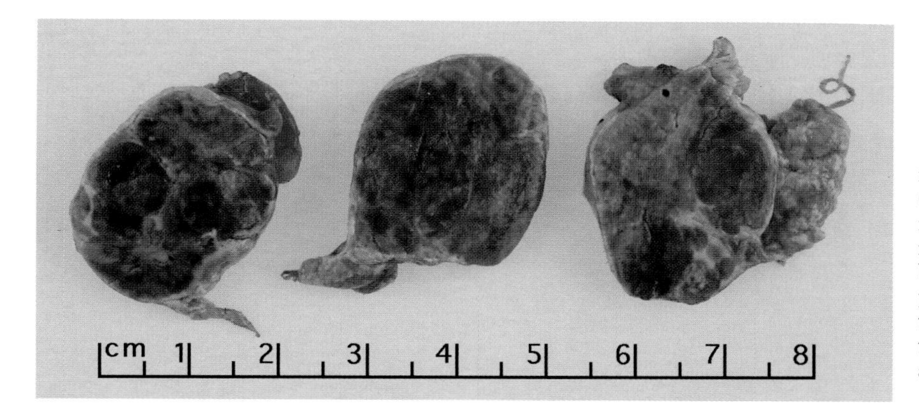

Figure 4-3
ADRENAL CORTICAL ADENOMA

This adrenal cortical adenoma is from a 35-year-old female with Cushing's syndrome. Note the marked atrophy of the attached adrenal cortex. Tumor has a confluent brown color due to cells with compact, eosinophilic cytoplasm and intracellular lipochrome pigment. The tumor weighed 16 g including the attached adrenal remnant.

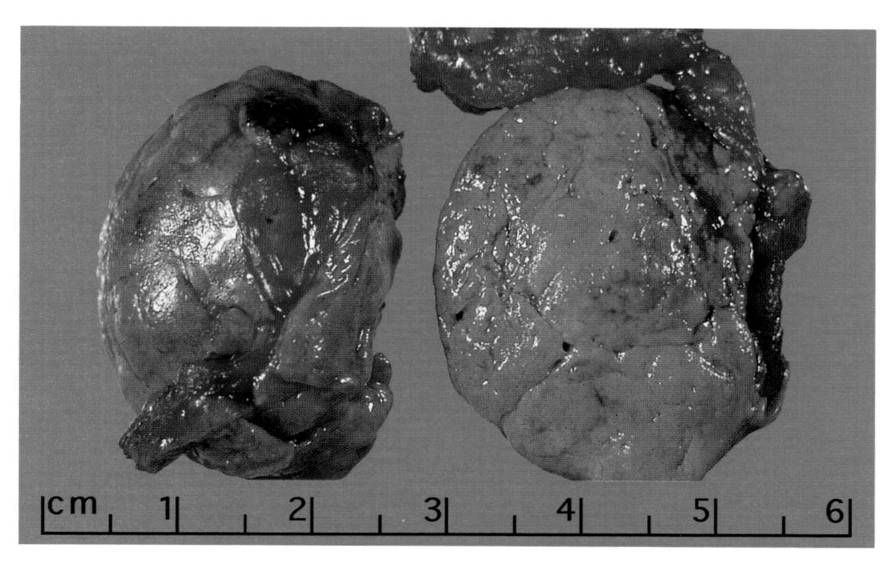

Figure 4-4
ADRENAL CORTICAL ADENOMA

This adrenal cortical adenoma is from a 33-year-old patient with Cushing's syndrome. The tumor is yellow-orange on cross section and has vague lobulations. It measured 3.5 x 3.0 x 2.5 cm.

alveolar arrangement (fig. 4-6, left), short cords, narrow interconnecting trabeculae (fig. 4-6, right), or a mixture of these patterns in the same tumor. Occasionally, the tumor cells are focally aligned in slender cords reminiscent of normal zona fasciculata. In rare instances, a small area with a spindle cell pattern is seen (fig. 4-7), but it should not pose a problem in diagnosis since more typical histology is almost always evident elsewhere in the tumor. When compared with normal cortical cells, ACA cells are usually larger, with a different quality of cytoplasm and variation in nuclear size and configuration. Most tumors have an abundance of cells with pale-staining, lipid-rich cytoplasm and relatively distinct cell borders similar to cells of the zona fasciculata (fig. 4-8). A few tumors have a virtually pure composition of lipid-rich cells, which gives the tumor a vivid yellow or yellow-orange hue. Many other tumors contain a variable component of compact lipid-poor cells with eosinophilic cytoplasm, sometimes with conspicuous lipochrome pigment (18). In some tumors there are cells with varied cytologic features, recalling the diversity of cell types in the normal adrenal cortex, although the neoplastic cells are usually larger. There may be cells that have intermediate or transitional cytologic features, sometimes in the same histologic field (fig. 4-9). Clusters of tumor cells with greatly enlarged lipid-rich cytoplasm, so-called balloon cells, stand out in stark contrast to cells with compact, eosinophilic cytoplasm (fig. 4-10). The pale-staining quality of the cytoplasm has been referred to as "clear," but on close examination of well-fixed specimens the cytoplasm is not optically clear or empty as in renal cell carcinoma, but is finely vacuolated due to dispersed intracytoplasmic lipid droplets of various

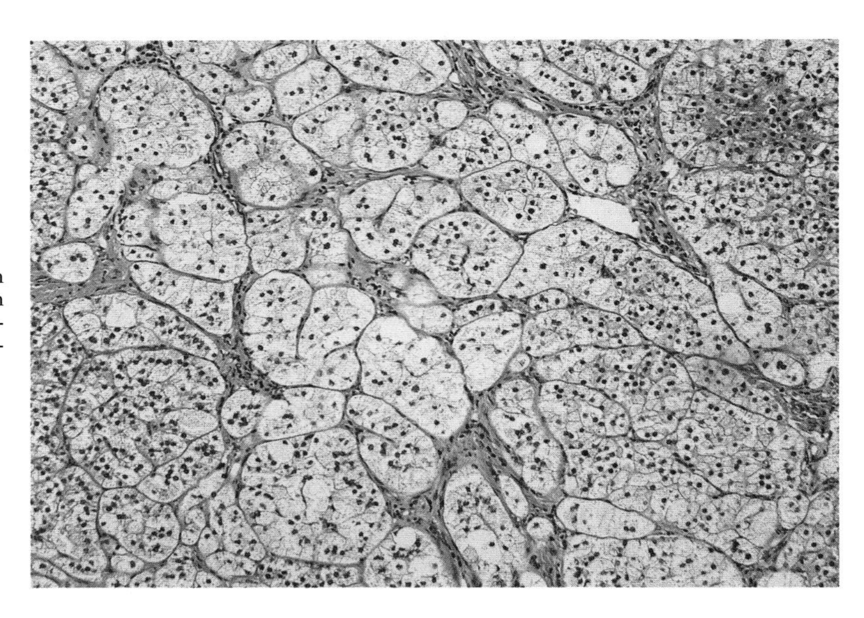

Figure 4-5
ADRENAL CORTICAL ADENOMA ASSOCIATED WITH CUSHING'S SYNDROME

The tumor cells are arranged in small clusters and short cords with pale-staining cytoplasm. Note the absence of nuclear enlargement and pleomorphism.

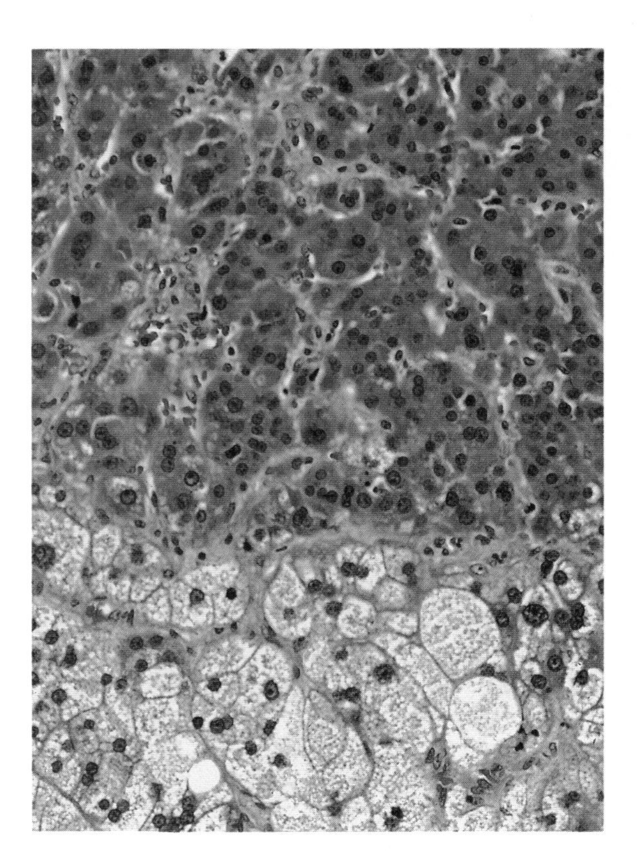

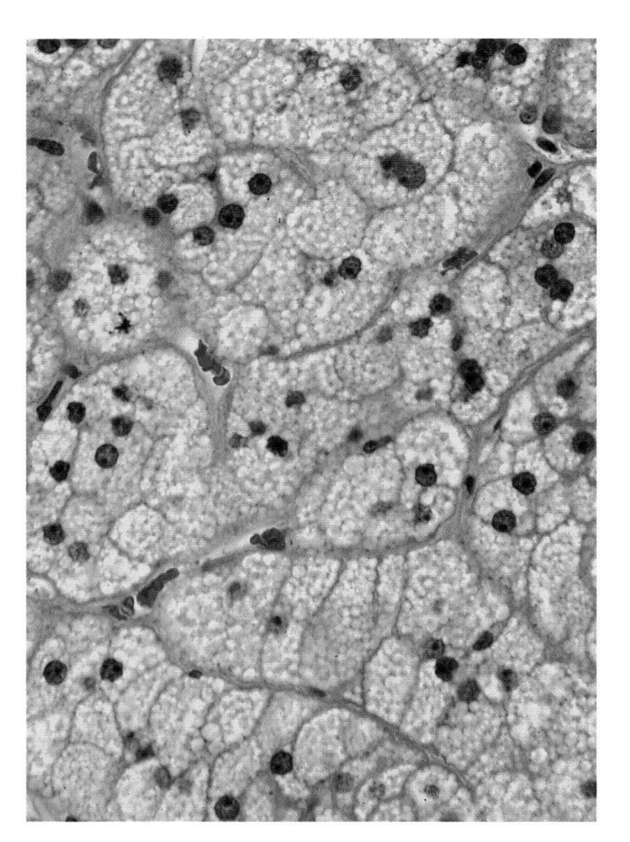

Figure 4-6
ADRENAL CORTICAL ADENOMA ASSOCIATED WITH CUSHING'S SYNDROME

Left: The tumor cells in this adrenal cortical adenoma are arranged in rounded to ovoid clusters or alveoli, with a delicate intersecting vasculature. There is gradation in cell size with the largest cells having abundant lipid.

Right: A different area of the same tumor with cells arranged in short cords. Some nuclei are densely pyknotic.

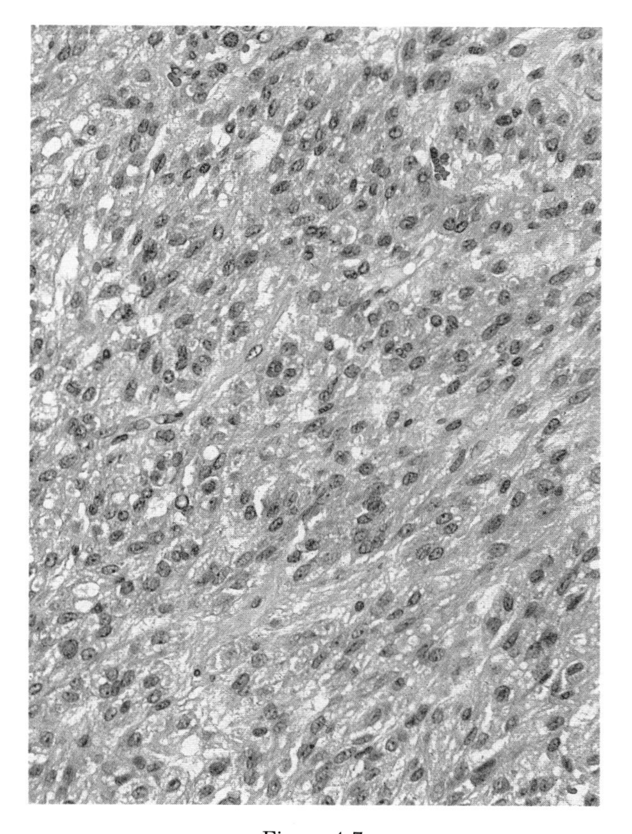

Figure 4-7
ADRENAL CORTICAL ADENOMA
This cortisol producing adrenal cortical adenoma has an ill-defined spindle cell pattern. More conventional histology was present in other fields.

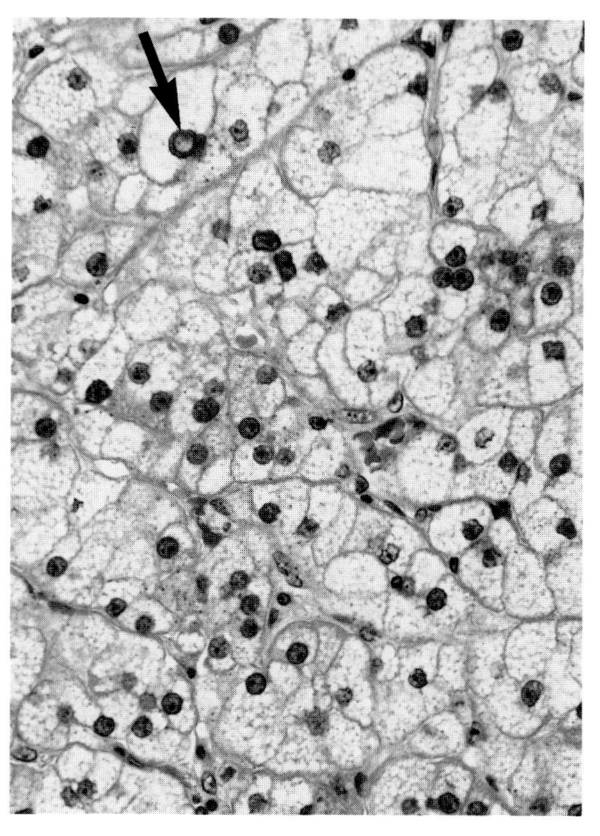

Figure 4-8
ADRENAL CORTICAL ADENOMA
ASSOCIATED WITH CUSHING'S SYNDROME
Individual tumor cells contain abundant lipid which appears as numerous clear vacuoles. The nuclei are fairly regular and round to oval, and most have a small dot-like nucleolus. Cytoplasmic borders are distinct. Note the nuclear "pseudoinclusion" (arrow).

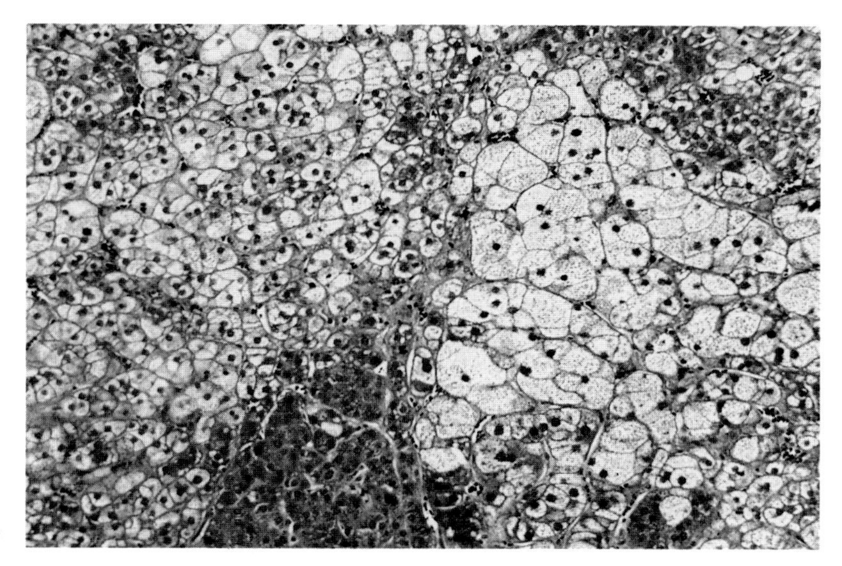

Figure 4-9
ADRENAL CORTICAL ADENOMA
A histologic field in a cortisol-producing adrenal cortical adenoma. There are nests of large lipid-rich cells (analogous to those of the zona fasciculata) along with smaller nests of cells resembling those of the zona glomerulosa, and cells having compact, eosinophilic cytoplasm resembling zona reticularis–type cells. Some cells in other fields had intermediate or transitional features.

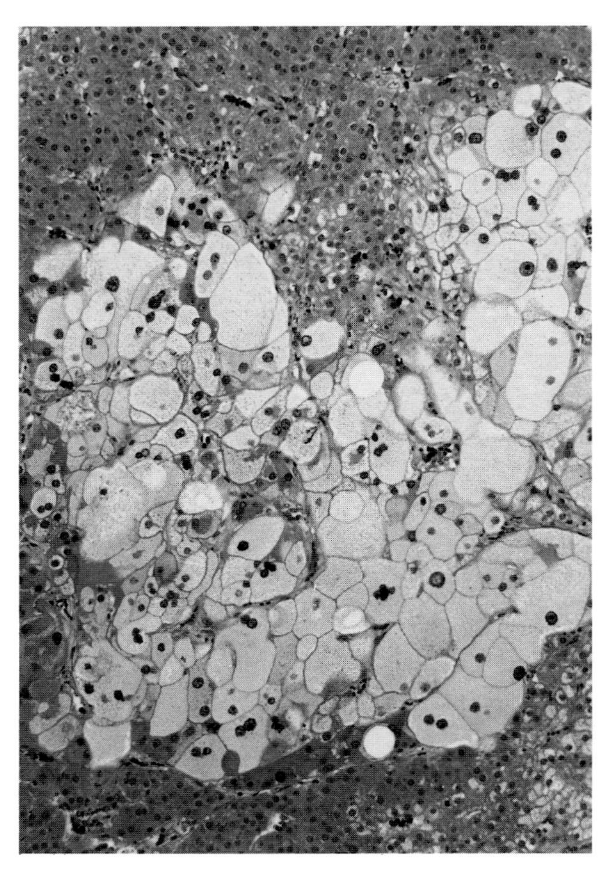

Figure 4-10
"BALLOON CELLS"
"Balloon cells" within an adrenal cortical adenoma from a patient with Cushing's syndrome. The enlarged cells have greatly expanded cytoplasm which is lipid rich. Some balloon cells are nearly 10-fold larger in diameter than the smaller cells within the adenoma.

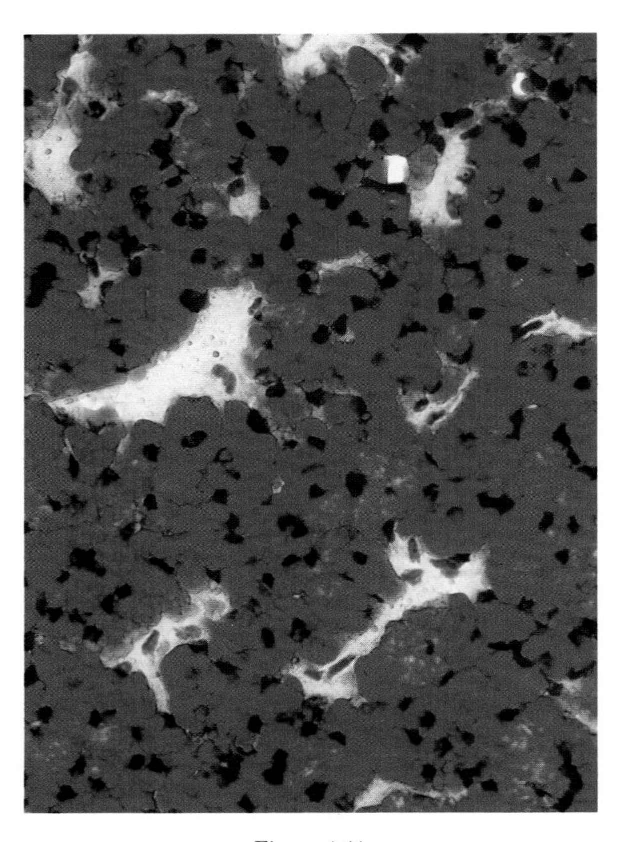

Figure 4-11
ADRENAL CORTICAL ADENOMA
Cells of this adrenal cortical adenoma contain abundant neutral lipid. (X220, oil red O stain)

sizes. Staining of fresh frozen tumor with oil red O demonstrates the abundant amount of intracytoplasmic lipid (fig. 4-11).

Tumor cell nuclei are usually single and round to oval; margination of chromatin along the nuclear membrane produces a vesicular appearance. Most nuclei contain a single dot-like nucleolus which is central or eccentric in location. There may be some nuclear enlargement and hyperchromasia, but these are usually focal in distribution and moderate in degree (fig. 4-12) (14). There may be a few nuclear "pseudoinclusions." These pseudoinclusions have the same quality and intensity of cytoplasmic staining as the rest of the cell or adjoining cells, or may be pale or vacuolated. There may be areas of lipomatous (fig. 4-13) or myelolipomatous metaplasia. On rare occasion monomorphous aggregates of mature lymphocytes can be observed (fig. 4-14), and it may be difficult to distinguish between a metaplastic process and an inflammatory reaction. Mitotic figures are quite rare, at least in ACAs occurring in adults, and atypical mitotic figures are exceptional. If several mitoses or atypical mitoses are present in consecutive high-power fields of a cortical neoplasm in an adult, these findings should be correlated with other clinical and pathologic features that indicate malignancy. An unusual finding in ACA is protrusion of tumor into venous tributaries of the central vein. An intact layer of endothelium over the tumor is usually due to intraluminal extension through discontinuities in the muscular wall of the vessel and not true vascular invasion. This phenomenon may or may not be apparent in the plane of section being observed (fig. 4-15). Similar

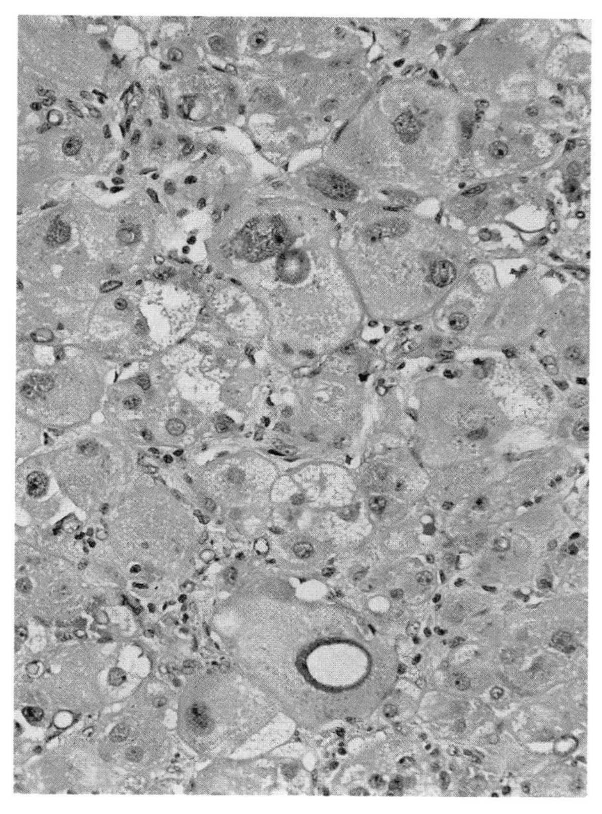

Figure 4-12
ADRENAL CORTICAL ADENOMA

Cells with compact eosinophilic cytoplasm have enlarged hyperchromatic nuclei, some with prominent nucleoli. Some cells show nearly a 5-fold variation in nuclear size. Some compact cells contain pigmented granular material representing lipofuscin. A prominent nuclear "pseudoinclusion" is present in the lower part of field.

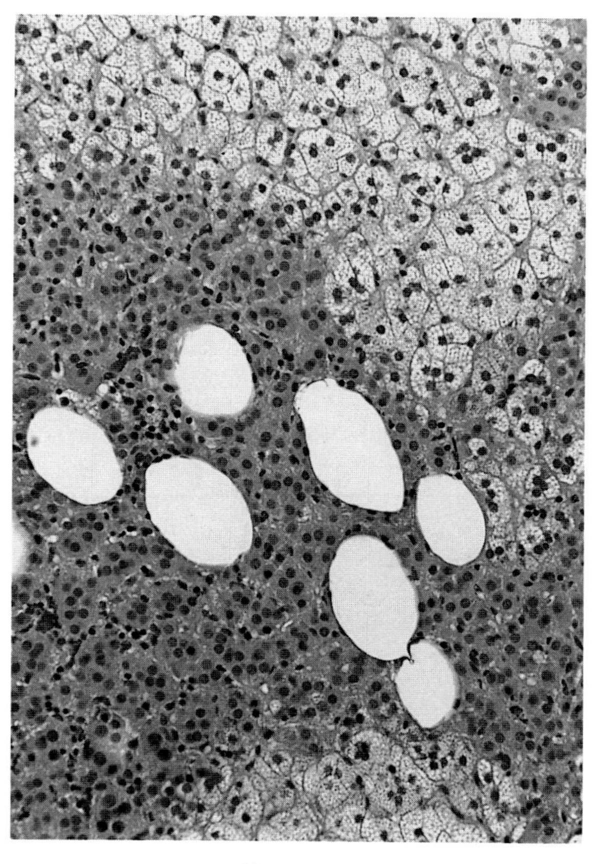

Figure 4-13
ADRENAL CORTICAL ADENOMA

Mixed composition of pale-staining, lipid-rich cells and cells with more compact, lipid-poor cytoplasm. Lipomatous metaplasia is also present.

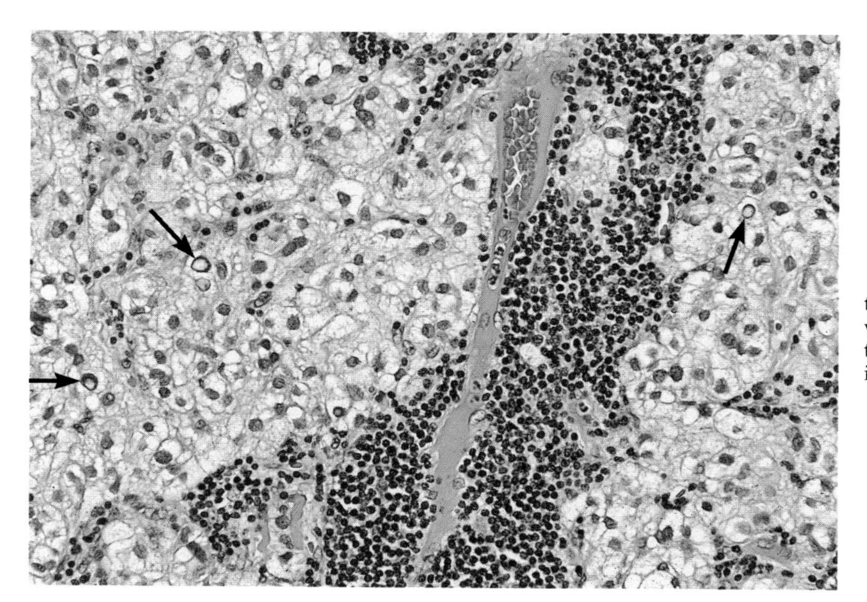

Figure 4-14
ADRENAL CORTICAL ADENOMA

This adrenal cortical adenoma contained collections of mature lymphocytes without hematopoietic cells or adipose tissue. There are a few nuclear "pseudoinclusions" (arrows).

to incidentally discovered adrenal nodules outlined in chapter 3, some ACAs have degenerative features such as fibrosis, organizing fibrin-rich thrombi within sinusoids (fig. 4-16, left), dystrophic calcification, or even metaplastic bone formation (fig. 4-16, right).

While these architectural and cytologic features are characteristic for ACAs associated with Cushing's syndrome, they are not pathognomonic, and clinical and endocrinologic correlation is needed to ascertain the associated endocrine syndrome (14). Without proper correlation it may not be possible to distinguish the ACA from an incidental dominant macronodule or nonhyperfunctional adenoma. Important clues can be provided by careful examination of the attached adrenal remnant (or the contralateral gland, as the case may be), since there is almost invariably some degree of adrenal cortical atrophy in association with Cushing's syndrome (fig. 4-17).

Pheochromocytomas with lipid degeneration are occasionally reported and can mimic an ACA grossly and microscopically (19,23). If the pheochromocytoma also happens to be ectopically producing adrenocorticotrophic hormone (ACTH) with Cushing's syndrome, the distinction may become even more difficult. A mixed ACA-pheochromocytoma (corticomedullary adenoma) has been reported in association with Cushing's syndrome (16). Other unusual associations include a separate nonfunctional ACA in the same adrenal gland with a pheochromocytoma (11); adrenal medullary hyperplasia associated with ACA, with or without Cushing's syndrome (7,13); ACA and ganglioneuroblastoma in a child with both Cushing's syndrome and virilization (9); and a case of pseudohermaphroditism in a woman with an ACA associated with both Cushing's syndrome and virilization (8). Exacerbation of autoimmune thyroid dysfunction has been reported after removal of an ACA in a patient with Cushing's syndrome; it was postulated to be related to a decrease in glucocorticoid secretion by the tumor (20).

Electron Microscopic Findings. Most tumor cells are remarkable for the abundant amount of intracytoplasmic lipid droplets, which vary in size and density from cell to cell (fig. 4-18). As might be suspected from the light microscopic heterogeneity of some of these tumors, some cells contain little or no lipid (fig. 4-19). As in the normal adrenal gland, there may be prominent microvillous projections along the cell borders. Smooth endoplasmic reticulum may be abundant, and occasional rudimentary intercellular attachments are seen (fig. 4-20). The nuclear "pseudoinclusion" is due to an irregularity in the nuclear membrane, with indentation and infolding of cell cytoplasm, often with the same complement and density of cellular organelles (fig. 4-21). Mitochondria may be prominent, and are usually round to oval although some may be elongated or distorted in shape. The mitochondrial cristae often have a tubular or vesicular profile (fig. 4-22) similar to cells of the zona fasciculata, or there may be lamellar cristae morphologically resembling zona reticularis cells (14,15,22).

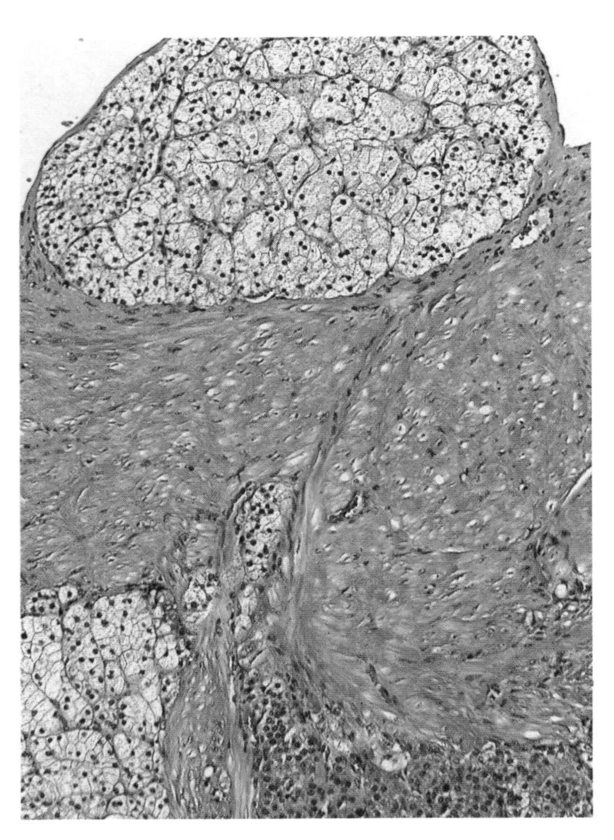

Figure 4-15
ADRENAL CORTICAL ADENOMA
This adrenal cortical adenoma weighed 17 g and measured 2.7 cm in diameter. Note the intraluminal vascular protrusion by tumor. Complete discontinuity in the smooth muscle bundles can account for this rare finding, but may not be apparent in the particular plane of section. This fortuitous finding does not constitute true vascular invasion.

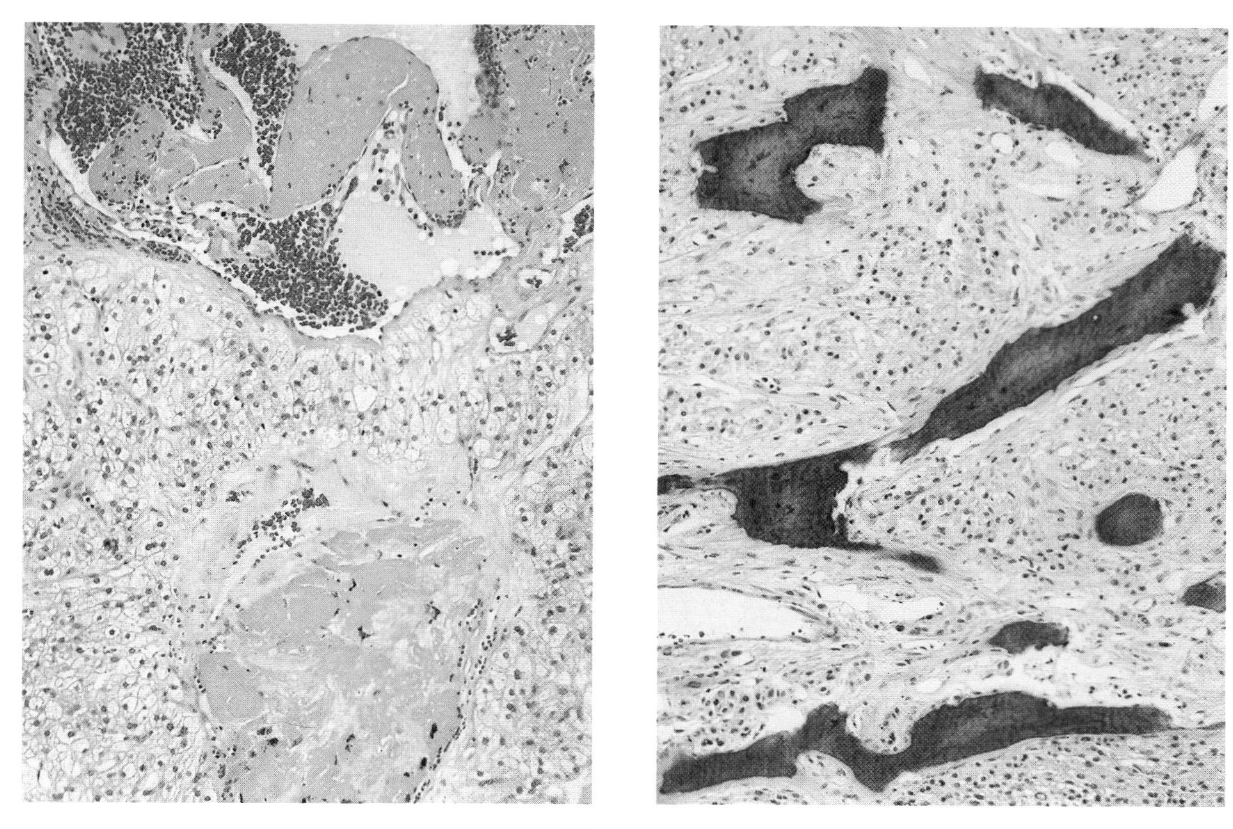

Figure 4-16
ADRENAL CORTICAL ADENOMA ASSOCIATED WITH CUSHING'S SYNDROME
Left: Central areas of adrenal cortical adenoma have irregular vascular spaces partially occluded by organizing fibrin-rich thrombi. Right: Another area in the same cortical adenoma shows metaplastic bone formation in association with fibrotic stroma.

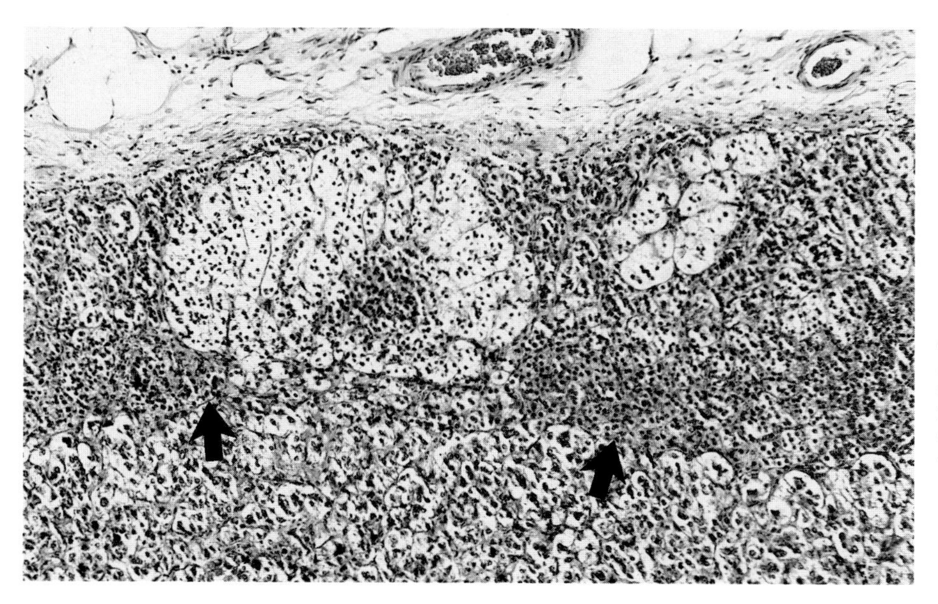

Figure 4-17
ATTACHED ADRENAL REMNANT IN CORTICAL ADENOMA ASSOCIATED WITH CUSHING'S SYNDROME
Note the marked degree of cortical atrophy. The cortex measures well under 1 mm in thickness throughout. Small micronodules are also seen. The cortical medullary junction is indicated by arrows.

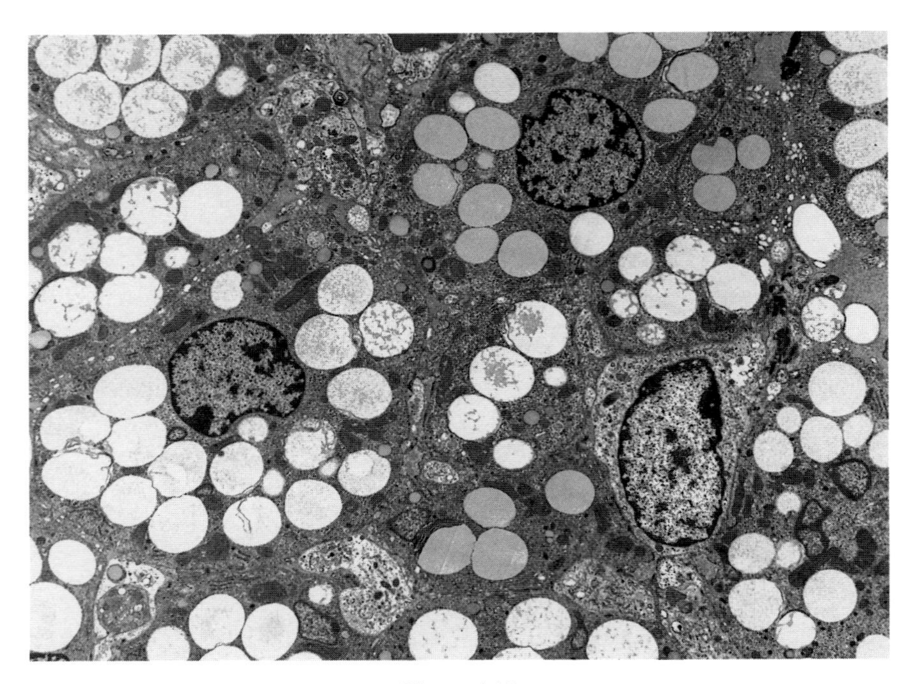

Figure 4-18

ADRENAL CORTICAL ADENOMA ASSOCIATED WITH CUSHING'S SYNDROME

The tumor cells contain prominent lipid droplets which vary slightly in size and electron density. Mitochondria are slightly pleomorphic. (X3,500)

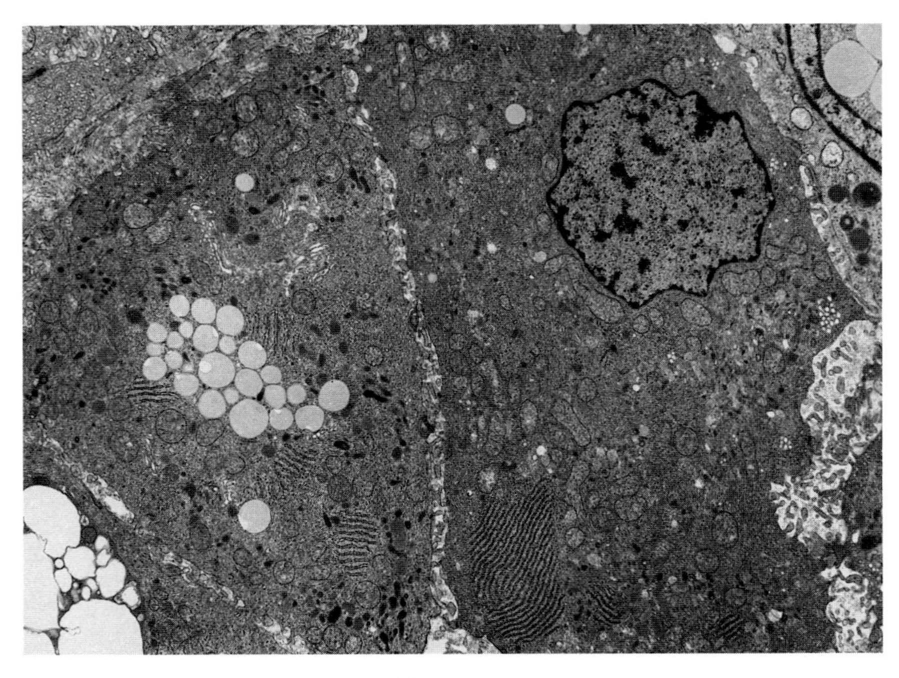

Figure 4-19

ADRENAL CORTICAL ADENOMA ASSOCIATED WITH CUSHING'S SYNDROME

The tumor cells contain only scant to minimal lipid droplets which are small in size relative to those in figure 4-18. Note the stacks of rough endoplasmic reticulum. The cells have prominent microvillous projections along cytoplasmic borders. Clusters of mildly pleomorphic dense granules probably represent primary lysosomes. (X3,500)

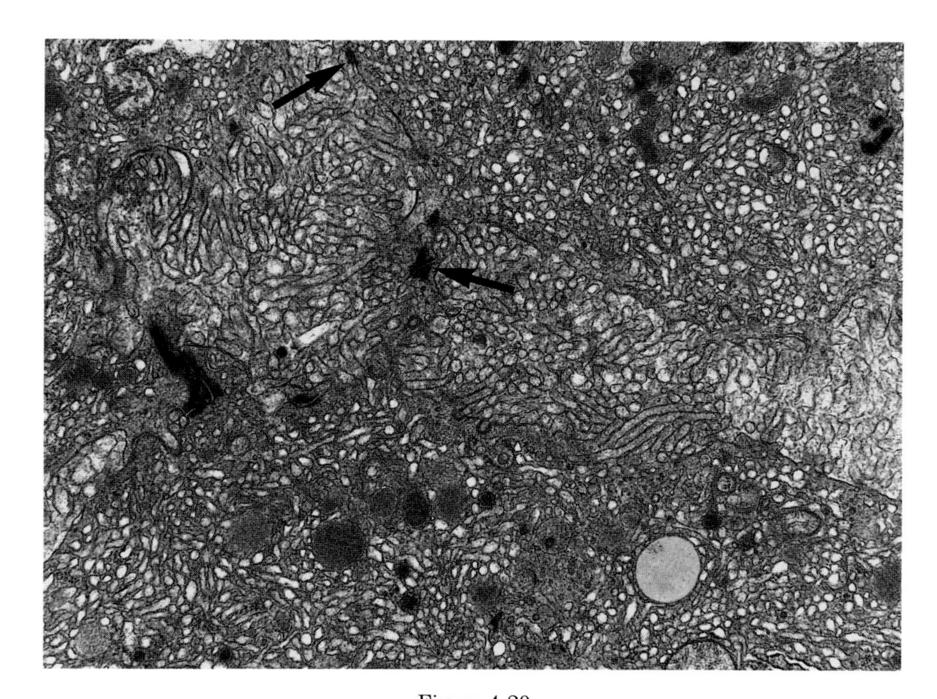

Figure 4-20

ADRENAL CORTICAL ADENOMA ASSOCIATED WITH CUSHING'S SYNDROME

The tumor cells contain abundant smooth endoplasmic reticulum which appears as tubular or vesicular profiles depending upon the plane of section. Note the few rudimentary intercellular attachments (arrows). (X14,000)

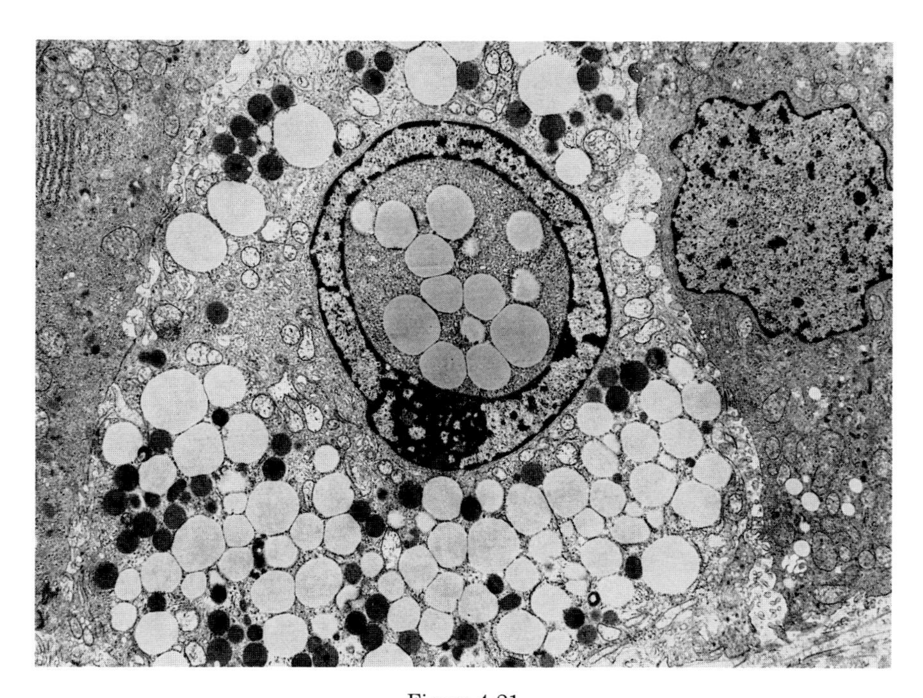

Figure 4-21

ADRENAL CORTICAL ADENOMA ASSOCIATED WITH CUSHING'S SYNDROME

Nuclear "pseudoinclusion" viewed en face in an adrenal cortical adenoma with Cushing's syndrome. The structure is nonspecific and results from irregular deep infolding of nuclear membrane. (X4,200)

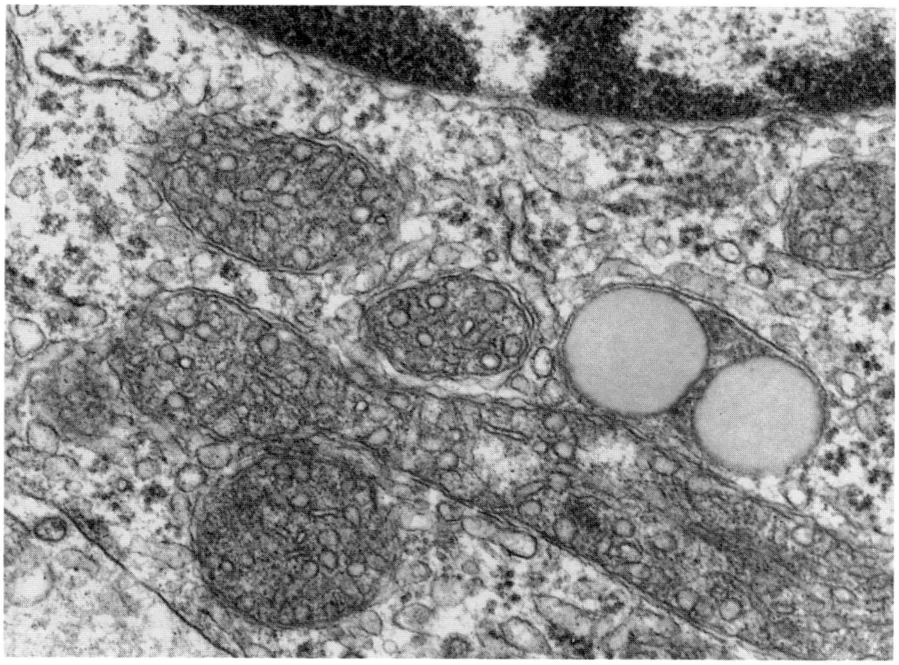

Figure 4-22
ADRENAL CORTICAL ADENOMA ASSOCIATED WITH CUSHING'S SYNDROME

Mitochondrial cristae have the tubular or vesicular profile typical of steroid-producing cells. Note the small components of rough endoplasmic reticulum and free polyribosomes. (X55,500)

FUNCTIONAL PIGMENTED ("BLACK") ADENOMA

Clinical Features. A diffusely pigmented or "black" adenoma is quite rare, particularly when small incidental pigmented nodules, many of which are not truly neoplastic in the classic sense, are excluded (29). Over 20 cases of black adenomas have been recorded in the literature, mostly as individual case reports, and most have been associated with Cushing's syndrome (28,29). Occasionally, these adenomas have resulted in primary hyperaldosteronism (24,25). There is a distinct predilection for female patients, and most tumors are diagnosed in the third to fifth decades of life. The tumors usually weigh less than 35 g, and measure 2 to 3 cm in diameter (29). Black ACAs have been reported to have a higher radiologic density with CT (27); this is probably due to a predominance of cells with compact, lipid-depleted cytoplasm and abundant lipofuscin (fig. 4-23). Some have proposed the designation "adrenal cortical adenoma with excess pigment deposition" (28) since there does not appear to be enough justification for separating these tumors from the more prevalent "yellow" adenomas.

Pathologic Findings. Black ACAs can present a striking gross appearance, which in the extreme, would seem to warrant a separate designation even if it is merely a descriptive one (fig. 4-24). Some tumors have been characterized as dark brown to yellowish (light) brown. When the pigmented adrenal mass is dark brown to black, other adrenal lesions enter into the differential diagnosis, such as adrenal hematoma and metastatic or primary malignant melanoma. Microscopically, the architectural patterns of black ACAs are comparable to other ACAs without excessive lipochrome pigment (fig. 4-25): most tumors are composed predominantly or entirely of cells with compact, eosinophilic cytoplasm similar to but larger than cells of the zona reticularis (fig. 4-25A). There is a variable amount of brown or golden brown pigment within the cytoplasm which may show some sparing of the immediate perinuclear zone. Clusters of pale-staining, lipid-rich cells may be found and occasionally there are foci of lipomatous or myelolipomatous metaplasia within the tumor (fig. 4-25B). The case illustrated in figure 4-25C also had striking lipomatous metaplasia in the atrophic attached cortex. Special stains can document the staining characteristics of lipofuscin: a positive argentaffin reaction

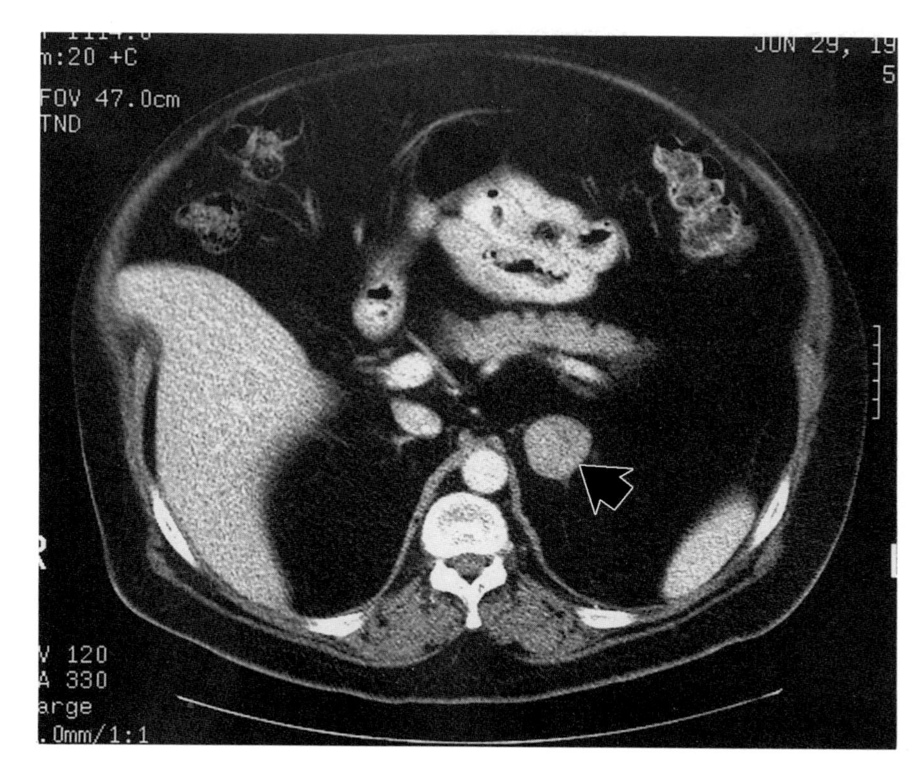

Figure 4-23
"BLACK" ADRENAL CORTICAL ADENOMA CAUSING CUSHING'S SYNDROME

The adrenal tumor on the left side (arrow) was mildly heterogeneous both before and after contrast enhancement. There is slight contrast enhancement on CT scan, raising the possibility of either primary or secondary malignancy. (Figures 4-23 and 4-24 are from the same case.)

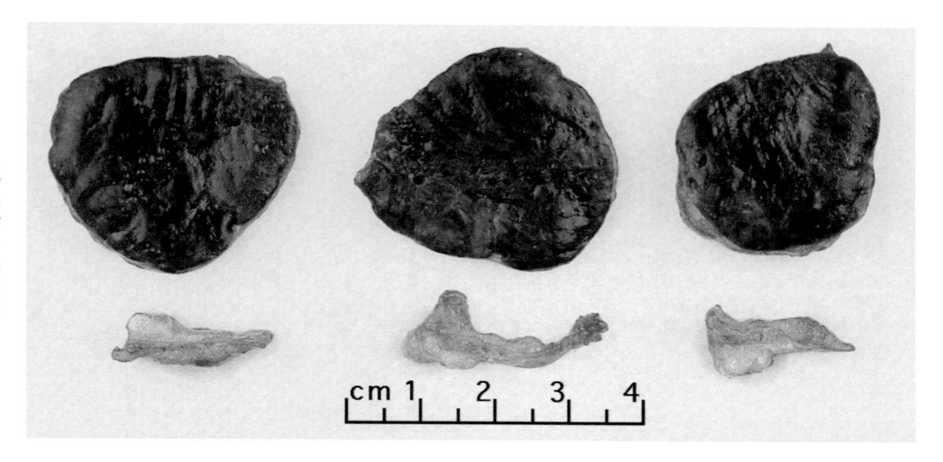

Figure 4-24
"BLACK" ADRENAL CORTICAL ADENOMA

This adenoma was resected from a 58-year-old man with Cushing's syndrome. The tumor weighed about 30 g and measured 2.9 x 2.8 x 2.5 cm. Cross sections of tumor became even darker after exposure of cut surface to air.

with the Fontana-Masson stain which is susceptible to bleaching procedures, a reddish-orange tint with periodic acid–Schiff (PAS) stain, and a negative reaction to iron stain (29). A recent study of "black pigmented adrenal nodules" (26) suggested that neuromelanin, similar to the pigment reported in the black thyroid syndrome, may be present (30).

Electron Microscopic Findings. On ultrastructural study, the tumor cells have a variable amount of cytoplasm; the cytoplasm is relatively poor in lipid droplets, and the lipid droplets that are present may be few in number and small in size. Some cells have such electron-dense cytoplasm that evaluation of cellular organelles such as mitochondria may be difficult in survey views. Tumor cells are polygonal or rounded with occasional simple intercellular attachments; there may be microvillous projections along cell borders (fig. 4-26). Most cells contain a variable

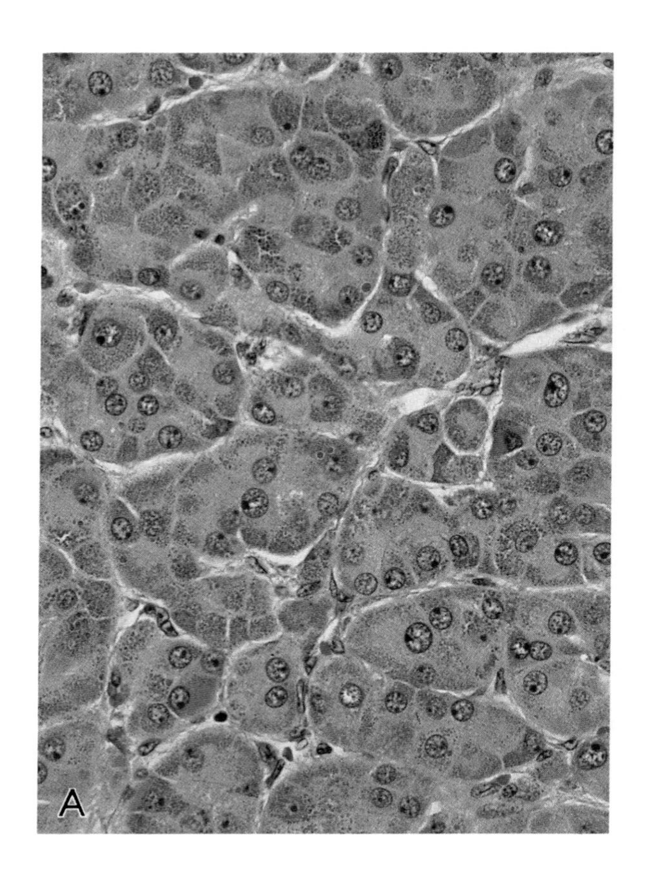

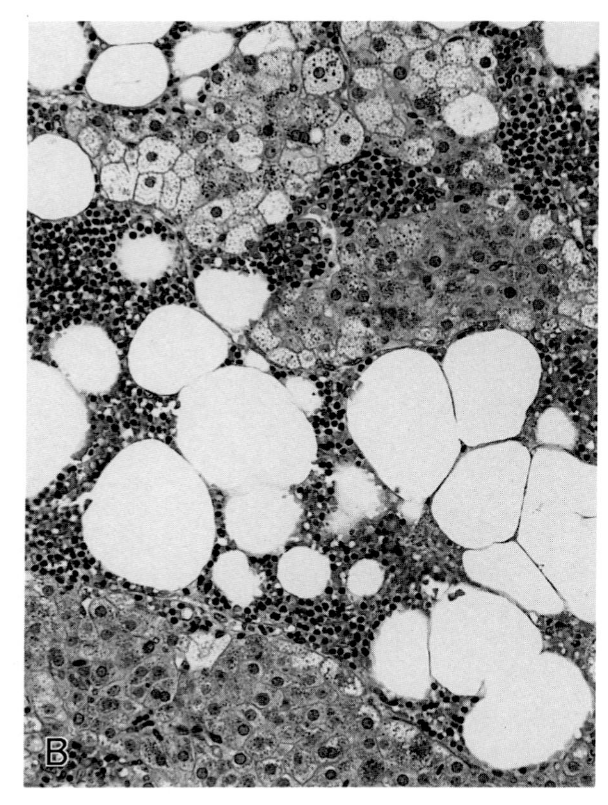

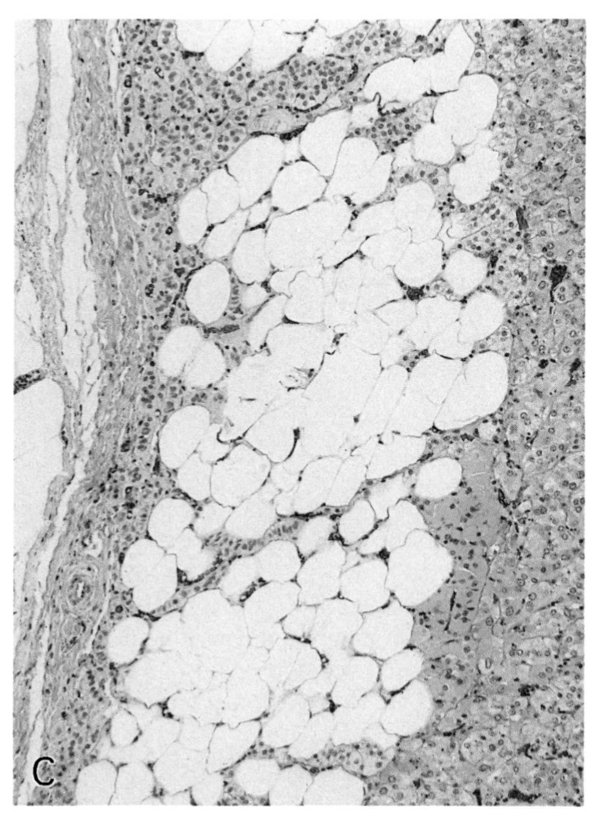

Figure 4-25
"BLACK" ADENOMA ASSOCIATED WITH CUSHING'S SYNDROME

A: The tumor cells have compact, eosinophilic cytoplasm and contain abundant lipofuscin. The nuclei have dispersed chromatin with small central to eccentric nucleoli. Cells are arranged in short cords and alveoli.

B: Areas of prominent myelolipomatous metaplasia were present.

C: The attached adrenal remnant shows marked cortical atrophy with prominent lipomatous metaplasia.

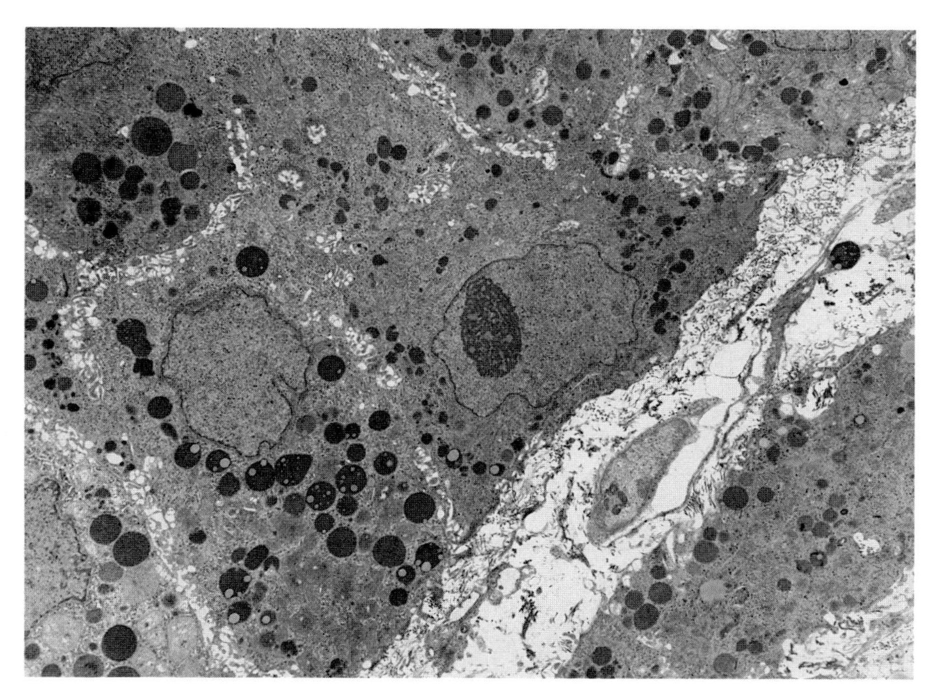

Figure 4-26
"BLACK" ADENOMA ASSOCIATED WITH CUSHING'S SYNDROME

The tumor cells contain abundant lipofuscin and have only sparse lipid droplets. Note the microvillous projections along cytoplasmic borders. (X3,500) (Figures 4-26 and 4-27 are from the same case.)

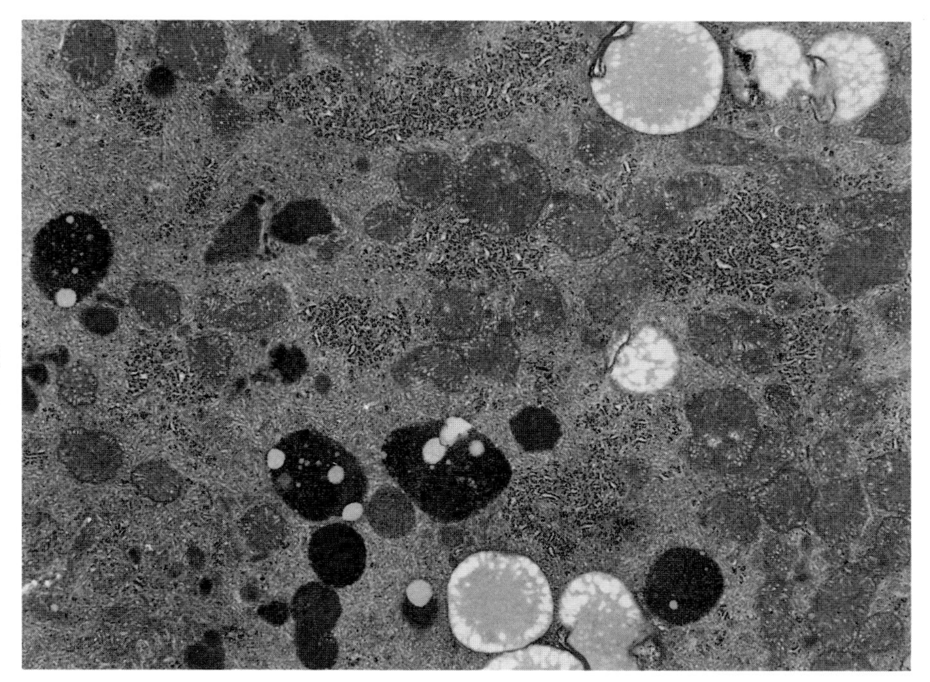

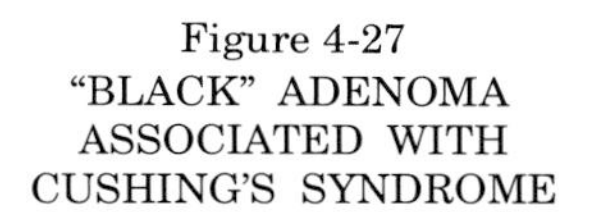

Figure 4-27
"BLACK" ADENOMA ASSOCIATED WITH CUSHING'S SYNDROME

The tumor cells have sparse lipid droplets. Note the abundant smooth endoplasmic reticulum with short profiles of rough endoplasmic reticulum and free polyribosomes. (X4,000)

number of electron-dense granules, often with a small lipid component, which is typical for lipofuscin. Some granules appear membrane bound. There are typically no pigment granules with ultrastructural features of melanosomes or premelanosomes. There may be prominent mitochondria, which are round or elongated, with irregular tubular (or lamellar) cristae. Profiles of rough and smooth endoplasmic reticulum may be found along with free ribosomes (fig. 4-27).

ADRENAL CORTICAL ADENOMA WITH PRIMARY HYPERALDOSTERONISM (CONN'S SYNDROME)

Conn described the clinical syndrome which came to bear his name in 1955 (41). It has classically been attributed to an underlying aldosterone-secreting ACA ("aldosteronoma"), although on occasion, the primary hyperaldosteronism can be due to an adrenal cortical carcinoma (61). Primary hyperaldosteronism occurs in about 2 percent of patients with systemic hypertension (53), although some estimate that the prevalence among unselected hypertensive patients is less than 1 percent (36). Conn suggested that primary hyperaldosteronism (due to an ACA) may be the cause of as much as 20 percent of all cases of essential hypertension (40). This was based in part on an autopsy study that reported ACAs of 1.5 cm or larger in as much as 20 percent of hypertensive patients (73). It is unclear whether the adrenal adenoma (or nodule) was the cause of the hypertension or a result of it (e.g., from localized ischemia due to capsular arteriopathy) (47). It has also been suggested that Conn's syndrome may exist for many years before symptoms or signs of potassium deficiency appear (40). Since some studies have shown that occasional patients may be normokalemic, measurement of serum potassium is not entirely reliable as a screening test (36,37,54). In patients with essential hypertension there is biochemical evidence that content of aldosterone and corticosterone in cortical nodules is similar to that of normal cortical tissue, and much less than that of aldosterone-producing ACAs (59,63). A variation in functional phenotype in vitro has also been reported with adenoma cells that predominantly produce cortisol under the influence of ACTH (64). One could argue that with time there is conversion of glomerulosa type cells to other types of cortical cells with different functional characteristics, and when the incidental ACA (or nodule) is discovered, without the expected biochemical profile of an aldosterone-secreting ACA, hypertension may already be established (61).

There are few population-based studies on the incidence rate of Conn's syndrome. In a recent study, the average annual incidence rate in the Danish National Registry was 0.8 per million population (33). Most series report a predilection for female patients with ACA (54), but the preponderance of females overall with primary hyperaldosteronism appears to be declining with increasing recognition of the idiopathic form of the disorder. Most aldosterone-producing ACAs are diagnosed in the third to fifth decades of life (61,65,66), whereas about 80 percent of incidental cortical nodules are seen in the 50- to 80-year-old age group (47).

Prevalence of Different Forms of Primary Hyperaldosteronism. Early data suggested that 60 to nearly 90 percent of cases of primary hyperaldosteronism were due to an aldosterone-producing ACA (37,68), but with increasing recognition of mild forms of the disorder different data have emerged. Prior to 1970, 70 percent of cases at the Mayo Clinic were due to an aldosterone-producing ACA and 26 percent due to bilateral adrenal hyperplasia, but from 1978 through 1987 ACA accounted for 54 percent of primary hyperaldosteronism cases and 45 percent were due to hyperplasia (76). A different source estimates that idiopathic bilateral hyperplasia of the zona glomerulosa may account for as much as 70 to 80 percent of cases of primary hyperaldosteronism (53).

Gross Findings. Aldosterone-producing ACA is usually a small, unicentric neoplasm measuring only a few centimeters in diameter (fig. 4-28) (61). In one study, 92 percent of tumors were less than 2 cm in diameter (68), while in the review by Conn et al. (43), 72 percent of tumors were less than 3 cm and 69 percent weighed less than 6 g, although it is not clear whether this represented the entire adrenal gland or just the neoplasm. One of the larger ACAs reported by Neville and Symington (69) weighed 75 g, but the recorded weights of most tumors were under 10 g; the largest tumor among the 18 patients with Conn's syndrome was an adrenal cortical carcinoma weighing over 2,000 g. In a recent study, the median size of ACAs was 1.7 cm, and the smallest tumor detected on abdominal CT was 0.7 cm (48). Most tumors are unilateral and solitary, but occasional bilateral ACAs have been reported in 1 percent (72) to 6 percent (62) of cases. Bilateral ACAs were recently reported in a patient who had concurrent hypersecretion of aldosterone and cortisol (67). In a small percentage of cases, ACAs have been described as multiple but still unilateral (68). Most tumors are

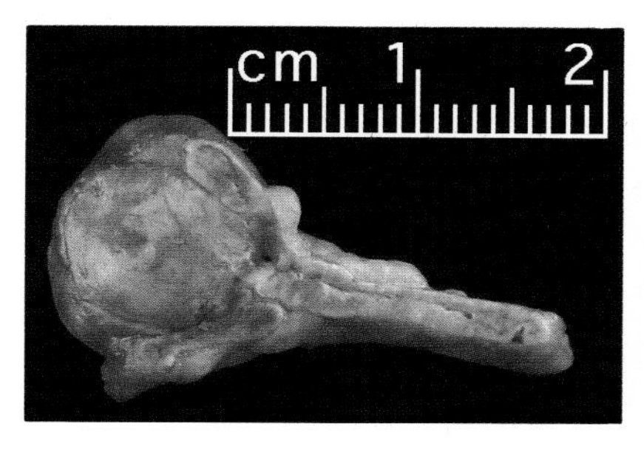

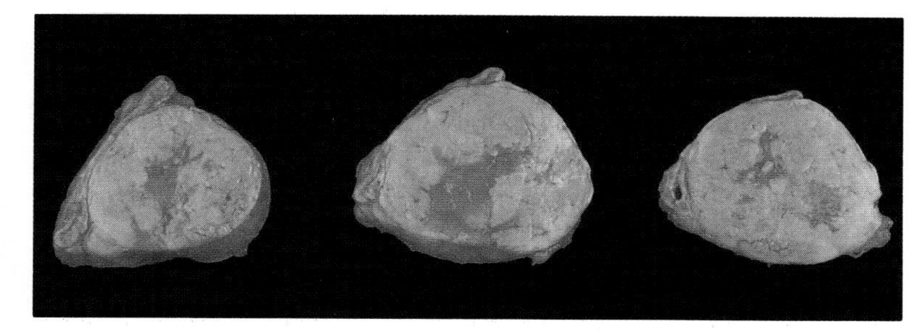

Figure 4-28
ALDOSTERONE-SECRETING ADRENAL CORTICAL ADENOMA

Left: The tumor is sharply demarcated and appears encapsulated, particularly where it expands the contours of the adrenal capsule (see MRI from figure 4-29). The remaining adrenal gland is grossly normal. The tumor measured only 1 cm in diameter.

Right: Resected right adrenal cortical adenoma in a different case measured 3 x 2.5 x 2 cm and on cross section is yellow-orange.

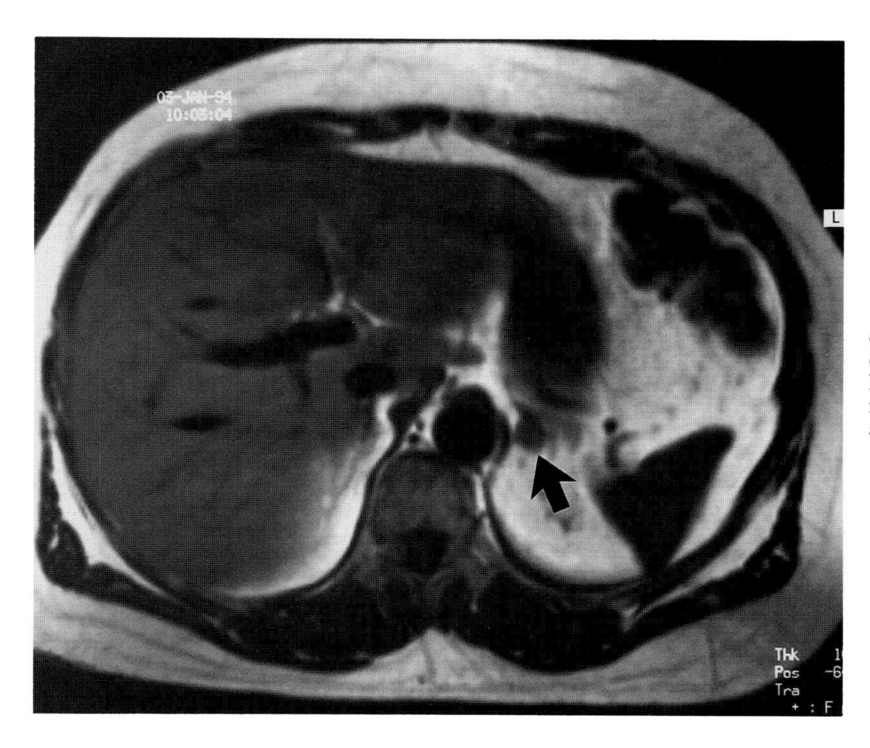

Figure 4-29
ALDOSTERONE-SECRETING ADRENAL CORTICAL ADENOMA

An aldosterone-secreting adrenal cortical adenoma was localized by abdominal MRI (left side, arrow). Patient had systemic hypertension, hypokalemia, and a small aldosterone-producing adrenal cortical adenoma.

large enough to be readily detected on abdominal CT scan or MRI (fig. 4-29); the sensitivity with CT scan is reported to be over 80 percent (48). The tumor may be obvious on gross examination of the intact gland, but occasionally it is difficult to appreciate because of its small size, and it may become apparent only after transverse sectioning of the gland. ACAs are usually round to ovoid, and sharply demarcated with what appears to be true encapsulation (fig. 4-28). The residual or attached adrenal cortex usually appears grossly normal without atrophy as is expected with Cushing's syndrome. ACAs have been described as homogenous, yellow-orange or "canary yellow" on cross section. Larger tumors may have areas of hemorrhage or cystic change (50,69). Adrenal venography has occasionally been complicated by venous thrombosis and marked intra-adrenal hemorrhage due to overzealous injection of contrast medium or wedging of the selective catheter; these complications are more likely in patients with Cushing's syndrome or

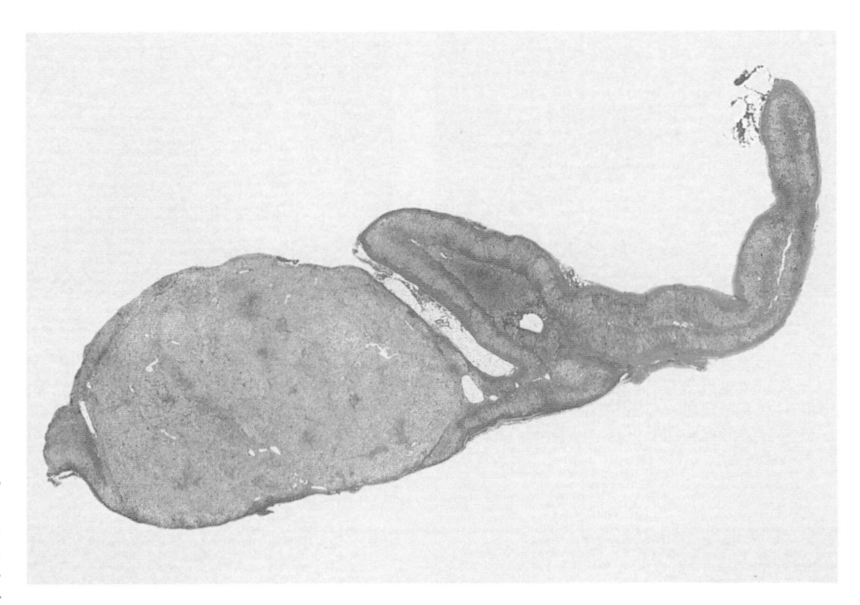

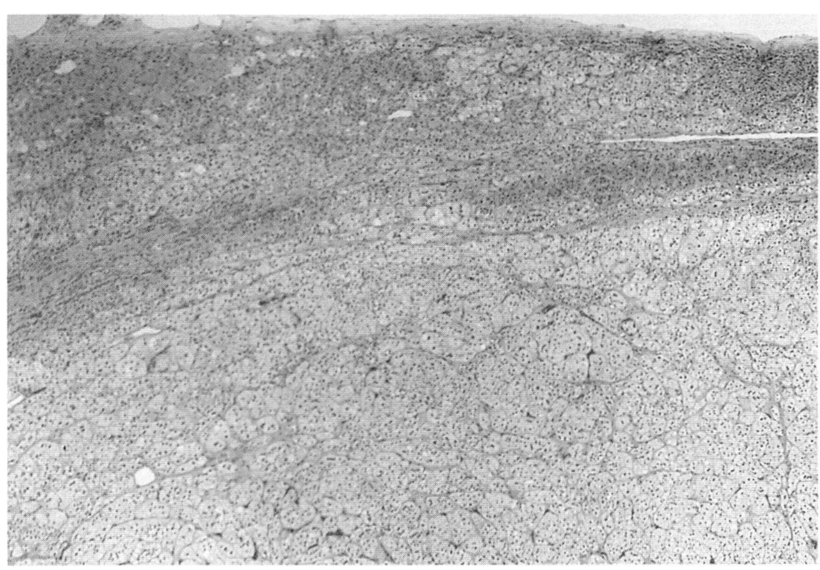

Figure 4-30
ALDOSTERONE-SECRETING ADRENAL CORTICAL ADENOMA

Top: Scanning view of an aldosterone-secreting adenoma. The tumor has expansile smooth borders with compression of adjacent adrenal parenchyma and expansion of adrenal capsule. Cross sectional aspect of the tumor may show some variation in staining density due to differences in lipid content of tumor cells.

Bottom: The borders of an aldosterone-secreting cortical adenoma compresses adjacent non-neoplastic cortical tissue.

Conn's syndrome due to excessive vascular fragility (46). On rare occasion, this vascular complication may result in prolonged remission from the manifestations of primary hyperaldosteronism (66). A heterotopic ACA in the lower pole of the kidney has also been reported to produce Conn's syndrome (51).

Microscopic Findings. In most instances, the gross impression of complete encapsulation is not borne out on low-power scanning of the pushing edges of the tumor (fig. 4-30). The ACA may appear partially (fig. 4-31) or even completely encapsulated, but often there is a compressed fibrous rim or fibrous "pseudocapsule" at the expansile borders of the tumor, or sometimes the tumor acquires part of its "capsule" from expansion of the adrenal capsule itself. A high incidence of associated small cortical nodules have been noted (58 percent) which may be related to the effects of hypertension rather than an additional cause of it (68). Tumor cells are arranged in a nesting or alveolar pattern (fig. 4-32, left), short cords, blunt anastomosing trabeculae (fig. 4-32, right), or mixtures of these architectural patterns.

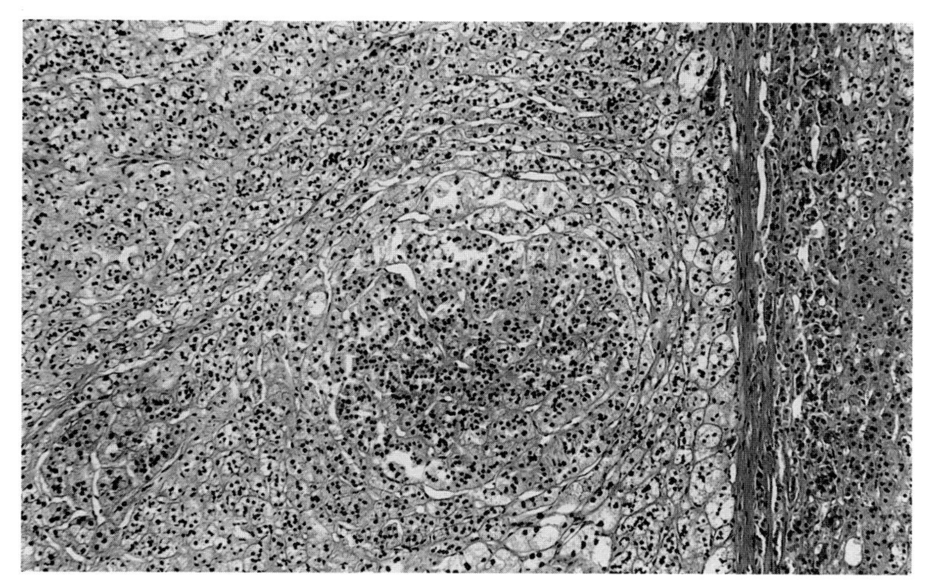

Figure 4-31
ALDOSTERONE-SECRETING ADRENAL CORTICAL ADENOMA

This aldosterone-secreting adrenal cortical adenoma has a thin fibrous capsule with compressed residual cortex on the right. There is faint micronodularity in this isolated field.

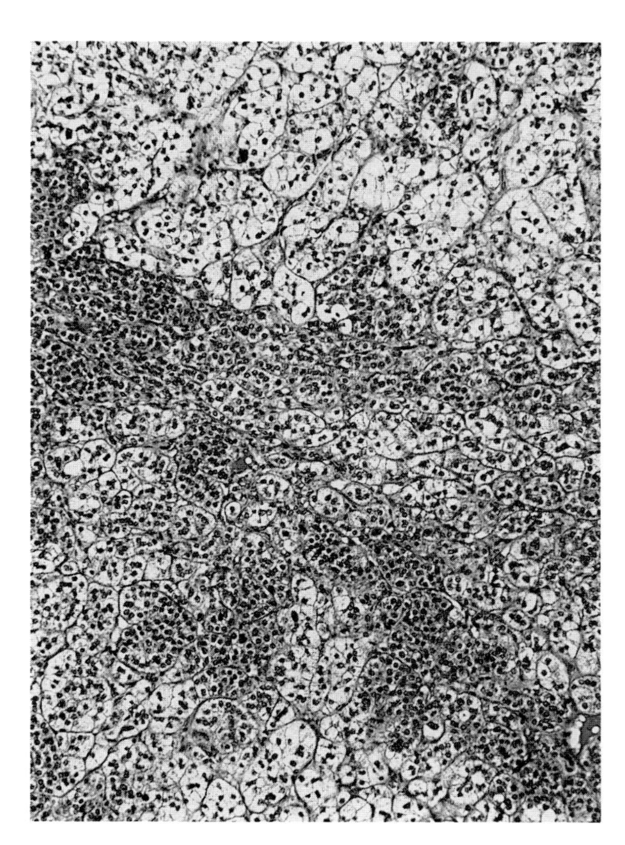

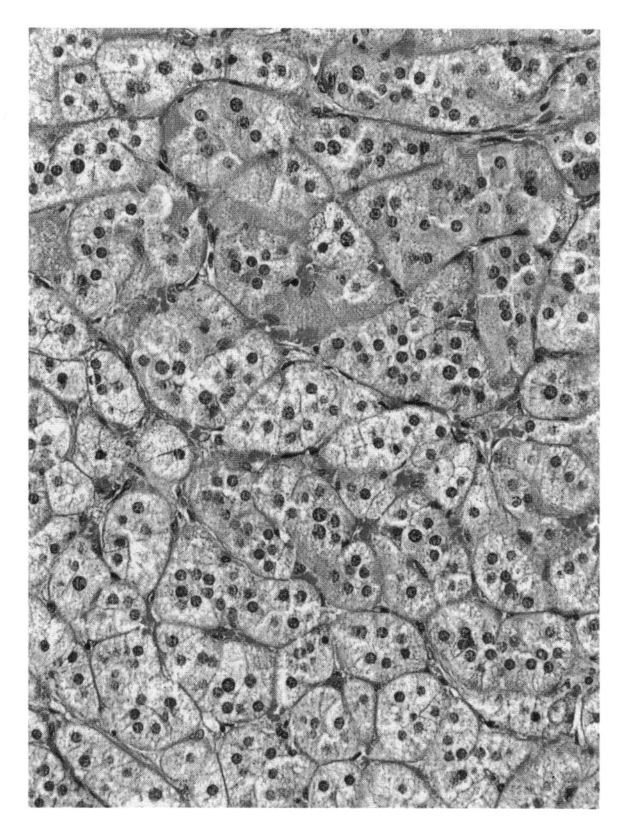

Figure 4-32
ALDOSTERONE-SECRETING ADRENAL CORTICAL ADENOMA

Left: The tumor cells have a nesting or alveolar pattern. Some cells are relatively small with diminutive lipid content while other larger cells have a moderate amount of lipid.

Right: The tumor cells are arranged in short cords and alveoli.

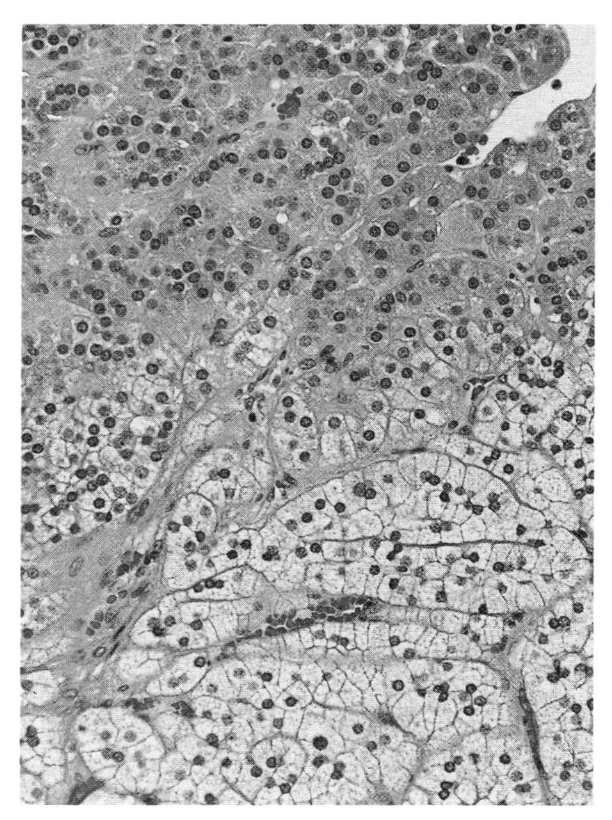

Figure 4-33
ALDOSTERONE-SECRETING
ADRENAL CORTICAL ADENOMA

Morphologically, there is a heterogeneous cell population ranging from cells which are large and lipid rich (analogous to those of zona fasciculata) to smaller cells with relatively sparse lipid (similar to those of zona glomerulosa) and cells with compact, eosinophilic cytoplasm resembling zona reticularis-type cells.

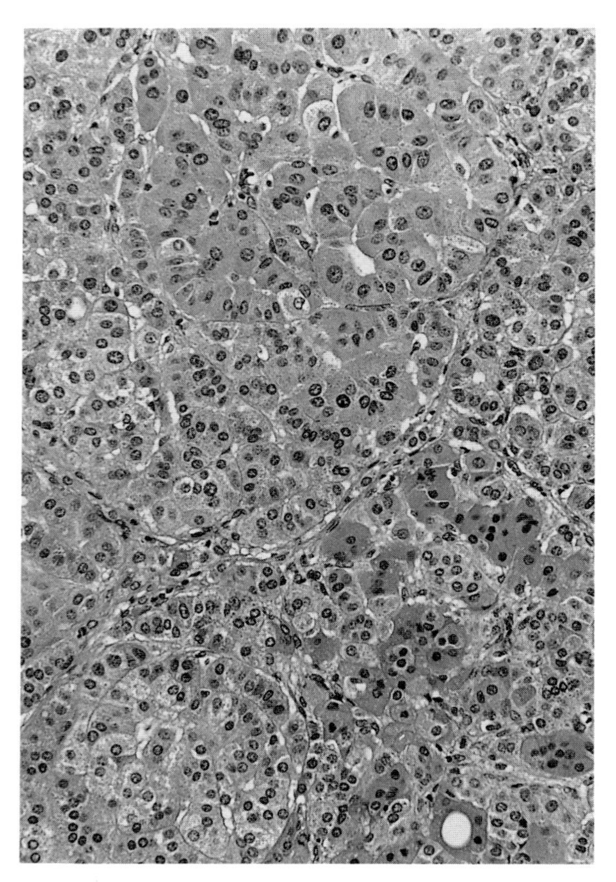

Figure 4-34
ALDOSTERONE-SECRETING
ADRENAL CORTICAL ADENOMA

Focal areas within the tumor consist of smaller, compact cells, some with sparse lipofuscin, as well as larger oncocytic cells with abundant granular pink cytoplasm.

Theoretically, most or all of the tumor should be composed of cells that strongly resemble those of the zona glomerulosa responsible for mineralocorticoid production, but such is far from the case. The morphology of individual cells may be quite heterogenous (fig. 4-33) (61). Four different types of cells have been recognized: 1) pale-staining, lipid-rich cells resembling, though larger than, zona fasciculata cells; 2) cells resembling zona glomerulosa cells with a higher nuclear/cytoplasmic ratio and only a small amount of vacuolated, lightly eosinophilic cytoplasm; 3) compact cells indistinguishable from those of the zona reticularis (although usually larger) or occasionally cells with oncocytic features (fig. 4-34); and 4) a group of cells designated as "hybrid" cells with cytologic features of both zona glomerulosa and zona fasciculata cells (69). Origin of ACA from a transitional or hybrid cell would be consistent with the functional behavior of these tumors, such as modulation of aldosterone secretion by ACTH, lack of responsiveness to angiotensin II, the ability to produce cortisol, and secretion of hybrid steroids. Some tumors probably arise from glomerulosa type cells (52). Some studies have reported that the zona glomerulosa–type cells and compact cells are more frequently present at the periphery of the tumor (69), whereas pale-staining cells are concentrated in more central areas (49,75). The large lipid-rich cells are most common; these cells coupled with the other lipid-rich cells give the tumor its characteristic golden yellow hue.

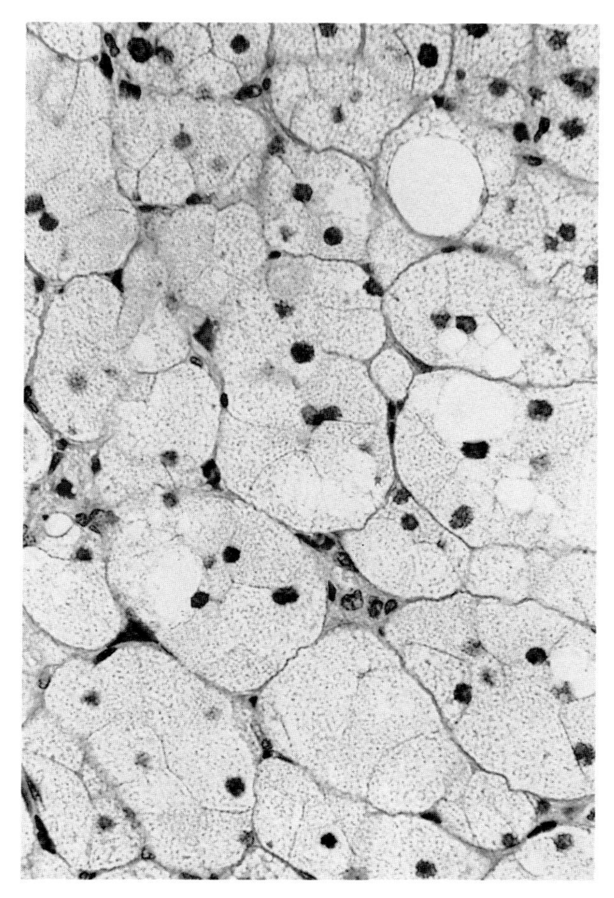

Figure 4-35
ALDOSTERONE-SECRETING
ADRENAL CORTICAL ADENOMA
This aldosterone-secreting adrenal cortical adenoma has areas with large lipid-rich "balloon cells."

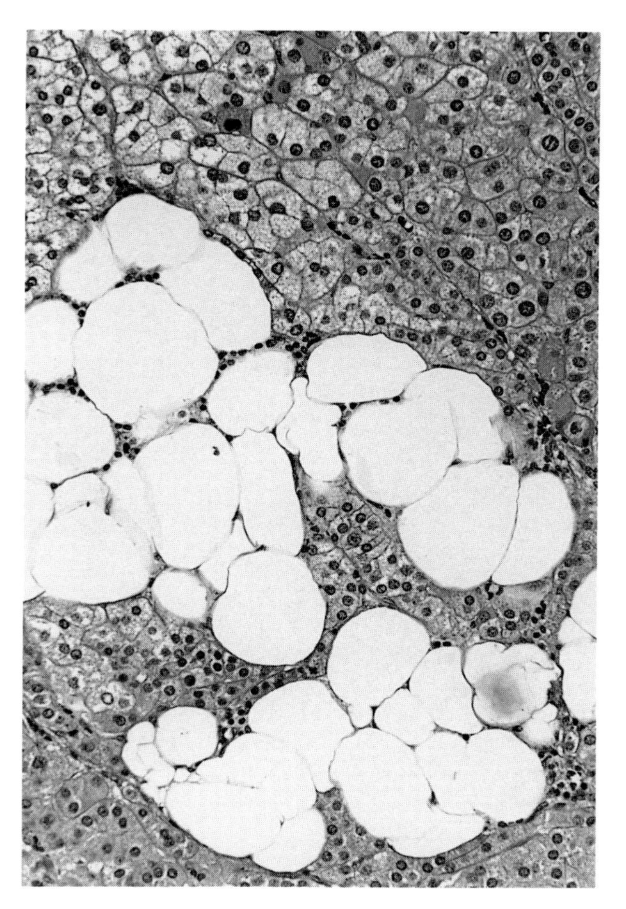

Figure 4-36
ALDOSTERONE-SECRETING
ADRENAL CORTICAL ADENOMA
Small areas of lipomatous metaplasia are present.

Occasionally there are small clusters of cells with abundant lipid-rich cytoplasm, so-called balloon cells, similar to those in ACAs associated with a different endocrine syndrome (fig. 4-35). The term hybrid cells, used to refer to the pale, lipid-rich cells of aldosterone-producing ACAs, emphasizes the capacity of these cells to elaborate hormones normally produced by either the zona glomerulosa (aldosterone) or the zona fasciculata (cortisol) (69). This is based upon the enzyme systems in the zona glomerulosa (18-oxidase system) and zona fasciculata (17-alpha–hydroxylase), and in vitro studies of tumors from patients with Conn's syndrome that produce cortisol, corticosterone, and aldosterone (34,35,38,44,63,70), which can also occur with ACTH stimulation (34,55).

Many cells have round to oval vesicular nuclei, often with a small, dot-like nucleolus. Some nuclei may be darkly pyknotic as seen in figure 4-35. There may also be a mild degree of nuclear pleomorphism in some tumors. Lipomatous or myelolipomatous metaplasia is an uncommon finding (fig. 4-36). Other unusual features include areas of interstitial fibrosis that are typically small and localized (fig. 4-37), chronic inflammatory infiltrates (fig. 4-38), and pseudoglandular foci with stringy basophilic material (fig. 4-39). These features are nonspecific, however, and one must correlate morphology with clinical and endocrinologic findings. A prominent infiltrate of mast cells has been reported in a large adrenal cortical tumor producing 11-deoxycorticosterone, with associated

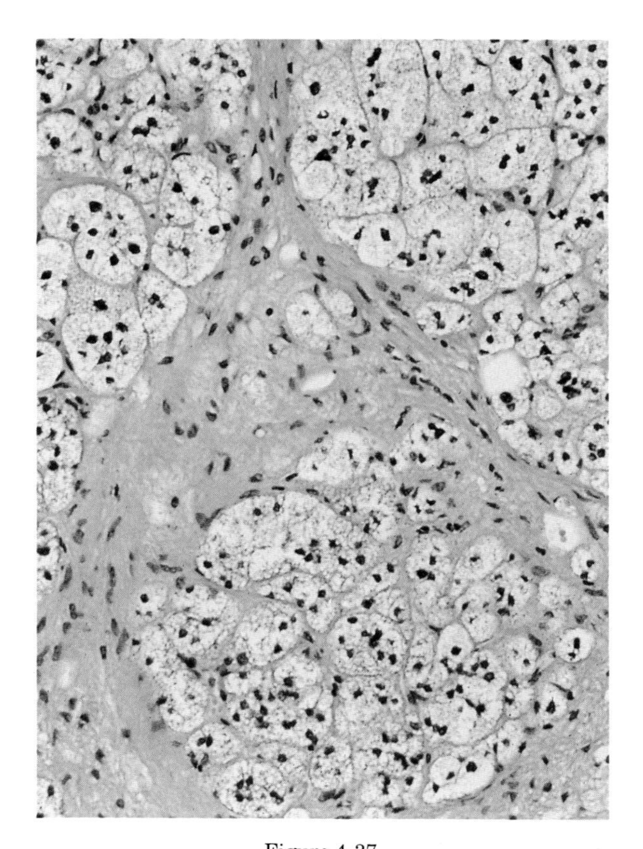

Figure 4-37
ALDOSTERONE-SECRETING
ADRENAL CORTICAL ADENOMA

Alveolar clusters of lipid-rich tumor cells are separated by bland fibrous connective tissue.

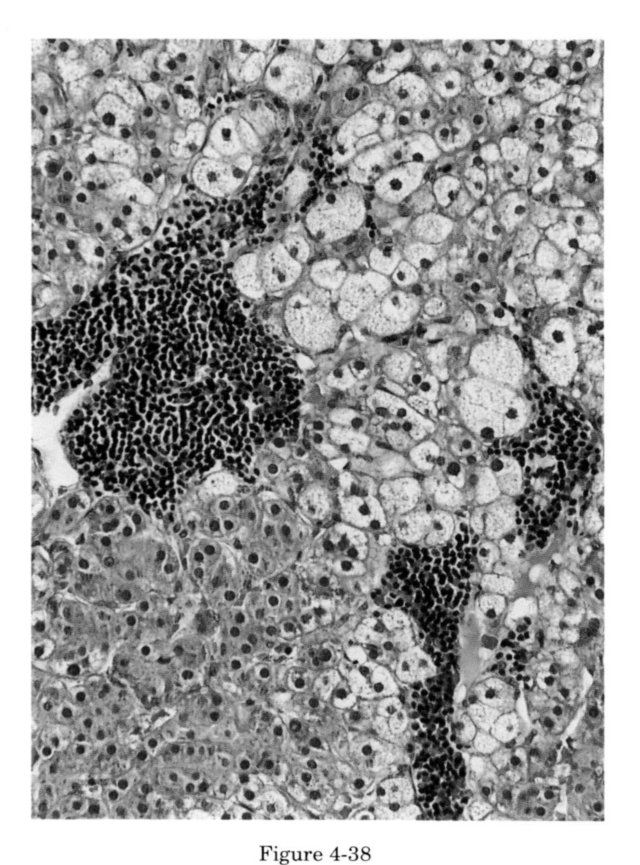

Figure 4-38
ALDOSTERONE-SECRETING
ADRENAL CORTICAL ADENOMA

This aldosterone-secreting adrenal adenoma contained a few aggregates of lymphocytes.

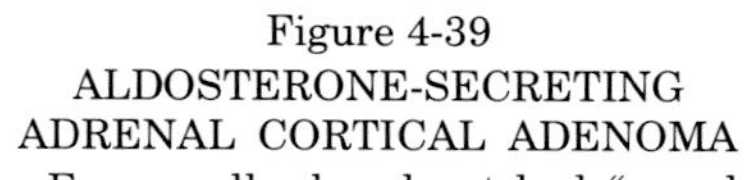

Figure 4-39
ALDOSTERONE-SECRETING
ADRENAL CORTICAL ADENOMA

Few small, sharply etched "pseudoglandular" spaces are present. No mucosubstances were identified with special stains.

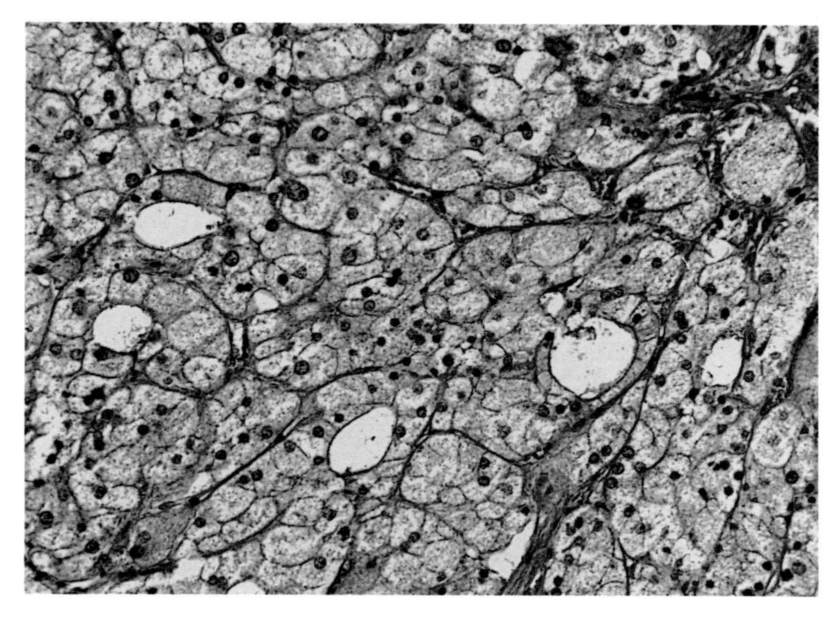

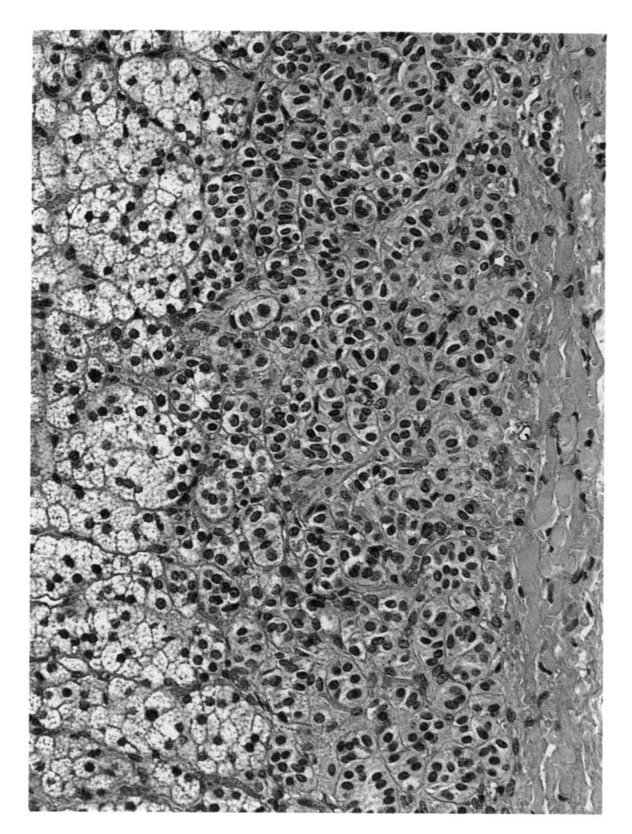

Figure 4-40
ALDOSTERONE-SECRETING
ADRENAL CORTICAL ADENOMA
A continuous zone of hyperplastic zona glomerulosa was evident in the non-neoplastic adrenal remnant.

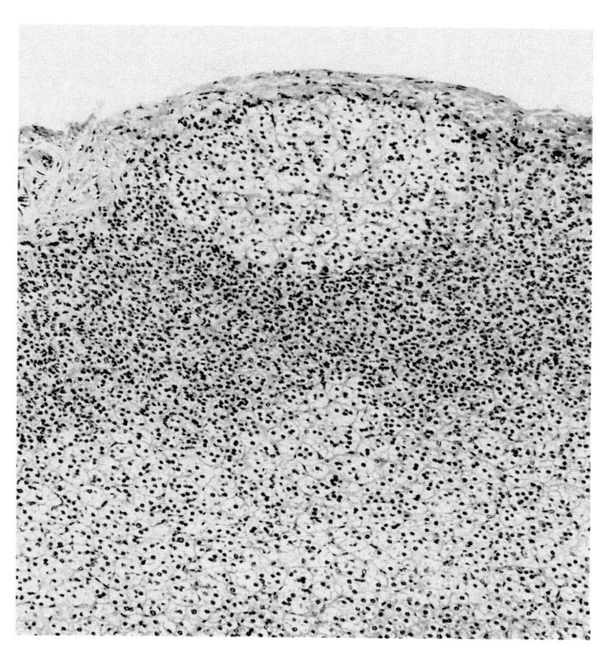

Figure 4-41
ALDOSTERONE-SECRETING
ADRENAL CORTICAL ADENOMA
Hyperplasia of the zona glomerulosa is both diffuse and focally micronodular. This section is from an adrenal remnant attached to an aldosterone-secreting adrenal cortical adenoma.

signs and symptoms of primary hyperaldosteronism (31), but ordinarily mast cells are inconspicuous in ACAs associated with primary hyperaldosteronism or other endocrine syndromes.

Hyperplasia of Zona Glomerulosa. Conn (41) first noted that the nontumorous zona glomerulosa was not atrophic in most cases, but often appeared wider than normal. The zona glomerulosa is said to be hypoplastic in some cases (53), but confirmation is difficult with routine morphology since this zone is normally quite thin and discontinuous. The hyperplastic zona glomerulosa may form a broad zone focally or a continuous thickened zone at the periphery of the entire cortex (fig. 4-40), sometimes with extension of small tongues of glomerulosa-type cells from the subcapsular region into the adjacent cortex. This is very different from the cortical atrophy which regularly occurs with Cushing's syndrome. Occasionally, there may be micronodules or macronodules in the tumor-bearing (fig. 4-41) or contralateral gland. Their presence might help explain some examples of multiple or bilateral tumors, but they could represent nonhyperfunctional cortical nodules possibly related to the underlying hypertension.

Electron Microscopic Findings. Ultrastructural studies document the presence of cellular heterogeneity (49). At the polar ends of the spectrum, cells with abundant or relatively sparse intracytoplasmic lipid (fig. 4-42) and cells which have essentially no lipid droplets analogous to cells of the zona reticularis are seen. The hybrid cell is as difficult to characterize at the ultrastructural level as by routine light microscopy. A smooth endoplasmic reticulum is prominent, often more so than the normal zona glomerulosa cell, and there may be short profiles of rough endoplasmic reticulum as well as free polyribosomes. Occasionally, concentric lamellar wraps of smooth endoplasmic reticulum associated with lipid material are seen (fig. 4-43).

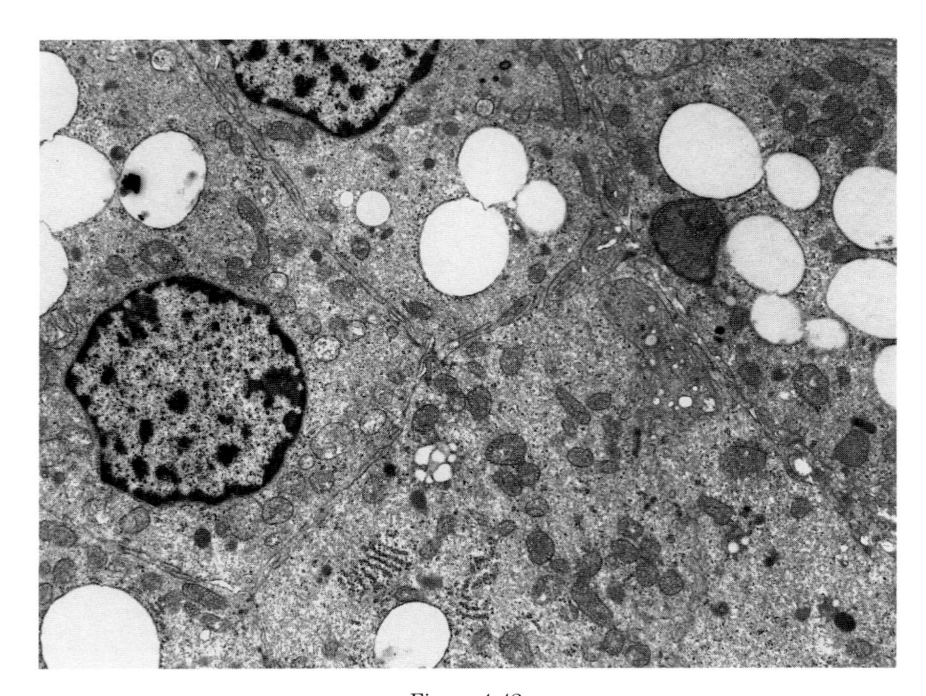

Figure 4-42
ALDOSTERONE-SECRETING ADRENAL CORTICAL ADENOMA
The tumor cells have much smooth endoplasmic reticulum and a few lipid droplets which vary in size. Microvillous cytoplasmic extensions are also evident. Mitochondria have tubulovesicular cristae. (X6,400)

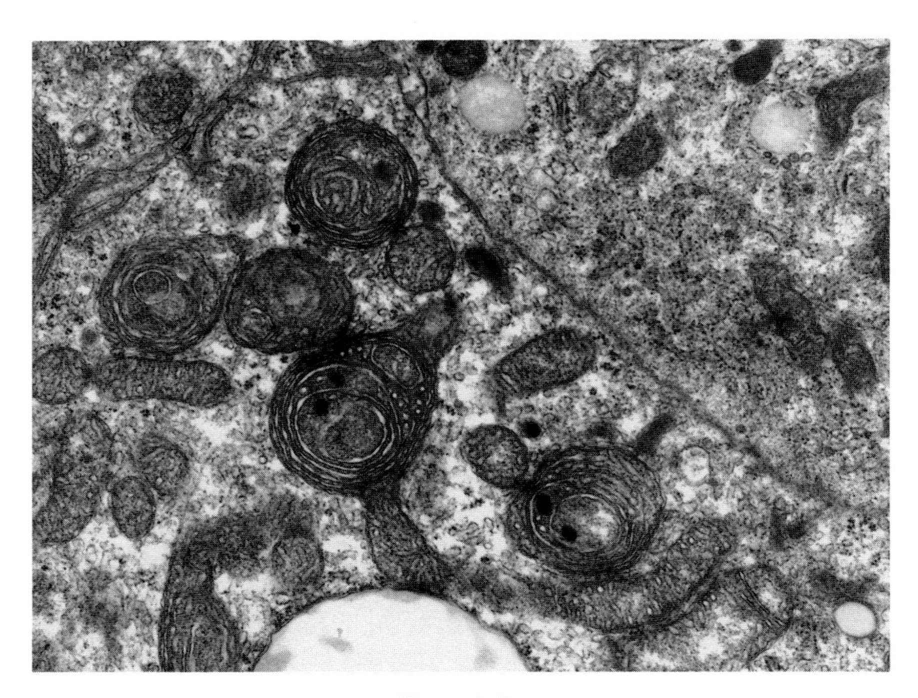

Figure 4-43
ALDOSTERONE-SECRETING ADRENAL CORTICAL ADENOMA
The mitochondria have tubular cristae, some of which are slightly dilated. A few lamellar, plate-like cristae can also be seen. Note the concentric wraps of smooth endoplasmic reticulum. (X20,000)

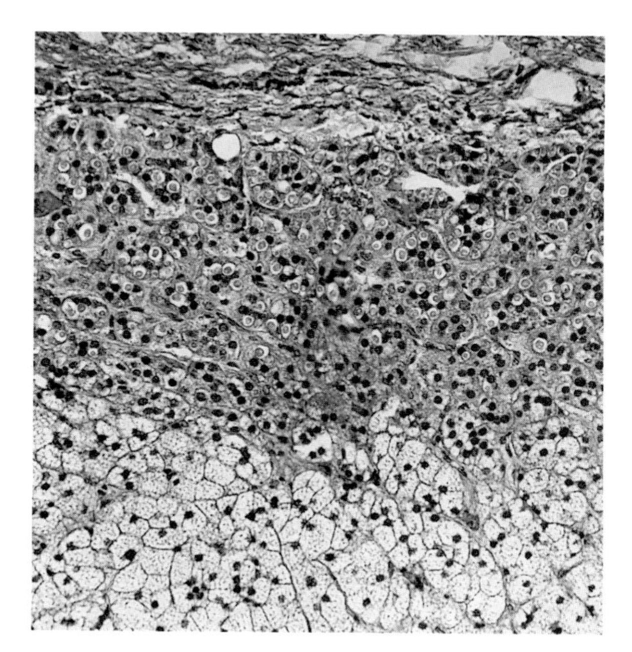

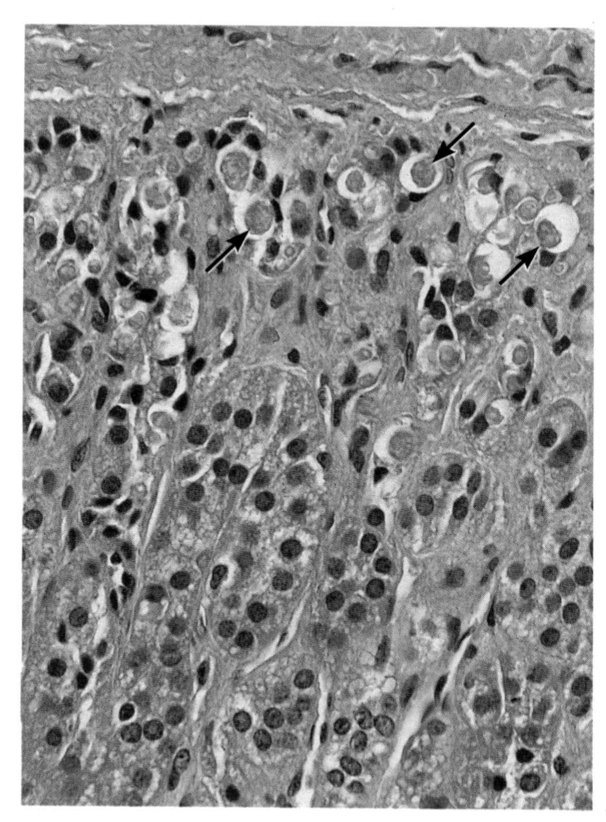

Figure 4-44
SPIRONOLACTONE BODIES

Left: This hyperplastic zona glomerulosa contains numerous cytoplasmic inclusions representing spironolactone bodies.
Right: Spironolactone bodies appear as eosinophilic laminated inclusions (arrows) within the cytoplasm of zona glomerulosa cells and may be surrounded by a clear halo. Occasional inclusions may be seen in what appears to be cells of the outer zona fasciculata.

Mitochondria are round to oval with short tubular or vesicular cristae, but abnormal shapes may be seen depending in large part on the plane of section. Some mitochondria have lamellar or plate-like cristae, a feature that is more characteristic of zona glomerulosa–type cells.

Spironolactone Bodies. Spironolactone bodies are characteristically small, intracytoplasmic inclusions that are lightly eosinophilic, with a laminated, scroll-like appearance (fig. 4-44). They develop in the cells of the zona glomerulosa (and sometimes cells deeper in the cortex) following treatment with the aldosterone antagonist spironolactone (45,58). These inclusions have been reported within tumor cells of aldosterone-producing ACAs (32,42,74), and zona glomerulosa cells in the nontumorous cortex, and can often be readily identified in zona glomerulosa cells in adrenal glands from patients who have been treated for secondary hyperaldosteronism. The inclusions are round to oval, measuring 2 to more than 12 µm in diameter, with 2 to 6 concentric rings, and are often demarcated from surrounding cytoplasm by a small clear halo. The spironolactone body is usually solitary within cells, and occurs mainly in cells with relatively compact eosinophilic cytoplasm (32). Due to their rich content of phospholipid, the inclusions may stain medium blue with the Luxol fast blue stain (fig. 4-45). Ultrastructurally, the spherical laminated whorls consist of a central core with amorphous electron-dense material surrounded by numerous smooth-walled concentric membranes continuous with the endoplasmic reticulum (60). Aldosterone has been demonstrated immunohistochemically in the concentric laminations (56).

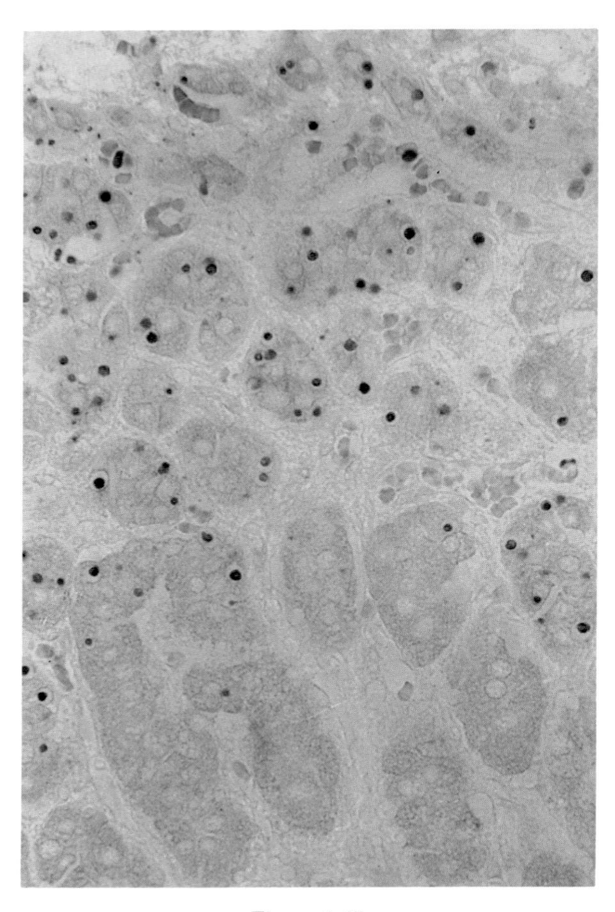

Figure 4-45
SPIRONOLACTONE BODIES
Spironolactone bodies appear as blue-black cytoplasmic inclusions in cells of the zona glomerulosa. (X350, Luxol-fast blue stain)

Carbonic anhydrase has been proposed as an immunochemical marker for zona glomerulosa cells of human adrenal glands and its localization suggests possible involvement in aldosterone biosynthesis or secretion (71).

Although there may be rare exceptions, intracytoplasmic inclusions are regarded as specific markers for spironolactone treatment (61). With time and continued administration of spironolactone, the inhibitory effect on aldosterone production by the ACA lessens or disappears, and spironolactone bodies also diminish or disappear (42). The frequency of occurrence of spironolactone bodies in ACA has been correlated positively with the number or percentage of zona glomerulosa–type cells in the ACA (39).

Treatment. The treatment options for patients with primary hyperaldosteronism depend largely on whether there is unilateral (e.g., ACA) or bilateral (e.g., hyperplasia) adrenal disease. Hypertension persists in most patients with bilateral adrenal hyperplasia who are treated surgically, therefore, the initial treatment is usually pharmacologic (76). The mean cure rate after unilateral or bilateral adrenalectomy for about 100 cases of idiopathic hyperaldosteronism reported in the literature was only 19 percent (76), compared with 70 to 80 percent for patients with an aldosterone-producing ACA (53,76). An unusual subset of primary aldosteronism, designated primary adrenal hyperplasia, also appears to be surgically correctable and resembles the rare ACTH-independent bilateral hyperplasia associated with autonomous cortisol production and Cushing's syndrome (57).

ADRENAL CORTICAL NEOPLASMS WITH VIRILIZATION OR FEMINIZATION

Adrenal cortical neoplasms causing virilization or feminization are uncommon, and they can be potentially malignant. In a series of 190 adrenal tumors collected over three decades, there were only 10 virilizing cortical tumors (5.3 percent) of which 7 were malignant (77). Correlation with pathologic features is essential. In a review of testosterone-producing adrenal cortical neoplasms in 47 adult females, the average tumor weight, when recorded, was 473 g (range, 13 to 1,500 g); at least 8 tumors (17 percent) were malignant, but follow-up in other cases was either limited or nonexistent (82). Most of the feminizing adrenal cortical neoplasms occurred in adults 25 to 45 years old, whereas virilizing tumors are more prevalent in the pediatric age group (79,81,86). In a review of 52 feminizing tumors, the average tumor weight, when recorded, was nearly 1,000 g (range, 175 to 2,650 g), and most tumors measured more than 12 cm in diameter (79). The feminizing adrenal cortical neoplasms are particularly ominous. In male patients gynecomastia is the most frequent presenting sign, with or without breast tenderness, and may be accompanied by testicular atrophy, decreased libido or potency, and feminizing hair changes.

Grossly, the tumors appear sharply circumscribed and even encapsulated, particularly the

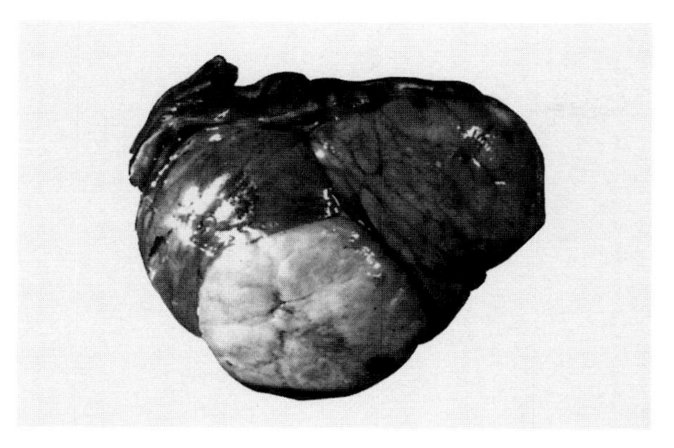

Figure 4-46
VIRILIZING ADRENAL CORTICAL ADENOMA
Virilizing adrenal cortical adenoma from a 40-year-old man who had undergone resection of bilateral interstitial (Leydig) cell tumors of the testes 1 year previously. The tumor measured 3.3 cm in diameter and weighed almost 25 g. Note the lobulated appearance on cross section with reddish tan areas. No Reinke crystalloids were identified on histologic study.

smaller neoplasms (fig. 4-46), but some of the larger neoplasms may have ominous features such as hemorrhage and necrosis. There may be a predominance of cells with compact, eosinophilic cytoplasm faintly resembling cells of the zona reticularis (which elaborate sex steroids) (fig. 4-47). Correlation with biochemical and endocrinologic data is essential since there are no reliable morphologic features (either gross or microscopic) that permit an accurate and reproducible prediction of the accompanying endocrine syndrome, if one exists at all (80). Because these tumors do not secrete excess glucocorticoids (if endocrinologically "pure"), the attached adrenal remnant or contralateral adrenal cortex would not be expected to be atrophic. Rare examples of virilizing adrenal neoplasms have been reported as Leydig cell adenomas of the adrenal gland, and although the cells specifically resemble lipid-depleted adrenal cortical cells, Reinke cystalloids have been identified (83–85). Recently, a case of testosterone-secreting ACA was reported with spironolactone body–like inclusions, but they were regarded as most likely representing focal cytoplasmic degeneration, particularly since the patient had no history of treatment with an aldosterone antagonist (78).

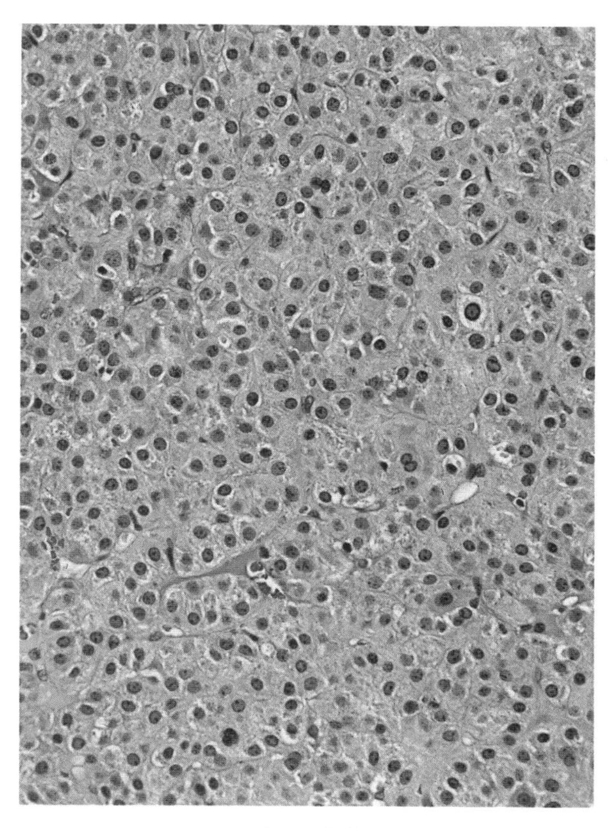

Figure 4-47
VIRILIZING ADRENAL CORTICAL ADENOMA
This virilizing adrenal cortical adenoma is composed of sheets of cells with compact, eosinophilic cytoplasm. No crystalloids of Reinke were identified.

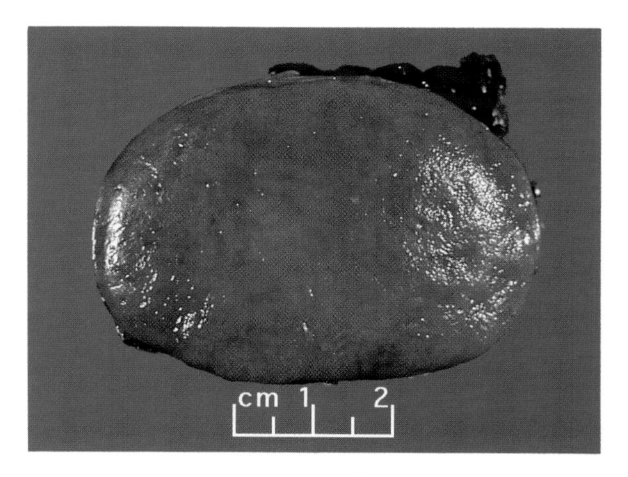

Figure 4-48
ONCOCYTIC ADRENAL CORTICAL ADENOMA
This oncocytic adrenal cortical adenoma ("oncocytoma") weighed 70 g and was 4 cm in diameter. The tumor was clinically nonfunctional. The tumor was mahogany brown on cross section. (Courtesy of Dr. Victor Reuter, New York, NY.)

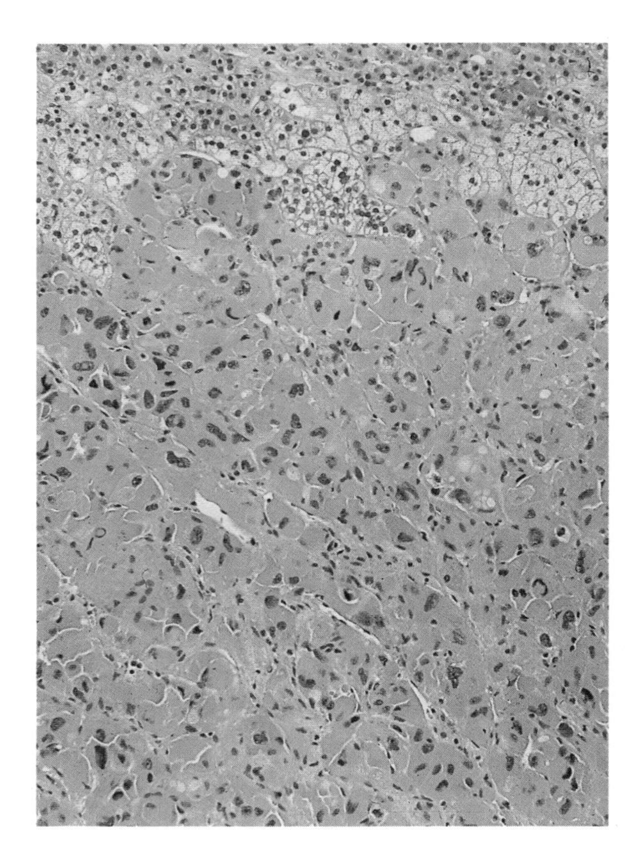

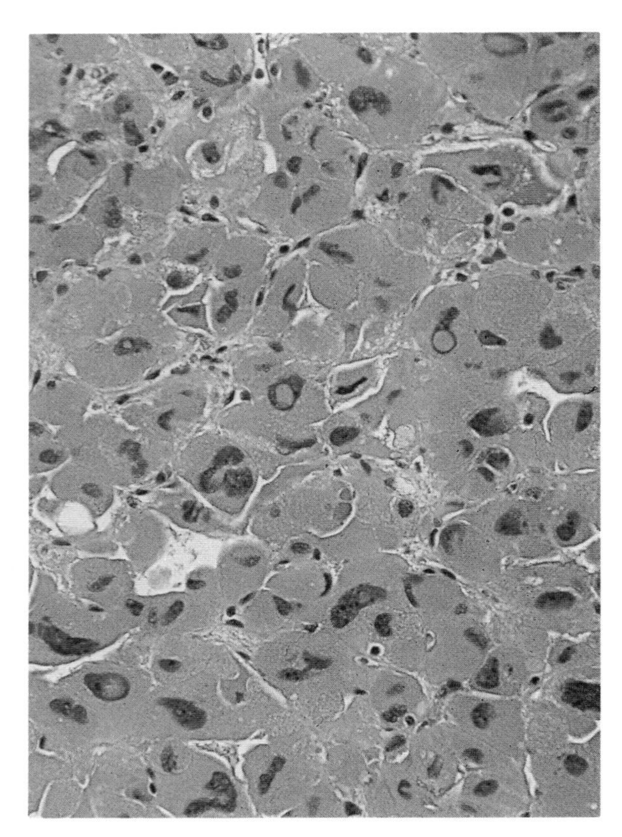

Figure 4-49
ONCOCYTIC ADRENAL CORTICAL ADENOMA

Left: Oncocytic adrenal cortical adenoma ("oncocytoma") weighed 12 g and measured 3 cm in diameter. It was discovered incidentally on abdominal CT scan in a 67-year-old man who underwent surgical resection of a colonic adenocarcinoma. The tumor compresses adjacent adrenal cortex.

Right: The tumor cells have an oncocytic appearance, with abundant, pink, granular cytoplasm. There is a marked degree of nuclear pleomorphism and numerous nuclear "pseudoinclusions." (Figures 4-49 and 4-50 are from the same case.)

ONCOCYTIC ADRENAL CORTICAL ADENOMA

Oncocytic ACA (or *adrenal cortical "oncocytoma"*) is composed of cells with abundant granular eosinophilic cytoplasm. The tumor may be dark tan or mahogany brown on gross examination (fig. 4-48), similar to oncocytomas in other anatomic sites. It is uncertain whether a tumor should be predominantly or entirely oncocytic (fig. 4-49) to merit the designation oncocytoma. Occasionally, an adrenal cortical neoplasm designated as adrenal cortical carcinoma can show focal areas of oncocytic change. The lipid content within these cells tends to be sparse or almost nonexistent. The oncocytic appearance of tumors in general is due to abundant mitochondria (fig. 4-50) (87). The term oncocytoma has been applied to a number of different neoplasms, but it is a relatively new concept for adrenal cortical tumors. Oncocytic adrenal cortical neoplasms have been reported both as adenoma (or "oncocytoma") (89–92), and in one case as adrenal cortical carcinoma (88). The small number of cases reported to date prevents any conclusive remarks regarding biologic behavior or even functional capacity. In a recent study of three cases, the tumors were considered to be truly nonfunctional with none expressing activity of enzymes involved in steroidogenesis (92).

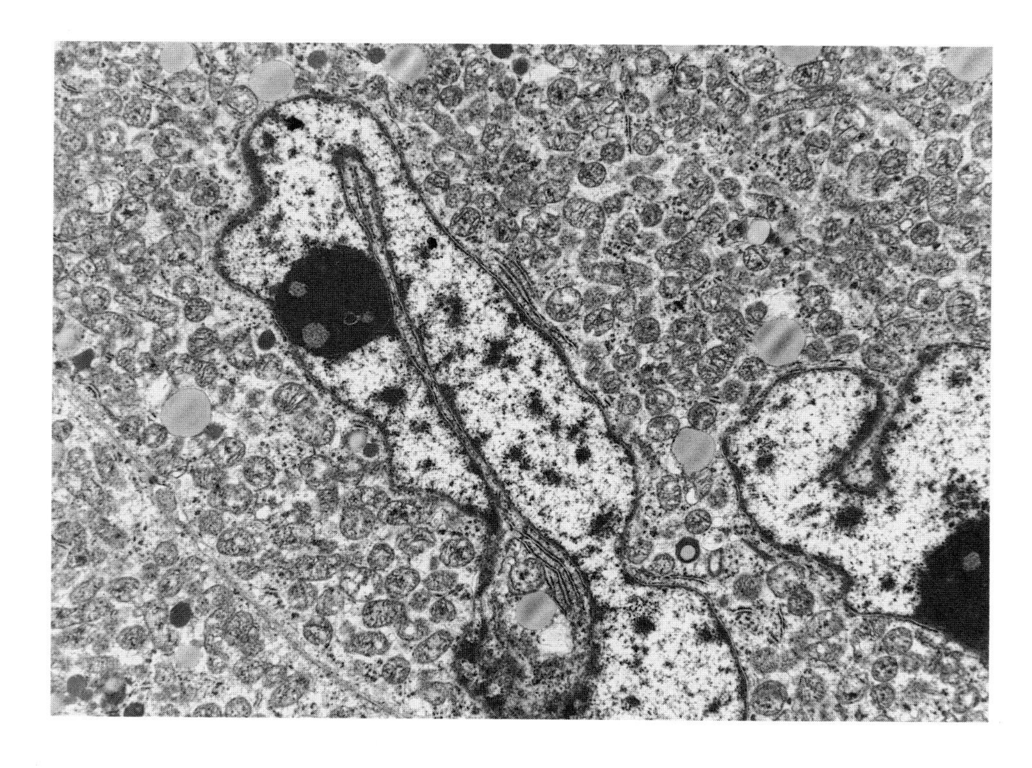

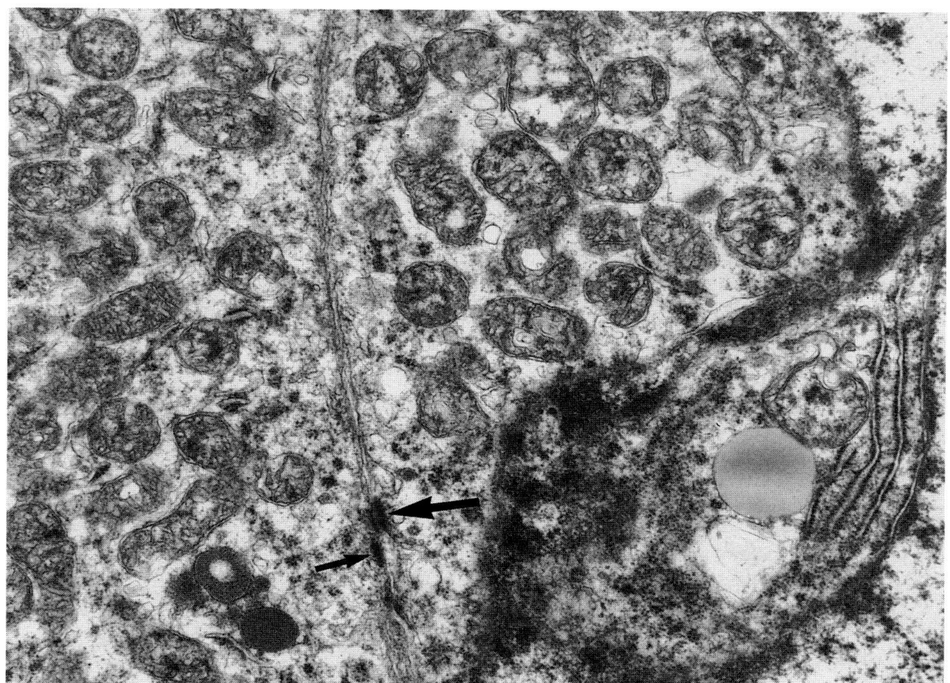

Figure 4-50
ONCOCYTIC ADRENAL CORTICAL ADENOMA

Top: This oncocytic adrenal cortical adenoma is composed of cells with numerous round to elongate mitochondria. The nuclear folds and clefts form nuclear "pseudoinclusions." (X7,000)

Bottom: The mitochondria have tubular and a few vesicular cristae. There are rudimentary intercellular attachments (arrows) and a few lysosomes. (X23,000) (Courtesy of Dr. J.M.B. Bloodworth, Madison, WI.)

REFERENCES

Adrenal Cortical Neoplasms, General

1. Bertagna C, Orth DN. Clinical and laboratory findings and results of therapy in 58 patients with adrenocortical tumors admitted to a single medical center (1951 to 1978). Am J Med 1981;71:855–75.
2. Gabrilove JL, Sharma DC, Wotiz HH, Dorfman RI. Feminizing adrenocortical tumors in the male. A review of 52 cases including a case report. Medicine 1965;44:37–79.
3. Lack EE, Travis WD, Oertel JE. Adrenal cortical neoplasms. In: Lack EE, ed. Pathology of the adrenal glands. New York: Churchill Livingston, 1990:115–71.
4. Tang CK, Gray GF. Adrenocortical neoplasms. Prognosis and morphology. Urology 1975;5:691–5.

Adrenal Cortical Adenoma with Cushing's Syndrome

5. Aiba M, Kawakami M, Ito Y, Fujimoto Y, Suda T, Demura H. Bilateral adrenocortical adenomas causing Cushing's syndrome. Report of two cases with enzyme histochemical and ultrastructural studies and a review of the literature. Arch Pathol Lab Med 1992;116:146–50.
6. Bertagna C, Orth DN. Clinical and laboratory findings and results of therapy in 58 patients with adrenocortical tumors admitted to a single medical center (1951 to 1978). Am J Med 1981;71:855–75.
7. Borrero E, Katz P, Lipper S, Chang JB. Adrenal cortical adenoma and adrenal medullary hyperplasia of the right adrenal gland—a case report. Angiology 1987;38:271–4.
8. Coslovsky R, Ashkenazy M, Lancet M, Barash A, Borenstein R. Female pseudohermaphroditism with adrenal cortical tumor in adulthood. J Endocrinol Invest 1985;8:63–5.
9. Dahms WT, Gray G, Vrana M, New MI. Adrenocortical adenoma and ganglioneuroblastoma in a child. A case presenting as Cushing syndrome with virilization. Am J Dis Child 1973;125:608–11.
10. Harrison JH, Mahoney EM, Bennett AH. Tumors of the adrenal cortex. Cancer 1973;32:1227–35.
11. Inoue J, Oishi S, Naomi S, Umeda T, Sato T. Pheochromocytoma associated with adrenocortical adenoma: case report and literature review. Endocrinal Jpn 1986;33:67–74.
12. Kato S, Masunaga R, Kawabe T, et al. Cushing's syndrome induced by hypersecretion of cortisol from only one of bilateral adrenocortical tumors. Metabolism 1992;41:260–3.
13. Kazama Y, Noguchi T, Kawabe T, et al. A case of Cushing's syndrome associated with possible adrenomedullary hyperplasia. Endocrinol Jpn 1985;32:355–9.
14. Lack EE, Travis WD, Oertel JE. Adrenal cortical neoplasms. In: Lack EE, ed. Pathology of the adrenal glands. New York: Churchill Livingstone, 1990:115–71.
15. Mackay A. Atlas of human adrenal cortex ultrastructure. In: Symington T, ed. Functional pathology of the human adrenal gland. Baltimore: Williams & Wilkins, 1969:346–484.
16. Mathison DA, Waterhouse CA. Cushing's syndrome with hypertensive crisis and mixed adrenal cortical adenoma-pheochromocytoma (corticomedullary adenoma). Am J Med 1969;47:635–41.
17. Neville AM, O'Hare MJ. Histopathology of the human adrenal cortex. Clin Endocrinol Metab 1985;14:791–820.
18. O'Leary TJ, Liotta LA, Gill JR. Pigmented adrenal nodules in Cushing's syndrome. Arch Pathol Lab Med 1982;106:257.
19. Ramsey JA, Asa SL, van Nordstrand AW, Hassaram ST, de Harven EP. Lipid degeneration in pheochromocytomas mimicking adrenal cortical tumors. Am J Surg Pathol 1987;11:480–6.
20. Takasu N, Komiya I, Nagasawa Y, Asawa T, Yamada T. Exacerbation of autoimmune thyroid dysfunction after unilateral adrenalectomy in patients with Cushing's syndrome due to an adrenocortical adenoma. N Engl J Med 1990;322:1708–12.
21. Tang CK, Gray GF. Adrenocortical neoplasms. Prognosis and morphology. Urology 1975;5:691–5.
22. Tannenbaum M. Ultrastructural pathology of the adrenal cortex. Pathol Annu 1973;8:109–56.
23. Unger PD, Cohen JM, Thung SN, Gordon R, Pertsemlidis D, Dikman SH. Lipid degeneration in a pheochromocytoma histologically mimicking an adrenal cortical tumor. Arch Pathol Lab Med 1990;114:892–4.

Functional Pigmented ("Black") Adenomas

24. Caplan RH, Virata RL. Functional black adenoma of the adrenal cortex. A rare cause of primary aldosteronism. Am J Clin Pathol 1974;62:97–103.
25. Cohen RJ, Brits R, Phillips JI, Botha JR. Primary hyperaldosteronism due to a functional black (pigmented) adenoma of the adrenal cortex. Arch Pathol Lab Med 1991;115:813–5.
26. Damron TA, Schelper RL, Sorensen L. Cytochemical demonstration of neuromelanin in black pigmented adrenal nodules. Am J Clin Pathol 1987;87:334–41.
27. Komiya I, Takasa N, Aizawa T, Yamada T, et al. Black (or brown) adrenal cortical adenoma: its characteristic features on computed tomography and endocrine data. J Clin Endocrinol Metab 1985;61:711–7.
28. Kovacs K, Horvath E, Feldman PS. Pigmented adenoma of adrenal cortex associated with Cushing's syndrome: light and electron microscopic study. Urology 1976;7:641–5.
29. Lack EE, Travis WD, Oertel JE. Adrenal cortical neoplasms. In: Lack EE, ed. Pathology of the adrenal glands. New York: Churchill Livingstone, 1990:115–71.
30. Landas SK, Schelper RL, Tio FO, Turner JW, Moore KC, Bennett-Gray J. Black thyroid syndrome: exaggeration of a normal process? Am J Clin Pathol 1986;85:411–8.

Adrenal Cortical Adenomas with Primary Hyperaldosteronism (Conn's Syndrome)

31. Aiba M, Iria H, Suzuki H, et al. Numerous mast cells in 11-deoxycorticosterone producing adrenocortical tumor. Histologic evaluation of benignancy and comparison with mast cell distribution in adrenal glands and neoplastic counterparts of 67 surgical specimens. Arch Pathol Lab Med 1985;109:357–60.
32. Aiba M, Suzuki H, Kageyama K, et al. Spironolactone bodies in aldosteronomas and in the attached adrenals. Enzyme histochemical study of 19 cases of primary aldosteronism and a case of aldosteronism due to bilateral diffuse hyperplasia of the zona glomerulosa. Am J Pathol 1981;103:404–10.
33. Anderson GS, Lund JO, Toftdahl D, Strandgaard S, Nielsen PE. Pheochromocytoma and Conn's syndrome in Denmark 1977-1981. Acta Medica Scand [Suppl] 1986–7;714:11–4.
34. Andreis PG, Mantero F, Armato U. The primary tissue culture of human adrenocortical Conn's adenomata. I. The synergistic stimulation of adenomatous cell growth by purine cyclic nucleatides and by ACTH 1-24 and angiotensin II. Path Res Pract 1981;173:66–81.
35. Bailey RE, Slade CI, Liberman AH, Luetscher JA. Steroid production by human adrenal adenomata and nontumorous adrenal tissue in vitro. J Clin Endocrinol 1960;20:457–65.
36. Bravo EL. Primary aldosteronism. Urol Clin N Am 1989;16:481–6.
37. Bravo EL, Tarazi RC, Dustan HP, et al. The changing clinical spectrum of primary aldosteronism. Am J Med 1983;74:641–51.
38. Brode E, Grant JK, Symington T. Biochemical and pathological investigation of adrenal tissues from patients with Conn's syndrome. Acta Endocr 1962;41:411–31.
39. Cohn D, Jackson RV, Gordon RD. Factors affecting the frequency of occurrence of spironolactone bodies in aldosteronomas and nontumorous cortex. Pathology 1983;15:273–7.
40. Conn JW. Plasma renin activity in primary aldosteronism. Importance in differential diagnosis and in research of essential hypertension. JAMA 1964;190:222–5.
41. Conn JW. Primary aldosteronism. J Lab and Clin Med 1955;45:661–4.
42. Conn JW, Hinerman DL. Spironolactone-induced inhibition of aldosterone biosynthesis in primary aldosteronism: morphological and functional studies. Metabolism 1977;26:1293–307.
43. Conn JW, Knopf RF, Nesbit RM. Clinical characteristics of primary aldosteronism from an analysis of 145 cases. Am J Surg 1964;107:159–72.
44. Davignon J, Tremblay G, Nowaczynski W, Korw E, Genest J. Parallel biochemical and histochemical studies of an adrenocortical adenoma from a patient with primary hyperaldosteronism. Acta Endocrinol 1961;38:207–19.
45. Davis DA, Medline NM. Spironolactone (aldactone) bodies: concentric lamellar formations in the adrenal cortices of patients treated with spironolactone. Am J Clin Pathol 1970;54:22–32.
46. Dedrick CG. Adrenal arteriography and venography. Urol Clin N Am 1989;16:515–26.
47. Dobbie JW. Adrenocortical nodular hyperplasia: the ageing adrenal. J Pathol 1969;99:1–18.
48. Dunnick NR, Leight GS Jr, Roubidoux MA, Leder RA, Paulson E, Kurylo L. CT in the diagnosis of primary aldosteronism: sensitivity in 29 patients. AJR Am J Roentgenol 1993;160:321–4.
49. Eto T, Kumamoto K, Kawasaki T, Omae T, Masaki Z, Yamamoto T. Ultrastructural types of cells in adrenal cortical adenoma with primary aldosteronism. J Path 1979;128:1–6.
50. Ferris JB, Beevers DG, Brown JJ, et al. Clinical, biochemical and pathological features of low-renin (primary) hyperaldosteronism. Am Heart J 1978;95:375–88.
51. Flanagan MJ, McDonald JH. Heterotopic adrenocortical adenoma producing primary aldosteronism. J Urol 1967;98:133–9.
52. Ganguly A. Cellular origin of aldosteronomas. Clin Investig 1992;70:392–5.
53. Gill JR Jr. Hyperaldosteronism. In: Becker KL, ed. Principles and practice of endocrinology and metabolism. Philadelphia: JB Lippincott, 1990:631–43.
54. Grant CS, Carpenter P, van Heerden JA, Hamberger B. Primary aldosteronism. Clinical management. Arch Surg 1984;119:585–90.
55. Honda M, Tsuchiya M, Tamura H, et al. In vivo and in vitro studies on steroid metabolism in a case of primary aldosteronism with multiple lesions of adenoma and nodular hyperplasia. Endocrinol Jpn 1982;29:529–40.
56. Hsu SM, Raine L, Martin HF. Spironolactone bodies. An immunoperoxidase study with biochemical correlation. Am J Clin Pathol 1981;75:92–5.
57. Irony I, Kater CE, Biglieri EG, Shackleton CH. Correctable subsets of primary aldosteronism. Primary adrenal hyperplasia and renin responsive adenoma. Am J Hypertens 1990;3:576–82.
58. Janigan DT. Cytoplasmic bodies in the adrenal cortex of patients treated with spironolactone. Lancet 1963;1:850–2.
59. Kaplan NM. The steroid content of adrenal adenomas and measurements of aldosterone production in patients with essential hypertension and primary aldosteronism. J Clin Invest 1967;46:728–34.
60. Kovacs K, Horvath E, Singer W. Fine structure and morphogenesis of spironolactone bodies in the zona glomerulosa of the human adrenal cortex. J Clin Path 1973;26:949–57.
61. Lack EE, Travis WD, Oertel JE. Adrenal cortical neoplasms. In: Lack EE, ed. Pathology of the adrenal glands. New York: Churchill Livingstone, 1990:115–71.
62. Lins PE, Adamson U. Primary aldosteronism. A follow-up study of 28 cases of surgically treated aldosterone-producing adenomas. Acta Med Scand 1987;221:275–82.
63. Louis LH, Conn JW. Primary aldosteronism: content of adrenocortical steroids in adrenal tissue. Rec Progr Horm Res 1961;17:415–36.
64. Matsuo K, Tsuchiyama H. Adrenocortical adenoma with primary aldosteronism in culture. Acta Pathol Jpn 1986;36:1659–68.
65. Melby JC. Diagnosis of hyperaldosteronism. Endocrinol Metab Clin North Am, 1991;20:247–55.
66. Melby JC. Identifying the adrenal lesion in primary aldosteronism. Ann Intern Med 1972;76:1039–41.

67. Nagae A, Murakami E, Hiwada K, Kubota O, Takada Y, Ohmori T. Primary aldosteronism with cortisol overproduction from bilateral multiple adrenal adenomas. Jpn J Med 1991;30:26–31.
68. Neville AM, O'Hare MJ. Histopathology of the human adrenal cortex. Clin Endocrinol Metab 1985;14:791–820.
69. Neville AM, Symington T. Pathology of primary aldosteronism. Cancer 1966;19:1854–68.
70. Pasqualini JR. Conversion of tritiated-18-hydroxycorticosterone to aldosterone by slices of human cortico-adrenal gland and adrenal tumour. Nature 1964;201:501.
71. Sasano H, Kato K, Nagura H, et al. Carbonic anhydrases in the human adrenal gland and its disorders: immunohistochemical and biochemical study of the enzymes. Endocr Pathol 1994;5:100–6.
72. Scott HW Jr, Sussman CR, Page DL, Thompson NW, Gross MD, Lloyd R. Primary hyperaldosteronism caused by adrenocortical carcinoma. World J Surg 1986;10:646–53.
73. Shamma AH, Goddard JW, Sommers SC. A study of the adrenal status in hypertension. J Chronic Dis 1958;8:587–95.
74. Shrago SS, Waisman J, Cooper PH. Spironolactone bodies in an adrenal adenoma. Arch Pathol 1975;99:416–20.
75. Tannenbaum M. Ultrastructural pathology of the adrenal cortex. Pathol Annu 1973;8:109–56.
76. Young WF Jr, Hogan MJ, Klee GG, Grant CS, van Heerden JA. Primary aldosteronism: diagnosis and treatment. Mayo Clin Proc 1990;65:96–110.

Adrenal Cortical Neoplasms with Virilization or Feminization

77. Del Gaudio A, Del Gaudio GA. Virilizing adrenocortical tumors in adult women. Report of 10 patients, 2 of whom each had a tumor secreting only testosterone. Cancer 1993;72:1997–2003.
78. Deng Y, Osamura Y, Tanaka M, Katsuoka Y, Kawamura N, Murakowshi M. A case of testerone-secreting adrenal cortical adenoma with spironolactone body-like inclusion. Acta Pathol Jpn 1990;40:67–72.
79. Gabrilove JL, Sharma DC, Wotiz HH, Dorfman RI. Feminizing adrenocortical tumors in the male. A review of 52 cases including a case report. Medicine 1965;44:37–79.
80. Lack EE, Travis WD, Oertel JE. Adrenal cortical neoplasms In: Lack EE, ed. Pathology of the adrenal glands. New York: Churchill Livingstone, 1990:115–71.
81. Lee PD, Winter RJ, Green OC. Virilizing adrenocortical tumors in childhood: eight cases and a review of the literature. Pediatrics 1985;76:437–44.
82. Mattox JH, Phelan S. The evaluation of adult females with testosterone producing neoplasms of the adrenal cortex. Surg Gynecol Obstet 1987;164:98–101.
83. Pollock WJ, McConnell CF, Hilton C, Lavine RL. Virilizing Leydig cell adenoma of adrenal gland. Am J Surg Pathol 1986;10:816–22.
84. Trost BN, Koenig MP, Zimmermann A, Zachmann M, Müller J. Virilization of a postmenopausal woman by a testosterone-secreting Leydig cell type adrenal adenoma. Acta Endocrinol (Copenh) 1981;98:274–82.
85. Vasiloff J, Chideckel EW, Boyd CB, Foshag LJ. Testosterone-secreting adrenal adenoma containing crystalloids characteristic of Leydig cells. Am J Med 1985;79:772–6.
86. Zerbini C, Kozakewich HP, Weinberg DS, Mundt DJ, Edwards JA III, Lack EE. Adrenocortical neoplasms in childhood and adolescence: analysis of prognostic factors including DNA content. Endocr Pathol 1992;3:116–28.

Oncocytic Adrenal Cortical Neoplasms

87. Chang A, Harawi SJ. Oncocytes, oncocytosis and oncocytic tumors. Pathol Annu 1992;27:263–304.
88. El-Naggar AK, Evans DB, Mackay B. Oncocytic adrenal cortical carcinoma. Ultrastr Pathol 1991;15:549–56.
89. Erlandson RA, Reuter VE. Oncocytic adrenal cortical adenoma. Ultrastr Pathol 1991;15:539–47.
90. Kakimoto S, Yushita Y, Sanefuji T, et al. Nonhormonal adrenocortical adenoma with oncocytoma-like appearance. Hinyokika Kiyo 1986;32:757–63.
91. Nguyen GK, Vriend R, Ronaghan D, Lakey WK. Heterotopic adrenocortical oncocytoma. A case report with light and electron microscopic studies. Cancer 1992;70:2681–4.
92. Sasano H, Suzuki T, Sano T, Kameya T, Sasano N, Nagura H. Adrenocortical oncocytoma. A true nonfunctioning adrenocortical tumor. Am J Surg Pathol 1991;15:949–56.

✧✧✧

5
ADRENAL CORTICAL CARCINOMA

Definition. Adrenal cortical carcinoma (ACC) is a malignant neoplasm arising from adrenal cortical cells, which may or may not have functional activity as evidenced by a clinically recognizable endocrine syndrome, biochemical abnormalities indicative of hypercorticalism, or both.

Incidence and Clinical Features. The estimated frequency of ACC in the United States is about one case per million population (5). This chapter deals almost solely with tumors in adult patients, although large clinical series often include a few patients in the pediatric age group. In adults, individuals in the fourth and fifth decades of life are most frequently affected, although ACC can occur at any age. A bimodal peak in age incidence has been reported in the first and fifth decades (48). There does not appear to be a significant racial predilection, although a recent epidemiologic study showed a trend of increased rate among blacks (5). Most large clinical series indicate a predilection for female patients, with a ratio of 1.5 to 1 (over 900 patients studied) (4,11,13,16,18,24–26,32,37,39,42,44,46); in several studies, however, there was a predilection for male patients (19,20,23,28) including one which reviewed all nonhormonal tumors (23). In a review of ACCs in the English language literature from 1952 to 1992, 58.6 percent of patients were female and 41.4 percent male (48). Rapaport et al. (33) reviewed a 20-year period from 1930 through 1949. In several series, female patients with ACC were diagnosed at an earlier age than males (4,11,17). The left adrenal gland is involved slightly more often than the right (52.8 versus 47.2 percent) (48). Bilateral ACC is extremely rare (6,39), although there may be metastases to the opposite adrenal gland in 1 percent (16) to 13 percent (27) of cases. In several large studies, metastases have been noted on initial presentation in 15 percent (4) to 38 percent (44) of patients. In a study by King and Lack (20), pulmonary (fig. 5-1), skeletal, or mediastinal metastases were noted on initial chest X ray in 24 percent of patients. An extraordinarily high incidence of metastases (67 percent) at the time of diagnosis has been reported (14).

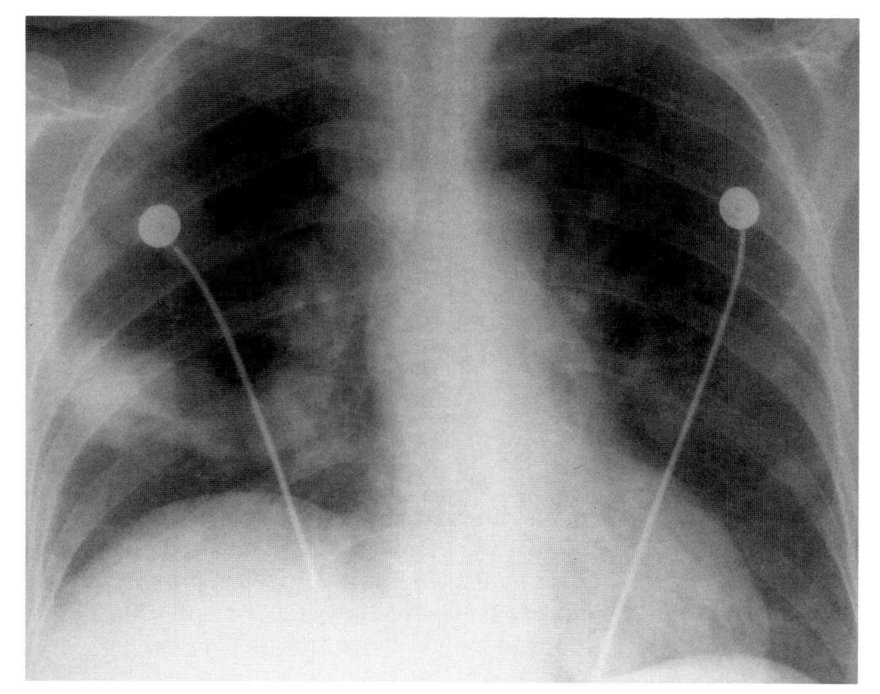

Figure 5-1
ADRENAL CORTICAL CARCINOMA

An adult female presented with abdominal and flank pain, and was found to have a large ACC on the right side. Multiple hepatic and pulmonary metastases were present at the time of diagnosis. Chest X ray shows multiple nodular densities representing metastatic ACC. The patient died within 9 months of diagnosis with widespread metastases.

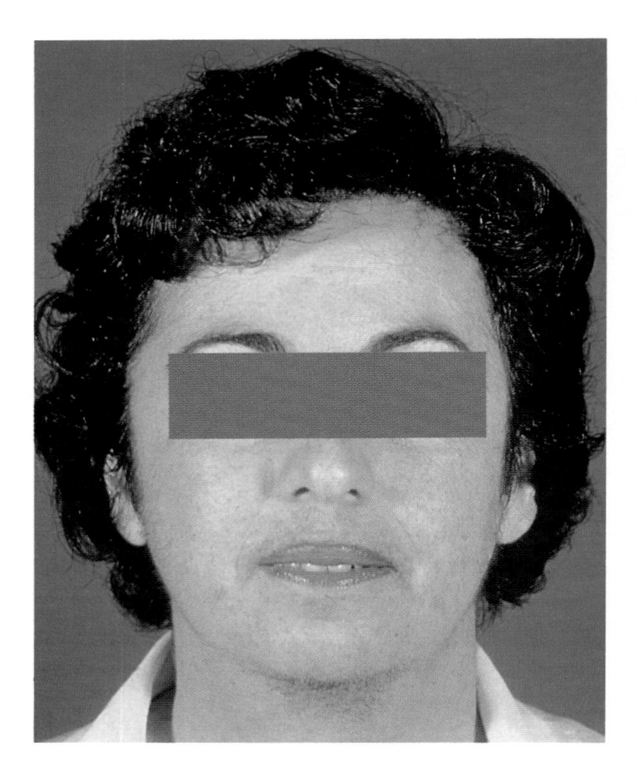

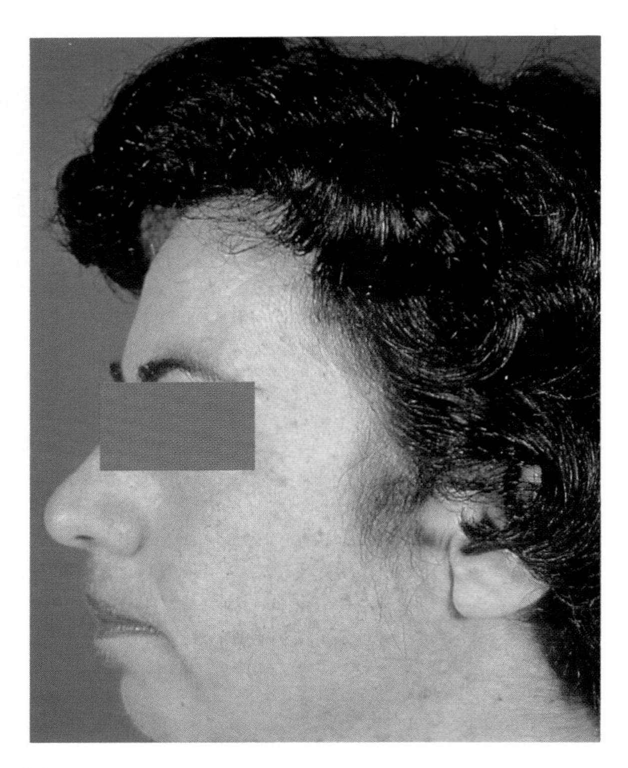

Figure 5-2
ADRENAL CORTICAL CARCINOMA
A 37-year-old woman presented with mixed endocrinopathy of Cushing's syndrome and virilization. The ACC measured 10 x 9 x 8 cm and weighed 300 g. The patient died of widespread ACC within a year of diagnosis, and at autopsy massive invasion of the inferior vena cava was seen.

The frequency of ACCs that function endocrinologically varies depending upon whether "function" is defined as a clinically recognizable "pure" syndrome, such as Cushing's syndrome; a "mixed" endocrine syndrome (fig. 5-2); or any biochemical evidence of excess steroid production. In 18 series, ACC was reported to be nonfunctional in 26 to 76 percent of cases (1,4,7,11,13,17–20, 24–28,32,39,42,43). In a review of nonhormonal adrenal cortical neoplasms, the tumors were considered capable of forming precursor steroids without hormonal activity and were, therefore, not actually nonfunctional (23). Data suggest that ACCs are less efficient in steroidogenesis due to decreased activity of 3-beta-hydroxysteroid dehydrogenase, 17-hydroxylase, and 17,20-desmolase (6). An immunohistochemical study has shown that some tumor cells in ACC do not express all the enzymes involved in steroidogenesis, whereas other cells do, suggesting that there may be malregulation in individual cells (36). These findings may help to explain the large size of ACC when signs or symptoms of hypercorticalism first appear. Culture of tumor cells in vitro has demonstrated multiple pathways of steroidogenesis, including formation of corticosteroids, mineralocorticoids, androgens, and estrogens, with all of the major enzyme systems required in their synthesis (9). A blunted or absent response to adrenocorticotrophic hormone (ACTH) has also been reported in malignant cells maintained in vitro (30). Feminization is an uncommon endocrine manifestation, and it is usually only recognized in the male patient as gynecomastia and sometimes decreased potency. Primary hyperaldosteronism is very uncommon in association with ACC (38,45).

The most common presenting complaints are abdominal or flank pain, discomfort, or fullness, and in a study involving 110 patients, 30 percent had a palpable abdominal mass (fig. 5-3) (44). Weight loss can also be a prominent feature.

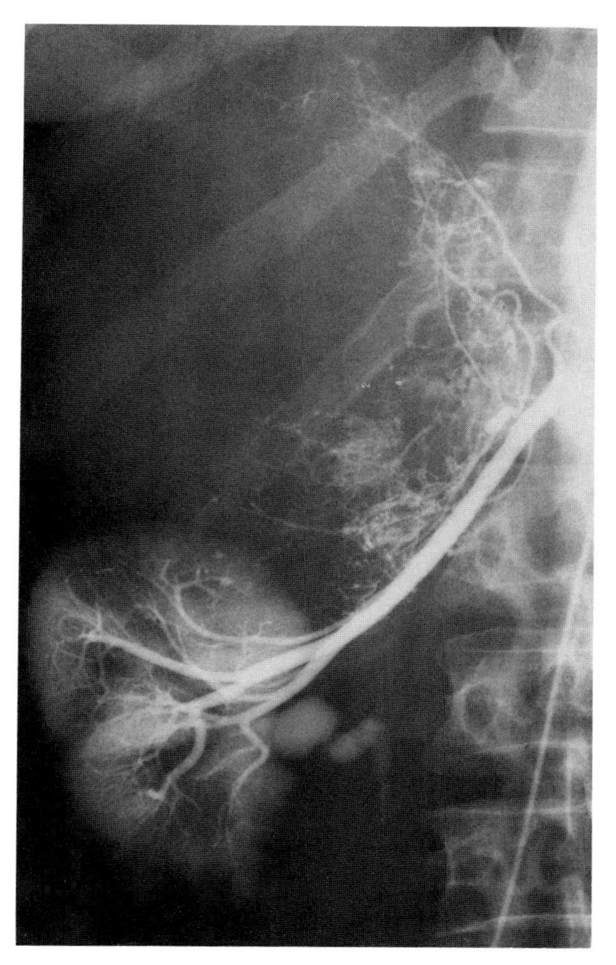

Figure 5-3
ADRENAL CORTICAL CARCINOMA
SIMULATING RENAL CELL CARCINOMA

A 57-year-old woman presented with abdominal pain, and had a large right upper quadrant mass on physical examination. Tumor could not be separated from kidney on imaging studies and the patient underwent radical nephrectomy since the tumor simulated a renal cell carcinoma. There were no signs or symptoms of an endocrine syndrome due to hypercorticalism. Abnormal tortuous vessels are seen in an early phase of selective arteriogram along with stretching of renal artery and its branches. (Figure 3-24 from Lack EE, Travis WD, Oertel JE. Adrenal cortical neoplasms. In: Lack EE, ed. Pathology of the adrenal glands. New York: Churchill Livingstone, 1990:115–71.) (Figures 5-3 and 5-4 are from the same case.)

Intermittent, low-grade fever has been reported in 15 percent (4) to 20 percent (20) of cases, and may be related to extensive tumor necrosis. Hypoglycemia and hypercalcemia have been reported in association with ACC, with the latter attributed to elaboration of a hypercalcemic hormone of malignancy (31).

Imaging Characteristics. On computed tomography (CT) scan ACCs are usually large with low intensity areas corresponding to necrosis; they have irregular contrast enhancement. Calcification may be present in the tumor. With magnetic resonance imaging (MRI), the tumor usually appears heterogeneous on T1-weighted images and has a signal intensity greater than fat on T2-weighted images. Enhancement may be very heterogeneous and there may be evidence of extension to retroperitoneal lymph nodes, renal vein, and inferior vena cava.

Gross Findings. ACC is often a bulky neoplasm, with the average weight in several series being 510 g (46), 714 g (18), 849 g (20), 1,190 g (4), and 1,210 g (43). Tumor weight has been reported to be an important prognostic factor (see also chapter 6): in the study by Tang and Gray (41), all tumors weighing 95 g or more were malignant, while tumors less than 50 g were benign. Clearly, there are exceptions since some tumors weighing less than 50 g metastasize (8,22,35), and some in excess of 1,000 g fail to do so on prolonged follow-up. Some tumors are 4,500 g or more (18,23). The average size of tumors recorded in several series was 12.0 cm (18), 12.4 cm (13,20), 14.0 cm (46), and 16.6 cm (4), but the range is wide: 3 to 40 cm (23).

On external examination and in cross section, ACCs often have a coarsely lobulated appearance, with soft, bulging nodules ranging from yellow-orange to tan. Necrotic areas appear pale tan or yellow-white with a putty-like consistency (fig. 5-4). Often there are areas of necrosis and hemorrhage (fig. 5-5). The nodularity may be related to intersecting broad fibrous bands. Areas of cystic degeneration may be seen. The overall appearance may be quite variegate, giving the unmistakable impression of malignancy on the basis of size, weight, and gross morphology; however, some of the smaller ACCs are not as heterogenous and don't look malignant. ACC can invade adjacent organs or tissues and en bloc surgical removal of involved structures may be necessary for total gross resection (fig. 5-6).

Microscopic Findings. *Architectural Patterns.* A variety of different architectural patterns can be found in ACC, and are sometimes admixed in the same neoplasm. One of the more characteristic is a broad trabecular growth pattern, with anastomosing columns and cords of cells, often 10 to 20 or more cells wide, separated by delicate,

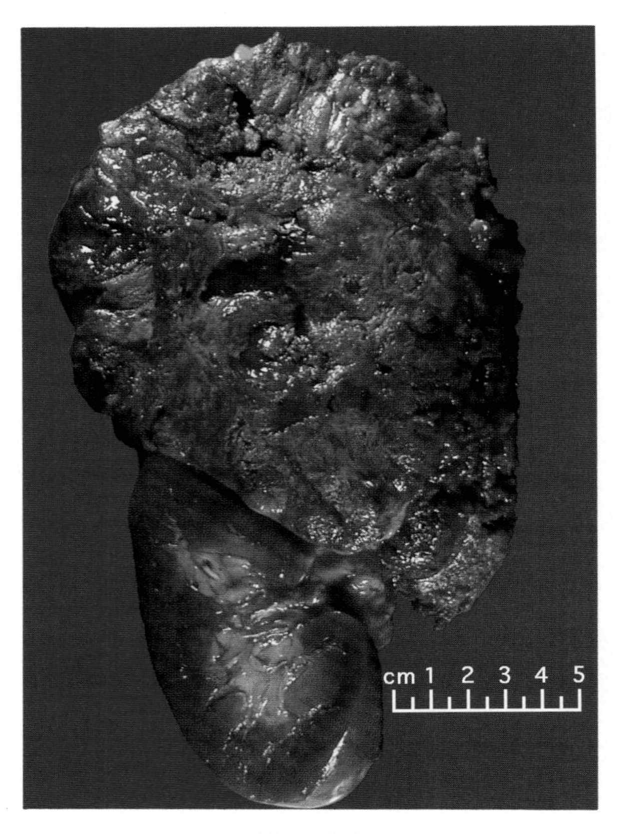

Figure 5-4
ADRENAL CORTICAL CARCINOMA

Large adrenal cortical carcinoma from a 57-year-old woman simulated a renal cell carcinoma. The patient had no recognizable endocrine syndrome. Over half the neoplasm was necrotic. (Same cases as fig. 5-3)

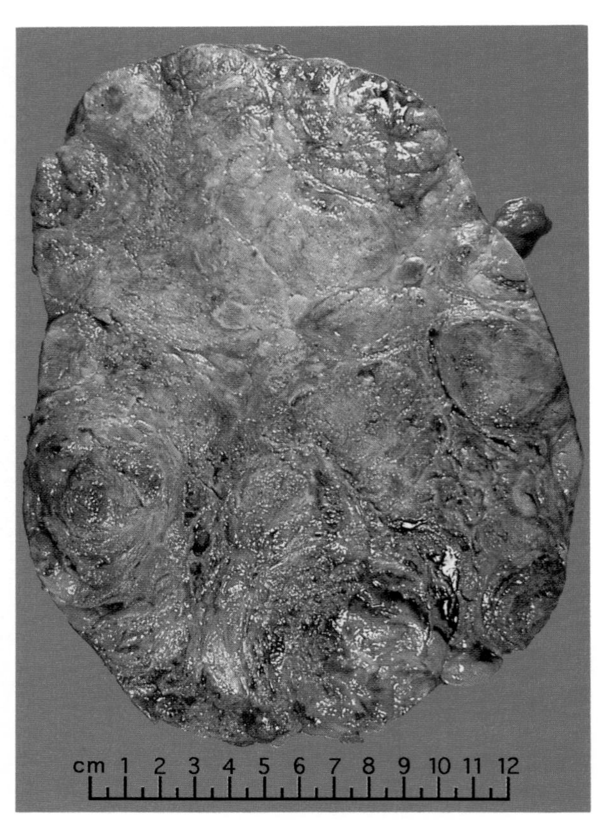

Figure 5-5
ADRENAL CORTICAL CARCINOMA

An adrenal cortical carcinoma from a 32-year-old female weighed 2,200 g and measured 21 cm in diameter. There were extensive areas of necrosis with foci of vascular invasion. The patient also had pulmonary metastases at the time of diagnosis.

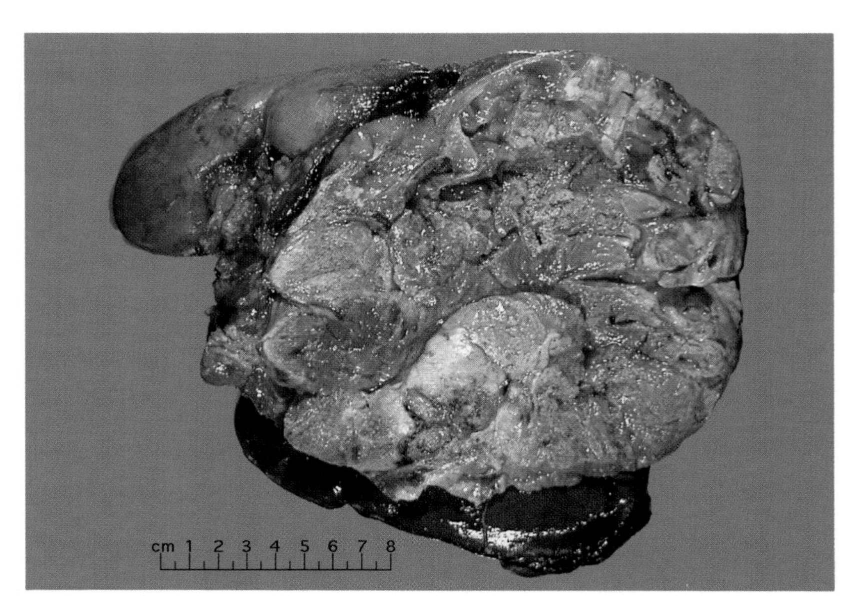

Figure 5-6
LARGE ADRENAL CORTICAL CARCINOMA

This large adrenal cortical carcinoma was resected from a 27-year-old female. The tumor measured 17 cm in diameter and invaded kidney and spleen which necessitated en bloc removal of these organs with tumor. Patient had evidence of virilization.

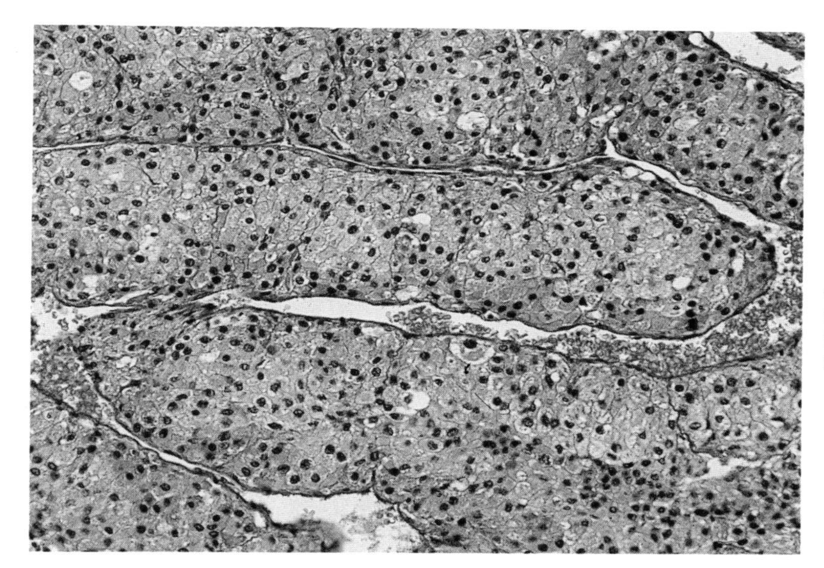

Figure 5-7
ADRENAL
CORTICAL CARCINOMA

Broad anastomosing trabecular pattern with intervening delicate sinusoids. Despite the lack of significant nuclear atypia, this histologic pattern may be associated with aggressive biologic behavior.

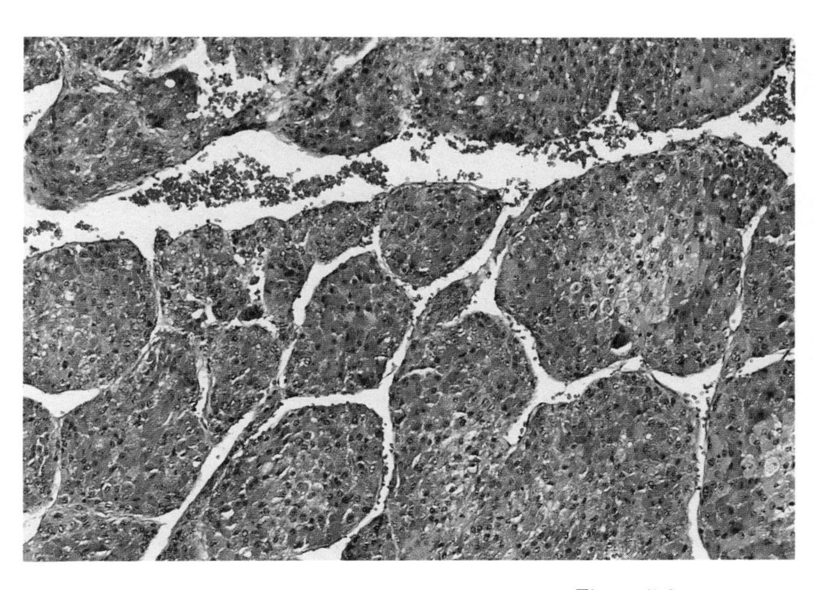

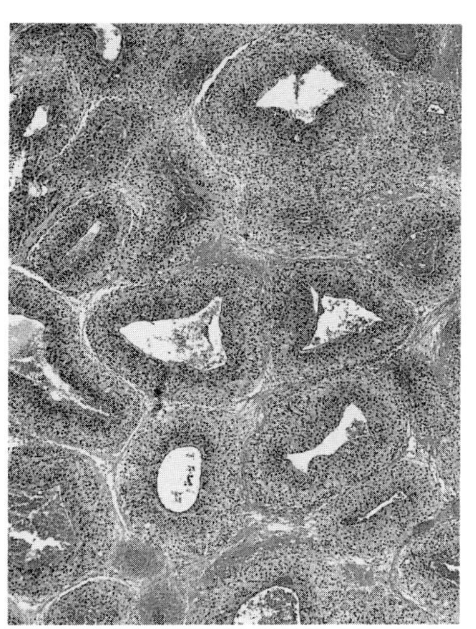

Figure 5-8
ADRENAL CORTICAL CARCINOMA

Left: Adrenal cortical carcinoma from an adult male who also had primary hyperaldosteronism. Occasional nests of tumor appear to be "free floating," but further sectioning may reveal sites of attachment. Sinusoidal sclerosis is absent and this area shows no significant cytologic or nuclear atypia.

Right: Perithelial distribution of tumor cells and intervening zones of necrosis.

gaping sinusoids lined by an attenuated endothelial layer (fig. 5-7). Occasionally, the trabeculae are oriented in a more parallel elongated array, or have a very irregular contour with daisy-like or clover leaf configuration, sometimes with areas of necrosis (fig. 5-8). The trabecular pattern can also be seen as an alignment of cells in slender elongated cords (fig. 5-9), sometimes with myxoid stromal change or fibrosis. In rare cases, there is a serpiginous arrangement of cells as might be seen in a carcinoid or islet cell tumor (fig. 5-10). A trabecular pattern, such as that seen in figure 5-7, is ominous even in the absence of other histologic features such as nuclear pleomorphism and with tumors which are large (i.e., several hundred grams), the diagnosis is rarely benign.

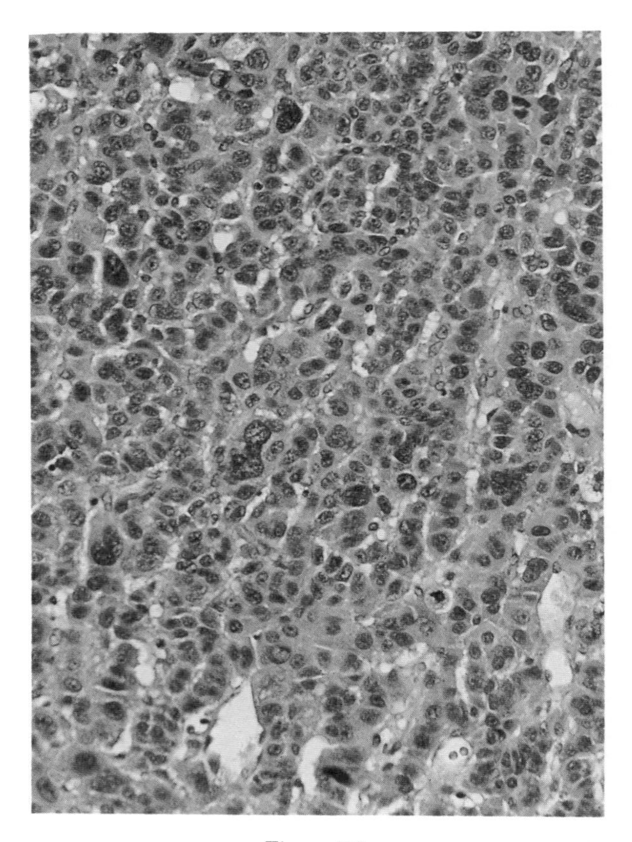

Figure 5-9
ADRENAL CORTICAL CARCINOMA
There is a mixed architectural pattern. In this field the tumor cells are closely aligned in narrow, elongate columns.

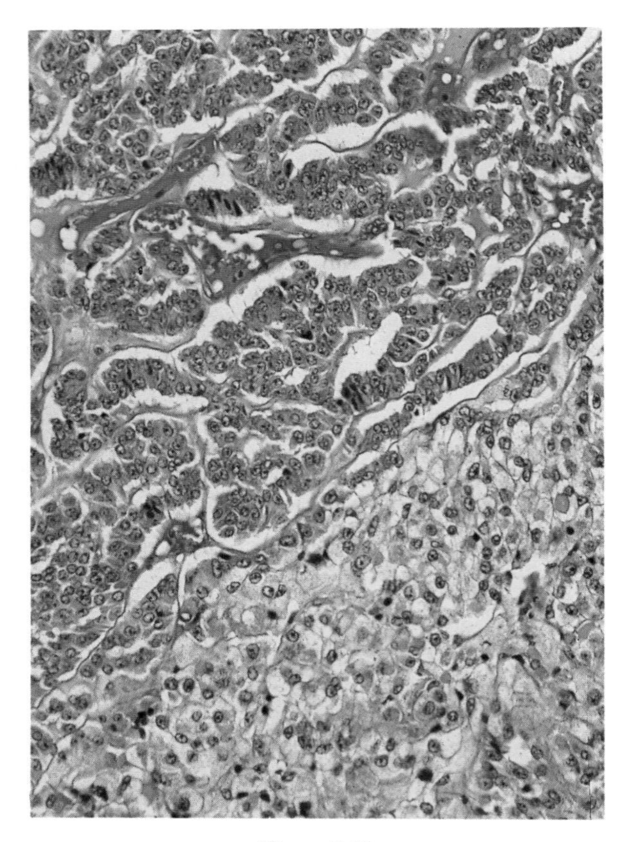

Figure 5-10
ADRENAL CORTICAL CARCINOMA
At the top are serpiginous cords of cells mimicking a carcinoid or islet cell tumor. Tumor cells in bottom half of field have a more diffuse or solid pattern with distinct cell borders and predominantly lipid-rich, pale-staining cytoplasm, but many cells had eosinophilic condensation of cell cytoplasm. No intracytoplasmic hyaline globules are evident.

Other architectural patterns can be found in tumors classified as ACC. A nesting or alveolar arrangement of cells can be present, and may be only focally distributed within a particular neoplasm (fig. 5-11); in areas this pattern may blend with the trabecular pattern noted above, which itself can be somewhat heterogeneous. There may be a diffuse or solid pattern which may be focal, or less commonly, diffuse in distribution, in which the endocrine nature of the tumor, and specifically an adrenal histogenesis, may not be obvious, particularly when coupled with significant cytologic pleomorphism (fig. 5-12). A spindle cell or frankly sarcomatous pattern in ACC is rare. Occasional myxoid foci may cause diagnostic problems either in the primary tumor or even in distant metastases. Superficially, this myxoid pattern may resemble a chordoma or other myxoid neoplasm (fig. 5-13) (42) and is usually focal within any particular tumor. A distinctive histologic pattern has been described in an ACC associated with hyperaldosteronism: an alveolar arrangement of cells separated by prominent, thick walled, dilated vascular spaces with zona glomerulosa type cells (29,40); this appearance, however, is nonspecific (see fig. 5-8, left).

Cellular Morphology. Most ACCs contain a predominance of cells with lipid-depleted or acidophilic, compact cytoplasm; however, this feature alone does not have a statistically significant bearing on prognosis. Occasionally, coarse granular pigment representing lipofuscin is seen within the cytoplasm (fig. 5-14). Some tumors, as seen in figure 5-11, contain an abundance of lipid-rich, pale-staining cells. The presence (focal or diffuse) of cells with compact, eosinophilic

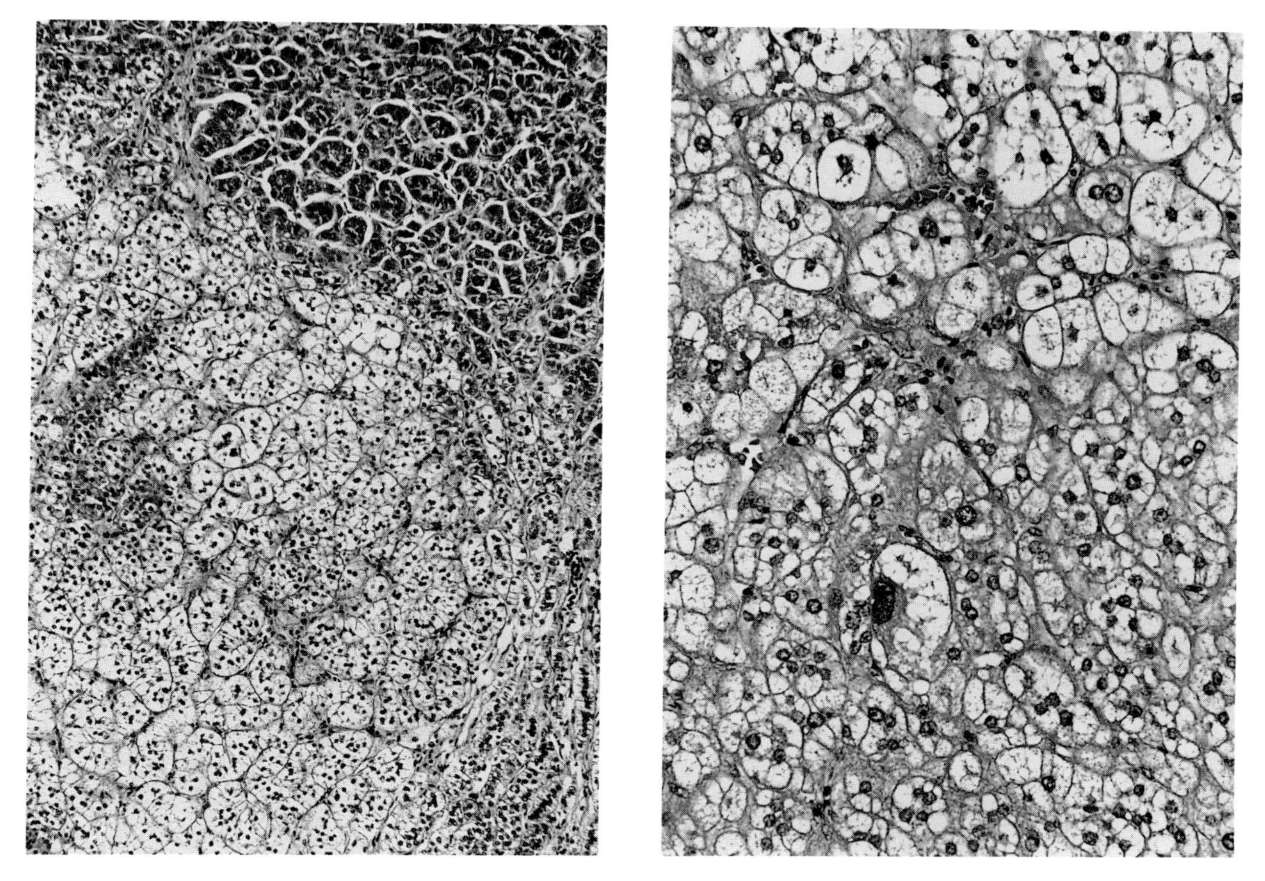

Figure 5-11
ADRENAL CORTICAL CARCINOMA

Left: Alveolar or nesting pattern was present, but there were other admixed patterns along with areas of extensive necrosis and foci of vascular invasion.

Right: Most cells in this field are arranged in round to ovoid nests, with individual cells having pale-staining, lipid-rich cytoplasm.

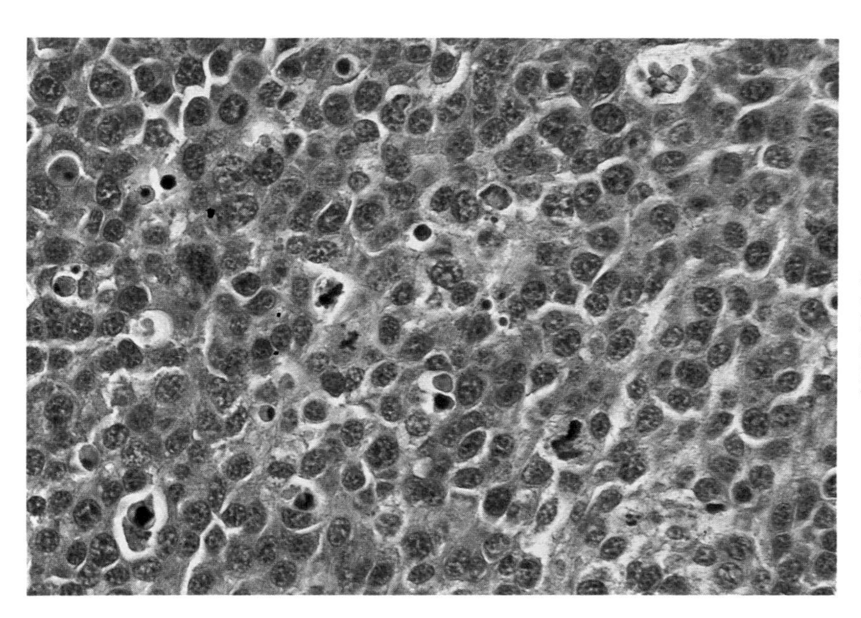

Figure 5-12
ADRENAL
CORTICAL CARCINOMA

The tumor has a diffuse or solid pattern of irregular pleomorphic cells which can cause diagnostic problems. Most tumor cells have moderate to abundant eosinophilic, compact cytoplasm. Mitotic figures were numerous with many atypical forms.

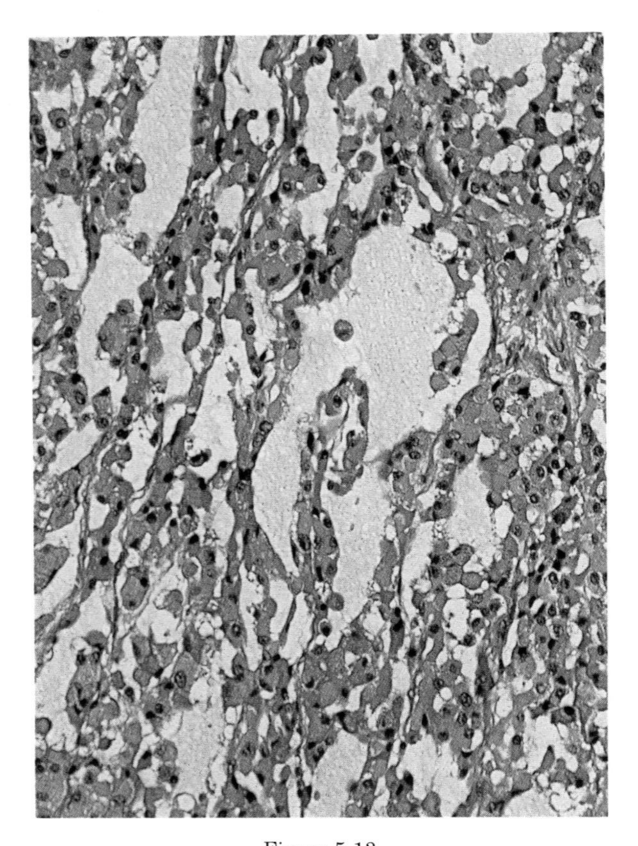

Figure 5-13
ADRENAL CORTICAL CARCINOMA
Areas of marked myxoid change separate cords of tumor cells with predominantly compact, eosinophilic cytoplasm.

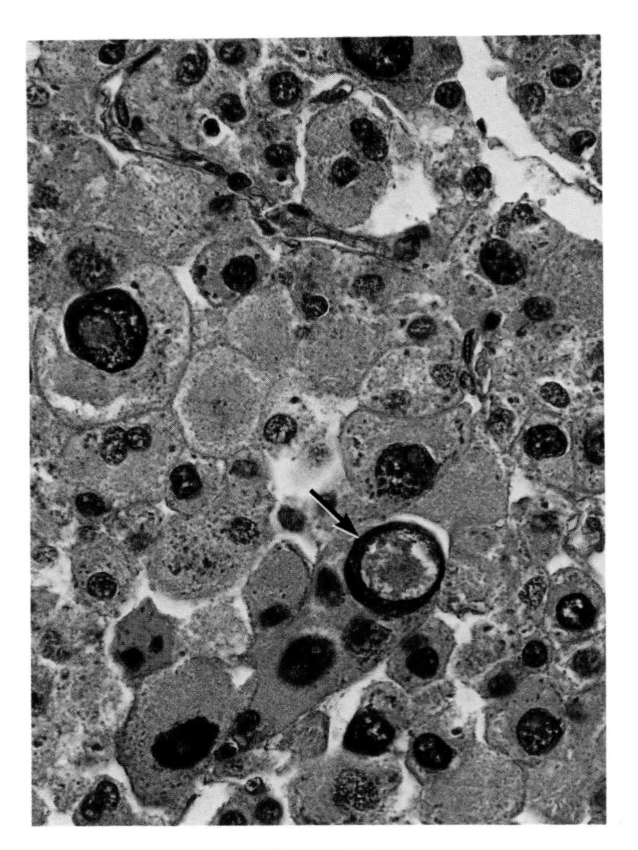

Figure 5-14
ADRENAL CORTICAL CARCINOMA
These tumor cells have a granular, compact cytoplasm. Some cells have granular pigment which is most likely lipofuscin. Note the large nuclear "pseudoinclusion" (arrow).

cytoplasm does not correlate with any particular endocrine syndrome. On rare occasion a tumor classified as ACC may have such abundant eosinophilic cytoplasm that a designation of "oncocytic" may be appropriate, but as noted in chapter 4, this variant of adrenal cortical neoplasm needs further characterization since both clinically benign and malignant forms have been reported. Cytologic borders of cells in ACC (and adenomas) are often fairly well defined.

Nuclear pleomorphism and hyperchromasia can be a striking feature in ACC (fig. 5-15), but nuclear atypia of similar degree can occasionally be seen in clinically benign tumors. The presence of this feature alone is not sufficient to classify an adrenal cortical neoplasm as malignant, and this may be important in interpretation of cytologic material obtained by fine-needle aspiration. On occasion, nuclei appear hyperlobated or multinucleated (fig. 5-16), or contain one or more prominent nucleoli (30). Nuclear "pseudoinclusions" can be found in some ACCs (fig. 5-14), as well as some cortical adenomas and pheochromocytomas. These may be solitary or multiple, and appear as sharply outlined structures which may stain identically as the remaining cell cytoplasm, or may show pallor or vacuolar change. These "pseudoinclusions" result from irregularities or infolding of the nuclear membrane with intranuclear extension of cell cytoplasm (see chapter 4, figs. 4-21, 4-50, top). An important feature in a few adrenal cortical tumors, both benign and malignant, is the presence of intracytoplasmic hyaline globules (fig. 5-17). These globules are round to oval, refractile, and deeply eosinophilic, and are identical by light microscopic morphology and special staining characteristics (i.e., periodic acid–Schiff

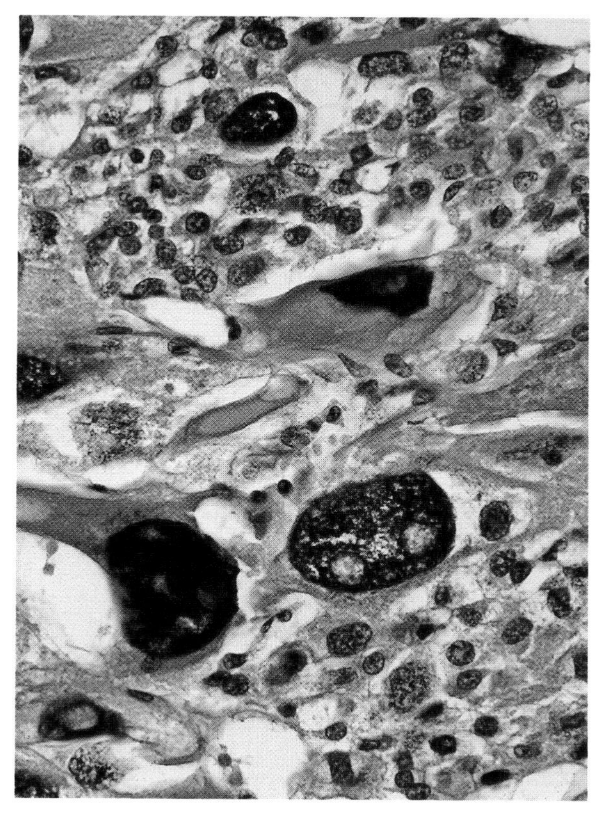

Figure 5-15
ADRENAL CORTICAL CARCINOMA
There is a marked degree of nuclear hyperchromasia, and great disparity in size and shape of nuclei. Compare these remarkable features with the smaller tumor cells, which in turn are larger than normal adrenal cortical cells.

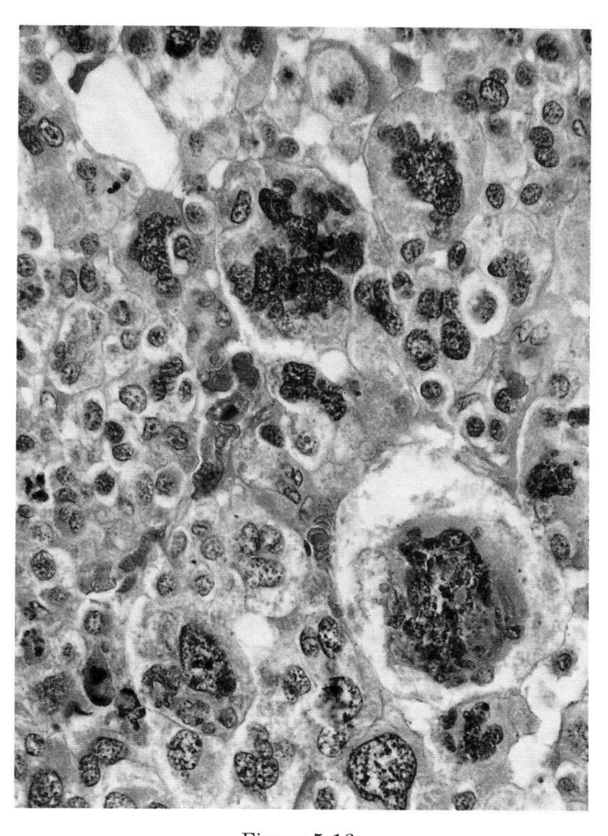

Figure 5-16
ADRENAL CORTICAL CARCINOMA
Focally, some tumor cells have enlarged, hyperlobated nuclei and some appear to be multinucleated.

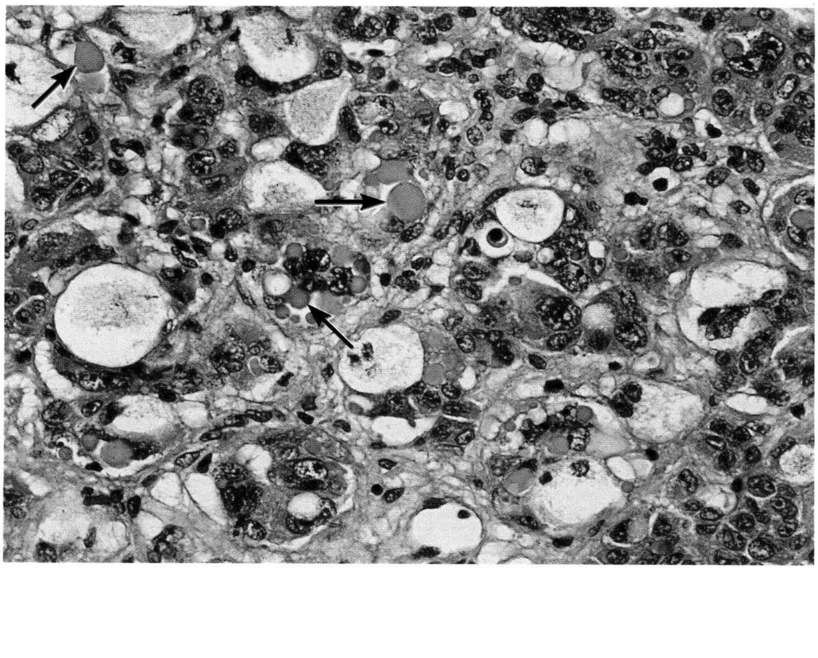

Figure 5-17
ADRENAL CORTICAL CARCINOMA
This adrenal cortical carcinoma is composed of cells with eosinophilic, granular cytoplasm. Note the presence of intracytoplasmic hyaline globules (arrows).

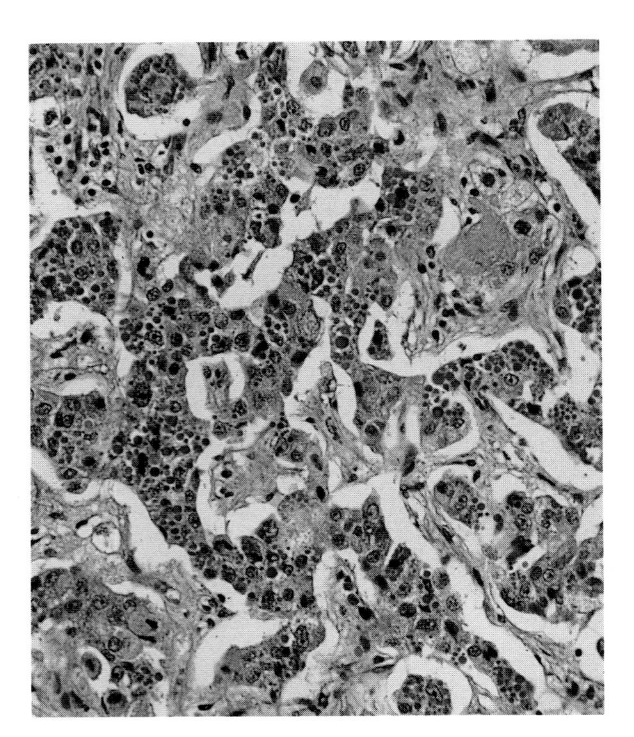

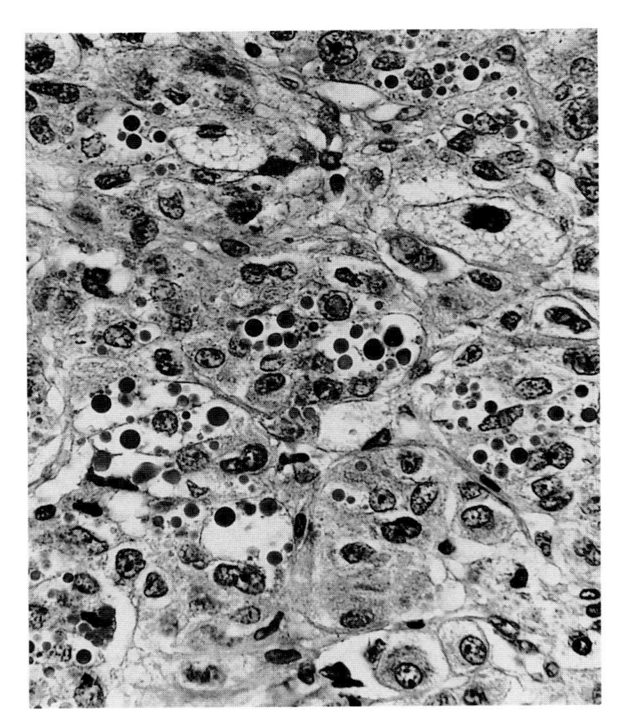

Figure 5-18
ADRENAL CORTICAL CARCINOMA

Left: The tumor had small areas with an anastomosing trabecular pattern and an extraordinary number of intracytoplasmic hyaline globules.

Right: Most of the intracytoplasmic globules are round and densely eosinophilic.

[PAS] positive and variably resistant to diastase predigestion) to globules that are seen much more frequently in pheochromocytomas. In rare instances, it may be very difficult to distinguish an adrenal cortical neoplasm from a pheochromocytoma, and differentiation may necessitate immunohistochemical stains (pheochromocytomas are positive for chromogranin) or even ultrastructural study to identify dense-core neurosecretory granules. An adrenal cortical tumor with an alveolar or anastomosing trabecular pattern and these globules can be confused with a pheochromocytoma (fig. 5-18).

Mitotic figures are relatively common in ACC, and atypical forms may be present. The presence of mitotic figures in several consecutive high-power fields (fig. 5-19) is suspicious for malignancy and other histologic and nonhistologic features that might be supportive should be sought. Weiss (46) found three histologic features specific to metastasizing or recurring adrenal cortical tumors: a mitotic rate of 6 or more per 50 high-power fields, atypical mitoses, and invasion of venous structures. These findings do not necessarily apply to adrenal cortical tumors in the pediatric age group (see chapter 6). A mitotic rate greater than 20 per 50 high-power fields in adults has been associated with a shortened median survival (14 months) compared with tumors having 20 or fewer mitoses (58 months median survival, $p<0.02$) (47).

Invasion. Vascular invasion is also an ominous finding in an adrenal cortical neoplasm. It is very unusual to recognize angioinvasion on gross examination of the resected tumor or in preoperative imaging studies, although some tumors have been reported as invading the inferior vena cava (2,34) and even extending on into the right atrium (3,10,15). Vascular invasion is usually seen in histologic sections as loose plugs of tumor within the lumen of large veins (fig. 5-20), or sometimes in smaller vascular spaces with some suggesting lymphatic channels. Invasion of the inferior vena cava can be associated with

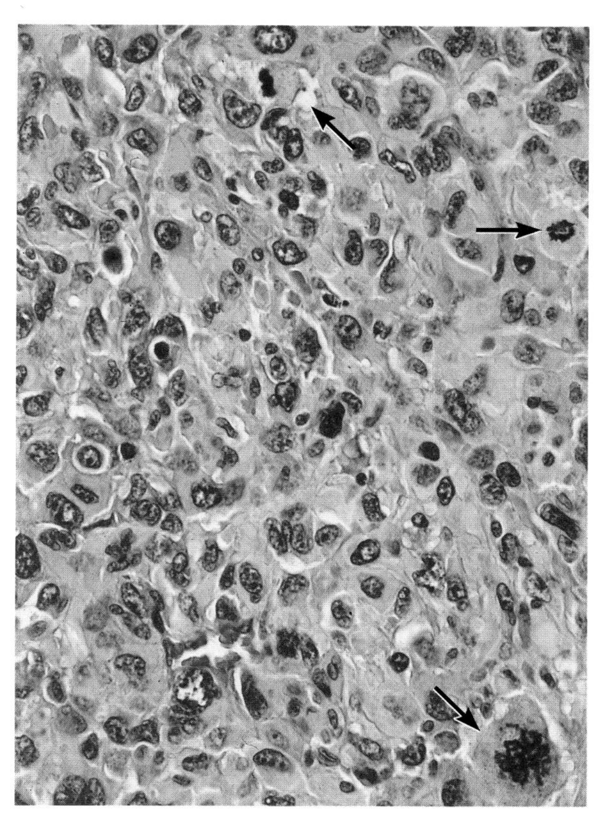

Figure 5-19
ADRENAL CORTICAL CARCINOMA
There is compact, eosinophilic cytoplasm and pleomorphic nuclei. Mitotic figures are numerous (arrows). Atypical mitotic figures were also present.

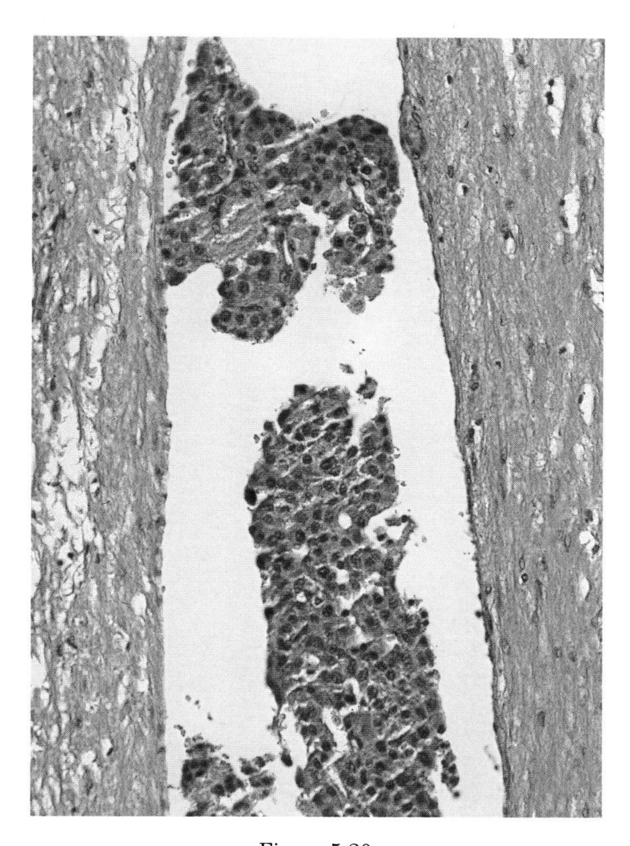

Figure 5-20
ADRENAL CORTICAL CARCINOMA
Tumor had several areas of large tumor plugs within venous channels.

malignant ascites and lower extremity edema and, if unrecognized, may pose a danger during surgical resection if intraoperative mechanical manipulation results in major tumor emboli. The tumor may extend in a sausage-like fashion into the vena cava without firm attachment to the vein wall (fig. 5-21).

Capsular invasion can be difficult to recognize in ACC since the expanded capsule (or fibrous pseudocapsule) may be, in part, preexisting adrenal capsule. This pattern of invasion may be apparent as one or more blunt extensions of tumor through the fibrous pseudocapsule (fig. 5-22). Invasion of adjacent soft tissues or organs such as kidney or liver is a priori evidence of malignancy with extension beyond the adrenal capsule. Identification of capsular invasion is seldom essential in establishing the malignant nature of the tumor.

Stromal Alterations and Changes in Attached Adrenal Gland. Broad fibrous bands may intersect the tumor, subdividing it into irregular macroscopic nodules. There may be broad confluent areas of necrosis, and occasionally most of the tumor may be necrotic as in figure 5-5. Irregular foci of dense dystrophic calcification may be present, which usually follows in the wake of tumor necrosis (fig. 5-23, left), and this may be detected on radiographic study of the abdomen. Hamper et al. (12) found that almost 20 percent of ACCs had calcification on sonographic evaluation as evidenced by a heterogeneous pattern of echopenic or echogenic zones. At times the calcification has a dust-like quality associated with individual necrotic cells (fig. 5-23, right). Other features include myxoid alteration of stroma and formation of lipomatous or myelolipomatous metaplasia. Occasionally, one can get important clues as to an associated

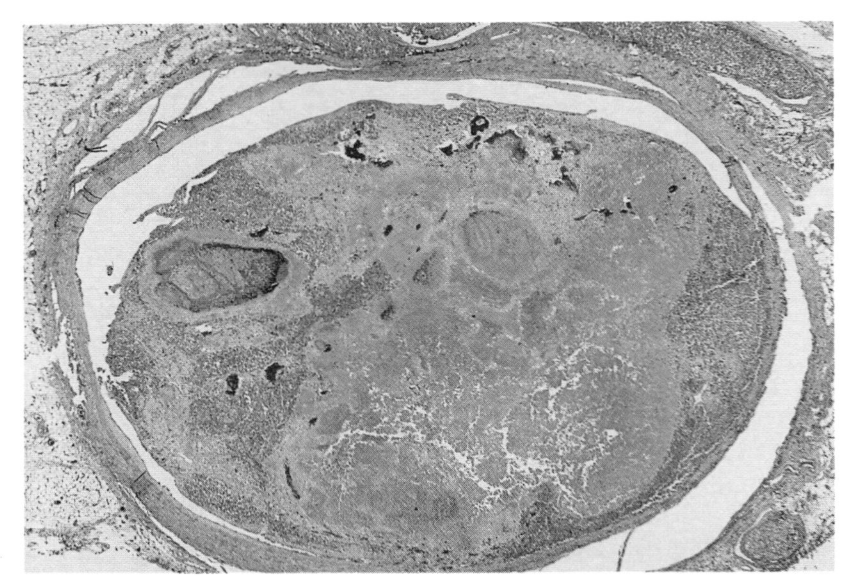

Figure 5-21
ADRENAL CORTICAL CARCINOMA
Invasion of the inferior vena cava by an adrenal cortical carcinoma caused almost complete occlusion of the lumen. Tumor shows extensive necrosis and, along one portion, is attached to the wall of the vein. A few areas of dystrophic calcification are also present.

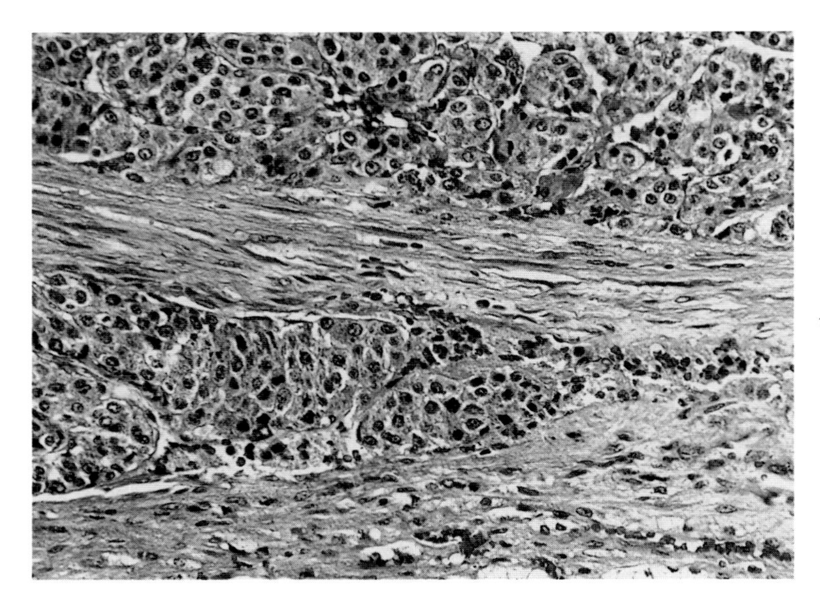

Figure 5-22
ADRENAL CORTICAL CARCINOMA
Blunt extensions of tumor project through the fibrous pseudocapsule.

endocrine syndrome, even when clinical features and endocrinologic data are not available for correlation. The presence of cortical atrophy usually indicates hypercortisolism with Cushing's syndrome or a mixed endocrine syndrome such as Cushing's syndrome and virilization. In the rare cases of ACC associated with primary hyperaldosteronism, there may be hyperplasia of the zona glomerulosa in the attached adrenal remnant.

Ultrastructural Findings. There is a range of ultrastructural features of ACC (49). As might be expected from the light microscopic findings, the abundance of cells with compact, eosinophilic cytoplasm indicates a cell population with few to no intracytoplasmic lipid droplets (fig. 5-24); this is in sharp contrast to neoplastic lipid-rich cortical cells and normal cortical cells of the zona fasciculata. The cytoplasmic eosinophilia seen by light microscopy may be contributed in part by a prominent smooth endoplasmic reticulum (fig. 5-25) and abundant mitochondria; the latter may give the cytoplasm a finely granular appearance. An overabundance of mitochondria can give the tumor cells an oncocytic

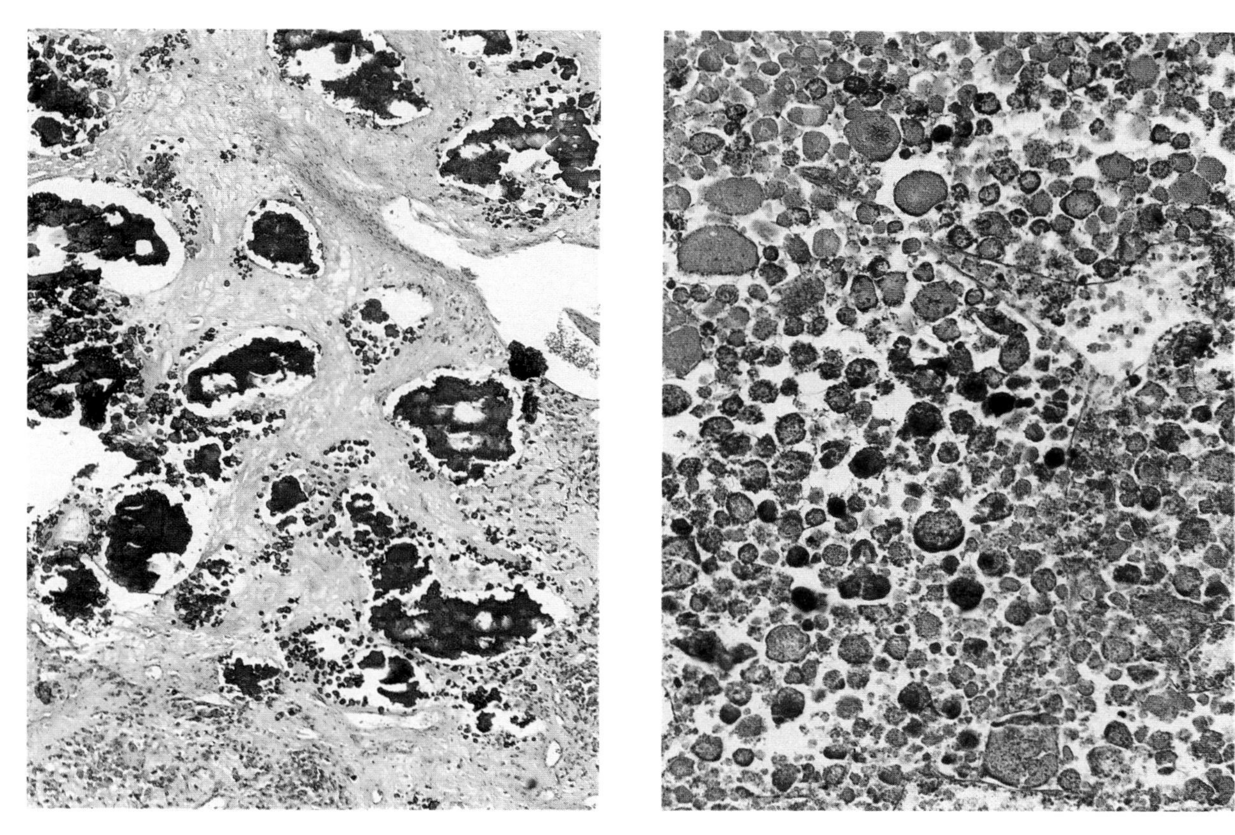

Figure 5-23
ADRENAL CORTICAL CARCINOMA
Left: Adrenal cortical carcinoma has areas of granular to coarse dystrophic calcification in a background of extensive tumor necrosis. Right: Most necrotic cells show granular, punctate to dust-like dystrophic mineralization.

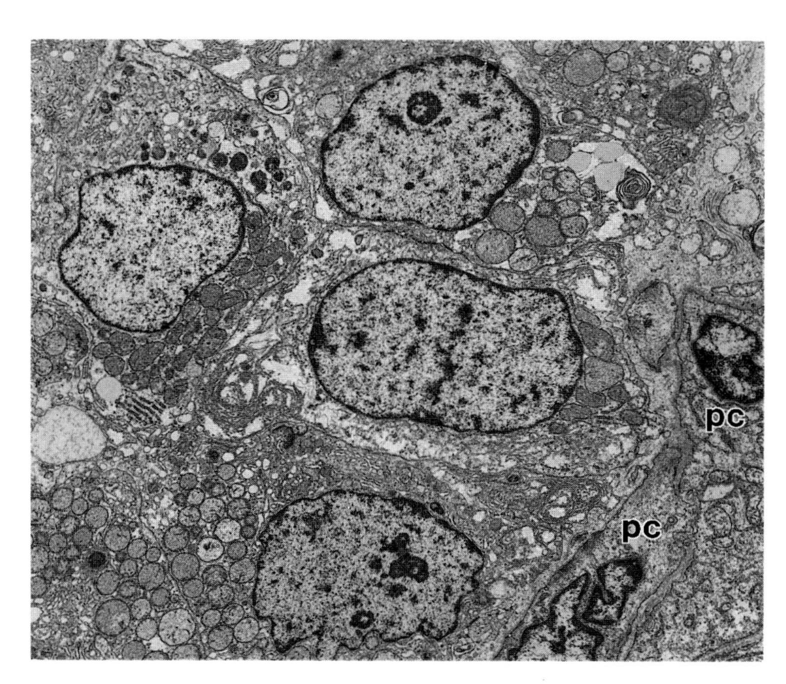

Figure 5-24
ADRENAL CORTICAL CARCINOMA

The cells contain sparse lipid droplets, and some have small, irregular microvillous extensions of cytoplasm along the cell border. The density and distribution of mitochondria vary. Cells contain both smooth and rough endoplasmic reticulum. Pericytes (pc) are seen in the right lower corner adjacent to the vascular channel just out of field. (X6,500)

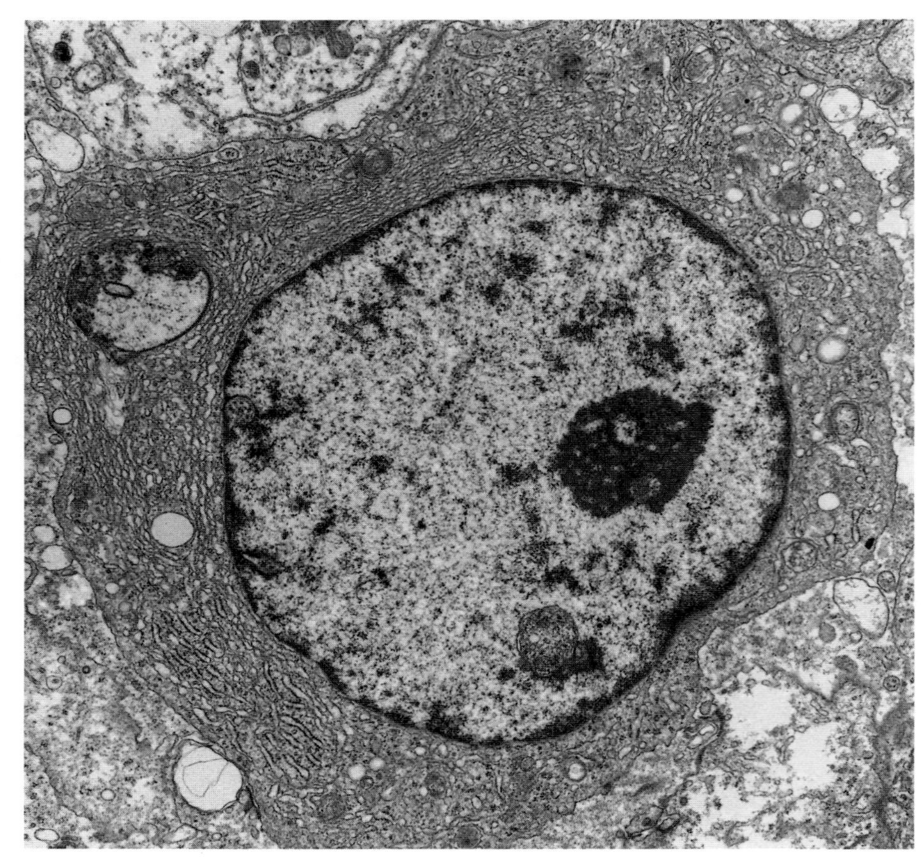

Figure 5-25
ADRENAL CORTICAL CARCINOMA

This cell contains abundant smooth endoplasmic reticulum and profiles of rough endoplasmic reticulum. Few primitive intercellular junctions were present. (X13,000) (Fig. 3-46 from Lack EE, Travis WD, Oertel JE. Adrenal cortical neoplasms. In: Lack EE, ed. Pathology of the adrenal glands. New York: Churchill Livingstone, 1990:115–71.)

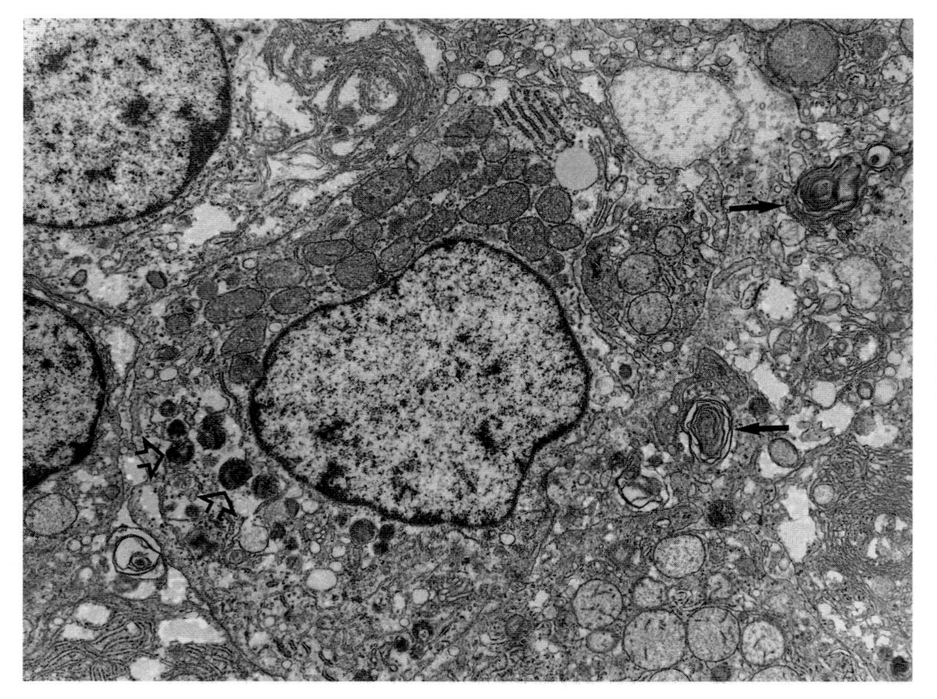

Figure 5-26
ADRENAL CORTICAL CARCINOMA

The cells have irregular cytoplasmic extensions as well as a few myelin figures (straight arrows). The dense granular material probably represents lipofuscin (open arrows). Parallel stacks of rough endoplasmic reticulum are present in the upper field. (X7,000)

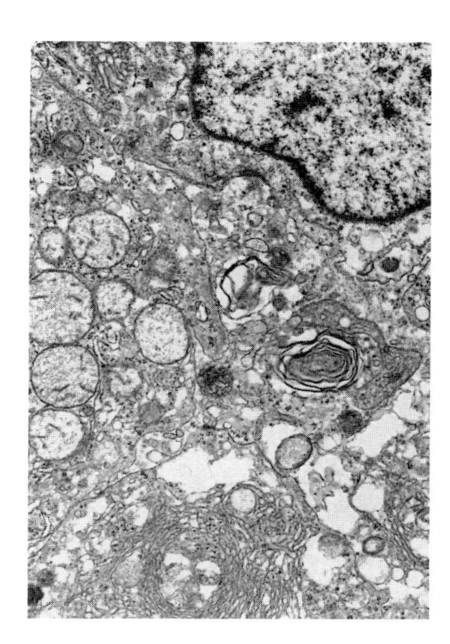
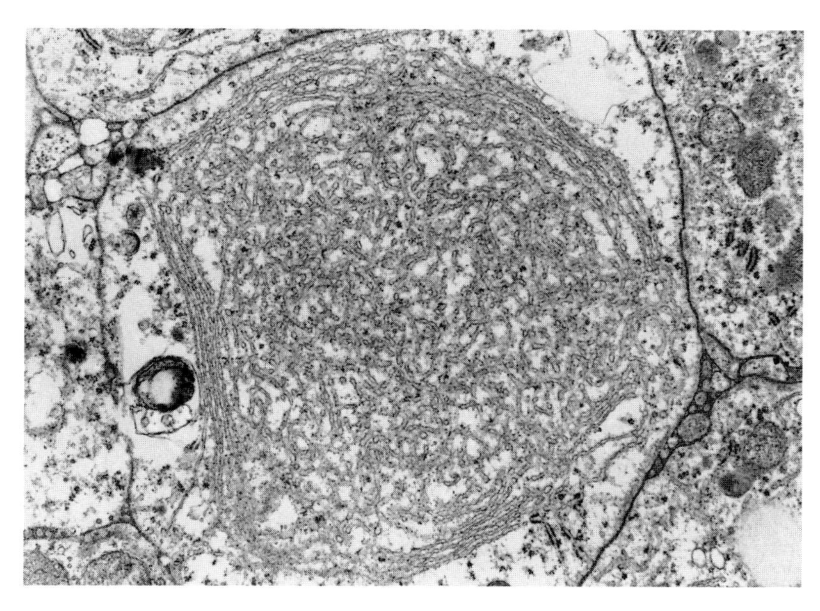

Figure 5-27
ADRENAL CORTICAL CARCINOMA

Left: There is a concentric whorl of smooth endoplasmic reticulum as well as a myelin figure. The mitochondria have sparse lamellar cristae. (X10,000)

Right: Adrenal cortical carcinoma with tangled skein of smooth endoplasmic reticulum forming a coarsely lamellar pattern. (X17,000)

appearance. In a recent study, about one third of ACCs failed to show convincing evidence of steroid cell differentiation (49). Most tumors contain cells with short, flattened profiles of rough endoplasmic reticulum; occasionally it is seen as small stacks (fig. 5-26) (49). The nucleus becomes a dominant feature in some cells, and may have dispersed chromatin with margination on the nuclear membrane or may be densely clumped. Tumor cells may have stubby, microvillous projections, but these are usually not as well developed as in adenomas (see chapter 4). Simple intercellular junctions are occasionally seen, but they tend to be sparse in number. The smooth endoplasmic reticulum may form concentric whorls (fig. 5-27), or there may be sparse lamellated structures resembling myelin figures.

Mitochondria may vary in size and shape, but are often small and round to oval. They may have a primitive cristal component which can be tubular, vesicular, or lamellar (shelf-like) (fig. 5-28). A granular matrix may be prominent within individual mitochondria. Cells of virilizing ACC can resemble the compact cells of the zona reticularis, with lamellar and tubular cristae, lipofuscin pigment, and scant lipid, but it is

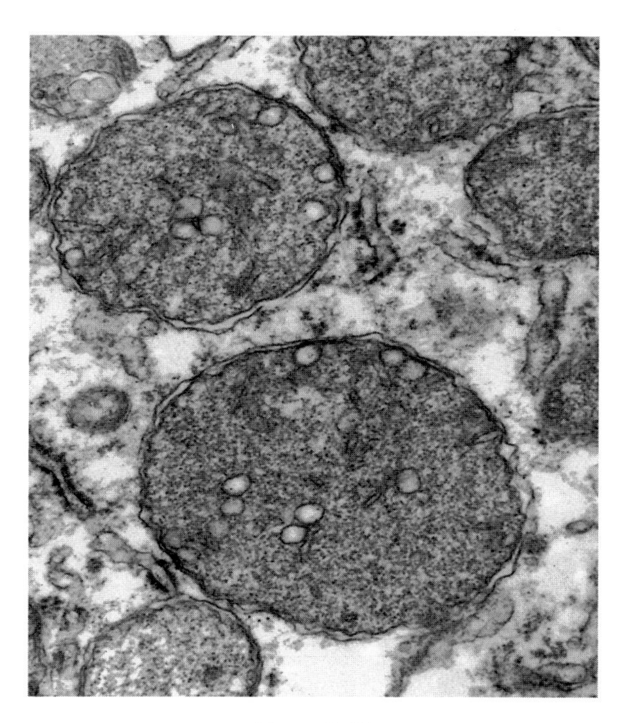

Figure 5-28
ADRENAL CORTICAL CARCINOMA

Mitochondrial cristae are relatively sparse with both vesicular and tubular profiles along with an abundant granular matrix. (X37,500)

virtually impossible to accurately predict the presence or absence of any particular endocrine syndrome solely from the ultrastructural appearance. Small intracytoplasmic lakes of glycogen have been reported in ACC, but are uncommon; in a recent study glycogen was noted in a metastatic ACC while the primary tumor did not show the same extensive accumulation of glycogen (49). Sparse, membrane-bound, dense-core granules have been reported, and in one recent report were considered consistent with neuroendocrine type granules even though the cells were not immunoreactive for chromogranin A (50).

Immunohistochemical Findings. At present there is no pathognomonic immunohistochemical profile for ACC, but even negative results can sometimes aid in a difficult differential diagnosis. ACCs are typically negative for cytokeratin (51,53,68,71), although occasional positive results may be obtained using fresh frozen tissue or sections pretreated with a protease such as trypsin (53,62,71). In a study by Schröder et al. (68), only 2 of 72 adrenal cortical neoplasms (57 adrenal cortical adenomas [ACAs] and 15 ACCs) stained for cytokeratin (1 ACA and 1 ACC); Cote et al. (51) reported positive results in normal cortical cells and ACA, but none of the ACC cells expressed cytokeratin. Nakano (63) reported 24 of 62 ACCs contained cytokeratin-positive cells, while all of the 42 ACAs were negative. In a recent study, 9 of 18 ACCs were positive for cytokeratin and in most cases less than 25 percent of cells were immunoreactive (55); none of the ACAs were immunoreactive for cytokeratin. Keratin staining was present in all of the normal adrenal cortices. Vimentin has been reported to be positive in tumor cells of ACC (fig. 5-29), but the frequency reported in the literature varies considerably: 8 percent among 57 ACAs and 15 ACCs (68); 65 percent (all ACCs) (53); 73 percent of ACCs (versus only 14 percent of ACAs) (63); and 100 percent of ACCs (51,55,62). Despite the variable results reported in the literature, as a general rule, a neoplasm that has the typical morphology, either in tissue sections or cytologic preparations, and features of an ACC (large size, suprarenal location, adverse imaging characteristics) would statistically be expected to be vimentin positive and cytokeratin negative (at least most tumor cells).

Differential Diagnosis. The differential diagnosis of ACC includes hepatocellular carcinoma (HCC), renal cell carcinoma (RCC), and metastatic carcinoma. Careful morphologic evaluation and close correlation with other features such as clinical presentation, location, or results of special stains for intracellular glycogen or mucosubstances often provide definitive information as to the correct diagnosis. In a few cases, however, there may be lingering uncertainty. Most RCCs are positive for cytokeratin and other epithelial markers, such as epithelial membrane antigen (EMA) (59,60,71). In one study, 33 of 33 HCCs (100 percent) were positive for cytokeratin and 6 (18 percent) were positive for vimentin, while 24 of 37 RCCs were positive for keratin (65 percent) and 22 of 37 were positive for vimentin (60 percent) (53). In another study, 94 percent of HCCs were positive for cytokeratin using the monoclonal antibody CAM 5.2 (56). It appears that the immunophenotypic overlap of ACC, RCC, and HCC may hinder interpretation of some cases, but careful scrutiny of morphology and use of basic special stains may resolve the dilemma. Expression of 3-beta-hydroxy-delta^5-steroid dehydrogenase activity, an enzyme involved in biosynthesis of all classes of adrenal cortical steroids, has not been shown to be a reliable discriminator between renal and adrenal cortical tumors since it has been identified in normal kidney including mRNA (64). Nuclear D11 immunoreactivity has been reported to allow accurate typing of benign and malignant adrenal cortical neoplasms (67), and distinguishes carcinomas metastatic to the adrenal, including RCC, as well as other primary tumors such as pheochromocytoma (58,70). A potentially important immunohistochemical finding is staining for synaptophysin in a significant proportion of ACCs (55,58,61, 68) which can lead to misdiagnosis unless attention is paid to routine morphology (fig. 5-30). In one study, 8 of 10 ACCs were positive, at least focally, and 3 showed extensive positivity of more than 30 percent of tumor cells (61). None of the ACCs were positive for chromogranin A or a variety of neuropeptides (58,61) and all tumors were negative for cytoplasmic argyrophilia (68). Chromogranin and somatostatin immunoreactivity is not detected in the normal adrenal cortex, ACA, or ACC (55). Clusters of dense-core granules have been identified ultrastructurally

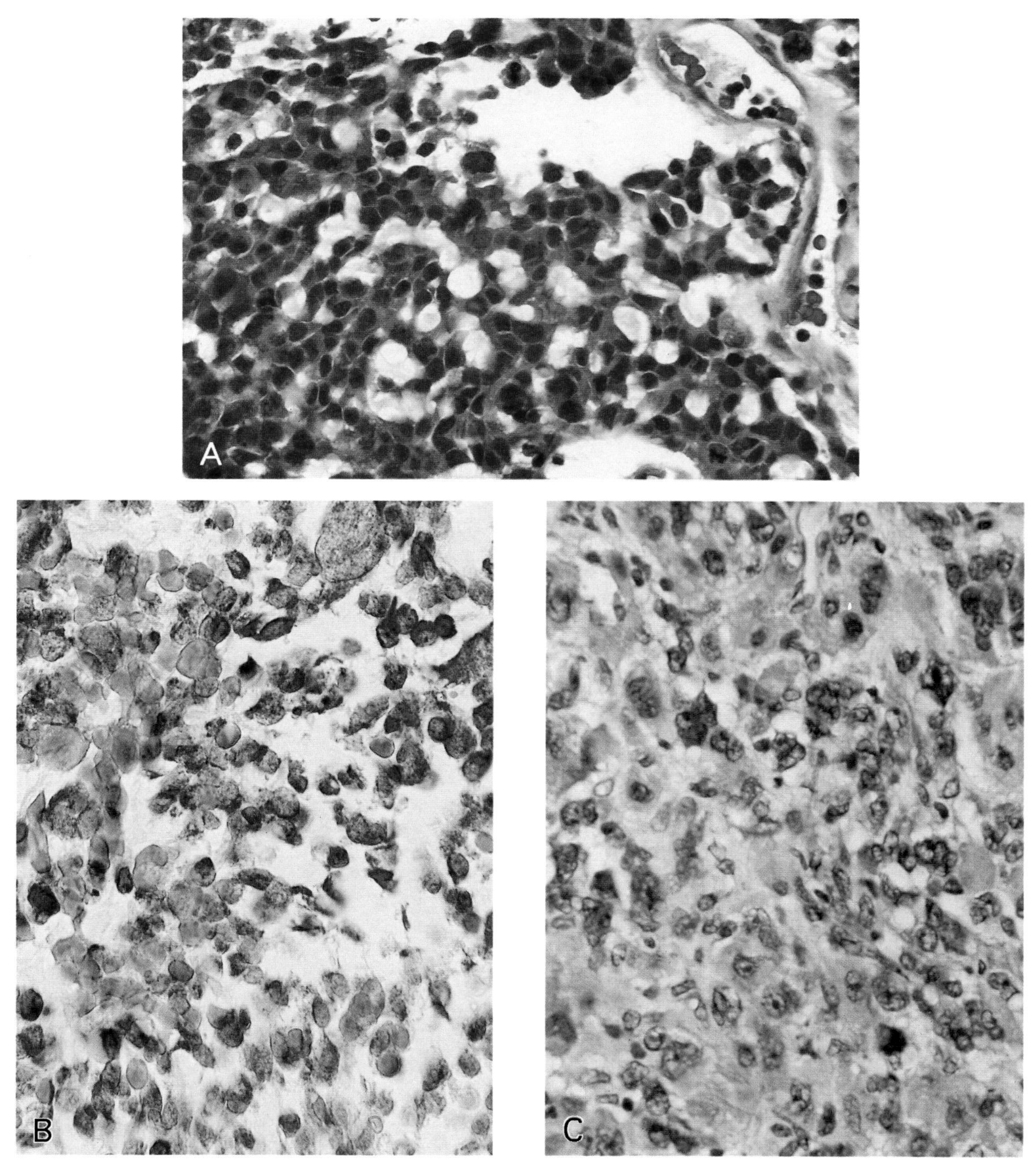

Figure 5-29
ADRENAL CORTICAL CARCINOMA

A: Cell block preparation from a fine-needle aspiration biopsy of a large ACC shows tumor cells with compact, eosinophilic cytoplasm and a mild degree of nuclear pleomorphism.

B: Tumor cells from the same case were negative for cytokeratin but positive for vimentin as seen here. Other special stains (e.g., PAS and mucicarmine) were also negative. Close correlation with clinical and radiographic findings is indicated (see figure 5-31). (X400, Streptavidin alkaline phosphatase method) (Figures 5-29A,B, 5-31, and 5-32 are from the same case.)

C: Tissue section from a different adrenal cortical carcinoma shows positive staining for vimentin. (X400, Peroxidase-antiperoxidase stain)

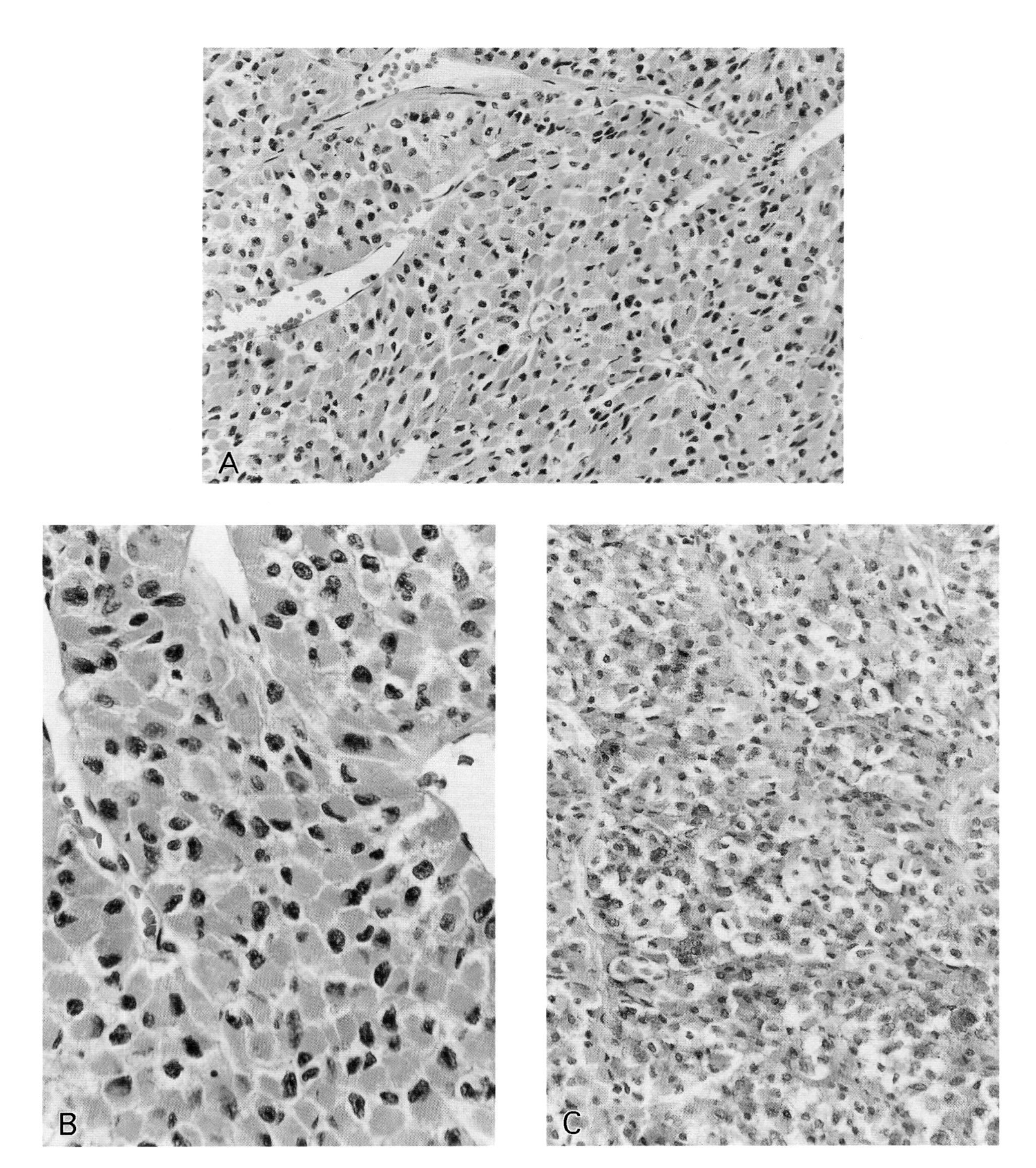

Figure 5-30
ADRENAL CORTICAL CARCINOMA IN AN ADULT PATIENT

A: This large tumor arose in the upper abdomen, and was immediately juxta-adrenal in location according to intraoperative findings. It was mistakenly interpreted as an extra-adrenal paraganglioma (organ of Zuckerkandl tumor).

B: Tumor has a well-developed trabecular pattern. The cells have compact, eosinophilic cytoplasm with relatively distinct cell borders and mild nuclear pleomorphism.

C: Many cells show positive immunostaining for synaptophysin. (X375, Peroxidase-antiperoxidase stain)

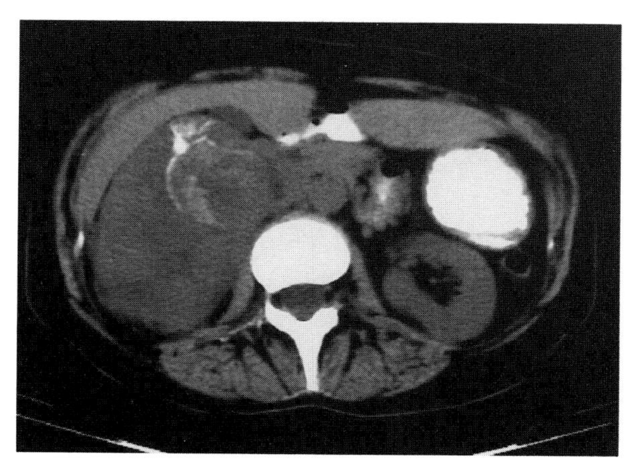

Figure 5-31
ADRENAL CORTICAL CARCINOMA

A 52-year-old woman presented with abdominal pain and a palpable mass. CT scan showed a large, suprarenal mass in the right upper quadrant which has nonuniform density and areas of dystrophic calcification. The patient underwent fine-needle aspiration.

in some tumors (61), but their distinction from primary lysosomes may be difficult.

An immunohistochemical study of markers of proliferative activity using a scoring system of proliferating cell nuclear antigen (PCNA) and Ki-67 has demonstrated a correlation with mitotic counts, histologic diagnosis, and clinical outcome (54). Suzuki et al. (69) found immunoreactivity for PCNA and epidermal growth factor receptor in all 6 ACAs and 15 ACCs, and concluded that only DNA ploidy determination and immunolocalization patterns of C-*myc* expression had any practical value in the pathologic evaluation of adrenal cortical tumors. Determination of nucleolar organizer regions (AgNORs) appears to offer little value in distinguishing between ACA and ACC, but may correlate with increased steroid hormone production (66). Similarly, lectin histochemical binding studies have not provided sufficient diagnostic information (65). Expression of epidermal growth factor receptors in ACC has been associated with tumor growth and metastatic potential (57). Another study reported no correlation between degree of reactivity for transforming growth factor-alpha and tumor grade, stage, or hormone content (52). Some of these markers may be important for tumor progression through autocrine stimulation and oncogene overexpression, but more investigation is needed.

Fine-Needle Aspiration. Percutaneous fine-needle aspiration is a very useful diagnostic procedure in the evaluation of an adrenal mass, particularly for staging an extra-adrenal primary malignancy. There are very few reports in which ACC was diagnosed by fine-needle aspiration (72,74,80,81), and an ACC may not be distinguished from a benign cortical neoplasm on the basis of cytologic findings alone. In several reported cases the malignant nature of the tumor was clearly evident with fine-needle biopsy, including one in which a pulmonary metastasis of ACC was diagnosed, but only after clinical correlation and comparison with the original primary tumor which had been resected a year earlier (79). Careful correlation with clinical and endocrinologic data is essential, as well as awareness of size, location, and imaging characteristics of the retroperitoneal mass (fig. 5-31). As noted in chapter 3, the chance of diagnosing an ACC in an incidentally discovered adrenal nodule are remote, particularly when the adrenal mass is small (3 cm or less). The cytologic features can be very atypical, with loosely cohesive clusters or individual cells having compact or vacuolated cytoplasm (fig. 5-32, left). The nucleus tends to dominate the cell thus giving a high nuclear/cytoplasmic ratio, and sometimes the nuclear enlargement and irregularity can be an outstanding feature (fig. 5-32, right). Additional information can be obtained by using special stains for intracytoplasmic glycogen or mucin (expect negative results in ACC), cytokeratin (typically negative), and vimentin (often positive). Unstained smears or cell block preparations can be utilized.

Occasionally, in aspirates of benign cortical nodules, one may see bare or "stripped" nuclei having no apparent cytoplasm; this may superficially mimic a small, round cell malignancy (fig. 5-33) (75,77). However, the nuclei tend to be relatively uniform, without molding, and there is typically no evidence of necrosis. Conversely, a pulmonary adenocarcinoma metastatic to the adrenal gland has been reported in which the aspirate of malignant cells closely resembled normal cortical cells (76). A large, upper quadrant mass can occasionally be difficult to distinguish from kidney or liver, and fine-needle aspiration of a primary renal or hepatic neoplasm might be confused with an adrenal cortical tumor. An adrenal metastasis from RCC was

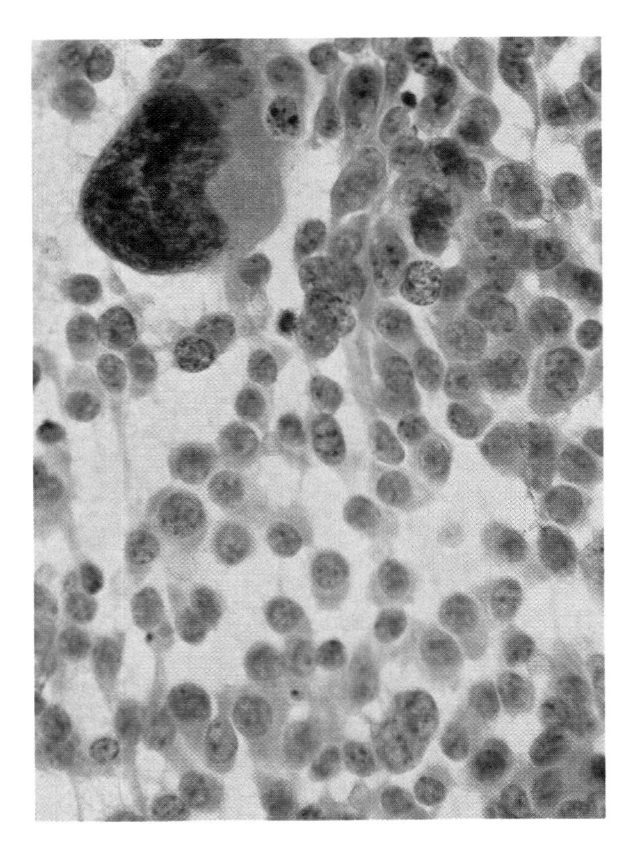

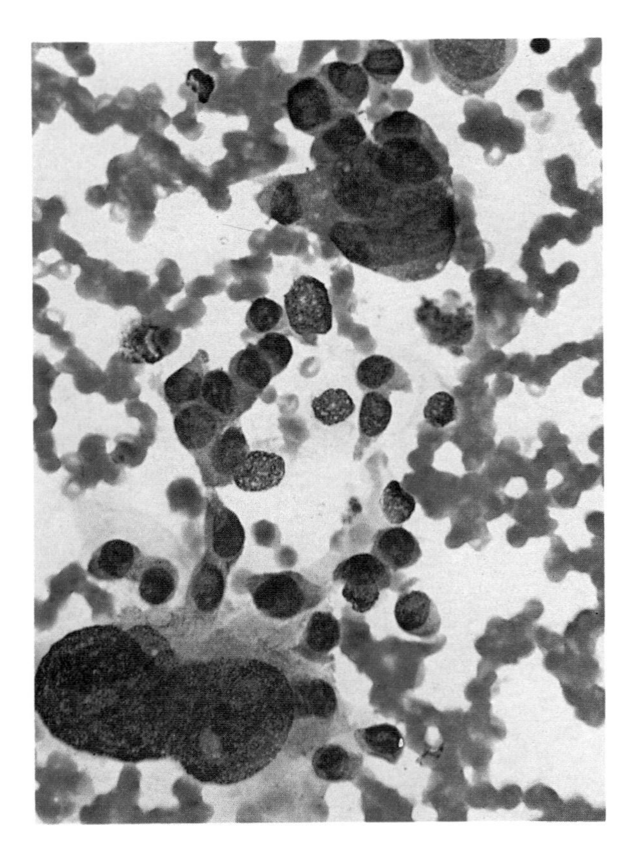

Figure 5-32
ADRENAL CORTICAL CARCINOMA

Left: Fine-needle aspirate from an adrenal tumor is quite cellular, with loosely dispersed malignant cells, some with gigantic hyperchromatic nuclei. Most cells have compact cytoplasm with a high nuclear/cytoplasmic ratio. (X400, Papanicolaou stain)

Right: Another field shows tremendous variation in nuclear shape and dimensions. Tumor cells are dispersed or loosely aggregated in small clusters. Nuclear detail tends to be less distinct compared with the Papanicolaou-stained specimen. (X400, Diff Quik stain)

Figure 5-33
BENIGN, INCIDENTAL "NONHYPERFUNCTIONAL" ADRENAL CORTICAL ADENOMA

A fine-needle aspirate from a benign, incidental "nonhyperfunctional" adrenal cortical adenoma (or nodule) in an adult patient. The cells are arranged in a loosely cohesive array with many having "bare" nuclei. Red blood cells are also present. This appearance resembles metastatic small cell carcinoma. Note the lack of nuclear molding and absence of necrotic background. (X400, Papanicolaou stain)

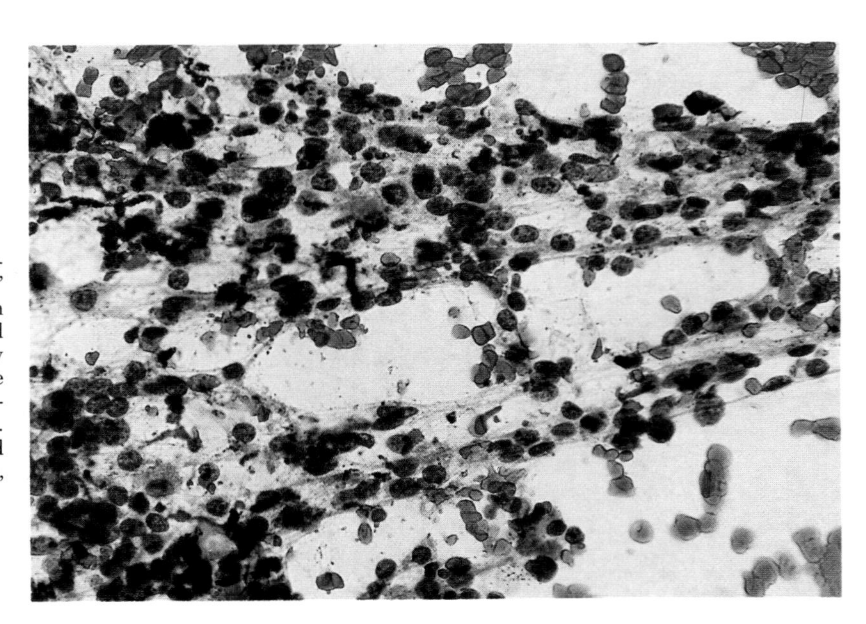

diagnosed by fine-needle aspiration, but required close correlation with clinical history and radiographic findings to distinguish it from an ACC (73). RCC has been reported to have eosinophilic globules on fine needle-aspiration (78), and potentially an ACC could present similar findings.

Cytogenetic Findings. There have been relatively few reported cytogenetic studies of ACA and ACC, but several cytogenetic numerical and structural abnormalities have been described (82–84,86,87). Yano et al. (87) reported rather consistent genetic changes on chromosomes 11p, 13q, and 17p with loss of alleles in 9 cases of primary ACC and metastases, but not in ACAs and hyperplasia. All patients with ACC whose normal somatic tissues were heterozygous for a locus on chromosome 17p lost one allele in the tumor, and a smaller proportion lost alleles on 11p and 13q. The development of homozygosity on chromosome 11 has also been shown in embryonal tumors in the pediatric age group such as hepatoblastoma, rhabdomyosarcoma (85), and Wilms' tumor (nephroblastoma) (83,85), and has also been reported in an ACA (82) and ACC (84) in patients with the Beckwith-Wiedemann syndrome. The loss of heterozygosity in region 11p15.5 in familial cases of ACC and Wilms' tumor suggests that there may be a nontissue-specific gene that could be involved in genetic predisposition (83).

DNA Quantitation and Ploidy Patterns. There are conflicting interpretations of the quantitative DNA profiles in adrenal cortical neoplasms. Most studies use flow cytometric analysis of material extracted from paraffin embedment (96,101) or static image analysis of Feulgen-stained sections. In a large study of adenomas of various endocrine organs, unequivocal evidence of DNA aneuploidy was reported in 29 percent of 44 pituitary adenomas, 25 percent of 49 thyroid, 35 percent of 54 parathyroid, and 53 percent of 17 ACAs; none of the tumors were malignant (98). In a recent study, 9 of 31 (29 percent) ACAs had aneuploid DNA (95). Quantitation of DNA content in the non-neoplastic adrenal gland with cytomegaly has also revealed considerable heterogeneity in the DNA profile, indicating that polyploidy (aneuploidy) is not a specific marker for neoplasia (92,94). Some studies report that DNA ploidy (nondiploid/aneuploid peaks) help distinguish benign from malignant adrenal cortical neoplasms in adults and children (89,97,99,100, 102,103). Of 52 ACCs analyzed by Hosaka et al. (97) by flow cytometry, in which DNA ploidy determination was restricted to patients undergoing curative resections, the number of patients with DNA diploid tumors was small and not statistically significant. A poor prognosis was associated with ACCs having two stem line DNA aneuploidy. Occasionally, different DNA profiles and aneuploid cell populations are identified by analyzing separate blocks of tumor (fig. 5-34).

Other studies, however, report no statistically significant correlation between aneuploidy or heterogeneous DNA content and biologic behavior (88,91,93,95), including two recent studies in children (90,104). In one study, DNA ploidy was correlated with tumor size, mitotic rate, and nuclear grade, but did not correlate with clinical outcome; aneuploid stem lines were identified in 9 of 13 ACCs (69 percent), but were also present in 6 of 30 ACAs (20 percent) (93). The literature regarding DNA ploidy in adrenal cortical neoplasms was briefly summarized by Zerbini et al. (104), who also noted that aneuploidy was relatively frequent in benign pediatric adrenal cortical tumors (fig. 5-35).

Criteria for Malignancy and Grading. Early studies of ACCs proposed various criteria for malignancy without rigorous testing using statistical methods. Features such as venous invasion, capsular invasion, documentation of distant metastases (105), extensive necrosis, and marked nuclear pleomorphism with one or more prominent nucleoli (113) were considered to be particularly useful in assessing malignant potential. Recent statistical analyses have identified histologic as well as nonhistologic parameters with prognostic value. Significant criteria for predicting malignant behavior include clinical evidence of weight loss, broad fibrous bands, diffuse growth pattern, vascular invasion, tumor necrosis, and increased tumor mass, although no single criterion is reliable for separating benign and malignant tumors (108). Weiss (116) reported three histologic features present only in metastasizing/recurring tumors: a mitotic rate of 6 or more per 50 high-power fields, atypical mitoses, and venous invasion; this series included 15 relatively small, innocuous ACAs associated with hyperaldosteronism which might skew the statistical analysis. A study using a histologic index identified tumor weight and mitotic activity as parameters

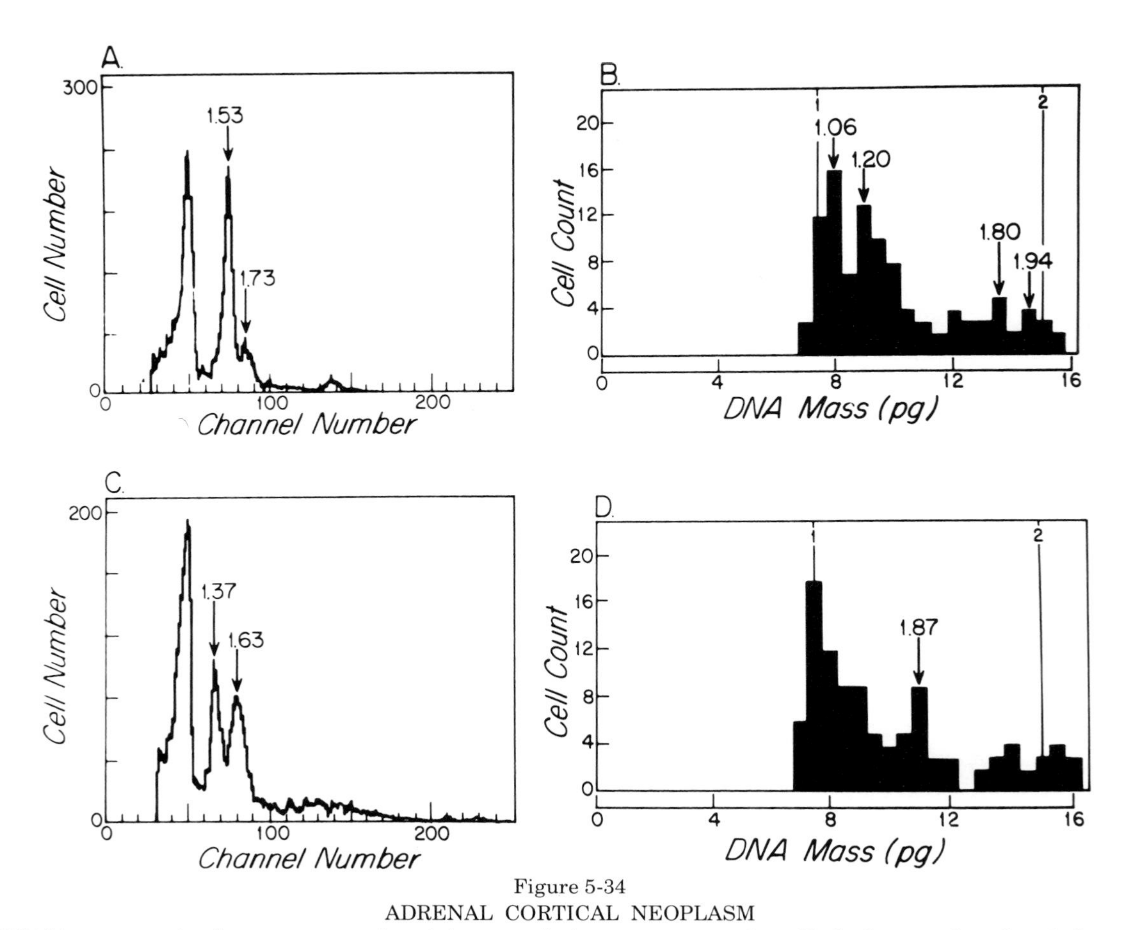

Figure 5-34
ADRENAL CORTICAL NEOPLASM

DNA histograms using flow cytometry and static image analysis on two separate tissue blocks from an adrenal cortical neoplasm (classified pathologically as an adenoma) from a 14-year-old female. Note the complex histograms and multiple aneuploid peaks in both flow cytometric and static image analysis. A: flow cytometry; B: image analysis of first block; C: flow cytometry; and D: image analysis of second block.

with the highest discriminating value (115). ACC can be reliably diagnosed in most cases, but there remains a small group in which it is extremely difficult to reliably predict biologic behavior, and in some cases use of the designation "adrenal cortical neoplasm of indeterminate malignant potential" may be appropriate (110). Long-term clinical follow-up may be the final arbiter in diagnosis of these troublesome cases. Although scintigraphic visualization of a unilateral adrenal cortical neoplasm with ^{131}I-6-beta-iodomethylnorcholesterol (NP-59) has been considered diagnostic of ACA, particularly in a patient with Cushing's syndrome, recent evidence indicates that this finding does not represent uniformly benign disease (114).

Grading of ACC has not been uniform due to the variability in criteria used. Grading has been based upon extent of cellular pleomorphism (anaplastic versus differentiated) (107), use of grades 1 through 3 (109,112), or overall level of differentiation, (e.g., Broder's grades 1 through 4) (106). More objective criteria have been proposed such as mitotic rate: ACCs having 20 or less mitoses per 50 high-power fields are low grade (median survival, 58 months), and tumors with more than 20 mitoses are high grade (median survival, 14 months) (111,117).

Prognosis and Patterns of Metastases. The mortality rate for adult patients with ACC ranges from 50 percent within 2 years (120) to 84 percent at 5 years (118) to 90 percent at 10 years (123); many large series report an overall mortality of 70 percent or greater (119). Death due to metastatic ACC often occurs within the first 12 months after diagnosis, but in some cases

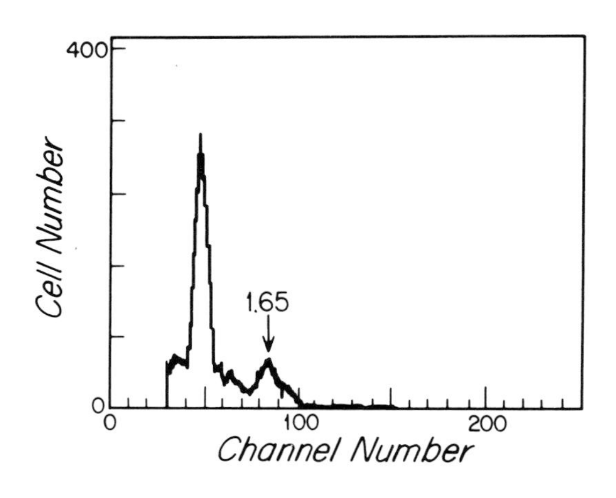

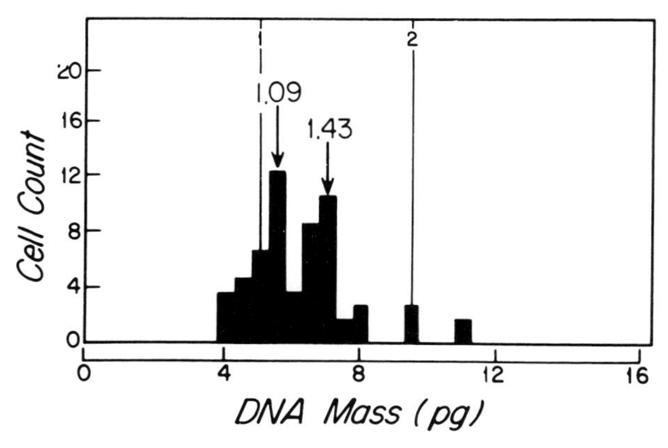

Figure 5-35
ANEUPLOID DNA HISTOGRAM FROM AN ADRENAL CORTICAL ADENOMA
The tumor (4 cm, 23 g) is from a 6-year old girl with Cushing's syndrome. The patient was alive and well 17 years later. Flow cytometric (top) and image analysis (bottom) histograms are shown. Note aneuploid and associated diploid peaks.

there may be a lingering course of up to a decade or more. In the study by van Slooten et al. (122), 93 percent of patients developed metastases within 10 years of diagnosis. The pattern of metastasis reflects both lymphatic and hematogenous avenues of spread, although there may be local intra-abdominal recurrence or peritoneal spread by tumor. Table 5-1 shows the distribution of metastases of ACCs among 50 patients autopsied at the National Institutes of Health (119). The most common sites of metastasis are liver (fig. 5-36), lung, retroperitoneum, and lymph nodes. The inferior vena cava may be invaded by tumor (see figure 5-21), sometimes causing obstruction manifested by lower extremity edema and ascites. Bony metastases are usually lytic (fig. 5-37). Metastases to brain (fig. 5-38) and skin are uncommon. Cutaneous involvement of scalp has been reported to simulate an angiosarcoma (121), but with clinical correlation there should be little problem in making the correct diagnosis (fig. 5-39).

Table 5-1

ANATOMIC SITES OF REGIONAL AND DISTANT METASTASES OF ADRENAL CORTICAL CARCINOMA

Distribution of Metastases in 50 Autopsies at the National Institutes of Health **Site**	**No. (%)**
Liver	46 (92)
Lung	39 (78)
Retroperitoneum	24 (48)
Inferior vena cava	14 (28)
Serosa of intestine	11 (22)
Lymph nodes:	
Abdominal	16 (32)
Thoracic	13 (26)
Bone	9 (18)
Peritoneum	8 (16)
Kidney	6 (12)
Diaphragm	6 (12)
Heart	6 (12)
Spleen	4 (8)
Pancreas	4 (8)
Thyroid	3 (6)
Brain	2 (4)
Skin	1 (2)

Staging of Adrenal Cortical Carcinoma. An extensive review by Wooten and King (127) using the staging criteria proposed by MacFarlane (125) and modified by Sullivan et al. (126), showed that most patients with ACC have relatively advanced disease at the time of diagnosis (Table 5-2). In the large series by Cohn et al. (124), only 30 percent of patients had tumor confined to the adrenal gland. Disease-free and overall survival rates have been strongly correlated with stage of ACC (124–127).

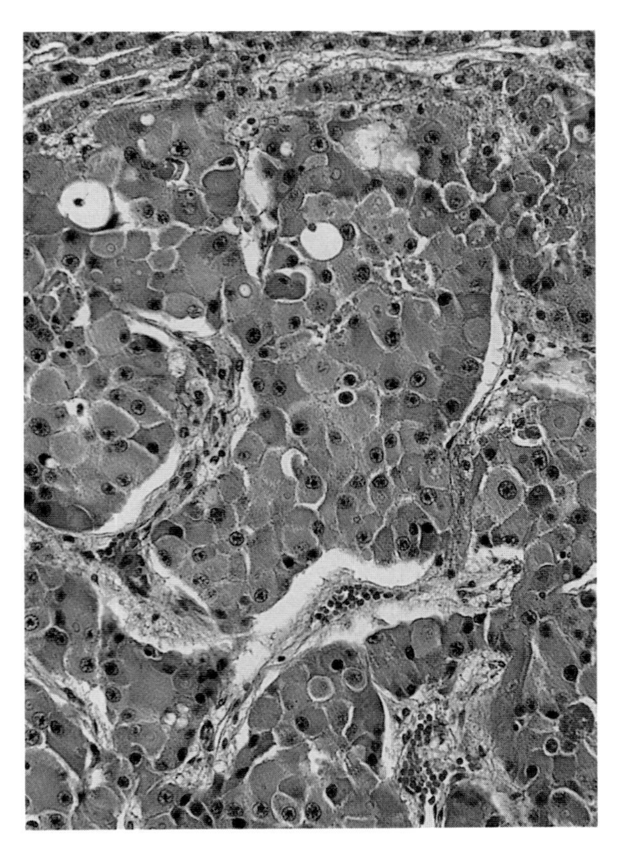

Figure 5-36
METASTATIC ADRENAL CORTICAL CARCINOMA TO LIVER

Fields such as this can simulate a hepatocellular carcinoma because of the trabecular pattern and large cells with compact, eosinophilic cytoplasm and prominent nucleoli. The residual liver is at the top of the field.

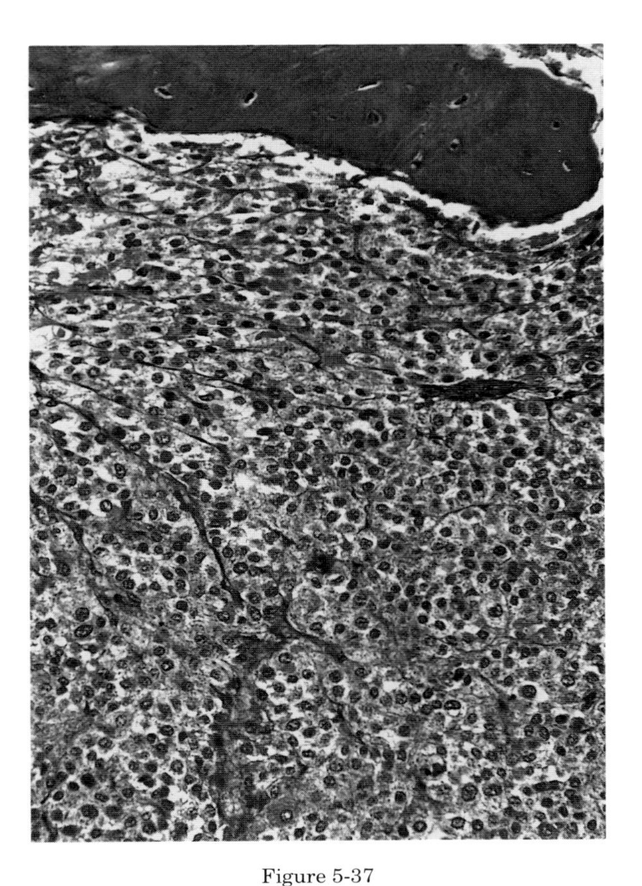

Figure 5-37
METASTATIC ADRENAL CORTICAL CARCINOMA TO BONE

The tumor cells have remarkably uniform nuclei.

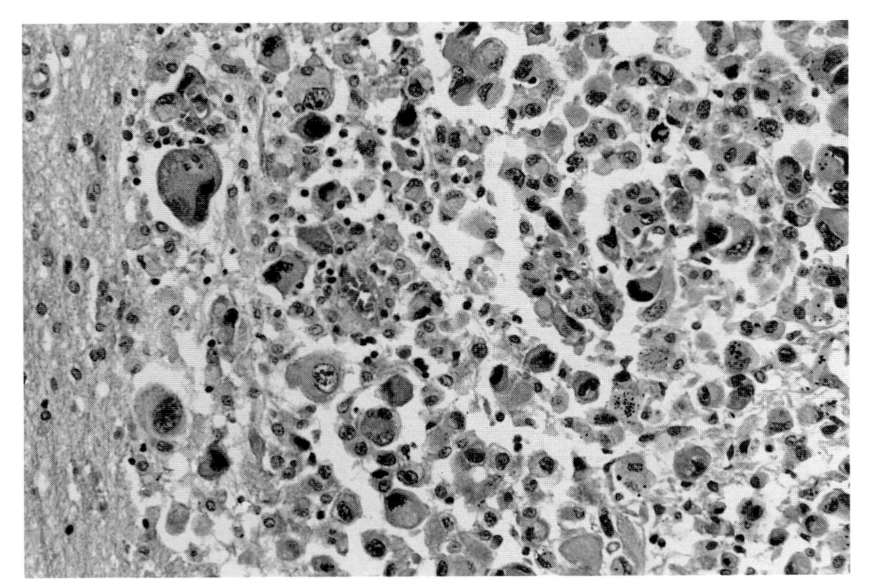

Figure 5-38
ADRENAL CORTICAL CARCINOMA METASTATIC TO BRAIN

The tumor is very pleomorphic, with large dyscohesive cells and a disorderly growth pattern. A specific diagnosis would be almost impossible without clinical correlation. Dark pigmented granules represent formalin.

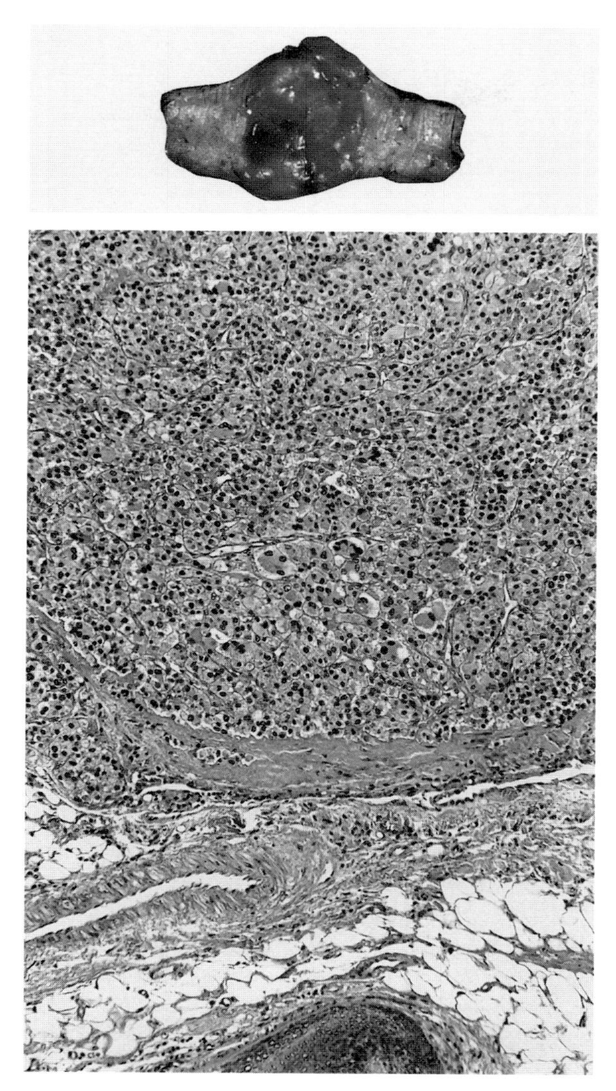

Figure 5-39
ADRENAL CORTICAL CARCINOMA
METASTATIC TO SCALP
Top: The tumor has a bulging surface with vague nodularity. Bottom: Portion of hair unit is present at bottom of field.

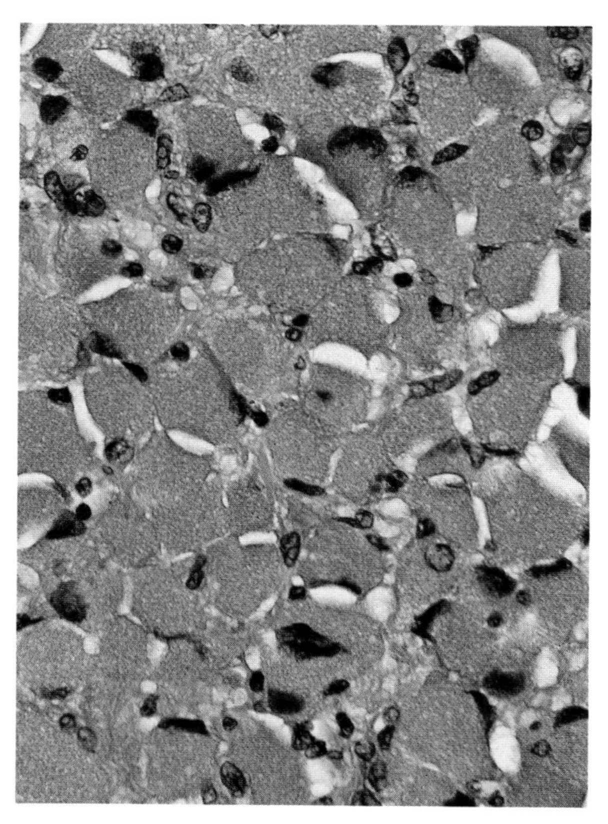

Figure 5-40
ADRENAL CORTICAL CARCINOMA
WITH ONCOCYTIC FEATURES
Adrenal cortical carcinoma with focal area of marked oncocytic features. The tumor cells have abundant, finely granular, eosinophilic cytoplasm.

UNUSUAL VARIANTS

Oncocytic Adrenal Cortical Carcinoma

Several examples of oncocytic adrenal cortical neoplasms have been reported; most are clinically benign and nonfunctional (oncocytoma; see chapter 4) (131,133,135,136), but on occasion the tumor may be malignant (130). These tumors contain cells rich in mitochondria. Oncocytic features are usually diffuse throughout. Occasionally, there are focal areas with sheets of oncocytic cells in an otherwise typical ACC (fig. 5-40).

Adrenal Carcinosarcoma

This is a rare adrenal malignancy which combines features of more conventional ACC with areas of sarcoma, including rhabdomyosarcoma (129,132), and areas showing osteogenic and chondroid differentiation (128). Embryologically, the adrenal cortex is of mesodermal origin, but growth of ACC in part as a sarcoma is exceptional.

Adrenal Cortical Blastoma

This unique tumor was reported recently in a young infant (see chapter 6) (134); however, it is not known whether tumors with this morphology are restricted to the pediatric age group.

Table 5-2

STAGING OF ADRENAL CORTICAL CARCINOMA*

Percent	Stage		Staging Criteria	
2.8	I	$T_1N_0M_0$	T_1	Tumor less than or equal to 5 cm, no invasion
			T_2	Tumor greater than 5 cm, no invasion
29.0	II	$T_2N_0M_0$	T_3	Tumor any size, locally invasive but not involving adjacent organs
			T_4	Tumor of any size with invasion of adjacent organs
19.3	III	$T_1N_1M_0$	N_0	Negative regional node
		$T_2N_1M_0$	N_1	Positive regional nodes
		$T_3N_0M_0$	M_0	No distant metastases
			M_1	Distant metastases
48.9	IV	Any T, any N, M_1		
		T_3, N_1		
		T_4		

*Data from references 124a, 126, and 127.

REFERENCES

Incidence, Clinical Aspects, and Pathology

1. Bertagna C, Orth DN. Clinical and laboratory findings and results of therapy in 58 patients with adrenocortical tumors admitted to a single medical center (1951-1978). Am J Med 1981;71:855–75.
2. Brabrand K, Soreide JA. Adrenal cortical carcinoma with invasion into the inferior vena cava. Br J Surg 1987;74:598–9.
3. Cheung PS, Thompson NW. Right atrial extension of adrenocortical carcinoma. Surgical management using hypothermia and cardiopulmonary bypass. Cancer 1989;64:812–5.
4. Cohn K, Gottesman L, Brennan M. Adrenocortical carcinoma. Surgery 1986;100:1170–7.
5. Correa P, Chen VW. Endocrine gland cancer. Cancer 1995;75:338–52.
6. D'Agata R, Malozowski S, Barkan A, Cassorla F, Loriaux D. Steroid biosynthesis in human adrenal tumors. Horm Metabol Res 1987;19:386–8.
7. Didolkar MS, Bescher RA, Elias EG, Moore RH. Natural history of adrenal cortical carcinoma: a clinicopathologic study of 42 patients. Cancer 1981;47:2153–61.
8. Gandour MJ, Grizzle WE. A small adrenocortical carcinoma with aggressive behavior. An evaluation of criteria for malignancy. Arch Pathol Lab Med 1986;110:1076–9.
9. Gazdar AF, Oie HK, Shackleton CH, et al. Establishment and characterization of a human adrenocortical carcinoma cell line that expresses multiple pathways of steroid biosynthesis. Cancer Res 1990;50:5488–96.
10. Godine LB, Berdon WE, Brasch RC, Leonidas JC. Adrenocortical carcinoma with extension into inferior vena cava and right atrium: report of 3 cases in children. Pediatr Radiol 1990;20:166–8.
11. Hajjar RA, Hickey RC, Samaan NA. Adrenal cortical carcinoma. A study of 32 patients. Cancer 1975; 35:549–54.
12. Hamper UM, Fishman EK, Hartman DS, Roberts JL, Sanders RC. Primary adrenocortical carcinoma: sonographic evaluation with clinical and pathologic correlation in 26 patients. AJR Am J Roentgenol 1987;148:915–9.
13. Henley DJ, van Heerden JA, Grant CS, Carney JA, Carpenter PC. Adrenal cortical carcinoma—a continuing challenge. Surgery 1983;94:926–31.
14. Hogan TF, Gilchrist KW, Westring DW, Citrin DL. A clinical and pathological study of adrenocortical carcinoma: therapeutic implications. Cancer 1980;45:2880–3.
15. Hugh TB, Jones RM, Shanahan MX. Intra-atrial extension of renal and adrenal tumors: diagnosis, management, and prognosis. World J Surg 1986;10:488–95.
16. Hutter AM, Kayhoe DE. Adrenal cortical carcinoma. Clinical features of 138 patients. Am J Med 1966;41:572–80.
17. Huvos AG, Hajdu SI, Brasfield RD, Foote FW Jr. Adrenal cortical carcinoma. Clinicopathologic study of 34 cases. Cancer 1970;25:354–61.
18. Icard P, Chapuis Y, Andreassian B, Bernard A, Proye C. Adrenocortical carcinoma in surgically treated patients: a retrospective study on 156 cases by the French Association of Endocrine Surgery. Surgery 1992;112:972–80.
19. Karakousis CP, Rao U, Moore R. Adrenal adenocarcinomas: histologic grading and survival. J Surg Oncol 1985;29:105–11.
20. King DR, Lack EE. Adrenal cortical carcinoma: a clinical and pathologic study of 49 cases. Cancer 1979;44:239–44.
21. Lack EE, Travis WD, Oertel JE. Adrenal cortical neoplasms. In: Lack EE, ed. Pathology of the adrenal glands. New York: Churchill Livingstone, 1990:115–71.
22. LeFevre M, Gerard-Marchant R, Gubler JP, Chaussain JL, Lemerle J. Adrenal cortical carcinoma in children: 42 patients treated from 1958 to 1980 at Villejuif. In: Humphreys GB, Grindey GB, Dehner LP, Acton RT, Pysher TJ, eds. Adrenal and endocrine tumors in children. Boston: Martinus Nijhoff, 1983:265–76.

23. Lewinsky BS, Grigor KM, Symington T, Neville AM. The clinical and pathologic features of non-hormonal adrenocortical tumors. Report of twenty new cases and review of the literature. Cancer 1974;33:778–90.
24. Lipsett MB, Hertz R, Ross GT. Clinical and pathophysiologic aspects of adrenocortical carcinoma. Am J Med 1963;35:374–83.
25. Luton JP, Cerdas S, Billaud L, et al. Clinical features of adrenocortical carcinoma, prognostic factors, and the effect of mitotane therapy. N Eng J Med 1990;322:1195–201.
26. MacFarlane DA. Cancer of the adrenal cortex. The natural history, prognosis and treatment in a study of fifty-five cases. Ann Royal Coll Surg Engl 1958;23:155–86.
27. Nader S, Hickey RC, Sellin RV, Samaan NA. Adrenal cortical carcinoma. A study of 77 cases. Cancer 1983;52:707–11.
28. Nakano M. Adrenal cortical carcinoma. A clinicopathological and immunohistochemical study of 91 autopsy cases. Acta Pathol Jpn 1988;38:163–80.
29. Neville AM, Symington T. Pathology of primary aldosteronism. Cancer 1966;19:1854–68.
30. O'Hare MJ, Monaghan P, Neville AM. The pathology of adrenocortical neoplasia: a correlated structural and functional approach to the diagnosis of malignant disease. Hum Pathol 1979;10:137–54.
31. Orland SM, Stewart AF, LiVolsi VA, Wein AJ. Detection of the hypercalcemic hormone of malignancy in adrenal cortical carcinoma. J Urol 1968;136:1000–2.
32. Pommier RF, Brennan MF. An eleven-year experience with adrenocortical carcinoma. Surgery 1992;112:963–71.
33. Rapaport E, Goldberg MB, Gordon GS, Hinman F Jr. Mortality in surgically treated adrenocortical tumors. II. Review of cases reported for the 20 year period 1930-1949, inclusive. Post Graduate Med 1952;11:325–53.
34. Ritchey ML, Kinard R, Novicki DE. Adrenal tumors: involvement of the inferior vena cava. J Urol 1987;138:1134–6.
35. Saracco S, Abramowsky C, Taylor S, Silverman RA, Berman BW. Spontaneous regressing adrenocortical carcinoma in a newborn. A case report with DNA ploidy analysis. Cancer 1988;62:507–11.
36. Sasano H, Suzuki T, Nagura H, Nishikawa T. Steroidogenesis in human adrenocortical carcinoma: biochemical activities, immunohistochemistry, and in situ hybridization of steroidogenic enzymes and histopathologic study in nine cases. Hum Pathol 1993;24:397–404.
37. Scott HW Jr, Abumrad NN, Orth DN. Tumors of the adrenal cortex and Cushing's syndrome. Ann Surg 1985;201:586–94.
38. Scott HW Jr, Sussman CR, Page DL, Thompson NW, Gross MD, Lloyd R. Primary aldosteronism caused by adrenocortical carcinoma. World J Surg 1986;10:646–53.
39. Sullivan M, Boileau M, Hodges CV. Adrenal cortical carcinoma. J Urol 1978;120:660–5.
40. Symington T. The adrenal cortex. In: Symington T, ed. Functional pathology of the human adrenal glands. Baltimore: Williams & Wilkins, 1969:3–216.
41. Tang CK, Gray GF. Adrenocortical neoplasms. Prognosis and morphology. Urology 1975;5:691–5.
42. Tang CK, Harriman BB, Toker C. Myxoid adrenal cortical carcinoma: a light and electron microscopic study. Arch Pathol Lab Med 1979;103:635–8.
43. van Slooten H, Schaberg A, Smeenk D, Moolenaar AJ. Morphologic characteristics of benign and malignant adrenocortical tumors. Cancer 1985;55:766–73.
44. Venkatesh S, Hickey RC, Sellin RV, Fernandez JF, Samaan NA. Adrenal cortical carcinoma. Cancer 1989;64:765–9.
45. Weinberger MH, Grim CE, Hollifield JW, et al. Primary aldosteronism: diagnosis, localization, and treatment. Ann Int Med 1979;90:386–95.
46. Weiss LM. Comparative histologic study of 43 metastasizing and nonmetastasizing adrenocortical tumors. Am J Surg Pathol 1984;8:163–9.
47. Weiss LM, Medeiros LJ, Vickery AL Jr. Pathologic features of prognostic significance in adrenocortical carcinoma. Am J Surg Pathol 1989;13:202–6.
48. Wooten MD, King DK. Adrenal cortical carcinoma. Epidemiology and treatment with mitotane and a review of the literature. Cancer 1993;72:3145–55.

Ultrastructure of Adrenal Cortical Carcinoma

49. Mackay B, El-Naggar A, Ordonez NG. Ultrastructure of adrenal cortical carcinoma. Ultrastruct Pathol 1994;18:181–90.
50. Miettinen M. Neuroendocrine differentiation in adrenocortical carcinoma. New immunohistochemical findings supported by electron microscopy. Lab Invest 1992;66:169–74.

Immunohistochemistry and Differential Diagnosis

51. Cote RJ, Cordon-Cardo C, Reuter VE, Rosen PP. Immunopathology of adrenal and renal cortical tumors. Coordinated change in antigen expression is associated with neoplastic conversion in the adrenal cortex. Am J Pathol 1990;136:1077–84.
52. Driman DK, Kobrin MS, Kudlow JE, Asa SL. Transforming growth factor-alpha in normal and neoplastic human endocrine tissues. Hum Pathol 1992;23:1360–5.
53. Gaffey MJ, Traweek ST, Mills SE, et al. Cytokeratin expression in adrenocortical neoplasia: an immunohistochemical and biochemical study with implications for the differential diagnosis of adrenocortical, hepatocellular and renal cell carcinoma. Hum Pathol 1992;23:144–53.
54. Goldblum JR, Shannon R, Kaldjian EP, et al. Immunohistochemical assessment of proliferative activity in adrenocortical neoplasms. Mod Pathol 1993;6:663–8.
55. Haak HR, Fleuren GJ. Neuroendocrine differentiation of adrenocortical tumors. Cancer 1995;75:860–4.
56. Johnson DE, Herndier BG, Medeiros LJ, Warnke RA, Roose RV. The diagnostic utility of the keratin profiles of hepatocellular carcinoma and cholangiocarcinoma. Am J Surg Pathol 1988;12:187–97.

57. Kamio T, Shigematsu K, Sou H, Kawai K, Tsuchiyama H. Immunohistochemical expression of epidermal growth factor receptors in human adrenocortical carcinoma. Hum Pathol 1990;21:277–82.
58. Komminoth P, Saremaslani P, Schröder S, Heitz PU, Roth J. Immunohistochemical marker profiles and polysialic acid expression in pheochromocytomas and adrenocortical carcinomas [Abstract]. Mod Pathol 1994;7:52.
59. Kumar D, Kumar S. Adrenal cortical adenoma and adrenal metastasis of renal cell carcinoma: immunohistochemical and DNA ploidy analysis. Mod Pathol 1993;6:36–41.
60. Medeiros LJ, Michie SA, Johnson DE, Warnke RA, Weiss LM. An immunoperoxidase study of renal cell carcinomas: correlation with nuclear grade, cell type and histologic pattern. Hum Pathol 1988;19:980–7.
61. Miettinen M. Neuroendocrine differentiation in adrenocortical carcinoma. New immunohistochemical findings supported by electron microscopy. Lab Invest 1992;66:169–74.
62. Miettinen M, Lehto VP, Virtanen I. Immunofluorescence microscopic evaluation of the intermediate filament expression of the adrenal cortex and medulla and their tumors. Am J Pathol 1985;118:360–6.
63. Nakano M. Adrenal cortical carcinoma. A clinicopathological and immunohistochemical study of 91 autopsy cases. Acta Pathol Jpn 1988;38:163–80.
64. Rank J, Pelletier G, Gown AM. 3-beta-hydroxy-delta-5-steroid dehydrogenase immunolocalization: a discriminator of adrenal vs. renal cell tumors? [Abstract] Mod Pathol 1994;7:55A.
65. Sasano H, Nose M, Sasano N. Lectin histochemistry in adrenocortical hyperplasia and neoplasms with emphasis on carcinoma. Arch Pathol Lab Med 1989;113:68–72.
66. Sasano H, Saito Y, Sato I, Sasano N, Nagura H. Nucleolar organizer regions in human adrenocortical disorders. Mod Pathol 1990;3:591–5.
67. Schröder S, Niendorf A, Achilles E, et al. Immunocytochemical differential diagnosis of adrenocortical neoplasms using the monoclonal antibody D11. Virchows Arch [A] 1990;417:89–96.
68. Schröder S, Padberg BC, Achilles E, Holl K, Dralle H, Klöppel G. Immunocytochemistry in adrenocortical tumors: a clinicopathological study of 72 neoplasms. Virchows Arch [A] 1992;420:65–70.
69. Suzuki T, Sasano H, Nisikawa T, Rhame J, Wilkinson DS, Nagura H. Discerning malignancy in human adrenocortical neoplasms: utility of DNA flow cytometry and immunohistochemistry. Mod Pathol 1992;5:224–31.
70. Tartour E, Caillou B, Tenenbaum F, et al. Immunohistochemical study of adrenocortical carcinoma. Predictive value of the D11 monoclonal antibody. Cancer 1993;72:3296–303.
71. Wick MR, Cherwitz DL, McGlennan RC, Dehner LP. Adrenocortical carcinoma. An immunohistochemical comparison with renal cell carcinoma. Am J Pathol 1986;122:343–52.

Fine-Needle Aspiration

72. Cochand-Priollet B, Jacquenod P, Warnet A. Adrenal cortical carcinoma: a case diagnosed by fine needle aspiration cytology [Letter]. Acta Cytol 1988;32:128–30.
73. Duggan MA, Forestell CF, Hanley DA. Adrenal metastases of renal-cell carcinoma 19 years after nephrectomy. Fine needle aspiration cytology of a case. Acta Cytopathol 1987;31:512–6.
74. Levin NP. Fine needle aspiration and histology of adrenal cortical carcinoma: a case report. Acta Cytol 1981;25:421–4.
75. Min KW, Song J, Boesenberg M, Acebey J. Adrenal cortical nodule mimicking small round cell malignancy on fine needle aspiration. Acta Cytol 1988;32:543–6.
76. Mitchell ML, Ryan FP Jr, Shermer RW. Pulmonary adenocarcinoma metastatic to the adrenal gland mimicking normal adrenal cortical epithelium on fine needle aspiration. Acta Cytol 1985;29:994–8.
77. Suen KC, McNeely TB. Adrenal cortical cells mimicking small cell anaplastic carcinoma in a fine-needle aspirate. Mod Pathol 1991;4:594–5.
78. Unger P, Hague K, Klein G, Gordon RE, Thung SN, Szporn A. Fine needle aspiration of a renal cell carcinoma with eosinophilic globules. A case report. Acta Cytol 1993;37:201–4.
79. Varma S, Amy RW. Adrenal cortical carcinoma metastatic to the lung: report of a case diagnosed by fine needle aspiration biopsy [Letter]. Acta Cytol 1990;34:104–5.
80. Wadih GE, Nance KV, Silverman JF. Fine needle aspiration cytology of the adrenal gland. Fifty biopsies in 48 patients. Arch Pathol Lab Med 1992;116:841–6.
81. Zornoza J, Ordonez N, Bernardino ME, Cohen MA. Percutaneous biopsy of adrenal tumors. Urology 1981;18:412–6.

Cytogenetics

82. Hayward NK, Little MH, Mortimer RH, Clouston WM, Smith PL. Generation of homozygosity at the c-Ha-ras-1 locus on chromosome 11p in an adrenal adenoma from an adult with Wiedemann-Beckwith syndrome. Cancer Genet Cytogenet 1988;30:127–32.
83. Henry I, Grandjouan S, Couillin P, et al. Tumor-specific loss of 11p15.5 alleles in del11p13 Wilms' tumor and in familial adrenocortical carcinoma. Proc Natl Acad Sci USA 1989;86:3247–51.
84. Henry I, Jeanpierre M, Couillin P, et al. Molecular definition of 11p15.5 region involved in Beckwith-Wiedemann syndrome and probably in predisposition to adrenocortical carcinoma. Hum Genet 1989;81:273–7.
85. Koufos A, Hansen MF, Copeland NG, Jenkins NA, Lampkin BC, Cavence WK. Loss of heterozygosity in three embryonal tumors suggests a common pathogenetic mechanism. Nature 1985;316:330–4.
86. Marks JL, Wyandt HE, Beazley RM, Milunsky JM, Sheahan K, Milunsky A. Cytogenetic studies of an adrenal cortical carcinoma. Cancer Genet Cytogenet 1992;61:96–8.
87. Yano T, Linehan M, Anglard P, et al. Genetic changes in human adrenocortical carcinomas. JNCI 1989;81:518–23.

DNA Quantitation and Ploidy Patterns

88. Amberson JB, Vaughan ED Jr, Gray GF, Naus GJ. Flow cytometry analysis of nuclear DNA from adrenocortical neoplasms. A retrospective study using paraffin-embedded tissue. Cancer 1987;59:2091–5.
89. Bowlby LS, DeBault LE, Abraham SR. Flow cytometric analysis of adrenal cortical tumor DNA. Relationship between cellular DNA and histopathologic classification. Cancer 1986;58:1499–505.
90. Bugg MF, Ribeiro RC, Roberson PK, et al. Correlation of pathologic features with clinical outcome in pediatric adrenocortical neoplasia. A study of a Brazilian population. Am J Clin Pathol 1994;101:625–9.
91. Camuto PM, Citrin D, Schinella R, Fredrickson G, Gilchrist K. Adrenal cortical carcinoma: flow cytometric study of 22 cases, an ECOG study. Urology 1991; 37:380–4.
92. Camuto PM, Wolman SR, Perle MA, Grecco MA. Flow cytometry of fetal adrenal glands with adrenocortical cytomegaly. Pediatr Pathol 1989;9:551–8.
93. Cibas ES, Medeiros LJ, Weinberg DS, Gelb AB, Weiss LM. Cellular DNA profiles of benign and malignant adrenocortical tumors. Am J Surg Pathol 1990;14:948–55.
94. Favara BE, Steele E, Grant JH, Steele P. Adrenal cytomegaly: quantitative assessment by image analysis. Pediatr Pathol 1991;11:521–36.
95. Haak HR, Cornelisse CJ, Hermans J, Cobben L, Fleuren GL. Nuclear DNA content and morphological characteristics in the prognosis of adrenocortical carcinoma. Br J Cancer 1993;68:151–5.
96. Hedley DW, Friedlander ML, Taylor IW, Musgrove EA. Method for analysis of cellular DNA content of paraffin-embedded pathological material using flow cytometry. J Histochem Cytochem 1983;31:1333–5.
97. Hosaka Y, Rainwater LM, Grant CS, et al. Adrenocortical carcinoma: nuclear deoxyribonucleic acid ploidy studied by flow cytometry. Surgery 1987;102:1027–34.
98. Joensuu H, Klemi PJ. DNA aneuploidy in adenomas of endocrine organs. Am J Pathol 1988;132:145–51.
99. Klein FA, Kay S, Ratliff JE, White FK, Newsome HH. Flow cytometric determination of ploidy and proliferation patterns of adrenal neoplasms: an adjunct to histological classification. J Urol 1985;134:862–6.
100. Klein FA, Miller NL, Hackler RH. Flow cytometry in feminizing adrenocortical carcinoma. J Urol 1985;134:933–5.
101. Stephenson RA, Gay H, Fair WR, Melamed MR. Effect of section thickness on quality of flow cytometric DNA content determinations in paraffin-embedded tissues. Cytometry 1986;7:41–4.
102. Suzuki T, Sasano H, Nisikawa T, Rhame J, Wilkinson DS, Nagura H. Discerning malignancy in human adrenocortical neoplasms: utility of DNA flow cytometry and immunohistochemistry. Mod Pathol 1992;5:224–31.
103. Taylor SR, Roederer M, Murphy RF. Flow cytometric DNA analysis of adrenocortical tumors in children. Cancer 1987;59:2059–63.
104. Zerbini C, Kozakewich HP, Weinberg DS, Mundt DJ, Edwards JA III, Lack EE. Adrenocortical neoplasms in childhood and adolescence: analysis of prognostic factors including DNA content. Endocr Pathol 1992;3:116–28.

Criteria for Malignancy and Grading

105. Heinbecker P, O'Neal LW, Ackerman LV. Functioning and nonfunctioning adrenal cortical tumors. Surg Gynecol Obstet 1957;105:21–33.
106. Henley DJ, van Heerden JA, Grant CS, Carney JA, Carpenter PC. Adrenal cortical carcinoma—a continuing challenge. Surgery 1983;94:926–31.
107. Hogan TF, Gilchrist KW, Westring DW, Citrin DL. A clinical and pathological study of adrenocortical carcinoma: therapeutic implications. Cancer 1980;45:2880–3.
108. Hough AJ, Hollifield JW, Page DL, Hartmann WH. Prognostic factors in adrenal cortical tumors. A mathematical analysis of clinical and morphologic data. Am J Clin Pathol. 1979;72:390–9.
109. Karakousis CP, Rao U, Moore R. Adrenal adenocarcinomas: histologic grading and survival. J Surg Oncol 1985;29:105–11.
110. Lack EE, Travis WD, Oertel JE. Adrenal cortical neoplasms. In: Lack EE, ed. Pathology of the adrenal glands. New York: Churchill Livingstone, 1990:115–71.
111. Medeiros LJ, Weiss LM. New developments in the pathologic diagnosis of adrenal cortical neoplasms. A review. Am J Clin Pathol 1992;97:73–83.
112. Nakano M. Adrenal cortical carcinoma. A clinicopathological and immunohistochemical study of 91 autopsy cases. Acta Pathol Jpn 1988;38:163–80.
113. O'Hare MJ, Monaghan P, Neville AM. The pathology of adrenocortical neoplasia: a correlated structural and functional approach to the diagnosis of malignant disease. Hum Pathol 1979;10:137–54.
114. Pasieka JL, McLeod MK, Thompson NW, Gross MD, Schteingart DE. Adrenal scintigraphy of well-differentiated (functioning) adrenocortical carcinomas: potential surgical pitfalls. Surgery 1992;112:884–90.
115. van Slooten H, Schaberg A, Smeenk D, Moolenaar AJ. Morphologic characteristics of benign and malignant adrenocortical tumors. Cancer 1985;55:766–73.
116. Weiss LM. Comparative histologic study of 43 metastasizing and nonmetastasizing adrenocortical tumors. Am J Surg Pathol 1984;8:163–9.
117. Weiss LM, Medeiros LJ, Vickery AL Jr. Pathologic features of prognostic significance in adrenocortical carcinoma. Am J Surg Pathol 1989;13:202–6.

Prognosis and Patterns of Metastases

118. Henley DJ, van Heerden JA, Grant CS, Carney JA, Carpenter PC. Adrenal cortical carcinoma—a continuing challenge. Surgery 1983;94:926–31.
119. Lack EE, Travis WD, Oertel JE. Adrenal cortical neoplasms. In: Lack EE, ed. Pathology of the adrenal glands. New York: Churchill Livingstone, 1990:115–71.

120. Lipsett MB, Hertz R, Ross GT. Clinical and pathophysiologic aspects of adrenocortical carcinoma. Am J Med 1963;35:374–83.
121. Milchgrub S, Wiley EL. Adrenal carcinoma presenting as a lesion resembling a cutaneous angiosarcoma. Cancer 1991;67:3087–92.
122. van Slooten H, Schaberg A, Smeenk D, Moolenaar AJ. Morphologic characteristics of benign and malignant adrenocortical tumors. Cancer 1985;55:766–73.
123. Venkatesh S, Hickey RC, Sellin RV, Fernandez JF, Samaan NA. Adrenal cortical carcinoma. Cancer 1989;64:765–9.

Staging of Adrenal Cortical Carcinoma

124. Cohn K, Gottesman L, Brennan M. Adrenocortical carcinoma. Surgery 1986;100:1170–7.
124a. Henley DJ, van Heerden JA, Grant CS, Carney A, Carpenter PC. Adrenal cortical carcinoma—a continuing challenge. Surgery 1993;94:926–31.
125. MacFarlane DA. Cancer of the adrenal cortex. The natural history, prognosis and treatment in a study of fifty-five cases. Ann Royal Coll Surg Engl 1958;23:155–86.
126. Sullivan M, Boileau M, Hodges CV. Adrenal cortical carcinoma. J Urol 1978;120:660–5.
127. Wooten MD, King DK. Adrenal cortical carcinoma. Epidemiology and treatment with mitotane and a review of the literature. Cancer 1993;72:3145–55.

Unusual Variants

128. Barksdale SK, Marincola FM. Carcinosarcoma of the adrenal cortex presenting with mineralocorticoid excess. Am J Surg Pathol 1993;17:941–5.
129. Decorato JW, Gruber H, Petti M, Levowitz BS. Adrenal carcinosarcoma. J Surg Oncol 1990;45:134–6.
130. El-Naggar AK, Evans DB, Mackay B. Oncocytic adrenal cortical carcinoma. Ultrastruct Pathol 1991;15:549–56.
131. Erlandson RA, Reuter VE. Oncocytic adrenal cortical adenoma. Ultrastruct Pathol 1991;15:539–47.
132. Fischler DF, Nunez C, Levin HS, McMahon JT, Sheeler LR, Adelstein DJ. Adrenal carcinosarcoma presenting in a woman with clinical signs of virilization. A case report with immunohistochemical and ultrastructural findings. Am J Surg Pathol 1992;16:626–31.
133. Kakimoto S, Yushita Y, Sanefuji T, et al. Nonhormonal adrenocortical adenoma with oncocytoma-like appearances. Hinyokika Kiyo 1986;32:757–63.
134. Molberg K, Vuitch F, Stewart D, Albores-Saavedra J. Adrenocortical blastoma. Hum Pathol 1992;23:1187–90.
135. Nguyen GK, Vriend R, Ronaghan D, Lakey WK. Heterotopic adrenocortical oncocytoma. A case report with light and electron microscopic studies. Cancer 1992;70:2681–4.
136. Sasano H, Suzuki T, Sano T, Kameya T, Sasano N, Nagura H. Adrenocortical oncocytoma. A true nonfunctioning adrenocortical tumor. Am J Surg Pathol 1991;15:949–56.

6

ADRENAL CORTICAL NEOPLASMS IN CHILDHOOD

Adrenal cortical neoplasms are uncommon in childhood. However, since they can differ significantly from similar neoplasms in adults with regard to epidemiology, clinical manifestations, and biologic behavior, particularly those of early infancy, they are described separately. The biologic behavior of some of these adrenal cortical neoplasms can be difficult to predict, even when the tumor has clearly adverse prognostic findings similar to those outlined in chapter 5 for tumors in adults.

Incidence and Epidemiology. Of 141 cases in the Manchester Children's Tumor Registry prior to 1973, 92 percent were classified as neuroblastoma, 6 percent as adrenal cortical carcinoma (ACC), and 2 percent as pheochromocytoma (47). Based upon the third National Cancer Survey carried out in 1969 through 1971 (53) and a recent update (35), ACC comprised 0.2 percent of all childhood malignancies in white patients under 15 years of age; about 13 new cases are diagnosed yearly in the United States. The annual incidence of all malignant neoplasms in children under 15 years of age was 124.5 per million whites and 97.8 per million blacks (53). Update of this cancer survey has continued in different regions of the United States as an ongoing monitor of cancer incidence in the form of the SEER (Surveillance, Epidemiology, and End Results) program of the National Cancer Institute (54). From 1973 through 1987, 28 ACCs were recorded in patients under age 20 years, indicating an estimated 19 new cases a year. The SEER program does not track benign neoplasms such as adrenal cortical adenoma (ACA), and assuming that about 26 percent of all adrenal cortical neoplasms are ACA (or classified pathologically as such), an estimated 25 adrenal cortical tumors occur each year in the United States in patients under 20 years of age (25). The annual incidence rate is about three per million children under 20 years; rates are slightly higher in females than males (fig. 6-1), but the sex difference appears to be limited to the first 5 years of life (25). Only 6 percent of ACCs occur under age 20 years (25), the age at which a modal peak is formed, in addition to that seen in adults (25,26). Daneman et al. (7), found that ACC comprised only 0.3 percent of all neoplasms at the Hospital for Sick Children in Toronto.

Age, Sex Distribution, and Laterality. In a recent study of 32 patients (19 female, 13 male) with adrenal cortical neoplasms, the average age at diagnosis was 8 years (range, 6 months to 19 years), with a median age of 5 years, and there was clustering of cases in the age group of 5 years or less (fig. 6-2) (55). In a study of 42 patients, two thirds were less than 5 years old at diagnosis (27). A recent literature review of adrenal cortical neoplasms in childhood indicated a predominance in girls (female to male ratio of 2.2 to 1) with the average age being 4.6 years (range, 5 days to 16.5 years); over half of the patients were diagnosed in the first 4 years of life (37). The median age at diagnosis in a study of Brazilian children with ACC by Ribeiro et al. (42) was 3.9 years, and over half were females; interestingly, ACC is apparently more common in Brazilian children than children in the United States. An uneven age distribution has been noted in the first two decades of life, with an "infantile group" having a peak incidence in the first year of life and an "adolescent group" with the incidence evenly distributed between 9 and 16 years (23). In a review by Lack et al. (25) 18 tumors arose in the right adrenal gland (60 percent) and 12 in the left (40 percent). Bilateral adrenal cortical tumors are extremely rare, as are ectopic tumors (37). A fascinating case of congenital ACC was reported in which the newborn had apparent spontaneous regression of cutaneous metastases and cerebral lesions (44).

Clinical Features. Most children with an adrenal cortical neoplasm have signs or symptoms of endocrine abnormality. In a review by Neblett et al. (37), nonfunctional cortical tumors were rare in children: only 17 were noted in over 200 cases. Most children present with virilization, followed by Cushing's syndrome which is often (60 percent) a mixed endocrine syndrome with virilization (25); pure Cushing's syndrome is uncommon. While obesity is reported by some to have a more truncal distribution in adults, in

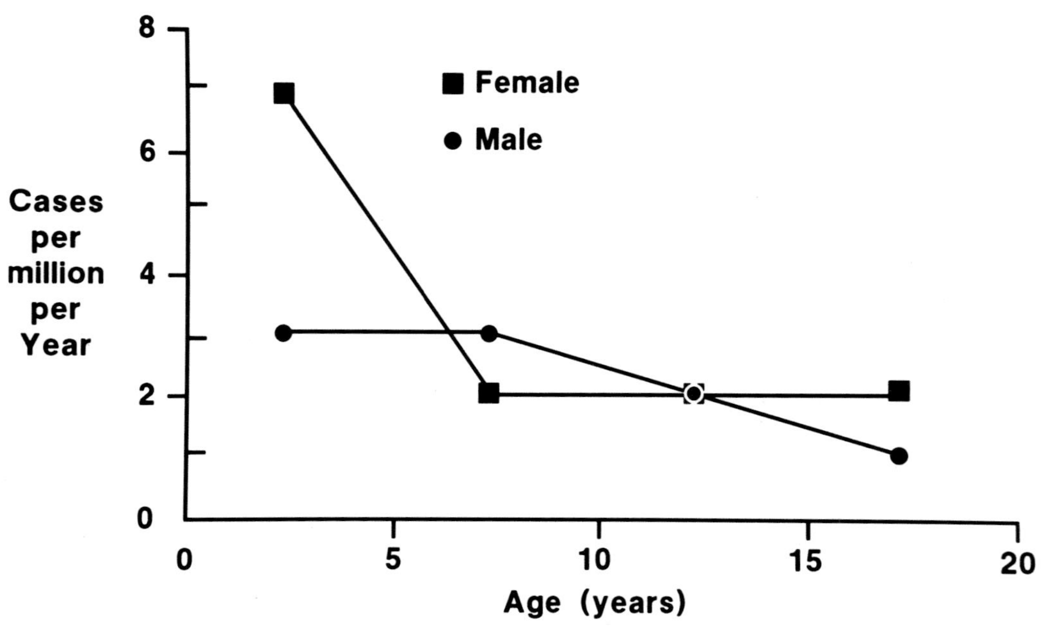

Figure 6-1
ADRENAL CORTICAL CARCINOMA

Sex and age-specific incidence of adrenal cortical carcinoma in the United States, 1973-1987. (Fig. 1 from Lack EE, Mulvihill JJ, Travis WD, Kozakewich HP. Adrenal cortical neoplasms in the pediatric and adolescent age group. Clinicopathological study of 30 cases with emphasis on epidemiological and prognostic factors. Pathol Annu 1992;27:1–53.)

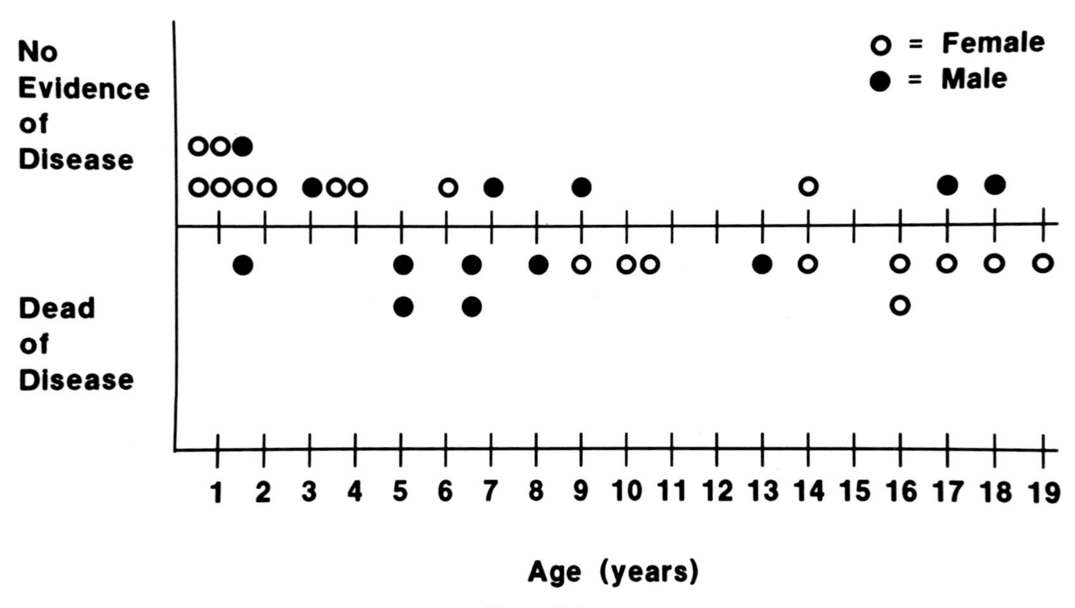

Figure 6-2
CLINICAL OUTCOME OF ADRENAL CORTICAL TUMORS

Age and sex distribution of 32 children and adolescents with adrenal cortical tumors plotted according to clinical outcome, i.e., no evidence of disease or dead of disease. One patient in group A (no evidence of recurrent or metastatic adrenal tumor) and one in group B (recurrent or metastatic tumor) developed second primary tumors and died. Another child in group A died suddenly 1 year after diagnosis. (Fig. 1 from Zerbini C, Kozakewich HP, Weinberg DS, et al. Adrenocortical neoplasms in childhood and adolescence: analysis of prognostic factors including DNA content. Endocr Pathol 1992;3:116–28.)

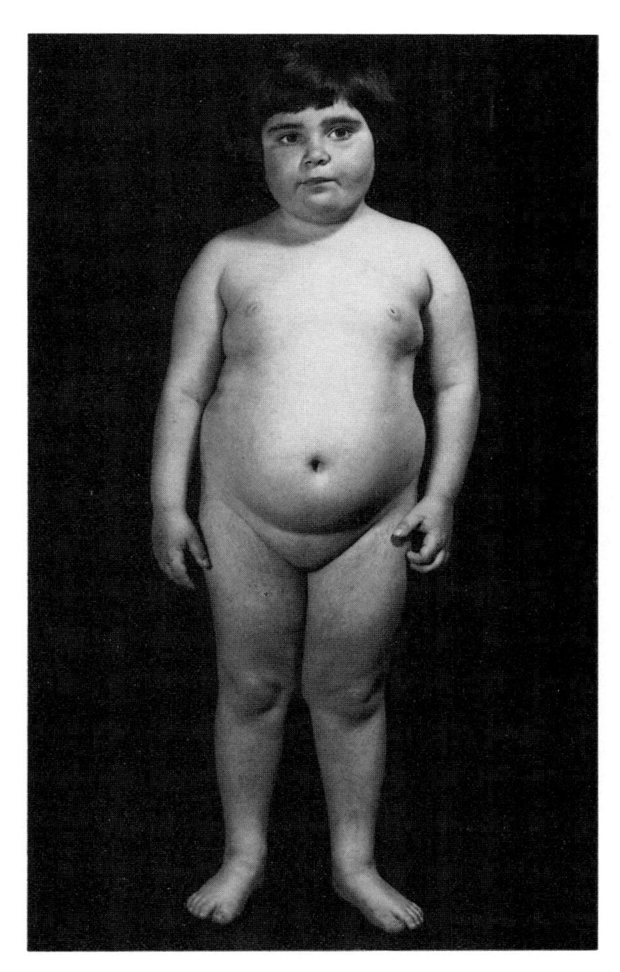

Figure 6-3
ADRENAL CORTICAL ADENOMA
WITH CUSHING'S SYNDROME

Six-year-old girl with "pure" Cushing's syndrome had an 11-month history of obesity, increasing abdominal girth, and hirsutism. The child had facial plethora and generalized obesity (more pronounced centrally). Cutaneous striae were also evident over upper thighs and lower abdomen. The patient was alive and well 17 years following right adrenalectomy. The resected tumor weighed 23 g and measured 4 cm in diameter.

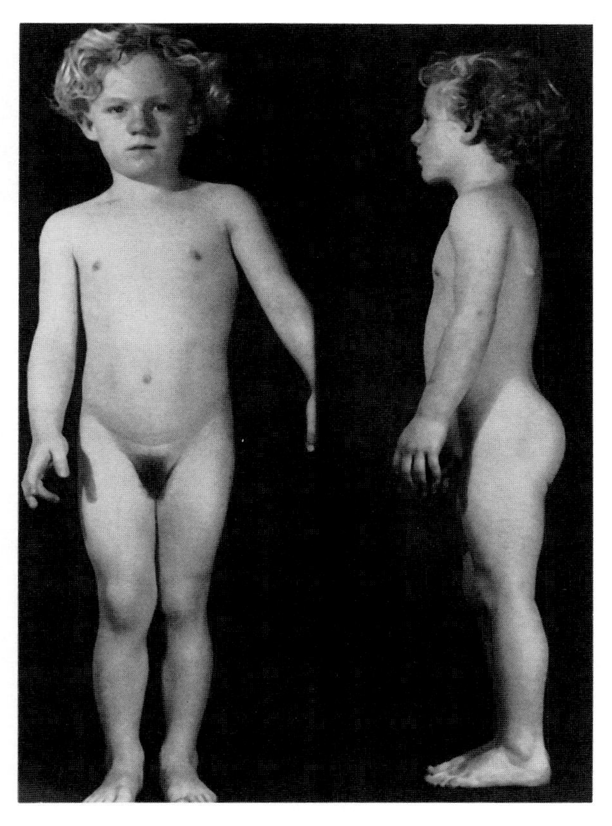

Figure 6-4
ADRENAL CORTICAL CARCINOMA

Virilization due to a right adrenal cortical tumor (classified pathologically as an adrenal cortical carcinoma) in a 3 1/2-year-old female. The tumor weighed 110 g and measured 7.5 cm in diameter. Clitoromegaly was noted shortly after birth. The child displayed remarkable development in terms of size and strength during the 2nd and 3rd years. She had a low-pitched voice, very well-developed musculature, and abundant pubic hair. The child died suddenly one year following surgical removal of the adrenal tumor, but there was no evidence of recurrence or metastasis. (Fig. 14 from Lack EE, Mulvihill JJ, Travis WD, Kozakewich HP. Adrenal cortical neoplasms in the pediatric and adolescent age group. Clinicopathological study of 30 cases with emphasis on epidemiological and prognostic factors. Pathol Annu 1992;27:1–53.) (Figs. 6-4, 6-5, and 6-14 are from the same case.)

infants it tends to be generalized, with involvement of the extremities as well as trunk (fig. 6-3) (15). Feminization is unusual, particularly in childhood (12,22,50), as is primary hyperaldosteronism (13,24,39,50). Features of virilization in females include increased muscle mass sometimes resulting in a "herculean" habitus (fig. 6-4), as well as clitoromegaly (fig. 6-5), facial hair, deepening of the voice, and the appearance of pubic hair (fig. 6-6). Excess androgen secretion in male patients usually causes isosexual precocity, with penile enlargement and pubic hair (fig. 6-7) (25). Conversion of an endocrine syndrome of virilization to feminization has been reported (17). Occasionally, the clinical presentation can mimic pheochromocytoma (fig. 6-8).

Gross Findings. Adrenal cortical tumors can range widely in size (2.4 to 19 cm) (25,41) and weight (18 to 6,000 g) (25). In a recent study of 32 adrenal cortical neoplasms in children and

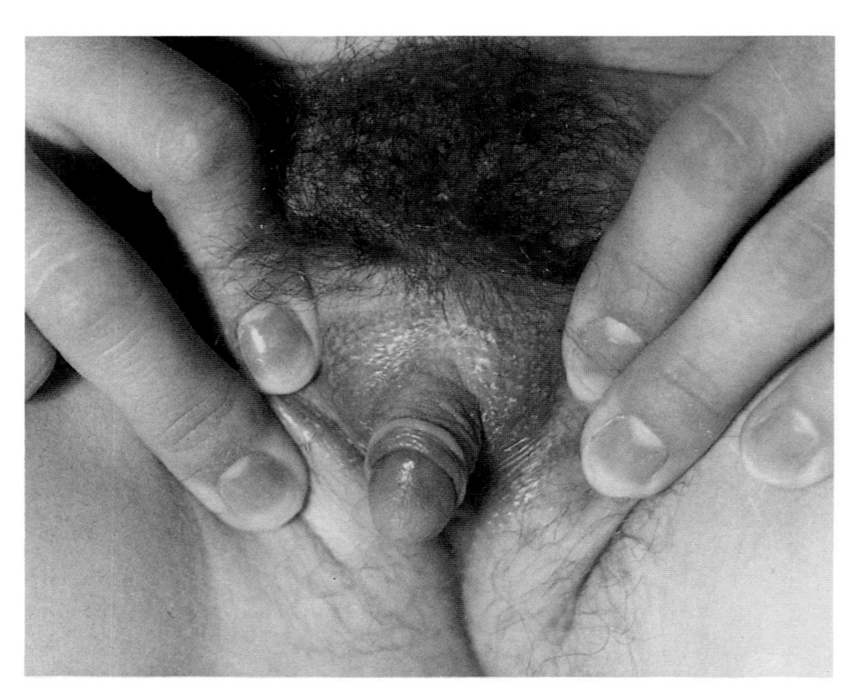

Figure 6-5
CLITOROMEGALY

The clitoris in a 3 1/2-year-old girl measured about 3.5 cm and the glans measured 1.4 x 1.5 cm. (Fig 14C from Lack EE, Mulvihill JJ, Travis WD, Kozakewich HP. Adrenal cortical neoplasms in the pediatric and adolescent age group. Clinicopathological study of 30 cases with emphasis on epidemiological and prognostic factors. Pathol Annu 1992;27:1–53.)

Figure 6-6
MIXED ENDOCRINE SYNDROME

One-year-old female with mixed endocrine syndrome consisting of virilization and Cushing's syndrome. Increased body hair is present over the pubic region, thighs, and lower abdomen. Child also had clitoral enlargement. A right adrenal tumor (classified pathologically as adrenal cortical carcinoma) weighed 44 g and measured 5 cm in diameter. The patient was alive and well 9 years later.

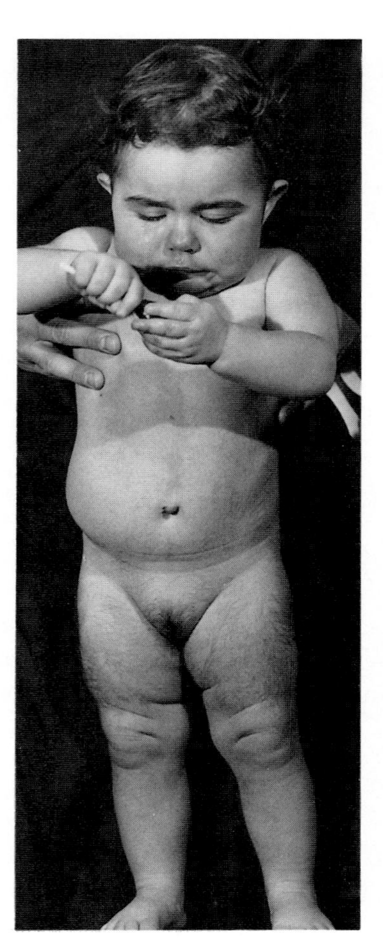

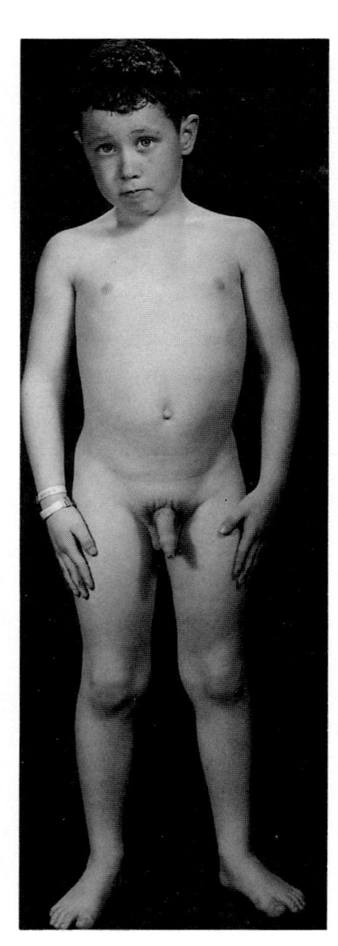

Figure 6-7
ADRENAL CORTICAL CARCINOMA WITH VIRILIZATION

A 6 1/2-year-old boy came to medical attention because of penile enlargement, appearance of pubic hair, and recent abdominal pain. Radiographs of hands and wrists showed advanced bone age. Child had pulmonary and hepatic metastases at presentation. The adrenal tumor weighed 475 g and measured 15 cm in diameter. The tumor invaded the inferior vena cava and the child died intraoperatively due to massive tumor embolization to right ventricle and main pulmonary artery. (Fig. 15 from Lack EE, Mulvihill JJ, Travis WD, Kozakewich HP. Adrenal cortical neoplasms in the pediatric and adolescent age group. Clinicopathological study of 30 cases with emphasis on epidemiological and prognostic factors. Pathol Annu 1992;27:1–53.)

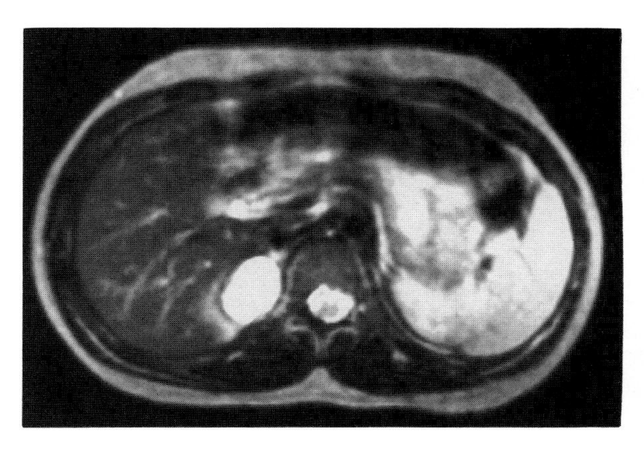

Figure 6-8
ADRENAL CORTICAL ADENOMA
A 9-year-old boy presented with hypertension and cardiomegaly documented on chest roentgenogram and ECG (see figure 6-9). There was also a history of blurred vision, headaches, sweating, palpitations, and intermittent facial flushing. Serum dopamine was slightly elevated, but levels of other catecholamines were normal. Magnetic resonance imaging of upper abdomen showed a right suprarenal mass. The tumor was "hyperintense" on T-2 weighted image and suggested a pheochromocytoma. The child was treated with alpha and beta adrenergic blockers and the tumor was successfully resected.

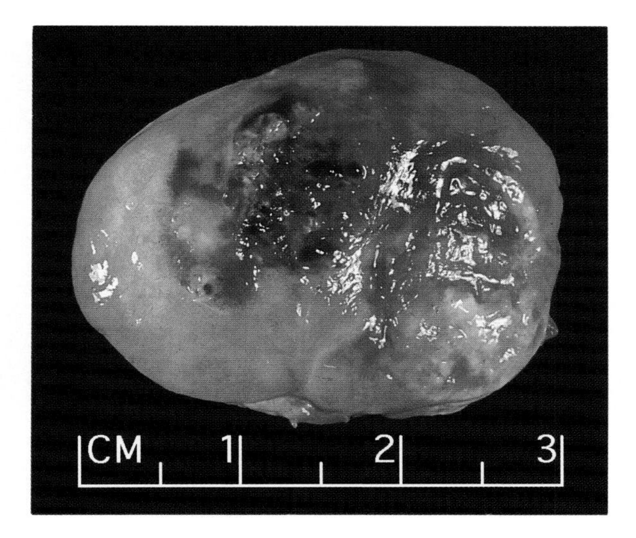

Figure 6-9
ADRENAL CORTICAL ADENOMA
This 12-g tumor had areas of necrosis and hemorrhage. There were 15 mitoses per 50 high-power fields as well as a few atypical mitotic figures. The patient was alive and well 5 years later. Tumor may have been secreting aldosterone, but laboratory work-up was not done since the neoplasm simulated a pheochromocytoma.

adolescents, patients were segregated into two general groups: group A (15 patients) consisted of patients who were alive (or died of other causes) without evidence of a recurrent or metastatic adrenal cortical neoplasm (i.e., clinically benign tumors); group B (17 patients) had documented metastases or fatal outcome due to tumor (i.e., clinically malignant tumors) (55). Included in group A were tumors classified on initial pathology review as ACA (5 tumors), ACC (9 tumors), or indeterminate malignant potential (1 tumor). The average size of tumors in group A was 5.8 cm (median weight of 44 g) (fig. 6-9), while tumors in group B were significantly larger (11.9 cm) with a median weight of 560 g. In the review by Neblett et al. (37), 27.9 percent of childhood adrenal cortical neoplasms were classified pathologically as ACA (average weight of 43.3 g, average diameter of 4.6 cm), and 72.1 percent as ACC (average weight of 466.8 g, average diameter of 8.6 cm); this classification was based upon gross and microscopic features and not on biologic behavior. The gross appearance of some tumors can easily lead to a presumptive diagnosis of ACC (fig. 6-10). Even some of the smaller tumors, however, which prove to be clinically benign, can show areas of tumor necrosis (figs. 6-9, 6-11), but seldom more than 25 percent in visual estimation of extent in histologic sections. The average weight of ACA in the study by Weatherby and Carney (50) was 54 g (range, 30 to 122 g).

Microscopic Findings. The histopathologic features of adrenal cortical tumors shown in Table 6-1 are from a recent review by Zerbini et al. (55), along with the number of tumors that were initially classified as ACC (including those in group A). From this table it is apparent that many tumors that prove to be clinically benign have adverse morphologic findings commonly associated with malignancy in tumors from adult patients. Most tumors have architectural patterns that can be classified as alveolar (or nesting), diffuse (or solid), trabecular, or an admixture of these major patterns. An alveolar or blunt cord-like pattern is most common in tumors classified pathologically as ACA (fig. 6-12). Nuclear pleomorphism and hyperchromasia can be found in both ACA (fig. 6-13) and ACC, and this finding alone is usually not helpful in distinguishing between the two. Rarely, a tumor has oncocytic features as evidenced by greatly enlarged cells with abundant granular, eosinophilic cytoplasm (fig. 6-14), or a

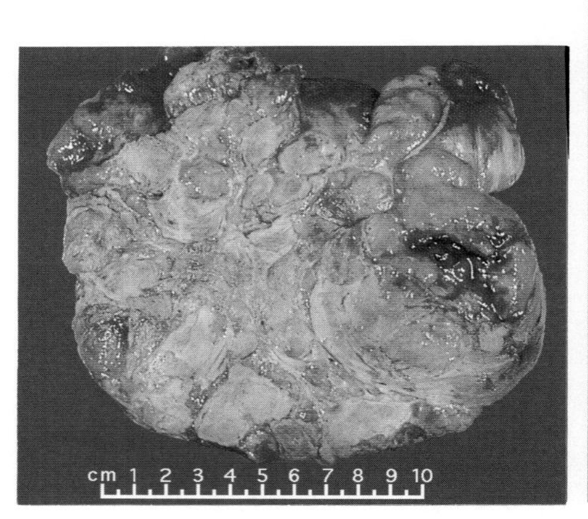

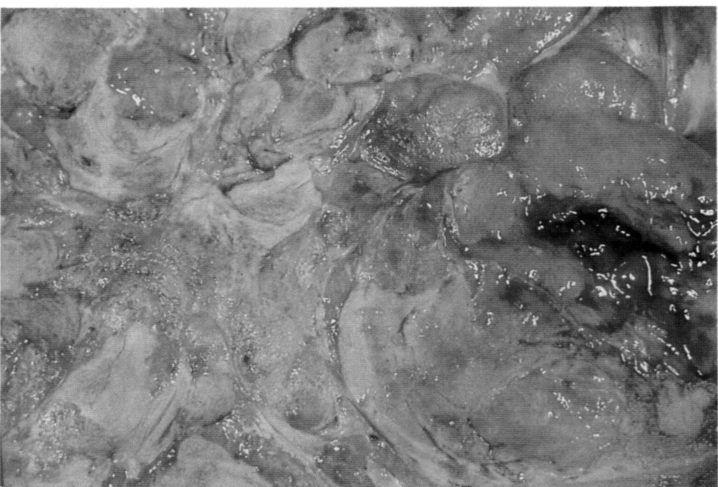

Figure 6-10
ADRENAL CORTICAL CARCINOMA

Left: Adrenal cortical carcinoma from a 16-year-old girl with virilization. The tumor weighed 1,250 g and measured 15.5 cm in diameter. The patient died 14 months following surgical resection, with massive intra-abdominal recurrence and metastases to lung, liver, and peritoneum. Neoplasm in cross section is coarsely nodular with most of the tumor being necrotic. Note confluent geographic zones of pale yellow tumor necrosis.

Right: Viable areas of the same tumor appear as bulging tan nodules.

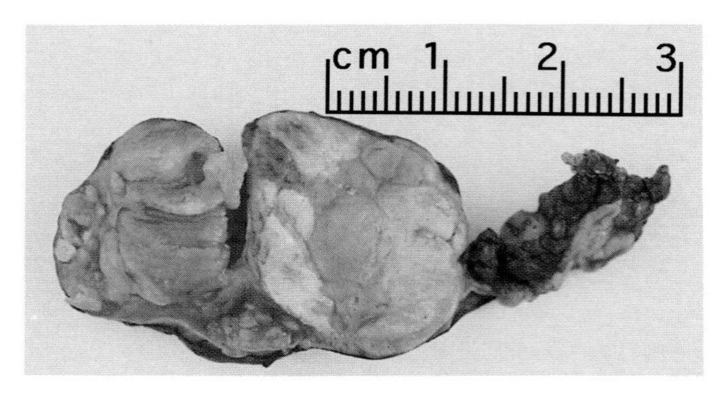

Figure 6-11
ADRENAL CORTICAL CARCINOMA

Adrenal cortical carcinoma in a 7-month-old female with virilization. The tumor weighed 27 g and had confluent areas of necrosis (25 percent) with dystrophic calcification, broad trabecular growth pattern, and about 10 mitoses per 50 high-power fields as well as atypical mitoses. The child was alive and well about 4 years later. India ink has been applied to the surgical margin of resection.

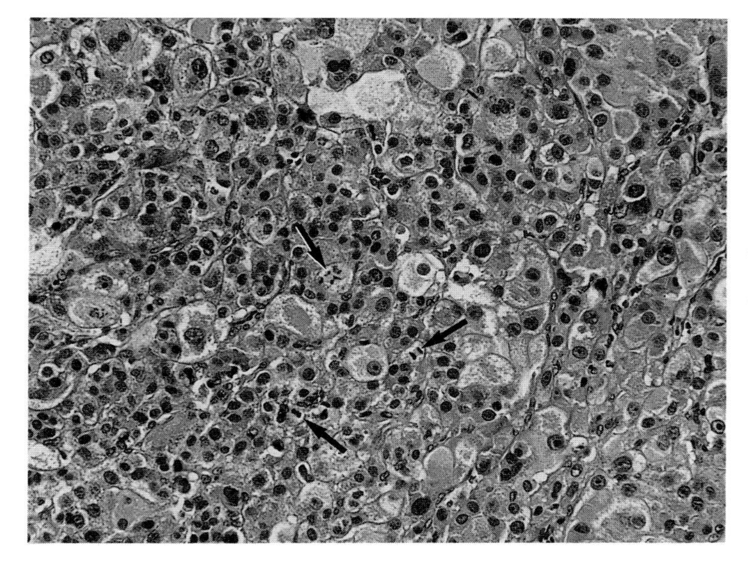

Figure 6-12
ADRENAL CORTICAL ADENOMA

This tumor in a young child is composed of cells with predominantly eosinophilic, compact cytoplasm arranged in short cords and ill-defined alveolar clusters. Three mitotic figures are in this field (arrows).

Table 6-1

HISTOPATHOLOGIC FEATURES OF ADRENAL CORTICAL TUMORS IN GROUP A AND GROUP B*

	Group A (n = 15)	Group B (n = 17)
Number initially classified as ACC	9/15 (60%)	17/17 (100%)
Number with mitotic figures	10/15 (67%)	16/17 (94%)
Average number mitoses (range)	11 per 50 high-power fields (1–61)	31 per 50 high-power fields (1–88)
Atypical mitoses	4/15 (27%)	5/17 (29%)
Tumor necrosis (number greater than 25%)	3/15 (20%) (7 of 17 tumors had necrosis)	10/17 (59%) (15 of 17 tumors had necrosis)
Vascular invasion	1/15 (7%)	4/17 (24%)
Capsular invasion	6/15 (37%)	6/17 (35%)
Broad fibrous bands	4/15 (27%)	7/17 (41%)
Calcifications	5/15 (33%)	11/17 (65%)

*Group A patients were alive (or dead of other causes) without evidence of recurrent or metastatic tumor; group B patients had documented metastasis, recurrence, or fatal outcome because of adrenal tumor. Note number of cases initially classified as ACC in group A (60%) and group B (100%). (Table 5 from Zerbini C, Kozakewich HP, Weinberg DS, Mundt DJ, Edwards JA III, Lack EE. Adrenocortical neoplasms in childhood and adolescence: analysis of prognostic factors including DNA content. Endocr Pathol 1992;3:116–28.)

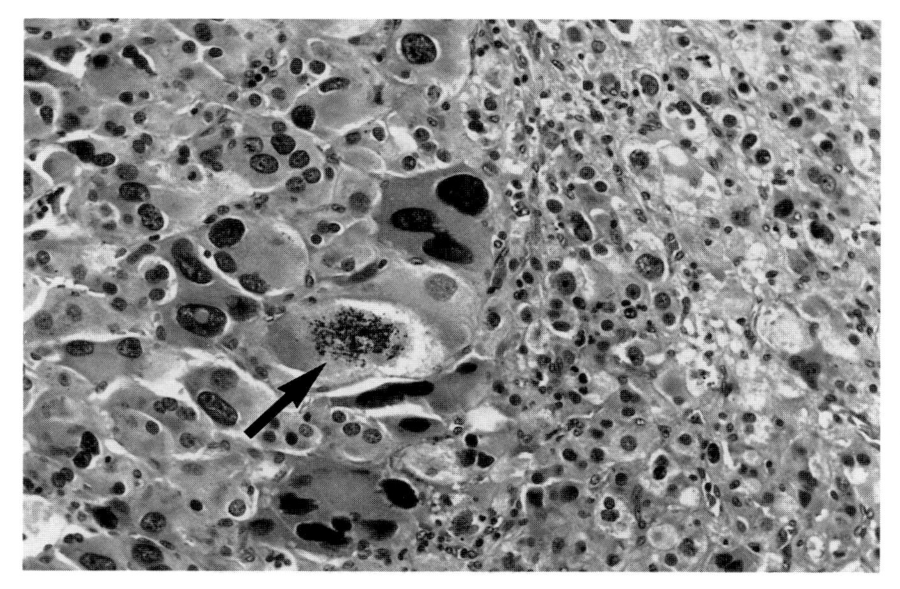

Figure 6-13
MASCULINIZING ADRENAL CORTICAL ADENOMA

The tumor in a 1 1/2-year-old male weighed 18 g and was 5 cm in diameter. Note the rather marked nuclear pleomorphism and hyperchromasia along with atypical mitotic figure (arrow). The patient was alive and well 17 years later, but eventually died of massive liposarcoma of retroperitoneum.

myxoid pattern (fig. 6-15). Occasionally, there appears to be capsular invasion in an otherwise clinically benign tumor (fig. 6-16); similar to cortical neoplasms in adults, capsular invasion may be difficult to recognize in histologic sections. At times a priori evidence of capsular invasion or extra-adrenal extension can be assumed by intraoperative assessment or gross examination.

Some tumors which prove to be clinically benign have areas of confluent necrosis (fig. 6-17), sometimes with small amounts of dystrophic calcification. Cagle et al. (4) found that clinically benign adrenal cortical tumors in children were significantly more likely to have mitoses, necrosis, broad fibrous bands, and moderate to marked pleomorphism. Significant necrosis (25 percent or

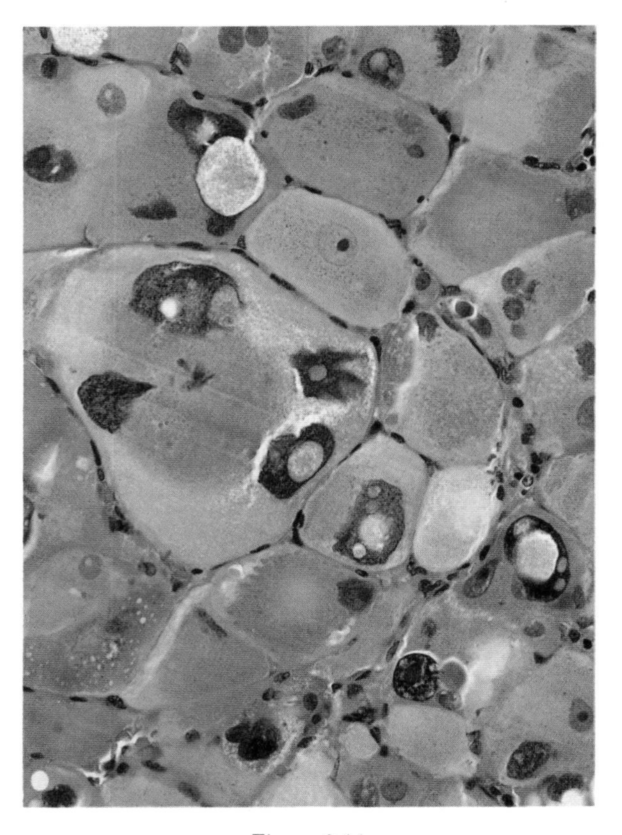

Figure 6-14
VIRILIZING ADRENAL CORTICAL NEOPLASM

This neoplasm from a 3 1/2-year-old female was classified initially as a carcinoma. The tumor cells have prominent oncocytic features along with numerous nuclear "pseudo-inclusions." (Same case as figure 6-4.)

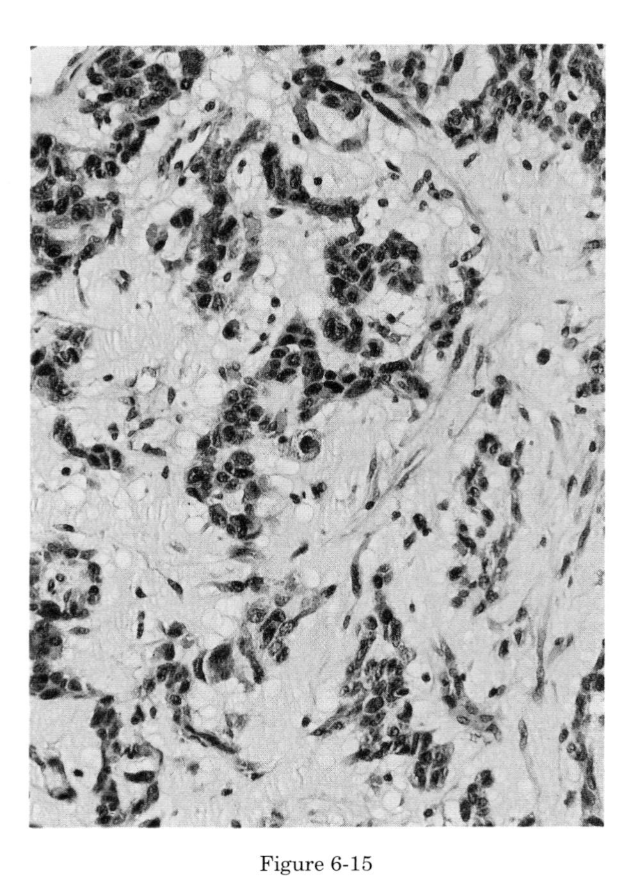

Figure 6-15
ADRENAL CORTICAL ADENOMA

Tumor from a young child with hypertension shows a marked myxoid stromal component.

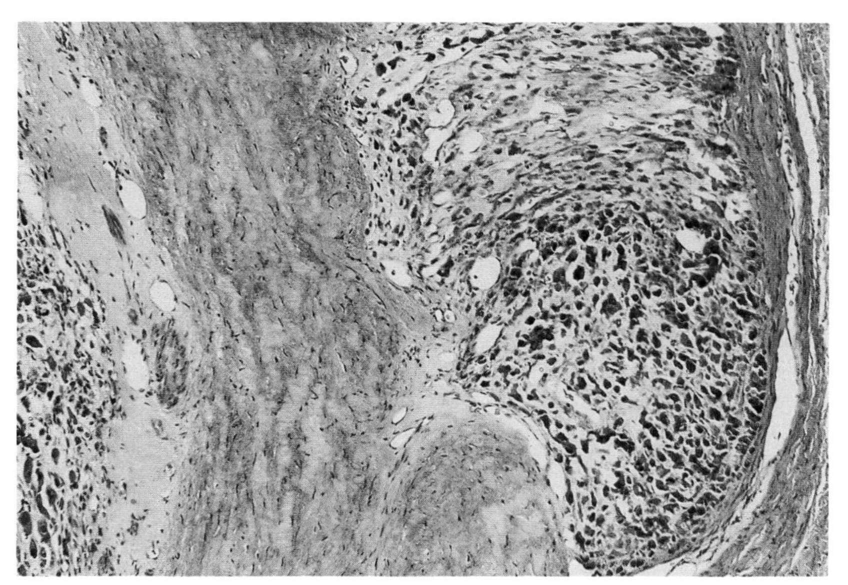

Figure 6-16
ADRENAL CORTICAL ADENOMA

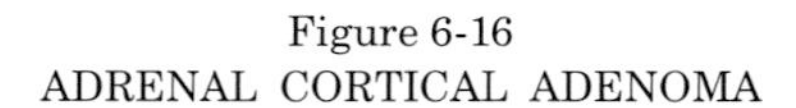

This fibrous capsule (or "pseudocapsule") was well developed except for a few areas where tumor extended into and almost through as blunt, tongue-like projections. A portion of connective tissue at right represents the capsule of the adrenal gland.

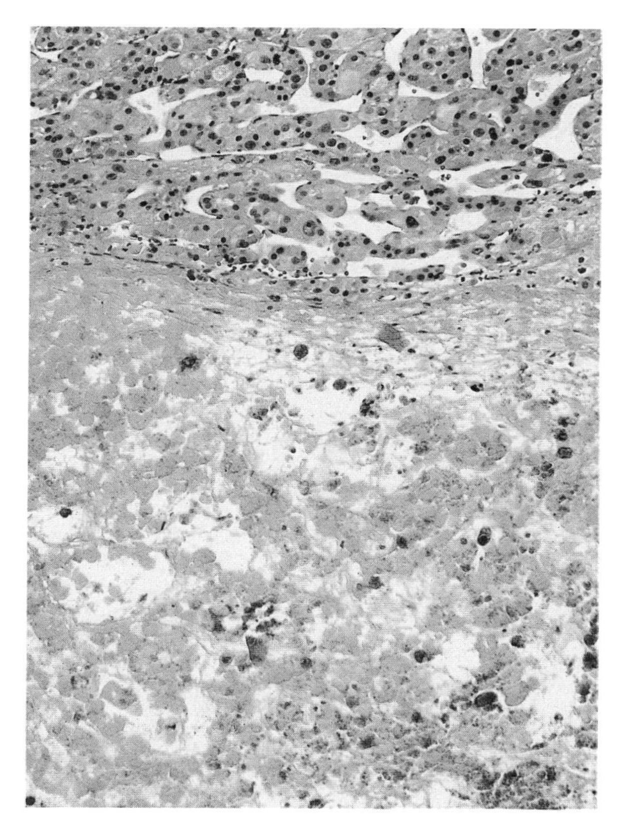

Figure 6-17
VIRILIZING ADRENAL CORTICAL NEOPLASM
This virilizing adrenal cortical neoplasm from a 7-month-old female was classified pathologically as carcinoma. Tumor had confluent areas of necrosis (25 percent total area in histologic sections) as well as spotty dystrophic calcification. This patient was alive and well 3 1/2 years later.

more by visual estimation in histologic sections), however, has been found to be an adverse prognostic finding (55). A broad anastomosing trabecular pattern can be found in both benign and malignant cortical neoplasms in childhood, although it is more prevalent in clinically malignant tumors. Occasionally, depending upon the plane of section, an attached (fig. 6-18, left) or what appears to be a free floating portion of tumor within a vascular sinusoid is seen (fig. 6-18, right); careful inspection may reveal a continuous layer of endothelial cells indicating that this is probably not true vascular invasion. This may be similar to the sinusoidal invasion referred to by Weiss (51). True vascular invasion usually appears as loose plugs within vascular channels, and when present indicates malignancy. Rarely, the tumor can propagate through the remaining gland via tributaries of the venous network. Extension of tumor into the inferior vena cava may result in malignant ascites or pose potential problems during surgery with mobilization of tumor thrombi (16). An occasional mitotic figure may not be an adverse feature (see fig. 6-13), but numerous mitoses (more than 31 per 50 high-power fields) is ominous, particularly if the tumor is large and the patient is in an older or "adolescent" age group (25,55). Intracytoplasmic hyaline globules are found in 10 percent of pediatric adrenal cortical neoplasms (both ACA and ACC) (25).

Prognostic Factors and Biologic Behavior. Because of the rarity of adrenal cortical neoplasms in the pediatric age group it is very difficult to draw definitive conclusions regarding the prognostic impact of morphologic features. The limited experience of most pathologists with these tumors in children may contribute to a tendency to overdiagnose these rare tumors as carcinoma (4,25,55). The study by Cagle et al. (4) concluded that in the pediatric age group adrenal cortical tumors are more likely to be benign than had previously been thought. Based in large part on data in the older literature, a relatively poor prognosis has been attached to adrenal cortical tumors in the pediatric age group (25). Of 222 cases of adrenal cortical tumors reported in children up to 1962, only 23 patients were recorded as surviving 2 or more years after treatment (19). There are a variety of factors contributing to this poor survival rate, such as far advanced disease, presentation in an era prior to availability of cortisone, and the varied experience of surgical and life support teams in management of the pediatric patient.

In some studies adverse histologic findings are present more often in clinically benign tumors in the pediatric age group (4) compared with tumors seen in adults (21,51). In a recent univariate statistical analysis of various prognostic factors, five were found to be statistically significant (Table 6-2) (55). With regard to age at diagnosis, the survival rate for patients older than 5 years with a pathologic diagnosis of ACC was only 13 percent, compared with 70 percent for children 5 years or younger (25); in a review by Humphrey et al. (23) the overall survival rate in the infantile group was 53 percent compared with 17 percent in the adolescent group. Although

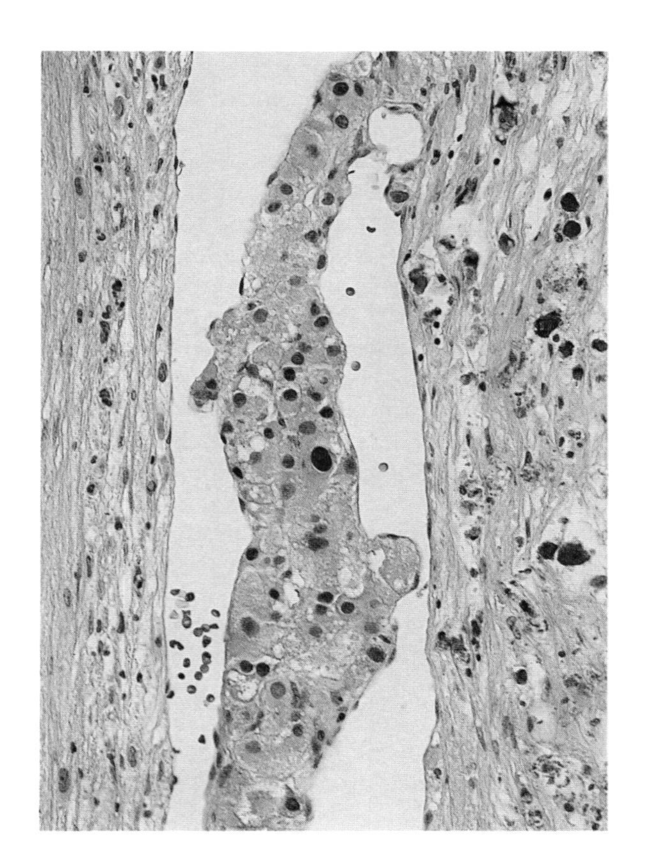

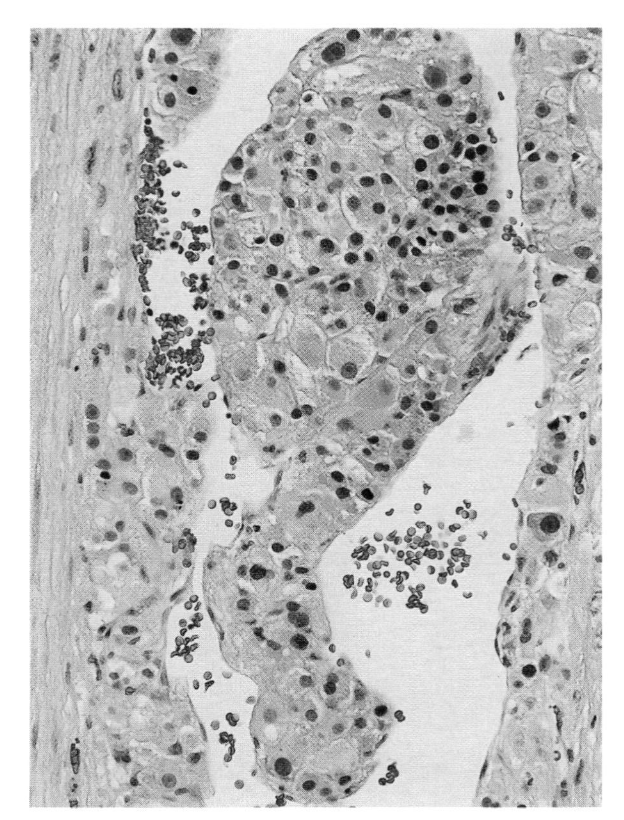

Figure 6-18
VIRILIZING ADRENAL CORTICAL NEOPLASM

Left: Areas showed occasional trabecula of tumor with small tenuous attachments and intact endothelial covering.

Right: Another area of same tumor shows a "free-floating" island of tumor adjacent to the capsule near the external aspect of tumor. While the tumor appears to be angioinvasive in this plane of section, a different plane of section may reveal attachment, as on the left. (Same case as figure 6-17.)

Table 6-2

ADVERSE PROGNOSTIC FACTORS*

Variables**	Overall	Group A	Group B	P Values
Age (years)	8.3	5.9	10.3	0.04
Average tumor size (cm)	8.6	5.8	11.9	0.0003
Median tumor weight (g)	210	44	560	0.0001
Mitotic count (per 50 high-power fields)	20	11	31	0.04
Tumor necrosis greater than or equal to 25% (visually estimated)	41%	20%	59%	0.03

*Table 4 from Zerbini C, Kozakewich HP, Weinberg DS, Mundt DJ, Edwards JA III, Lack EE. Adrenocortical neoplasms in childhood and adolescence: analysis of prognostic factors including DNA content. Endocr Pathol 1992;3:116–128.

**Parameters with statistically significant predictive value relating to prognosis.

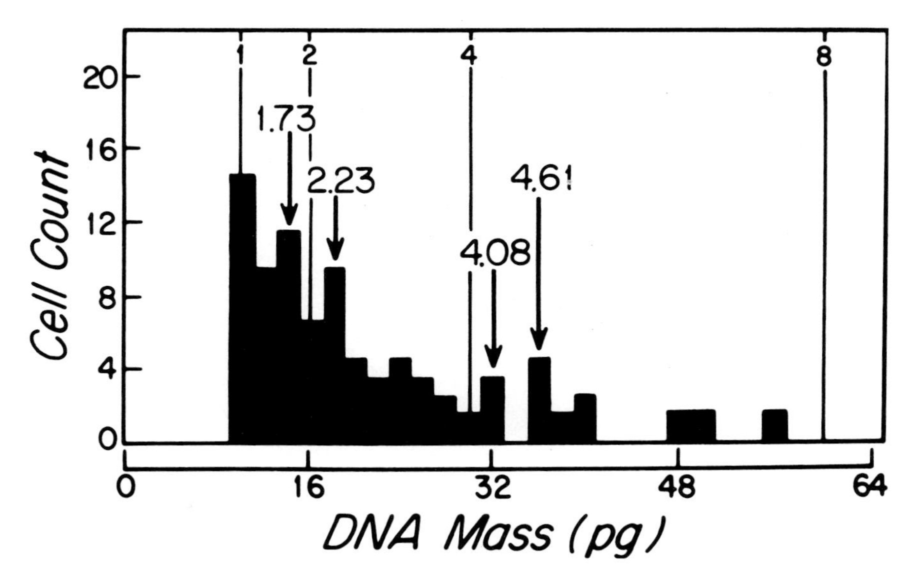

Figure 6-19
ADRENAL CORTICAL ADENOMA

DNA histogram by static image analysis shows multiple aneuploid peaks. The tumor weighed only 12 g. The child was alive and well 4 1/2 years later.

mitotic rate may be useful in distinguishing low-grade (20 mitoses or less per 50 high-power fields) from high-grade ACC (more than 20 mitoses) in adults (52), a recent study of pediatric adrenal cortical neoplasms found mitoses not to be a significant prognostic indicator (55). Clinically malignant adrenal cortical tumors are often much larger than benign tumors (25,37), although exceptions occur. Cagle et al. (4) found tumor weight to be the only reliable morphologic predictor of malignant behavior in the pediatric age group, with all tumors over 500 g being malignant. Similarly, Ribeiro et al. (42), in a univariate statistical analysis, reported that age 3.5 years or older at diagnosis, tumor weight more than 100 g, and size greater than 200 cm^3 were associated with an unfavorable outcome. A recent study found that tumor weight of 100 g or more was an adverse prognostic finding along with histologic typing of tumors as low-grade and high-grade ACC; tumor diameter was not significantly predictive of biologic behavior, but this parameter was available in relatively few cases (3). Exceptions exist regarding weight criteria and prognosis: rare tumors of more than 1,000 g prove to be clinically benign, and rare tumors under 40 g (22 g [27] and 35 g [44]) are malignant with metastases. Biochemical evidence of a deficiency of 11-beta-hydroxylase has also been reported in childhood ACC (8), but its significance in terms of predicting biologic behavior is not known.

The recent review by Zerbini et al. (55) summarizes data from nine different studies of DNA ploidy in adrenal cortical tumors; in their own study, 23 tumors (14 clinically benign and 9 clinically malignant) were analyzed by static image analysis (10 tumors) and by both static image analysis and flow cytometry (13 tumors). There was no discrepancy between results of DNA ploidy analysis in tumors studied by both methods. Twelve of 14 clinically benign tumors were aneuploid (4 with multiple aneuploid peaks) (fig. 6-19), compared with 5 of 9 clinically malignant tumors (one with multiple aneuploid peaks); 4 of 9 clinically malignant tumors had a diploid DNA value (fig. 6-20). The results indicate no statistically significant association between clinical outcome and DNA ploidy pattern. A recent study of over 50 adrenal cortical tumors in the pediatric age group also concluded that ploidy does not reliably predict outcome: 21 of 29 patients with aneuploid tumors were disease-free following diagnosis (median, 1.75 years) (3). A relatively high incidence of aneuploidy was noted by Taylor et al. (48) (4 of 4 cases), but it was also apparent in one tumor that was clinically benign.

Most deaths caused by ACC occur within 1 (25) to 2 years (23) following diagnosis, but some patients survive longer with recurrent or metastatic tumor. The most frequent sites of metastasis are lung (figs. 6-21, 6-22) followed by liver. Invasion of the inferior vena cava was reported in 6 of 17

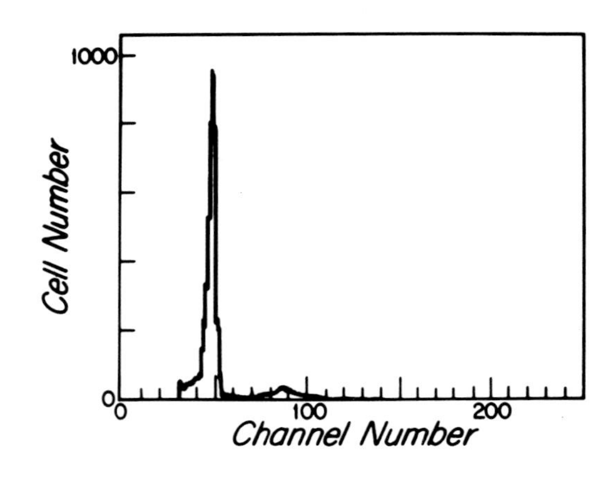

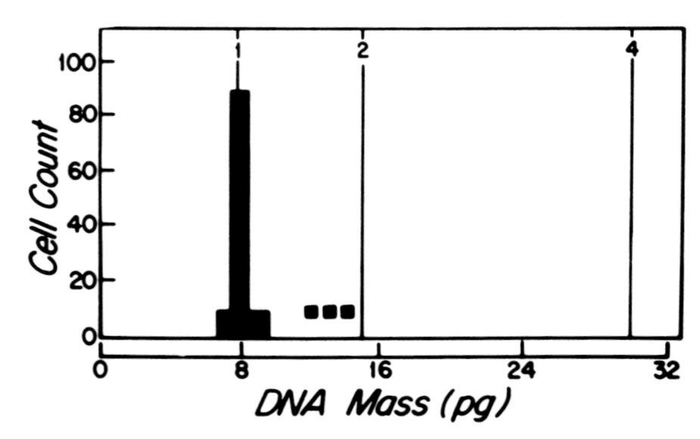

Figure 6-20
ADRENAL CORTICAL CARCINOMA
AND VIRILIZATION

Flow cytometric histogram (top) and image analysis histogram (bottom) of ACC in a 16-year-old girl. Tumor had diploid DNA content, but patient died of massive intra-abdominal recurrence and metastases a little over 1 year after diagnosis.

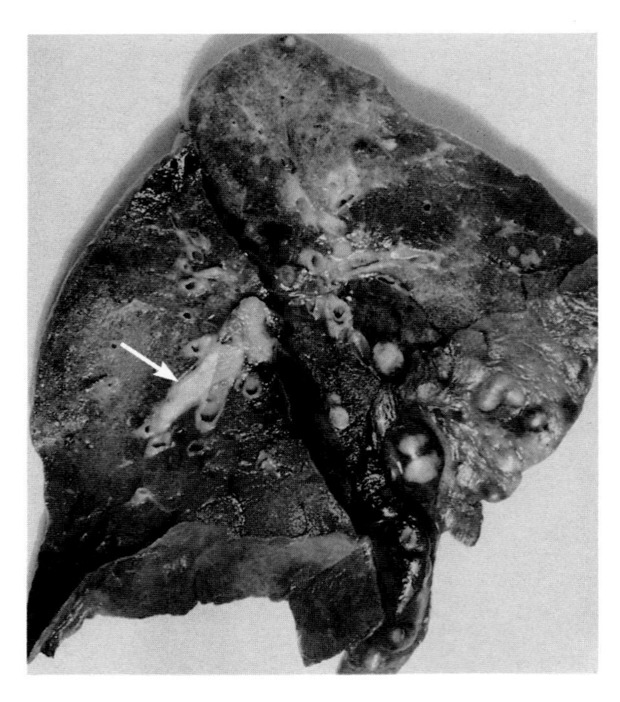

Figure 6-21
ADRENAL CORTICAL CARCINOMA

Adrenal cortical carcinoma in a 6 1/2-year-old male with masculinization. There were metastases to liver and lungs along with invasion of inferior vena cava. Left lung has numerous metastases, some of which are pleural based. Arrow indicates large tumor embolus straddling branches of pulmonary artery.

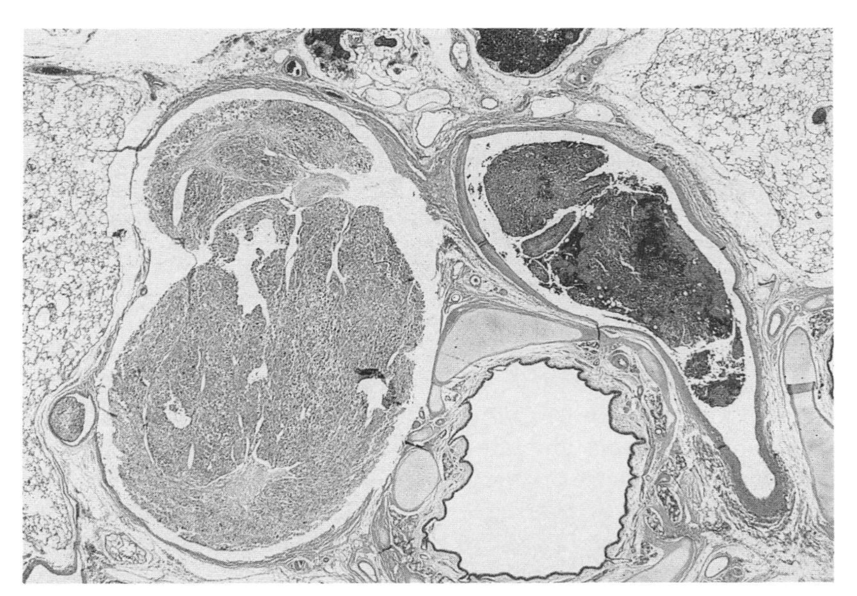

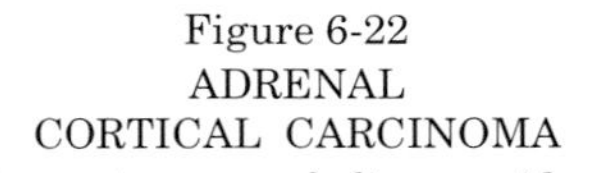

Figure 6-22
ADRENAL
CORTICAL CARCINOMA

Large tumor emboli are evident in venous channels of lung.

patients with clinically malignant adrenal cortical neoplasms (35 percent), with obstruction in a number of instances resulting in lower extremity and truncal edema (25). Other sites of metastasis include peritoneum (29 percent), pleura and/or diaphragm (24 percent), abdominal lymph nodes (24 percent), and kidney (18 percent) (25).

Hemihypertrophy and Other Abnormalities

In 1967, Fraumeni and Miller (10) highlighted the association between adrenal cortical neoplasms and hemihypertrophy in the pediatric age group. In a clinical chart review of 62 children with adrenal cortical neoplasms from 12 different hospitals, 46 tumors were designated pathologically as ACC (74.2 percent) and 16 as ACA (25.8 percent); of all of these patients, 2 (3 percent) had congenital hemihypertrophy (fig. 6-23). The adrenal cortical tumors are not necessarily located on the same side as the hemihypertrophy. Other pediatric tumors reported in association with hemihypertrophy include nephroblastoma (Wilms' tumor) (9), hepatoblastoma (10,11), malignant pheochromocytoma (45), and one patient with ACA and medullary sponge kidney (49). Urinary tract abnormalities have also been noted in children with adrenal cortical tumors, such as duplication of the collecting system and polycystic kidney. Adrenal cortical neoplasms have rarely been reported in association with ganglioneuroma (14) and ganglioneuroblastoma (6).

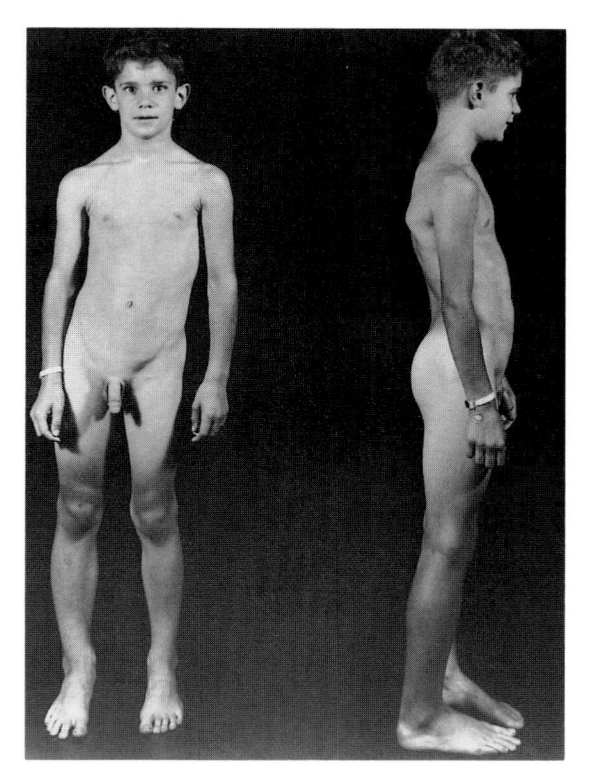

Figure 6-23
VIRILIZING ADRENAL CORTICAL ADENOMA
In infancy this 7-year-old boy had hemihypertrophy on right side. Evaluation revealed advanced skeletal age, onset of acne, deepening of voice, enlarged genitalia, and appearance of pubic hair. The resected adrenal tumor weighed 40 g and measured 7 cm in diameter. Patient was alive and well 5 years later. (Fig. 2 from Lack EE, Mulvihill JJ, Travis WD, Kozakewich HP. Adrenal cortical neoplasms in the pediatric and adolescent age group. Clinicopathological study of 30 cases with emphasis on epidemiological and prognostic factors. Pathol Annu 1992;27:1–53.)

Beckwith-Wiedemann Syndrome and Adrenal Cytomegaly

Adrenal cytomegaly is a characteristic feature of Beckwith-Wiedemann syndrome which has an association with adrenal cortical neoplasms as well as other tumors, both benign and malignant (see chapter 2). Intra-abdominal nephroblastoma is the main associated neoplasm followed by ACC and hepatoblastoma. A case of congenital metastasizing ACC was reported in which cytomegaly was present in the fetal adrenal cortex and elsewhere (46).

Cancer Family Syndrome (Li-Fraumeni or SBLA Syndrome)

In 1969 a remarkable familial aggregation of cancers was defined as a possible syndrome by Li and Fraumeni (29) based upon a review of hospital records of children with rhabdomyosarcoma. The acronym SBLA (sarcoma; breast and brain tumors; leukemia, laryngeal carcinoma, and lung cancer; and adrenal cortical carcinoma) cancer syndrome was later proposed based upon the complex of tumors (31). An autosomal dominant mode of inheritance has been reported with soft tissue sarcomas, bone sarcomas, and breast carcinoma (28–30). ACC comprised 10 percent of neoplasms other than sarcomas and breast cancer in the 0 to 44-year-old age group, whereas in the United States for all ages, ACC accounts for less than 1 percent of malignant neoplasms (30). In many cases of the Li-Fraumeni syndrome, alterations in the p53 tumor suppressor gene

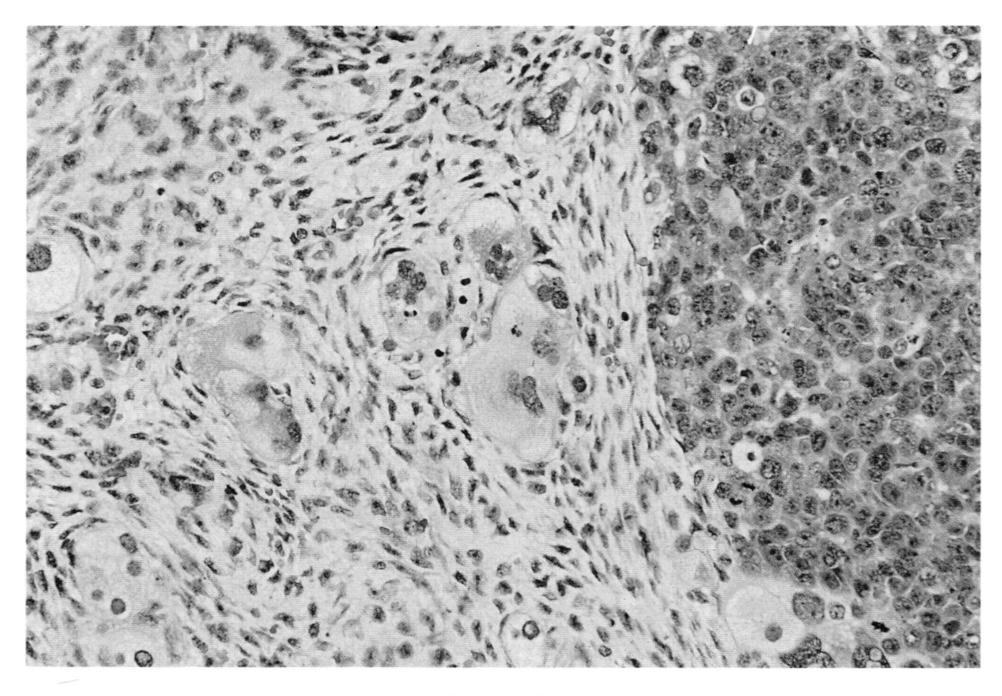

Figure 6-24
ADRENAL CORTICAL BLASTOMA
Tumor contains small nests of pleomorphic cells and more primitive spindle cells.

have been detected (34,43); the gene is located on the short arm of human chromosome 17 band 13, and encodes a 53 kD nuclear phosphoprotein that appears to function as a negative regulator of cell growth and proliferation (33). Loss of heterozygosity limited to region 11p15.5 was reported in a case of familial ACC; study of family pedigree showed additional tumors (osteosarcoma and breast cancer) (20).

Congenital Adrenal Hyperplasia

Adrenal cortical neoplasms, both ACA and ACC, have rarely been reported in association with congenital adrenal hyperplasia (CAH), also known as the adrenogenital syndrome (see chapter 2). At least three examples of ACA occurred in children with CAH; two of these were associated with virilization (5,32,40). A virilizing ACC was reported in a 10-year-old child with CAH (1), and two other ACCs were reported in patients 32 (2) and 37 (18) years of age. Another case of ACC raises the possibility of untreated CAH that later became neoplastic (38). Testicular "tumors" of adrenal cortical type are not infrequent in CAH, but large tumors (usually bilateral) necessitating orchiectomy are uncommon. It has been suggested that persistent trophic stimulation of adrenal cortical tissues by ACTH might induce neoplastic transformation, but this remains speculative (25).

Adrenal Cortical Blastoma

A unique case of a virilizing malignant adrenal cortical tumor was reported by Molberg et al. (36) as an adrenal cortical blastoma in a 21-month-old infant with increased serum alpha-fetoprotein. The tumor contained a mixture of immature epithelial and mesenchymal elements (fig. 6-24), as well as occasional foci of vascular invasion (fig. 6-25), but no metastases were evident at the time of autopsy. The tumor focally recapitulated the morphology of the developing fetal cortex.

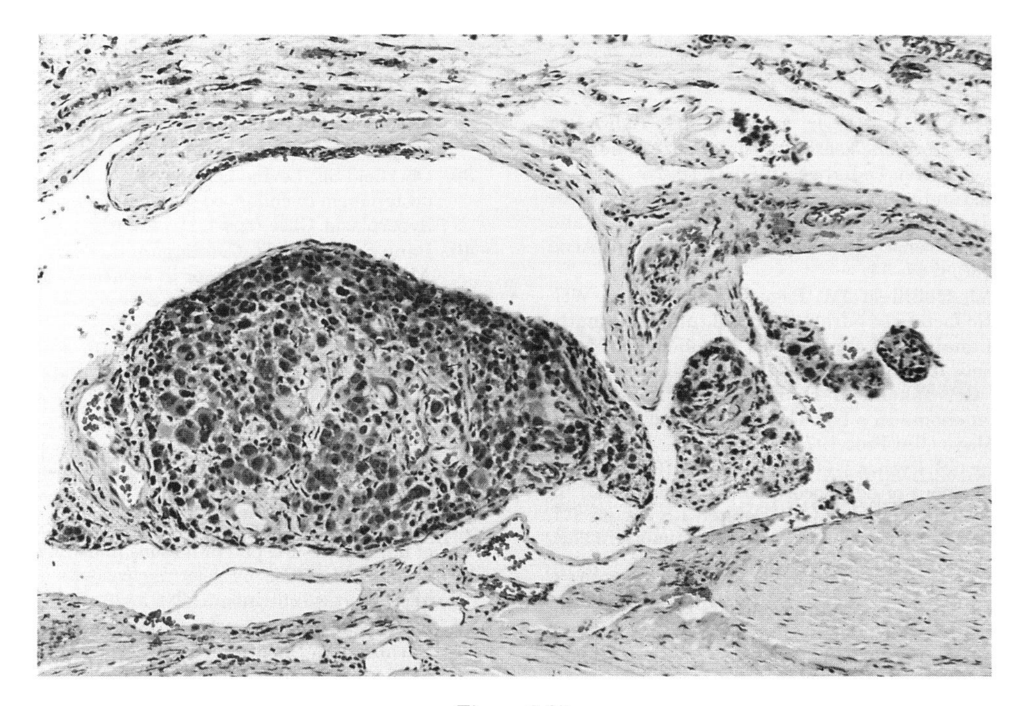

Figure 6-25
ADRENAL CORTICAL BLASTOMA
Large area of vascular (venous or lymphatic) invasion is apparent.

REFERENCES

1. Bauman A, Bauman CG. Virilizing adrenocortical carcinoma. Development in a patient with salt-losing congenital adrenal hyperplasia. JAMA 1982;248:3140–1.
2. Bratrud TE, Thompson WH. Congenital hyperplasia of adrenals. Staff meeting. Bull Hosp Univ Minn 1943;15:25–43.
3. Bugg MF, Ribeiro RC, Roberson PK, et al. Correlation of pathologic features with clinical outcome in pediatric adrenocortical neoplasia. A study of a Brazilian population. Am J Clin Pathol 1994;101:625–29.
4. Cagle PT, Hough AJ, Pysher TJ, et al. Comparison of adrenal cortical tumors in children and adults. Cancer 1986;57:2235–7.
5. Daeschner GL. Adrenal cortical adenoma arising in a girl with congenital adrenogenital syndrome. Pediatrics 1965;36:140–2.
6. Dahms WT, Gray G, Vrana M, New MI. Adrenocortical adenoma and ganglioneuroblastoma in a child. A case presenting as Cushing syndrome with virilization. Am J Dis Child 1973;125:608–11.
7. Daneman A, Chan HS, Martin J. Adrenal carcinoma and adenoma in children: a review of 17 patients. Pediatr Radiol 1983;13:11–8.
8. Doerr HG, Sippell WG, Drop SL, Bidlingmaier F, Knorr D. Evidence of 11-β-hydroxylase deficiency in childhood adrenocortical tumors. The plasma corticosterone/11-deoxycorticosterone ratio as a possible marker for malignancy. Cancer 1987;60:1625–9.
9. Fraumeni JF Jr, Geiser CF, Manning MD. Wilms' tumor and congenital hemihypertrophy: report of five new cases and review of literature. Pediatrics 1967;40:886–99.
10. Fraumeni JF Jr, Miller RW. Adrenocortical neoplasms with hemihypertrophy, brain tumors and other disorders. J Pediatr 1967;70:129–38.
11. Fraumeni JF Jr, Miller RW, Hill JA. Primary carcinoma of the liver in childhood: an epidemiologic study. JNCI 1968;40:1087–99.
12. Gabrilove JL, Sharma DC, Wotiz HH, Dorfman RI. Feminizing adrenocortical tumors in the male. A review of 52 cases including a case report. Medicine 1965;44:37–79.
13. Ganguly A, Bergstein J, Grim CE, Yum MN, Weinberger MH. Childhood primary aldosteronism due to an adrenal adenoma: preoperative localization by adrenal vein catheterization. Pediatrics 1980;65:605–9.
14. Gershanik JJ, Elmore M, Levkoff AH. Congenital concurrence of adrenal cortical tumor, ganglioneuroma and toxoplasmosis. Pediatrics 1973;51:705–9.
15. Gilbert MG, Cleveland WW. Cushing's syndrome in infancy. Pediatrics 1970;46:217–29.
16. Godine LB, Berdon WE, Brasch RC, Leonidas JC. Adrenocortical carcinoma with extension into inferior vena cava and right atrium: report of 3 cases in children. Pediatr Radiol 1990;20:166–8.
17. Halmi KA, Lascari AD. Conversion of virilization to feminization in a young girl with adrenal cortical carcinoma. Cancer 1971;27:931–5.

18. Hamwi GJ, Serbin RA, Kruger FA. Does adrenocortical

37. Neblett WW, Frexes-Steed M, Scott HW Jr. Experience

Tumors of the Adrenal Gland and Extra-Adrenal Paraganglia

Figure 7-2
DISSEMINATED HISTOPLASMOSIS
Transverse section of an enlarged adrenal gland from a patient with disseminated histoplasmosis. The gland is expanded by broad zones of caseous necrosis. (Courtesy of Dr. Daniel H. Connor, Washington, DC.)

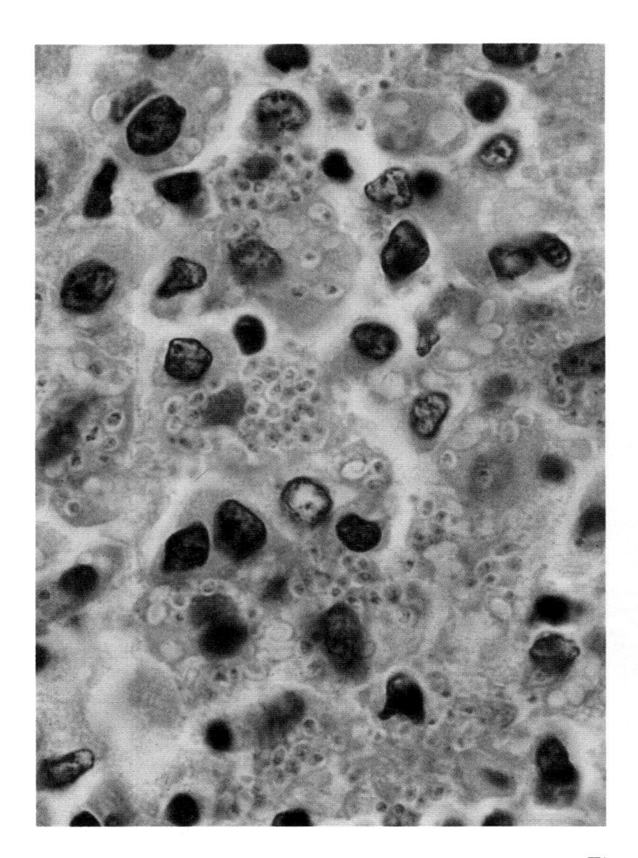

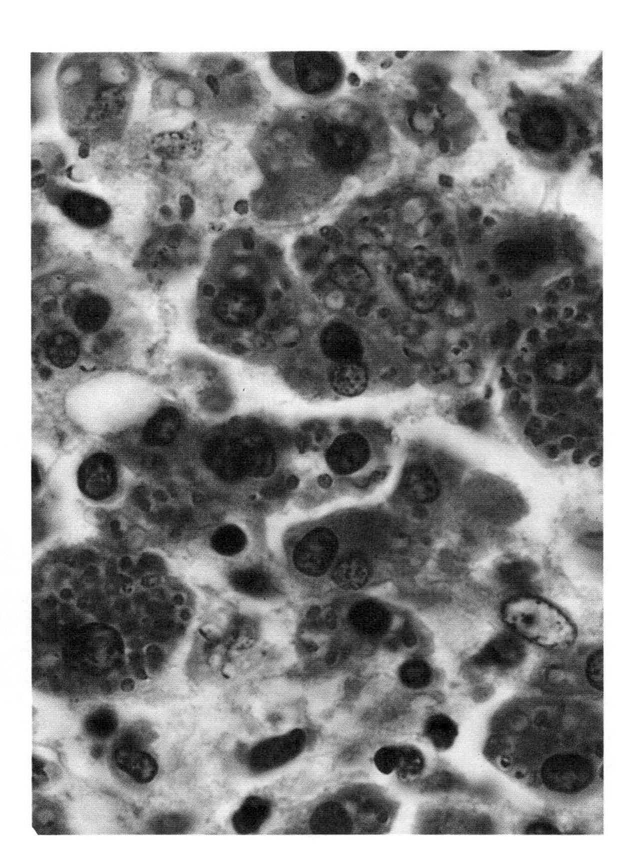

Figure 7-3
ADRENAL HISTOPLASMOSIS
Left: Numerous organisms typical for *Histoplasma capsulatum* distend the cytoplasm of histiocytes within sinusoids of adrenal cortex.
Right: Intracytoplasmic organisms are better delineated with PAS stain. (X1,000, Periodic acid–Schiff stain)

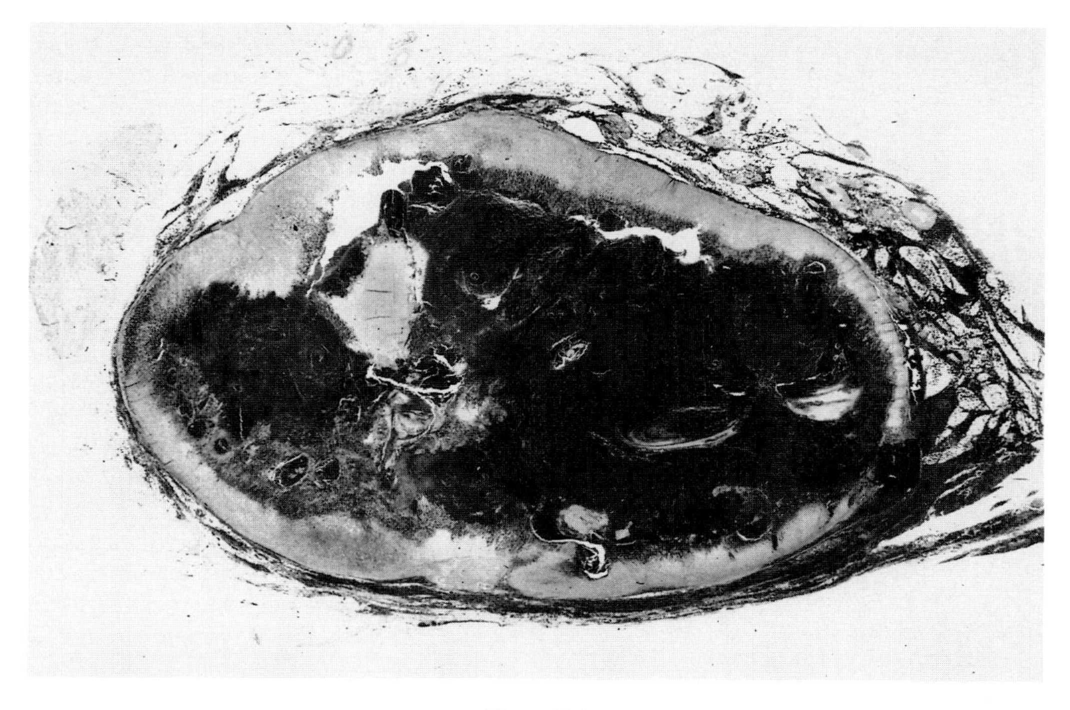

Figure 7-4
WATERHOUSE-FRIDERICHSEN SYNDROME IN AN ADULT PATIENT
Adrenal gland shows extensive necrosis and hemorrhage, with hematoma formation and extension into periadrenal adipose tissue.

by bacteria, usually *Escherichia coli,* followed by Group B *Streptococcus* and *Bacteroides,* is attributable to hematogenous dissemination. Malakoplakia of the adrenal gland has also been reported in association with *E. coli* infection (2).

ADRENAL ENLARGEMENT DUE TO HEMORRHAGE AND HEMATOMA FORMATION

Adrenal hemorrhage in adults can present antemortem as unilateral or bilateral adrenal enlargement. It is associated with a wide variety of factors including mechanical trauma, sepsis with (fig. 7-4) or without Waterhouse-Friderichsen syndrome, coagulopathies, steroid or adrenocorticotrophic hormone (ACTH) administration, primary or metastatic tumors, adrenal vein thrombosis, and as a complication of adrenal venography (10). Adrenal enlargement due to hemorrhage may be detected on abdominal imaging studies such as CT scan. Acute adrenal hemorrhage appears as a hyperintense mass with "streaky infiltration" of periadrenal tissues; older lesions appear as a nonspecific mass. On MRI, subacute hemorrhage has a high signal intensity in most cases on both T1- and T2-weighted images. This imaging modality may be useful in estimating the age of the hematoma. Only rarely is an adrenal hematoma removed as a surgical specimen simulating a nonfunctional adrenal tumor (8). Over time the adrenal hematoma may shrink or even resolve, with dystrophic calcification and possibly cyst formation (10). Neonatal adrenal hemorrhage has been associated with complicated delivery or asphyxia, and is most often confined to the right adrenal gland (fig. 7-5). It can be confused, radiographically, with neuroblastoma complicated by hemorrhage (fig. 7-6) (7).

Adrenal hemorrhage can be focal or diffuse, range in size from only a few millimeters to 15 cm, and involve up to 2 L of blood (11). There is fresh or clotted blood in various stages of organization, and the adjacent adrenal cortex or medulla may be necrotic. Adrenal hemorrhage can be complicated by adrenal insufficiency, secondary infection with abscess formation, or retroperitoneal

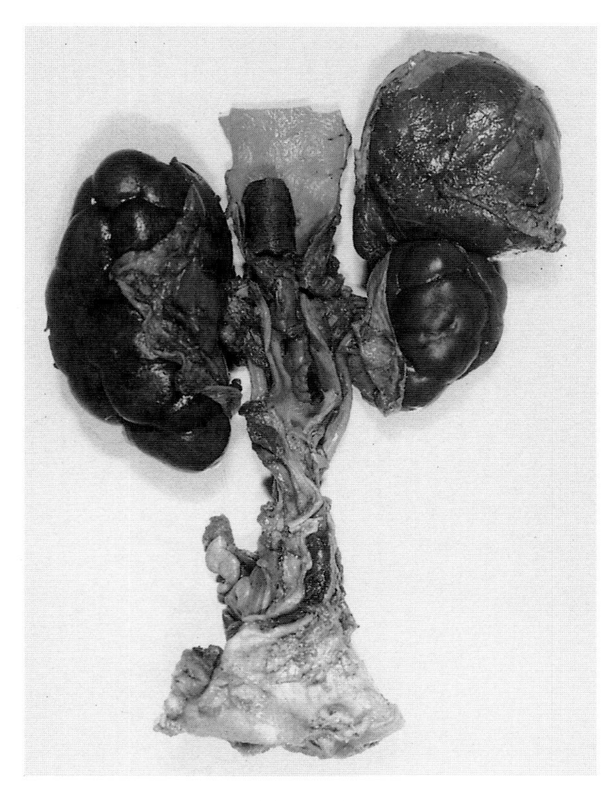

Figure 7-5
RIGHT ADRENAL HEMORRHAGE
Right adrenal hemorrhage and large hematoma formation complicate extensive thromboemboli in the aorta in a 3-week-old infant. The child had a ductus arteriosus aneurysm and probably multiple emboli.

hemorrhage; it may be life-threatening in some patients who have associated sepsis, malignancy, history of anticoagulant or steroid treatment, or major surgery (6). The peculiar susceptibility of the adrenal gland to massive hemorrhage has been attributed to its vascular supply and preeminent role in physiologic response to stress; likened to a "vascular dam," any rise in adrenal venous pressure (e.g., vasoconstriction during shock) can lead to hemorrhage into the gland (9).

ADRENAL CYSTS

Adrenal cysts are rare tumefactive lesions which can occur at any age, but are more commonly seen in the fifth and sixth decades of life (12,23). Less than 5 percent of adrenal cysts occur in children, and these lesions are rare in the neonatal period (13,20). In the review by Abeshouse (12), there was a three-fold greater incidence in female patients. The adrenal cyst is most often unilateral; only 5 to 8 percent are bilateral (12,15). It was detected at autopsy in 45 percent of cases and during surgery in 55 percent in one review (15). In another series of 13,996 cases, the frequency of adrenal cysts at autopsy was 0.06 percent; three were considered to arise from adrenal adenoma (24). Signs and symptoms when present are usually vague and nonspecific, and include dull flank pain, various gastrointestinal complaints such as epigastric distress or indigestion, and a palpable abdominal mass (23). Occasionally, there may be constitutional symptoms such as malaise and weakness. Fever with leukocytosis is rare. Intracystic hemorrhage can result in anemia and a slowly growing abdominal mass (12). Rarely, an adrenal cyst can mimic metastatic disease.

Adrenal cysts have been classified into four major types (12,15): 1) *parasitic cysts* (7 percent), which are usually ecchinococcal and discovered incidentally at autopsy; 2) *epithelial cysts* (9 percent), which are divided into true glandular or retention cysts, embryonal cysts, and cystic adrenal tumors such as cystic pheochromocytoma (19); 3) *endothelial cysts* (45 percent), usually lymphangiomatous, but occasionally angiomatous; and 4) *adrenal "pseudocysts"* (39 percent), which are the most common clinically recognized type of adrenal cyst encountered during surgery. The adrenal pseudocyst may be a heterogenous subtype as well since some have an apparent vascular origin (21), which has been supported immunohistochemically by positive staining for endothelial markers (16,18). A mesothelial origin has recently been reported for an adrenal cyst (22) with pathogenesis analogous to the proposed origin of some splenic cysts (14).

The adrenal pseudocyst is discovered with increased frequency due to improved imaging procedures. The characteristics of the cyst on CT scan provide valuable information (fig. 7-7): they are usually well-defined with near water density; the cyst wall has areas of calcification or is enhanced following contrast administration, and there are often internal septations. It may be difficult to distinguish a low-density adrenal cortical adenoma from a cyst. On MRI, adrenal cysts usually have a low signal intensity on T1-weighted images and have a high signal intensity on T2-weighted images with enhancement

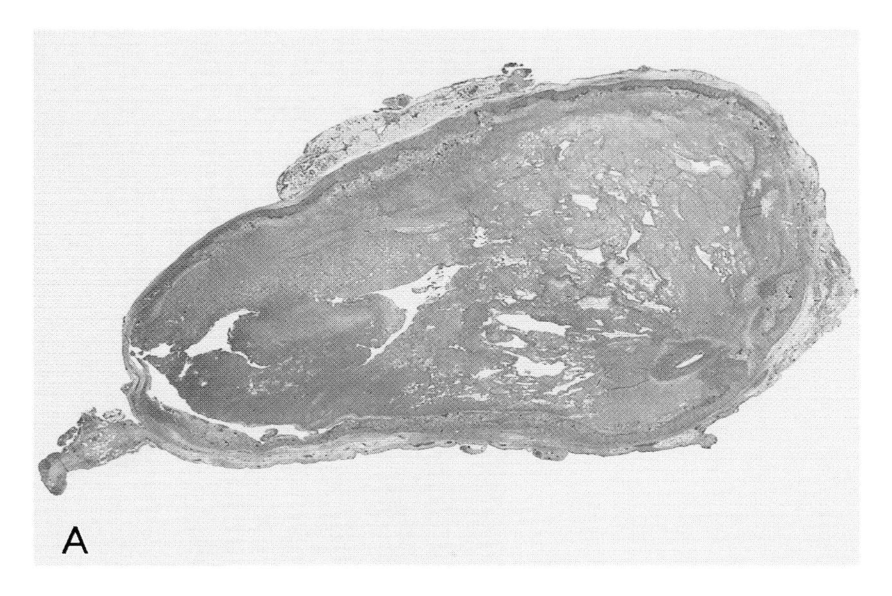

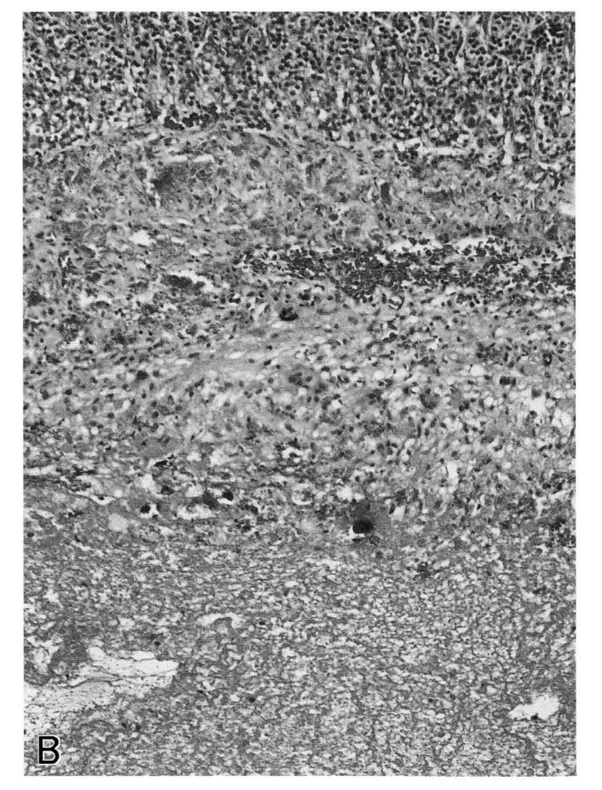

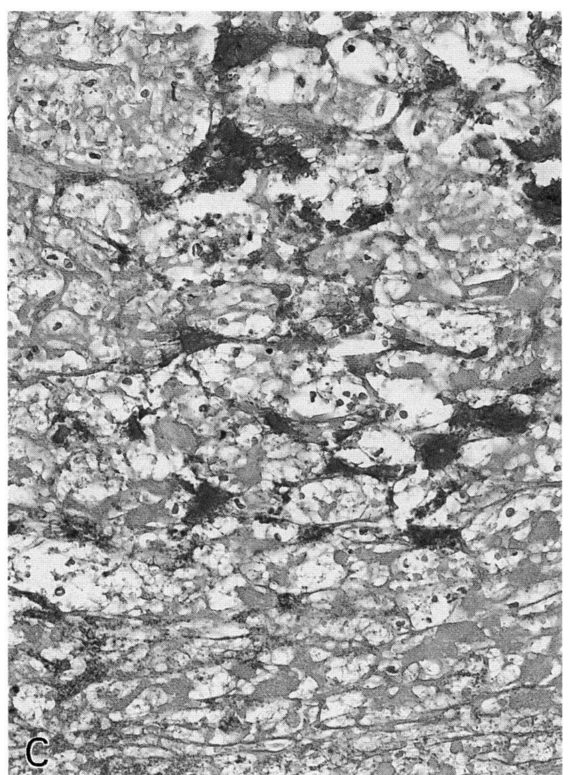

Figure 7-6
RIGHT ADRENAL HEMORRHAGE

A: Right adrenal hemorrhage and necrosis in a newborn with nonspecific abdominal symptoms. Abdominal roentgenogram showed a mass effect and ultrasound revealed an adrenal mass which did not decrease in size on repeat study. There also was an elevated serum ferritin level which heightened suspicion for a neuroblastoma. Adrenalectomy was performed.

B: Adrenal hemorrhage and necrosis affects mainly fetal or provisional cortex. The fetal zone is largely necrotic and replaced by amorphous matter.

C: Dystrophic calcification is seen in the outer aspect of necrotic fetal cortex. Hemosiderin deposition was also present and indicated old hemorrhage.

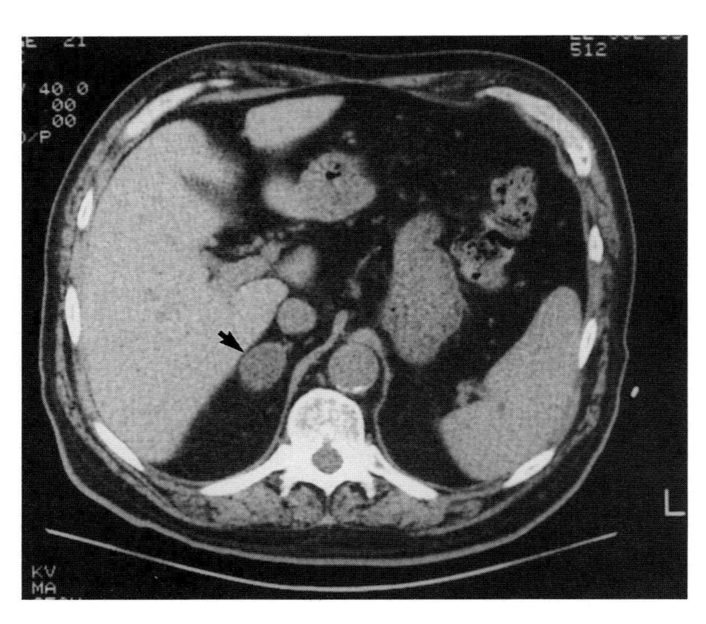

Figure 7-7
RIGHT ADRENAL CYST
A 2.5-cm right adrenal cyst (arrow) was discovered incidentally on abdominal CT scan in a 66-year-old man who was evaluated for abdominal pain. The cyst appears isodense and fine-needle aspiration yielded only amber liquid. (Courtesy of Dr. Calvin Neithamer, Alexandria, VA.)

characteristics similar to those on CT scan. As with MRI scans in general, small areas of calcification are usually not detected. The median cyst size in a recent study was 6 cm (range, 1.8 to 10 cm) (21), but there are reports in which the cyst filled most of the abdomen, reaching a size of 33 cm, weighing 20.5 kg, and containing about 12 L of mahogany brown fluid (15). The major finding on roentgenogram of the abdomen is peripheral curvilinear calcification (fig. 7-8). Grossly, the adrenal pseudocyst is unilocular, has a wall usually 1 to 5 mm thick, and is filled with yellow-brown or bloody amorphous material. The lining is smooth or shaggy (fig. 7-8C), and may contain elevated nodules or plaques. The dense, fibrous connective tissue capsule may be hyalinized with spotty areas of calcification, and on close inspection mottled, yellow areas representing residual adrenal cortex may be seen. The cyst lining may have a partially organized, fibrinoid appearance without any apparent cellular lining when observed by routine light microscopy (fig. 7-9). In some cases, a flat to cuboidal endothelial cell lining may be focally identified (23). Some have reported smooth muscle in the wall continuous with the smooth muscle of the adrenal vein (21). Unusual variants of adrenal pseudocysts have been reported with intracystic fat, myelolipomatous metaplasia (17), and even a rare example of mammary carcinoma manifesting as an intracystic metastasis (16,17).

MYELOLIPOMA

Adrenal myelolipoma is a benign tumor-like lesion composed of mature adipose tissue admixed with hematopoietic elements of various proportions (46). While most of these lesions arise in the adrenal glands, extra-adrenal myelolipomas have been reported, usually in the presacral area of the retroperitoneum (32,36,38,39), but also in unusual sites such as perirenal (27), mediastinum, liver (40), stomach, leptomeninges, and lung (38). Myelolipoma has also been reported in a heterotopic adrenal gland (30). The age range of patients with adrenal myelolipoma from a study by Plaut (42) is 17 to 93 years, and the average age at diagnosis is about 50 years (32). It is rare in individuals under 30 years of age. Almost all adrenal myelolipomas are unilateral and solitary with equal distribution on either side; only rarely is the lesion bilateral (32). There is a roughly equal sex distribution. The estimated incidence at autopsy varies from 0.08 to 0.2 percent (47); in one study it was 0.01 percent for the age group between 36 and 65 years of age (42). With the increasing use of sensitive imaging techniques such as CT scan (fig. 7-10), a larger number of asymptomatic patients with adrenal myelolipoma may be diagnosed during life. On CT scan myelolipomas are usually well-circumscribed, with a variable appearance depending upon the amount of fat present. The lesions may

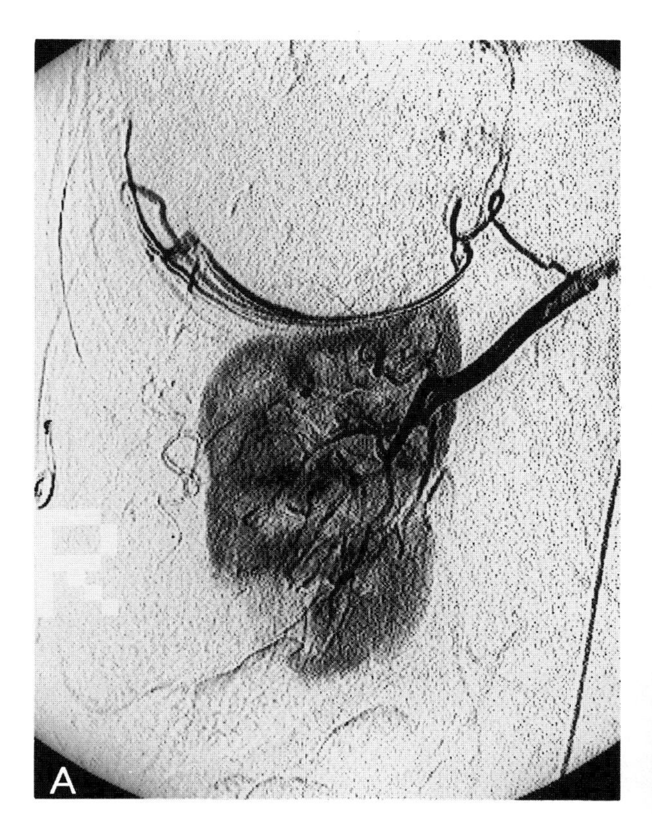

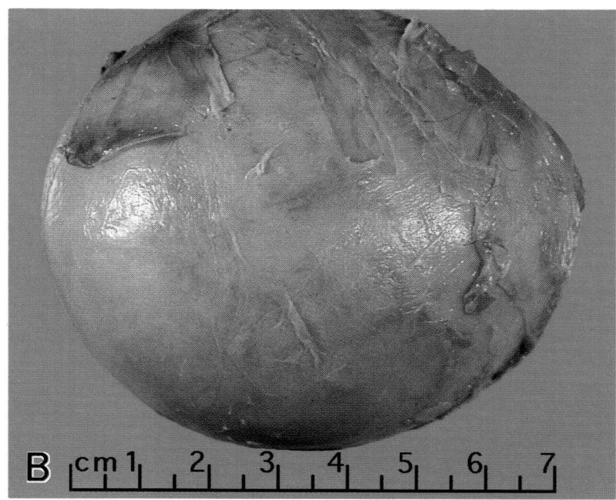

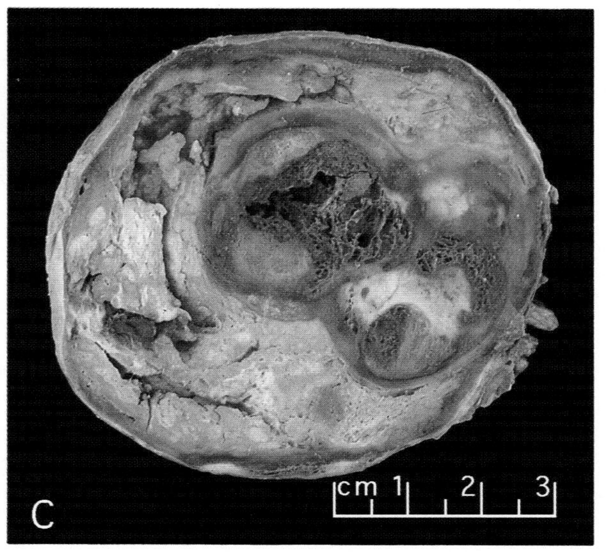

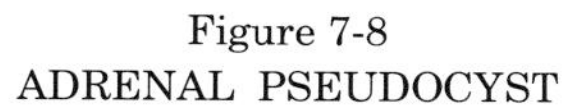

Figure 7-8
ADRENAL PSEUDOCYST

A: Adrenal pseudocyst in a 36-year-old woman. An early phase of selective arteriogram shows a large, suprarenal mass on the right side which had a faint peripheral rim of calcification. (Courtesy of Dr. Calvin Neithamer, Alexandria, VA.) (Figures A and C are from the same case.)

B: Adrenal pseudocyst measured 9 x 7 x 7 cm. The external surface had yellowish areas consistent with residual adrenal cortex.

C: The contents of this adrenal pseudocyst were creamy and curd-like. The cyst wall averaged about 0.2 cm in thickness and contained foci of calcification.

show internal enhancement or low attenuation due to fat content. Lesions with little or no adipose tissue may be difficult to distinguish from other adrenal tumors (similar to MRI). On MRI, myelolipomas tend to have an appearance based upon high fat signal on T1-weighted images, with heterogeneous enhancement following contrast (fig. 7-11).

Roughly half of the patients undergoing surgical resection of an adrenal myelolipoma are asymptomatic while others have a variety of complaints or findings such as abdominal or flank pain, hematuria, a palpable mass, and hypertension, or rarely, the patient presents with a near calamitous episode of retroperitoneal hemorrhage (46). Myelolipomas have been associated with a variety of endocrine disturbances including Cushing's syndrome (combined with an adrenal cortical adenoma) (47), pituitary-dependent Cushing's disease (25), Addison's disease, virilism, and pseudohermaphroditism (42). Adrenal myelolipomas have also been reported in association with congenital adrenal hyperplasia due to 21-hydroxylase (26) and 17-hydroxylase deficiency (29). There is

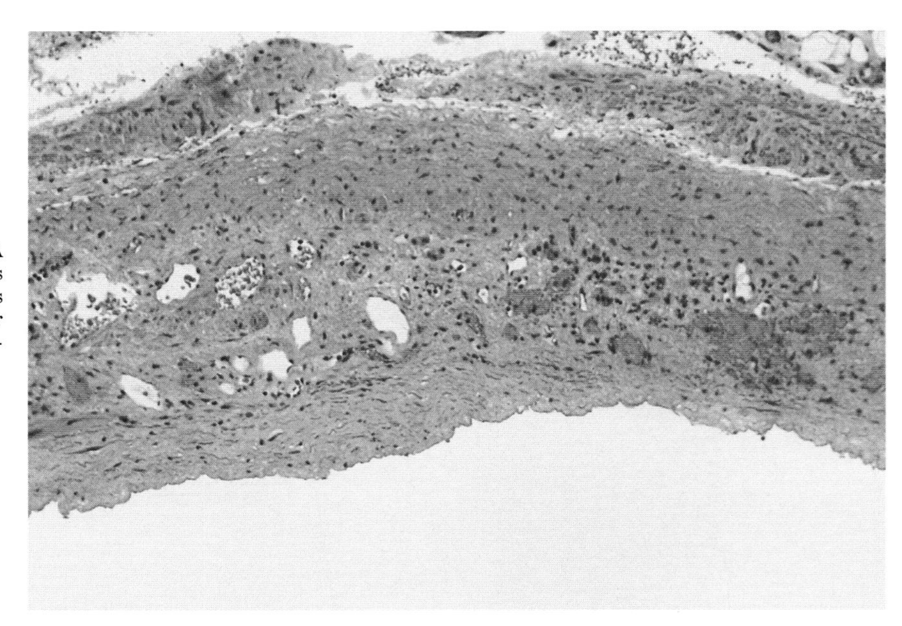

Figure 7-9
ADRENAL PSEUDOCYST

In the same case as figure 7-8A and C, the adrenal cortex at top has a thick, fibrous wall and amorphous contents. There was no epithelial or endothelial lining identified. Cholesterol clefts were also seen.

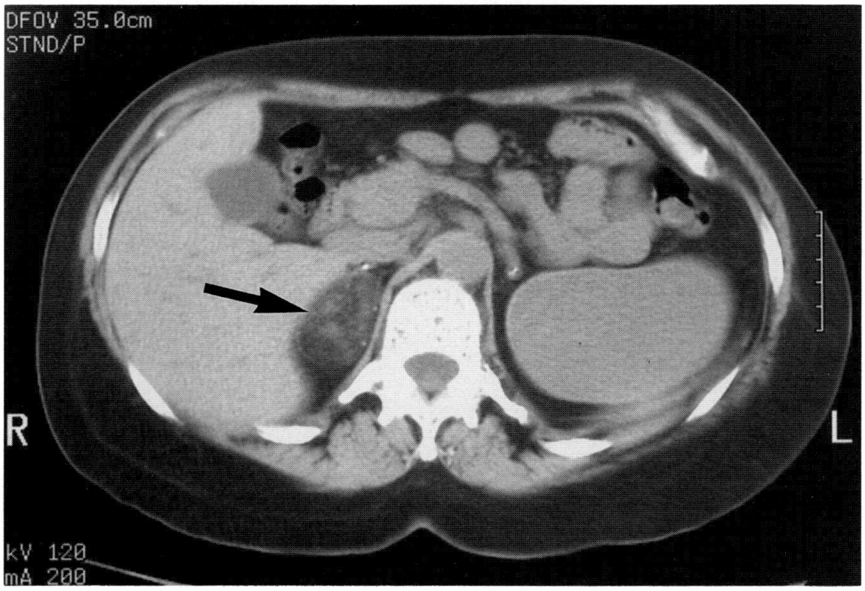

Figure 7-10
ADRENAL MYELOLIPOMA

A 53-year-old female had a right adrenal mass on CT scan (arrow). The lesion is well-circumscribed with areas of low attenuation suggesting a fatty component. Fine-needle aspiration yielded material diagnostic of myelolipoma.

no relationship to anemia or other disturbance of the hematopoietic system (42). Some studies indicate a higher incidence in obese patients (41). Adrenal myelolipomas are occasionally associated with hypertension, and rarely, may simulate a pheochromocytoma (28,43). A case of alimentary tract ganglioneuromatosis-lipomatosis, adrenal myelolipomas, pancreatic telangiectasia, and multinodular goiter has been reported as a possible neuroendocrine syndrome (37). An adrenal myelolipoma has also been reported in association with Castleman's disease (45).

Adrenal myelolipomas vary considerably in size, ranging from the small lesion discovered incidentally at autopsy (fig. 7-12) to an immense mass measuring up to 34 cm and weighing 5,900 g (26). The lesion is well circumscribed on gross inspection, but is rarely encapsulated. The color varies from pale yellow to deep red or red-brown depending upon the relative proportions of

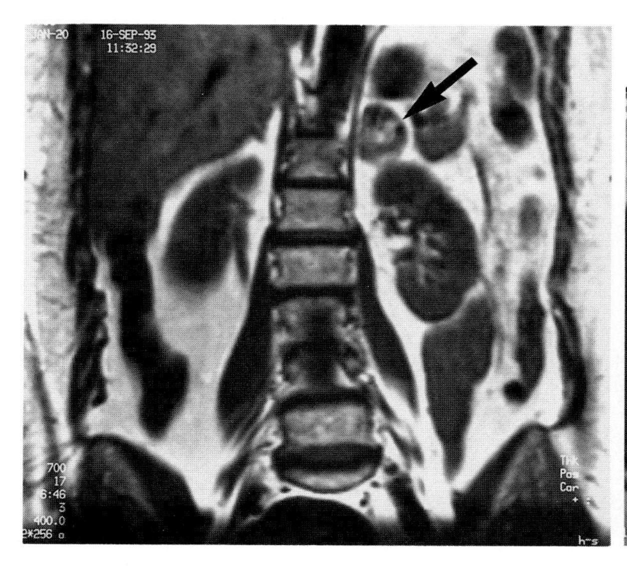

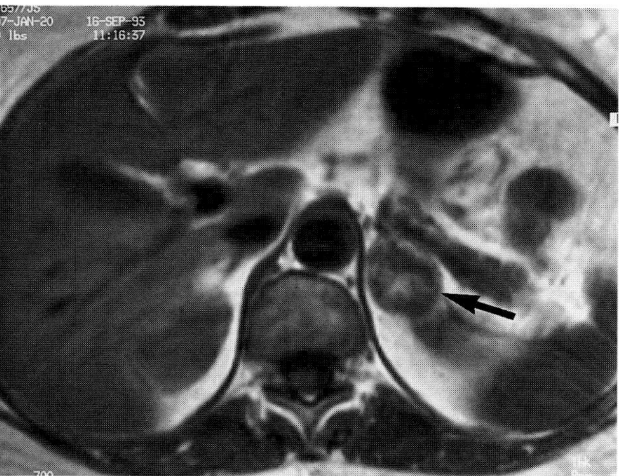

Figure 7-11

LEFT ADRENAL MYELOLIPOMA IN A 73-YEAR-OLD FEMALE

Left: Adrenal myelolipoma in coronal plane (arrow). The T-1 weighted image on MRI shows a high central signal from a fatty component.

Right: Adrenal myelolipoma in transverse plane (arrow). High central signal is due to the fatty component. T-1 weighted "fat saturation" image showed selective nulling of the fat signal, proving the fatty content of tumor. (Courtesy of Dr. Richard Patt, Washington, DC.)

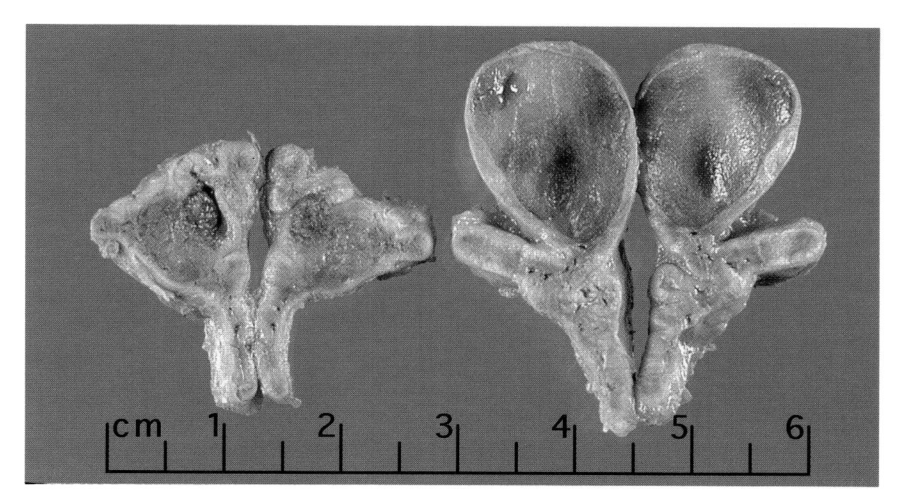

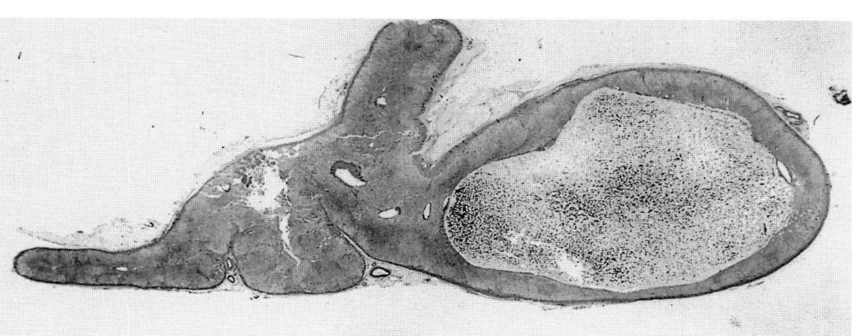

Figure 7-12

INCIDENTAL ADRENAL MYELOLIPOMA

Top: This incidental adrenal myelolipoma was discovered at autopsy.

Bottom: Whole mount section of an incidental myelolipoma discovered at autopsy of an adult patient. One wing or ala of the gland is expanded by myelolipoma. (Fig. 10-12 from Travis WD, Oertel JE, Lack EE. Miscellaneous tumors and tumefactive lesions of the adrenal gland. In: Lack EE, ed. Pathology of the adrenal glands. New York: Churchill Livingstone, 1990:351–78.)

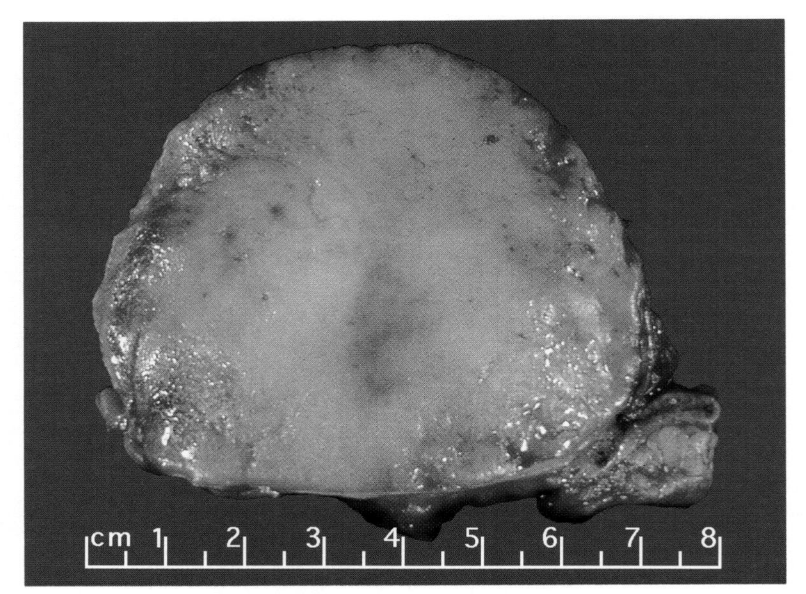

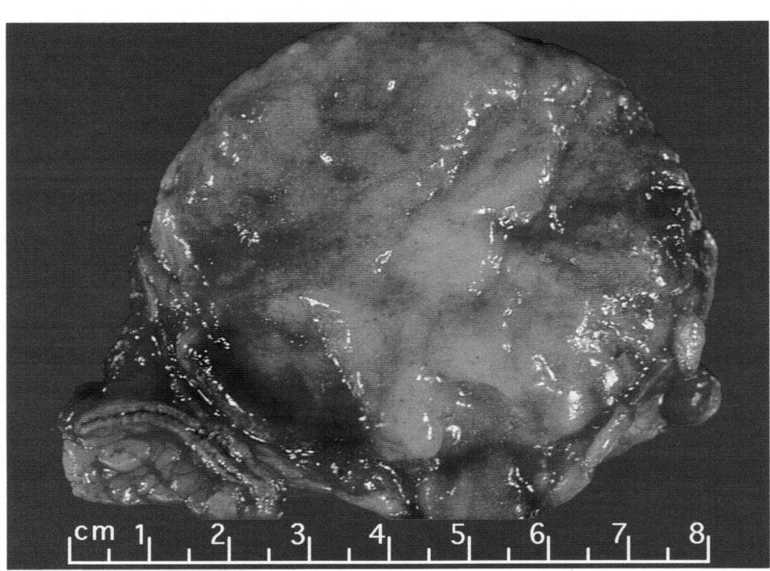

Figure 7-13
ADRENAL MYELOLIPOMA

Top: Cross section of adrenal myelolipoma shows a yellow, fatty tumor.

Bottom: Different section of the same adrenal myelolipoma showing darker zones representing concentrated areas of hematopoietic tissue.

fat and hematopoietic elements (fig. 7-13). The contour of the adrenal myelolipoma is smooth, wavy, or irregular and may show intermingling of cortical cells with elements of the myelolipoma. The surrounding cortical cells can be relatively normal in appearance (fig. 7-14A) or compressed. There is a variable mixture of mature fat with hematopoietic elements, often with full representation of the major cell lines (fig. 7-14B). Occasionally, infarction or hemorrhage occurs with secondary hematoma formation or fibrosis (46). Rarely, foci of ossification are seen (fig. 7-14C and D). The diagnosis can sometimes be established by fine-needle aspiration cytology in conjunction with a typical appearance on imaging studies (fig. 7-15) (31,35).

The etiology of myelolipoma is obscure. Foci of lipomatous and myelolipomatous metaplasia can be found in a variety of adrenal cortical disorders, many characterized by cortical hyperfunction such as adrenal cortical hyperplasia and neoplasia. A number of theories have been proposed for the origin of fat and hematopoietic cells in the adrenal gland: 1) bone marrow embolization by the

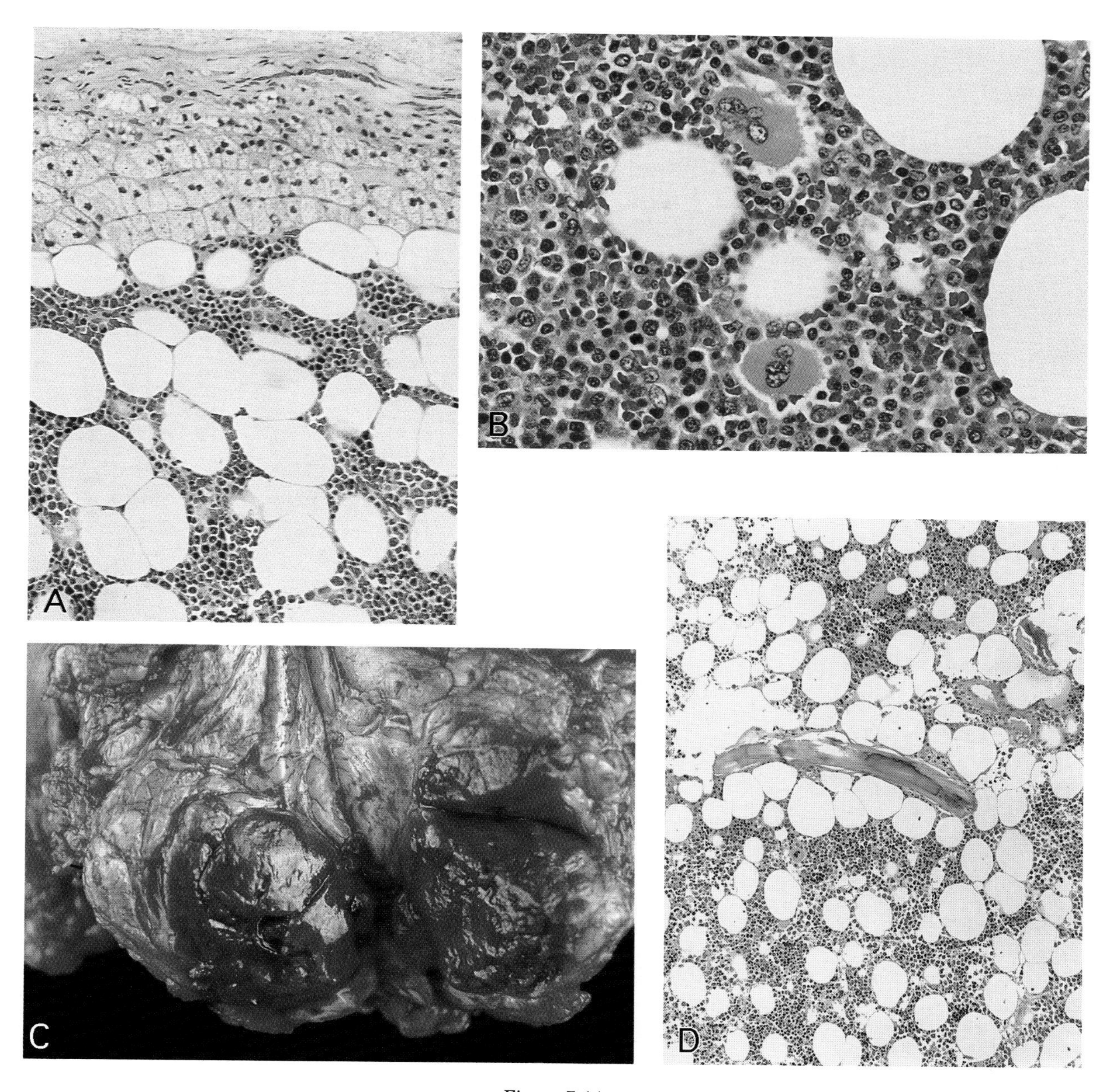

Figure 7-14
ADRENAL MYELOLIPOMA

A: The adrenal capsule (top of field) has an underlying rim of swollen, lipid-rich cortical cells.

B: In this juxta-adrenal myelolipoma, trilinear hematopoietic elements are evident with predominance of myeloid cells along with a few clusters of erythroid cells and occasional megakaryocytes.

C: This extra-adrenal myelolipoma arose in the retroperitoneum adjacent to, but separate from, the adrenal gland.

D: Histologic section of same myelolipoma as C shows foci of bony trabeculae.

hematogous route; 2) intra-adrenal embryonic rests of bone marrow; 3) metaplasia of adrenal cortical cells; and 4) metaplasia of uncommitted or pluripotential adrenal stromal cells (33,46). Lipomatous and myeloid transformation has been induced experimentally in the rat by administration of methyltestosterone and crude pituitary extracts rich in ACTH (44).

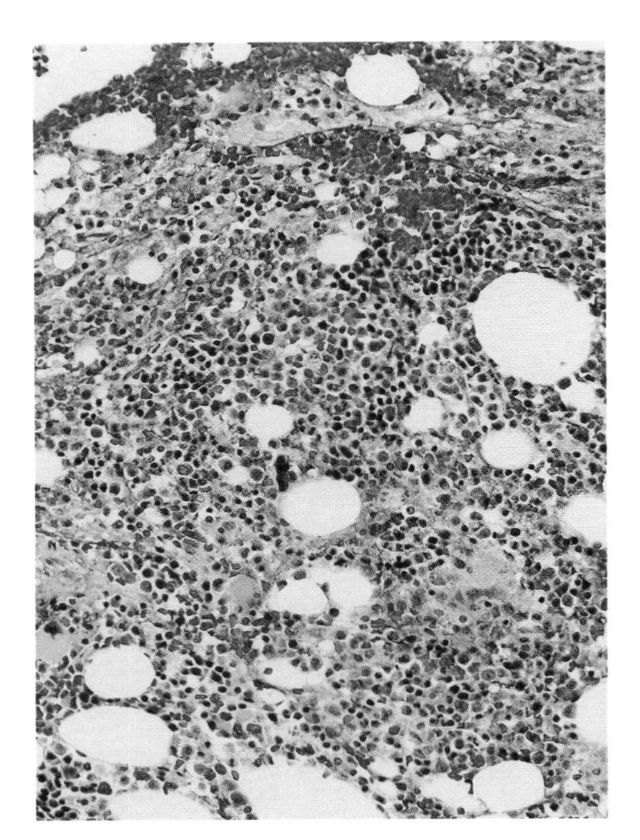
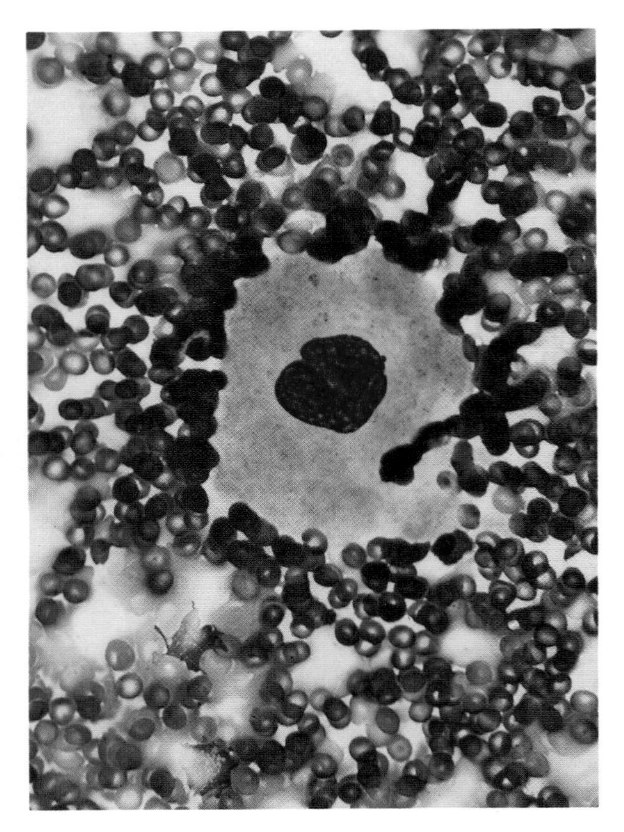

Figure 7-15
ADRENAL MYELOLIPOMA
Left: Fine-needle aspiration of lesion shown in figure 7-10. Aspirate consisted of blood with a few small tissue fragments composed of hematopoietic elements and mature fat.
Right: An occasional megakaryocyte is present in the fine-needle aspirate of adrenal myelolipoma.

PRIMARY MALIGNANT MELANOMA

Primary malignant melanoma of the adrenal gland is extremely uncommon. Proposed diagnostic criteria include: presence of malignant melanoma in only one adrenal gland; no prior or current pigmented lesions of skin, mucosal surfaces, or eye; no history of removal of pigmented skin or eye lesions; and failure to detect an extra-adrenal primary by a thorough autopsy (48). A recent review of primary malignant melanoma of the adrenal gland identified six cases since 1946, and proposed an origin from pheochromocytes, hence these tumors are regarded as melanotic pheochromocytomas and not true melanocytic tumors (50). Melanin or melanin-like pigment has rarely been reported in pheochromocytomas (49,54), although it may be difficult to distinguish from neuromelanin, a pigment related to altered lipofuscin. Neuromelanin has also been detected in ganglioneuroblastomas (51,52,55) and ganglioneuromas (53). A distinguishing feature of melanocytic melanin pigment is the presence of typical melanosomes or premelanosomes on ultrastructural study.

The author has encountered only one case of malignant melanoma primary in the adrenal gland, in a patient who had no evidence of malignant melanoma in any other site following a rigorous investigation using a multidisiplinary approach (fig. 7-16). Grossly, the tumor is brown to black (fig. 7-17), but the degree of pigmentation varies and some tumors are amelanotic. There may be hemorrhage and focal necrosis. Grossly, the mass may look like another tumor, such as pheochromocytoma. The histology is typical for malignant melanoma arising in more conventional sites (fig. 7-18); confirmation includes

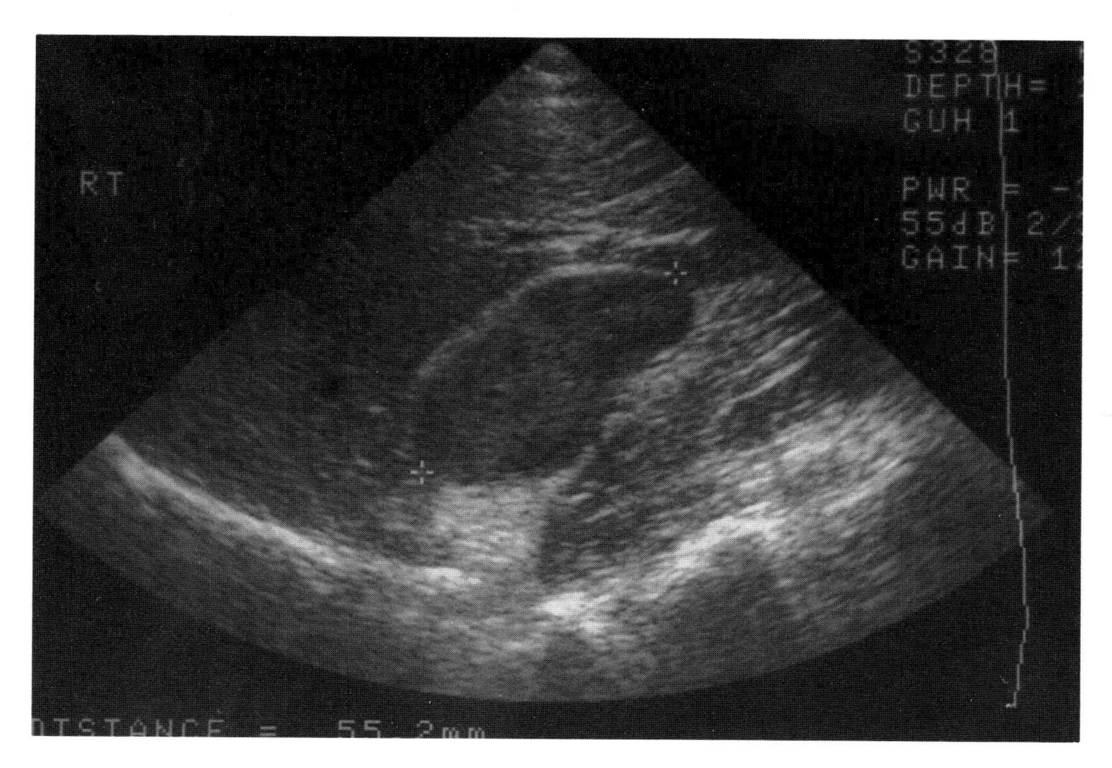

Figure 7-16
PRIMARY MALIGNANT MELANOMA OF ADRENAL GLAND

A 48-year-old female complained of abdominal pain and imaging studies of the upper abdomen revealed a right adrenal mass. Ultrasound showed an ovoid mass measuring about 5.5 cm in diameter. There was no history of a mucocutaneous pigmented "lesion," and intensive investigation failed to reveal a primary source. (Figures 7-16 through 7-19 are from the same case.)

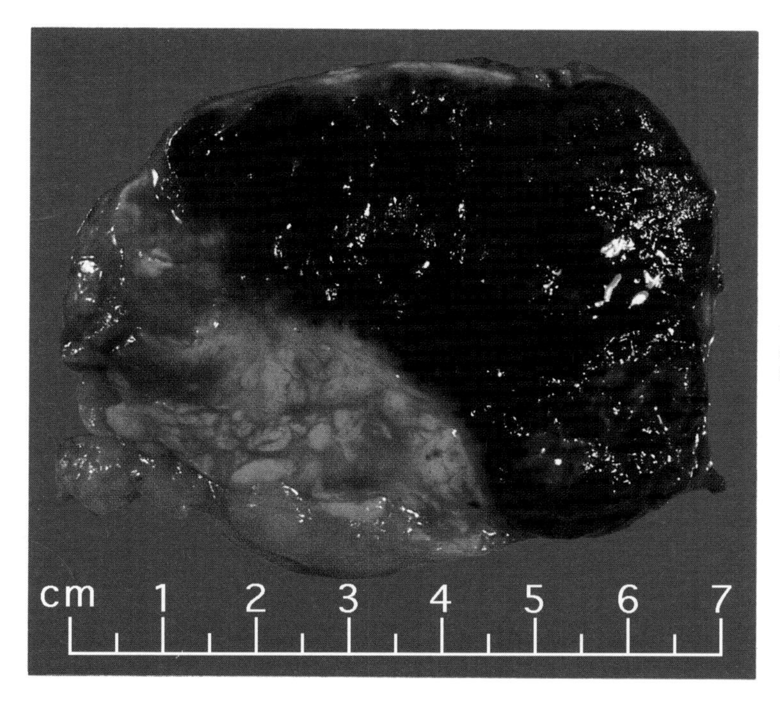

Figure 7-17
PRIMARY MALIGNANT MELANOMA OF ADRENAL GLAND

In cross section, much of the tumor is black, with coarse nodularity. Periadrenal adipose tissue is attached to the tumor. The tumor measured about 6 cm in diameter.

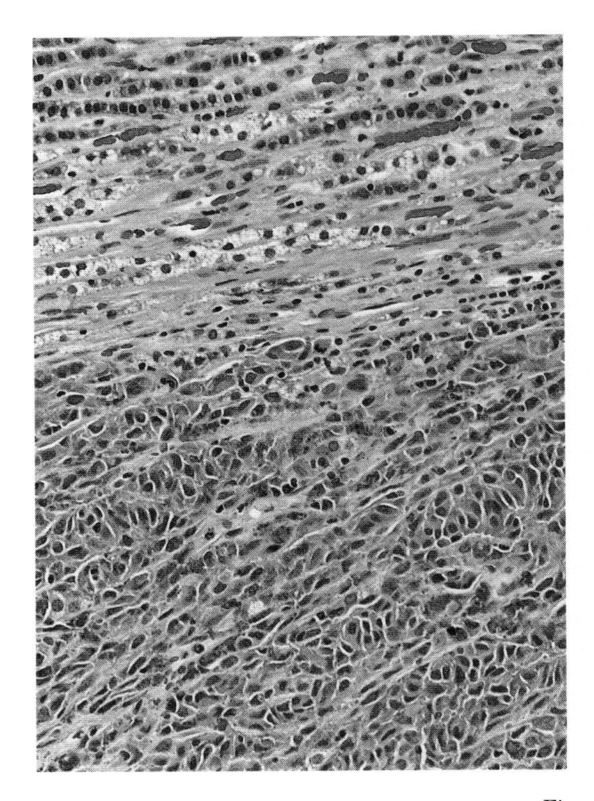

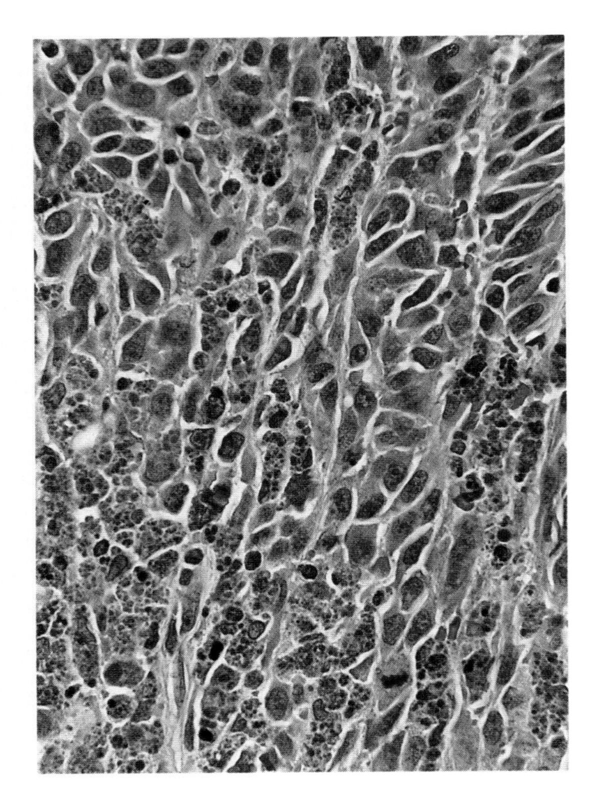

Figure 7-18
PRIMARY MALIGNANT MELANOMA OF RIGHT ADRENAL GLAND
Left: Tumor compresses the residual cortex in top portion of field.
Right: Abundant melanin pigment and pleomorphic cells with prominent nucleoli are shown.

immunohistochemical staining for S-100 protein and HMB-45, and ultrastructural presence of premelanosomes or melanosomes. Primary malignant melanoma of the adrenal gland may have diagnostic features on fine-needle aspiration (fig. 7-19). Other "pigmented" adrenal lesions, such as adrenal hematoma with hemosiderin-laden macrophages, pigmented (black) adenomas, and even pigmented pheochromocytomas are part of the differential diagnosis. Primary malignant melanoma of the adrenal gland is highly malignant and usually fatal within 2 years of diagnosis (50).

PRIMARY MALIGNANT LYMPHOMA

Malignant lymphoma has been reported on rare occasion to be primary in the adrenal gland (56–58), but adrenal involvement almost always occurs with more widespread disease. This is covered further in chapter 8.

PRIMARY MESENCHYMAL TUMORS

Vascular Neoplasms

Hemangioma. Hemangiomas of the adrenal gland are extremely rare; most are discovered incidentally at autopsy (fig. 7-20). The files of the Armed Forces Institute of Pathology listed one adrenal angioma for every 10,000 autopsy protocols accessioned between 1943 and 1958 (frequency of 0.01 percent) (71). Very few adrenal hemangiomas have been detected during life as a surgical lesion (61,70,74), and only rarely do patients present with symptoms related to a mass effect by the adrenal tumor (68). The age range is the third to the eighth decades of life; in 11 surgically treated cases, 9 patients were females (61,70,74). The size of adrenal hemangioma discovered at autopsy is usually less than 2 cm while those removed surgically are usually much larger, measuring up to 22 cm in diameter. Most are

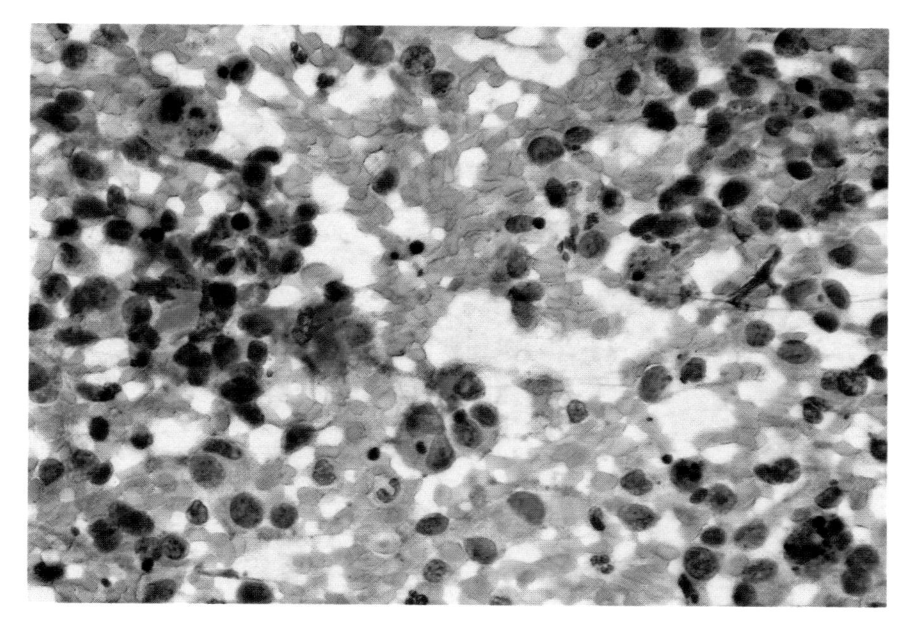

Figure 7-19
PRIMARY ADRENAL MALIGNANT MELANOMA IN FINE-NEEDLE ASPIRATION

Many tumor cells have partially disrupted cytoplasm. The abundant pigment is melanin. On ultrastructural study of a subsequent adrenalectomy specimen, typical melanosomes were present. (X400, Papanicolaou stain)

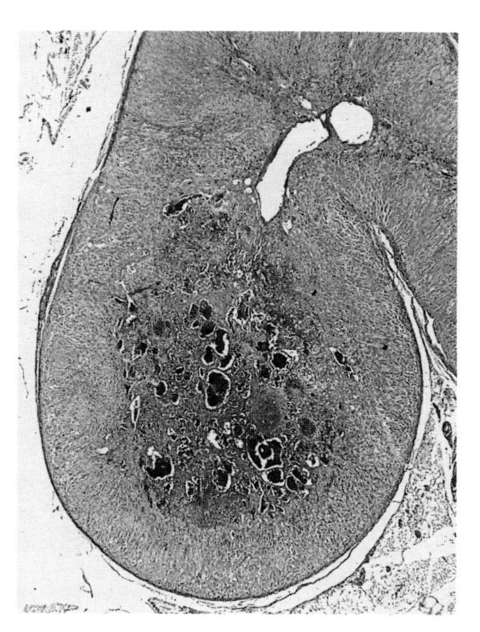

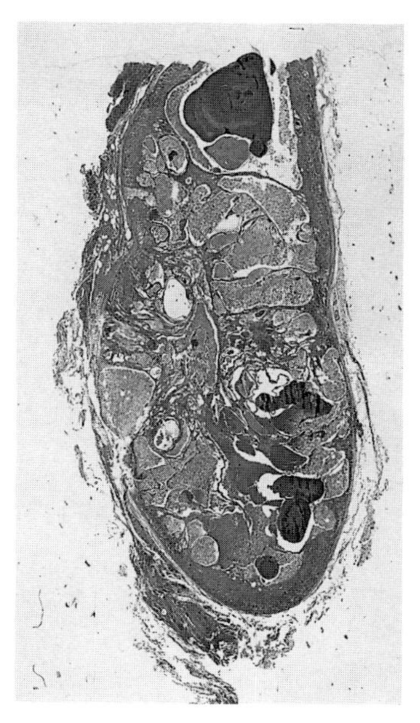

Figure 7-20
INCIDENTAL ADRENAL HEMANGIOMA

Left: Incidental adrenal hemangioma in a 50-year-old man who died of pulmonary tuberculosis. The lesion is composed of small to medium-sized vessels with some areas suggesting communication with tributaries of the central adrenal vein.

Right: Adrenal gland from a 19-year old male who died of a gunshot wound through the neck. The adrenal gland is expanded by a cavernous hemangioma. Most vascular spaces were filled with blood and a few contained phleboliths. (Fig. 1 from Plaut A. Hemangiomas and related lesions of the adrenal gland. Arch Pathol 1962;335:345–55.)

unilateral and solitary, but occasional bilateral hemangiomas have been reported (73). Although visceral hemangiomas and telangiectasias occur in the setting of hereditary hemorrhagic telangiectasia, involvement of the adrenal glands is rare (66). Most adrenal hemangiomas are of the cavernous type. The author has seen one case of multifocal juvenile hemangioma (benign hemangioendothelioma of infancy) in which the newborn infant had a large hepatic hemangioma as well as a much smaller adrenal tumor with identical histology (fig. 7-21); the child also had the Kasabach-Merritt syndrome and died of high output cardiac failure.

Lymphangioma. Lymphangioma of the adrenal gland has been reported, but is exceedingly rare. Two of the three cases reported by Plaut (72) would be best classified as adenomatoid tumor.

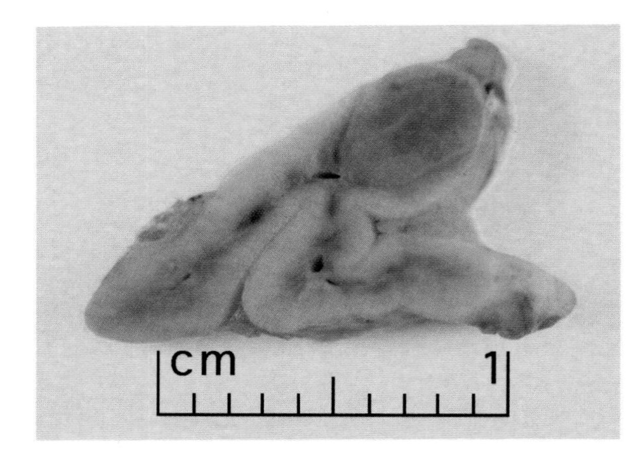

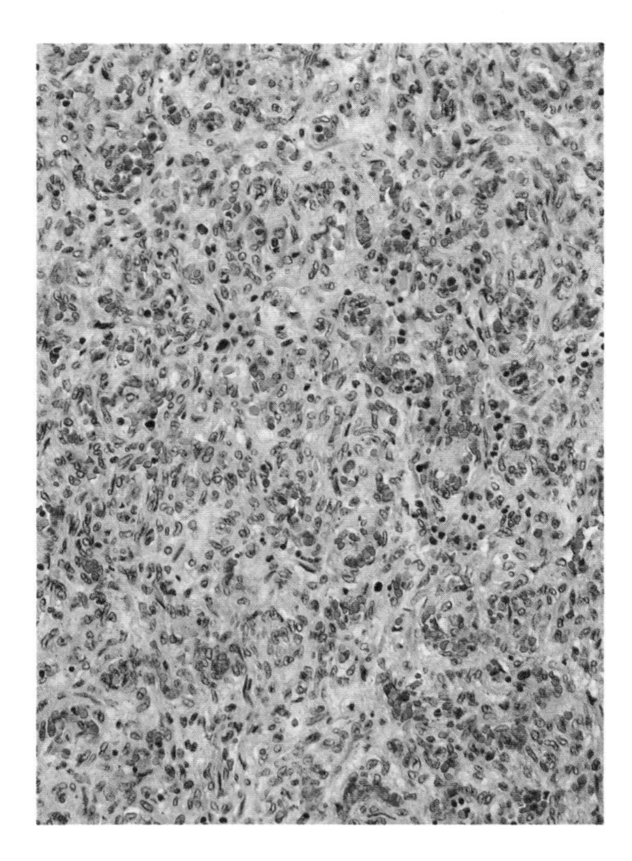

Figure 7-21
JUVENILE HEMANGIOMA OF ADRENAL GLAND

Gross and histologic appearance of a small juvenile hemangioma of adrenal gland in a newborn child. There were numerous cutaneous lesions and a large liver tumor of identical histology. The adrenal tumor is uniformly tan, 5 mm in diameter, and is present in the ridge or crista of the gland. The child also had the Kasabach-Merritt syndrome with thrombocytopenia.

Angiosarcoma. Angiosarcoma is another rare primary mesenchymal tumor of the adrenal gland (fig. 7-22). Over a dozen cases have been reported (59,60,63,65,67,75), one coexisting with an adrenal hemangioma (67). A case of an epithelioid angiosarcoma was reported in a 59-year-old male who worked as a vineyard cultivator, and the tumor in this case was presumed to be related to a long history of exposure to arsenicals (65). One case was reported in association with mesenteric fibromatosis (60). Adrenal angiosarcoma esually presents little difficulty in diagnosis when there is a clear vasoformative pattern (fig. 7-22B), but problems arise when the tumor has more of a solid epithelioid pattern, as seen focally in figure 7-22C. Recently, nine epithelioid angiosarcomas of the adrenal gland were reported by Wenig et al. (75). Endothelial differentiation was confirmed by immunohistochemistry (including factor-VIII–related antigen, CD-34, and *Ulex europaeus* lectin binding) and by ultrastructural features; immunoreactivity for cytokeratin was reported in seven of the cases. A recent adrenal angiosarcoma grossly resembled an adrenal pseudocyst (59), and a massive hemorrhagic adrenal cortical adenoma mimicked an angiosarcoma (62).

Smooth Muscle Neoplasms

Leiomyoma. Primary adrenal leiomyoma is a very rare tumor associated with the adrenal vein or its tributaries. It is often an incidental finding at autopsy (69). Histologically, adrenal leiomyoma has features identical to benign smooth muscle tumors occurring in other sites (fig. 7-23).

Leiomyosarcoma. Only a few cases of primary adrenal leiomyosarcoma have been reported (64) including a recent case in a man with acquired immunodeficiency syndrome (AIDS) (75a). The tumor most likely arises from smooth muscle associated with the central adrenal vein and its tributaries. Macroscopically, the tumor can have large areas of hemorrhage and necrosis (fig. 7-24). Microscopically, residual adrenal gland is seen, particularly in sections taken from the periphery of the tumor (fig. 7-25, left). The mitotic rate is high (fig. 7-25, right), and the tumor is quite cellular, similar to leiomyosarcomas in other sites. Electron microscopy or immunohistochemistry (fig. 7-26) can confirm the smooth muscle nature of the sarcoma.

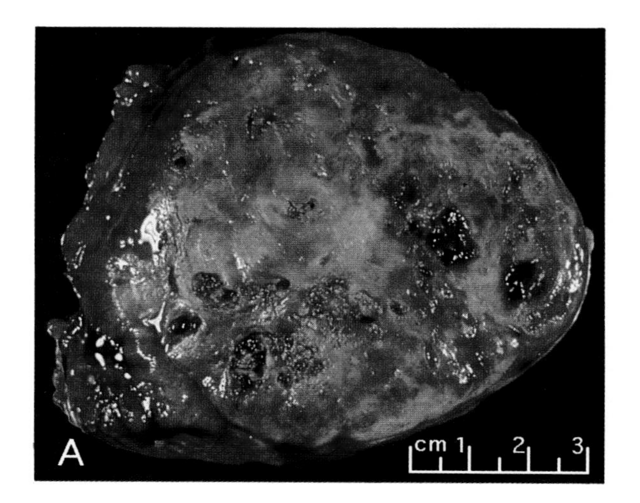

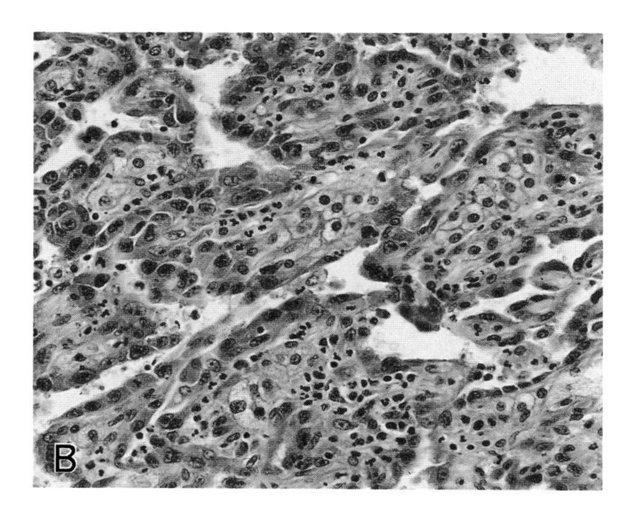

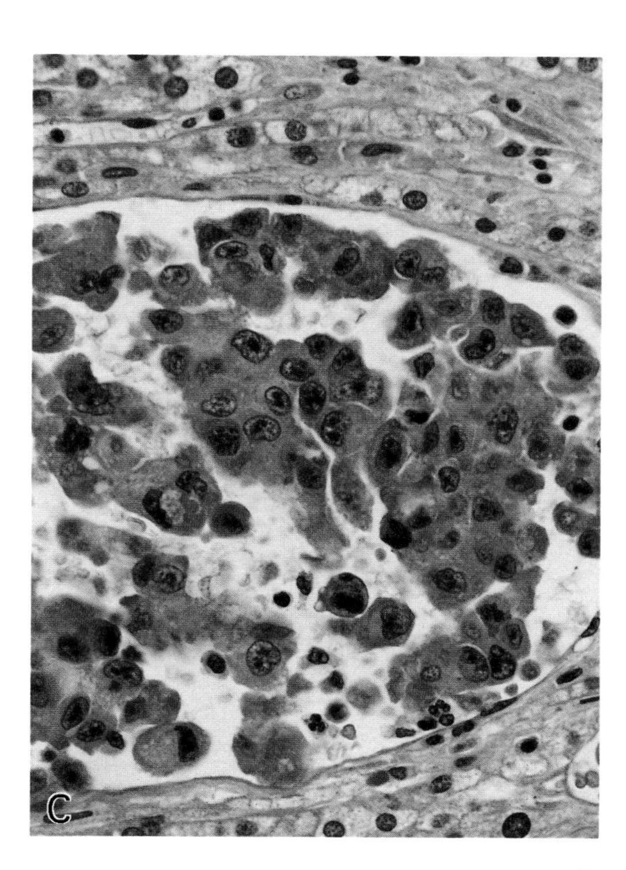

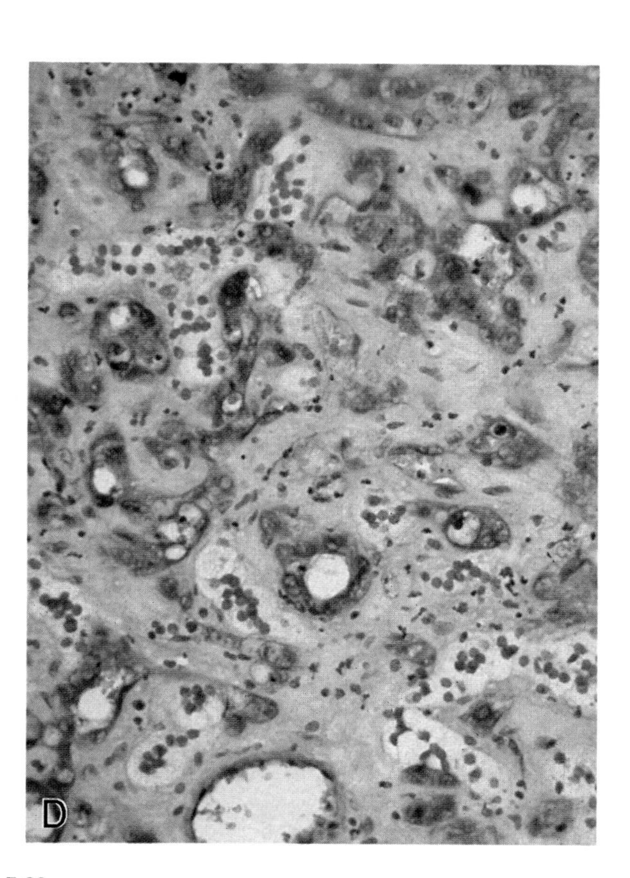

Figure 7-22

PRIMARY ADRENAL ANGIOSARCOMA

A: Tumor in cross section is markedly variegate and has areas of hemorrhage. The tumor was about 8 cm in diameter.

B: Primary adrenal angiosarcoma (different case than A). Note the well-developed vasoformative architecture with growth in sinusoids between cords of vacuolated cortical cells. Acute inflammation is also present.

C: Primary adrenal angiosarcoma (same case as B) seen growing in part as a high-grade tumor with epithelioid features. Residual adrenal cortical cells are seen.

D: Immunostain of primary adrenal angiosarcoma is markedly positive for factor VIII-related antigen. (X350, Peroxidase-antiperoxidase stain) (A and D courtesy of Dr. Sambasiva Rao, Chicago, IL.)

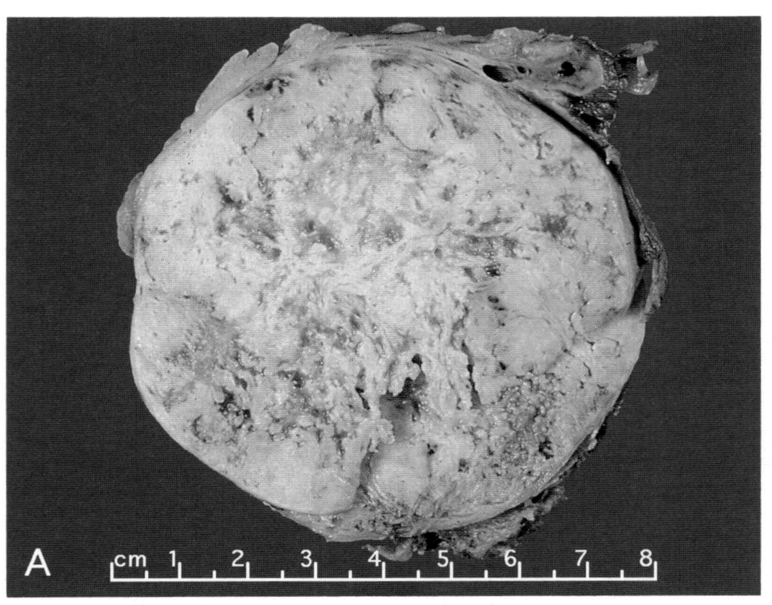

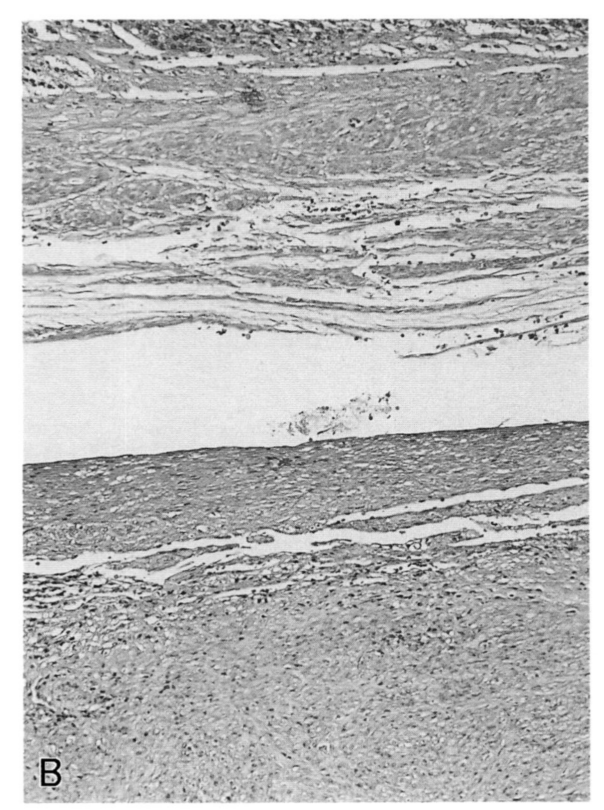

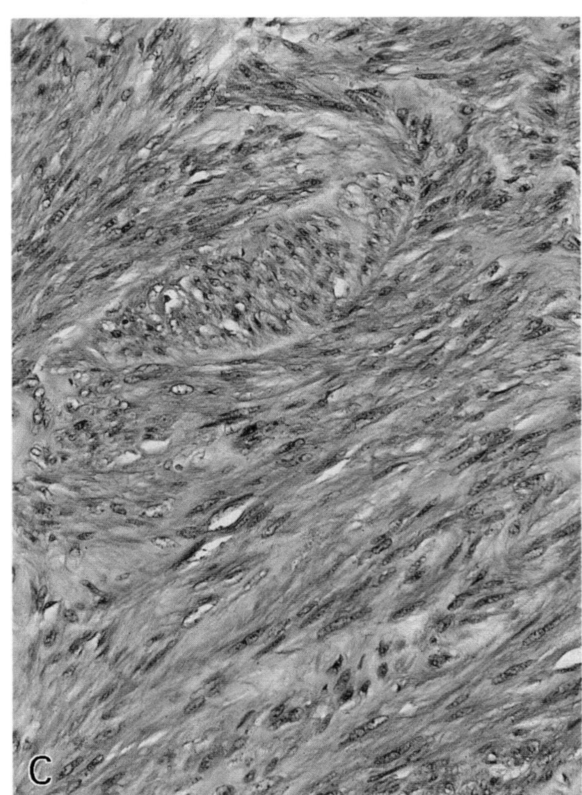

Figure 7-23
PRIMARY LEIOMYOMA OF ADRENAL GLAND

A: Surgical resection specimen of a primary leiomyoma of the adrenal gland. Tumor in cross section has a small portion of attached residual adrenal gland (right upper corner).

B: This primary adrenal leiomyoma was surgically excised. Residual adrenal cortex is present at top of field.

C: Tumor is composed of interlacing fascicles of spindle cells in various planes of section. No mitotic figures were identified and there was no necrosis. (Courtesy of Dr. Manuel Marcial, San Juan, Puerto Rico.)

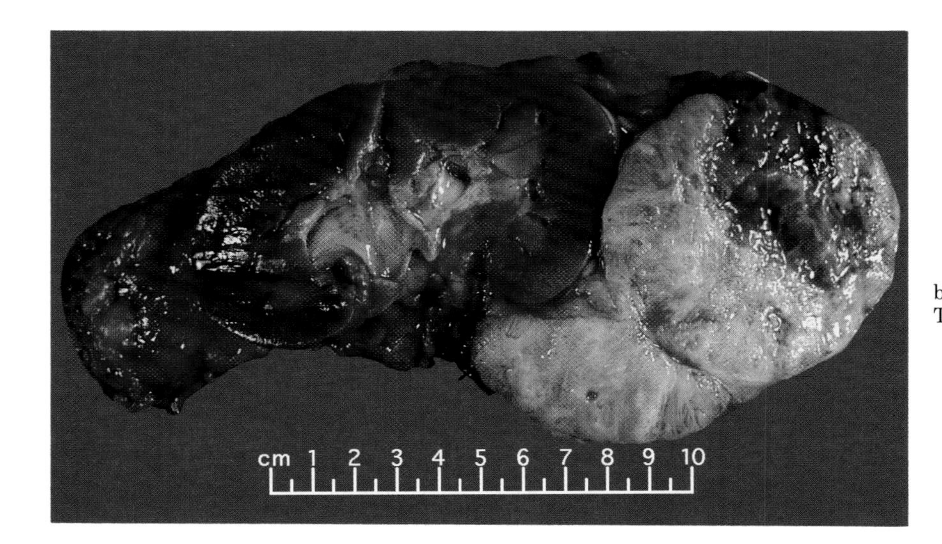

Figure 7-24
PRIMARY LEIOMYOSARCOMA OF RIGHT ADRENAL GLAND

Tumor and kidney have been bisected in the coronal plane. Tumor measured 11 x 8 x 7.5 cm.

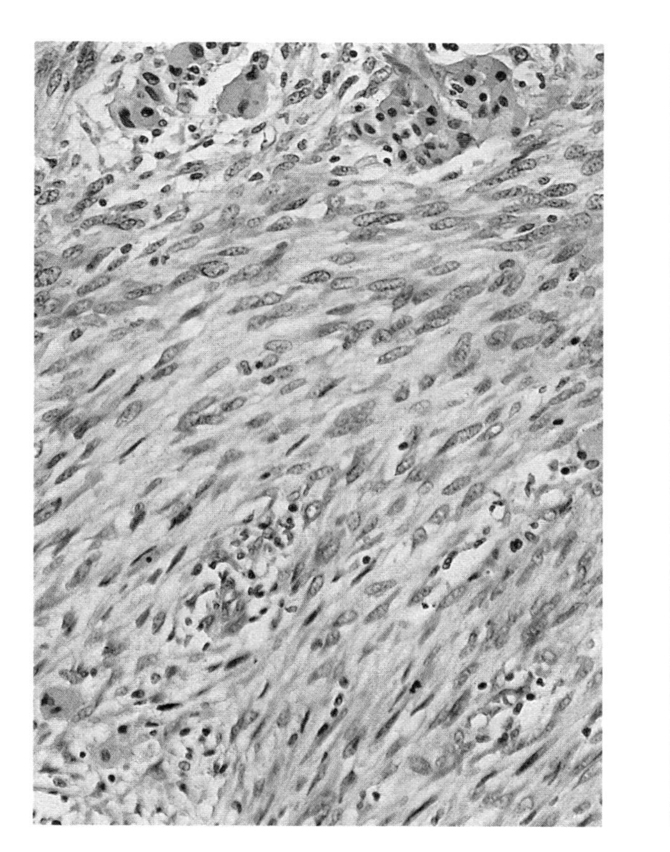

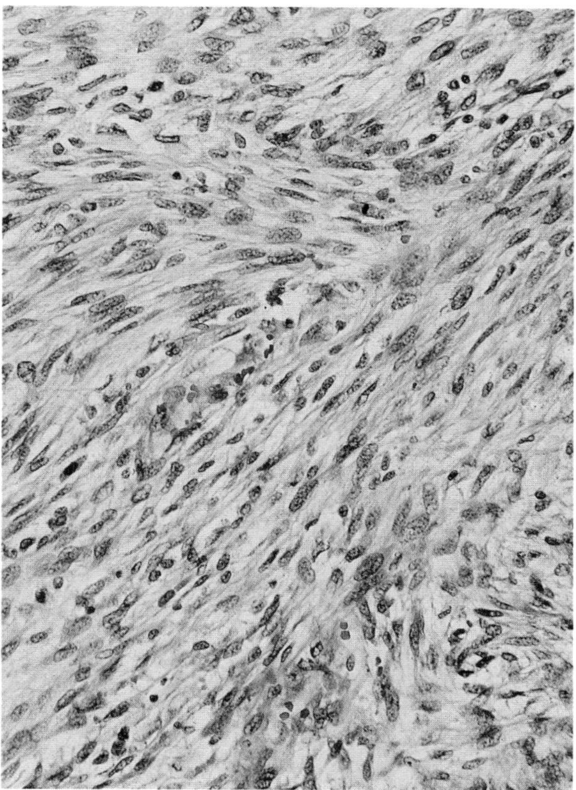

Figure 7-25
PRIMARY ADRENAL LEIOMYOSARCOMA

Left: Residual adrenal cortex is seen at top of field.

Right: Tumor had areas of confluent necrosis. The mitotic rate averaged 15 per 10 high-power fields in some of the more active areas. Electron microscopy confirmed the smooth muscle nature of the tumor.

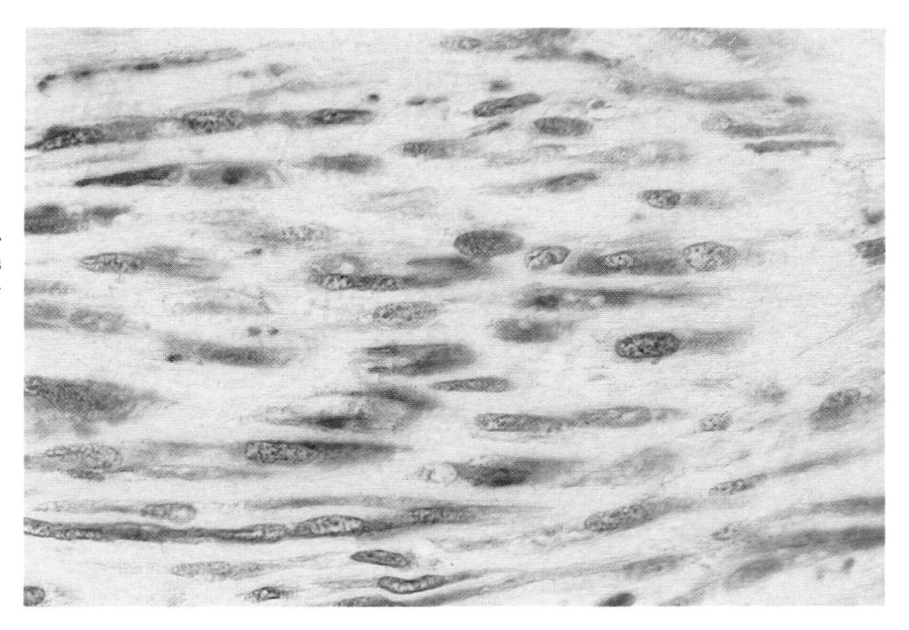

Figure 7-26
PRIMARY ADRENAL LEIOMYOSARCOMA
Tumor cells are positive for smooth muscle actin which stains dark red. (X400, Streptavidin-alkaline phosphatase method)

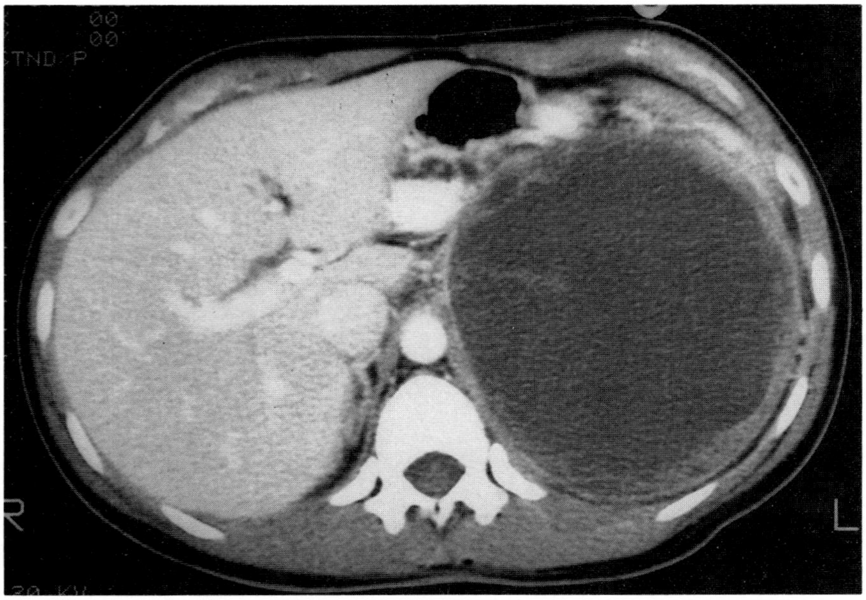

Figure 7-27
LARGE PRIMARY CYSTIC ADRENAL SCHWANNOMA
The large primary cystic adrenal schwannoma in a 29-year-old female measured 14 cm in diameter. CT scan shows the marked cystic change in the tumor (left side). At surgery the cystic mass contained abundant clotted and altered blood.

OTHER UNUSUAL PRIMARY ADRENAL TUMORS

Neural Tumors

Primary adrenal (78,79) or *juxta-adrenal* (76, 89) *schwannomas* have been documented. The author has seen a large schwannoma that presented as a large left upper quadrant cystic mass in a 29-year-old woman (fig. 7-27). The tumor was surgically resected, and while the adrenal gland was difficult to identify, random sections clearly revealed it as an attenuated structure over the surface of portions of the tumor (fig. 7-28). Although the adrenal gland is a rare primary site for schwannoma, it should not be totally unexpected given the neural innervation of the gland (see chapter 1). *Adrenal neurofibroma* has also been reported (fig. 7-29) (79,95). Equally

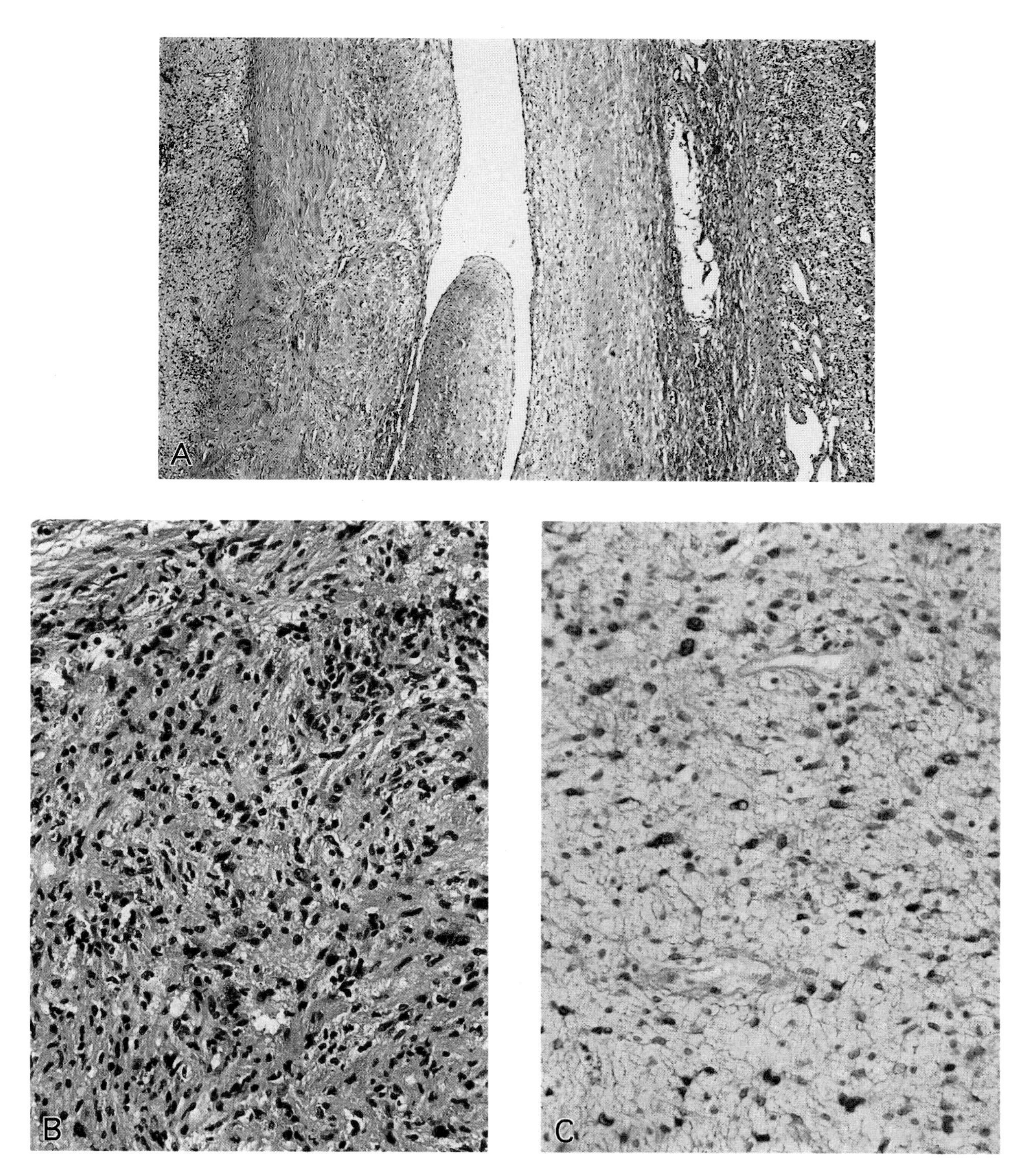

Figure 7-28
PRIMARY ADRENAL SCHWANNOMA

A: Residual adrenal gland is present on the right, portion of central adrenal vein in center, and schwannoma on the left side.
B: Primary adrenal schwannoma shows a mild degree of nuclear pleomorphism. There were a few areas with Antoni A pattern with poorly formed Verocay bodies.
C: Virtually all nuclei as well as small cytoplasmic extensions stain strongly for S-100 protein. (X175, Peroxidase-antiperoxidase stain)

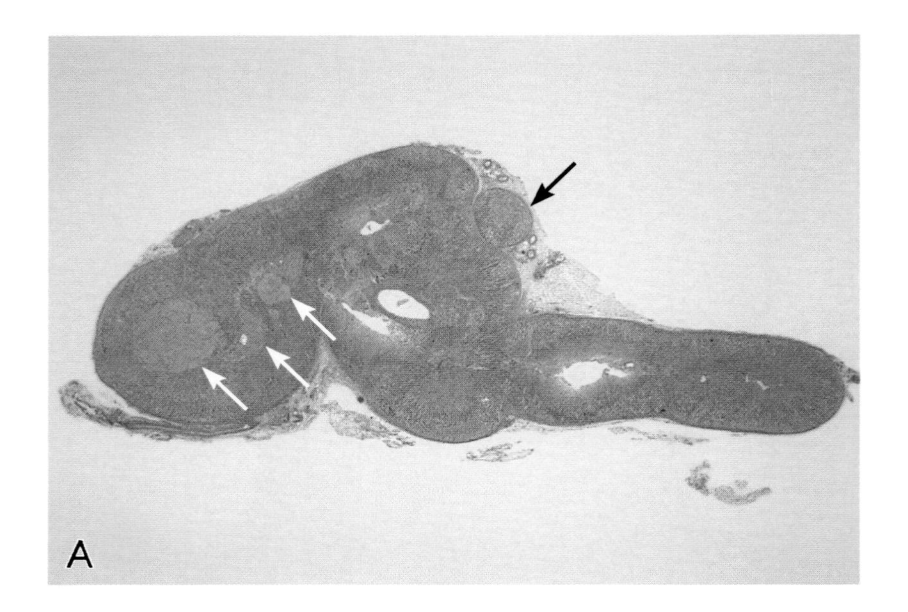

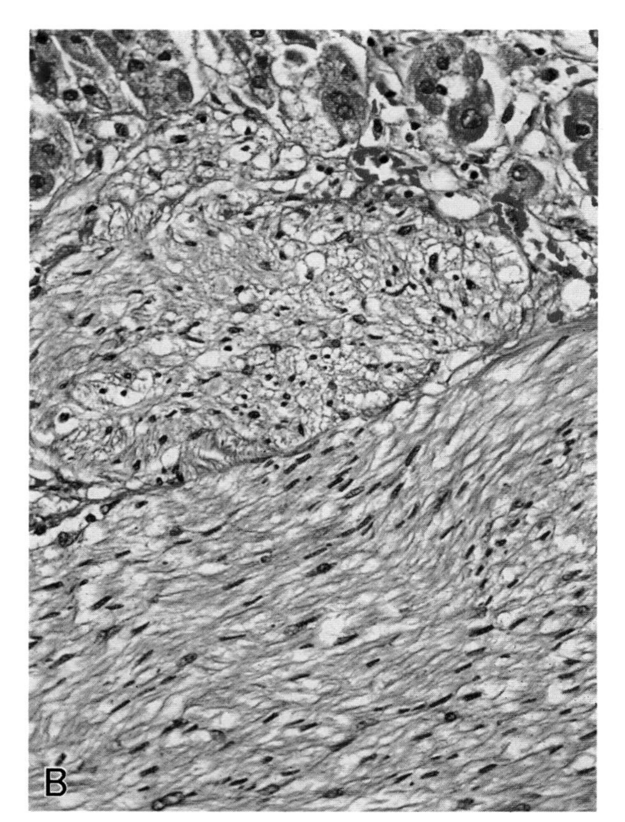

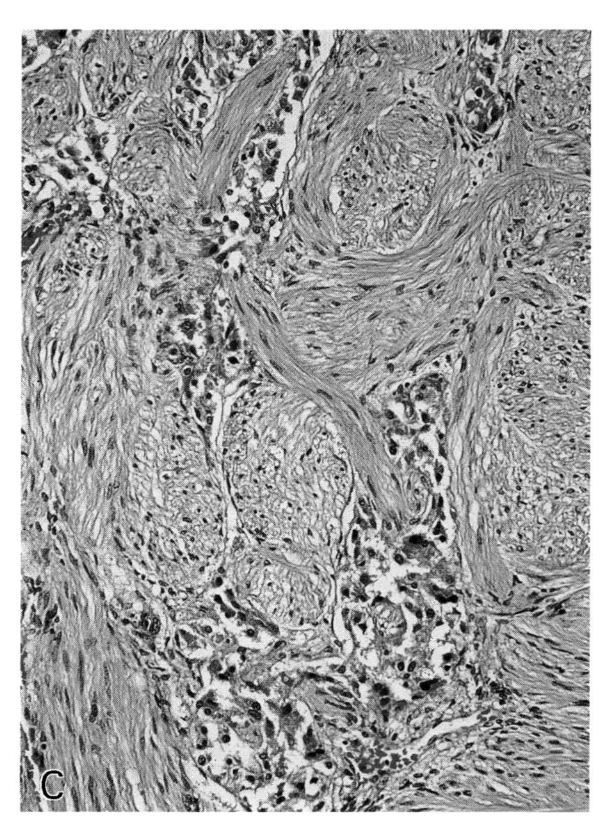

Figure 7-29
ADRENAL NEUROFIBROMA

A: Adrenal gland from an adult at autopsy shows neurofibroma growing in multiple small foci (white arrows). Cortical extrusion is also present (black arrow).

B: This small adrenal neurofibroma (same case as A) was an incidental finding at autopsy of an adult patient who had no history of von Recklinghausen's disease. Tumor was relatively circumscribed but unencapsulated.

C: Areas of the same tumor show fascicles of spindle cells intersected with clusters of normal chromaffin cells.

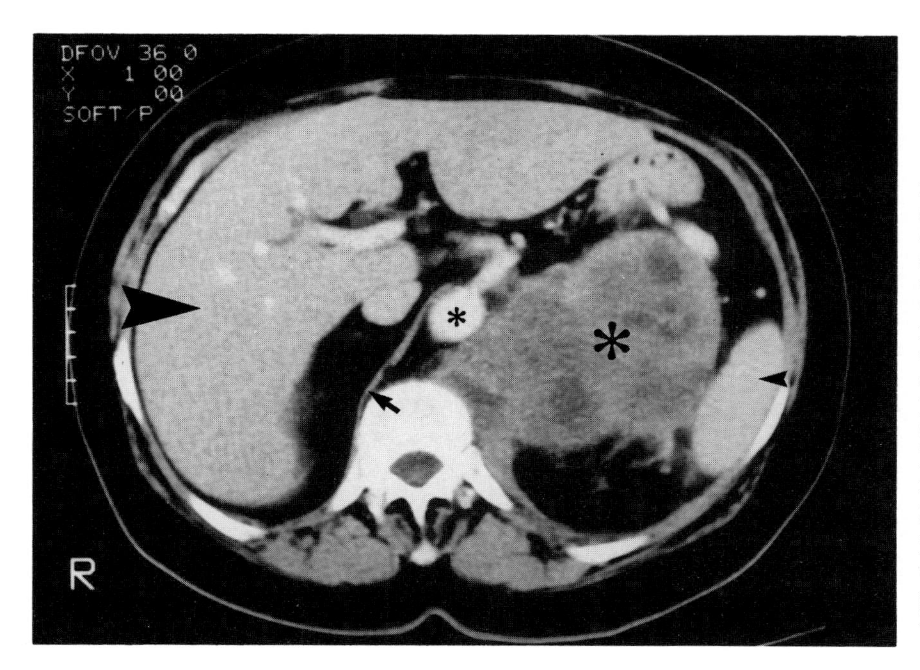

Figure 7-30
MALIGNANT PERIPHERAL NERVE SHEATH TUMOR

Primary malignant peripheral nerve sheath tumor of left adrenal gland of a 60-year-old female. CT scan shows an 8 x 7 x 7 cm left suprarenal mass (*) which is nonhomogeneous. The tumor abuts upon the paravertebral (psoas) muscles medially and the spleen (small arrowhead). It also invades and obliterates the right crus of the diaphragm (small arrow). Upper abdominal aorta is seen (small asterisk) as well as liver (large arrowhead). (Fig. 1A from Ayala GE, Ettinghausen SE, Epstein AH, Travis WD, Lack EE. Primary malignant peripheral nerve sheath tumor of the adrenal gland. Case report and literature review. J Urol Pathol 1994;2:265–72.)

rare is the *primary adrenal malignant schwannoma* or *malignant peripheral nerve sheath tumor* (fig. 7-30) (77,83). One example occurred in association with an ipsilateral pheochromocytoma, an example of a rare composite tumor (88), while another arose in an adrenal ganglioneuroma in an adult male homosexual who was HIV positive (80). A patient was recently reported with neurofibromatosis type 1 who had bilateral composite pheochromocytoma and malignant peripheral nerve sheath tumor (92b). Histologic features of adrenal malignant schwannoma are shown in figure 7-31 (77). Identification of tumor cells positive for S-100 protein by immunohistochemistry can help in diagnosis (fig. 7-32).

Adenomatoid Tumor

Primary adenomatoid tumor of the adrenal is also rare. Two examples have recently been reported (93,94). Two of the three cases reported by Plaut (92) as "locally invasive lymphangioma" of adrenal gland also appear to be adenomatoid tumors, and both were discovered at autopsy. On gross examination the tumor appears smooth, white, and homogeneous. On microscopic examination the tumor is not truly encapsulated (fig. 7-33), hence Plaut's term "locally invasive." This rare tumor is of mesothelial origin and has the classic histomorphology of adenomatoid tumors, with a sieve-like appearance due to cytoplasmic vacuoles and gland-like spaces (fig. 7-34, left). Nuclei have a vesicular quality, often with a single, small, dot-like nucleolus (fig. 7-34, right). There is usually a small amount of interlacing connective tissue. A mesothelial origin can be confirmed by immunohistochemical staining for cytokeratin (fig. 7-35), and ultrastructural demonstration of characteristic long, "bushy" cytoplasmic microvilli (94).

Other Rare Primary Tumors

Other rarely described adrenal tumors include lipoma (86), granulosa cell tumor (90), adrenal Leydig cell tumor (91,96), and adrenal adenoma containing crystalloids of Reinke with masculinization (97). Ovarian thecal metaplasia, which has been covered in chapter 1, morphologically might have a sex-cord stromal derivation. Leydig cells are rare within the adrenal gland, but the existence of these cells and tumors derived from them can be explained, in part, by the close embryologic relationship between the developing gonad and the adrenal primordium. The presence of crystalloids of Reinke provides definitive evidence for Leydig cells. Many of the masculinizing adrenal cortical neoplasms contain abundant cells superficially resembling Leydig cells due to their compact, finely granular,

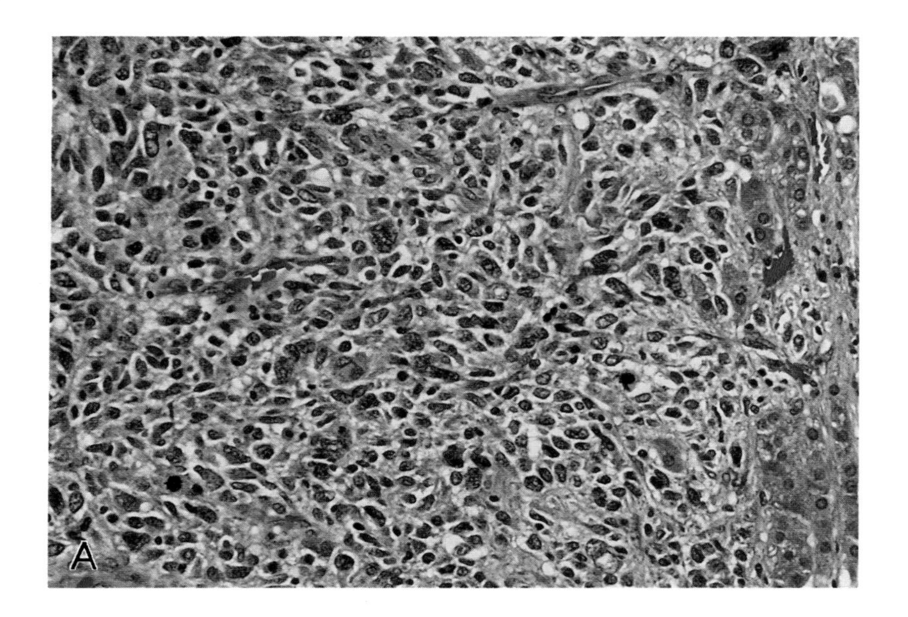

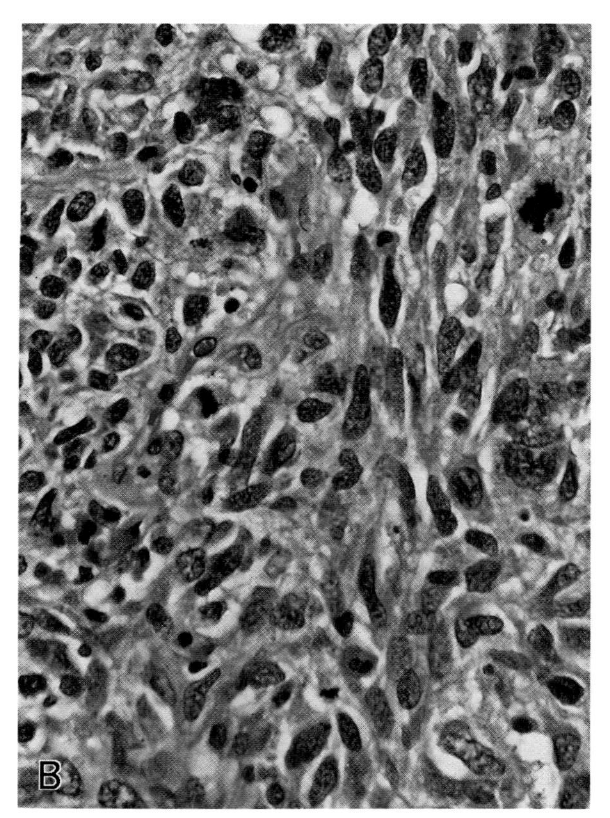

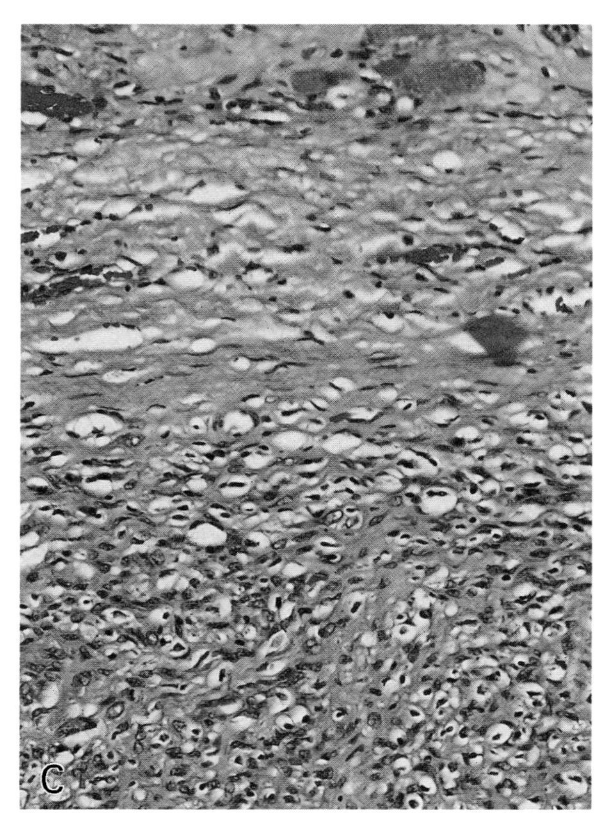

Figure 7-31

PRIMARY ADRENAL MALIGNANT PERIPHERAL NERVE SHEATH TUMOR

A: Primary malignant peripheral nerve sheath tumor of adrenal gland with residual cortex (right side).

B: Tumor had areas which were densely cellular, and in selected fields there were 1 to 2 mitoses per high-power field. Many tumor cells were positive for S-100 protein.

C: Tumor also involved several nerve trunks immediately adjacent to the adrenal tumor. Residual compressed nerve and ganglion cells are present at top of field.

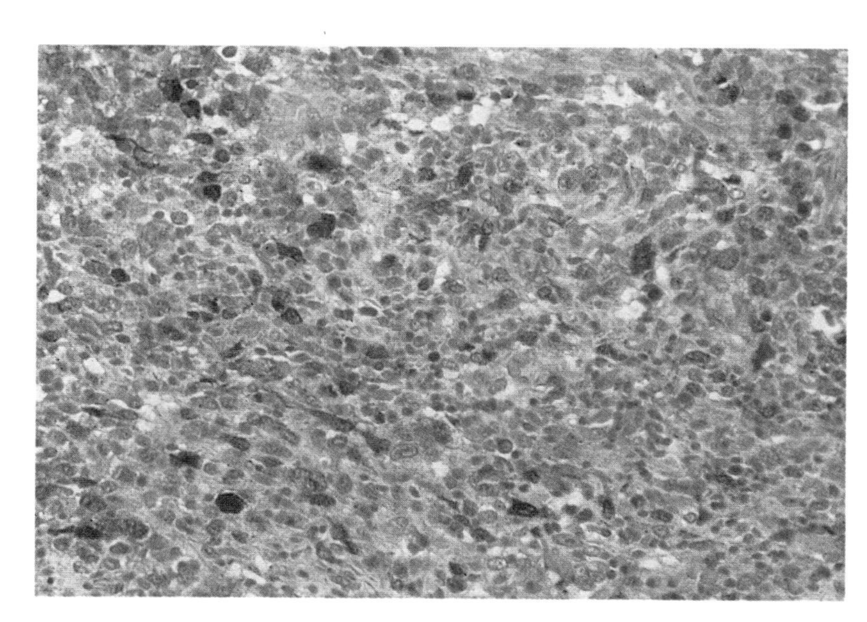

Figure 7-32
PRIMARY ADRENAL MALIGNANT PERIPHERAL NERVE SHEATH TUMOR
Numerous cells are immunoreactive for S-100 protein. (X200, Streptavidin-alkaline phosphatase method)

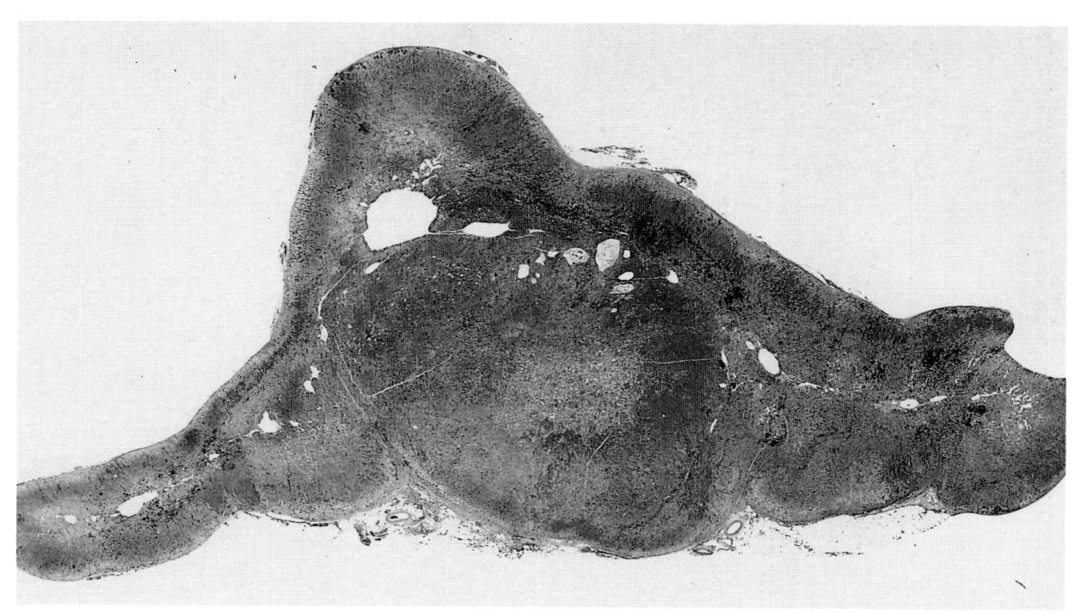

Figure 7-33
ADENOMATOID TUMOR OF THE ADRENAL GLAND
Unilateral, solitary adenomatoid tumor of adrenal gland in a patient with ectopic ACTH syndrome. The tumor expands the mid-portion of the gland and is ill-demarcated on low-power examination. Note expansile but unencapsulated edges of tumor, which measured about 1 cm in diameter. Adrenalectomy was done to rule out ectopic ACTH production by small pheochromocytoma.

eosinophilic cytoplasm, but crystalloids of Reinke are usually not a feature. On only one occasion has the author observed hilus (or Leydig) cells within the adrenal cortex, in a case of an adult female with an aldosterone-producing adrenal cortical adenoma (fig. 7-36) (85). Intra-adrenal Leydig-like cells have also been reported in a patient with ectopic ACTH syndrome (84). Spindle-shaped cells with crystalline inclusions bearing ultrastructural similarity to Reinke crystalloids have been identified in the adrenal cortex of male patients (87).

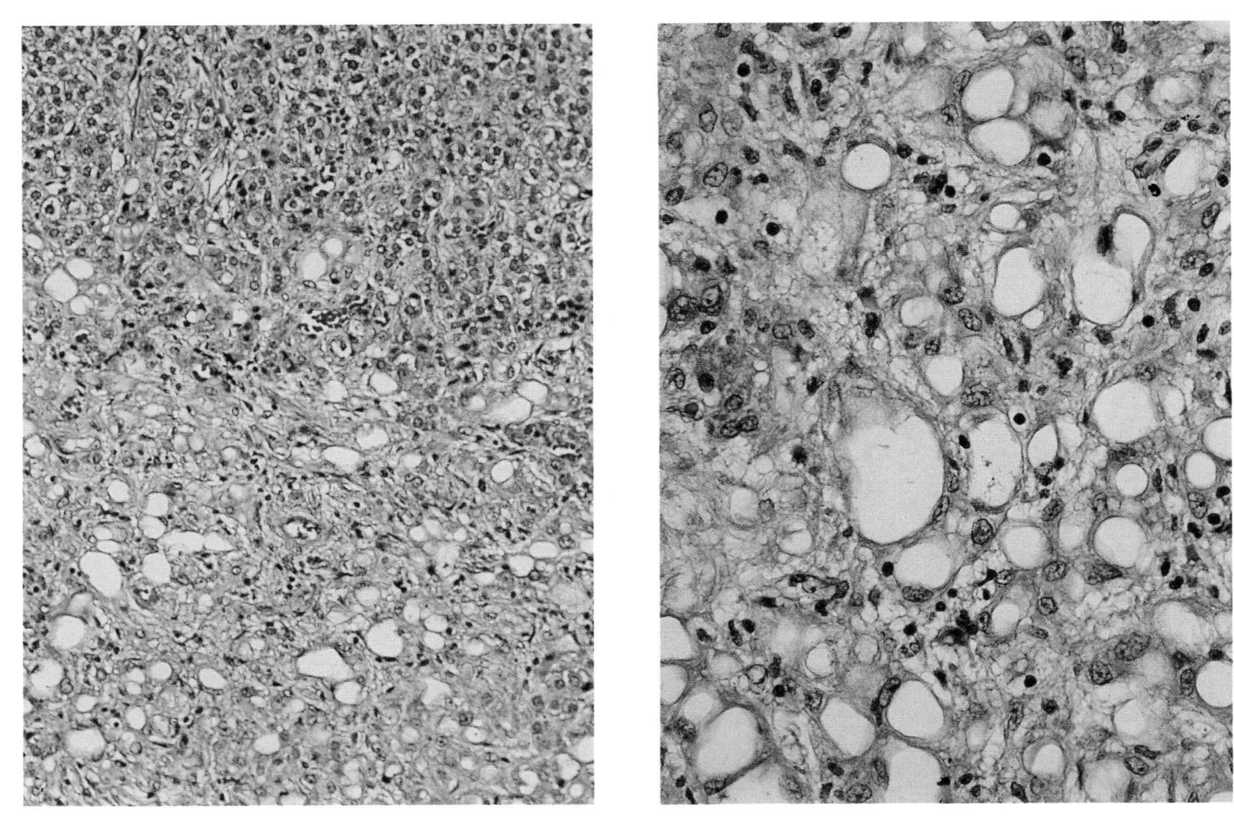

Figure 7-34
PRIMARY ADRENAL ADENOMATOID TUMOR

Left: This primary adrenal adenomatoid tumor has numerous small gland-like spaces. The tumor had enveloped small nests of adrenal cortical cells with compact eosinophilic cytoplasm.

Right: Cells have light, eosinophilic cytoplasm with vacuoles of various sizes.

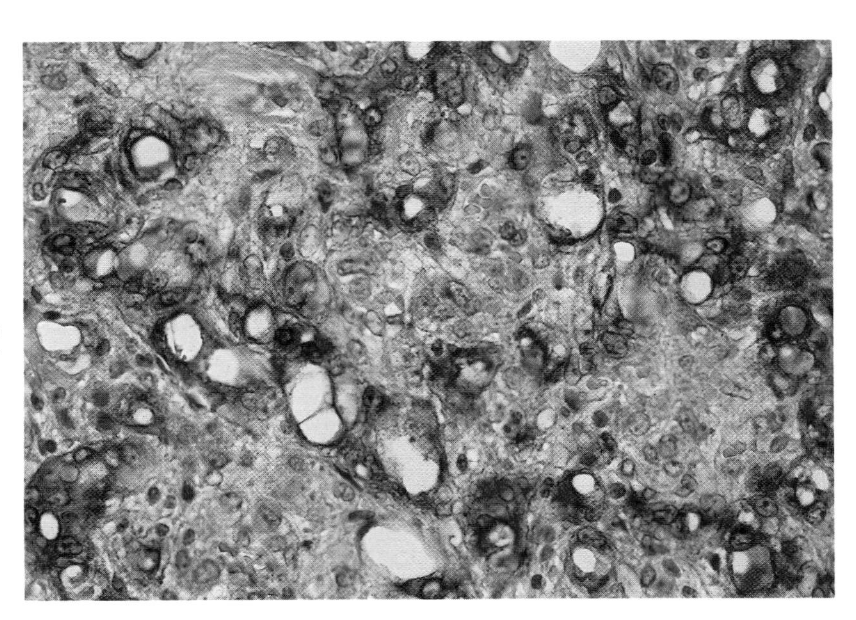

Figure 7-35
PRIMARY ADRENAL ADENOMATOID TUMOR

Primary adenomatoid tumor of adrenal gland is positive for cytokeratin. Staining reaction highlights cells extending out into adjacent cortex. (X200, Streptavidin-alkaline phosphatase method)

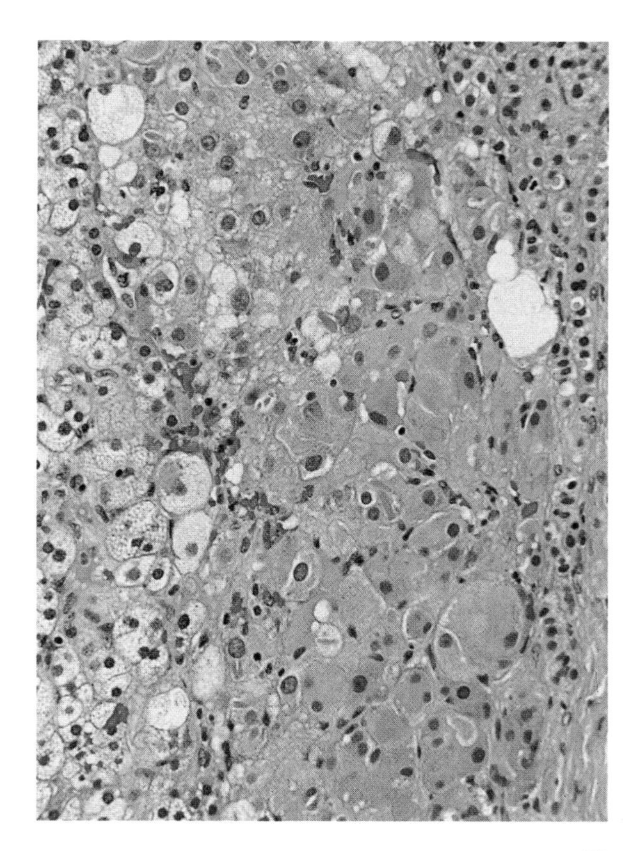

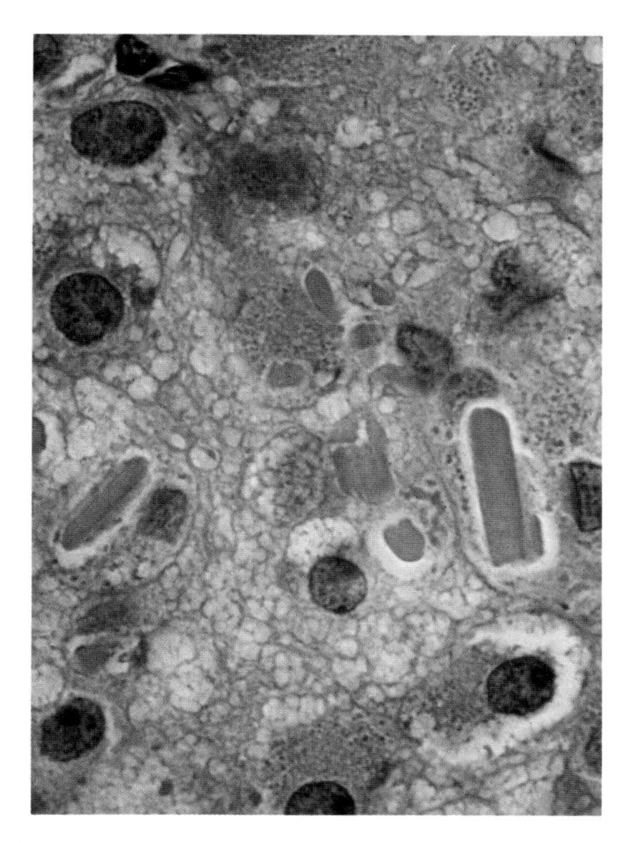

Figure 7-36
ALDOSTERONE-PRODUCING ADRENAL CORTICAL ADENOMA

Left: A 49-year-old female with aldosterone-producing adrenal cortical adenoma. The adrenal cortex adjacent to the adenoma contains a cluster of hilus (or Leydig) cells replete with numerous crystalloids of Reinke. Some cells of adjacent zona glomerulosa contain "spironolactone bodies." Patient had been treated with spironolactone for primary hyperaldosteronism.

Right: Several intra-adrenal hilus cells contain typical crystalloids of Reinke.

Castleman's disease of the adrenal gland has also been reported (81). There is an unusual example of retroperitoneal bronchogenic cyst presenting as an adrenal mass, but the lesion was found to be in an immediate juxta-adrenal location at surgery and the gland was left intact (82). A poorly differentiated neuroendocrine carcinoma (or primitive neuroectodermal tumor [PNET] different from neuroblastoma) presenting as a suprarenal mass without clear evidence of a primary tumor elsewhere may be an adrenal primary, remote as it may seem. Some cases may be a metastasis from another site and careful follow-up is indicated. Recently a primary adrenal neoplasm with morphologic features of an extrarenal Wilms' tumor (nephroblastoma) was reported in a 4-year-old boy (92c). A solitary fibrous tumor of the adrenal gland has also recently been described (92a). The author has recently seen a large, partially necrotic mesenchymal tumor of the adrenal gland with features of a malignant fibrous histiocytoma.

REFERENCES

Adrenal Infection and Abscess Formation

1. Atkinson GO Jr, Kodroff MB, Gay BB Jr, Ricketts RR. Adrenal abscess in the neonate. Radiology 1985; 155:101–4.
2. Benjamin E, Fox H. Malakoplasia of the adrenal gland. J Clin Pathol 1981;34:606–11.
3. Goodwin RA Jr, Shapiro JL, Thurman GH, Thurman SS, Des Prez RM: Disseminated histoplasmosis: clinical and pathological correlations. Medicine (Baltimore) 1980;59:1–33.
4. Slavin RE, Walsh TJ, Pollack AD: Late generalized tuberculosis: a clinical pathological analysis and comparison of 100 cases in the preantibiotic and antibiotic eras. Medicine (Baltimore) 1980;59:352–66.
5. Travis WD, Oertel JE, Lack EE. Miscellaneous tumors and tumefactive lesions of the adrenal gland. In: Lack EE, ed. Pathology of the adrenal glands. New York: Churchill Livingstone, 1990:351–78.

Adrenal Hemorrhage and Hematoma Formation

6. Clark OH, Hall AD, Schambelan M. Clinical manifestations of adrenal hemorrhage. Am J Surg 1974; 128:219–24.
7. Eklöf O, Mortensson W, Sandstedt B. Suprarenal hematoma versus neuroblastoma complicated by haemorrhage. A diagnostic dilemma in the newborn. Acta Radiol [Diagn] (Stockholm) 1986;27:3–10.
8. Moore MA, Riggs PJ. Unilateral adrenal hemorrhage. An unusual presentation. Southern Med J 1985;78:989–92.
9. Rao RH, Vagnucci AH, Amico JA. Bilateral massive adrenal hemorrhage: early recognition and treatment. Ann Int Med 1989;110:227–35.
10. Travis WD, Oertel JE, Lack EE. Miscellaneous tumors and tumefactive lesions of the adrenal gland. In: Lack EE, ed. Pathology of the adrenal glands. New York: Churchill Livingstone, 1990:351–78.
11. Xarli VP, Steele AA, Davis PJ, Buescher ES, Rios CN, Garcia-Bunuel R. Adrenal hemorrhage in the adult. Medicine (Baltimore) 1978;57:211–21.

Adrenal Cysts

12. Abeshouse GA, Goldstein RB, Abeshouse BS. Adrenal cysts: review of the literature and report of three cases. J Urol 1959;81:711–9.
13. Barron SH, Emanuel B: Adrenal cyst. A case report and review of the pediatric literature. J Pediatr 1961; 59:592–9.
14. Bürrig KF. Epithelial (true) splenic cysts. Pathogenesis of the mesothelial and so-called epidermoid cyst of the spleen. Am J Surg Pathol 1988;12:275–81.
15. Foster DG. Adrenal cysts. Arch Surg 1966;92:131–43.
16. Gaffey MJ, Mills SE, Fechner RE, Bertholf MF, Allen MS Jr. Vascular adrenal cysts. Review of the literature and report of a case. A clinicopathologic and immunohistochemical study of endothelial and hemorrhagic (pseudocystic) variants. Am J Surg Pathol 1989;13:740–7.
17. Gaffey MJ, Mills SE, Medeiros LJ, Weiss LM. Unusual variants of adrenal pseudocysts with intracystic fat, myelolipomatous metaplasia, and metastatic carcinoma. Am J Clin Pathol 1990;94:706–13.
18. Groben PA, Roberson JB Jr, Anger SR, Askin FB, Price WG, Siegal GP. Immunohistochemical evidence for the vascular origin of primary adrenal pseudocysts. Arch Pathol Lab Med 1986;110:121–3.
19. Kearney GP, Mahoney EM, Maher E, Harrison JH. Functioning and nonfunctioning cysts of the adrenal cortex and medulla. Am J Surg 1977;134:363–8.
20. Levin SE, Collins DL, Kaplan GW, Weller MH. Neonatal adrenal pseudocyst mimicking metastatic disease. Ann Surg 1974;179:186–9.
21. Medeiros LJ, Lewandrowski KB, Vickery AL Jr. Adrenal pseudocyst: a clinical and pathologic study of eight cases. Hum Pathol 1989;20:660–5.
22. Medeiros LJ, Weiss LM, Vickery AL Jr. Epithelial-lined (true) cyst of the adrenal gland: a case report. Hum Pathol 1989;20:491–2.
23. Travis WD, Oertel JE, Lack EE. Miscellaneous tumors and tumefactive lesions of the adrenal gland. In: Lack EE, ed. Pathology of the adrenal glands. New York: Churchill Livingstone, 1990:351–78.
24. Wahl HR. Adrenal cysts [Abstract]. Am J Pathol 1951;27:758.

Myelolipoma

25. Bennett BD, McKenna TJ, Hough AJ, Dean R, Page DL. Adrenal myelolipoma associated with Cushing's disease. Am J Clin Pathol 1980;73:443–7.
26. Boudreaux D, Waisman J, Skinner DG, Low R. Giant adrenal myelolipoma and testicular interstitial cell tumor in a man with congenital 21-hydroxylase deficiency. Am J Surg Pathol 1979;3:109–23.
27. Brietta LK, Watkins D. Giant extra-adrenal myelolipoma. Arch Pathol Lab Med 1994;118:188–90.
28. Case records of the Massachusetts General Hospital: Case 46-1988. N Engl J Med 1988;319:1336–43.
29. Condom E, Villabona CM, Gómez JM, Carrera M. Adrenal myelolipoma in a woman with congenital 17-hydroxylase deficiency. Arch Pathol Lab Med 1985;109:1116–7.
30. Damjanov I, Katz SM, Catalano E, Mason D, Schwartz AB. Myelolipoma in a heterotopic adrenal gland: light and electron microscopic findings. Cancer 1979;44:1350–6.
31. deBlois GG, DeMay RM. Adrenal myelolipoma diagnosis by computed tomography-guided fine-needle aspiration. A case report. Cancer 1985;55:848–50.
32. Del Gaudio A, Solidaro G. Myelolipoma of the adrenal gland: report of two cases and a review of the literature. Surgery 1986;99:293–301.

33. Dieckman KP, Hamm B, Pickartz H, Jonas D, Bauer HW. Adrenal myelolipoma: clinical, radiologic, and histologic features. Urology 1987;29:1–8.
34. Escuin F, Gomez P, Martinez I, Pérez-Fontan M, Selgas R, Sanchez-Sicilia L. Angiomyelolipoma associated with bilateral adrenocortical hyperplasia and hypertension. J Urol 1985;133:655–7.
35. Evans GW, Olinde HD, Kozdereli E. Extraadrenal myelolipoma. A lesion that can be diagnosed by fine needle aspiration biopsy. Acta Cytologica 1990;34:536–8.
36. Grignon DJ, Shkrum MJ, Smout MS. Extra-adrenal myelolipoma. Arch Pathol Lab Med 1989;113:52–4.
37. Hegstrom JL, Kircher T. Alimentary tract ganglioneuromatosis-lipomatosis, adrenal myelolipomas, pancreatic telangiectasias, and multinodular thyroid goiter. A possible neuroendocrine syndrome. Am J Clin Pathol 1985;83:744–7.
38. Hunter SB, Schemankewitz EH, Patterson C, Varma VA. Extraadrenal myelolipoma. A report of two cases. Am J Clin Pathol 1992;97:402–4.
39. Massey GS, Green JB, Marsh WL Jr. Presacral myelolipoma. Cancer 1987;60:403–6.
40. Nishizaki T, Kanematsu T, Matsumata T, Yasunaga C, Kakizoe S, Sugimachi K. Myelolipoma of the liver. A case report. Cancer 1989;63:930–4.
41. Noble MJ, Montague DK, Levin HS. Myelolipoma: an unusual surgical lesion of the adrenal gland. Cancer 1982;49:952–8.
42. Plaut A. Myelolipoma in the adrenal cortex (myeloadipose structures). Am J Pathol 1958;34:487–503.
43. Schellen RA. Myelolipoma of the adrenal gland: case report and review of the literature. J Am Osteopath Assoc 1986;86:26–30.
44. Selye H, Stone H. Hormonally induced transformation of adrenal into myeloid tissue. Am J Pathol 1950;26:211–33.
45. Seniuta P, Cazenave-Mahe JP, Le Treut A, Trojani M. Adrenal myelolipoma and Castleman's pseudotumor. A case of association in a retroperitoneal tumor. J Urol (Paris) 1989;95:511–4.
46. Travis WD, Oertel JE, Lack EE. Miscellaneous tumors and tumefactive lesions of the adrenal gland. In: Lack EE, ed. Pathology of the adrenal glands. New York: Churchill Livingstone, 1990:351–78.
47. Vyberg M, Sestoft L. Combined adrenal myelolipoma and adenoma associated with Cushing's syndrome. Am J Clin Pathol 1986;86:541–45.

Malignant Melanoma

48. Carstens PH, Kuhns JG, Ghazi C. Primay malignant melanomas of the lung and adrenal. Hum Pathol 1984;15:910–14.
49. Chetty R, Clark SP, Taylor DA. Pigmented pheochromocytomas of the adrenal medulla. Hum Pathol 1993;24:420–3.
50. Dao AH, Page DL, Reynolds VH, Adkins RB Jr. Primary malignant melanoma of the adrenal gland. A report of two cases and review of the literature. Am Surg 1990;56:199–203.
51. Gonzalez-Crussi F, Hsueh W. Bilateral adrenal ganglioneuroblastoma with neuromelanin. Clinical and pathologic observations. Cancer 1988;61:1159–66.
52. Hahn JF, Netsky MG, Butler AB, Sperber EE. Pigmented ganglioneuroblastoma: relation of melanin and lipofuscin to schwannomas and other tumors of neural crest origin. J Neuropath Exp Neurol 1976;35:393–403.
53. Lack EE. Pathology of adrenal and extra-adrenal paraganglia. Major problems in pathology, Vol 29, Philadelphia: WB Saunders, 1994.
54. Landas SK, Leigh C, Bonsid SM, Layne K. Occurrence of melanin in pheochromocytoma. Mod Pathol 1993;6:175–8.
55. Mullins JD. A pigmented differentiating neuroblastoma: a light and ultrastructural study. Cancer 1980;46:522–8.

Malignant Lymphoma

56. Choi GH, Durishin M, Garbudawala ST, Richard J. Non-Hodgkin's lymphoma of the adrenal gland. Arch Pathol Lab Med 1990;114:883–5.
57. Harris GJ, Tio FO, Von Hoff DD. Primary adrenal lymphoma. Cancer 1989;63:799–803.
58. Schnitzer B, Smid D, Lloyd RV. Primary T-cell lymphoma of the adrenal glands with adrenal insufficiency. Hum Pathol 1986;17:634–6.

Primary Mesenchymal Tumors

59. Ansari SJ, Ordonez NG, Romsdahl MM, Ro JY. Primary angiosarcoma mimicking adrenal pseudocyst. Am J Surg Pathol (in press).
60. Ben-Izhak O, Auslander L, Rabinson S, Lichtig C, Sternberg A. Epithelioid angiosarcoma of the adrenal gland with cytokeratin expression. Report of a case with accompanying mesenteric fibromatosis. Cancer 1992;69:1808–12.
61. Goren E, Bensal D, Reif RM, Eidelman A. Cavernous hemangioma of the adrenal gland. J Urol 1986;135:341–2.
62. Granger JK, Houn HY, Collins C. Massive hemorrhagic functional adrenal adenoma histologically mimicking angiosarcoma. Report of a case with immunohistochemical study. Am J Surg Pathol 1991;15:699–704.
63. Kareti LR, Katlein S, Siew S, Blauvelt A. Angiosarcoma of the adrenal gland. Arch Pathol Lab Med 1988;112:1163–5.
64. Lack EE, Graham CW, Azumi N, et al. Primary leiomyosarcoma of the adrenal gland. Case report with immunohistochemical and ultrastructural study. Am J Surg Pathol 1991;15:899–905.
65. Livaditou A, Alexiou G, Floros D, Filippidis T, Dosios T, Bays D. Epithelioid angiosarcoma of the adrenal gland associated with chronic arsenical intoxication? Path Res Pract 1991;187:284–9.
66. Mellor JA. Hereditary haemorrhagic telangiectasia. Br J Clin Pract 1983;37:234–6.

67. Nakagawa N, Takahashi M, Maeda K, Fujimura N, Yufu M. Case report: adrenal haemangioma coexisting with malignant haemangioendothelioma. Clin Radiol 1986;37:97–9.
68. Orringer RD, Lynch JA, McDermott WV. Cavernous hemangioma of the adrenal gland. J Surg Oncol 1983;22:106–8.
69. Page DL, DeLellis RA, Hough AJ Jr. Tumors of the adrenal. Atlas of Tumor Pathology, 2nd series, Fascicle 23. Washington, D.C.: Armed Forces Institute of Pathology, 1986.
70. Päivänsalo M, Siniluoto T, Seppänen U. Cavernous hemangioma of the adrenal gland. Diagn Imag Clin Med 1986;55:168–71.
71. Plaut A. Hemangiomas and related lesions of the adrenal gland. Virchows Arch [A] 1962;335:345–55.
72. Plaut A. Locally invasive lymphangioma of adrenal glands. Cancer 1962;15:1165–9.
73. Travis WD, Oertel JE, Lack EE. Miscellaneous tumors and tumefactive lesions of the adrenal gland. In: Lack EE, ed. Pathology of the adrenal glands. New York: Churchill Livingstone, 1990:351–78.
74. Vargas AD. Adrenal hemangioma. Urology 1980;16:389–90.
75. Wenig BM, Abbondanzo SL, Heffess CS. Epithelioid angiosarcoma of the adrenal glands. A clinicopathologic study of nine cases with a discussion of the implications of finding epithelial-specific markers. Am J Surg Pathol 1994;18:62–73.
75a. Zetler PJ, Filipenko JD, Bilbey JH, Schmidt N. Primary adrenal leiomyosarcoma in a man with acquired immunodeficiency syndrome (AIDS). Further evidence for an increase in smooth muscle tumors related to Epstein-Barr infection in AIDS. Arch Pathol Lab Med 1995;119:1164–7.

Other Unusual Primary Adrenal Tumors

76. Andreu J, Alegret X, Perez C, Llauger J. Cystic schwannoma mimicking adrenal tumor. Comput Med Imaging Graph 1988;12:183–5.
77. Ayala GE, Ettinghausen SE, Epstein AH, Travis WD, Lack EE. Primary malignant peripheral nerve sheath tumor of the adrenal gland. Case report and literature review. J Urol Pathol 1994;2:265–72.
78. Bedard YC, Horvath E, Kovacs K. Adrenal schwannoma with apparent uptake of immunoglobulins. Ultrastr Pathol 1986;10:505–13.
79. Billaud L, Benabed K, Requeda E, et al. Lésions tumorales et pseudo-tumorales de la loge surrénalienne à ne pas méconnaitre. Presse Médicale 1987;16:1405–9.
80. Chandrasoma P, Shibata D, Radin R, Brown LP, Koss M. Malignant peripherial nerve sheath tumor arising in an adrenal ganglioneuroma in an adult male homosexual. Cancer 1986;57:2022–5.
81. Debatin JF, Spritzer CE, Dunnick NR. Castleman's disease of the adrenal gland: MR imaging features. AJR Am J Roentgenol 1991;157:781–3.
82. Foerster HM, Sengupta EE, Montag AG, Kaplan EL. Retroperitoneal bronchogenic cyst presenting as an adrenal mass. Arch Pathol Lab Med 1991;115:1057–9.
83. Harach HR, Laidler P. Adrenal spindle-cell sarcoma with features of malignant peripheral nerve sheath tumor. Endocr Pathol 1993;4:222–5.
84. Horvath E, Chalvardjian A, Kovacs K, Singer W. Leydig-like cells in the adrenals of a woman with ectopic ACTH syndrome. Hum Pathol 1980;11:284–7.
85. Lack EE, Nauta RJ. Intracortical Leydig cells in a patient with an aldosterone-secreting adrenal cortical adenoma. J Urol Pathol 1993;1:411–8.
86. Lam KY. Adrenal tumours in Chinese. Virchows Arch [A] 1992;421:13–6.
87. Magalhaes MC. A new crystal-containing cell in human adrenal cortex. J Cell Biol 1972;55:126–33.
88. Min KW, Clemens A, Bell J, Dick H. Malignant peripheral nerve sheath tumor and a pheochromocytoma. A composite tumor of the adrenal. Arch Pathol Lab Med 1988;112:266–70.
89. Oliver WR, Reddick RL, Gillespie GY, Siegal GP. Juxtadrenal schwannoma: verification of the diagnosis by immunohistochemical and ultrastructural studies. J Surg Oncol 1985;30:259–68.
90. Orselli RC, Bassler TJ. Theca granulosa cell tumor arising in adrenal. Cancer 1973;31:474–7.
91. Pollock WJ, McConnell CF, Hilton C, Lavine RL. Virilizing Leydig cell adenoma of adrenal gland. Am J Surg Pathol 1986;10:816–22.
92. Plaut A. Locally invasive lymphangioma of adrenal glands. Cancer 1962;15:1165–9.
92a. Prévot S, Penna C, Imbert JC, Wendum D, de Saint-Maur PP. Solitary fibrous tumor of the adrenal gland. Modern Pathol 1996;9:1170–4.
92b. Sakaguchi N, Sano K, Ito M, Baba T, Fukuzawa M, Hotchi M. A case of von Recklinghausen disease with bilateral pheochromocytoma—malignant peripheral nerve sheath tumors of the adrenal and gastrointestinal autonomic nerve tumors. Am J Surg Pathol 1996;20:889–97.
92c. Santonja C, Diaz MA, Dehner LP. A unique dysembryonic neoplasm of the adrenal gland composed of nephrogenic rests in a child. Am J Surg Pathol 1996;20:118–24.
93. Simpson PR. Adenomatoid tumor of the adrenal gland. Arch Pathol Lab Med 1990;114:725–7.
94. Travis WD, Lack EE, Azumi N, Tsokos M, Norton J. Adenomatoid tumor of the adrenal gland with ultrastructural and immunohistochemical demonstration of a mesothelial origin. Arch Pathol Lab Med 1990;114:722–4.
95. Travis WD, Oertel JE, Lack EE. Miscellaneous tumors and tumefactive lesions of the adrenal gland. In: Lack EE, ed. Pathology of the adrenal glands. New York: Churchill Livingstone, 1990:351–78.
96. Trost BN, Koenig MP, Zimmermann A, Zachmann M, Müller J. Virilization of a post-menopausal woman by a testosterone-secreting Leydig cell type adrenal adenoma. Acta Endocrinol 1981;98:274–82.
97. Vasiloff J, Chideckel EW, Boyd CB, Foshag LJ. Testosterone-secreting adrenal adenoma containing crystalloids characteristic of Leydig cells. Am J Med 1985;79:772–6.

8
TUMORS METASTATIC TO ADRENAL GLANDS

INCIDENCE AND PRIMARY SITES OF TUMORS METASTATIC TO ADRENAL GLANDS

While much discussion has been devoted to primary adrenal tumors of various types, including the uncommon and rare neoplasms in chapter 7, the adrenal glands are more frequently involved by metastatic tumors from other primary sites. Per unit weight the adrenal glands are the organs most frequently involved by metastases (5), and as a specific anatomic site are reported to be the fourth most common site of spread, surpassed in frequency only by lung, liver, and bone (10). In an autopsy study by Abrams et al. (1) involving 1,000 carcinomas, the adrenal glands were secondarily involved in 27 percent of cases; the leading sources of adrenal metastases were breast (53.9 percent), lung (35.6 percent) (fig. 8-1), kidney (24 percent), stomach (21 percent), pancreas (19 percent), ovary (17 percent), and colon (14.4 percent). The pattern of adrenal blood supply (three-fold source of arterial supply) with high flow and sinusoidal vasculature has been offered as an explanation for the high incidence of metastases despite the relatively small size of the adrenal gland. Spread of tumor within sinusoids of the involved adrenal gland may be evident adjacent to the main site of metastasis, and may extend into small capsular extrusions of cortex (fig. 8-2). Bilateral adrenal metastases have been reported in 41 percent of patients with metastatic cancer involving the adrenals (9). Recent autopsy studies have shown that the frequency of adrenal metastases decreases with age in patients with mammary carcinoma (4), and there appears to be a lower frequency in patients with small cell carcinoma of lung who have received chemotherapy and radiation therapy (3). Metastases from extra-adrenal primary malignancies have been reported rarely in primary adrenal neoplasms; neoplasm to neoplasm metastases have been reported for pheochromocytoma (6) as well as adrenal cortical adenoma (7,8).

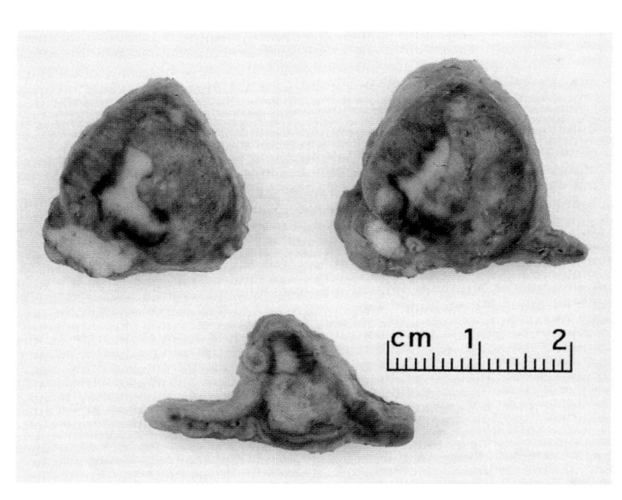

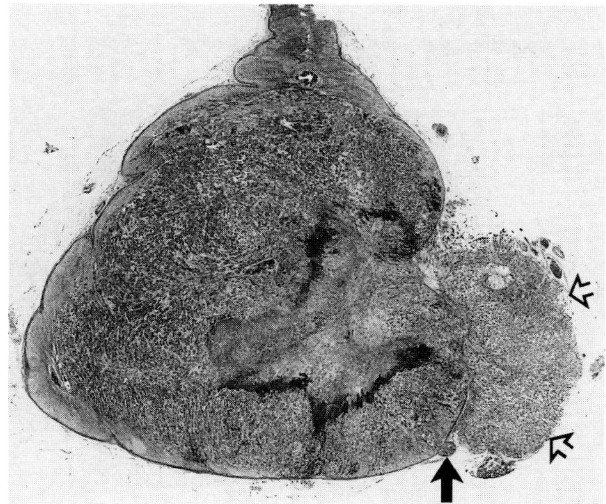

Figure 8-1
ADENOCARCINOMA METASTATIC TO ADRENAL GLAND

Left: Poorly differentiated adenocarcinoma metastatic to adrenal gland in a 58-year-old man with bronchogenic carcinoma. Opposite gland was less extensively involved. Tumor is grey to cream colored, with few areas of confluent necrosis.

Right: Metastatic pulmonary adenocarcinoma replaces much of the adrenal gland with extension outside the gland into periadrenal fat (open arrows). Portions of cortex are compressed and stretched over the periphery of the tumor. Small capsular extrusion (straight arrow) is also involved by metastatic carcinoma.

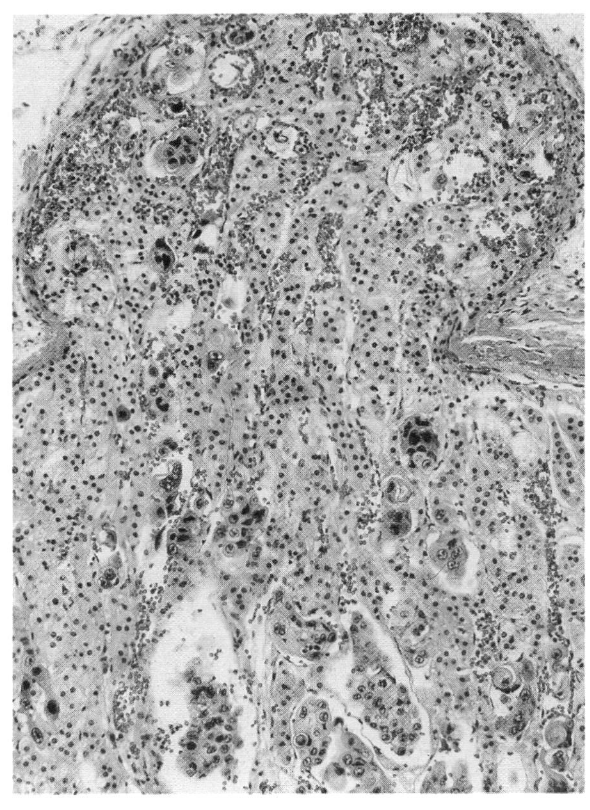

Figure 8-2
ADENOCARCINOMA METASTATIC TO ADRENAL GLAND
Sinusoidal invasion by metastatic bronchogenic carcinoma with involvement of capsular extrusion at top.

With the aid of high resolution imaging studies such as computed tomography (CT) and magnetic resonance imaging (MRI), adrenal metastases are more frequently being recognized during life. In a recent study, the prevalence of adrenal metastases in 91 autopsied lung cancer patients was 35 percent, with adenocarcinoma and squamous cell carcinoma the most frequent, and metastases were bilateral in 23 percent; although the sensitivity of CT scan varied from 20 percent to 41 percent, the specificity was 85 percent or more (2). During the staging work-up for patients with a known malignancy elsewhere the finding of an adrenal mass can prove to be very significant in terms of prognosis. In this setting, CT or ultrasound-guided fine-needle aspiration biopsy of the adrenal mass is a very useful method for distinguishing between a metastasis and a primary adrenal tumor (figs. 8-3, 8-4). On occasion, a metastatic carcinoma can clinically and pathologically simulate a primary adrenal cortical carcinoma. With lung carcinoma, for example, there may be marked unilateral adrenal enlargement (fig. 8-5) and multiple pulmonary nodules suggesting metastases from a primary adrenal cortical carcinoma. There may be involvement of tributaries of the central adrenal vein (fig. 8-6), which with overgrowth of the adrenal vascular system, may result in retrograde extension into the inferior vena cava (fig. 8-5). Occasionally,

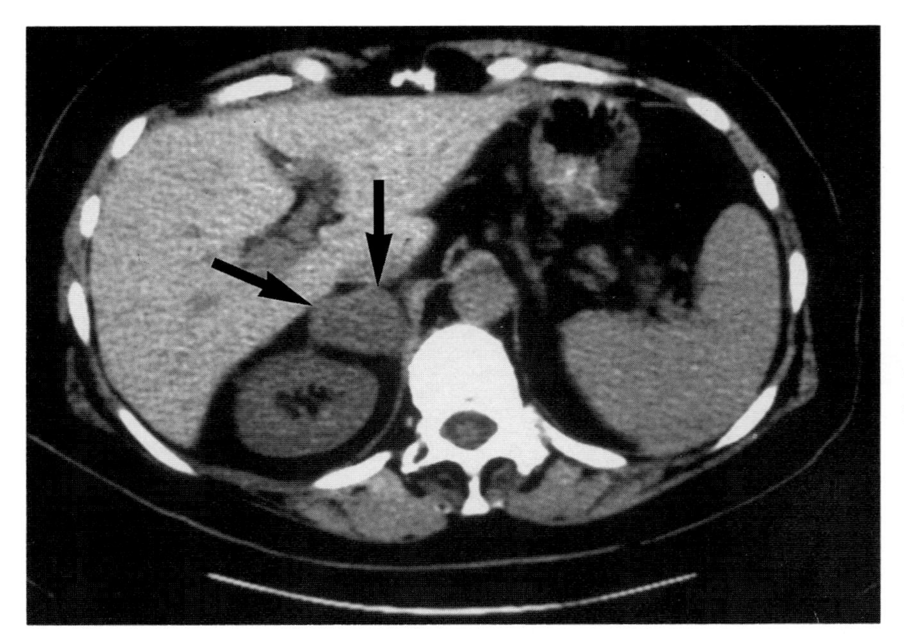

Figure 8-3
ADENOCARCINOMA METASTATIC TO ADRENAL GLAND
A right adrenal mass was detected on CT scan of the abdomen (arrows) in a 61-year-old woman with a history of pulmonary adenocarcinoma diagnosed 7 months earlier. (Courtesy of Dr. Calvin Neithamer, Alexandria, VA.)

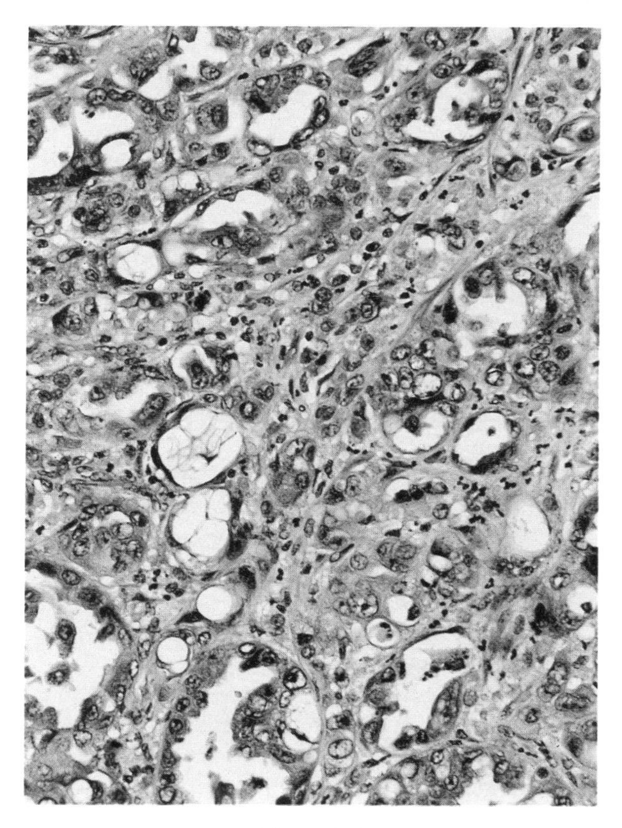

Figure 8-4
ADENOCARCINOMA METASTATIC TO ADRENAL GLAND

Cell block preparation of fine-needle aspirate shows moderately differentiated adenocarcinoma metastatic to adrenal gland, most consistent with a pulmonary primary.

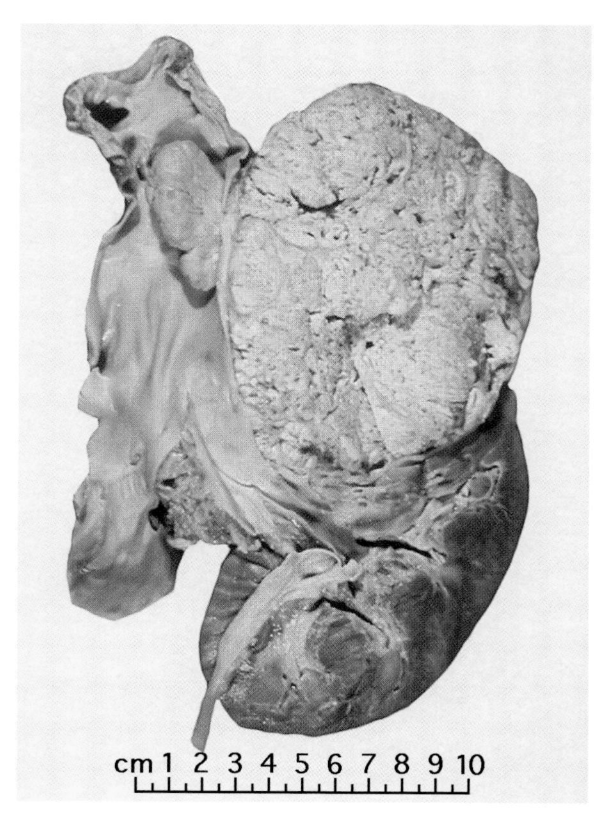

Figure 8-5
ADENOCARCINOMA METASTATIC TO ADRENAL GLAND

Patient had large suprarenal mass on left side and multiple pulmonary nodules. At autopsy the gross appearance of the tumor with extension into the inferior vena cava suggested an adrenal cortical carcinoma. Tumor proved to be a metastatic poorly differentiated adenocarcinoma of pulmonary origin.

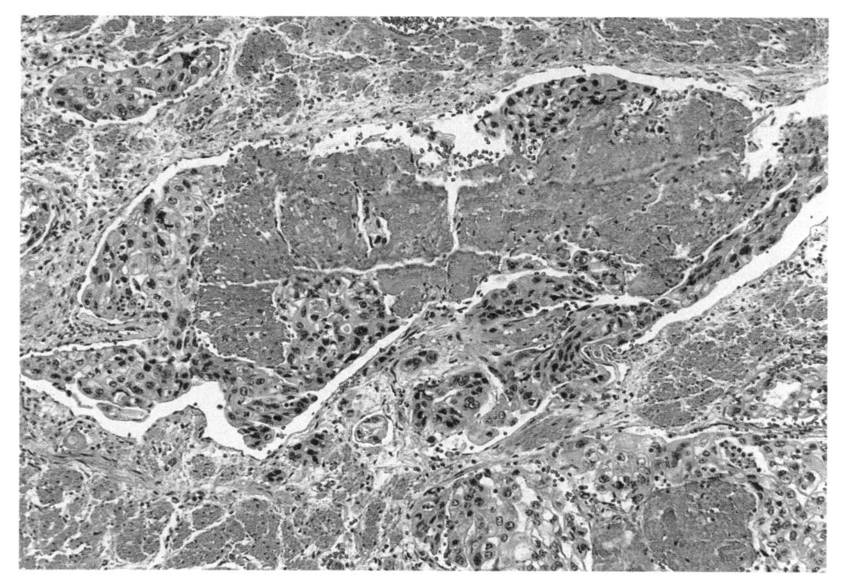

Figure 8-6
ADENOCARCINOMA METASTATIC TO ADRENAL GLAND

Poorly differentiated bronchogenic adenocarcinoma metastatic to adrenal gland with involvement of a tributary of the central adrenal vein. Tumor shows a confluent zone of necrosis and molds to the contour of venous channel.

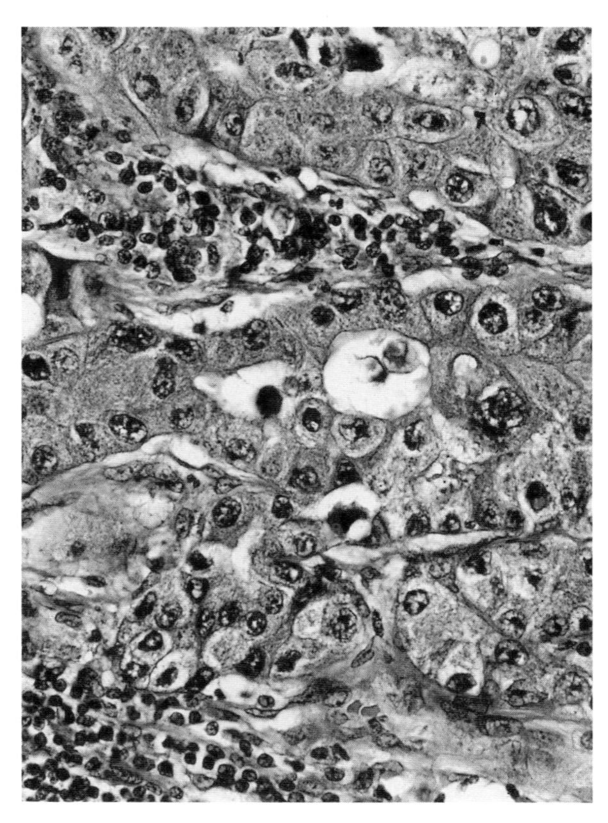

Figure 8-7
POORLY DIFFERENTIATED ADENOCARCINOMA METASTATIC TO ADRENAL GLAND

The patient had undergone adrenalectomy for clinically suspected adrenal cortical carcinoma. Many other areas of tumor were growing in solid sheets or tightly packed cords of cells. There is a chronic inflammatory infiltrate and a few areas of glandular differentiation.

surgical resection of the adrenal mass is performed. Large cell carcinoma and poorly differentiated adenocarcinoma may cause difficulties in interpretation of biopsies or even adrenalectomy specimens obtained surgically (fig. 8-7).

SECONDARY ADRENAL CORTICAL INSUFFICIENCY (ADDISON'S DISEASE)

Bilateral metastases to the adrenal glands may lead to latent (borderline) or overt adrenal cortical insufficiency or Addison's disease (13,15, 16,19). It has been estimated that 80 to 90 percent of the adrenal gland must be replaced or destroyed before adrenal insufficiency is detected (14), which attests to the remarkable endocrine reserve of the adrenal glands with regard to cortical function; however, a variety of physiological or "stress-related" factors play a pivotal role in borderline cases in this adrenoprival state such as superimposed illness or surgery. Thomas Addison in his classic monograph in 1855 (11) first drew attention to a peculiar "bronzing" of the skin along with progressive weakness and other symptoms (such as "irritability of stomach") occurring in association with extensive destruction of the adrenal glands (or "supra-renal capsules"). Most of the 11 cases in his 39-page monograph were due to tuberculosis with near complete destruction of the adrenal glands and "conversion into a mass of strumous disease"; there were several examples due to metastatic carcinoma to the adrenal glands (cases VII: breast carcinoma, VIII: gastric carcinoma, and XI: carcinoma most likely pulmonary in origin). In two of these cases, extensive replacement of only one gland was noted at autopsy while the state of the opposite gland was not given in detail.

The true incidence of Addison's disease due to metastases to the adrenal glands is difficult to determine since the relatively nonspecific symptoms of adrenal insufficiency may be confused with cachexia or the fluid and electrolyte imbalance associated with cancer in some cases; often there is no endocrinologic testing for adrenal reserve in patients with metastases and bilateral adrenal enlargement (21). Two recent studies reported adrenal insufficiency in 19 to 33 percent of patients with known metastatic tumor and CT evidence of bilateral adrenal enlargement (17,18). A wide variety of primary malignancies can cause Addison's disease by massive adrenal replacement, most commonly metastatic lung (18) and breast carcinomas (18,20); others include renal cell carcinoma, gastric carcinoma, colonic adenocarcinoma, seminoma, pancreatic carcinoma, transitional cell carcinoma (12), and malignant melanoma (fig. 8-8) (21). Adrenal cortical carcinoma has also been reported to cause Addison's disease due to bilateral adrenal involvement (20).

Imaging Characteristics. On CT scan the involved adrenal gland is variable in size; sometimes the changes are bilateral. The involved gland is usually round or oval and may have smooth or lobulated contours. Most glands involved by metastatic tumor are of soft tissue density unless large and necrotic. Variable enhancement is evident on

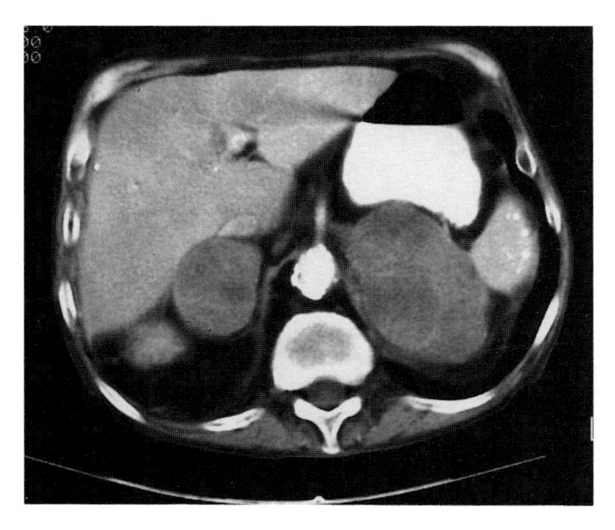
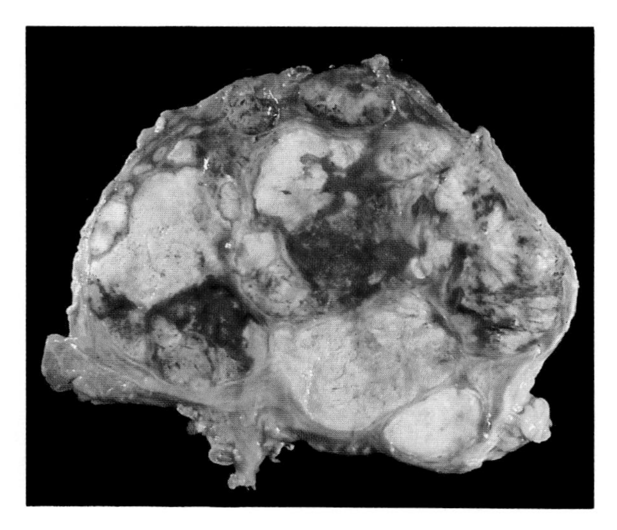

Figure 8-8
MALIGNANT MELANOMA METASTATIC TO ADRENAL GLANDS

Left: A 73-year-old man had amelanotic malignant melanoma of the right nostril diagnosed about 4 years previously. Huge bilateral adrenal masses were seen on CT scan. The patient presented with weakness, dehydration, and hyponatremia probably due in part to acute Addisonian crisis. The patient was septicemic. There was also a remote history of disseminated histoplasmosis (note calcified areas in spleen and one in liver).

Right: Both adrenal glands were completely replaced by metastatic malignant melanoma which was coarsely nodular with extensive areas of necrosis. (Photograph by Dr. Daniel H. Connor, Washington, DC.)

CT scan. On MRI, the involved adrenal gland usually has a heterogeneous signal intensity on T2-weighted images and sometimes on T1-weighted images as well, in which the adrenal gland may appear isointense or hypointense in comparison to liver. If the metastatic tumor hemorrhages internally there is usually a high signal on T1- and T2-weighted images. An adrenal metastasis may appear like an adrenal cortical adenoma on CT scan, so MRI should be performed on any solitary adrenal mass discovered in a patient with known malignancy and no other signs or symptoms of metastasis.

Pathology and Differential Diagnosis. Grossly, a metastatic malignancy (rarely seen as a surgically resected specimen) is gray-white, with or without zones of tumor necrosis (see fig. 8-1, left), and usually lacks the yellow-orange hue of an adrenal cortical primary. Gross black to brown pigmentation may arouse suspicion for a metastatic malignant melanoma. There is usually no problem in making the histologic or cytologic diagnosis of metastatic carcinoma, although some tumors, such as large cell lung carcinoma, renal cell carcinoma, or even hepatocellular carcinoma (fig. 8-9), can simulate an adrenal cortical carcinoma. Adrenal metastases from renal cell carcinoma have been reported in 5.5 percent of patients undergoing nephrectomy (fig. 8-10) (29), and in 19 percent of autopsy cases (22). Renal cell carcinoma can involve the ipsilateral adrenal gland by direct extension, and although metastasis is usually to the ipsilateral gland, contralateral metastasis can occur and potentially cause confusion with an adrenal neoplasm. Rarely, renal cell carcinoma presents with contralateral (figs. 8-11, 8-12) (24) or bilateral adrenal metastases (31). There can also be an alveolar or nesting pattern similar to that of an adrenal cortical neoplasm, but the optical clarity of the cytoplasm differs from the finely vacuolated cytoplasm seen in many adrenal cortical nodules and tumors. Correlation of clinical, radiologic, and endocrinologic data or intraoperative findings are important for a correct diagnosis. The adrenal gland also may be involved by metastatic pancreatic islet cell carcinoma which might mimic a pheochromocytoma or even an adrenal cortical carcinoma.

There are occasional diagnostic pitfalls in fine-needle aspiration of an adrenal mass. Metastatic adenocarcinoma has been reported mimicking normal adrenal cortical cells (27), and

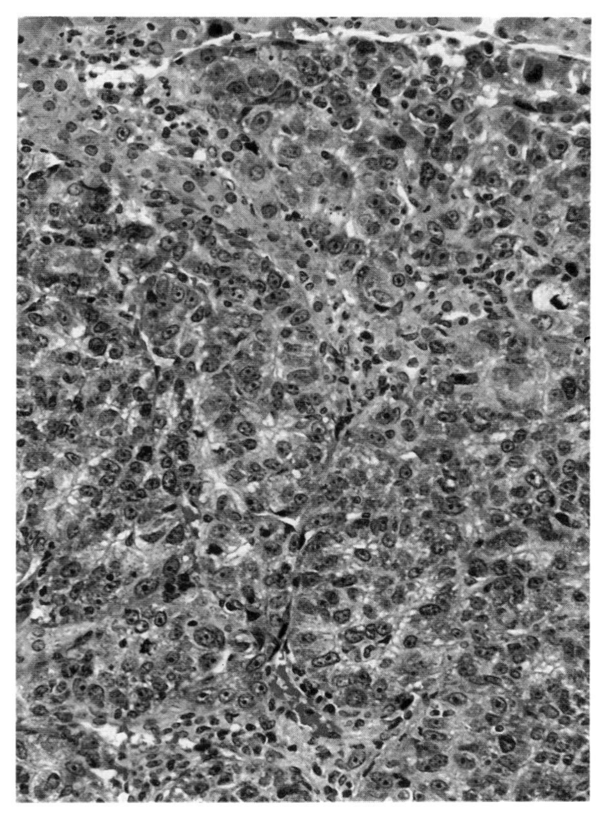

Figure 8-9
HEPATOCELLULAR CARCINOMA
METASTATIC TO ADRENAL GLAND

Hepatocellular carcinoma metastatic to adrenal gland simulated a primary adrenal tumor. The metastasis has a vague trabecular pattern and tumor cells have prominent nucleoli.

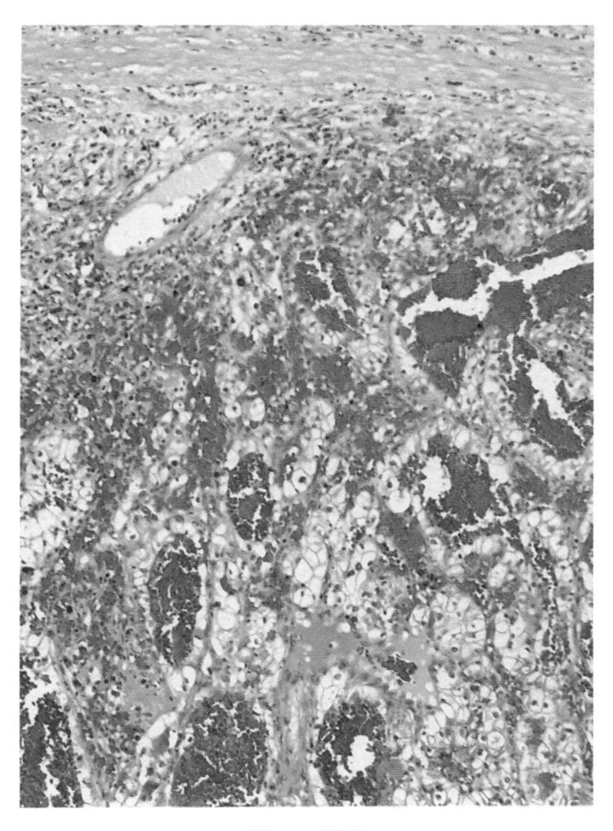

Figure 8-10
RENAL CELL CARCINOMA
METASTATIC TO ADRENAL GLAND

Small solitary adrenal metastasis from ipsilateral renal cell carcinoma. The patient had undergone radical nephrectomy for a large renal cell carcinoma.

Figure 8-11
RENAL CELL CARCINOMA
METASTATIC TO
CONTRALATERAL
ADRENAL GLAND

A 55-year-old man underwent left radical nephrectomy, including the left adrenal gland, for a large renal cell carcinoma measuring 11 cm in diameter. The tumor invaded the renal vein but was entirely resected. Note the tight, solid nesting pattern of the primary renal tumor. Most cells have optically clear cytoplasm.

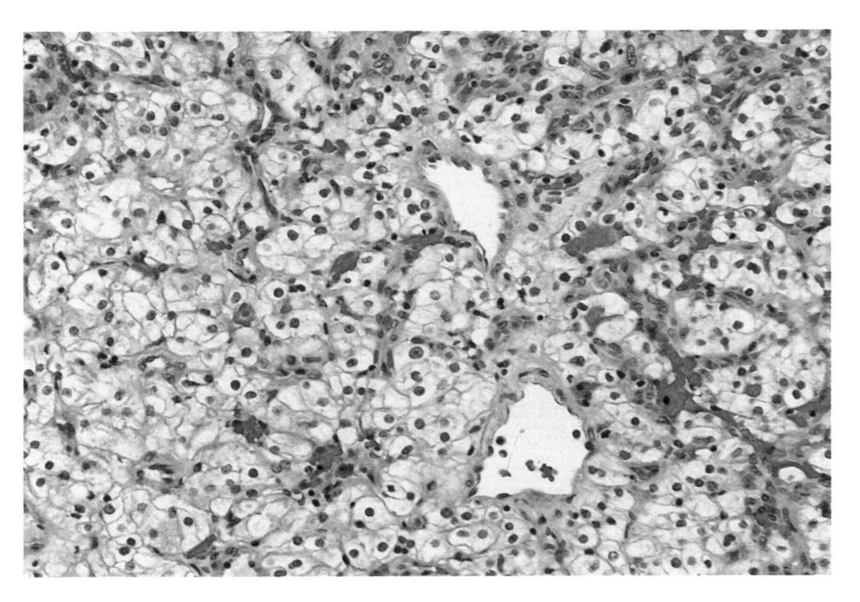

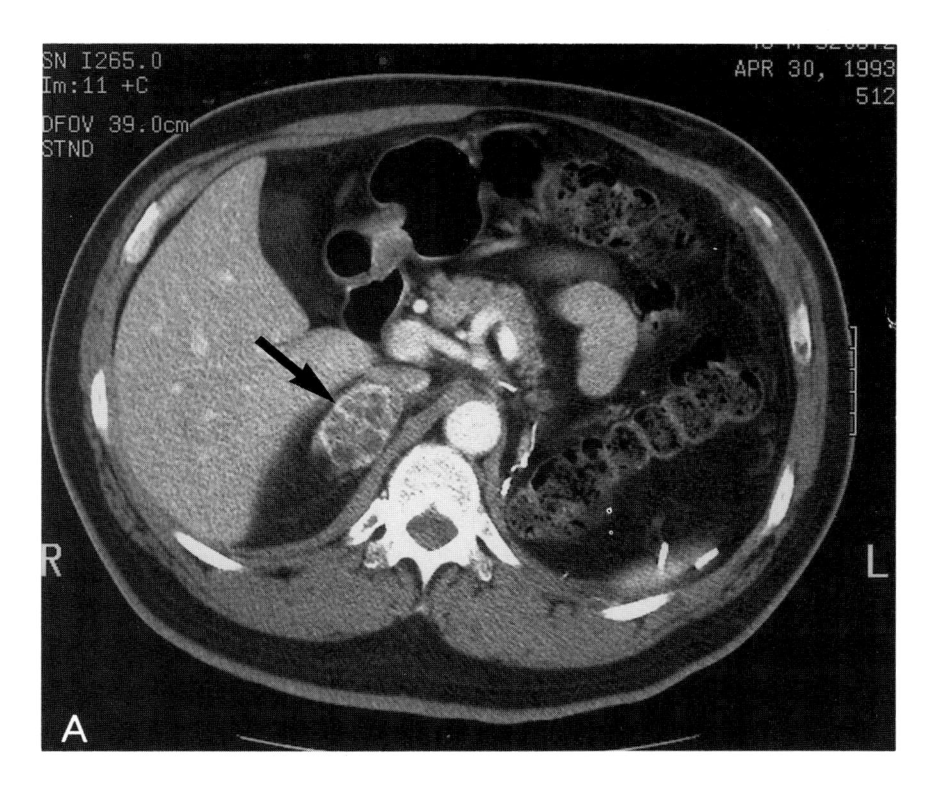

Figure 8-12
RENAL CELL CARCINOMA METASTATIC TO CONTRALATERAL ADRENAL GLAND

A: Ten months later the same patient (fig. 8-11) was found to have a contralateral right adrenal mass on CT scan which was nonhomogeneous (arrow). The few metal clips mark the surgical bed on the opposite side. There was no evidence of metastases elsewhere.

B: Cell block preparation shows small nests of metastatic renal cell carcinoma with a prominent bloody background.

C: Separate core biopsy done at same time as fine-needle aspiration shows metastatic renal cell carcinoma virtually identical to that seen 10 months earlier.

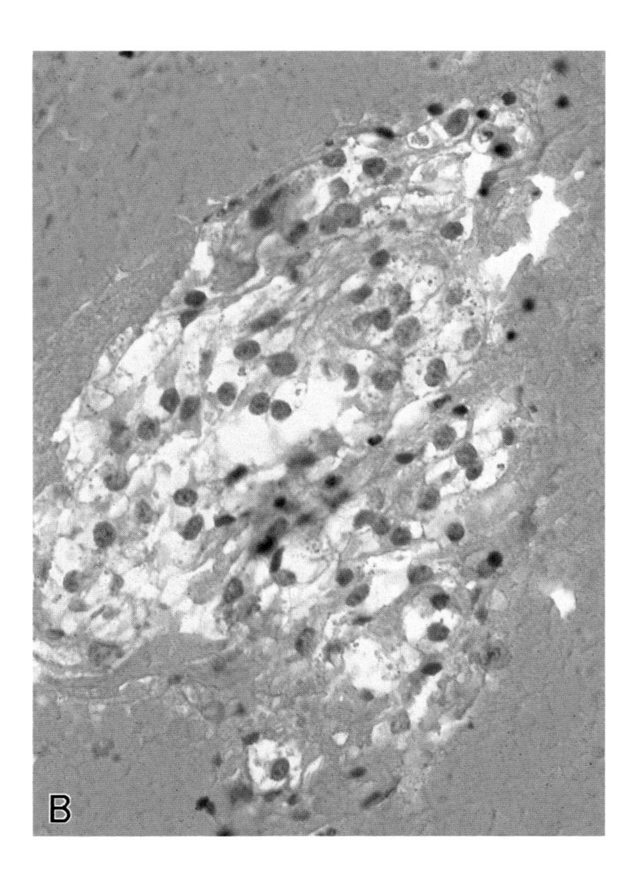

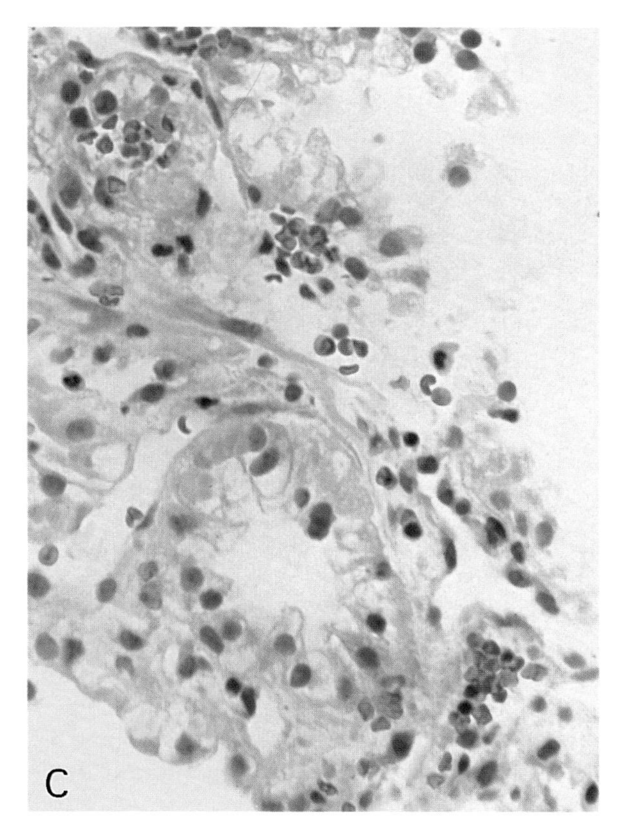

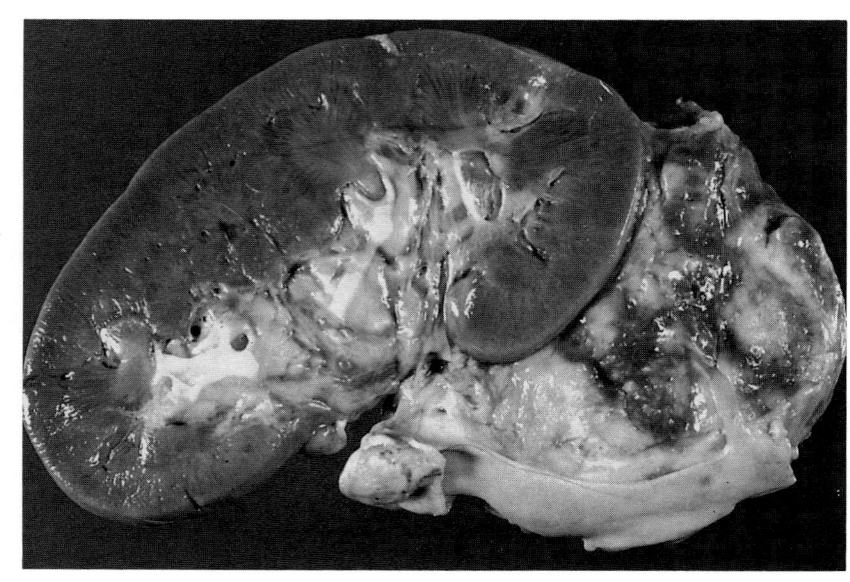

Figure 8-13
MASSIVE ADRENAL INVOLVEMENT BY MALIGNANT LYMPHOMA

This tumor was found at autopsy of a patient with disseminated lymphoma. The bulging, lobulated surface was soft and creamy white on section. (Fig. 10-4A from Travis WD, Oertel JE, Lack EE: Miscellaneous tumors and tumefactive lesions of the adrenal gland. In: Lack EE, ed. Pathology of the adrenal glands. New York: Churchill Livingstone, 1990:351–78.)

conversely, aspiration of an adrenal cortical nodule can mimic a small cell malignancy (see figure 5-33) (26). Immunohistochemical stains may help distinguish a metastatic carcinoma from a primary adrenal cortical neoplasm: adrenal cortical carcinoma is usually positive for vimentin, but some studies report a relatively low rate of positivity (28,30), and immunostains for epithelial markers such as cytokeratin and epithelial membrane antigen are usually nonreactive (23,25,32), although there may be exceptions in some cases (25,30,32).

INVOLVEMENT OF ADRENAL GLANDS BY MALIGNANT LYMPHOMA AND LEUKEMIA

Secondary involvement of the adrenal glands by malignant lymphoma is seen at autopsy in 18 to 25 percent of patients (41,42), usually those with disseminated disease (fig. 8-13). Unilateral adrenal involvement by malignant lymphoma was found in 5.5 percent of patients with Hodgkin's disease and 8 percent of patients with non-Hodgkin's malignant lymphoma; bilateral adrenal involvement has been reported in 9 percent of patients with Hodgkin's disease, and 12 percent with non-Hodgkin's malignant lymphoma (41). CT scans have demonstrated adrenal involvement by non-Hodgkin's malignant lymphoma in 3 to 4 percent of patients during their disease course (37,39). Massive bilateral involvement can result in Addison's disease, and this may be a presenting manifestation, although rarely (44). The adrenal insufficiency has been reported to resolve following treatment with combination chemotherapy. Only rarely have extranodal malignant lymphomas presented in the adrenal gland without detectable involvement elsewhere (34,36,43).

Intravascular lymphomatosis, a peculiar type of non-Hodgkin's malignant lymphoma with destructive angiotropism, can involve the adrenal glands (fig. 8-14) and cause gross enlargement detectable on CT scan. The disorder was originally felt to be a primary endothelial malignancy, hence the term malignant angioendotheliomatosis, but it was shown to be a malignant lymphoma of large cell or immunoblastic type, with B-cell or less commonly T-cell phenotype (33,35,45). The malignant cells proliferate within small vessels in most organs (fig. 8-15), but have an affinity for the central nervous system, with varied neurologic manifestations. There may be massive involvement of adrenal glands (fig. 8-14B) which can result in Addison's disease (40), and may account for the fever, hypotension, and electrolyte abnormalities frequently seen in these patients (45).

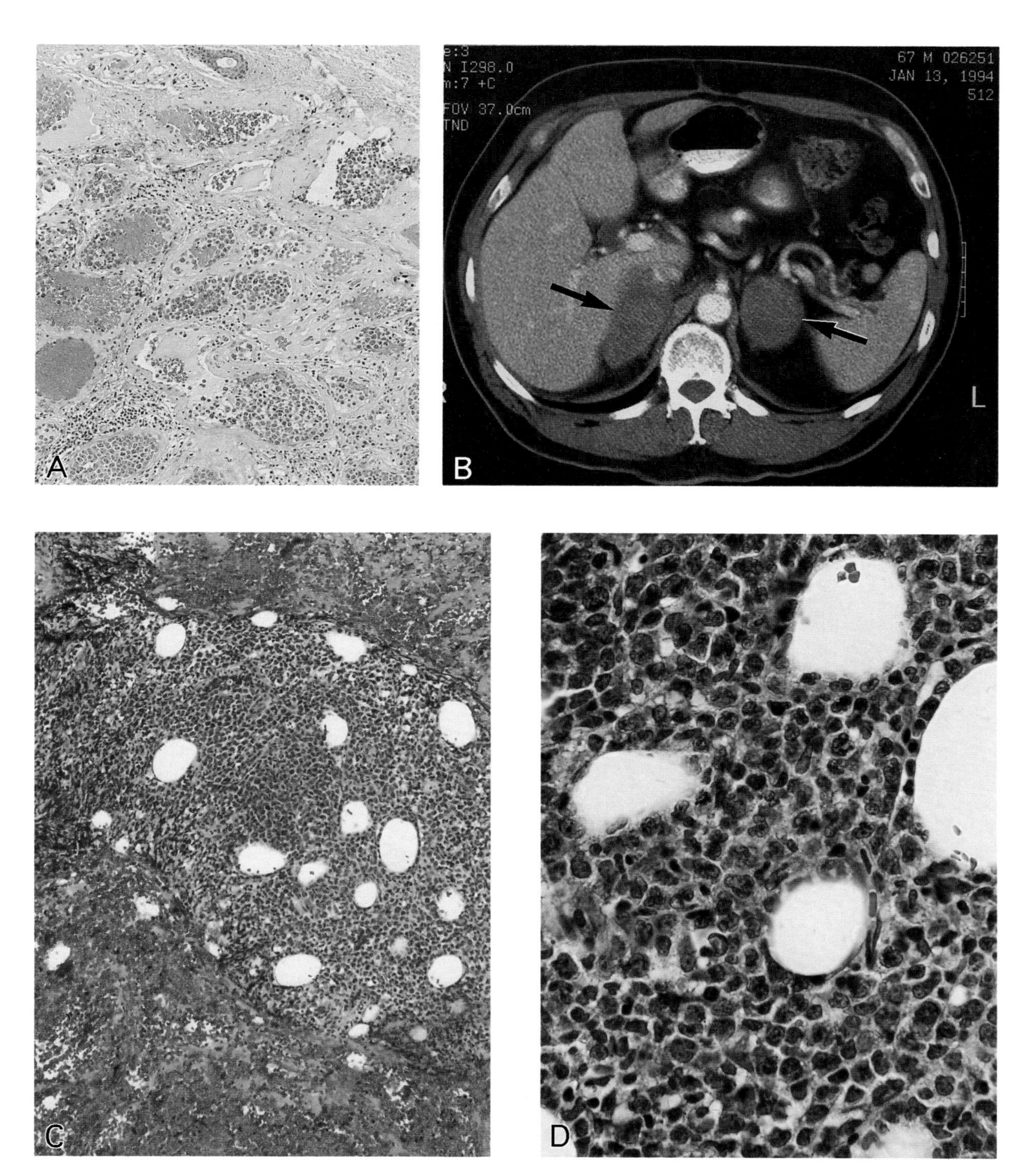

Figure 8-14
INTRAVASCULAR "LYMPHOMATOSIS" INVOLVING ADRENAL GLAND

A: An adult male patient presented with cutaneous cavernous hemangiomas involved by malignant lymphoma, non-Hodgkin's type (intravascular lymphomatosis).

B: Later, bilateral suprarenal masses (arrows) obliterating both adrenal glands were found.

C: Fine-needle aspiration in same case as A yielded small fragments of malignant lymphoma in cell block preparations.

D: A closer view shows malignant lymphoma, large cell ("histiocytic") type.

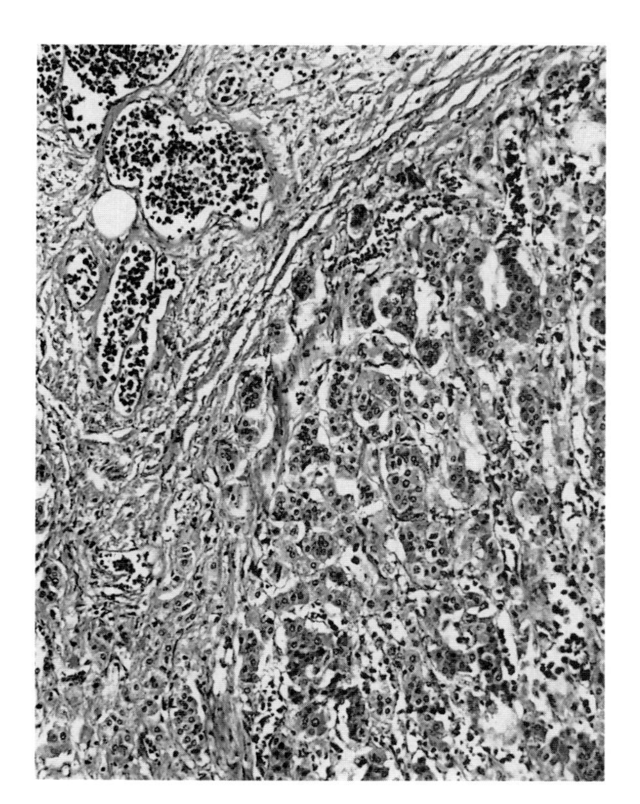

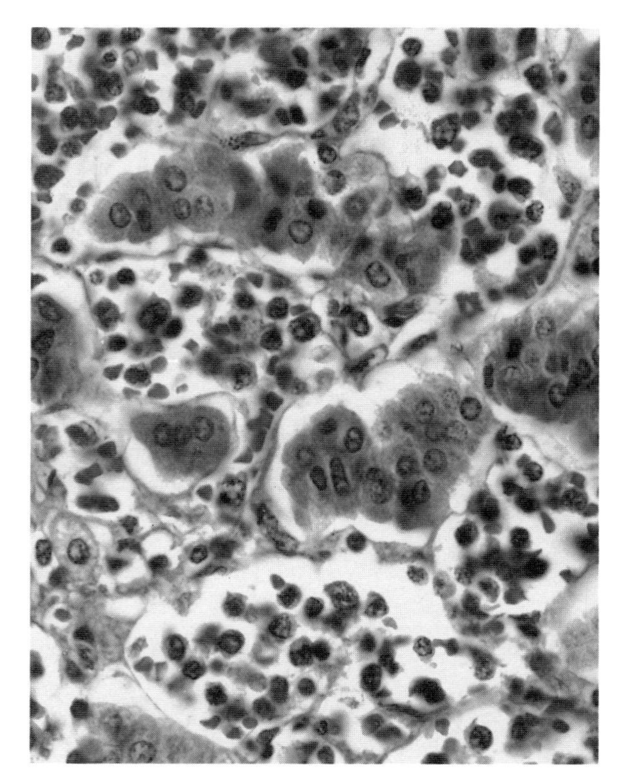

Figure 8-15

INTRAVASCULAR "LYMPHOMATOSIS" INVOLVING ADRENAL GLAND

Left: Adrenal gland from a patient with disseminated intravascular malignant lymphoma (intravascular lymphomatosis). Note the loosely cohesive malignant cells within vascular spaces in periadrenal connective tissue and within sinusoids of the adrenal cortex.

Right: Higher power view shows cytologically malignant cells distending sinusoids, with intervening short cords of cortical cells. (Fig. 10-5 from Travis WD, Oertel JE, Lack EE. Miscellaneous tumors and tumefactive lesions of the adrenal gland. In: Lack EE, ed. Pathology of the adrenal glands. New York: Churchill Livingstone, 1990:351–78.)

Plasmacytoma presenting primarily in the adrenal gland is rare (38), and the possibility of a low-grade malignant lymphoma with plasmacytoid features should be considered. The diagnosis of adrenal involvement by malignant lymphoma can be confirmed on fine-needle aspiration biopsy. Problems in differential diagnosis (e.g., metastatic undifferentiated carcinoma) can usually be resolved by immunohistochemical stains (immunopositive for leukocyte common antigen and negative for epithelial markers). Involvement of adrenal glands by leukemia is almost always an incidental finding at autopsy (fig. 8-16).

SECONDARY INVOLVEMENT BY OTHER MALIGNANT TUMORS

The adrenal glands are only rarely involved secondarily by mesenchymal neoplasms. The author has observed one case of metastatic leiomyosarcoma to the adrenal gland (unilateral and under 2 cm) from a primary arising in the duodenum (fig. 8-17). Angiosarcoma can also involve the adrenal gland secondarily. There may also be incidental involvement of the adrenal glands by Kaposi's sarcoma (fig. 8-18) as a manifestation of more widely disseminated tumor in the acquired immunodeficiency syndrome (AIDS). Both angiosarcoma and Kaposi's sarcoma have a sinusoidal pattern with extension between residual columns and cords of cortical cells and there may be extension outside the gland into periadrenal fat. As a final cautionary note, liver tissue should not be mistaken for adrenal tissue on fine-needle aspiration biopsy, since small portions of liver parenchyma can mimic adrenal cortical tissue either in aspirate smears or cell block preparations (fig. 8-19).

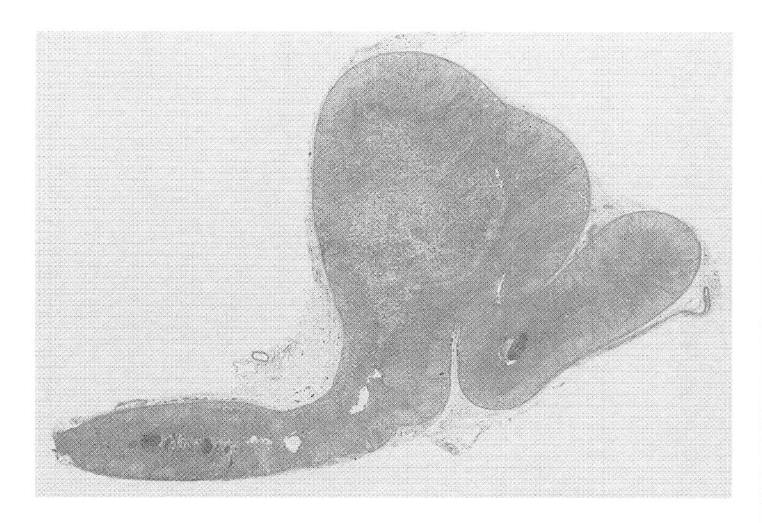

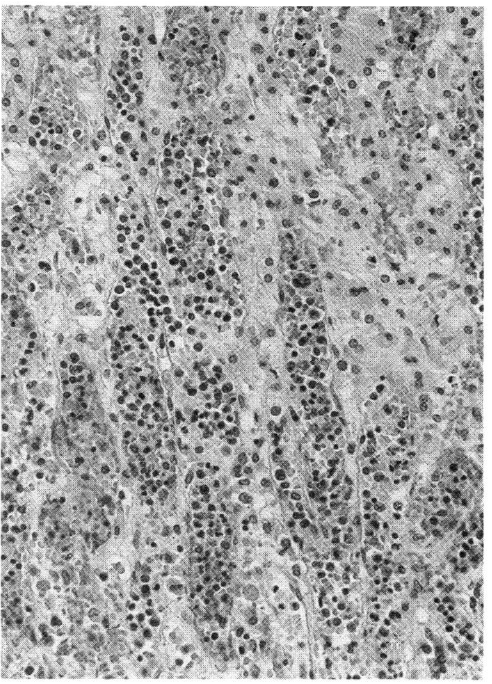

Figure 8-16
ACUTE LEUKEMIA INVOLVING ADRENAL GLAND

Left: A 51-year-old male with a history of myelofibrosis developed acute leukemic transformation and died of sepsis. Right adrenal gland weighed 18 g and was heavily infiltrated by acute leukemia.

Right: Same case showing infiltration of sinusoids by acute leukemia. Patchy areas of dystrophic calcification were also present in other areas.

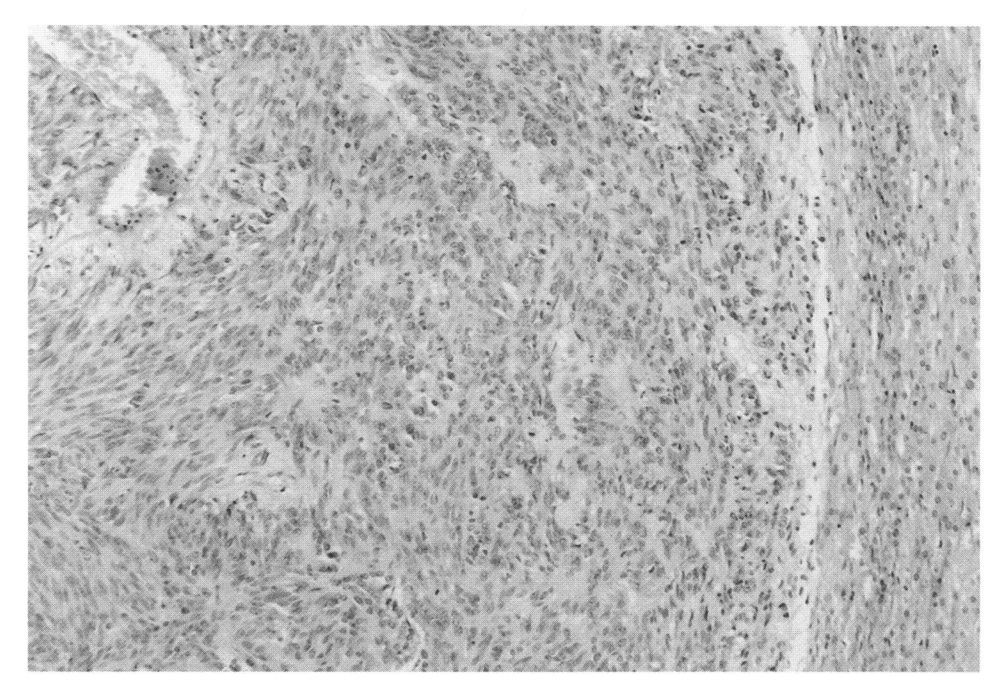

Figure 8-17
LEIOMYOSARCOMA METASTATIC TO ADRENAL GLAND

Metastatic leiomyosarcoma to adrenal gland from a primary tumor of the duodenum.

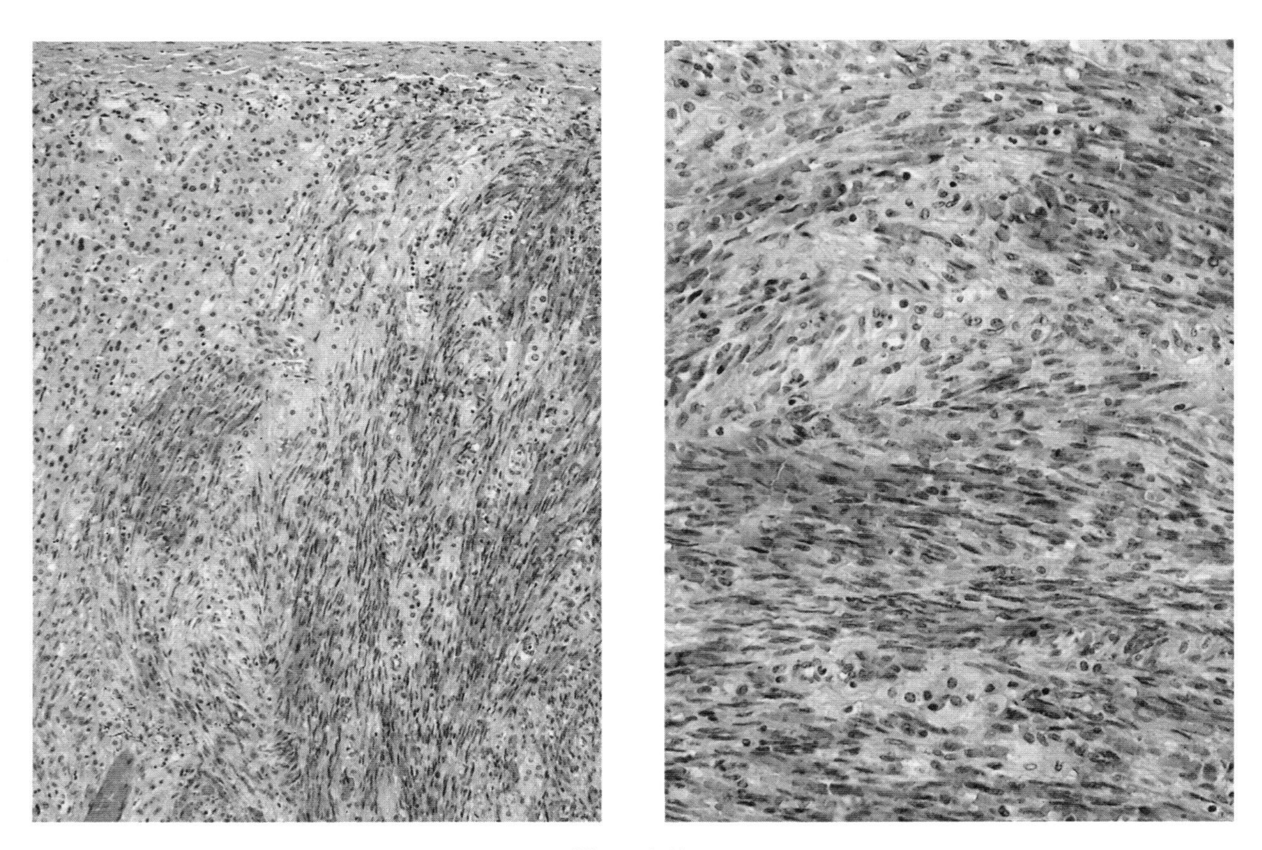

Figure 8-18
KAPOSI'S SARCOMA INVOLVING ADRENAL GLAND

Left: Kaposi's sarcoma involving adrenal gland in an adult male with acquired immunodeficiency syndrome (AIDS).
Right: Residual compressed cortical cells are widely separated by Kaposi's sarcoma. Rare hyaline globules were present.

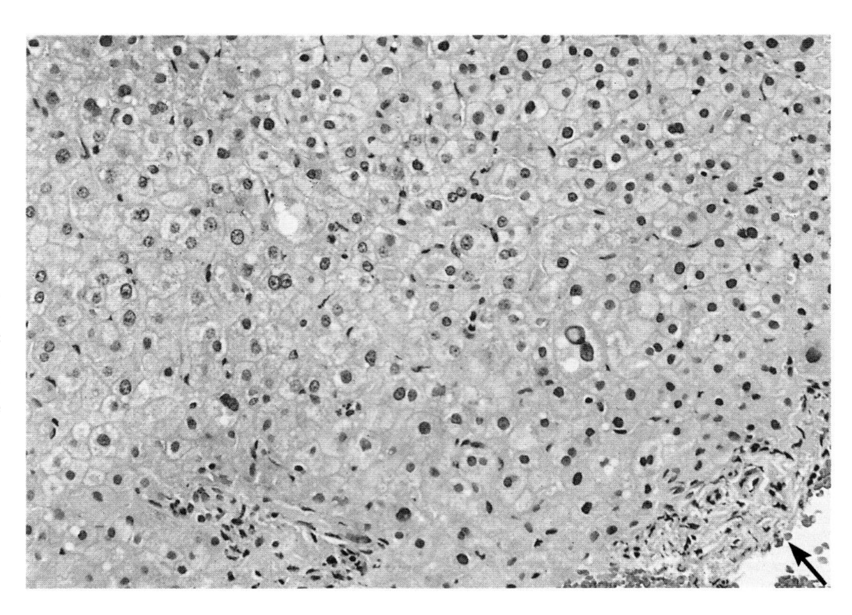

Figure 8-19
HEPATIC PARENCHYMA MIMICKING ADRENAL CORTICAL NEOPLASM

The patient had a putative adrenal mass and underwent fine-needle aspiration biopsy. The cell block shows hepatic parenchyma which had initially been regarded as a possible adrenal cortical neoplasm. Note the small portal tract in the right lower corner (arrow).

REFERENCES

Incidence and Primary Sites

1. Abrams HL, Spiro R, Goldstein N. Metastases in carcinoma. Analysis of 1,000 autopsied cases. Cancer 1950;3:74–85.
2. Allard P, Yankaskas BC, Fletcher RH, Parker LA, Halvorsen RA Jr. Sensitivity and specificity of computed tomography for the detection of adrenal metastatic lesions among 91 autopsied lung cancer patients. Cancer 1990;66:457–62.
3. de la Monte SM, Hutchins GM, Moore GW. Altered metastatic behavior of small cell carcinoma of the lung after chemotherapy and radiation. Cancer 1988;61:2176–82.
4. de la Monte SM, Hutchins GM, Moore GW. Influence of age on the metastatic behavior of breast carcinoma. Hum Pathol 1988;19:529–34.
5. Glomset DA. The incidence of metastasis of malignant tumors to the adrenals. Am J Cancer 1938;32:57–61.
6. Lack EE. Pathology of adrenal and extra-adrenal paraganglia. Major problems in pathology, Vol 29. Philadelphia: WB Saunders, 1994.
7. McMahon RF. Tumour-to-tumour metastasis: bladder carcinoma metastasizing to an adrenocortical adenoma. Br J Urol 1991;67:216–7.
8. Moriya T, Manabe T, Yamashita K, Arita S. Lung cancer metastasis to adrenocortical adenomas. A chance occurrence or a predilected phenomenon? Arch Pathol Lab Med 1988;112:286–9.
9. Sahagian-Edwards A, Holland JF. Metastatic carcinoma to the adrenal glands with cortical hypofunction. Cancer 1954;7:1242–5.
10. Willis RA. The spread of tumors in the human body. 3rd ed. London: Butterworth, 1973.

Adrenal Cortical Insufficiency (Addison's Disease)

11. Addison T. On the constitutional and local effects of disease of the supra-renal capsules. London: Samuel Highley, 1855.
12. Kennedy RL, Ball RY, Dixon AK, Apsimon AT. Metastatic transitional cell carcinoma of the bladder causing Addison's disease. J Urol 1987;137:986–8.
13. Kung, AW, Pun, KK, Lam, K, Wang, C, Leung, Y. Addisonian crisis as presenting feature in malignancies. Cancer 1990;65:177–9.
14. Lack EE, Kozakewich HP. Embryology, developmental anatomy, and selected aspects of non-neoplastic pathology In: Lack EE, ed. Pathology of the adrenal glands. New York: Churchill Livingstone, 1990:1–74.
15. Omoigui NA, Cave WT Jr, Chang AY. Adrenal insufficiency. A rare initial sign of metastatic colon carcinoma. J Clin Gastroenterol 1987;9:470–4.
16. Prayson RA, Segal GH, Stoler MH, Licata AA, Tubbs RR. Angiotropic large-cell lymphoma in a patient with adrenal insufficiency. Arch Pathol Lab Med 1991;115:1039–41.
17. Redman BG, Pazdur R, Zingas AP, Loredo R. Prospective evaluation of adrenal insufficiency in patients with adrenal metastasis. Cancer 1987;60:103–7.
18. Seidenwurm DJ, Elmer EB, Kaplan LM, Williams EK, Morris DG, Hoffman AR. Metastasis to the adrenal glands and the development of Addison's disease. Cancer 1984;54:552–7.
19. Serrano S, Tejedor L, Garcia B, Hallal H, Polo JA, Alguacil G. Addisonian crisis as the presenting feature of bilateral primary adrenal lymphoma. Cancer 1993;71:4030–3.
20. Sheeler LR, Myers JH, Eversman JJ, Taylor HC. Adrenal insufficiency secondary to carcinoma metastatic to the adrenal gland. Cancer 1983;52:1312–6.
21. Travis WD, Oertel JE, Lack EE. Miscellaneous tumors and tumefactive lesions of the adrenal gland. In: Lack EE, ed. Pathology of the adrenal glands. New York: Churchill Livingstone, 1990:351–78.

Pathology and Differential Diagnosis

22. Campbell CM, Middleton RG, Rigby OF. Adrenal metastasis in renal cell carcinoma. Urology 1983;21:403–5.
23. Cote RJ, Cordon-Cardo C, Reuter VE, Rosen PP. Immunopathology of adrenal and renal cortical tumors. Coordinated change in antigen expression is associated with neoplastic conversion in the adrenal cortex. Am J Pathol 1990;136:1077–84.
24. Foucar E, Dehner LP. Renal cell carcinoma occurring with contralateral adrenal metastasis. A clinical and pathological trap. Arch Surg 1979;114:959–63.
25. Gaffey MJ, Traweek ST, Mills SE, et al. Cytokeratin expression in adrenocortical neoplasia: an immunohistochemical and biochemical study with implications for the differential diagnosis of adrenocortical, hepatocellular and renal cell carcinoma. Hum Pathol 1992;23:144–53.
26. Min KW, Song J, Boesenberg M, Acebey J. Adrenal cortical nodule mimicking small round cell malignancy on fine needle aspiration. Acta Cytol 1988;32:543–6.
27. Mitchell ML, Ryan FP Jr, Shermer RW. Pulmonary adenocarcinoma metastatic to the adrenal gland mimicking normal adrenal cortical epithelium on fine needle aspiration. Acta Cytol 1985;29:994–8.
28. Miettinen M, Lehto VP, Dahl D, Virtanen I. Immunofluorescence microscopic evaluation of the intermediate filament expression of the adrenal cortex and medulla and their tumors. Am J Pathol 1985;118:360–6.
29. O'Brien WM, Lynch JH. Adrenal metastases by renal cell carcinoma. Incidence at nephrectomy. Urology 1987;29:605–7.
30. Schröder S, Padberg BC, Achilles E, Hull K, Dralle H, Klöppel G. Immunocytochemistry in adrenocortical tumors: a clinicomorphological study of 72 neoplasms. Virchows Arch [A] 1992;420:65–70.
31. Selli C, Carini M, Barbanti G, Barbagli G, Turini D. Simultaneous bilateral adrenal involvement by renal cell carcinoma: experience with 3 cases. J Urol 1987;137:480–2.
32. Wick MR, Cherwitz DL, McGlennan RC, Dehner LP. Adrenocortical carcinoma. An immunohistochemical comparison with renal cell carcinoma. Am J Pathol 1986;122:343–52.

Secondary Involvement by Malignant Lymphoma, Leukemia, and Other Malignant Tumors

33. Carrol TJ Jr, Schelper RL, Goeken JA, Kemp JD. Neoplastic angioendotheliomatosis: immunopathologic and morphologic evidence for intravascular malignant lymphomatosis. Am J Clin Pathol 1986;85:169–75.
34. Choi CH, Durishin M, Garbudawala ST, Richard J. Non-Hodgkin's lymphoma of the adrenal gland. Arch Pathol Lab Med 1990;114:883–5.
35. Glass J, Hochberg FH, Miller DC. Intravascular lymphomatosis. A systemic disease with neurologic manifestations. Cancer 1993;71:3156–64.
36. Harris GJ, Tio FO, Von Hoff DD. Primary adrenal lymphoma. Cancer 1989;63:799–803.
37. Jafri SZ, Francis IR, Glazer GM, Bree RL, Amendola MA. CT detection of adrenal lymphoma. J Comput Assist Tomogr 1983;7:254–6.
38. Page DL, DeLellis RA, Hough AJ Jr. Tumors of the adrenal. Atlas of Tumor Pathology. 2nd Series, Fascicle 23. Washington, D.C.: Armed Forces Institute of Pathology, 1986.
39. Paling MR, Williamson BR. Adrenal involvement in non-Hodgkin lymphoma. AJR Am J Roentgenol 1983;141:303–5.
40. Prayson RA, Segal GH, Stoler MH, Licata AA, Tubbs RR. Angiotropic large-cell lymphoma in a patient with adrenal insufficiency. Arch Pathol 1991;115:1039–41.
41. Richmond J, Sherman RS, Diamond HD, Craver LF. Renal lesions associated with malignant lymphomas. Am J Med 1962;32:184–207.
42. Rosenberg SA, Diamond HD, Jaslowitz B, Craver LF. Lymphosarcoma. A review of 1269 cases. Medicine 1961;40:31–84.
43. Schnitzer B, Smid D, Lloyd RV. Primary T-cell lymphoma of the adrenal glands with adrenal insufficiency. Hum Pathol 1986;17:634–6.
44. Serrano S, Tejedor L, Garcia B, Hallal H, Polo JA, Alguacil G. Addisonian crisis as the presenting feature of bilateral primary adrenal lymphoma. Cancer 1993;71:4030–3.
45. Wick MR, Mills SE, Scheithauer BW, Cooper PH, Davitz MA, Parkinson K. Reassessment of malignant angioendotheliomatosis. Evidence in favor of its reclassification as intravascular lymphomatosis. Am J Surg Pathol 1986;10:112–23.

9

ADRENAL MEDULLARY HYPERPLASIA AND MULTIPLE ENDOCRINE NEOPLASIA (MEN) SYNDROME TYPE II

Definition. Adrenal medullary hyperplasia (AMH) is defined as an increase in the number of chromaffin cells, with expansion of the medullary compartment into areas of the gland where it is not normally present. Expansion in volume of the medullary compartment may result in increased gland size and weight as well as increased proportion of medulla relative to cortex when viewed in transverse section. AMH may be diffuse, nodular, or a combination of both. The morphologic features may be symmetric or asymmetric.

General Features. AMH may be accompanied by clinical and biochemical evidence of hyperfunction, i.e., excess secretion of catecholamines. AMH should not be an unexpected entity since hyperplasia is identified in virtually all other endocrine tissues. AMH is usually seen in association with multiple endocrine neoplasia (MEN) syndrome types IIa and IIb, but it has also been reported in other settings where it can mimic a pheochromocytoma. Hyperplasia of extra-adrenal paraganglia of the sympathoadrenal neuroendocrine system is rare although it has been noted in the Beckwith-Wiedemann syndrome (2,3,21). Anatomic documentation of AMH necessitates careful dissection and weighing of the gland and use of morphometric techniques (see chapter 1).

SPORADIC ADRENAL MEDULLARY HYPERPLASIA

There is mounting evidence that AMH exists as a distinct entity, but accurate identification may depend upon rigid morphometric criteria or close correlation with clinical and endocrinologic data (14). The clinical picture may resemble that of pheochromocytoma, with paroxysmal hypertension, diaphoresis, and tachycardia, yet no pheochromocytoma or extra-adrenal paraganglioma is found on laparotomy (1,6–8,13,15,16, 18,20,22–24). AMH, therefore, is part of the differential diagnosis of pseudopheochromocytoma (14). AMH may be complicated by catecholamine "acute abdomen" with ileus, abdominal distension, and pain (6). Many patients with sporadic AMH experience amelioration of signs or symptoms of excess catecholamine secretion following surgical resection of one or both adrenal glands. Biochemical documentation of increased catecholamine secretion is a prerequisite for a diagnosis of AMH for some (10). In a review of 15 patients with sporadic (simple) AMH, 7 experienced marked improvement following surgery, and 5 had partial reduction in hypertension; 2 of the 3 patients who experienced no benefit from surgery died of cerebral hemorrhage or thrombosis (23).

AMH has been noted in some patients with cystic fibrosis (fig. 9-1), and elevated catecholamine levels (mainly epinephrine) were seen with quantitative analysis of medullary tissue at autopsy (5). In this study, a single transverse section from each adrenal gland from six patients with cystic fibrosis proved positive for AMH, although no specific morphometric techniques were described. An enlarged "mass" of chromaffin cells was reported in the adrenal medullae of victims of sudden infant death syndrome (SIDS), and has been used as evidence supporting chronic alveolar hypoventilation, along with increased musculature in small pulmonary arteries, abnormal retention of brown fat, and extramedullary hematopoiesis (17). Adrenal corticomedullary hyperplasia has been demonstrated in rats exposed to hypobarism at a simulated altitude of 5,500 m, and is reported to closely resemble some pheochromocytomas (9). There is some suggestion that extra-adrenal chromaffin cells may secrete catecholamines in response to hypoxemia (11), but currently there is no evidence of increased medullary activity in humans acclimatized to high altitude (9). AMH presumably reflects an ongoing need for catecholamines in chronic hypoxemia, but does not necessarily indicate an underlying direct chemoreceptor function (9). Sporadic AMH has also been considered a cause of hypertension in the pediatric age group (4). It has been reported in association with Cushing's syndrome due to an adrenal cortical adenoma, and may contribute to the hypertension (12).

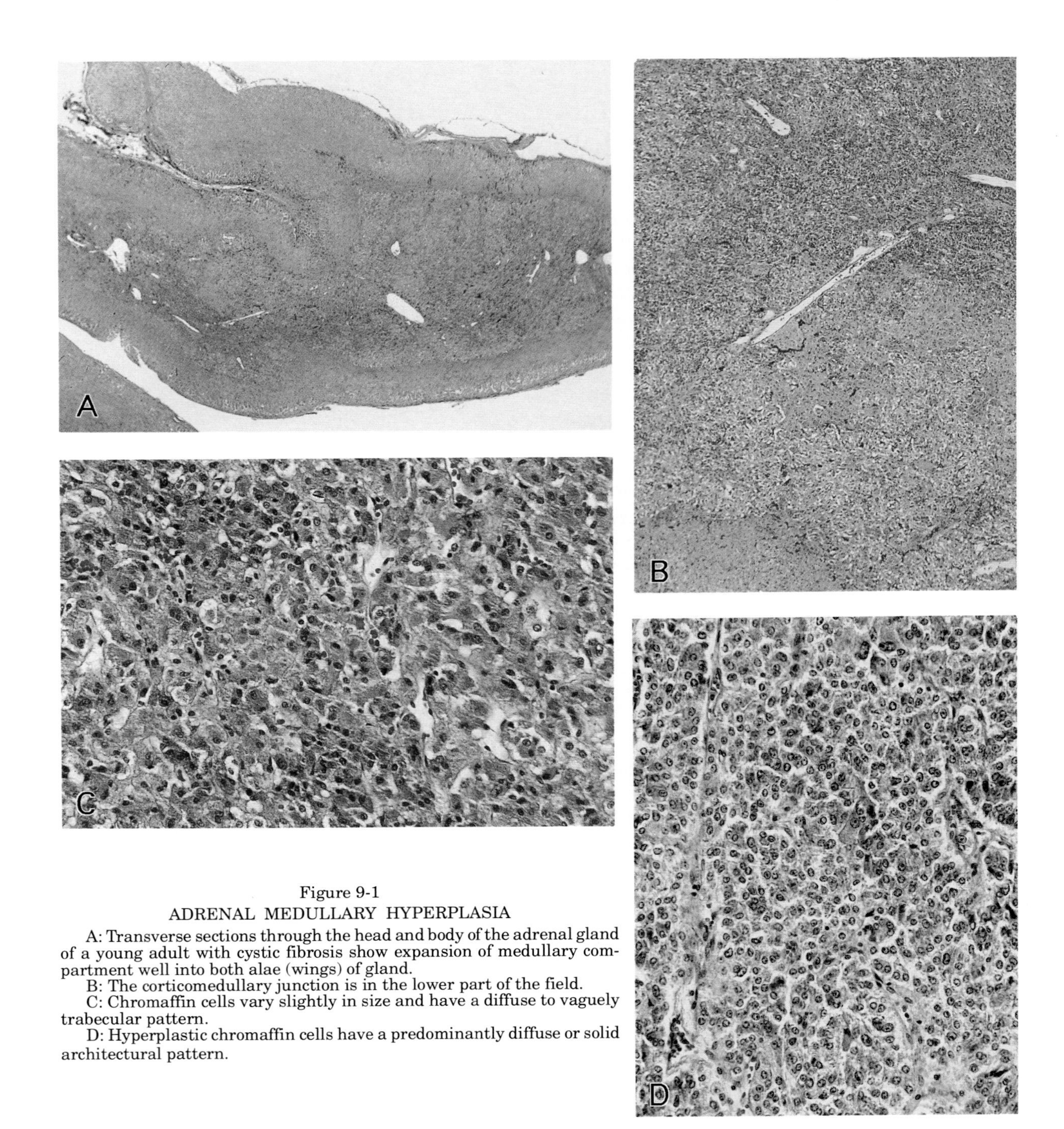

Figure 9-1
ADRENAL MEDULLARY HYPERPLASIA

A: Transverse sections through the head and body of the adrenal gland of a young adult with cystic fibrosis show expansion of medullary compartment well into both alae (wings) of gland.

B: The corticomedullary junction is in the lower part of the field.

C: Chromaffin cells vary slightly in size and have a diffuse to vaguely trabecular pattern.

D: Hyperplastic chromaffin cells have a predominantly diffuse or solid architectural pattern.

AMH has been reported in the Beckwith-Wiedemann syndrome (see fig. 2-22) (2,21); 85 percent of these cases are sporadic in nature (14). Five of six infants studied by Beckwith (3) had AMH, and in one case there was "definite hyperplasia" of extra-adrenal paraganglia. The adrenal medulla and extra-adrenal paraganglia may show an inappropriate degree of development for the infantile age group. A case of malignant giant pheochromocytoma has been reported in association with hemihypertrophy (19).

FAMILIAL ADRENAL MEDULLARY HYPERPLASIA

AMH has been well established as a pathologic entity in the MEN syndrome types IIa and IIb, and is regarded as the precursor of pheochromocytomas in these disorders (27,28,30). The Beckwith-Wiedemann syndrome can also occur in a familial manner. There may be other familial settings in which pheochromocytomas arise, such as von Recklinghausen's disease and von Hipple-Lindau disease, but the precursor lesion (presumably AMH) has not been as well characterized as in MEN type II (39).

Multiple Endocrine Neoplasia (MEN) Syndromes

In 1961 Sipple (43) first noted a significant increase in the incidence of thyroid carcinoma in patients with pheochromocytoma; in 1965 it was shown independently by two groups that the thyroid malignancy was medullary thyroid carcinoma (MTC) (42,47), a distinctive thyroid malignancy recognized in 1951 by Horn (34) and more fully characterized by Hazard et al. in 1959 (33). C-cell hyperplasia was subsequently shown to be the precursor of MTC in this familial disorder (49). The characteristic neuromas of the oral mucosa were noted by Williams and Pollock (48) along with ganglioneuromatosis of the gastrointestinal tract. It was suggested by Steiner et al. (44) that the combination of MTC, pheochromocytoma, and parathyroid disease be referred to as MEN type II, and the multiple mucosal neuroma complex be designated MEN type IIb or MEN type III. The presence of AMH and its relation to pheochromocytoma as a precursor lesion is consistent with Knudson's "two mutational event or hit" theory for initiation of neoplasia, with AMH being the first or genetic mutational event (29,38).

MEN Syndrome Type IIa (Sipple's Syndrome). MEN syndrome type IIa has an autosomal dominant mode of inheritance with a high degree of penetrance. The syndrome includes pheochromocytoma, MTC, and parathyroid hyperplasia. About 25 percent of patients have clinical or biochemical evidence of hyperparathyroidism (25); in some patients the enlarged parathyroids are noted during surgery for thyroid cancer (36). A parathyroid mitogenic factor has been detected in the plasma from patients with MEN type I, but it has not been found in patients with MEN type II, thus suggesting a different mechanism for promoting parathyroid hyperplasia (26). The MTC is usually the most prominent component of the syndrome, and almost invariably precedes development of the pheochromocytoma. Some patients with MEN type IIa also have Hirschsprung's disease; 9 percent of individuals in one family were affected (46).

MEN Syndrome Type IIb. MEN syndrome type IIb also has an autosomal dominant mode of inheritance, but many cases occur in isolated or sporadic fashion. Explanations for this apparent sporadic occurrence include lack of a careful pedigree analysis and systematic screening of family members or a new genetic mutation that is fatal before the patient passes the syndrome on to a future generation (37). The phenotypic expression of MEN type IIb is distinctive (see chapter 10), and important to recognize early in the disorder; the syndrome may have gastrointestinal manifestations, ophthalmologic findings, and the characteristic neuromatous proliferation within mucosa of lips, tongue, and other mucosal sites including gastrointestinal tract.

Pathology of AMH and Distinction from Pheochromocytoma

The pathologic diagnosis of AMH sometimes requires rigorous application of morphometric criteria (see chapter 1), particularly when morphologic changes are borderline or subtle; at other times the diagnosis is easily made on gross examination of the gland following transverse sectioning (fig. 9-2). Removal of periadrenal connective tissue and fat and sectioning of the gland at narrow intervals in the transverse plane permits more precise evaluation of the amount, character, and distribution of chromaffin tissue. Nodular or diffuse hyperplasia is a characteristic feature of MEN types IIa and IIb, and the pheochromocytomas are frequently multicentric and bilateral. AMH can be nodular, diffuse, or both, with symmetric or asymmetric involvement of the adrenal glands (fig. 9-3), or, in a small proportion of cases, the glands may appear normal. In a study of adrenal glands from 19 patients with MEN type II (6 had MEN type IIb), 14 had symmetric involvement (multilobular pheochromocytoma, nodular or diffuse AMH, or normal gland), 4 had asymmetric involvement, and 1 had only unilateral changes (27).

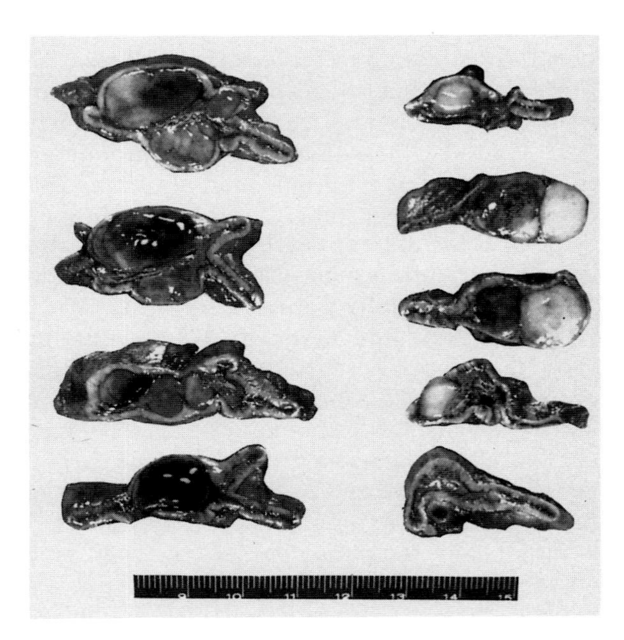

Figure 9-2
NODULAR HYPERPLASIA AND
MEN SYNDROME TYPE IIA

Transverse sections of bilateral adrenalectomy specimens from a 36-year-old man with MEN syndrome type IIa (Sipple's syndrome). Left adrenal weighed 15 g and right 15.4 g. Both glands show numerous nodules of hyperplastic chromaffin cells with some representing small pheochromocytomas using the "1-cm rule." Nodules vary in color from gray-white to deeply congested red-brown. (Fig. 11-3 from Lack EE. Pathology of adrenal and extra-adernal paraganglia. Major problems in pathology, Vol 29. Philadelphia: WB Saunders Co, 1994:224.)

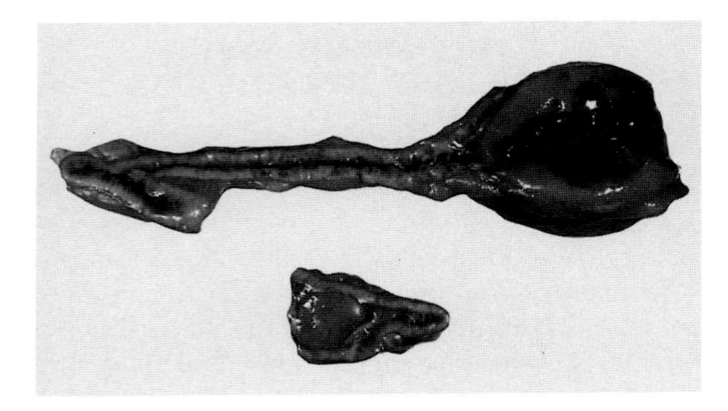

Figure 9-3
NODULAR HYPERPLASIA AND
MEN SYNDROME TYPE IIA

Transverse sections of adrenal gland from a patient with MEN syndrome type IIa. Nodular and diffuse adrenal medullary hyperplasia (AMH) are evident along with a small pheochromocytoma using the "1-cm rule."

Nodules of AMH may be pale gray to tan and fleshy, but some vary in color and texture (fig. 9-2). On low-power magnification there is often a mixed pattern of diffuse and nodular hyperplasia, with expansion of the medullary compartment into one or both alae (fig. 9-4), or into the tail of the gland. There may be compression and distortion of adjacent cortex by nodular expansion of the medulla. An invasive or frankly infiltrative pattern is not seen, but there is typically no histologic evidence of true encapsulation, and sometimes there may be intermingling of cortical and medullary cells. Some nodules of hyperplastic chromaffin cells are partially molded one to the other with merging patterns (fig. 9-5), and some may present a more complicated pattern with vague nodules within a larger nodule, suggesting different clones of proliferating chromaffin cells (39). Various architectural patterns can be found in AMH that are similar to those in pheochromocytoma, such as nesting or alveolar arrangement of cells (fig. 9-6A), anastomosing trabeculae (fig. 9-6B), a solid or diffuse growth, or even a spindle cell component (fig. 9-6C). Diffuse hyperplasia may antedate nodular hyperplasia, and represent the earliest morphologic correlate of chromaffin cell hyperfunction.

Hyaline globules can be conspicuous in AMH in MEN type II (fig. 9-7), and there may also be large numbers of vacuolated or granular cells, possibly reflecting increased secretory activity (39). There may be marked nuclear hyperchromasia and pleomorphism (fig. 9-8), and mitotic figures are found in some cases, although they are not numerous. In one study, enlarged nuclei were often seen in the juxtacortical area (30). A recent study of the DNA content in AMH and pheochromocytoma reported diploid or euploid histograms in normal and hyperplastic glands while 33 of 38 clinically benign pheochromocytomas (87 percent) and all 5 malignant pheochromocytomas were aneuploid or nondiploid (40).

The distinction between AMH and pheochromocytoma is arbitrary, and it may be very difficult at times to distinguish between the two, particularly when the AMH is nodular (fig. 9-9). Carney et al. (27) designated nodules 1 cm or larger as pheochromocytoma and nodules smaller than 1 cm as nodular AMH; this arbitrary designation was based upon the lower limit in size of pheochromocytoma as defined in the first series Armed

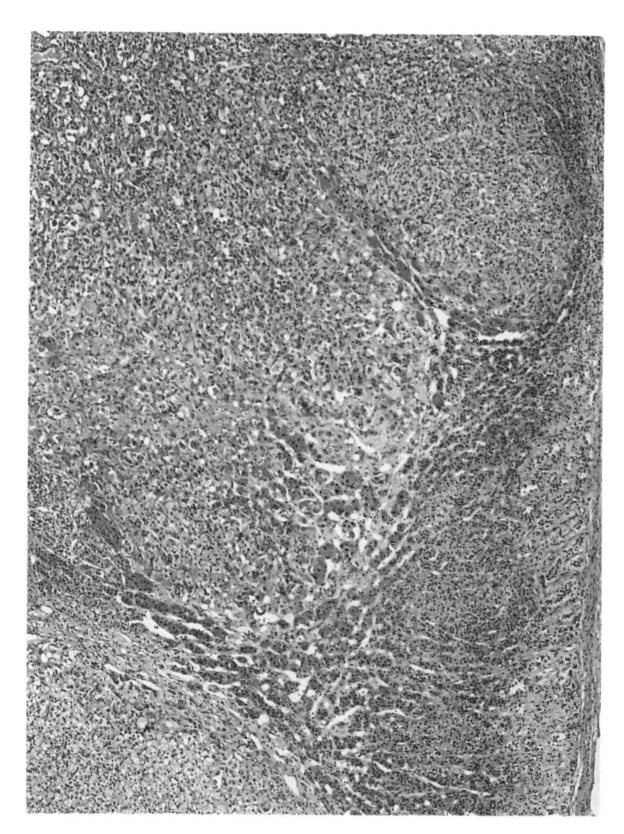

Figure 9-4
NODULAR AND DIFFUSE AMH IN MEN TYPE IIA
Nodular and diffuse AMH in adrenal gland from a patient with MEN syndrome type IIa. Smoothly contoured nodular expansions of chromaffin cells compress the adjacent cortex, with some intermingling of lipid-depleted cortical cells. Occasional hyaline globules were evident.

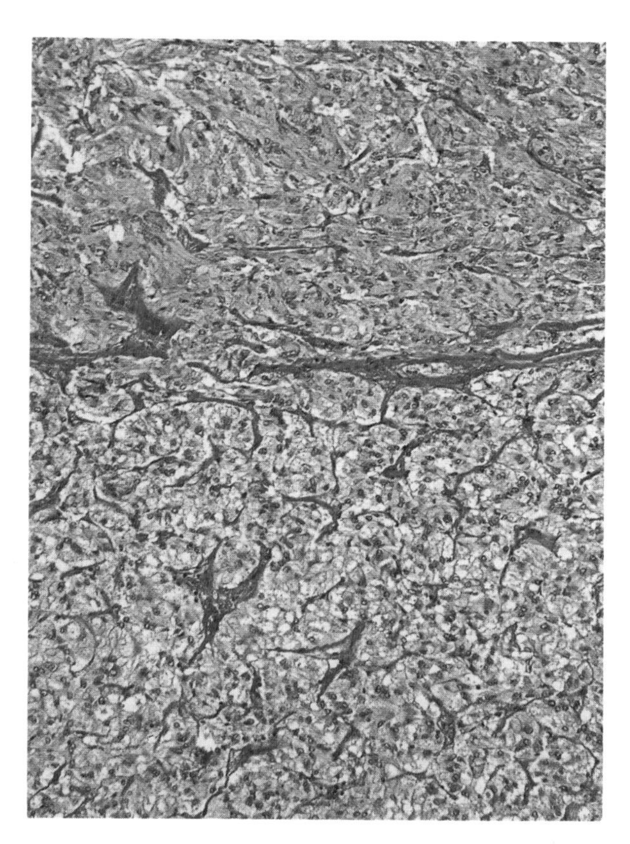

Figure 9-5
NODULAR AMH IN PATIENT WITH MEN SYNDROME TYPE IIA
Two juxtaposed nodules without any encapsulation are seen. Nodule at the top has a spindle cell component while the nodule on the bottom has nesting (alveolar) and trabecular patterns.

Forces Institute of Pathology Fascicle on adrenal neoplasms published in 1950 (35). Pheochromocytomas in MEN type II are discussed in chapter 10. Some regard pheochromocytoma as representing an extreme degree of hyperplasia rather than a true neoplasm (30). In MEN syndrome type II there may be advanced pathology of the adrenal medulla, without clinical evidence of disease, and laboratory testing may yield variable results (27). The tumors may not even respond to the usual provocative tests which have been used for diagnosing pheochromocytomas (41). One of the early indications of adrenal medullary hyperfunction in MEN type II is an elevated ratio of epinephrine to norepinephrine in urine (30,31), or increased levels of epinephrine in tissues of AMH; this is in contrast to sporadic pheochromocytoma where norepinephrine predominates (27,31,32,42). When adrenal medullary disease has been detected in a patient with MEN type II, some have recommended bilateral total adrenalectomy (27). Functional as well as anatomic evidence of adrenal medullary abnormalities can be detected in some patients with ^{131}I-metaiodobenzylguanidine scintigraphy (45).

PROLIFERATIVE LESIONS OF ADRENAL MEDULLA IN RATS

Diffuse and nodular AMH can develop spontaneously in various strains of aging rats or be induced experimentally by exogenous xenobiotic agents such as drugs (reserpine, nicotine, growth hormone, estrogen, and retinoids) (51,53, 54,58) and irradiation (60). The most important

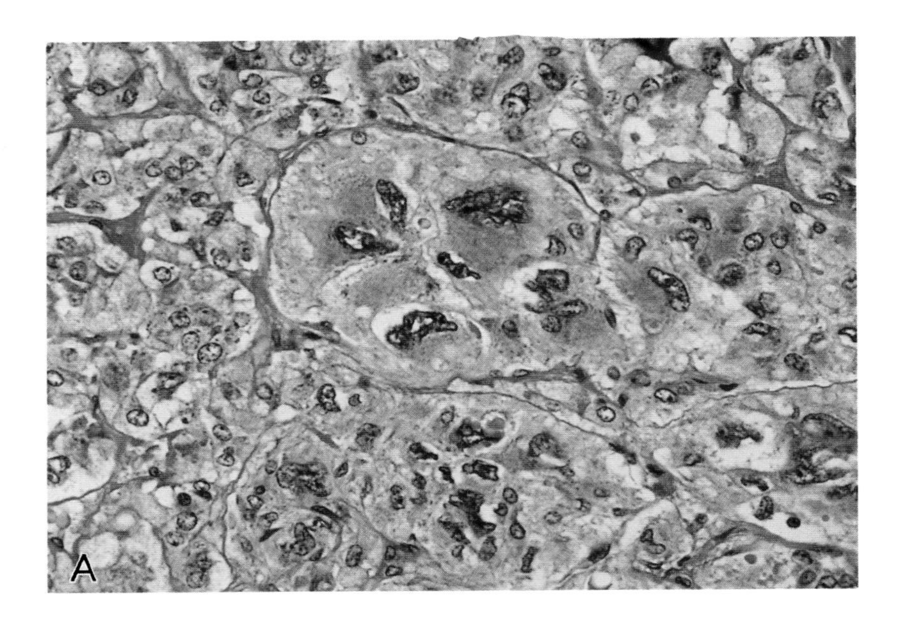

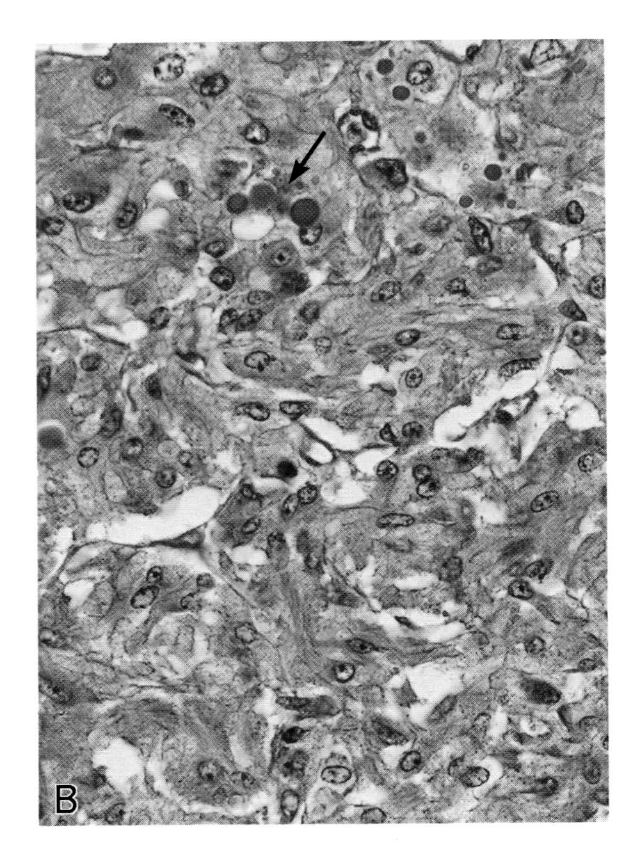

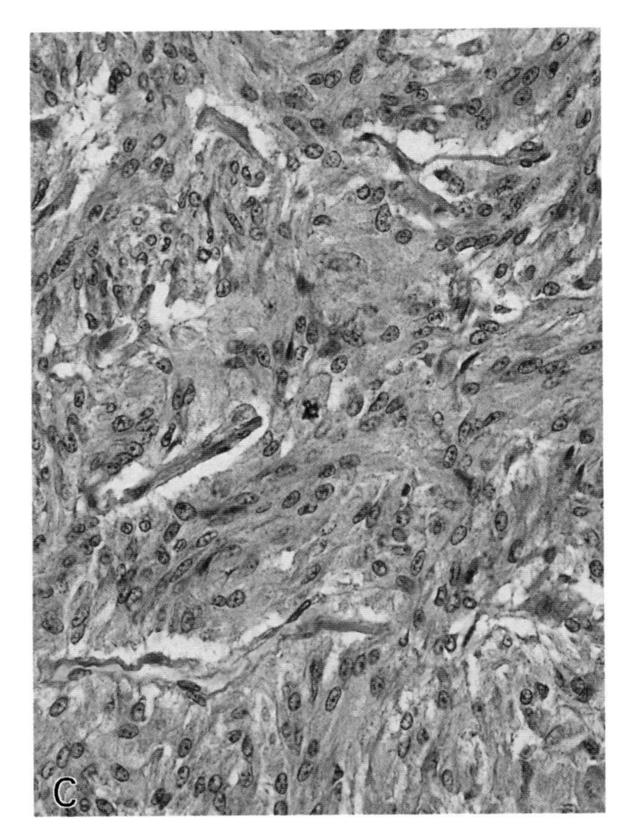

Figure 9-6
NODULAR AMH IN MEN TYPE IIA

A: Nesting or alveolar pattern with moderate degree of nuclear enlargement and hyperchromasia.
B: Anastomosing trabecular pattern in nodular AMH. Cells have pale to compact cytoplasm. Note the large hyaline globules (arrow).
C: Spindle cell pattern in nodular AMH. Most nuclei are also elongate in the same axis.

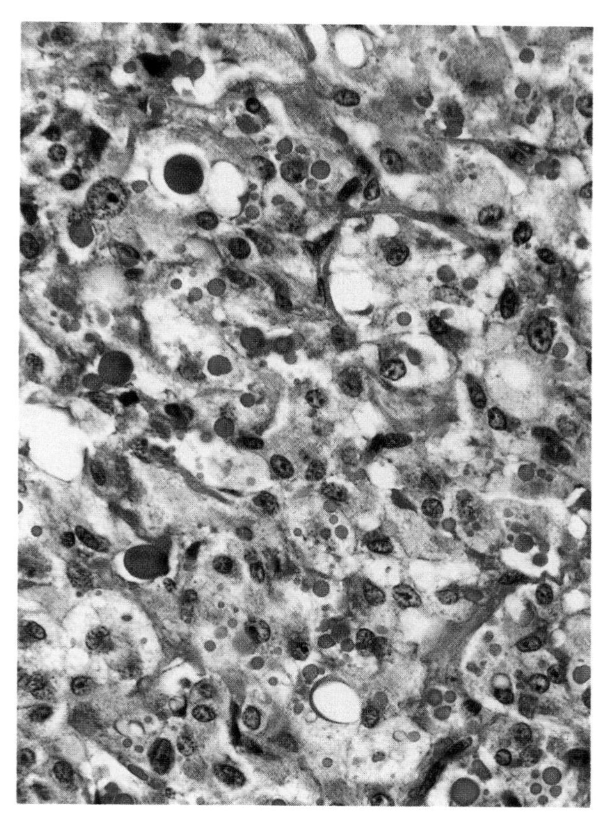

Figure 9-7
NODULAR AND DIFFUSE AMH IN MEN TYPE IIA
Hyperplastic chromaffin cells contain abundant eosinophilic hyaline globules. Some globules appear to reside within the extracellular space but this is probably artifact.

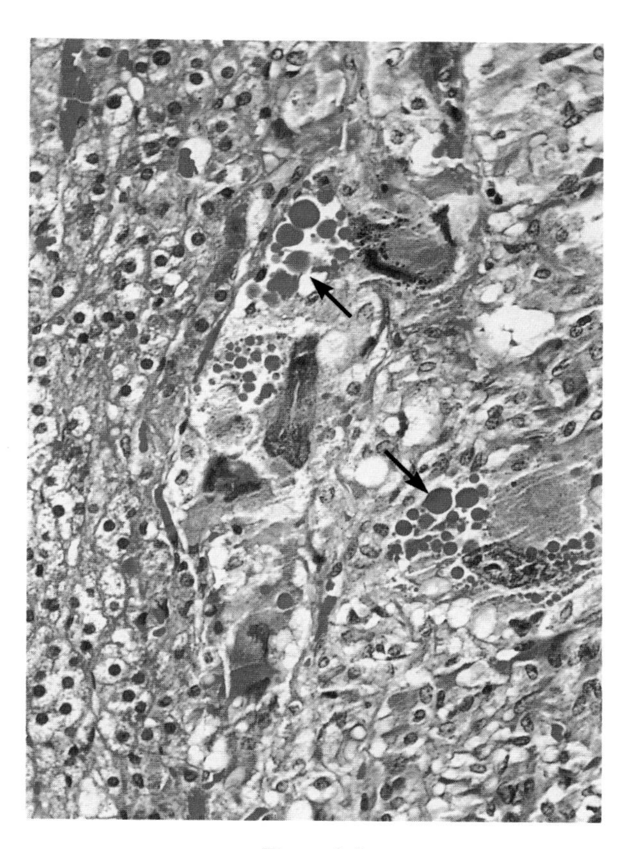

Figure 9-8
NODULAR AMH IN MEN TYPE IIA
Chromaffin cells near adjacent cortex (left) have enlarged pleomorphic nuclei and intracytoplasmic hyaline globules (arrows).

endogenous factor appears to be a genetic predisposition (52,53). Proliferation of extra-adrenal paraganglia has also been reported in older animals (50), although this has not been seen by other investigators (55). Chromaffin cells of the adult rat adrenal gland proliferate in vivo in response to neurally derived signals; proliferation in vitro occurs after stimulation by nerve growth factor or by activators of adenylate cyclase or protein kinase C which mimic effects of neurotransmitters in adrenal medullary nerve endings (57). The highest frequency of medullary proliferative lesions occurs in Wistar rats (86 percent of males and 74 percent of females) (52), but variation in incidence may be related to age at sacrifice of the animal and vagaries in tissue sampling (53). Accurate classification of these spontaneous or induced lesions as AMH versus pheochromocytoma are relevant for drug licensing applications (53). Similar to AMH in humans with MEN type II, it may be very difficult to distinguish AMH in rats from pheochromocytoma (59). Spontaneous or drug-induced pheochromocytomas in rats are almost invariably norepinephrine producing, and the inability to produce epinephrine may be due to absence or inactivity of phenylethanolamine N-methyl transferase. Most adrenal medullary proliferative lesions in the rat are of the chromaffin cell lineage, with an estimated 2 percent ultimately metastasizing; neuroblastoma and ganglioneuroblastoma are rare in this experimental animal (53). There is an apparent lower responsiveness in human chromaffin cells to mitogenic signals or responses to different types of signals, and this may contribute to a lower frequency of AMH and pheochromocytoma in humans (56).

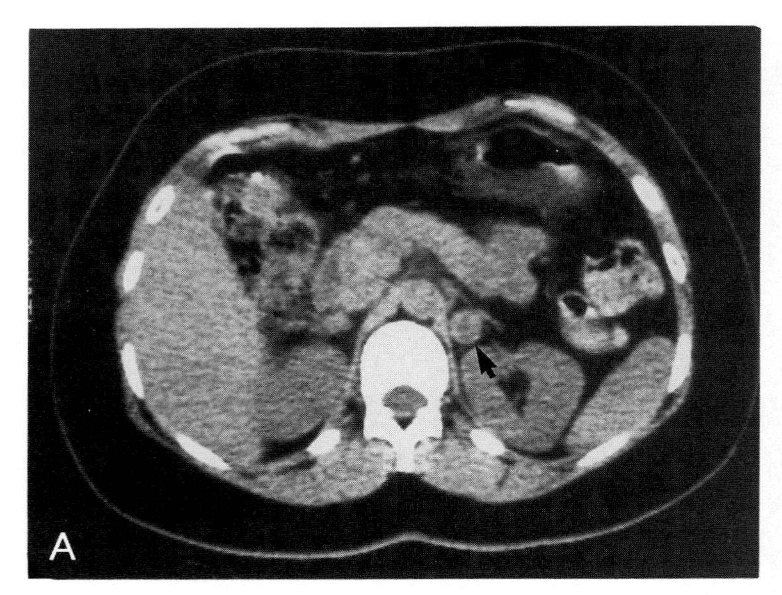

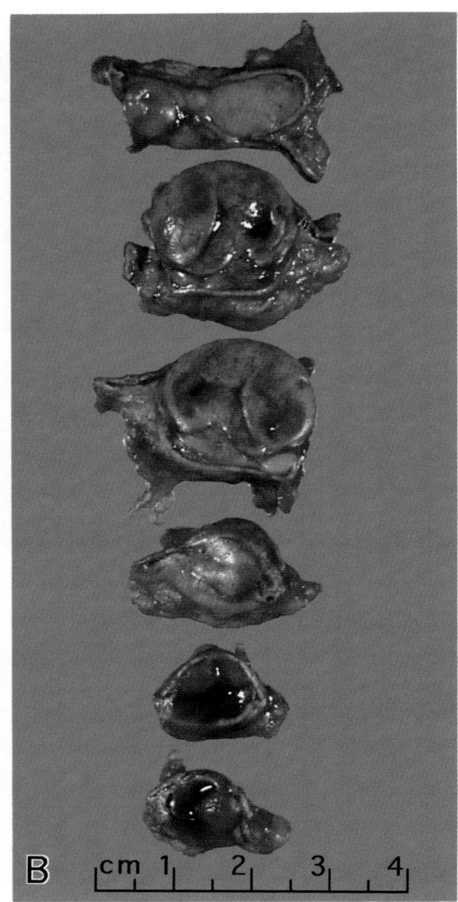

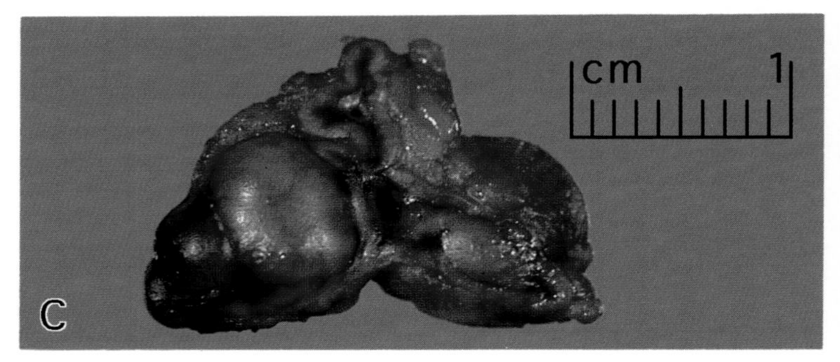

Figure 9-9

NODULAR AMH AND EARLY PHEOCHROMOCYTOMAS IN MEN TYPE IIA

A: Bilateral adrenal enlargement was apparent on abdominal CT scan in a 31-year-old woman with MEN type IIa. Enlargement of left adrenal gland is apparent in transverse cut at this level (arrow); right adrenal was also enlarged. Patient underwent bilateral adrenalectomy.

B: Transverse sections of left adrenal gland show multinodular AMH, with the largest nodule measuring 1.5 cm in diameter (i.e., a small pheochromocytoma using the "1-cm rule"). Some nodules have a complex pattern with smaller nodules arising within larger ones.

C: Nodules on the left compress and distort overlying cortex.

REFERENCES

Sporadic Adrenal Medullary Hyperplasia

1. Bauman A. Unilateral adrenal catecholamine excess. Pheochromocytoma or possible sporadic medullary hyperplasia. Arch Intern Med 1982;142:377–8.
2. Beckwith JB. Extreme cytomegaly of the adrenal fetal cortex, omphalocele, hyperplasia of kidneys and pancreas, and Leydig-cell hyperplasia another syndrome? Presented at Annual Meeting of Western Society for Pediatric Research, Los Angeles, November 11, 1963.
3. Beckwith JB. Macroglossia, omphalocele, adrenal cytomegaly, gigantism, and hyperplastic visceromegaly. Birth Defects 1969;5:188–96.
4. Bialestock D. Hyperplasia of the adrenal medulla in hypertension of children. Arch Dis Child 1961;36:465–73.
5. Bongiovanni AM, Yakovac WC, Steiker DD. Study of adrenal glands in childhood: hormonal content correlated with morphologic characteristics. Lab Invest 1961;10:956–67.
6. Chen SX, Zhong-quan Z, Jing-Shen Z, Shu-zhen W. Catecholamine acute abdomen. A case of adrenal medullary hyperplasia accompanied by acute abdomen. Chin Med J 1989;102:811–3.

7. Dralle H, Schröder S, Gratz KF, Grote R, Padberg B, Hesch RD. Sporadic unilateral adrenomedullary hyperplasia with hypertension cured by adrenalectomy. World J Surg 1990;14:308–16.
8. Dupont AG, Vanderniepen P, Gerlo E. A case of unilateral adrenal epinephrine excess: adrenal medullary hyperplasia? Acta Clin Belg 1985;40:230–5.
9. Gosney JR. Adrenal corticomedullary hyperplasia in hypobaric hypoxia. J Pathol 1985;146:59–64.
10. Harrison TS, Gann DS. Adrenal medullary hyperplasia: an opinion. Surgery 1979;85:353–4.
11. Hervonen A, Korkala O. The effect of hypoxia on the catecholamine content of human fetal abdominal paraganglia and adrenal medulla. Acta Obstet Gynecol Scand 1972;51:7–24.
12. Kazama Y, Noguchi T, Kawabe T, et al. A case of Cushing's syndrome associated with possible adrenomedullary hyperplasia. Endocrinol Jpn 1985;32:355–9.
13. Kurihara K, Mizuseki K, Kondo T, Ohoka H, Mannami M, Kawai K. Adrenal medullary hyperplasia. Hyperplasia—pheochromocytoma sequence. Acta Pathol Jpn 1990;40:683–6.
14. Lack EE. Pathology of adrenal and extra-adrenal paraganglia. Major problems in pathology, Vol 29. Philadelphia: WB Saunders, 1994.
15. Maki Y, Irie S, Ohashi T, Ohmori H. A case of unilateral adrenal medullary hyperplasia. Acta Med Okayama 1989;43:311–5.
16. Montalbano FP, Baronofsky ID, Ball H. Hyperplasia of the adrenal medulla. A clinical entity. JAMA 1962;182:264–7.
17. Naeye RL. Brain-stem and adrenal abnormalities in the sudden infant death syndrome. Am J Clin Pathol 1976;66:526–30.
18. Rudy FR, Bates RD, Cimorelli AJ, Hill GS, Engleman K. Adrenal medullary hyperplasia: a clinicopathologic study of four cases. Hum Pathol 1980;11:650–7.
19. Schnakenburg K, Müller M, Dörner K, et al. Congenital hemihypertrophy and malignant giant pheochromocytoma—a previously undescribed coincidence. Europ J Pediat 1976;122:263–73.
20. Visser JW, Axt R. Bilateral adrenal medullary hyperplasia: a clinicopathologic entity. J Clin Path 1975;28:298–304.
21. Wiedemann HR. Complexe malformatif familial avec hernie ombilicale et macroglossie—un syndrome nouveau? J Genet Hum 1964;13:223–32.
22. Wu CP. Adrenal medullary hyperplasia. Natl Med J Chin 1977;57:331–3.
23. Wu JP, Xu FJ, Zéng ZP. Adrenal medullary hyperplasia. Long-term follow up of 15 patients. Chin Med J (Engl) 1984;97:653–6.
24. Zhang ZX, Yu ST. Analysis of 17 cases of adrenal medullary hyperplasia. Natl Med J Chin 1979;59:95–7.

Familial Adrenal Medullary Hyperplasia

25. Baylin SB. The multiple endocrine neoplasm syndromes: implications for the study of inherited tumors. Semin Oncol 1978;5:35–45.
26. Brandi ML, Aurbach GD, Fitzpatrick LA, et al. Parathyroid mitogenic activity in plasma from patients with familial multiple endocrine neoplasia type I. N Engl J Med 1986;314:1287–93.
27. Carney JA, Sizemore GW, Sheps SG. Adrenal medullary disease in multiple endocrine neoplasia, type 2: pheochromocytoma and its precursors. Am J Clin Pathol 1976;66:279–90.
28. Carney JA, Sizemore GW, Tyce GM. Bilateral adrenal medullary hyperplasia in multiple endocrine neoplasia, type 2: the precursor of bilateral pheochromocytoma. Mayo Clin Proc 1975;50:3–10.
29. Cerny JC, Jackson CE, Talpos GB, Yott JB, Lee MW. Pheochromocytoma in multiple endocrine neoplasia type II: an example of the two–hit theory of neoplasia. Surgery 1982;92:849–52.
30. DeLellis RA, Wolfe HJ, Gagel RT, et al. Adrenal medullary hyperplasia. A morphometric analysis in patients with familial medullary thyroid carcinoma. Am J Pathol 1976;83:177–90.
31. Gagel RF, Tashjian AH Jr, Cummings T, et al. The clinical outcome of prospective screening for multiple endocrine neoplasia type 2a. An 18-year experience. N Engl J Med 1988;318:478–84.
32. Hamilton BP, Landsberg L, Levine RJ. Measurement of urinary epinephrine in screening for pheochromocytomas in multiple endocrine neoplasia type II. Am J Med 1978;65:1027–32.
33. Hazard JB, Hawk WA, Crile G Jr. Medullary (solid) carcinoma of the thyroid —a clinicopathological entity. J Clin Endocrinol Metab 1959;19:152–61.
34. Horn RC Jr. Carcinoma of the thyroid: description of a distinctive morphological variant and report of seven cases. Cancer 1951;4:697–707.
35. Karsner HT. Tumors of the adrenal. Atlas of Tumor Pathology, 1st Series, Fascicle 29. Washington, D.C.: Armed Forces Institute of Pathology, 1950.
36. Keiser HR, Beaven MA, Doppman J, Wells S Jr, Buja LM. Sipple's syndrome: medullary thyroid carcinoma, pheochromocytoma, and parathyroid disease. Studies in a large family. NIH conference. Ann Int Med 1973;78:561–79.
37. Khairi MR, Dexter RN, Burzynski NJ, Johnston CC Jr. Mucosal neuroma, pheochromocytoma and medullary thyroid carcinoma: multiple endocrine neoplasia type 3. Medicine 1975;54:89–112.
38. Knudson AG Jr, Strong LC. Mutation and cancer: neuroblastoma and pheochromocytoma. Am J Hum Genet 1972;24:514–32.
39. Lack EE. Pathology of adrenal and extra-adrenal paraganglia. Major problems in pathology, Vol 29. Philadelphia: WB Saunders, 1994.
40. Padberg BC, Garbe E, Achilles E, Dralle H, Bressel M, Schröder S. Adrenomedullary hyperplasia and pheochromocytoma. DNA cytophotometric findings in 47 cases. Virchows Arch [A] 1990;416:443–6.
41. Schimke RN. Multiple endocrine adenomatosis syndromes. Adv Intern Med 1976;21:249–65.
42. Schimke RN, Hartmann WH. Familial amyloid-producing medullary thyroid carcinoma and pheochromocytoma. A distinct genetic entity. Ann Int Med 1965;63:1027–39.
43. Sipple JH. The association of pheochromocytoma with carcinoma of the thyroid gland. Am J Med 1961;31:163–5.

44. Steiner AL, Goodman AD, Powers SR. Study of a kindred with pheochromocytoma, medullary thyroid carcinoma, hyperparathyroidism and Cushing's disease: multiple endocrine neoplasia, type 2. Medicine 1968;47:371–409.
45. Valk, TW, Frager, MS, Gross, MD, et al. Spectrum of pheochromocytoma in multiple endocrine neoplasia. A scintigraphic portrayal using 131I-metaiodobenzylguanidine. Ann Int Med 1981;94:762–7.
46. Verdy M, Weber AM, Roy CC, Morin CL, Cadotte M, Brochu P. Hirschsprung's disease in a family with endocrine neoplasia type 2. J Pediatr Gastroenterol Nutr 1982;1:603–7.
47. Williams ED. A review of 17 cases of carcinoma of the thyroid and phaeochromoctyoma. J Clin Pathol 1965;18:288–92.
48. Williams ED, Pollock DJ. Multiple mucosal neuromata with endocrine tumors: a syndrome allied to von Recklinghausen's disease. J Pathol Bacteriol 1966;91:71–7.
49. Wolfe HJ, Melvin KE, Cervi-Skinner SJ, et al. C-cell hyperplasia preceding medullary thyroid carcinoma. N Engl J Med 1973;289:437–41.

Proliferative Lesions of Adrenal Medulla in Rats

50. Partanen M, Chiveh CC, Rapaport SL. Age-related increase in catecholamine-containing paraganglia in male Fischer-344 rats. Anat Rec 1981;201:563–6.
51. Tischler AS. Cell proliferation in the adult adrenal medulla. Chromaffin cells as a model of indirect carcinogenesis. In: Pathology of laboratory animals, endocrine system. ILSI Monograph. New York: Springer-Verlag, 1994.
52. Tischler AS, Coupland RE. Changes in structure and function of the adrenal medulla In: Pathology of the aging rat, Vol 2. 1994:245–68.
53. Tischler AS, DeLellis RA. The rat adrenal medulla: II. Proliferative lesions. J Am Coll Toxicol 1988;7:23–44.
54. Tischler AS, DeLellis RA, Nunnemacher G, Wolfe HJ. Acute stimulation of chromaffin cell proliferation in the adult rat adrenal medulla. Lab Invest 1988;58:733–5.
55. Tischler AS, DeLellis RA, Perlman RL, et al. Spontaneous proliferative lesions of the adrenal medulla in aging Long-Evans rats. Comparison to PC12 cells, small granule-containing cells, and human adrenal medullary hyperplasia. Lab Invest 1985;53:486–98.
56. Tischler AS, Riseberg JC. Different responses to mitogenic agents by adult rat and human chromaffin cells in vitro. Endocr Pathol 1993;4:15–9.
57. Tischler AS, Riseberg JC, Cherington V. Mitogenic signalling pathways in normal and neoplastic chromaffin cells [Abstract]. Mod Pathol 1994;7:58A.
58. Tischler AS, Ruzicka LA, Donahue SR, DeLellis RA. Chromaffin cell proliferation in the adult rat adrenal medulla. Int J Devl Neurosci 1989;7:439–48.
59. Tischler AS, Ruzicka LA, Van Pelt CS, Sandusky GE. Catecholamine-synthesizing enzymes and chromogranin proteins in drug-induced proliferative lesions of the rat adrenal medulla. Lab Invest 1990;63:44–51.
60. Warren S, Grozdev L, Gates O, Chute RN. Radiation-induced adrenal medullary tumors in the rat. Arch Pathol 1966;82:115–8.

✧✧✧

10
PHEOCHROMOCYTOMA

Definition. Pheochromocytoma is a paraganglioma arising from chromaffin cells of the adrenal medulla. This tumor is also referred to as *adrenal medullary paraganglioma.*

Paragangliomas are named according to their anatomic site of origin; adrenal medullary paraganglioma is referred to as pheochromocytoma. The term pheochromocytoma is also used for extra-adrenal tumors of the sympathoadrenal neuroendocrine system, and given the great overlap in morphology, immunohistochemical profile, and ultrastructure of pheochromocytoma and extra-adrenal paraganglioma differentiation may be difficult. Accurate designation of the paraganglioma based upon anatomic location and correlation with clinical signs and symptoms may offer some prognostic information since extra-adrenal retroperitoneal tumors tend to have a greater malignant potential than pheochromocytomas.

Incidence. Using population-based data, the average annual incidence of pheochromocytoma is 8 per million person-years in the United States; this increases to 9.5 per million with the inclusion of two additional familial cases (2). In Sweden, the average annual incidence rate is 2.1 cases per million population (6), and in Denmark it is 1.9 per million (1). In a review of population-based data from the SEER (Surveillance, Epidemiology, and End Results) registries of 1973 to 1987, the age-specific incidence rate for pheochromocytoma for any age group never exceeded 0.1 per 100,000 population (3). Pheochromocytomas are uncommon neoplasms and especially rare in children (5). Some have suggested that for every pheochromocytoma diagnosed during life, two would be discovered incidentally at autopsy. In a review of 54 autopsy-proven cases of pheochromocytoma over a 50-year period at the Mayo Clinic, 24 percent had been diagnosed correctly during life while 76 percent had not been suspected clinically; 75 percent of patients in the latter group died suddenly from either myocardial infarction or cardiovascular catastrophe, with one third of the sudden deaths occurring during or immediately after an unrelated surgical procedure (7). These findings cast serious doubt on the theory that most tumors are "nonfunctional." Heightened clinical awareness and the availability of more sophisticated diagnostic, biochemical, and imaging procedures may lead to more accurate diagnosis during life. In one review, 53 percent of pheochromocytomas seen before 1962 were undiagnosed prior to surgery or autopsy while since 1962 only 18 percent of tumors were clinically unsuspected (4).

Age, Sex, and Laterality. The peak age at diagnosis is in the fifth decade of life, but pheochromocytomas can affect any age group (14,16, 24). Most series report a roughly equal sex incidence, but some show a slight predilection for either males or females. In some of the larger studies, the right adrenal gland is involved slightly more often than the left, perhaps reflecting the greater amount of chromaffin tissue that has been reported on that side (21).

Pheochromocytomas have been dubbed the "10 percent tumor": 10 percent bilateral, 10 percent extra-adrenal, 10 percent malignant, and about 10 percent occurring in childhood, but these figures are only an approximation and must be correlated with variables such as proportion of familial cases in any particular series, location of tumor, and age group studied (16). In a sporadic setting, about 95 percent of pheochromocytomas are solitary, about 5 percent are bilateral, and 5 percent to 10 percent are extra-adrenal (Table 10-1) (16). In the familial setting, over 50 percent of tumors are bilateral, and patients tend to be diagnosed at an earlier age (22). In the pediatric age group there is an increased incidence of bilateral pheochromocytomas as well as multicentric and extra-adrenal tumors (14).

Patterns of Catecholamine Secretion. The clinical signs and symptoms of patients with pheochromocytoma vary considerably (Table 10-2), but the triad which is most diagnostic is paroxysmal hypertension, headaches, and diaphoresis (11,15,18). Norepinephrine-secreting tumors are usually associated with sustained hypertension, while tumors secreting relatively large quantities of epinephrine along with norepinephrine

Table 10-1

INCIDENCE OF SOLITARY AND BILATERAL PHEOCHROMOCYTOMAS AND EXTRA-ADRENAL PARAGANGLIOMAS

	Solitary Adrenal	Bilateral Adrenal	Extra-Adrenal
Sporadic (~90% of total)	95%	5%	5–10%
Familial (5–10% of total)	<50%	>50%	<10%
Childhood (5–10% of total)	50%	20–25%	15–20%

Table 10-2

SIGNS AND SYMPTOMS OF PHEOCHROMOCYTOMA*

Signs	Frequency	Symptoms	Frequency
Hypertension	76–100%	Headaches	76–100%
Tachycardia or reflex bradycardia	51–75%	Palpitations	51–75%
Postural hypotension	51–75%	Sweating	51–75%
Paroxysmal hypertension	26–50%	Anxiety/nervousness	26–50%
Weight loss	26–50%	Tremulousness	26–50%
Pallor	26–50%	Nausea/emesis	26–50%
Hypermetabolism	26–50%	Pain in chest/abdomen	26–50%
Fasting hyperglycemia	26–50%	Weakness/fatigue	26–50%
Tremor	26–50%	Dizziness	1–25%
Increased respiratory rate	26–50%	Heat intolerance	1–25%
Decreased GI motility	26–50%	Paresthesias	1–25%
Psychosis (rare)	1–25%	Constipation	1–25%
Flushing, paroxysmal (rare)	1–25%		

*Table 5-1 from Keiser HR, Doppman JL, Robertson CN, Linehan WM, Averbuch SD. Diagnosis, localization, and management of pheochromocytoma. In: Lack EE, ed. Pathology of the adrenal glands. New York: Churchill Livingstone, 1990:237–55. Data from references 1,5,16.

are associated with paroxysmal or episodic hypertension (11). Pure epinephrine-secreting tumors may cause hypotension (11) and may require precise measurement of epinephrine excretion, particularly in patients with multiple endocrine neoplasia (MEN) syndrome type II (8). In some normotensive patients, the tumor (which is most often extra-adrenal) secretes mainly dopamine, presumably due to decreased activity of dopamine beta-hydroxylase (12,13,20), and this profile may be associated with malignancy (13). The non-neoplastic adrenal medulla is able to take up ^{131}I-metaiodobenzylguanidine (MIBG) in the presence of a pheochromocytoma with excess catecholamine secretion (9). On rare occasion, spontaneous retroperitoneal hemorrhage by pheochromocytoma occurs (17).

Preoperative Localization and Imaging Characteristics. Preoperative localization of pheochromocytoma and extra-adrenal paraganglioma can be accomplished by the use of high resolution computed tomography (CT) (fig. 10-1) or magnetic resonance imaging (MRI). These have almost eliminated the need for selective arteriography except in rare instances where it is necessary to delineate the blood supply to the tumor; in those unusual cases it should be done only in patients who are adequately treated with

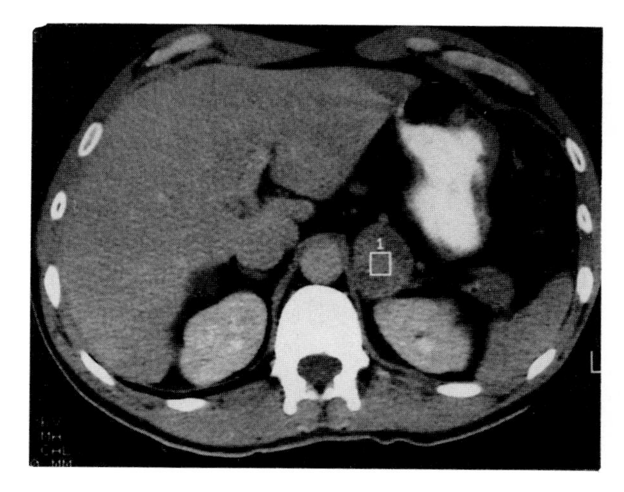

Figure 10-1
PHEOCHROMOCYTOMA
Pheochromocytoma of left adrenal gland in an adult patient is well demonstrated by computed tomography (CT scan) of abdomen.

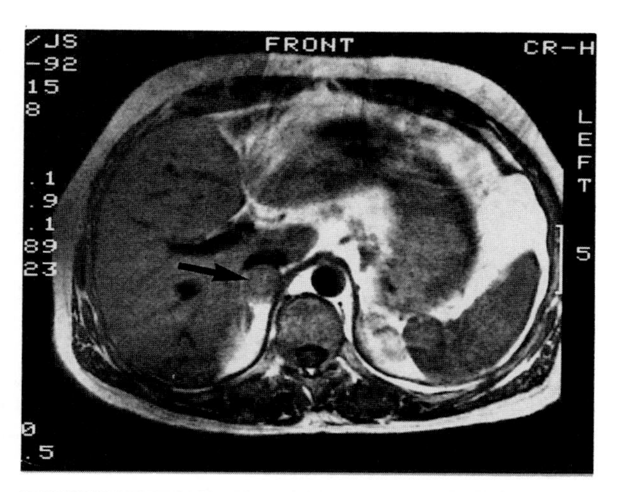

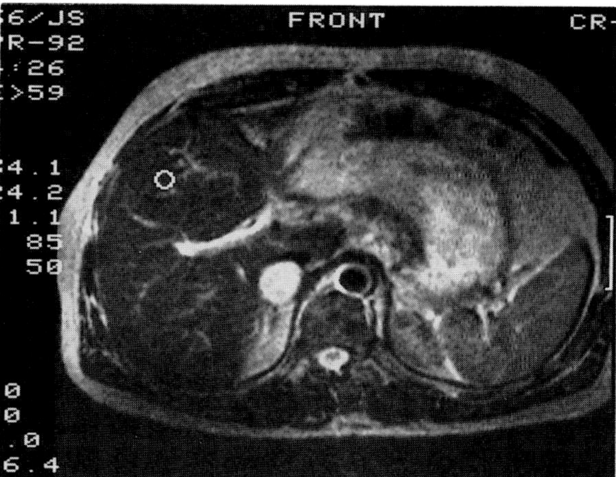

Figure 10-2
PHEOCHROMOCYTOMA
Top: Magnetic resonance imaging (MRI) of abdomen in a 38-year-old man shows a rounded pheochromocytoma on the right side (arrow) with a low signal intensity in T1-weighted image.

Bottom: Tumor shows a bright signal on T2-weighted image with MRI. The study was prompted by a hypertensive episode during laparoscopic cholecystectomy. The patient was also noted to have "cardiomyopathy" with atrial fibrillation.

adrenergic blockade to prevent a hypertensive crisis (15). On CT scan the tumor is usually greater than 3 cm in diameter and has a homogeneous soft tissue density. Necrosis may be present and larger tumors have a central low density on scan. Contrast enhancement may show heterogeneity better. Sometimes calcifications are seen. On MRI, pheochromocytomas (and other extra-adrenal paragangliomas) tend to show a very high signal intensity on T2-weighted images (fig. 10-2), which are isointense compared to liver on T1-weighted images. Adrenal cortical carcinomas tend to have an intermediate signal intensity and adrenal cortical adenomas a low intensity (15). The imaging on MRI may be nonspecific if hemorrhage occurs within the tumor. Localization using ^{131}I-MIBG depends upon uptake of a radiolabeled analogue of guanethidine (fig. 10-3) within the intracellular storage granules (23), but a wide range of neuroendocrine tumors, such as neuroblastoma, medullary thyroid carcinoma, and carcinoid tumors, can also be localized with this technique. Uptake of ^{131}I-MIBG does not appear to correlate with catecholamine secretion as measured in plasma or urine (9,10,19,25), but a direct proportional correlation has been reported between the percentage uptake by the tumor and the number of neurosecretory type granules (10).

SPORADIC PHEOCHROMOCYTOMA

Gross Findings. Pheochromocytoma in the sporadic or nonfamilial setting typically presents as a rounded, unicentric mass with distortion of the gland, which is usually apparent as an attached remnant (fig. 10-4, left) or splayed over the surface of the tumor (fig. 10-4, right). Identification of an adrenal remnant may be difficult with extremely large tumors. Most pheochromocytomas measure 3 to 5 cm in diameter (38), but there is a

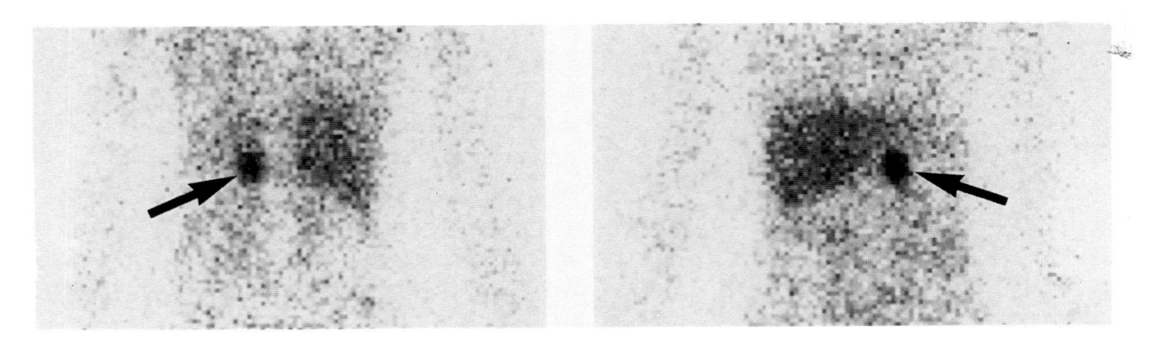

Figure 10-3
PHEOCHROMOCYTOMA
Pheochromocytoma (arrows) of left adrenal gland is visualized scintigraphically using ^{131}I-metaiodobenzylguanidine.

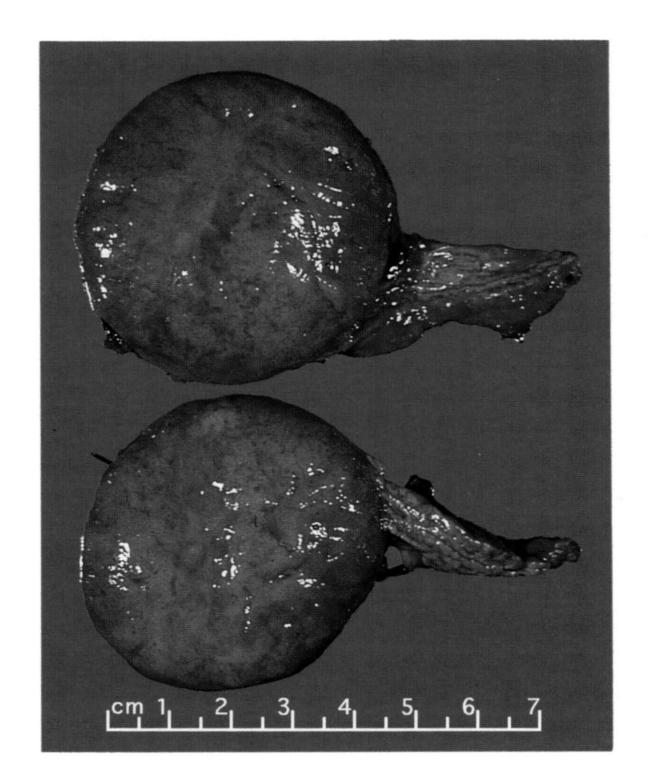

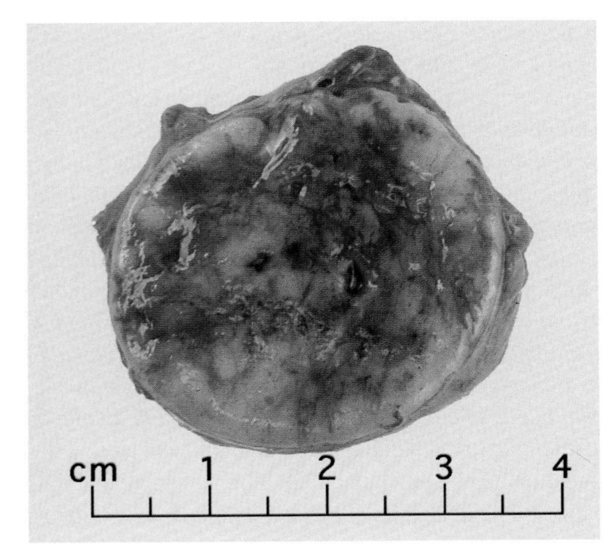

Figure 10-4
PHEOCHROMOCYTOMA
Left: The pheochromocytoma is well-circumscribed with a bulging pale-gray surface. Attached adrenal remnant is also present.
Right: The pheochromocytoma measures about 3 cm in diameter and on cross section is glistening gray-white, with an irregular pattern of congestion. There was a strong chromaffin reaction after tumor immersion in Zenker's fixative.

wide range of from 1 to 10 cm or more. The average weight of pheochromocytomas in several large series (most classified as benign) was 73 g (35), 85 g (26), 90 g (42), 113 g (40), and 156.5 g (36); clinically malignant tumors tend to be heavier than benign pheochromocytomas (average 176 g [40], 383 g [35], and 759 g [36]). Given the greater concentration of chromaffin tissue in the head and body of the gland, one would expect most pheochromocytomas to arise in these regions, but in most cases this is impossible to determine with certainty (31).

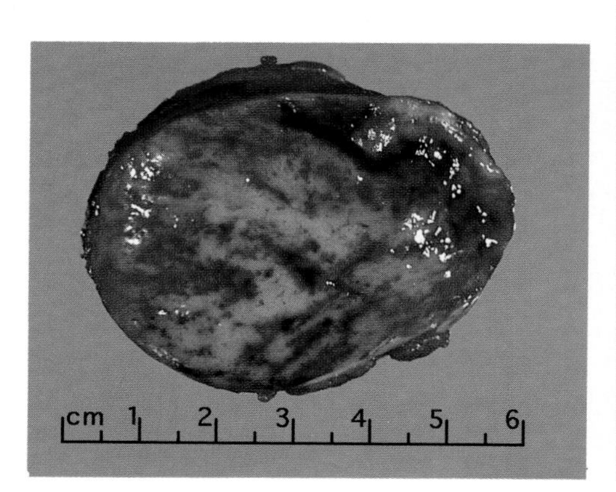

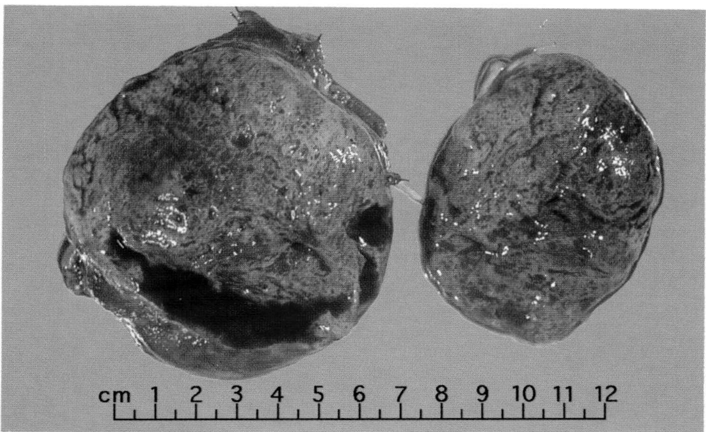

Figure 10-5
PHEOCHROMOCYTOMA
Left: In cross section this pheochromocytoma shows mottled to confluent areas of hemorrhage.
Right: A pheochromocytoma from a different patient is extensively congested and hemorrhagic, with areas of cystic degeneration.

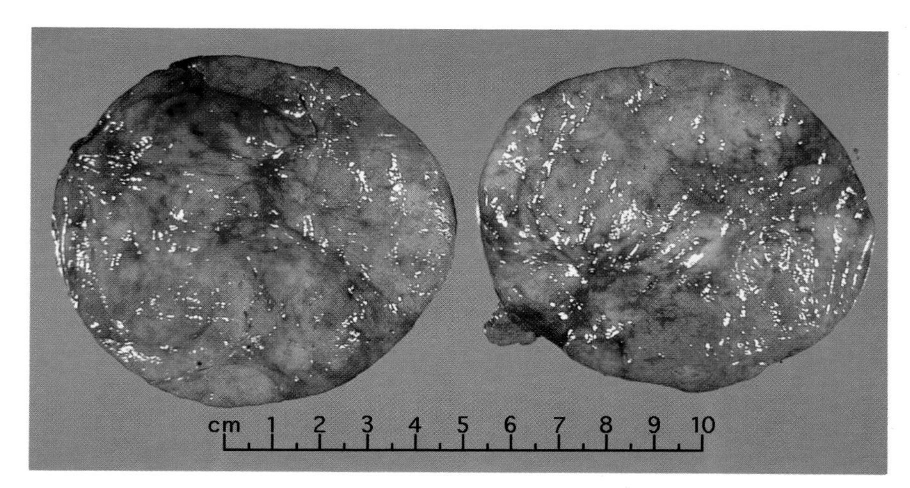

Figure 10-6
PHEOCHROMOCYTOMA
In cross section, the tumor is gray-white to tan, with a finely nodular appearance due to vascular channels cut in various planes with slight retraction beneath the surface.

On cross section, the tumor is usually sharply circumscribed and may even appear encapsulated, but close inspection may reveal a fibrous pseudocapsule or expansion of the adrenal capsule itself. Pheochromocytomas are usually resiliently firm and gray-white, similar to the texture and color of the normal adrenal medulla, but there may be areas of mottled to confluent congestion (fig. 10-5), or frank hemorrhage within the tumor sometimes extending out into surrounding adipose tissue. In extreme examples, the tumor grossly resembles a hematoma. Careful inspection of the cut surface of the tumor in cross section may reveal punctate or curvilinear foci, often retracted slightly beneath the surface, which represent vascular structures of various size (fig. 10-6). Central degenerative changes can be seen, particularly in larger tumors, and may appear as zones of remote necrosis, fibrosis, or cystic change (fig. 10-7). The cystic degeneration may appear as nonhomogeneous areas on CT scan (fig. 10-8, above) or ultrasound (fig. 10-8, right). Extreme examples of cystic degeneration are very unusual and in such cases it may be difficult to identify remnants of the tumor (fig. 10-9). Cyst contents range from thin, blood-tinged fluid to more grumous, red-brown material. Occasionally, a pheochromocytoma may

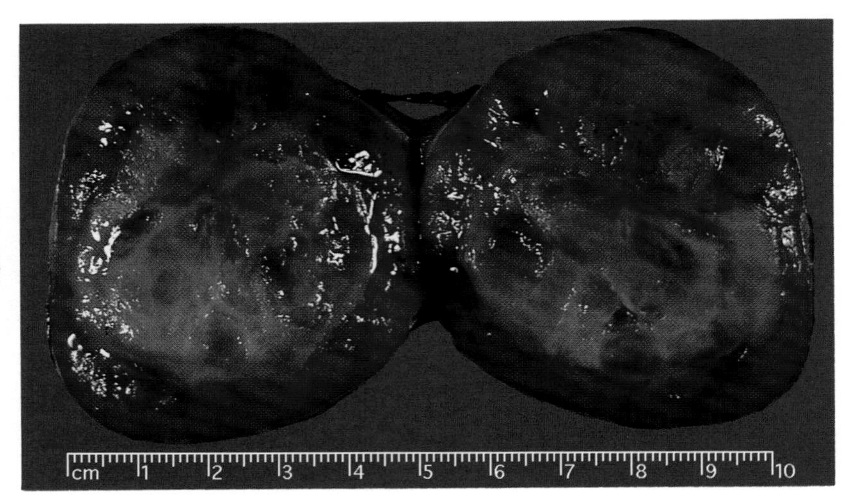

Figure 10-7
PHEOCHROMOCYTOMA

A bisected pheochromocytoma shows a large central area of degenerative change with fibrosis, edema, and cystic change. The peripheral portion of tumor is resiliently firm and brown.

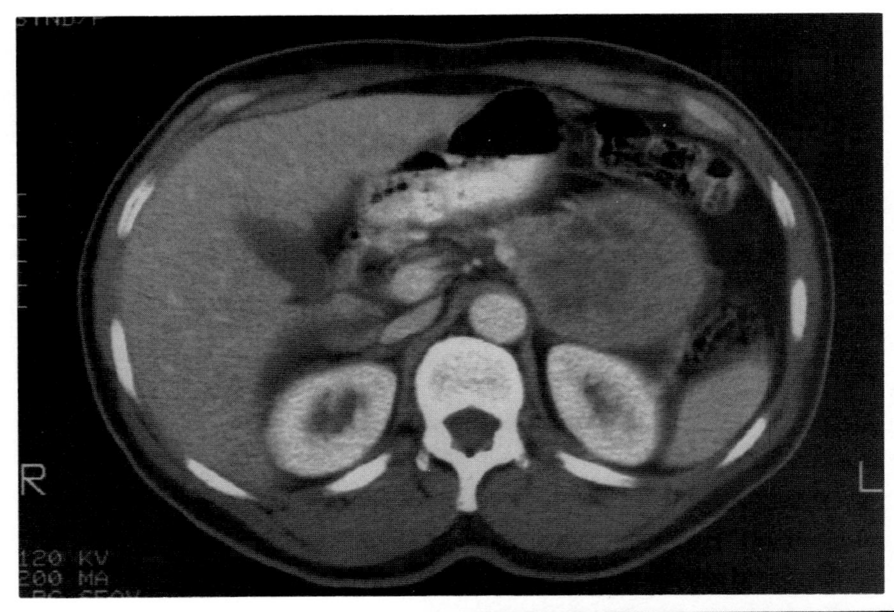

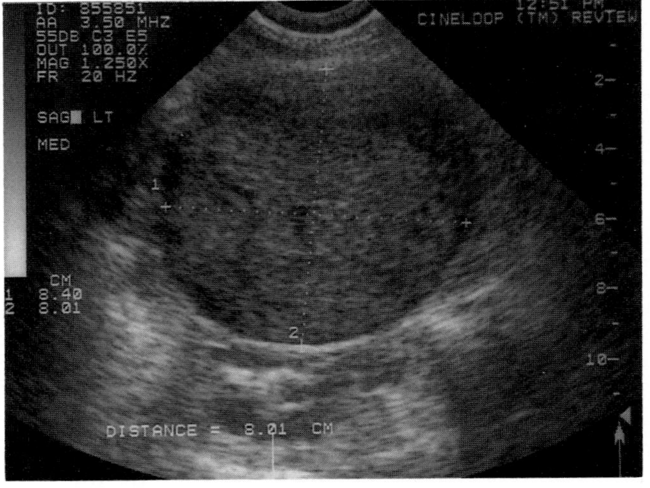

Figure 10-8
PHEOCHROMOCYTOMA

Above: A large pheochromocytoma is apparent on the left side in an abdominal CT scan of a 55-year-old man who presented with flank pain. Tumor is nonhomogeneous on CT scan after intravenous and gastrointestinal contrast enhancement.

Right: Ultrasonograph in same case shows a sharply demarcated mass which is roughly spherical (8.01 x 8.40 cm).

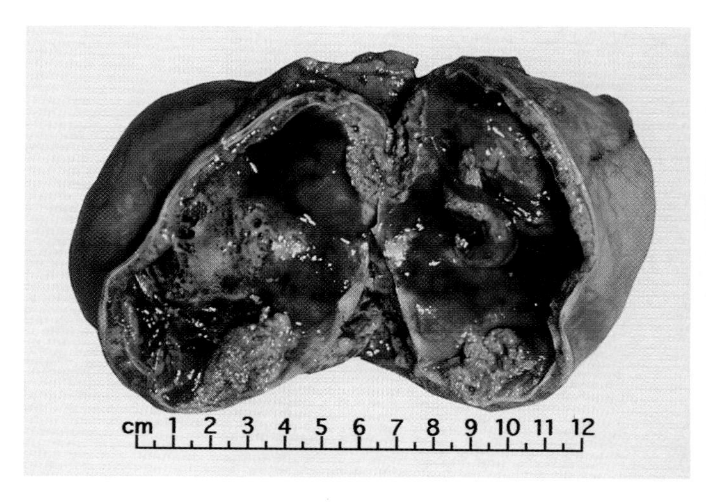

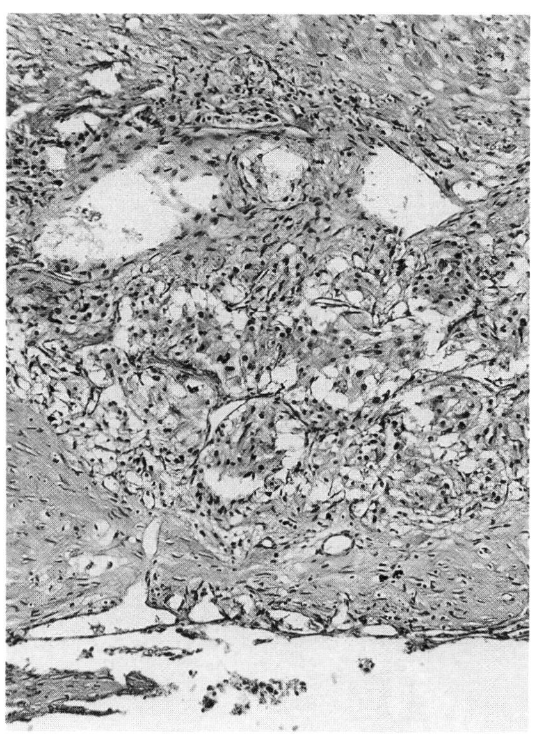

Figure 10-9
PHEOCHROMOCYTOMA

Above: A markedly cystic pheochromocytoma resected from an adult. The inner aspect of the cystic tumor has a smooth to shaggy appearance. The tumor contained amber, blood tinged fluid with amorphous material.

Right: In a different cystic pheochromocytoma, representative sections through cyst wall show residual pheochromocytoma. Note the fibrosis with fibrinous matter on the inner aspect of cyst.

have areas of dystrophic calcification which may be detected on plain films of the abdomen (31).

Pheochromocytomas also can become adherent to adjacent structures such as kidney or liver, and frank invasion of adjacent organs or tissues may be an indication of malignancy (31,32). They occasionally extend into the inferior vena cava (30,43) and even into the right atrium (41); in one case the tumor caused symptoms of recurrent pulmonary emboli (30). The tumor can theoretically gain access to tributaries of the central adrenal vein through discontinuities in the medial smooth muscle (see chapter 1) and cause hemorrhage and infarction (fig. 10-10). Intracaval extension is not necessarily a bad prognostic finding, but may be associated with local recurrence (43).

Microscopic Findings. *Architectural Patterns.* Pheochromocytomas usually have a limited array of architectural patterns; one may predominate in a particular tumor or there may be an admixture in the same neoplasm (31,32). The architectural patterns observed in 98 sympathoadrenal paragangliomas (mostly pheochromocytomas) included a mixture of alveolar and trabecular patterns (36 percent), a predominantly alveolar (nesting or "zellballen") pattern (35 percent) (fig. 10-11), and a predominantly trabecular arrangement of cells (27 percent) (fig. 10-12) (35). A spindle cell pattern has been reported in about 2 percent of tumors (35,40), but it is usually not prominent throughout the tumor. In areas with a spindle cell pattern, the tumor cells have a rounded to ovoid nucleus, or a nucleus elongated in the long axis of the cell (fig. 10-13). A stain for reticulum can accentuate the alveolar (fig. 10-14, left) or anastomosing trabecular patterns (fig. 10-14, right). Nests of tumor cells may vary considerably in size and shape, and occasional central degenerative change or necrosis is seen (fig. 10-15). Some pheochromocytomas have areas in which the growth pattern is more solid or diffuse (fig. 10-16).

Sections from the periphery of the tumor may reveal a junction between the pheochromocytoma and residual cortex which is curvilinear or sinuous in contour without any evidence of an intervening fibrous capsule (fig. 10-17, left). Careful examination of these areas may reveal an intermingling of non-neoplastic cortical cells among the tumor cells (fig. 10-17, right). In some tumors, the cytoarchitectural features can be quite similar to the adjacent non-neoplastic cortex (fig. 10-18, left)

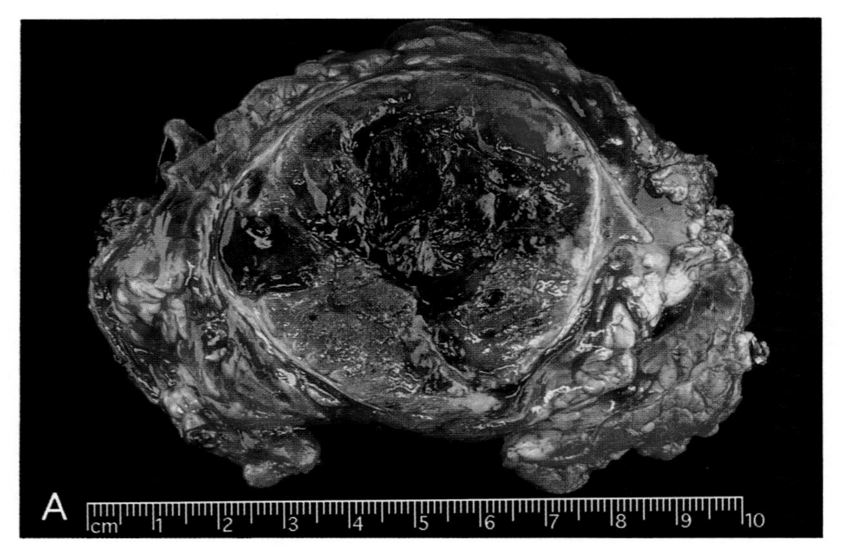

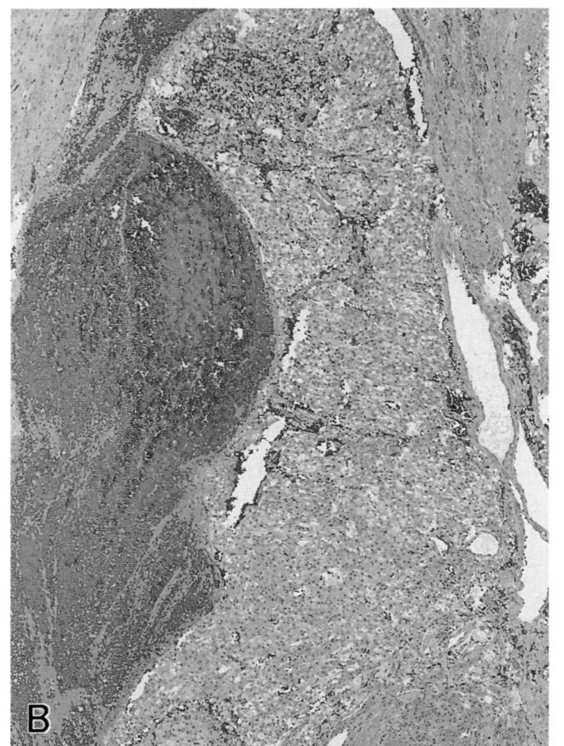

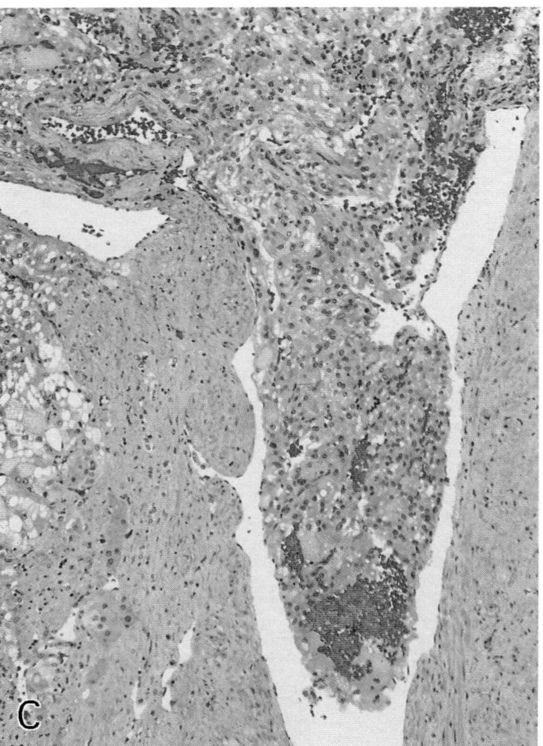

Figure 10-10
PHEOCHROMOCYTOMA

A: Pheochromocytoma from a 32-year-old man shows confluent areas of hemorrhage and necrosis. Note the hemorrhage into periadrenal adipose tissue. The patient presented with headaches, abdominal pain, and hypertensive crisis. He later underwent total thyroidectomy for medullary thyroid carcinoma. The patient and related family members were undergoing evaluation for MEN syndrome type II.

B: Areas of same tumor show intravascular protrusion by pheochromocytoma associated with fresh thrombus. A portion of the wall of the central vein is present.

C: Same case showing intravascular protrusion by tumor. An intact layer of endothelium is over the tumor and portions of the muscular wall of the central adrenal vein are on either side. Intravascular growth of this type may be related to discontinuities in medial smooth muscle of the central adrenal vein and its tributaries. The patient was alive and well 5 years later.

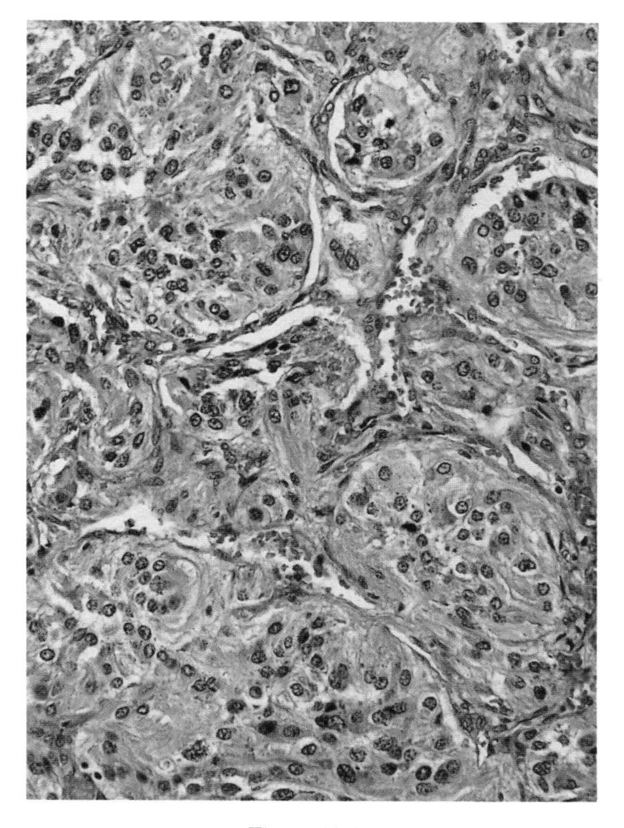

Figure 10-11
PHEOCHROMOCYTOMA
Pheochromocytoma with alveolar or nesting arrangement of tumor cells.

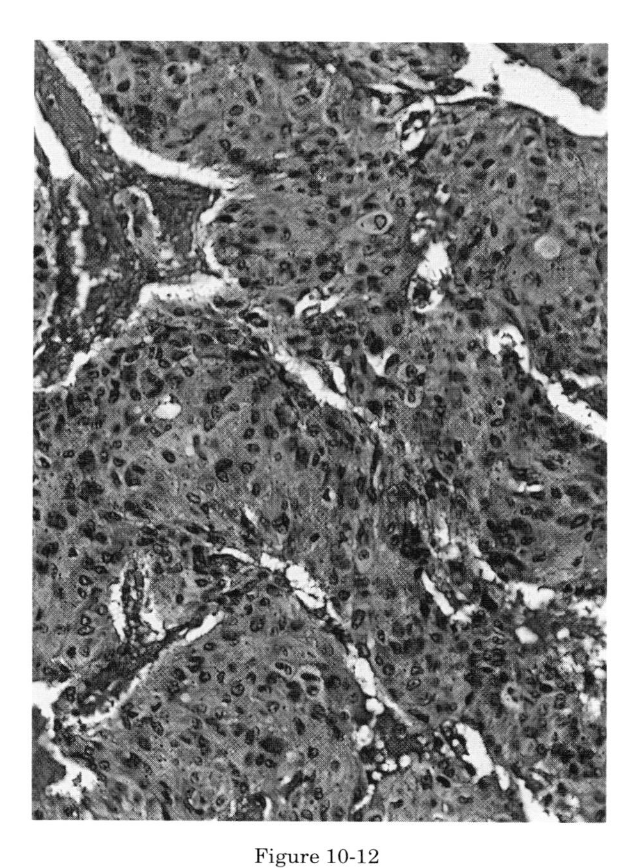

Figure 10-12
PHEOCHROMOCYTOMA
Pheochromocytoma with an anastomosing trabecular pattern.

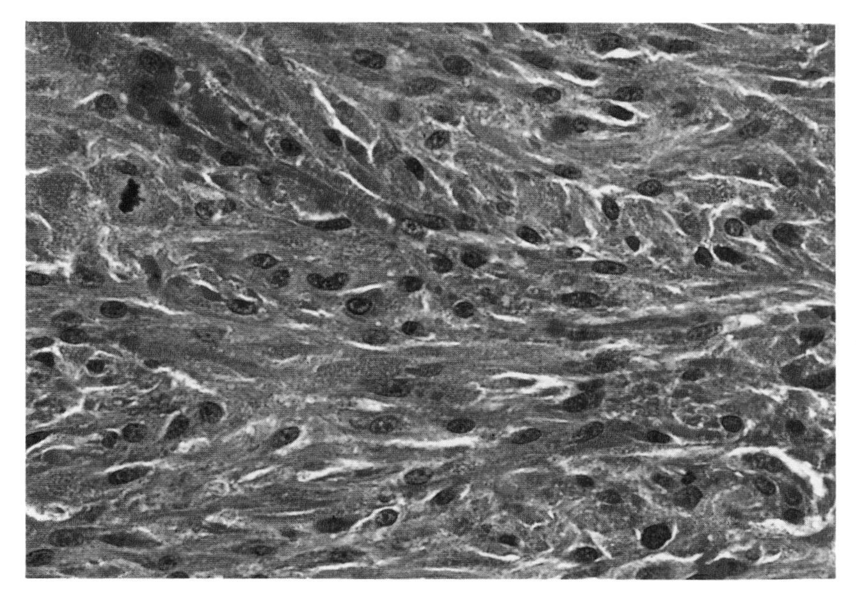

Figure 10-13
PHEOCHROMOCYTOMA
Pheochromocytoma with spindle cells oriented along the long axis of interconnecting trabeculae. Many tumor cells have nuclei that are elongate in the same axis. Note mitotic figure in left upper corner.

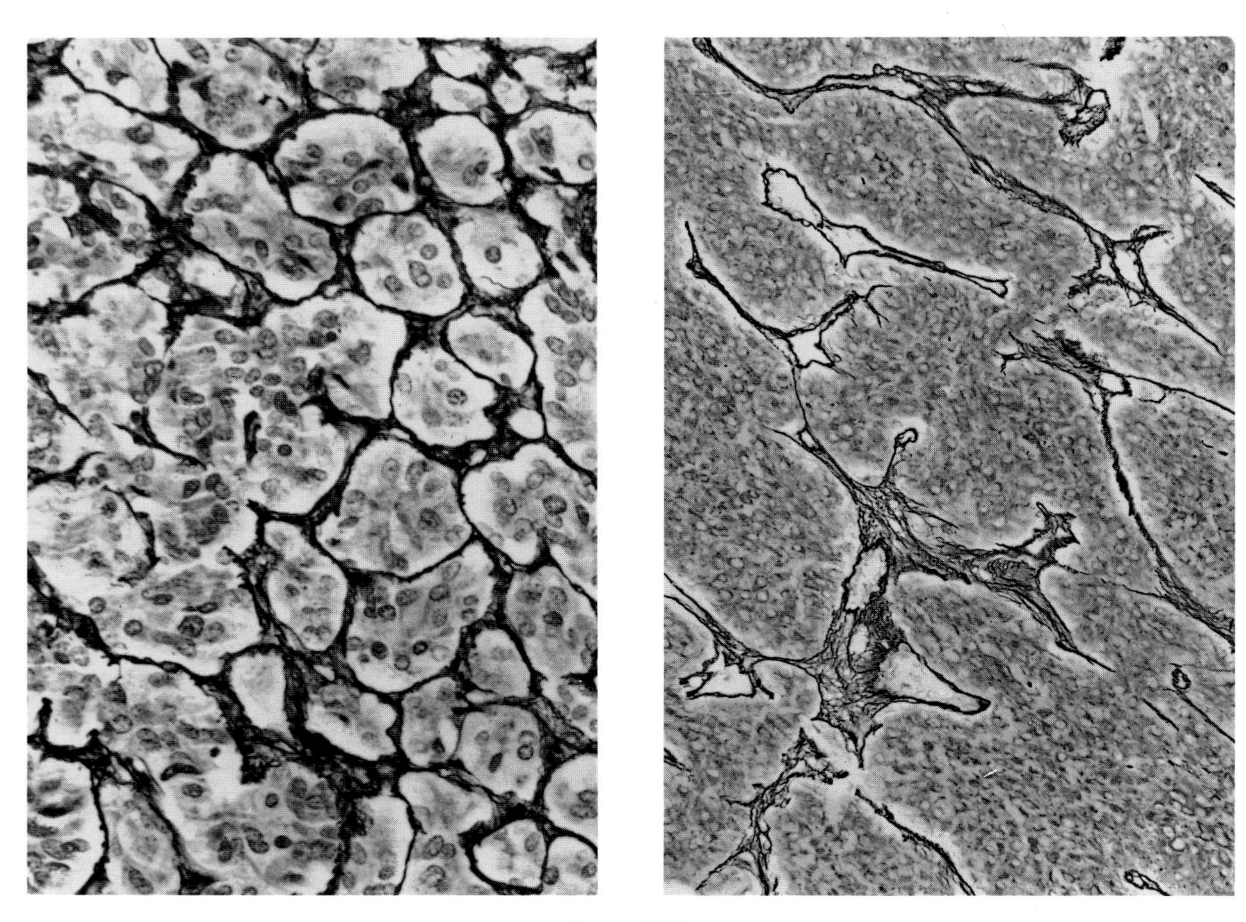

Figure 10-14
PHEOCHROMOCYTOMA
Left: Stain for reticulum clearly accentuates the alveolar pattern with distinct nests of cells ("zellballen"). (X200, Reticulum stain)
Right: Pheochromocytoma showing an interconnecting or anastomosing trabecular pattern. (X200, Reticulum stain)

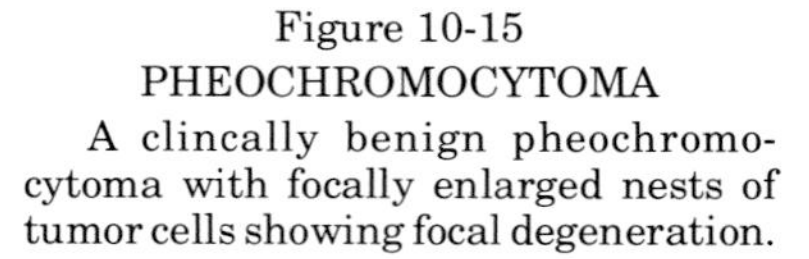

Figure 10-15
PHEOCHROMOCYTOMA
A clincally benign pheochromocytoma with focally enlarged nests of tumor cells showing focal degeneration.

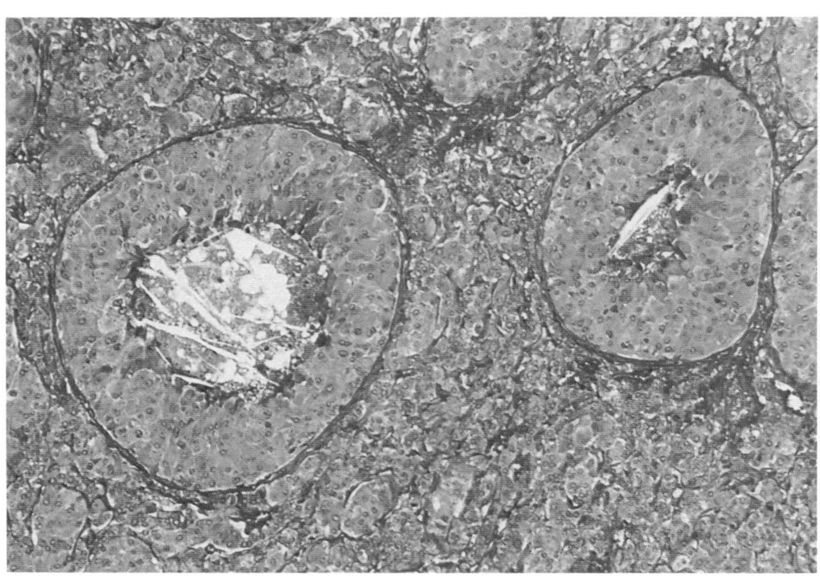

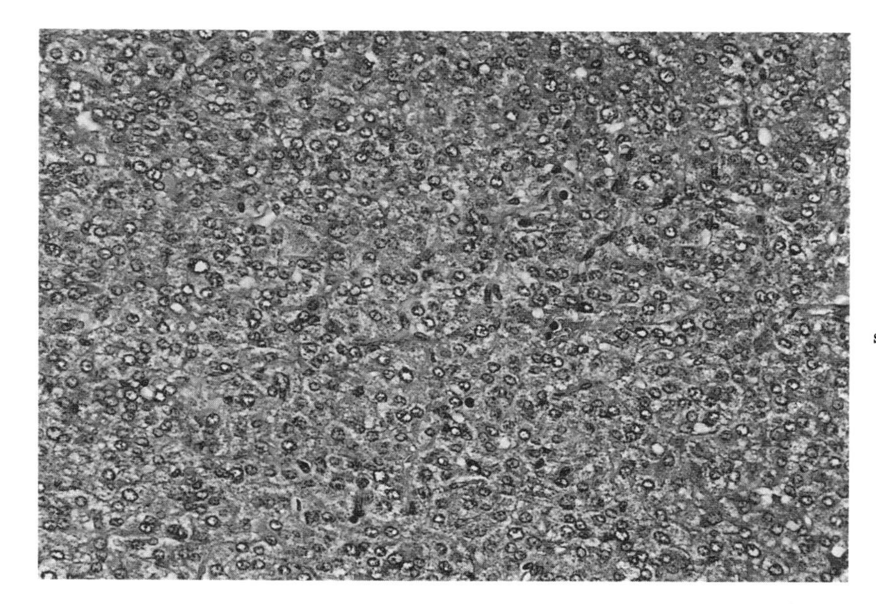

Figure 10-16
PHEOCHROMOCYTOMA
This pheochromocytoma has a more solid or diffuse pattern.

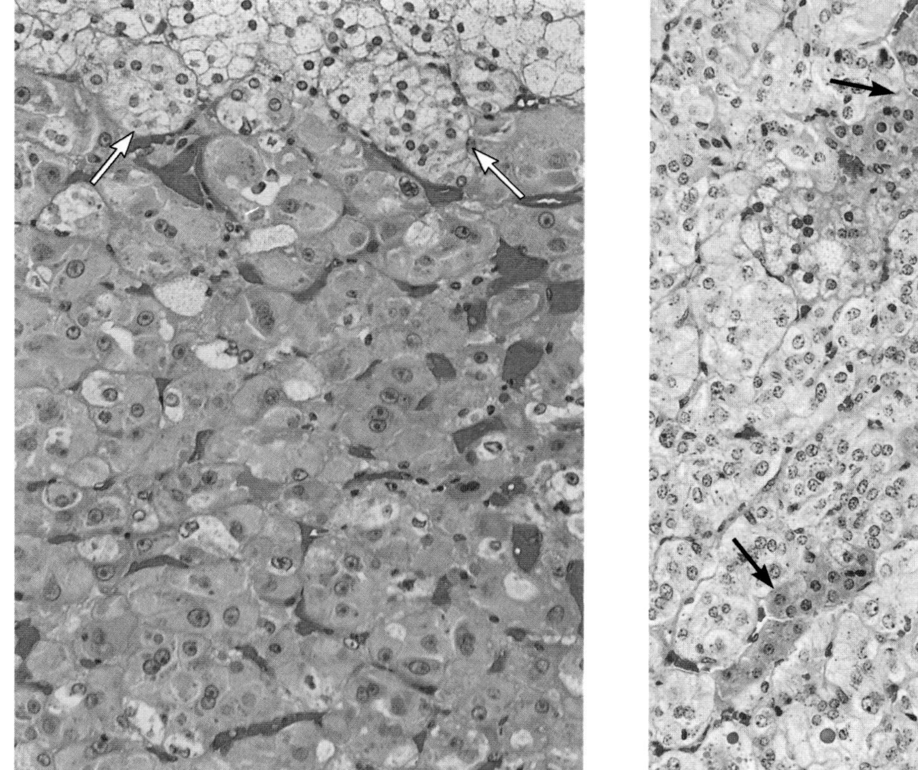

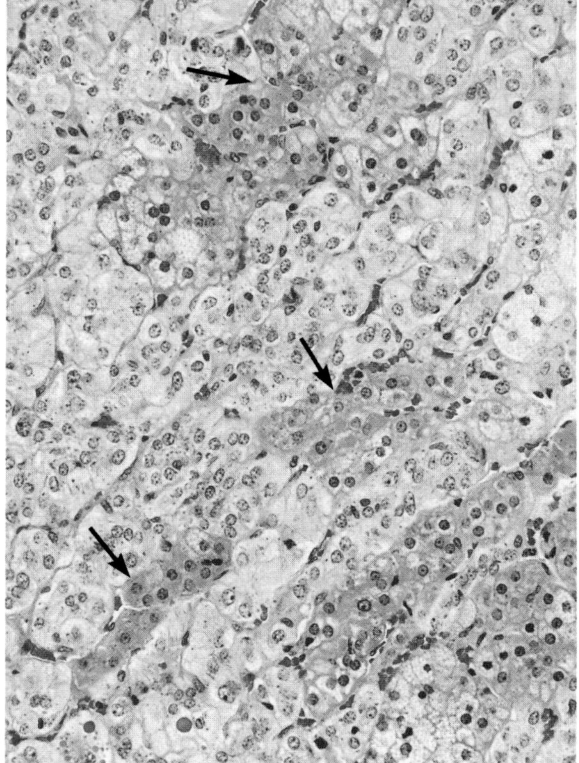

Figure 10-17
PHEOCHROMOCYTOMA
Left: The junction between pheochromocytoma and adjacent adrenal cortex (open arrows, top of field) is seen. There is no evidence of encapsulation.
Right: A different pheochromocytoma has a pushing border adjacent to cortex without any evidence of encapsulation. Cortical cells intermingle within the tumor (straight arrows).

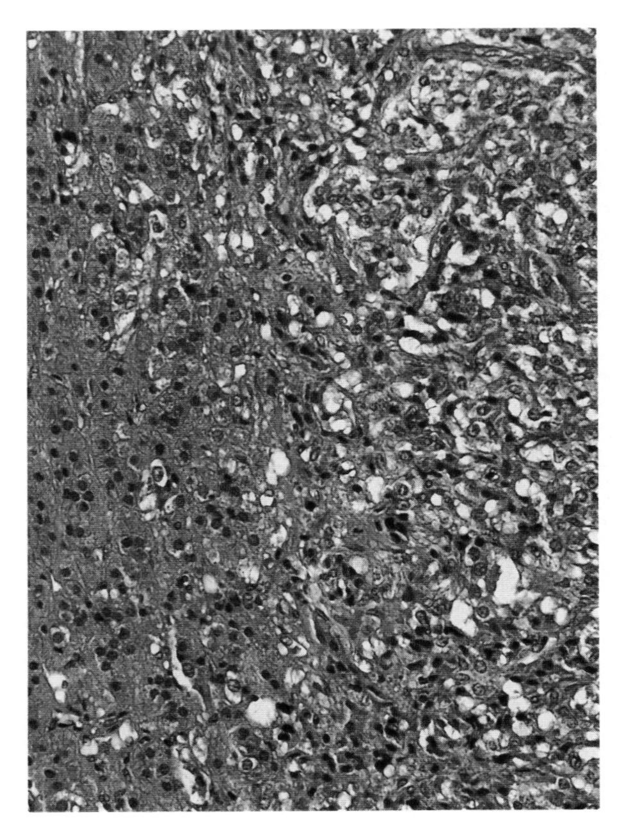

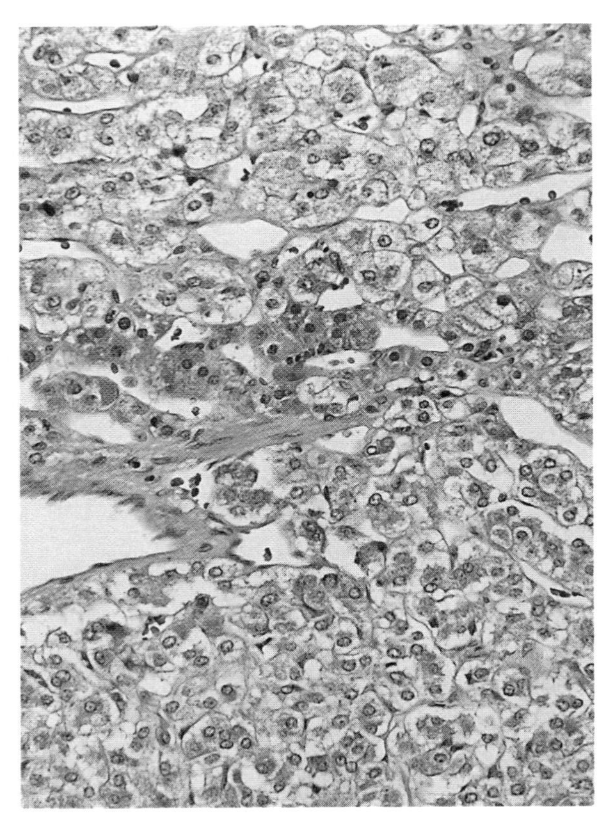

Figure 10-18
PHEOCHROMOCYTOMA

Left: Cells of pheochromocytoma (right portion of field) and cortex (left) have a similar appearance. On rare occasion it may be difficult to distinguish adrenal cortical and medullary neoplasms in routinely stained sections.

Right: Pheochromocytoma in lower half of field resembles non-neoplastic adrenal medulla at top. A thin zone of residual adrenal cortex is present near the center of the field.

or even the residual adrenal medulla (fig. 10-18, right). Occasionally, the similarity in morphology between some pheochromocytomas and adrenal cortical neoplasms can result in misdiagnosis in routine sections. A tumor may also undergo what appears to be spontaneous hemorrhagic necrosis with extensive disruption of the architecture of much of the tumor making accurate diagnosis difficult without the aid of ancillary stains (fig. 10-19).

Cellular Morphology. The cytoplasm of tumor cells is often lightly eosinophilic and finely granular, but it is sometimes amphophilic to basophilic or may even have a lavender hue with a myriad of minute punctate granules that can barely be seen by light microscopy (fig. 10-20). Tumor cells may be polygonal with sharply defined cell borders, or the cells may interdigitate with indistinct cytoplasmic outlines. Some cells may contain large vacuoles which resemble the "pseudoacini" seen in some carotid body type paragangliomas; in many instances this feature does not appear to be an artifact of fixation or processing (fig. 10-21). A potentially confusing picture has been ascribed to lipid degeneration (39,45) in which the tumor can mimic an adrenal cortical neoplasm with abundant intracytoplasmic lipid (fig. 10-22). Some tumor cells contain such abundant and densely eosinophilic cytoplasm that the tumor has oncocytic features (fig. 10-23). Variation in staining intensity, sometimes in routinely stained sections, gives the impression of a dimorphic population of "light" and "dark" types of cells (fig. 10-24), but this has no known significance.

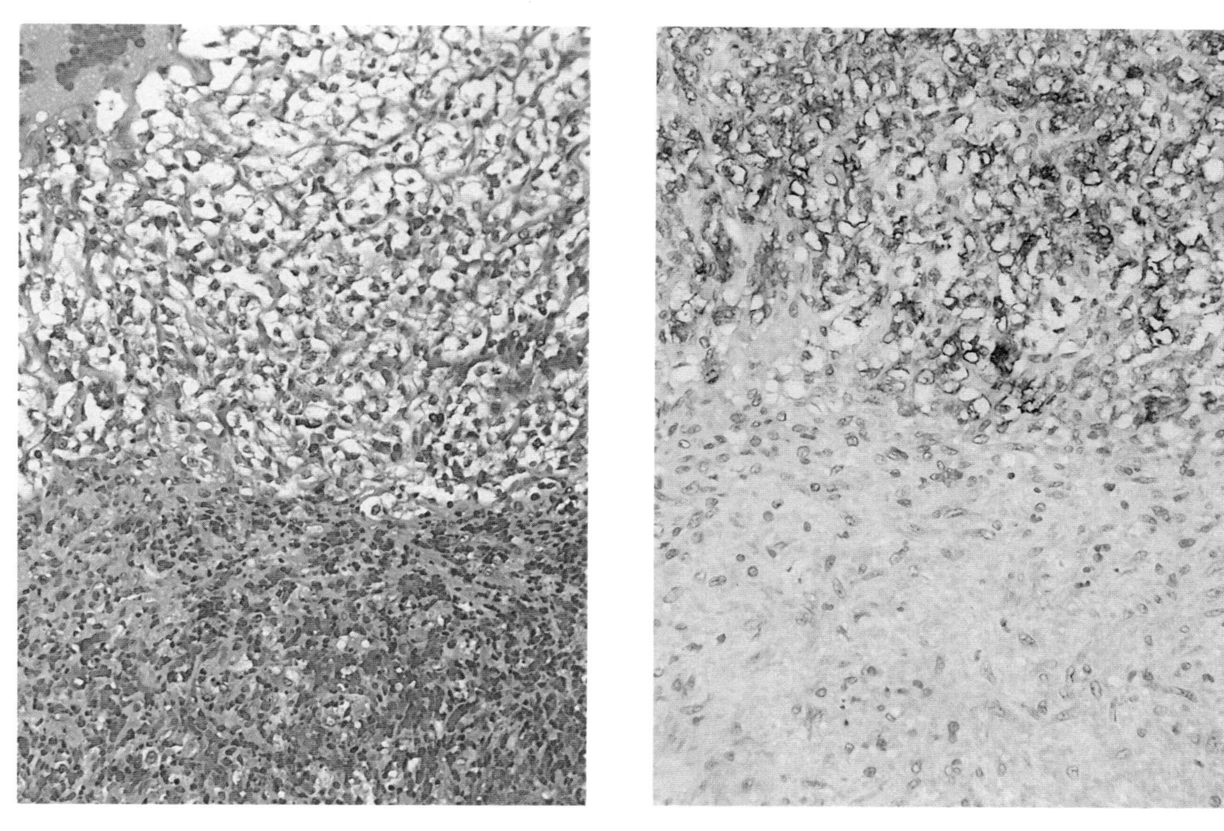

Figure 10-19
PHEOCHROMOCYTOMA

Left: A pheochromocytoma with extensive "spontaneous" hemorrhage and necrosis. Much of the tumor had areas of granulation tissue with organization. Viable tumor is present at top of field. Grossly, the tumor simulated a hematoma.

Right: Residual tumor is strongly immunoreactive for chromogranin A. An area of organizing granulation tissue is in lower half of field. (X200, Peroxidase-antiperoxidase stain)

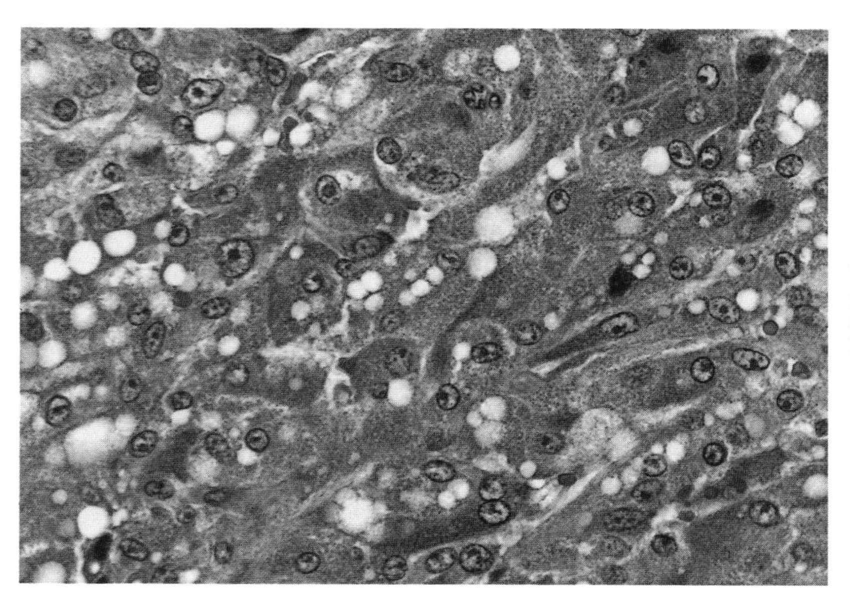

Figure 10-20
PHEOCHROMOCYTOMA

The tumor cells have indistinct cell borders and contain numerous small pinpoint granules. When granules are numerous the cytoplasm may acquire a lavender tint.

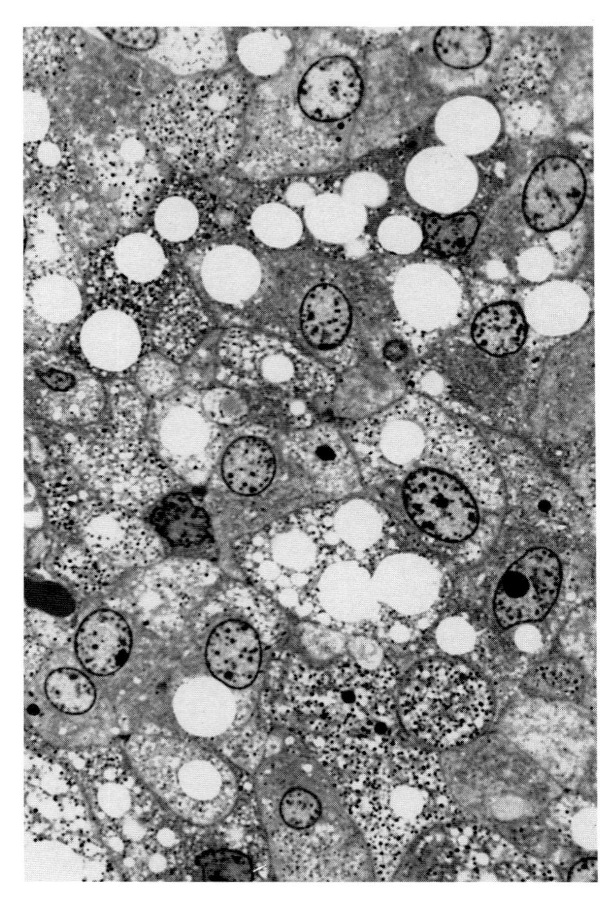

Figure 10-21
PHEOCHROMOCYTOMA

The tumor cells have numerous vacuolar spaces within the cytoplasm (so called pseudoacini). There are punctate blue-black granules of variable density, most of which were dense-core neurosecretory granules on ultrastructural study. Some cells vary in overall staining of cytoplasm giving the impression of "light" and "dark" cells. The tumor specimen was fresh and electron microscopy showed that it was excellently preserved. (X1,000, Toluidine blue stain)

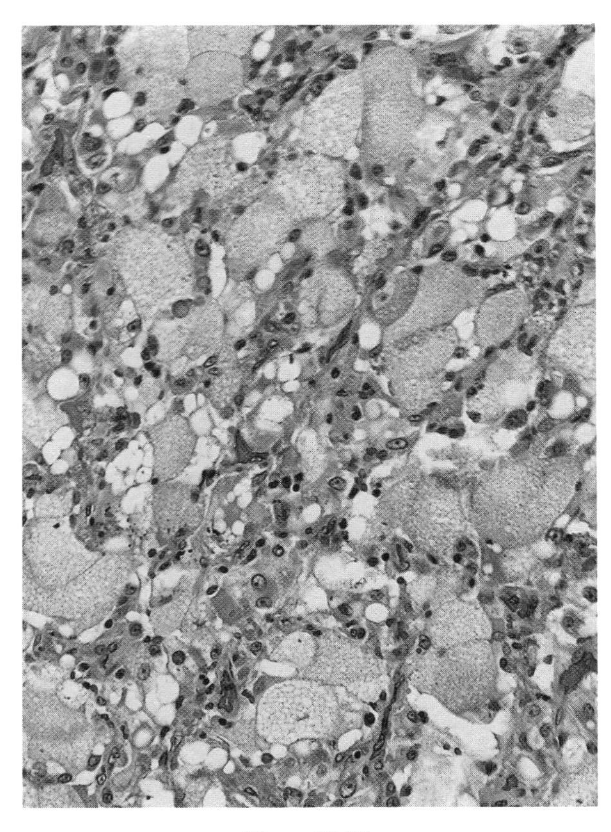

Figure 10-22
PHEOCHROMOCYTOMA

This pheochromocytoma had areas of "lipid degeneration," with enlarged cells having finely vacuolated cytoplasm.

The nuclei of some cells contain one or more "pseudoinclusions" which usually appear as a solitary, round to oval structure of variable size having the same tinctorial staining as the remaining cytoplasm (fig. 10-25). These are irregular folds or indentations of the nuclear membrane with invagination of cell cytoplasm (29). Nuclear pseudoinclusions may be central or eccentric when viewed en face, with a smooth or occasionally notched border. There may be a difference in density of cellular organelles within the pseudoinclusion resulting in variation in staining intensity, and sometimes there are one or more vacuoles. Rarely, there is more than one pseudoinclusion, and in some areas with excessive nuclear folding the process may be viewed in profile.

There may be intracytoplasmic hyaline globules which are periodic acid–Schiff (PAS) positive and resistant to diastase predigestion; these globules are identical to those observed in the normal (28) and hyperplastic adrenal medulla. The globules may be numerous (fig. 10-26), or sparse in number and very difficult to identify on casual inspection. In one study, globules were detected in 38 of 64 clinically benign and only 8 of 34 malignant sympathoadrenal paragangliomas (35). They have been related to secretory activity in some way, but their functional significance is not clear (37). It is important to remember that intracytoplasmic hyaline globules have also been reported in about 10 percent of adrenal cortical neoplasms, both benign and malignant (33).

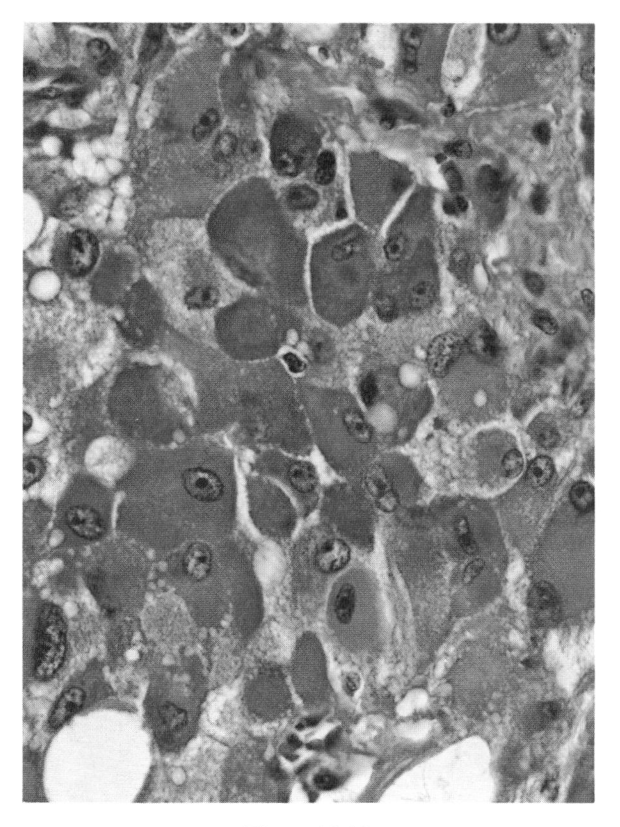

Figure 10-23
PHEOCHROMOCYTOMA
Tumor cells have copious cytoplasm which is densely eosinophilic and finely granular, giving the cells an "oncocytic" appearance.

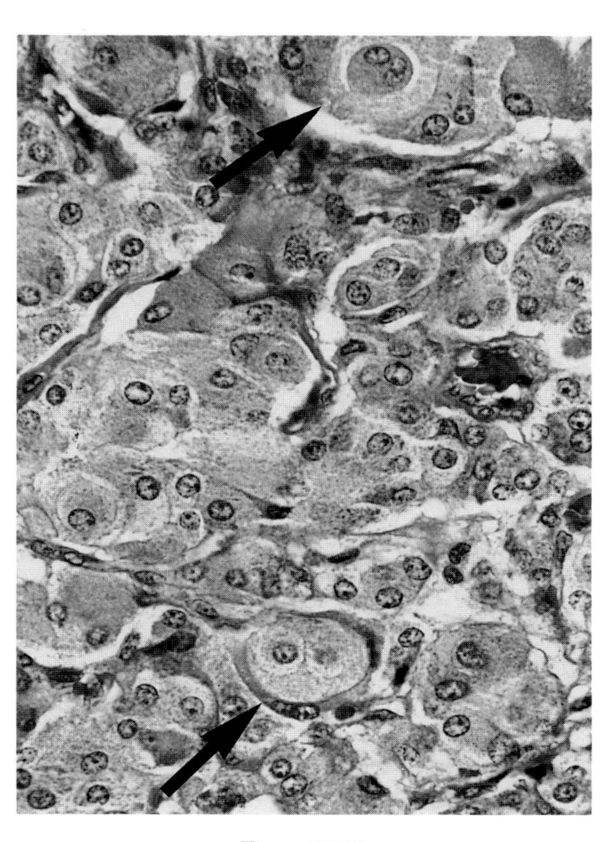

Figure 10-24
PHEOCHROMOCYTOMA
Some tumor cells vary in overall density of cytoplasmic staining suggesting a dimorphic ("light" and "dark") cell population. Note that some cells (arrows) partially envelop other cells ("cell embracing").

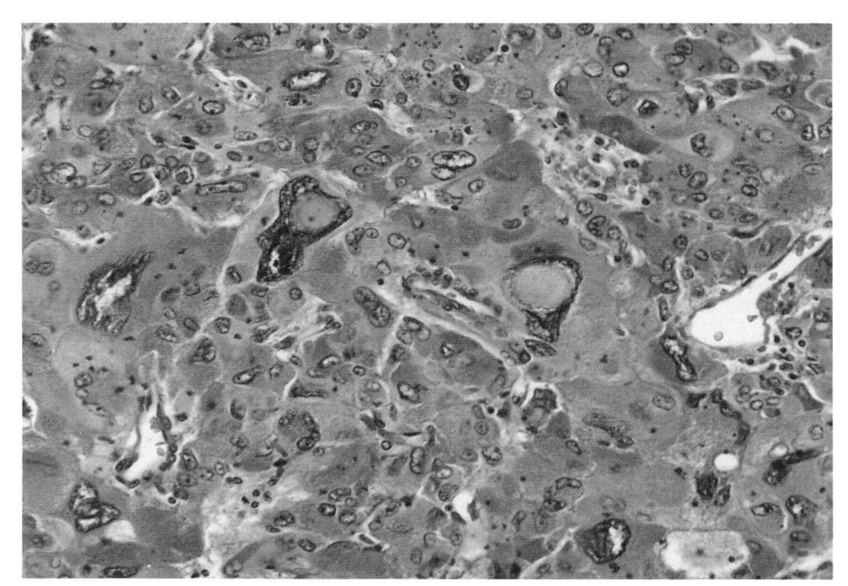

Figure 10-25
PHEOCHROMOCYTOMA
Two tumor cells having large nuclear "pseudoinclusions." There is a moderate degree of nuclear pleomorphism and hyperchromasia.

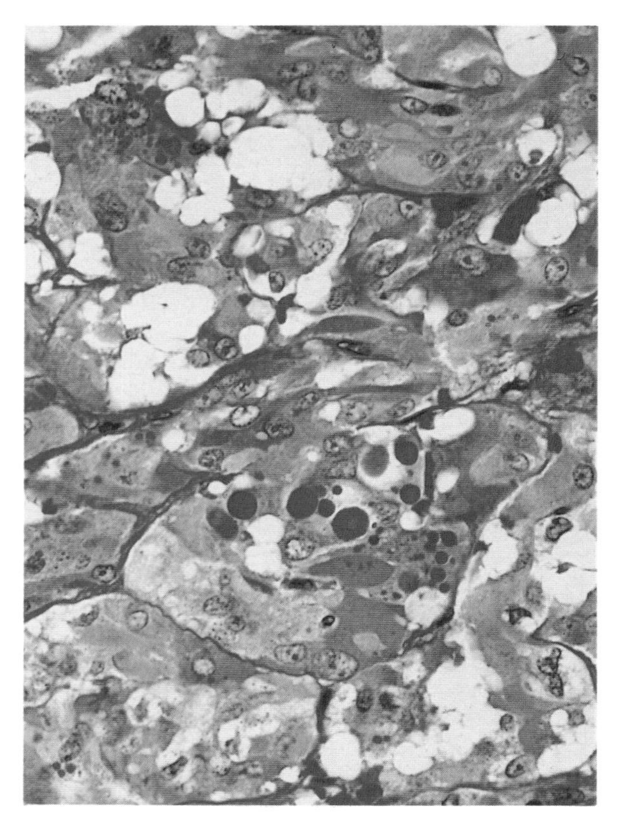

Figure 10-26
PHEOCHROMOCYTOMA
A few tumor cells in this field contain numerous eosinophilic hyaline globules which vary considerably in size. Some appear to reside in an extracellular location, but this is probably an artifact.

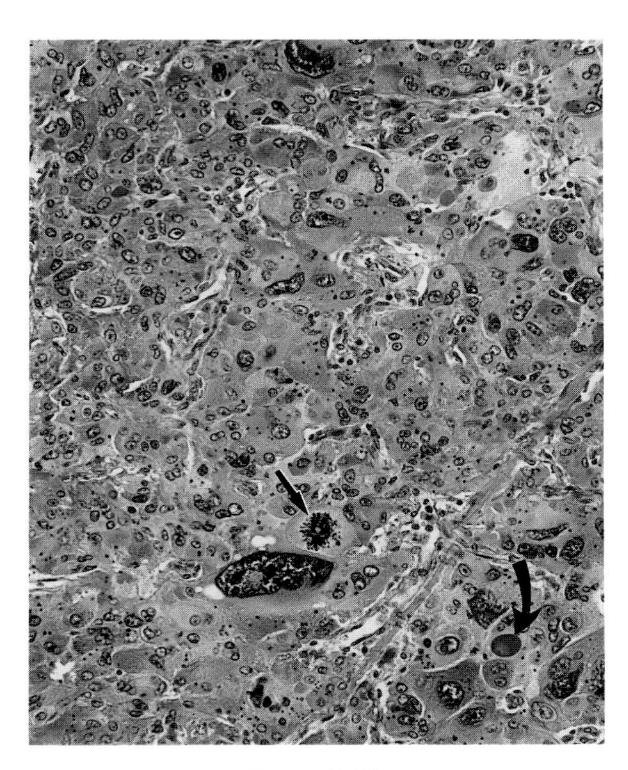

Figure 10-27
PHEOCHROMOCYTOMA
There is a marked degree of nuclear pleomorphism and hyperchromasia, a rare mitotic figure (straight arrow), and an occasional hyaline globule (curved arrow).

Some tumors contain cells with moderate to marked nuclear enlargement and hyperchromasia (fig. 10-27), and occasionally this nuclear pleomorphism can be a spectacular histologic feature. In several recent studies, nuclear atypia or pleomorphism has not been shown to have a significant impact on prognosis. Occasional mitotic figures can be identified in tumors which prove to be clinically benign. In the study by Linnoila et al. (35), an average of one mitosis per 30 high-power fields was found in clinically benign sympathoadrenal paragangliomas. Occasionally, cells within an otherwise typical pheochromocytoma may have cytologic features resembling neuronal or ganglion cells, with tapering cell processes, eccentric nucleus with nucleolus, and even granular basophilic material at the edge of the cell resembling Nissl substance (fig. 10-28). These and other neural features may be seen in tumors classified as composite pheochromocytomas.

The cytoplasm of pheochromocytoma cells (and other paraganglioma cells) is typically argyrophilic (fig. 10-29), and the specificity of the Grimelius stain for neurosecretory granules has been demonstrated by ultrastructural study (46). Melanin-like pigment has recently been reported in pheochromocytomas (27,34); ultrastructurally melanosomes and premelanosomes were found, but alternative interpretations for this pigment include neuromelanin, lipofuscin, or products related to catecholamine oxidation (34). The pigment is argentaffin positive with the Fontana-Masson stain and labile to bleaching procedures using permanganate or picric acid (27,34). These are rare tumors and common embryogenesis along with melanocytes from the neural crest should not negate the possibility of a shared morphologic phenotype. An example of

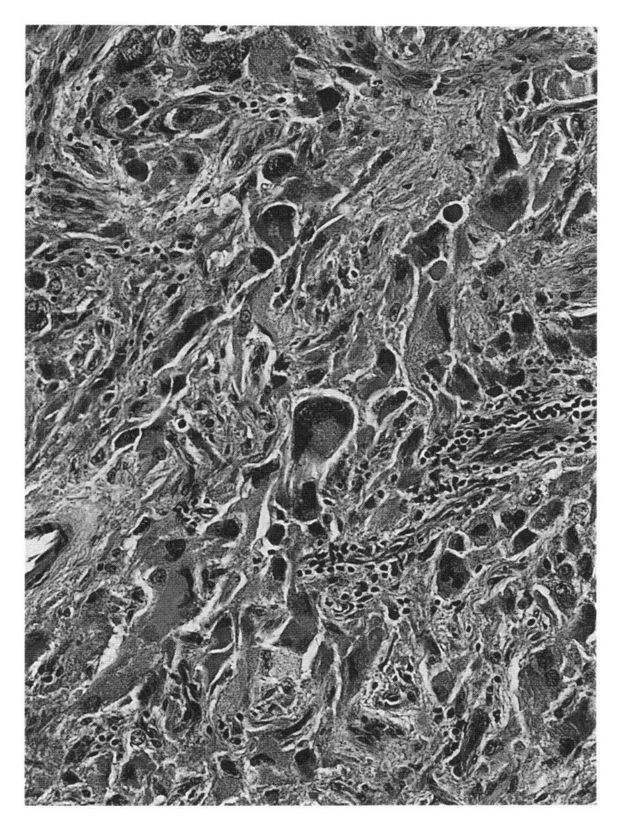

Figure 10-28
PHEOCHROMOCYTOMA
Areas of tumor contain cells with ganglionic or neuronal features. Some cells had prominent nucleoli, and basophilic material in peripheral cytoplasm resembling Nissl substance.

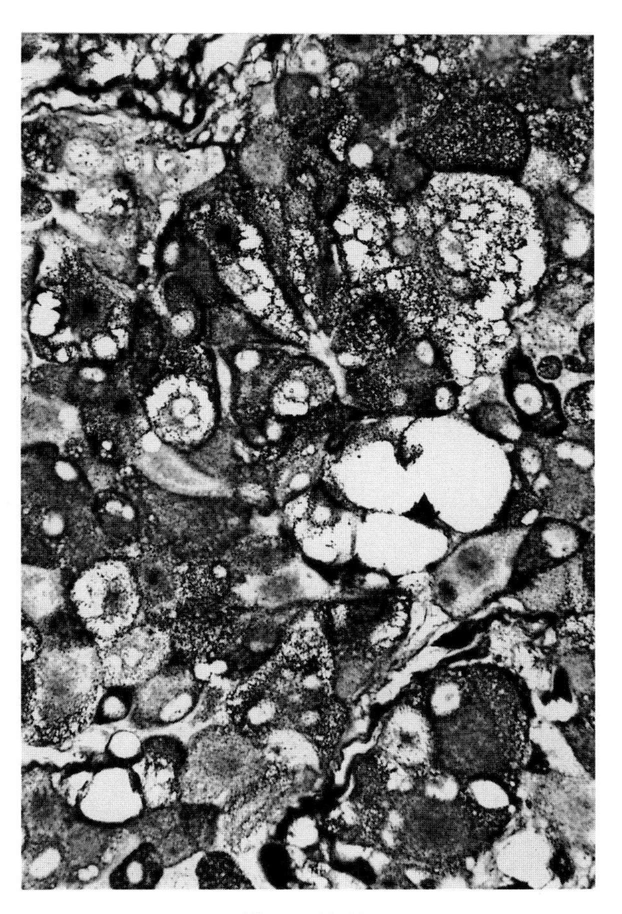

Figure 10-29
PHEOCHROMOCYTOMA
There is strong cytoplasmic argyrophilia with a myriad of pinpoint granules. (X375, Grimelius stain)

a pigmented extra-adrenal paraganglioma of the retroperitoneum is illustrated in chapter 12.

Stromal Alterations. Some pheochromocytomas exhibit remarkable alterations in connective tissue stroma, and this may cause problems in diagnosis. Areas of sclerosis may be prominent (fig. 10-30), sometimes in association with cystic degeneration. Amyloid has been identified in pheochromocytomas (36,44); in a recent study it was found in 70 percent of pheochromocytomas and in most cases was considered abundant (44). The amyloid was detected by Congo red stain, but the ultrastructural features were not illustrated (36, 44). In this author's experience, stromal changes suggesting amyloid are less frequent and almost never abundant. A recent study identified amyloid deposits in 9 percent of pheochromocytomas (37a). At times, sclerosis can have a sinusoidal distribution with accentuation of the alveolar or trabecular pattern of tumor cells (fig. 10-31, left). In some tumors the fibrosis can severely distort the shape of entrapped tumor cells (fig. 10-31, right). A prominent vascular component with plump endothelial cells may be confused with a vasoformative neoplasm (fig. 10-32). Pheochromocytomas (and other paragangliomas) are characteristically highly vascular neoplasms, and hemorrhage within a tumor may artifactually separate clusters of tumor cells. Lakes of eosinophilic proteinaceous material can be seen in occasional pheochromocytomas which have clear vacuoles at the periphery (fig. 10-33); this most likely represents a secondary or degenerative change within the tumor. Rarely, there may

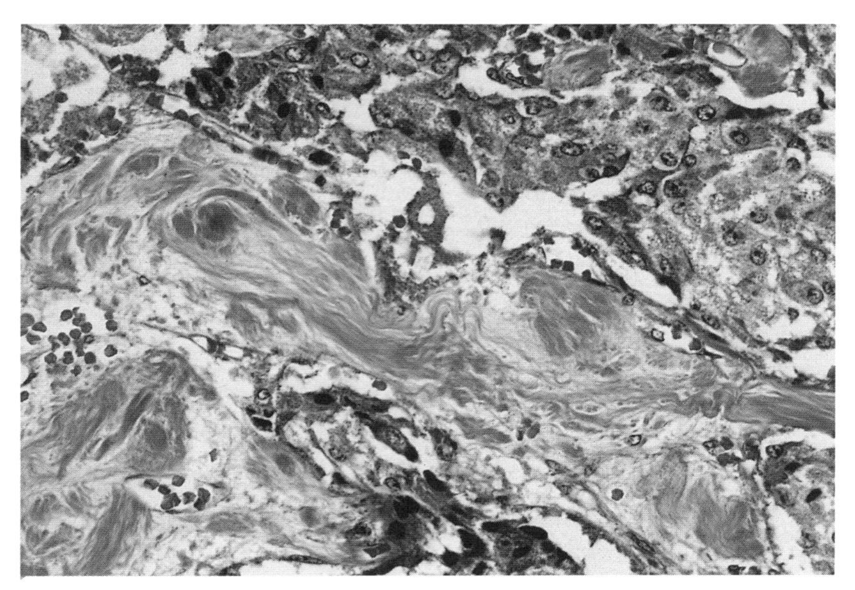

Figure 10-30
PHEOCHROMOCYTOMA
Areas of dense sclerosis incorporate small nests of tumor cells. The fibrotic matrix has a fibrillar quality in areas. The stain for collagen was strongly positive.

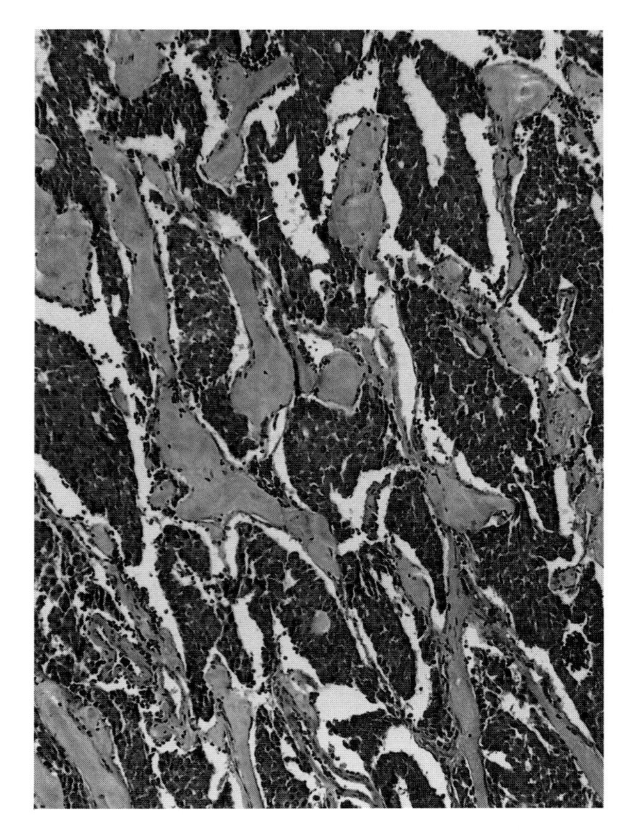

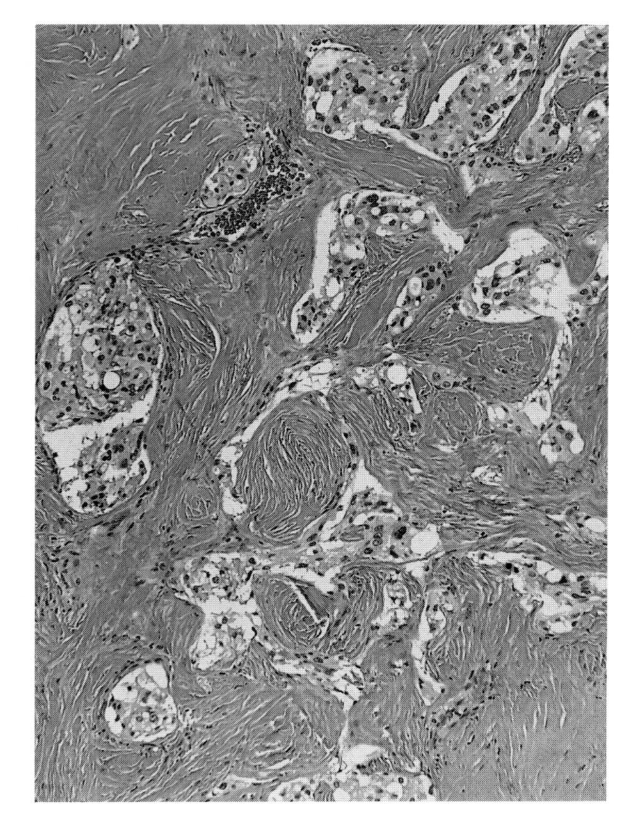

Figure 10-31
PHEOCHROMOCYTOMA
Left: The fibrosis within a pheochromocytoma has a sinusoidal pattern with accentuation of anastomosing trabeculae of tumor cells.
Right: Dense fibrosis within a pheochromocytoma with compression and distortion of tumor cells. The hyalinized stroma resembles amyloid.

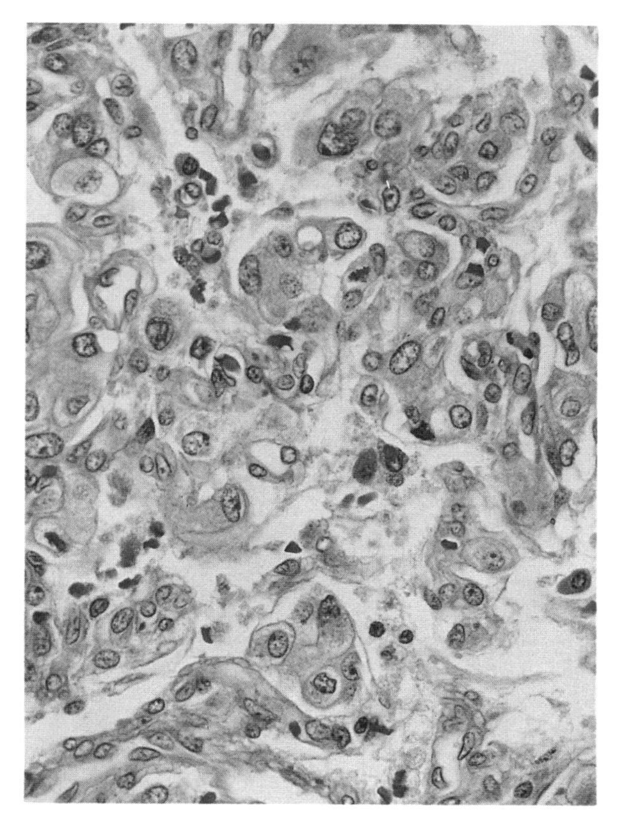

Figure 10-32
PHEOCHROMOCYTOMA
There is a prominent microvasculature with plump endothelial cells. Occasional mast cells are also present.

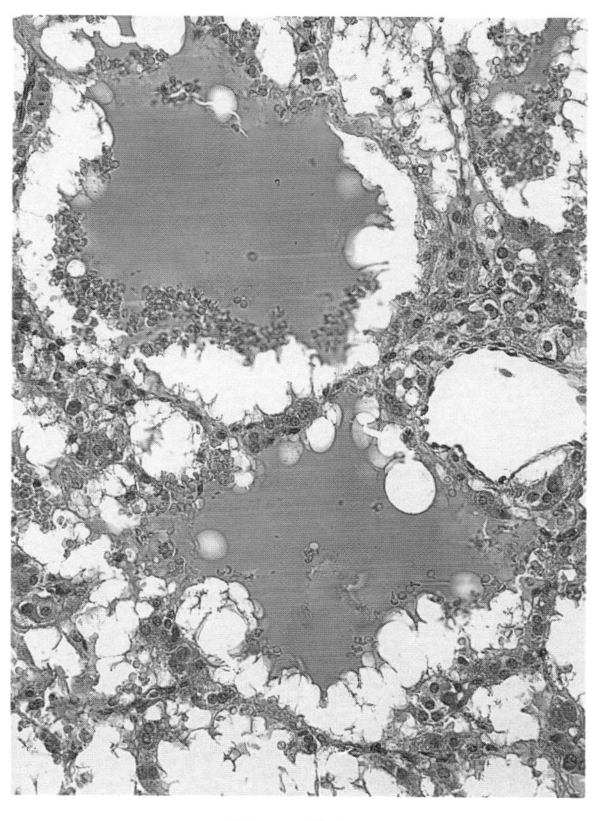

Figure 10-33
PHEOCHROMOCYTOMA
Proteinaceous lakes in a pheochromocytoma with peripheral vacuoles or "scalloping." This is probably a degenerative change.

be gaping sinusoids with a broad anastomosing trabecular arrangement of cells (fig. 10-34), but this should not be confused with the broad trabecular pattern seen in some adrenal cortical carcinomas.

The Chromaffin Reaction. The chromaffin reaction is due to oxidation of catecholamines to form adrenochrome pigments. It was described in 1865 (47), and has sometimes been referred to as the "Henle chromoreaction"; Sherwin and Rosen (49) credit Joesteu in 1864 with an earlier description of the chromaffin reaction. Dichromate-containing fixatives may produce the chromaffin reaction on fresh tumor tissue with a resulting dark brown color (fig. 10-35). At one time the gross chromoreaction was considered the most valuable single procedure in the diagnosis of pheochromocytoma, but currently, with the availability of more sophisticated modern technology, the chromaffin reaction is mainly of historic interest (48). The chromaffin reaction can also be detected microscopically, but with prolonged fixation in aqueous fixatives it may become quite weak due to aqueous extraction of catecholamines. The fixative solution may turn dark brown or the color of cider over time.

Periadrenal Brown Fat. An increased prevalence of periadrenal brown adipose tissue (BAT) has been reported in association with 50 to 88 percent of pheochromocytomas (fig. 10-36) (58,59, 62). It has been suggested that catecholamines play a significant role in the transformation of periadrenal fat into BAT (53,61). Reactivation of intra-abdominal fat in the presence of high circulating norepinephrine levels may contribute to the weight loss often observed in patients with

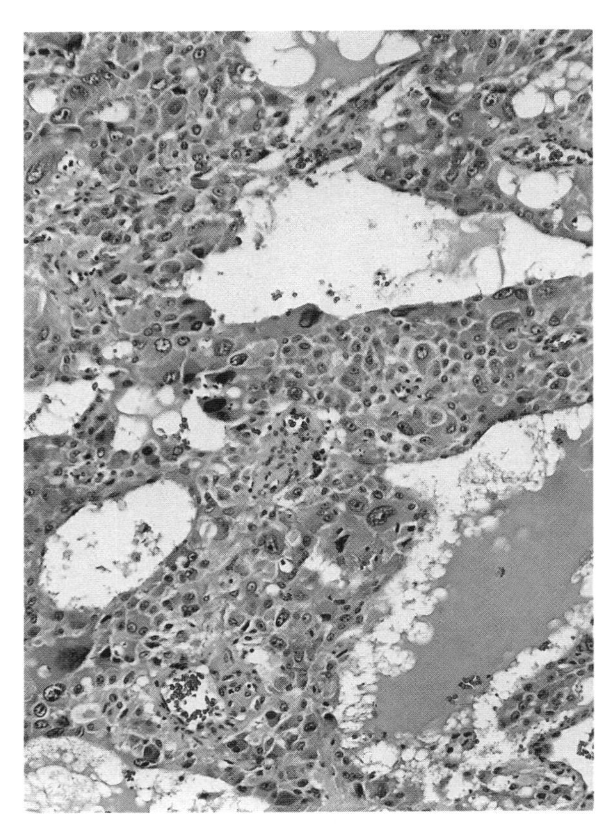

Figure 10-34
PHEOCHROMOCYTOMA
Pheochromocytoma with dilated vascular spaces. The tumor could be mistaken for an adrenal cortical carcinoma.

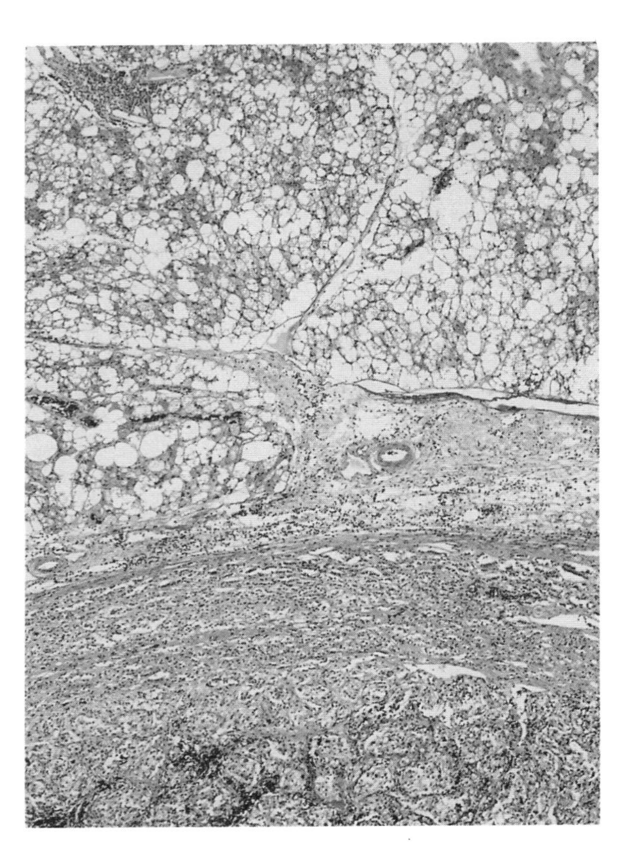

Figure 10-36
PHEOCHROMOCYTOMA
There is abundant periadrenal brown adipose tissue. In the lower half of the field there is a fibrous pseudocapsule and an investing adrenal capsule.

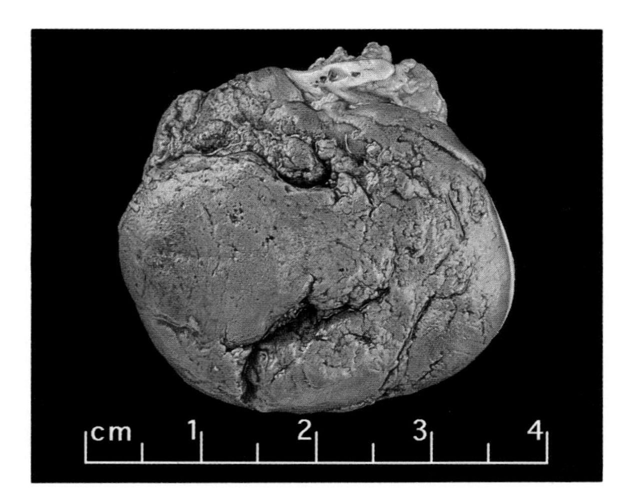

Figure 10-35
PHEOCHROMOCYTOMA
A positive chromaffin reaction followed immersion in Zenker's fixative. The same tumor is seen in a fresh, unfixed state in figure 10-4, right. The chromaffin reaction is apparent as a dark, mahogany brown color which deepened slightly on exposure to air.

pheochromocytoma (53). Pheochromocytomas have also been reported in association with tumors of brown or fetal fat ("hibernomas") (51,54). Heat production due to uncoupling of oxidative phosphorylation has been proposed as a mechanism for the fevers that some patients with pheochromocytoma experience, and following surgical resection the patient may become afebrile due to decreased adrenergic hyperactivity (52). A recent study showed no significant difference in the prevalence of BAT in control patients (51 percent) and those with a pheochromocytoma (53 percent) (57), but additional studies need to be done using more critical quantitative evaluation.

Other Associated Abnormalities. Catecholamine-associated cardiomyopathy can occur in patients with pheochromocytoma, with associated arrhythmias, cardiac failure, and occasionally even sudden death. There may be myocardial lesions (active catecholamine myocarditis) showing focal degeneration and necrosis of myocardium along with mild inflammation, particularly involving the inner two thirds of the left ventricular myocardium (63). Other associated abnormalities include fibromuscular dysplasia (55), renal artery stenosis, multiple intracranial aneurysms (50), cholelithiasis (23 percent of patients reported by ReMine et al. [60]) and a variety of constitutional and metabolic abnormalities covered in greater detail elsewhere (56).

FAMILIAL PHEOCHROMOCYTOMA

Familial occurrence of pheochromocytomas has been reported in about 10 percent of cases (88), but the incidence varies depending upon the series examined, referral patterns, and other factors (93). Familial pheochromocytomas are most notable in MEN syndrome types IIa and IIb, but can occur with von Recklinghausen's disease and von Hippel-Lindau disease. About 5 percent of cases of pheochromocytoma are reported in association with von Recklinghausen's disease (86,87), although some estimate the frequency of association is probably 1 percent or less (108). Some reports indicate a higher association of pheochromocytoma in patients with von Recklinghausen's disease who have coexisting hypertension (92). Recently a case of bilateral composite pheochromocytoma-ganglioneuroma was reported in a patient with type 1 neurofibromatosis (77), as well as another case with bilateral pheochromocytoma-malignant peripheral nerve sheath tumor (109a). Pheochromocytomas have been reported in 10 percent (90) to 21 percent (64,105) of patients with von Hippel-Lindau disease, and there is an increased incidence of bilateral tumors (64,111). There appears to be no firm evidence linking pheochromocytoma with tuberous sclerosis or Sturge-Weber disease (86). Pheochromocytomas can also occur in a familial setting without any other associated disease (88). Patients with familial pheochromocytoma in the setting of MEN syndrome type II and von Hippel-Lindau disease tend to be younger at diagnosis than those with sporadic pheochromocytomas (105).

Pheochromocytomas in MEN Syndrome Types IIa and IIb

Pheochromocytomas develop in 30 to 50 percent of patients with MEN type II (76,84,113); the tumors are bilateral or multifocal in about 60 percent (119) to 70 percent of cases (67,113) or even higher (97). Patients may be asymptomatic (75), and the pheochromocytoma may not respond to the usual provocative tests (112). The tumors tend to produce more epinephrine in contrast to sporadic pheochromocytomas in which norepinephrine is the predominant catecholamine secreted (82,85, 89,112). A case of Cushing's syndrome due to ectopic adrenocorticotrophic hormone (ACTH) production by bilateral pheochromocytomas has been reported (103). A kindred has also been reported with symmetric pruritic skin lesions, but the etiology was unclear (66).

When the pheochromocytoma is small there is often extratumoral adrenal medullary hyperplasia, but when the tumor is large it may not be possible to evaluate the non-neoplastic medulla (fig. 10-37). Extra-adrenal paragangliomas have been reported in the MEN type II syndrome (96,98), but they appear to be uncommon. The gross morphologic features alone may be sufficiently distinctive that the surgical pathologist is alerted to the possibility of MEN type IIa or IIb (117).

Cytogenetic studies in patients with MEN IIa and IIb indicate a genetic linkage to a locus near the centromere of chromosome 10 (91,99,116), and the availability of sensitive DNA probes has permitted screening of individuals at risk at any age with a high level of certainty (95). There may also be a deletion of a hypervariable region of DNA on the short arm of chromosome 1, but it does not represent the site of inherited mutation in MEN type II (100). The *ret* proto-oncogene, located in the DNA segment 10q11.2, is reported to be consistently expressed in patients with pheochromocytoma and medullary thyroid carcinoma (MTC) (110), and missense mutations of this oncogene have been identified in a high proportion of families with MEN IIa (110) and MEN IIb (68). Although MEN syndrome types I and IIa are considered distinct separate entities, there may be rare exceptions (93,94).

The biologic behavior of pheochromocytomas in MEN IIa and IIb varies from series to series (93). Some have suggested that these tumors are

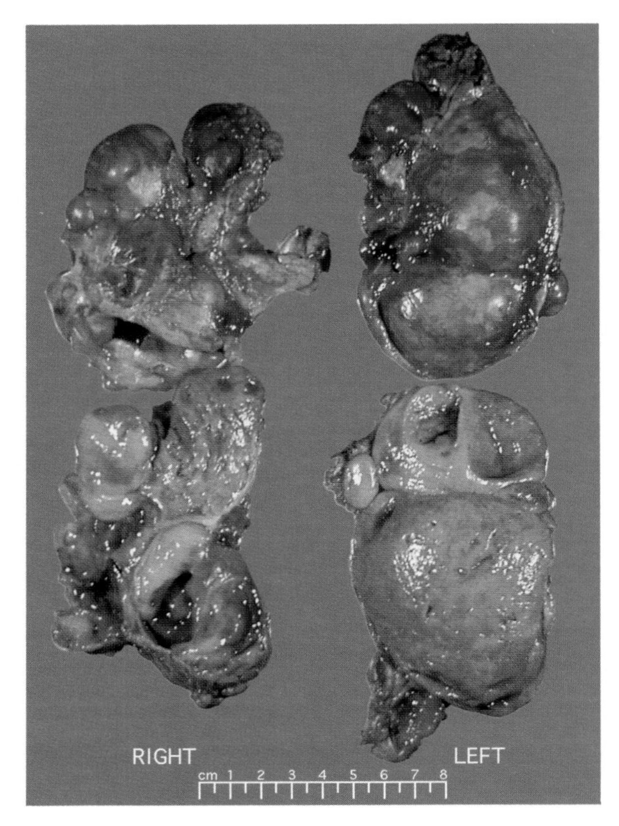

Figure 10-37
BILATERAL PHEOCHROMOCYTOMA
Cross section of bilateral pheochromocytomas from a 30-year-old man with MEN syndrome type IIa. The right adrenal tumor weighed 168 g and the left 220 g. Note the distinct multinodular, multicentric pattern of growth on both sides.

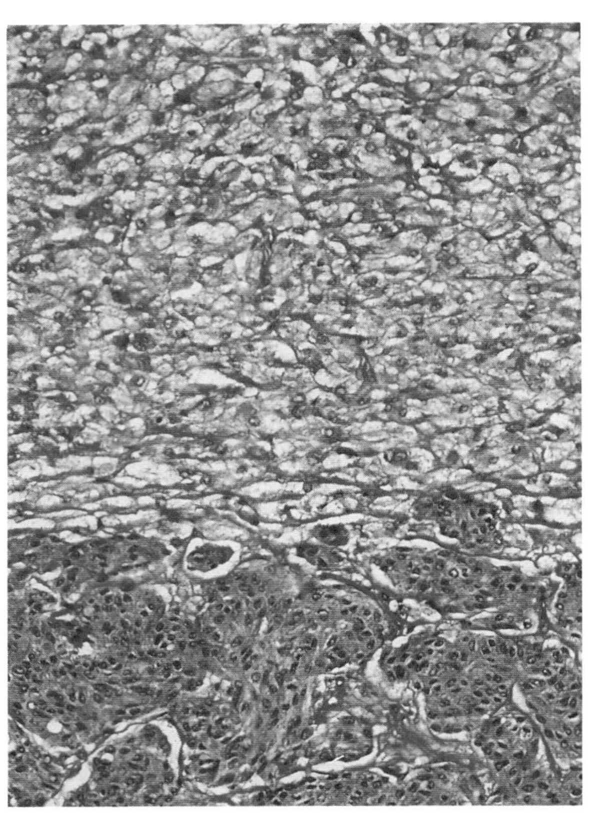

Figure 10-38
MEDULLARY THYROID CARCINOMA
METASTATIC TO A PHEOCHROMOCYTOMA
Medullary thyroid carcinoma (MTC) (bottom of field) metastatic to a pheochromocytoma (top of field) in a patient with MEN syndrome type IIa. Metastatic MTC was diffusely and strongly positive for thyrocalcitonin.

extreme examples of adrenal medullary hyperplasia (79,82). Some data suggest that malignant pheochromocytomas are relatively rare in MEN type II (67,78,105) and possibly the von Hipple-Lindau disease (105). In a study by Carney et al. (75), 5 of 19 patients (6 MEN IIb, 13 MEN IIa) died as a direct result of the pheochromocytoma (29 percent): 1 due to intracerebral hemorrhage, 2 due to hypotensive crises, and 2 because of pulmonary metastases; 4 patients developed metastases to lung, liver, or bone (21 percent). In a recent review of 10 series of patients with MEN type II the incidence of malignant pheochromocytoma was 4.4 percent (84). Rare tumor to tumor metastases have occurred from medullary thyroid carcinoma to pheochromocytoma (fig. 10-38) (82,93,101,114).

MEN Syndrome Type IIb

The phenotypic expression of MEN type IIb is very distinctive. The various abnormalities are listed in Tables 10-3 and 10-4. Although this syndrome also has an autosomal dominant pattern of inheritance similar to MEN IIa, not infrequently cases may appear to be isolated or sporadic. Mucosal neuromas of the oral and labial mucosae are often the first manifestation, usually in the first decade of life (87). The tongue has multiple nodular or hemispheric fleshy protrusions characteristically studding the anterior portion and extending along the lateral borders (fig. 10-39) (93,94). The lips may be thickened and nodular giving a "blubbery" appearance. The nasal, laryngeal, pharyngeal, and conjunctival

Table 10-3

MULTIPLE ENDOCRINE NEOPLASIA (MEN) SYNDROME TYPE IIB: PHENOTYPIC MANIFESTATIONS

Upper Aerodigestive Tract/Gastrointestinal Tract
Neuromatous proliferation in oral, lingual, and other mucosal sites in upper aerodigestive tract
Ganglioneuromatosis of gastrointestinal tract
Variety of manifestations: motility disorders including megacolon, cholecystitis (calculous or acalculous)

Ocular
Thickened corneal nerves, perilimbal neuromas, keratoconjunctivitis sicca, failing vision (rare)
Conjunctival/eyelid neuromas

Neuromuscular
Marfanoid habitus, asthenia with muscular atrophy, somatic and autonomic neuropathy

Musculoskeletal Abnormalities
Elongated facies, dolichocephaly, micrognathia, laxity of joints, congenital dislocation of hip, lordosis, kyphosis, genu valgum, slipped femoral capital epiphysis, cox valga, pes cavus

Table 10-4

MULTIPLE ENDOCRINE NEOPLASIA (MEN) SYNDROME TYPE IIB: ENDOCRINE MANIFESTATIONS

Medullary Thyroid Carcinoma
Aggressive tumor with metastasis/recurrence: most pernicious component of syndrome

Adrenal Medullary Disease
(Hyperplasia and pheochromocytoma) Adrenal medullary disease (34%) with bilateral pheochromocytomas (68%)

Parathyroid Enlargement/Hyperplasia
Very low incidence of clinical/biochemical hyperfunction (4%)

mucosae can also be involved. The neural lesions are composed of circumscribed but unencapsulated aggregates of hypertrophied, elongated nerves (fig. 10-40), occasionally with some interstitial edema or myxoid stroma. The lesions only superficially resemble "traumatic" or "amputation" neuromas (93,94). The term *mucosal ganglioneuromatosis* has been used because these lesions may represent just the "tip of the iceberg" in terms of gastrointestinal involvement (69,74); ganglion cells, however, are usually not seen in these superficial mucosal lesions (93,94).

The ocular manifestations are also distinctive and include neuromatous nodules on lid and conjunctiva; thickening of lids, sometimes with eversion; thickened perilimbal neuromas; and the presence of thickened corneal nerves within a clear corneal stroma (fig. 10-41). Visual impairment due to hypertrophied corneal nerves occasionally occurs (83). A variety of neurologic signs and symptoms may result from involvement of somatic and sensory nerves or the autonomic nervous system (83). Ganglioneuromatosis of the urinary bladder has been reported with secondary bladder

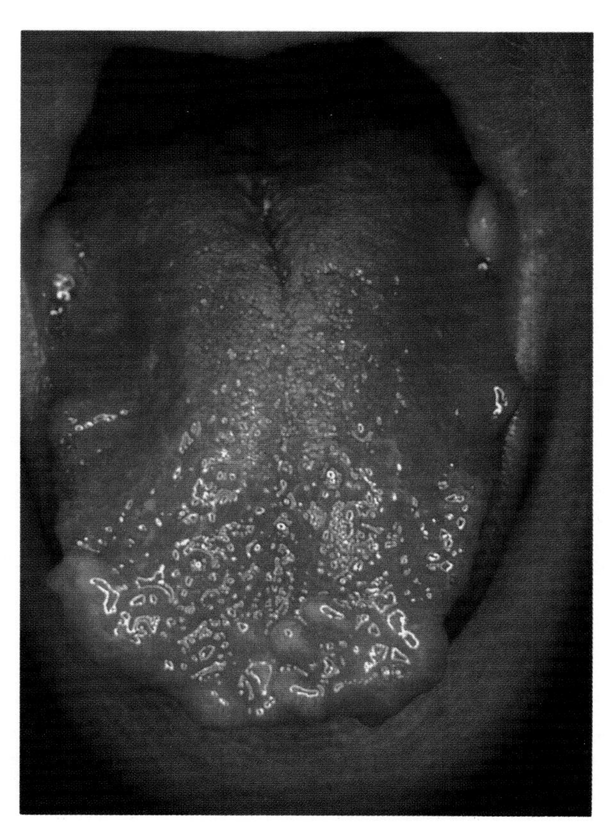

Figure 10-39
MEN SYNDROME TYPE IIB
Young female with MEN syndrome type IIb has grotesque mucosal neuromatous nodules. The patient died of widely metastatic medullary thyroid carcinoma. No other immediate family members had MEN IIb.

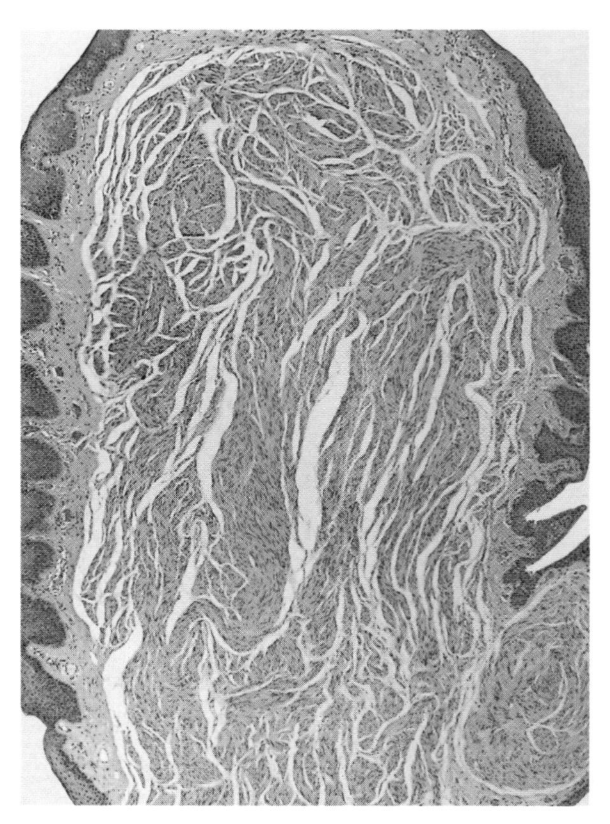

Figure 10-40
MEN SYNDROME TYPE IIB
Polypoid lesion of eyelid from patient with MEN syndrome type IIb. Irregular bundles of myelinated nerve with slight interstitial edema are seen. No ganglion cells were identified.

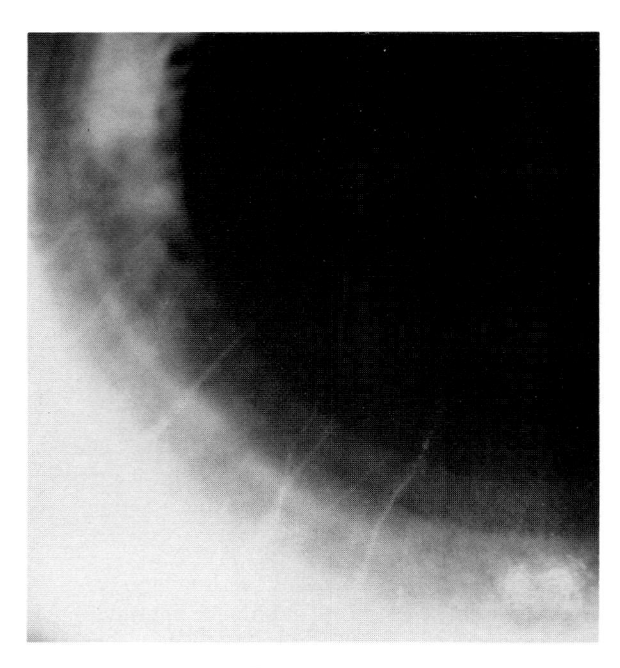

Figure 10-41
MEN SYNDROME TYPE IIB
Young female with MEN syndrome type IIb has thickened elongated nerves coursing from the limbus in clear corneal stroma. (Fig. 4-57 from Lack EE. Adrenal medullary hyperplasia and pheochromocytoma. In: Lack EE, ed. Pathology of the adrenal glands. New York: Churchill Livingstone, 1990:173–235.)

infections (109). There is a low incidence of parathyroid disease in MEN IIb (4 percent) (73), and most descriptions of parathyroid hyperplasia are not accompanied by hyperfunction (71).

The gastrointestinal manifestations in MEN IIb are important to recognize since they form a prominent component of the syndrome and often antedate the endocrine neoplasms (65,69,70,80). Manifestations include intestinal dysmotility with constipation, intestinal pseudo-obstruction, borborygmi, projectile vomiting, or a clinical picture mimicking megacolon or diverticulitis. Ganglioneuromatosis involves much of the gastrointestinal tract and all layers to a variable extent. It can involve other sites as well such as pancreas, salivary gland, adrenal gland (73), and gallbladder. The ganglioneuromatosis consists of a hamartomatous proliferation of Schwann cells, neurites, and ganglion cells, and it has been implicated in motility disturbances. Intestinal ganglioneuromatosis (mainly mucosal) can also be found in patients without MEN IIb but with juvenile polyposis (102,107), colonic polyps (115, 118), colonic adenocarcinoma, von Recklinghausen's disease (81), and rarely, as a nonspecific finding in inflamed bowel.

The most life-threatening component of MEN IIb is medullary thyroid carcinoma (MTC) which is often aggressive with fatal outcome (72,73,106). In the review by Carney et al. (72,73), 22 percent of 69 patients with MTC died at an average age of 21 years, and it was suggested that most patients would die of metastatic MTC unless total thyroidectomy was performed at an early age. Adrenal medullary disease was diagnosed in 34 percent of patients at an average age of 25 years, and 68 percent of pheochromocytomas were bilateral. Once a diagnosis of adrenal medullary disease is made, total adrenalectomy is recommended (73).

Table 10-5

OTHER ENDOCRINE DISORDERS ASSOCIATED WITH PHEOCHROMOCYTOMA

Chemodectoma, bronchial carcinoid tumor, pituitary adenoma, hyperplasia of parathyroid glands, and duodenal gastrin-producing cells
Pituitary adenoma, parathyroid hyperplasia, and multiple functioning extra-adrenal paragangliomas
Medullary thyroid carcinoma, multiple parathyroid adenomas, adrenal cortical adenoma, and small cell carcinoma of bronchus
Bilateral pheochromocytoma and pancreatic islet cell tumor
Familial pheochromocytoma and pancreatic islet cell tumor
Pituitary adenoma and pheochromocytoma
Pituitary adenoma, papillary thyroid carcinoma, bilateral carotid body paraganglioma (CBP), parathyroid hyperplasia, gastric leiomyoma, and systemic amyloidosis
von Recklinghausen's disease, pheochromocytoma, and duodenal carcinoid tumor
von Recklinghausen's disease, pheochromocytoma, jugulotympanic paraganglioma (JTP), and pulmonary paragangliomas
Pheochromocytoma and papillary thyroid carcinoma

Other Associated Endocrine Disorders

Other endocrine tumors (or hyperplasias) have occurred in association with pheochromocytoma (or other paragangliomas), usually in a sporadic setting. Some have been regarded as a distinct MEN syndrome or variant of MEN (120). A list of some of these associations is given in Table 10-5.

THE TRIAD OF GASTRIC EPITHELIOID LEIOMYOSARCOMA, PULMONARY CHONDROMA, AND FUNCTIONING EXTRA-ADRENAL PARAGANGLIOMA

This rare but interesting association of three unusual tumors occurs most often in young females, but has no established etiology and no known Mendelian inheritance pattern (121–124). Most of the paragangliomas are extra-adrenal, in the head and neck region and base of heart, but pheochromocytomas have also been documented, although the tumor may be periadrenal (126). The gastric tumors may have an organoid pattern reminiscent of a paraganglioma (125). A recent update of this rare association identified 59 patients (51 females, 8 males) distributed worldwide, with 51 cases diagnosed in the first two decades of life (86 percent). A provisional diagnosis is possible if two of the three tumors are present, especially if one or both are multicentric and the affected patient is young and female; a definitive diagnosis is warranted if all three tumors are present (124).

COMPOSITE PHEOCHROMOCYTOMA

This is a designation for a tumor that is composed, in part, of typical pheochromocytoma, but also has a component resembling neuroblastoma (NB), ganglioneuroblastoma (GNB), or typical ganglioneuroma (131,133,134). In the series by Linnoila et al. (135), 3 percent of the sympathoadrenal paragangliomas were classified as composite pheochromocytomas (fig. 10-42). A bilateral composite pheochromocytoma-ganglioneuroma has been reported in type 1 neurofibromatosis (129). Rare examples have been reported in an intra-abdominal extra-adrenal location (140). Another distinctive, but even rarer type of composite pheochromocytoma is one that has a component of malignant peripheral nerve sheath tumor (malignant schwannoma) (138, 139,139a). Rarely, malignant schwannoma can occur as a primary adrenal tumor (128). Composite pheochromocytoma usually includes tumors that have common embryologic ancestry from the neural crest (fig. 10-43),

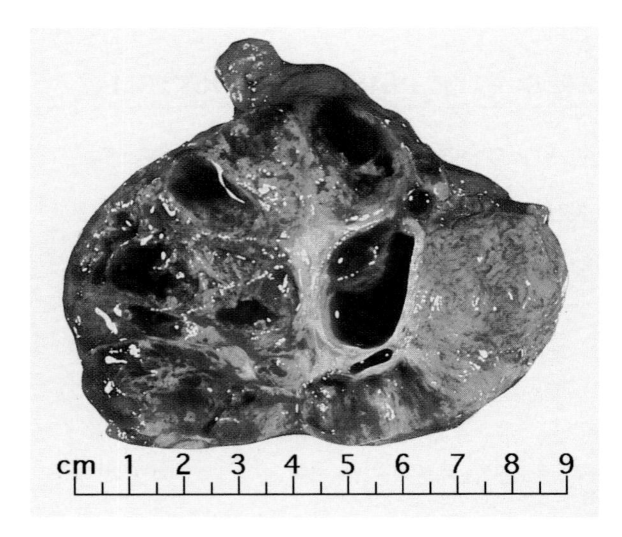

Figure 10-42
COMPOSITE PHEOCHROMOCYTOMA
This cross section of a composite pheochromocytoma has many areas which microscopically resemble ganglioneuroblastoma. The tumor was resected from a 42-year-old woman who presented with signs and symptoms of excess catecholamine secretion. There are irregular areas of cystic degeneration along with congestion and hemorrhage.

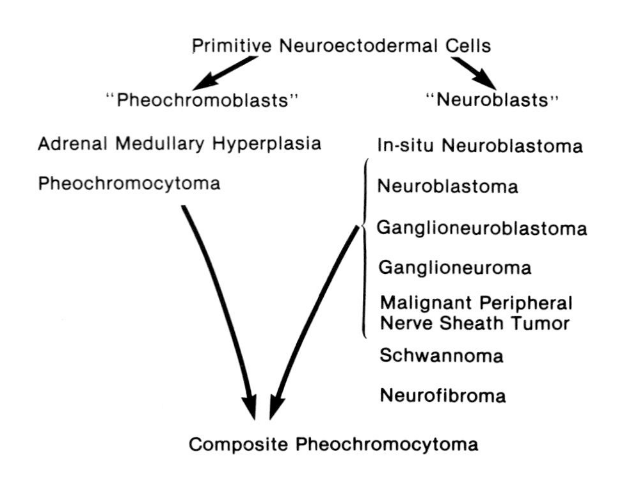

Figure 10-43
COMPOSITE PHEOCHROMOCYTOMA
The fate of the primitive neuroectodermal cells within the developing adrenal is variable, but two major lines of cellular differentiation can be envisioned as well as possible types of tumors which may develop. Composite pheochromocytoma combines dual neural and endocrine composition in various combination.

but there are other rare combinations of tumors: mixed adrenal cortical adenoma-pheochromocytoma (corticomedullary adenoma) (136), concurrent adrenal cortical adenoma and pheochromocytoma in the same gland (130, 132,141), and composite pheochromocytoma-ganglioneuroma with cortical adenoma (127).

Histologically, composite pheochromocytomas may have areas resembling ganglioneuroblastoma (fig. 10-44), with neuronal or ganglion cell features admixed with loose fibrillar matrix resembling neuropil. Transition between the different patterns may be gradual or abrupt. Ganglionic cells may contain granular basophilic material corresponding to Nissl substance. The Nissl substance in these ganglionic (or neuronal) cells may have an uneven distribution in the perikaryon and occasionally may not even be appreciated in the particular plane of section. These cells are characterized by relatively abundant light pink cytoplasm with distinct borders and rounded eccentric nuclei, sometimes with a prominent nucleolus (fig. 10-44B). In some fields the ganglionic cells appear suspended in a complex web of matted neuropil (fig. 10-44C). There may be a more primitive small cell component resembling neuroblastoma (fig. 10-45).

Composite pheochromocytoma-ganglioneuroma is also a rare tumor. The histologic features of both tumors are admixed together, often with abrupt transition (fig. 10-46, left). Ganglion cells may be few and widely scattered, but their presence, coupled with the prominent Schwann cells, are diagnostic (fig. 10-46, right). The pheochromocytoma may grow as small clusters of cells within the neural component of the tumor (fig. 10-47, left), and can readily be detected by staining for cytoplasmic argyrophilia or immunohistochemical stains for neuroendocrine differentiation such as chromogranin A (fig. 10-47, right).

Many of the composite pheochromocytomas reported to date have been functionally active, with excess catecholamine secretion. These tumors occasionally have been associated with a watery diarrhea syndrome due to the secretion of vasoactive intestinal peptide (VIP) (137,145). Elaboration of VIP has been associated with a neuronal or ganglionic morphologic phenotype, but this is not absolute (133); in vitro study of cultured human pheochromocytoma cells has also demonstrated a dissociation between VIP production and outgrowth of neuronal processes

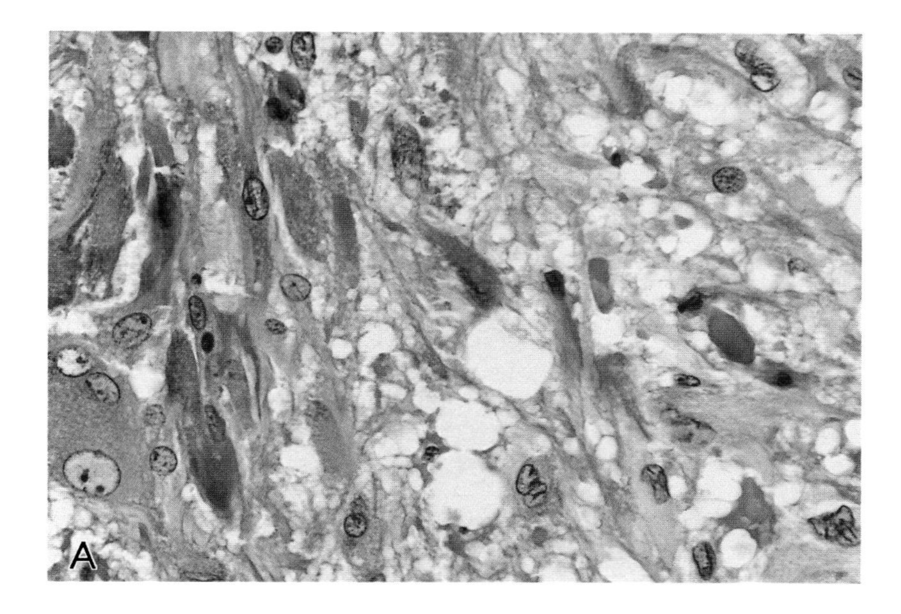

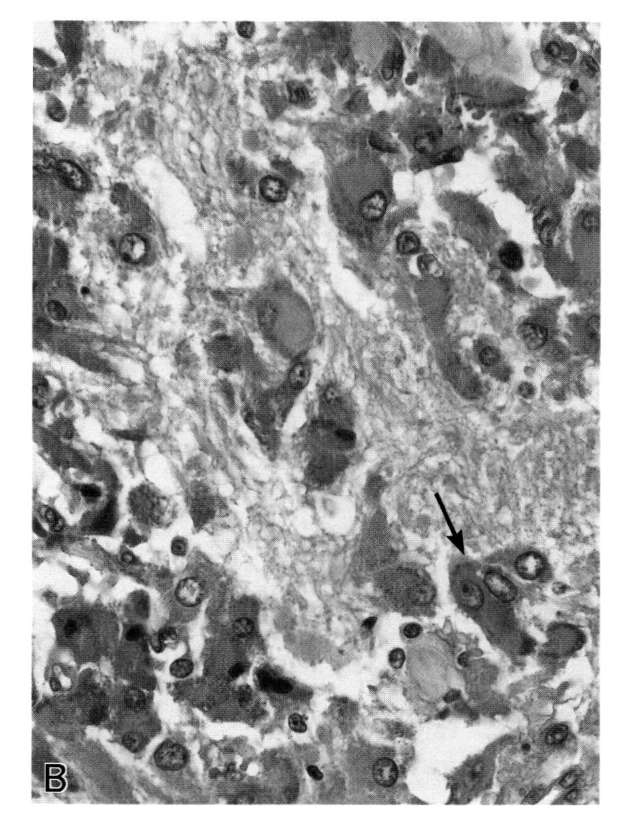

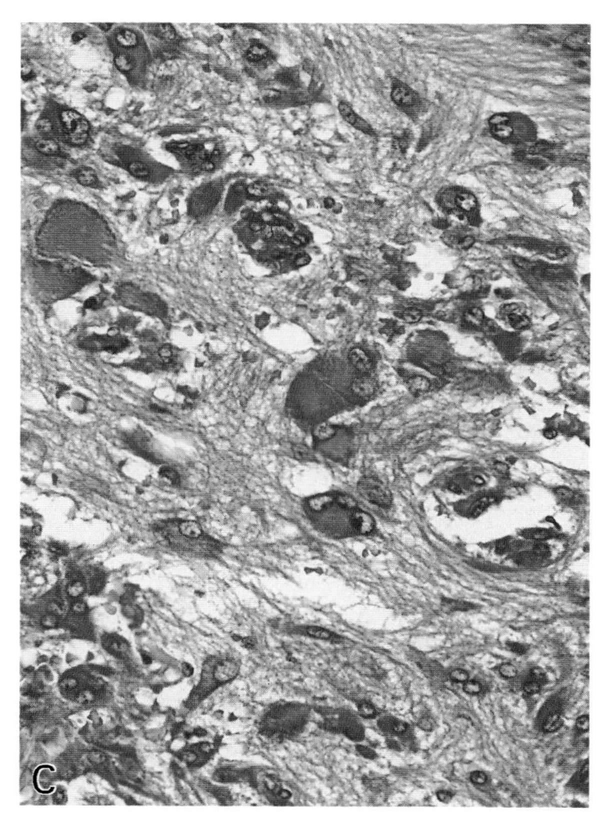

Figure 10-44
COMPOSITE PHEOCHROMOCYTOMA

A: Tumor cells of the pheochromocytoma have neuronal or ganglionic features. In the right half of the field there is background of fibrillary matrix representing intertwined neuritic cell processes.

B: Some cells with eccentric nuclei have compact cytoplasm with well-defined borders and basophilic staining near edge resembling Nissl substance (arrow).

C: Ganglion-type cells in a background rich in neuropil-like fibrillary matrix.

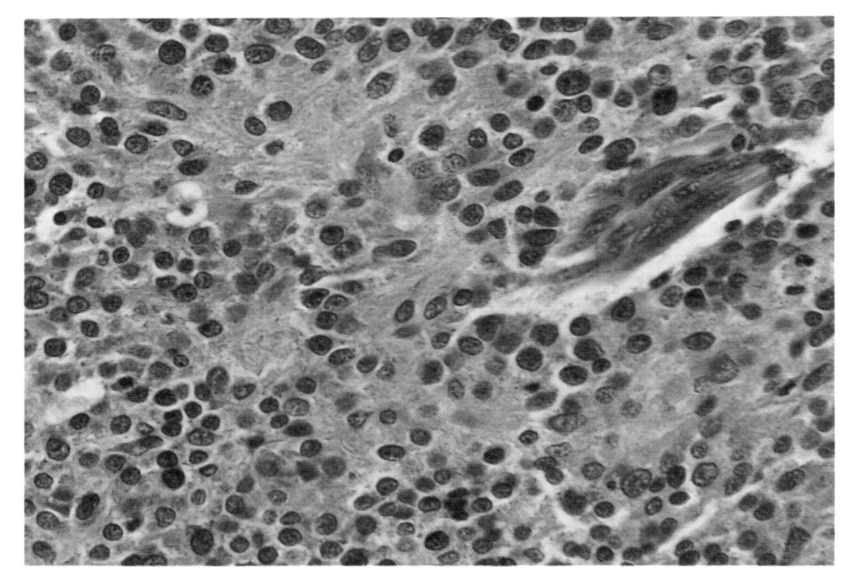

Figure 10-45
COMPOSITE PHEOCHROMOCYTOMA

Small immature cells with fibrillary matrix representing neuritic cell processes are seen. The pattern resembles neuroblastoma. Other areas showed morphology typical for pheochromocytoma.

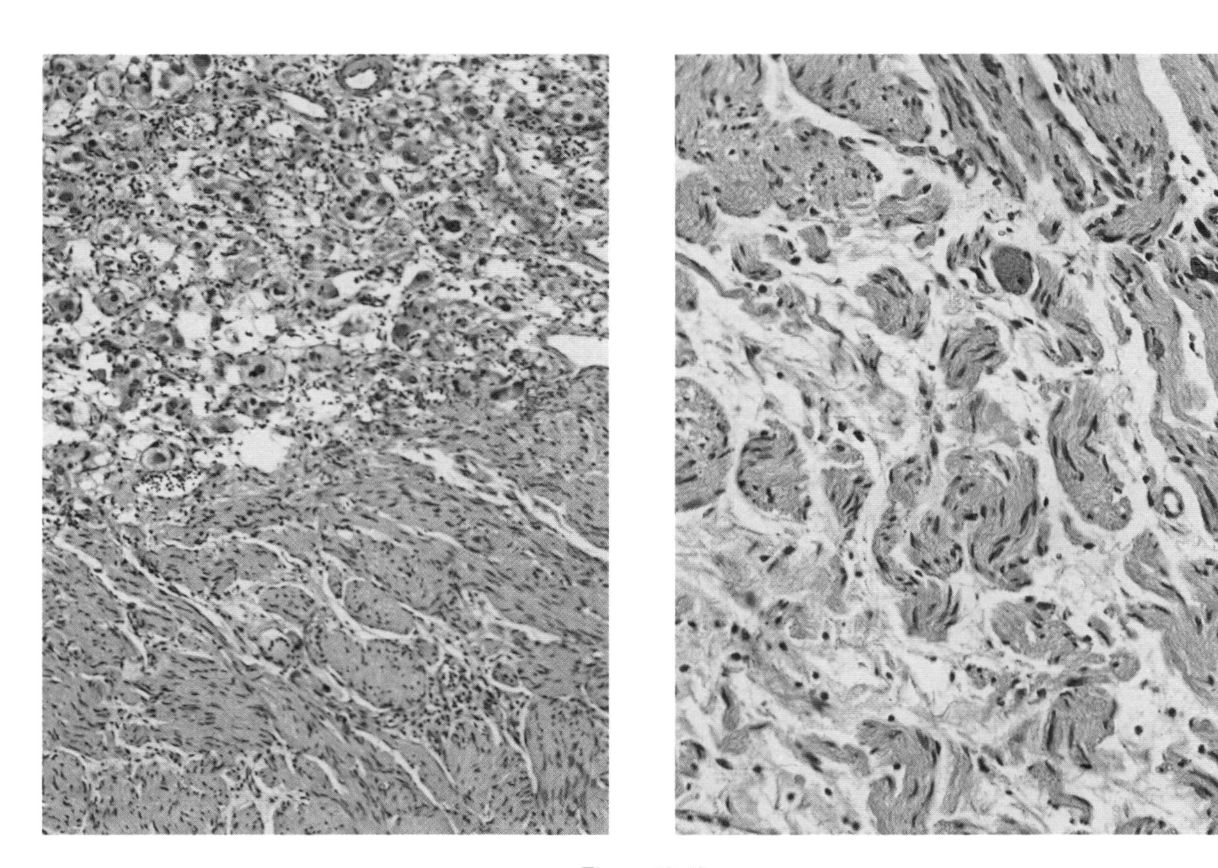

Figure 10-46
COMPOSITE PHEOCHROMOCYTOMA WITH GANGLIONEUROMA

Left: Half of the tumor is ganglioneuroma (lower half) and half (top) is pheochromocytoma. The tumor was clinically malignant with metastasis to para-aortic lymph nodes.

Right: Same tumor showing component of ganglioneuroma and a few ganglion cells. (Figures 10-46–10-48 are from the same case.)

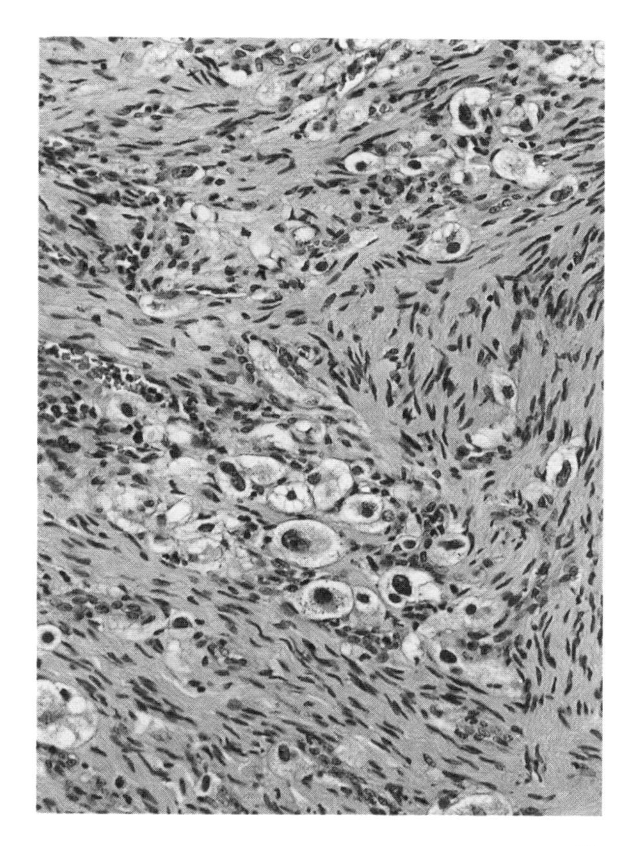

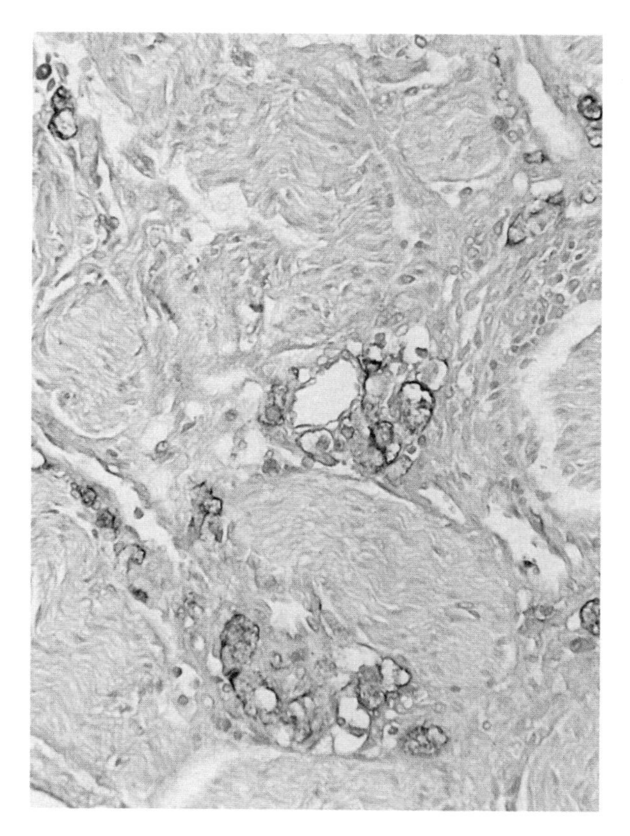

Figure 10-47
COMPOSITE PHEOCHROMOCYTOMA WITH GANGLIONEUROMA
Left: Small nests of pheochromocytoma cells are present between fascicles of Schwann cells.
Right: Immunostain for chromogranin A highlights small nests of cells of pheochromocytoma. (X200, Peroxidase-antiperoxidase stain)

(144). Intense immunostaining for VIP was reported in non-neuronal cells, and overall the pattern for VIP reactivity among tumors is less predictable (142). The existence of pheochromocytomas with composite neural and endocrine features is fascinating; they may be the in vivo counterpart of the neuronal phenotype which can be spontaneous or induced in cultures of human pheochromocytoma cells (143,144). The biologic behavior of composite pheochromocytomas may be as difficult to predict as more traditional pheochromocytomas; based upon the paucity of cases reported to date the presence of areas resembling ganglioneuroblastoma or neuroblastoma does not necessarily indicate a poorer prognosis. Some may behave in a malignant fashion with metastasis by a component of the tumor which has neural features (fig. 10-48).

PHEOCHROMOCYTOMAS IN CHILDHOOD

Pheochromocytomas are uncommon in the pediatric age group. In a review of the first 100 cases reported in children up to 15 years of age, the average age was 11 years and the youngest child was 5 months old (149). Bilateral pheochromocytomas have been diagnosed in a newborn infant (148). In one series, the tumor was bilateral (fig. 10-49), multicentric (fig. 10-50), or extra-adrenal in 32 percent of cases (148). Multicentric paragangliomatosis has been reported in a teenager who had 21 paragangliomas (adrenal and extra-adrenal) resected surgically between 13 and 17 years of age, and still had clinical evidence of additional tumors (147). Bilateral pheochromocytomas have been reported in 19 percent

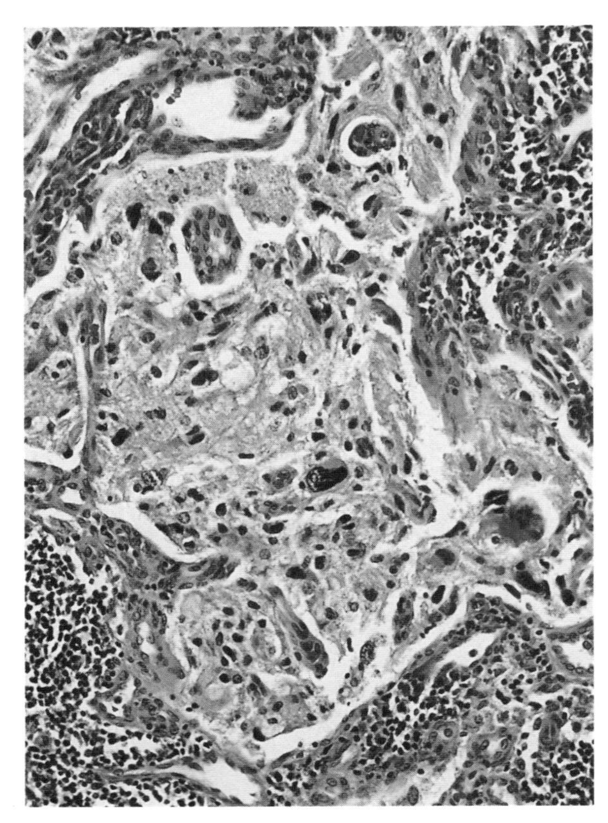

Figure 10-48
CLINICALLY MALIGNANT COMPOSITE PHEOCHROMOCYTOMA WITH GANGLIONEUROMA

Regional lymph node metastasis from same tumor as in figures 10-46 and 10-47. Metastatic tumor has neural features.

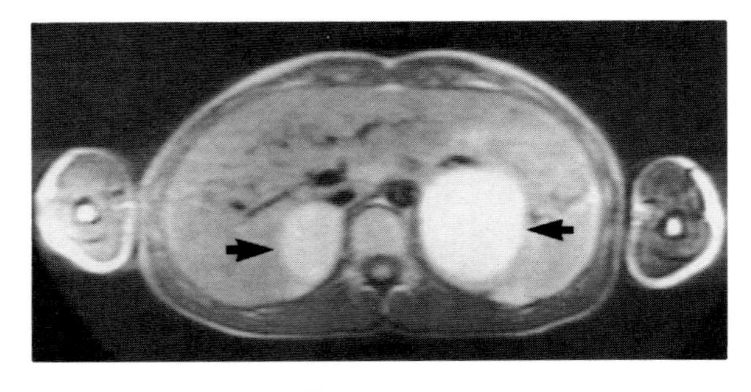

Figure 10-49
BILATERAL PHEOCHROMOCYTOMAS

A 16-year-old boy with history of back pain, nausea, vomiting, and headaches has bilateral pheochromocytomas. The tumor on the left side has some cystic degeneration. Bilateral pheochromocytomas show an intense signal on T2-weighted MRI. (Fig. 4-43B from Lack EE. Adrenal medullary hyperplasia and pheochromocytoma. In: Lack EE, ed. Pathology of the adrenal glands. New York: Churchill Livingstone, 1990:173–235.)

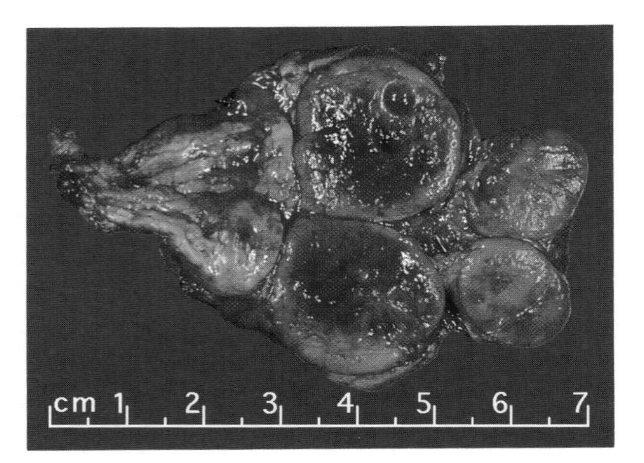

Figure 10-50
BIVALVED PHEOCHROMOCYTOMA

Bivalved pheochromocytoma from a child. Two distinct (multicentric) foci of tumor are apparent, with larger tumor having mild cystic degeneration.

(148) to 24 percent (146) of cases. Familial occurrence of some tumors may help to explain the higher incidence of bilaterality. The incidence of malignancy is similar to adults: only 2 of 85 cases (2.4 percent) were malignant in a review by Hume (146).

PSEUDOPHEOCHROMOCYTOMA

This term is used for the rare patient who presents with typical signs or symptoms of a pheochromocytoma, but has no adrenal or extra-adrenal tumor upon surgical exploration. Adrenal medullary hyperplasia enters into the differential diagnosis, and careful morphometric study may be necessary to exclude this possibility. There may also be biochemical abnormalities with elevated catecholamines. Pathologic anatomic lesions with features similar to pseudopheochromocytoma include adrenal myelolipoma (152), renal cyst (157), coarctation of abdominal aorta (154), fibrosarcoma of pulmonary artery (158), and astrocytoma (153). Acute mercury poisoning (acrodynia) can also mimic pheochromocytoma (155). An unusual cause of pseudopheochromocytoma is surreptitious administration of epinephrine (151) or isoproterenol (156). Pseudopheochromocytoma has also been attributed to overactivity of adrenergic receptors (150). Rarely, adrenal cortical tumors

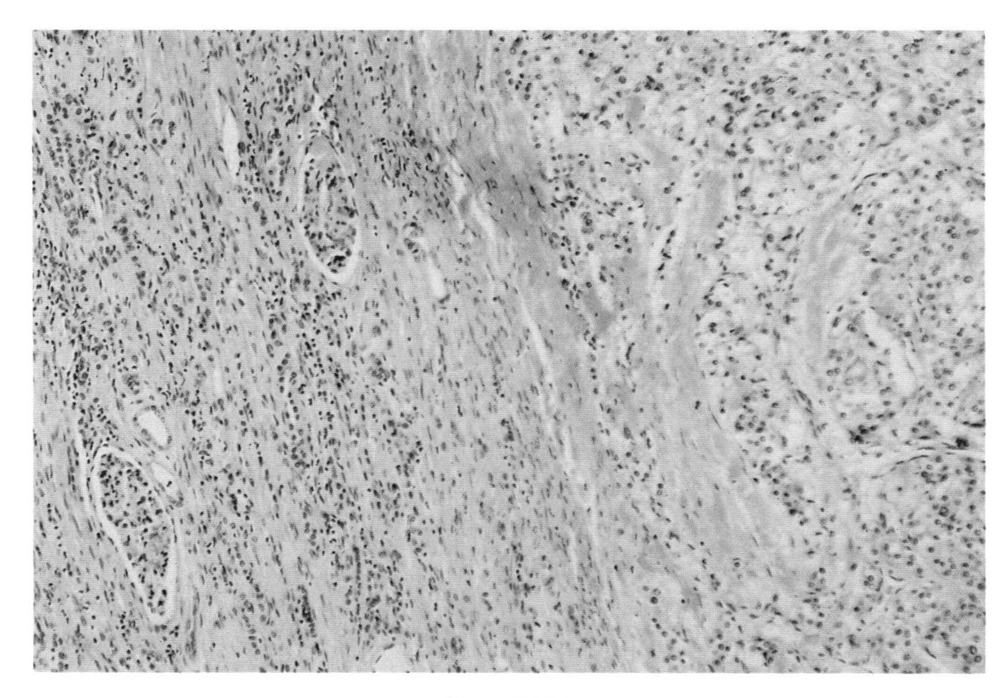

Figure 10-51
PHEOCHROMOCYTOMA REMOVED EN BLOC WITH NEPHRECTOMY
The tumor invaded the renal parenchyma, and was regarded as malignant based upon extensive local invasion.

can clinically mimic a pheochromocytoma with biochemical evidence of elevated catecholamine secretion in serum or urine (149a).

MALIGNANT PHEOCHROMOCYTOMA

Clinically malignant pheochromocytomas are uncommon. Diagnosis is based on evidence of extensive local invasion, or more reliably, documentation of metastasis to one or more sites where non-neoplastic chromaffin tissue is not normally present (167). Early reviews indicate a 2.5 percent (169) to 2.8 percent (160) rate of malignancy in adults and 2.4 percent in children (160). Some of the more recent series report an incidence of malignancy of 2.4 percent (165), 7 percent (166), 8 percent (159), 13 percent (168), and 14 percent (170). Intra-abdominal, extra-adrenal paragangliomas should be excluded since these tumors tend to be more aggressive clinically (161,162). The intraoperative or perioperative mortality rate in older reports should not be confused with clinically malignant tumors (162).

The 5-year survival rate for patients with malignant pheochromocytoma was 44 percent (168) and 53 percent (170) in two sequential series from the Mayo clinic. The pathologic distinction between clinically benign and malignant pheochromocytomas can be virtually impossible to make. In a study of a large number of sympathoadrenal paragangliomas, only four factors were found to have significant statistical correlation with malignancy: 1) extra-adrenal location; 2) coarse nodularity of the primary tumor; 3) confluent tumor necrosis; and 4) absence of hyaline globules (163). Compared with benign tumors, malignant tumors are larger (383 g versus 73 g); have a higher mitotic count (average, 3 per 30 high-power fields versus 1); and have extensive local (fig. 10-51) or vascular invasion. They also express fewer neuropeptides on immunohistochemical study than benign tumors (164). Some tumors have a lingering or indolent course, thus mandating prolonged follow-up. Pheochromocytomas can metastasize by lymphatic or hematogenous pathways, with involvement of liver, lymph node (fig. 10-52), lung, and bone (161,162). Rarely, a patient may present with an isolated lytic bone metastasis (161,162).

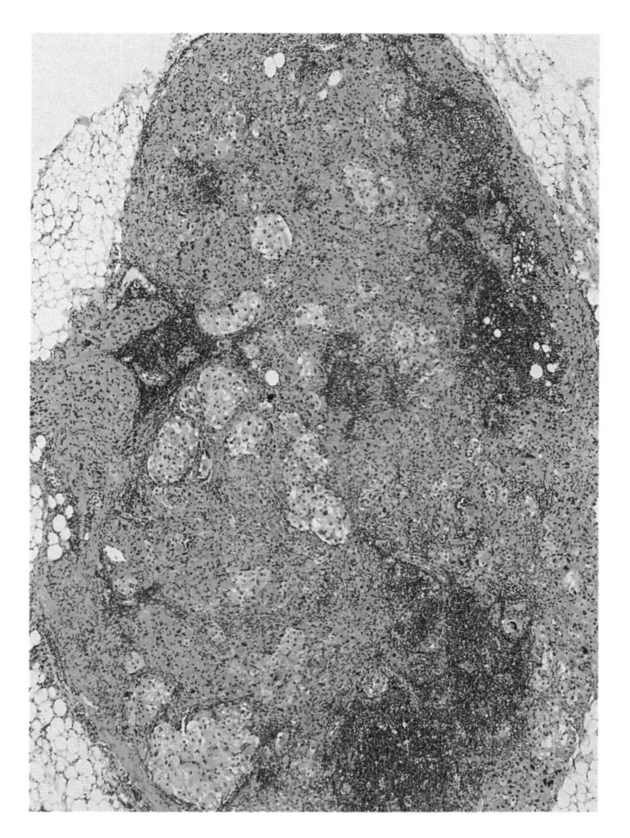

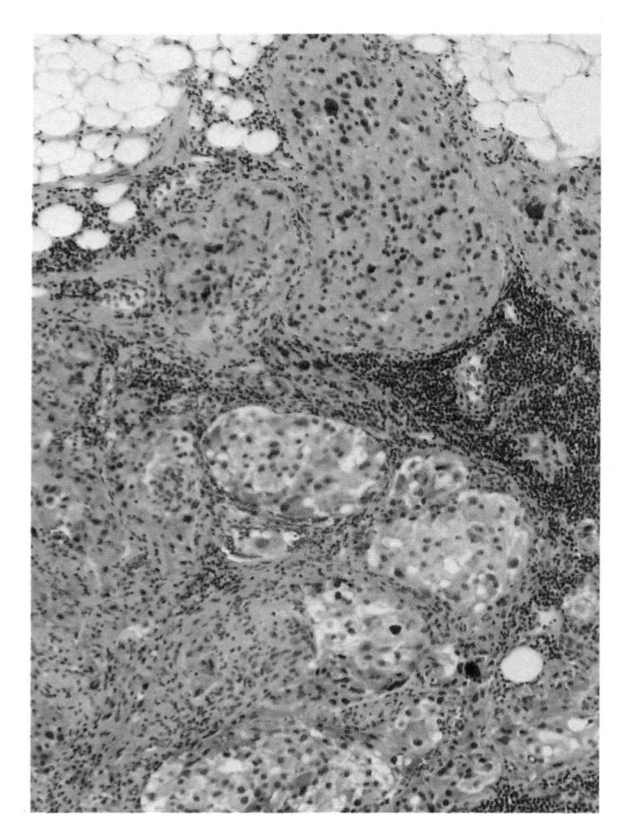

Figure 10-52
METASTATIC PHEOCHROMOCYTOMA

Left: Pheochromocytoma metastatic to supraclavicular lymph node in a young adult with a history of pheochromocytoma resected several years before.

Right: Higher magnification view.

REFERENCES

Incidence of Pheochromocytoma

1. Andersen GT, Lund JO, Toftdahl D, Strandgaard S, Nielsen PE. Pheochromocytoma and Conn's syndrome in Denmark 1977-1981. Acta Medica Scand (suppl) 1986:717–20.
2. Beard CM, Sheps SG, Kurland LT, Carney JA, Lie JT. Occurrence of pheochromocytoma in Rochester, Minnesota, 1950 through 1979. Mayo Clin Proc 1983;58:802–4.
3. Correa P, Chen VW. Endocrine gland cancer. Cancer 1995;75:338–52.
4. Krane NK. Clinically unsuspected pheochromocytomas. Experience at Henry Ford Hospital and a review of the literature. Arch Intern Med 1986;146:54–7.
5. Stackpole RH, Melicow MM, Uson AC. Pheochromocytoma in children. Report of 9 cases and review of the first 100 published cases with follow-up studies. J Pediatr 1963;63:315–30.
6. Stenström G, Svärdsudd K. Pheochromocytoma in Sweden 1958-1981. An analysis of the National Cancer Registry data. Acta Med Scand 1986;220:225–32.
7. St. John Sutton MG, Sheps SG. Prevalence of clinically unsuspected pheochromocytoma. Review of a 50-year autopsy series. Mayo Clin Proc 1981;56:354–60.

Clinical Features and Patterns of Catecholamine Secretion

8. Backmann AW, Hawkins PG, Gordon RD. Phaeochromocytomas secreting adrenaline but not noradrenaline do not cause hypertension and require precise adrenaline measurement for diagnosis. Clin Exp Pharmacol Physiol 1989;16:275–9.
9. Bomanji J, Bouloux PM, Levison DA, et al. Observations on the function of normal adrenomedullary tissue in patients with phaeochromocytomas and other paragangliomas. Eur J Nucl Med 1987;13:86–9.

10. Bomanji J, Levison DA, Flatman WD, et al. Uptake of iodine-123MIBG by pheochromocytomas, paragangliomas and neuroblastomas: a histopathological comparison. J Nucl Med 1987;28:973–8.
11. Bravo EL. Pheochromocytoma: new concepts and future trends [clinical conference]. Kidney Int 1991;40:544–56.
12. Feldman JM, Blalock JA, Zern RT, et al. Deficiency of dopamine-beta-hydroxylase. A new mechanism for normotensive pheochromocytomas. Am J Clin Pathol 1979;72:175–85.
13. Florkowski CM, Fairlamb DJ, Freeth MG, et al. Raised dopamine metabolites in a case of malignant paraganglioma. Postgrad Med J 1990;66:471–3.
14. Hume DM. Pheochromocytoma in the adult and in the child. Am J Surg 1960;99:458–96.
15. Keiser HR, Doppman JL, Robertson CN, Linehan WM, Averbuch SD. Diagnosis, localization, and management of pheochromocytoma. In: Lack EE, ed. Pathology of the adrenal glands. New York: Churchill Livingstone, 1990:237–55.
16. Lack EE. Pathology of adrenal and extra-adrenal paraganglia. In: Major problems in pathology, Vol 29. Philadelphia: WB Saunders, 1994.
17. Lee PH, Blute R Jr, Malhotra R. A clinically silent pheochromocytoma with spontaneous hemorrhage. J Urol 1987;138:1429–32.
18. Manger WM, Gifford RW Jr. Pheochromocytoma. New York: Springer-Verlag, 1977.
19. McEwan AJ, Shapiro B, Sisson JC, Beierwaltes WN, Ackery DM. Radio-iodobenzylguanidine for the scintigraphic location and therapy of adrenergic tumors. Sem Nucl Med 1985;15:132–53.
20. Proye C, Fossati P, Fontaine P, et al. Dopamine-secreting pheochromocytoma: an unrecognized entity? Classification of pheochromocytomas according to their type of secretion. Surgery 1986;100:1154–61.
21. Quinan C, Berger AA. Observations on human adrenals with especial reference to the relative weight of the normal medulla. Ann Intern Med 1933;6:1180–92.
22. Samaan NA, Hickey RC, Shutts PE. Diagnosis, localization, and management of pheochromocytoma. Pitfalls and follow-up in 41 patients. Cancer 1988;62:2451–60.
23. Sisson JC, Frager MS, Valk TW, Gross MD, et al. Scintigraphic localization of pheochromocytoma. N Engl J Med 1981;305:12–7.
24. Stackpole RH, Melicow MM, Uson AC. Pheochromocytoma in children. Report of 9 cases and review of the first 100 published cases with follow-up studies. J Pediatr 1963;63:315–30.
25. Von Moll L, McEwan AJ, Shapiro B, et al. Iodine-131MIBG scintigraphy of neuroendocrine tumors other than pheochromocytoma and neuroblastoma. J Nucl Med 1987;28:979–88.

Pathology of Pheochromocytoma

26. Aguilo F, Tamayo N, Vazquez-Quintana E, et al. Pheochromocytoma: a twenty year experience at the University Hospital. PR Health Sci J 1991;10:135–42.
27. Chetty R, Clark SP, Taylor DA. Pigmented pheochromocytomas of the adrenal medulla. Hum Pathol 1993;24:420–3.
28. Dekker A, Oehrle JS. Hyaline globules of the adrenal medulla of man. A product of lipid peroxidation? Arch Path 1971;91:353–64.
29. DeLellis RA, Suchow E, Wolfe HJ. Ultrastructure of nuclear inclusions in pheochromocytoma and paraganglioma. Hum Pathol 1980;11:205–7.
30. Dicke TE, Henry ML, Minton JP. Intracaval extension of pheochromocytoma simulating pulmonary embolism. J Surg Oncol 1987;34:160–4.
31. Lack EE. Adrenal medullary hyperplasia and pheochromocytoma. In: Lack EE, ed. Pathology of the adrenal glands. New York: Churchill Livingstone, 1990:173–235.
32. Lack EE. Pathology of adrenal and extra-adrenal paraganglia. Major problems in pathology, Vol 29. Philadelphia: WB Saunders, 1994.
33. Lack EE, Mulvihill JJ, Travis WD, Kozakewich HP. Adrenal cortical neoplasms in the pediatric and adolescent age group. Clinicopathologic study of 30 cases with emphasis on epidemiological and prognostic factors. Pathol Annu 1992;27:1–53.
34. Landas SK, Leigh C, Bonsib SM, Layne K. Occurrence of melanin in pheochromocytoma. Mod Pathol 1993;6:175–8.
35. Linnoila RI, Keiser HR, Steinberg SM, Lack EE. Histopathology of benign versus malignant sympathoadrenal paragangliomas: clinicopathologic study of 120 cases including unusual histologic features. Hum Pathol 1990;21:1168–80.
36. Medeiros LJ, Wolf BC, Balogh K, Federman M. Adrenal pheochromocytoma: a clinicopathologic review of 60 cases. Hum Pathol 1985;16:580–9.
37. Mendelsohn G, Olson JL. Pheochromocytoma [Letter]. Hum Pathol 1978;9:607–8.
37a. Miranda RN, Wu CD, Nayak RN, Kragel PJ, Medeiros LJ. Amyloid in adrenal gland pheochromocytomas. Arch Pathol Lab Med 1995;119:827–30.
38. Page DL, DeLellis RA, Hough AJ Jr. Tumors of the adrenal. Atlas of Tumor Pathology, 2nd Series, Fascicle 23. Washington, D.C.: Armed Forces Institute of Pathology, 1986.
39. Ramsay JA, Asa SL, van Nostrand AW, Hassaram ST, deHarven EP. Lipid degeneration in pheochromocytomas mimicking adrenal cortical tumors. Am J Surg Pathol 1987;11:480–6.
40. ReMine WH, Chong GC, van Heerden JA, Sheps SG, Harrison EG Jr. Current management of pheochromocytoma. Ann Surg 1974;179:740–7.
41. Rote AR, Flint LD, Ellis FH Jr. Intracaval recurrence of pheochromocytoma extending into right artrium. Surgical management using extracorporeal circulation. N Engl J Med 1977;296:1269–71.
42. Sherwin RP. Histopathology of pheochromocytoma. Cancer 1959;12:861–77.
43. Smith EJ, McPherson GA, Lynn J. Inferior vena cava involvement by a phaeochromocytoma. Br J Surg 1987;74:597.
44. Steinhoff MM, Wells SA Jr, DeSchryver-Kecskemeti K. Stromal amyloid in pheochromocytomas. Hum Pathol 1992;23:33–6.
45. Unger PD, Cohen JM, Thung SN, Gordon R, Pertsemlidis D, Dikman SH. Lipid degeneration in a pheochromocytoma histologically mimicking an adrenal cortical tumor. Arch Pathol Lab Med 1990;114:892–4.
46. Vassallo G, Capella C, Solcia E. Grimelius' silver stain for endocrine cell granules as shown by electron microscopy. Stain Technol 1971;46:7–13.

The Chromaffin Reaction

47. Henle J. Ueber das gewebe der nebenniere und der hypophyse. Ztschr rat Med 1865;24:143–52.
48. Lack EE. Pathology of adrenal and extra-adrenal paraganglia. Major problems in pathology, Vol 29. Philadelphia: WB Saunders, 1994.
49. Sherwin RP, Rosen VJ. New aspects of the chromoreactions for the diagnosis of pheochromocytoma. Am J Clin Path 1965;43:200–6.

Periadrenal Brown Fat and Other Abnormalities

50. DeSouza TG, Berlad L, Shapiro K, Walsh C, Saenger P, Shinnar S. Pheochromocytoma and multiple intracerebral aneurysms. J Pediatr 1986;108:947–9.
51. English JT, Patel SK, Flanagan MJ. Association of pheochromocytomas with brown fat tumors. Radiology 1973;107:279–81.
52. Klausner JM, Nakash R, Inbar M, Gutman M, Lelcuk S, Rozin RR. Prolonged fever as a presenting symptom in adrenal tumors. Oncology 1988;45:15–7.
53. Lean ME, James WP, Jennings G, Trayhurn P. Brown adipose tissue in patients with phaeochromocytoma. Int J Obesity 1986;10:219–27.
54. Leiphart CJ, Nudelman EJ. Hibernoma masquerading as a pheochromocytoma. Radiology 1970;95:659–60.
55. Lüscher TF, Lie JT, Stanson AW, Houser OW, Hollier LH, Sheps SG. Arterial fibromuscular dysplasia. Mayo Clin Proc 1987;62:931–52.
56. Manger WM, Gifford RW Jr. Pheochromocytoma. New York: Springer-Verlag, 1977.
57. Medeiros LJ, Katsas GG, Balogh K. Brown fat and adrenal pheochromocytoma: association or coincidence? Hum Pathol 1985;16:970–2.
58. Medeiros LJ, Wolf BC, Balogh K, Federman M. Adrenal pheochromocytoma: a clinicopathologic review of 60 cases. Hum Pathol 1985;16:580–9.
59. Melicow MM. Hibernating fat and pheochromocytoma. Arch Pathol Lab Med 1957;63:367–2.
60. ReMine WH, Chòng GC, van Heerden JA, Sheps SG, Harrison EG Jr. Current management of pheochromocytoma. Ann Surg 1974;179:740–7.
61. Rona G. Changes in adipose tissue accompanying pheochromocytoma. Can Med Assoc J 1964;91:303–5.
62. Sherwin RP. Histopathology of pheochromocytoma. Cancer 1952;12:861–77.
63. Van Vliet PD, Burchell, HB, Titus, JL. Focal myocarditis associated with pheochromocytoma. N Engl J Med 1966;274:1102–8.

Familial Pheochromocytoma

64. Atuk NO, McDonald T, Wood T, et al. Familial pheochromocytoma, hypercalcemia, and von Hippel-Lindau disease. A ten year study of a large family. Medicine 1979;58:209–18.
65. Barwick KW. Gastrointestinal manifestations of multiple endocrine neoplasia, type IIB. J Clin Gastroenterol 1983;5:83–7.
66. Bugalho MJ, Limbert E, Sobrinho LG, et al. A kindred with multiple endocrine neoplasia type 2a associated with pruritic skin lesions. Cancer 1992;70:2664–7.
67. Cance WG, Wells SA Jr. Multiple endocrine neoplasia. Type IIa. Curr Probl Surg 1985;22:8–56.
68. Carlson KM, Dan S, Chi D, et al. Single missense mutation in the tyrosine kinase catalytic domain of the RET protooncogene is associated with multiple endocrine neoplasia type 2B. Proc Natl Acad Sci USA 1994;91:1579–83.
69. Carney JA, Go VL, Sizemore GW, Hayles AB. Alimentary-tract ganglioneuromatosis. A major component of the syndrome of multiple endocrine neoplasia, type 2b. N Engl J Med 1976;295:1287–91.
70. Carney JA, Hayles AB. Alimentary tract manifestations of multiple endocrine neoplasia, type 2b. Mayo Clin Proc 1977;52:543–8.
71. Carney JA, Roth SI, Heath H III, Sizemore GW, Hayles AB. The parathyroid glands in multiple endocrine neoplasia, type 2b. Am J Pathol 1980;99:397–400.
72. Carney JA, Sizemore GW, Hayles AB. C-cell disease of the thyroid gland in multiple endocrine neoplasia, type 2b. Cancer 1979;44:2173–83.
73. Carney JA, Sizemore GW, Hayles AB. Multiple endocrine neoplasia, type 2b. Pathobiol Annu 1978;8:105–53.
74. Carney JA, Sizemore GW, Lovestedt SA. Mucosal ganglioneuromatosis, medullary thyroid carcinoma, and pheochromocytoma: multiple endocrine neoplasia, type 2b. Oral Surg Oral Med Oral Pathol 1976;41:739–52.
75. Carney JA, Sizemore GW, Sheps SG. Adrenal medullary disease in multiple endocrine neoplasia, type 2. Pheochromocytoma and its precursors. Am J Clin Pathol 1976;66:279–90.
76. Carney JA, Sizemore GW, Tyce GM. Bilateral adrenal medullary hyperplasia in multiple endocrine neoplasia, type 2: the precursor of bilateral pheochromocytoma. Mayo Clin Proc 1975;50:3–10.
77. Chetty R, Duhig JD. Bilateral pheochromocytoma-ganglioneuroma of the adrenal in type 1 neurofibromatosis. Am J Surg Pathol 1993;17:837–41.
78. Chevinsky AH, Mintou JP, Falko JM. Metastatic pheochromocytoma associated with multiple endocrine neoplasia syndrome type II. Arch Surg 1990;125:935–8.
79. Cho KJ, Freier DT, McCormick TL, et al. Adrenal medullary disease in multiple endocrine neoplasia type II. AJR Am J Roentgenol 1980;134:23–9.
80. Cope R, Schleinitz PF. Multiple endocrine neoplasia, type 2b, as a cause of megacolon. Am J Gastroenterol 1983;78:802–5.
81. d'Amore ES, Manivel JC, Pettinato G, Niehans GA, Snover DC. Intestinal ganglioneuromatosis: mucosal and transmural types. A clinicopathologic and immunohistochemical study of six cases. Hum Pathol 1991;22:276–86.
82. DeLellis RA, Wolfe HJ, Gagel RF, et al. Adrenal medullary hyperplasia. A morphometric analysis in patients with familial medullary thyroid carcinoma. Am J Pathol 1976;83:177–90.
83. Dyck PJ, Carney JA, Sizemore GW, Okazaki H, Brimijoin WS, Lambert EH. Multiple endocrine neoplasia type 2b. Phenotype recognition: neurological features and their pathologic basis. Ann Neurol 1979;6:302–14.
84. Evans DB, Lee JE, Merrell RC, Hickey RC. Adrenal medullary disease in multiple endocrine neoplasia type 2. Appropriate management. Endocrinol Metab Clin N Am 1994;23:167–76.

85. Gagel RF, Tashjian AH Jr, Cummings T, et al. The clinical outcome of prospective screening for multiple endocrine neoplasia type 2a. An 18-year experience. N Engl J Med 1988;318:478–84.
86. Glushien AS, Mansuy MM, Littman DS. Pheochromocytoma: its relationship to the neurocutaneous syndromes. Am J Med 1953;14:318–27.
87. Gorlin RJ, Mirkin BL. Multiple mucosal neuromas, pheochromocytoma, medullary carcinoma of the thyroid and marfanoid body build with muscle wasting. Syndrome of hyperplasia and neoplasia of neural crest derivatives—an unitarian concept. Z Kinderheilk 1972;113:313–25.
88. Greene JP, Guay AT. New perspectives in pheochromocytomas. Urol Clin N Am 1989;16:487–503.
89. Hamilton BP, Landsberg L, Levine RJ. Measurement of urinary epinephrine in screening for pheochromocytomas in multiple endocrine neoplasia, type II. Am J Med 1978;65:1027–32.
90. Horton WA, Wong V, Eldridge R. Von Hippel-Lindau disease: clinical and pathological manifestations in nine families with 50 affected members. Arch Int Med 1976;136;769–77.
91. Jackson CE, Norum RA, Boyd SB, et al. Hereditary hyperparathyroidism and multiple ossifying jaw fibromas: a clinically and genetically distinct syndrome. Surgery 1990;108:1006–13.
92. Kalff V, Shapiro B, Lloyd R, et al. The spectrum of pheochromocytoma in hypertensive patients with neurofibromatosis. Arch Intern Med 1982;142:2092–8.
93. Lack EE. Adrenal medullary hyperplasia and pheochromocytoma. In: Lack EE, ed. Pathology of the adrenal glands. New York: Churchill Livingstone, 1990:173–235.
94. Lack EE. Pathology of adrenal and extra-adrenal paraganglia. Major problems in pathology, Vol 29. Philadelphia: WB Saunders, 1994.
95. Lips CJ, Landsvater RM, Höppener JW, et al. Clinical screening as compared with DNA analysis in families with multiple endocrine neoplasia type 2A. N Engl J Med 1994;331:825–35.
96. Lips CJ, Minder WH, Leo JR, Alleman A, Hackeng WH. Evidence of multicentric origin of the multiple endocrine neoplasia syndrome type 2a (Sipple's syndrome) in a large family in the Netherlands. Diagnostic and therapeutic implications. Am J Med 1978;64:569–78.
97. Lips CJ, van der Sluys Veer J, Struyvenberg A, et al. Bilateral occurrence of pheochromocytoma in patients with the multiple endocrine neoplasia syndrome type 2a (Sipple's syndrome). Am J Med 1981;70:1051–60.
98. Marks AD, Channick BJ. Extra-adrenal pheochromocytoma and medullary thyroid carcinoma with pheochromocytoma. Arch Intern Med 1974;134:1106–9.
99. Mathew CG, Chin KS, Easton DF, et al. A linked genetic marker for multiple endocrine neoplasia type 2A on chromosome 10. Nature 1987;328:527–8.
100. Mathew CG, Smith BA, Thorpe K, et al. Deletion of genes on chromosome 1 in endocrine neoplasia. Nature 1987;328:524–6.
101. Mendelsohn G, Baylin SB, Eggleston JC. Relationship of metastatic medullary thyroid carcinoma to calcitonin content of pheochromocytomas: an immunohistochemical study. Cancer 1980;45:498–502.
102. Mendelsohn G, Diamond MP. Familial ganglioneuromatous polyposis of the large bowel. Report of a family with associated juvenile polyposis. Am J Surg Pathol 1984;8:515–20.
103. Mendonca BB, Arnhold IJ, Nicolau W, Avancini VA, Boise W. Cushing's syndrome due to ectopic ACTH secretion by bilateral pheochromocytomas in multiple endocrine neoplasia type 2a [Letter]. N Engl J Med 1988;319:1610–1.
104. Mulligan LM, Kwok JB, Healey CS, et al. Germ-line mutations of the RET proto-oncogene in multiple endocrine neoplasia type 2A. Nature 1993;363:458–60.
105. Neumann HP, Berger DP, Sigmund G, et al. Pheochromocytomas, multiple endocrine neoplasia type 2, and von Hipple-Lindau disease. N Engl J Med 1993;329:1531–8.
106. Norton JA, Froome LC, Farrell RE, Wells SR Jr. Multiple endocrine neoplasia type IIb: the most aggressive form of medullary thyroid carcinoma. Surg Clin N Am 1979;59:109–18.
107. Pham BN, Villanueva RP. Ganglioneuromatous proliferation associated with juvenile polyposis coli. Arch Pathol Lab Med 1989;113:91–4.
108. Riccardi VM. Von Recklinghausen neurofibromatosis. N Engl J Med 1981;305:1617–27.
109. Rougier PH, Caillou B, Parmentier C, Lemerle J. Multiple endocrine neoplasia type 2b: experience at Villejuif. In: Humphrey GB, Grindey GB, Dehner LP, Acton RT, Pysher TJ, eds. Adrenal and endocrine tumors in children, Boston: Martinus Nijhoff, 1983:343–7.
109a. Sakaguchi N, Sano K, Ito M, Baba T, Fukuzawa M, Hotchi M. A case of von Recklinghausen's disease with bilateral pheochromocytoma-malignant peripheral nerve sheath tumors of the adrenal and gasdrointestinal autonomic nerve tumors. Am J Surg Pathol 1996;20:889–97.
110. Santoro M, Rosati R, Greico M, et al. The ret proto-oncogene is consistently expressed in human pheochromocytomas and thyroid medullary carcinomas. Oncogene 1990;5:1595–8.
111. Sato Y, Waziri M, Smith W, et al. Hippel-Lindau disease: MR imaging. Radiology 1988;166:241–6.
112. Schimke RN. Multiple endocrine adenomatosis syndromes. Adv Intern Med 1976;21:249–65.
113. Schimke RN. The multiple endocrine neoplasia syndromes. In: Humphrey GB, Grindey GB, Dehner LP, Acton RT, Pysher TJ, eds. Adrenal and endocrine tumors in children. Boston: Martinus Nijhoff, 1983:249–64.
114. Schimke RN, Hartmann WH, Prout TE, Rimoin DL. Syndrome of bilateral pheochromocytoma, medullary thyroid carcinoma and multiple neuromas. A possible regulatory defect in the differentiation of chromaffin tissue. N Engl J Med 1968;279:1–7.
115. Shekitka KM, Sobin LH. Ganglioneuromas of the gastrointestinal tract. Relation to von Recklinghausen disease and other multiple tumor syndromes. Am J Surg Pathol 1994;18:250–7.
116. Simpson NE, Kidd KK, Goodfellow PJ, et al. Assignment of multiple endocrine neoplasia type 2A to chromosome 10 by linkage. Nature 1987;328:528–30.
117. Webb TA, Sheps SG, Carney JA. Differences between sporadic pheochromocytoma and pheochromocytoma in multiple endocrine neoplasia, type 2. Am J Surg Pathol 1980;4:121–6.
118. Weidner N, Flanders DJ, Mitros FA. Mucosal ganglioneuromatosis associated with multiple colonic polyps. Am J Surg Pathol 1984;8:779–86.
119. Wilson RA, Ibanez ML. A comparative study of 14 cases of familial and nonfamilial pheochromocytomas. Hum Pathol 1978;9:181–8.

Other Associated Endocrine Disorders

120. Lack EE. Pathology of adrenal and extra-adrenal paraganglia. Major problems in pathology, Vol 29. Philadelphia: WB Saunders, 1994.

Triad of Gastric Epithelioid Leiomyosarcoma, Pulmonary Chondroma, and Functioning Extra-adrenal Paraganglioma

121. Carney JA. The triad of gastric epithelioid leiomyosarcoma, functioning extra-adrenal paraganglioma, and pulmonary chondroma. Cancer 1979;43:374–82.
122. Carney JA. The triad of gastric epithelioid leiomyosarcoma, pulmonary chondroma, and functioning extra-adrenal paraganglioma: a five-year review. Medicine 1983;62:159–69.
123. Carney JA. The triad of gastric epithelioid leiomyosarcoma, pulmonary chondroma, and functioning extra-adrenal paraganglioma [Abstract]. Mod Pathol 1994;7:324.
124. Carney JA, Sheps SG, Go VL, Gordon H. The triad of gastric leiomyosarcoma, functioning extra-adrenal paraganglioma and pulmonary chondroma. N Engl J Med 1977;296:1517–8.
125. Lack EE. Pathology of adrenal and extra-adrenal paraganglia in major problems in pathology, Vol 29. Philadelphia: WB Saunders, 1994.
126. Margulies KB, Sheps SG. Carney's triad: guidelines for management. Mayo Clin Proc 1988;63:496–502.

Composite Pheochromocytoma

127. Aiba M, Hirayama A, Ito Y, et al. A compound adrenal medullary tumor (pheochromocytoma and ganglioneuroma) and a cortical adenoma in the ipsilateral adrenal gland. A case report with enzyme histochemical and immunohistochemical studies. Am J Surg Pathol 1988;12:559–66.
128. Ayala G, Ettinghausen SE, Tsokas MG, Travis WD, Lack EE. Primary malignant schwannoma of the adrenal gland. Case report and literature review. J Urol Pathol 1994;2:265–72.
129. Chetty R, Duhig JD. Bilateral pheochromocytoma-ganglioneuroma of the adrenal in type 1 neurofibromatosis. Am J Surg Pathol 1993;17:837–41.
130. Cope O, Labbe JP, Raker JW, Bland EF. Pheochromocytoma and adrenal cortical adenoma. Report of case with both tumors and discussion of their relation. J Clin Endocrinol 1952;12:875–80.
131. Franquemont DW, Mills SE, Lack EE. Immunohistochemical detection of neuroblastomatous foci in composite adrenal pheochromocytoma-neuroblastoma. Am J Clin Pathol 1994;102:163–70.
132. Inoue J, Oishi S, Naomi S, Umeda T, Sato T. Pheochromocytoma associated with adrenocortical adenoma: case report and literature review. Endocrinol Jpn 1986;33:67–74.
133. Lack EE. Adrenal medullary hyperplasia and pheochromocytoma. In: Lack EE, ed. Pathology of the adrenal glands. New York: Churchill Livingstone, 1990:173–235.
134. Lack EE. Pathology of adrenal and extra-adrenal paraganglia. Major problems in pathology, Vol 29. Philadelphia: WB Saunders, 1994.
135. Linnoila RI, Keiser HR, Steinberg SM, Lack EE. Histopathology of benign versus malignant sympathoadrenal paragangliomas: clinicopathologic study of 120 cases including unusual histologic features. Hum Pathol 1990;21:1168–80.
136. Mathison DA, Waterhouse CA. Cushing's syndrome with hypertensive crisis and mixed adrenal cortical adenoma-pheochromocytoma (corticomedullary adenoma). Am J Med 1969;47:635–41.
137. Mendelsohn G, Eggleston JC, Olson JL, Said SI, Baylin SB. Vasoactive intestinal peptide and its relationship to ganglion cell differentiation in neuroblastic tumors. Lab Invest 1979;41:144–9.
138. Miettinen M, Saari A. Pheochromocytoma combined with malignant schwannoma: unusual neoplasm of the adrenal medulla. Ultrastr Pathol 1988;12:513–27.
139. Min KW, Clemens A, Bell J, Dick H. Malignant peripheral nerve sheath tumor and pheochromocytoma. A composite tumor of the adrenal. Arch Pathol Lab Med 1988;112:266–70.
139a. Sakaguchi N, Sano K, Ito M, Baba T, Fukuzawa M, Hotchi M. A case of von Recklinghausen's disease with bilateral pheochromocytoma-malignant peripheral nerve sheath tumors of the adrenal and gastrointestinal autonomic nerve tumors. Am J Surg Pathol 1996; 20:889–97.
140. Sclafani LM, Woodruff JM, Brennan MF. Extra-adrenal retroperitoneal paragangliomas: natural history and response to treatment. Surgery 1990;108:1124–30.
141. Sparagana M, Feldman JM, Molnar Z. An unusual pheochromocytoma associated with an androgen secreting adrenocortical adenoma. Evaluation of its polypeptide hormone, catecholamine, and enzyme characteristics. Cancer 1987;60:223–31.
142. Tischler AS, Dayal Y, Balogh K, Cohen RB, Connolly JL, Tallberg K. The distribution of immunoreactive chromogranins, S-100 protein, and vasoactive intestinal peptide in compound tumors of the adrenal medulla. Hum Pathol 1987;18:909–17.
143. Tischler AS, Dichter MA, Biales B, DeLellis RA, Wolfe H. Neural properties of cultured human endocrine tumor cells of proposed neural crest origin. Science 1976;192:902–4.
144. Tischler AS, Lee YC, Perlman RL, Costopoulos D, Slayton VW, Bloom SR. Production of "ectopic" vasoactive intestinal peptide-like and neurotensin-like immunoreactivity in human pheochromocytoma cell cultures. J Neurosci 1984;4:1398–404.
145. Trump DL, Livingstone JN, Baylin SB. Watery diarrhea syndrome in an adult with ganglioneuroma-pheochromocytoma: identification of vasoactive intestinal peptide, calcitonin, and catecholamines and assessment of their biologic activity. Cancer 1977;40:1526–32.

Pheochromocytoma In Childhood

146. Hume DM. Pheochromocytoma in the adult and in the child. Am J Surg 1960;99:458–96.
147. Karasov RS, Sheps SG, Carney JA, van Heerden JA, DeQuattro V. Paragangliomatosis with numerous catecholamine-producing tumors. Mayo Clinic Proc 1982;57:590–5.
148. Kaufman BH, Telander RL, van Heerden JA, Zimmerman D, Sheps SG, Dawson B. Pheochromocytoma in the pediatric age group: current status. J Ped Surg 1983;18:879–84.
149. Stackpole RH, Melicow MM, Uson AC. Pheochromocytoma in children. Report of 9 cases and review of the first 100 published cases with follow-up studies. J Pediatr 1963;63:315–30.

Pseudopheochromocytoma

149a. Alsabeh R, Mazoujian G, Goates J, Medeiros LJ, Weiss LM. Adrenal cortical tumors clinically mimicking pheochromocytoma. Am J Clin Pathol 1995;104:382–90.
150. Blum I, Weinstein R, Sztern M, Lahav M. Adrenergic receptor hyperactivity—a cause for pseudopheochromocytoma? Med Hypotheses 1987;22:89–96.
151. Brandenburg RO Jr, Gutnik LM, Nelson RL, Abboud CF, Edis AJ, Sheps SG. Factitial epinephrine-only secreting pheochromocytoma. Ann Int Med 1979;90:795.
152. Case Records of the Massachusetts General Hospital. Case 46-1988. N Engl J Med 1988;319:1336–43.
153. Evans CH, Westfall V, Atuk NO. Astrocytoma mimicking the features of pheochromocytoma. N Engl J Med 1972;286:1397–9.
154. Goldzieher JW, McMahon HE, Goldzieher MA. Coarctation of the abdominal aorta simulating pheochromocytoma. Arch Int Med 1951;88:835–9.
155. Henningsson C, Hoffmann S, Mcgonigle L, Winter JS. Acute mercury poisoning (acrodynia) mimicking pheochromocytoma in an adolescent. J Ped 1993;122:252–3.
156. Lurvey A, Yussin A, DeQuattro V. Pseudopheochromocytoma after self-administered isoproterenol. J Clin Endocrinol Metab 1973;36:766–9.
157. Weaver JC, Kawata N, Hinman F Jr. Renal cyst simulating pheochromocytoma. Post Grad Med 1952; 11:294–8.
158. Wolf PL, Dickenman RC, Langston JD. Fibrosarcoma of the pulmonary artery, masquerading as a pheochromocytoma. Am J Clin Pathol 1960;34:146–54.

Malignant Pheochromocytoma

159. Aguilo F, Tamayo N, Vazquez-Quintana E, et al. Pheochromocytoma: a twenty year experience at the University Hospital. PR Heath Sci J 1991;10:135–42.
160. Hume DM. Pheochromocytoma in the adult and in the child. Am J Surg 1960;99:458–69.
161. Lack EE. Adrenal medullary hyperplasia and pheochromocytoma. In: Lack EE, ed. Pathology of the adrenal glands. New York: Churchill Livingstone, 1990: 173–235.
162. Lack EE. Pathology of adrenal and extra-adrenal paraganglia. Major problems in pathology, Vol 29. Philadelphia: WB Saunders, 1994.
163. Linnoila RI, Keiser HR, Steinberg SM, Lack EE. Histopathology of benign versus malignant sympathoadrenal paragangliomas. Clinicopathologic study of 120 cases including unusual histologic features. Hum Pathol 1990;21:1168–80.
164. Linnoila RI, Lack EE, Steinberg SM, Keiser HR. Decreased expression of neuropeptides in malignant paragangliomas: an immunohistochemical study. Hum Pathol 1988;19:41–50.
165. Melicow MM. One hundred cases of pheochromocytoma (107 tumors) at the Columbia-Presbyterian Medical Center, 1926-1976: a clinicopathological analysis. Cancer 1977;40:1987–2004.
166. Modlin IM, Farndon JR, Shepherd A, et al. Phaeochromocytomas in 72 patients: clinical and diagnostic features, treatment and long term results. Br J Surg 1979;66:456–65.
167. Neville AM. The adrenal medulla. In: Symington T, ed. Functional pathology of the human adrenal glands. Baltimore: Williams & Wilkins, 1969:219–324.
168. ReMine WH, Chong GC, van Heerden JA, Sheps SG, Harrison EG Jr. Current management of pheochromocytoma. Ann Surg 1974;179:740–7.
169. Symington T, Goodall AL. Studies in phaeochromocytoma. I. Pathological aspects. Glas Med J 1953; 34:75–96.
170. van Heerden JA, Sheps SG, Hamberger B, Sheedy PF II, Poston JG, ReMine WH. Pheochromocytoma: current status and changing trends. Surgery 1982;91:367–73.

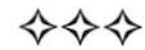

11

EXTRA-ADRENAL PARAGANGLIA OF THE SYMPATHOADRENAL NEUROENDOCRINE SYSTEM

Definition and Anatomy. The sympathoadrenal neuroendocrine system is an integrated complex composed of the sympathetic nervous system, with postganglionic neurons mediating effector responses via the neurotransmitter norepinephrine, and the adrenal medullae, which synthesize and secrete the hormones epinephrine and in lesser amounts norepinephrine (18,19). Extra-adrenal paraganglia of the neuroendocrine system are distributed along the paravertebral and para-aortic axis, closely paralleling the distribution of the sympathetic nervous system (fig. 11-1) (4); tumors arise from the sympathoadrenal paraganglia along this axis. The adrenal medullae are the largest compact collection of paraganglia in this system, and the most common site of paragangliomas (pheochromocytomas).

The nomenclature of extra-adrenal paragangliomas is based upon anatomic site of origin. Glenner and Grimley (9) recognized four families of extra-adrenal paraganglia: branchiomeric, intravagal, aorticosympathetic, and visceral-autonomic; these families are based upon anatomic distribution, innervation, and microscopic structure. The visceral-autonomic paraganglia are poorly defined, and occur in association with visceral organs and blood vessels.

Gross Findings. Extra-adrenal paraganglia are usually tiny structures, and recognizable only with aid of a microscope; an exception are some of the paraganglia described by Zuckerkandl in 1901 (fig. 11-2) (23,24). These paraganglia were identified in the human fetus and newborn on either side of the aorta, with the cephalic component near the origin of the superior mesenteric artery or the renal arteries, and the caudal portion at or just above the aortic bifurcation; they were referred to as aortic bodies (24). In 14.8 percent of cases, these extra-adrenal paraganglia are united by an isthmus lying anterior to the aorta just below the superior mesenteric artery (fig. 11-2, right); they are multiple separate collections in other cases (fig. 11-2, left) The multiplicity of these extra-adrenal paraganglia argues against use of the term *"organ" of Zuckerkandl.* With close inspection some of these paraganglia can be detected macroscopically in the fetus and newborn. In Zuckerkandl's experience, the average length of the right aortic body was 11.6 mm and left, 8.8 mm; the number of extra-adrenal paraganglia in the abdominal plexuses varied from 12 to 26 (23).

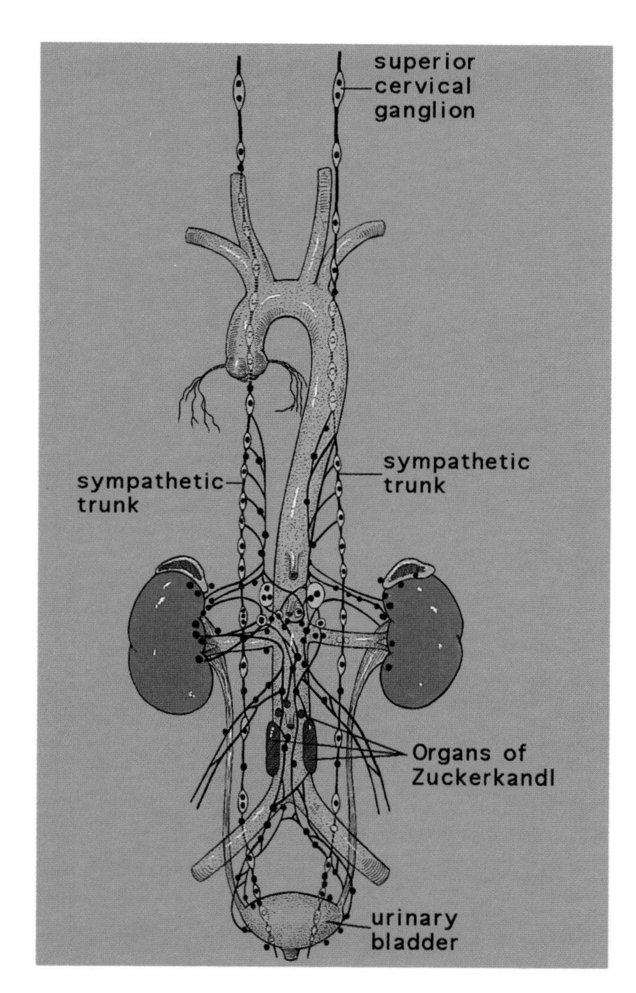

Figure 11-1
ANATOMIC DISTRIBUTION OF SYMPATHOADRENAL PARAGANGLIA

The paraganglia extend from the neck down to the base of the pelvis. (Modified from fig. 64 from Coupland RE. The natural history of the chromaffin cell. Boston: Little, Brown and Co, 1965:194.)

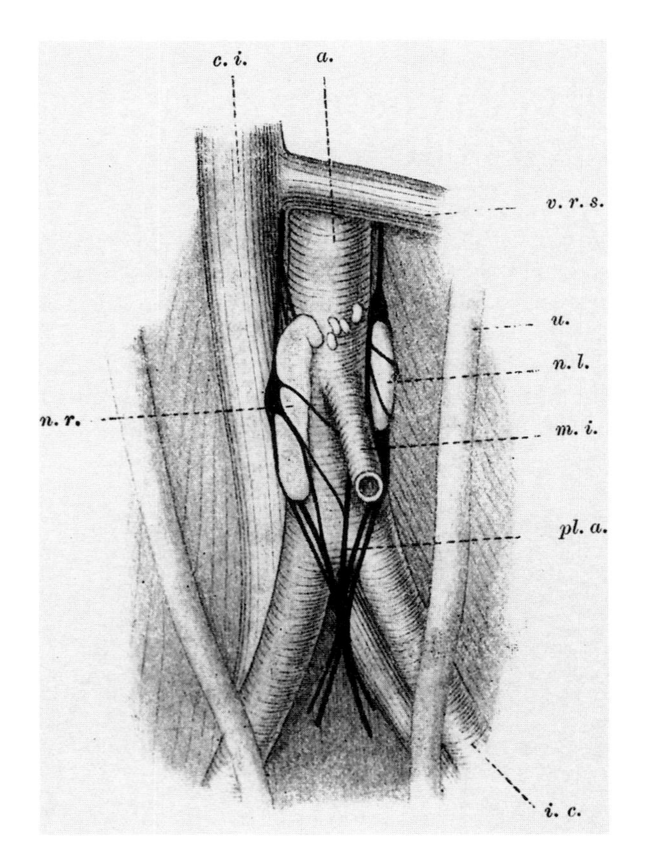

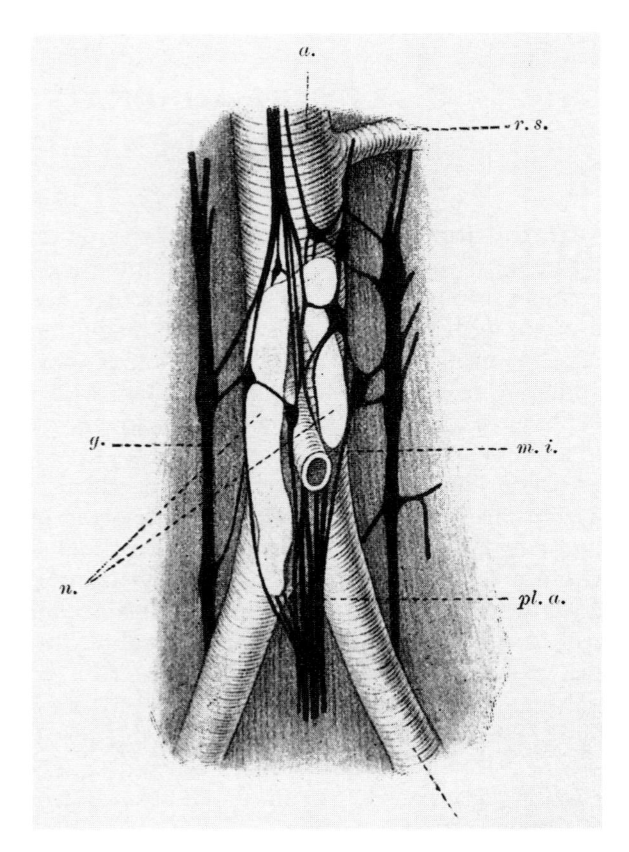

Figure 11-2
ORGANS OF ZUCKERKANDL

Left: Organs of Zuckerkandl in most cases appear as multiple discrete collections of paraganglia on either side of the aorta. Right: In a minority of cases a paraganglion is apparent as a continuous structure forming a partial collarette about the origin of the inferior mesenteric artery. (Figs. 1 and 2 from Zuckerkandl E. Ueber nebenorgane des sympathicus im retroperitonaealraum des menschen. Verh Dtsch Anat Ges 1901;15:95–107.)

Microscopic Anatomy. The spatial distribution of the organs of Zuckerkandl is shown in figure 11-3 in a human fetus of about 11 weeks' gestational age. It is notable in the human fetus that extra-adrenal paraganglia such as these are much more prominent than the developing adrenal medulla. These elongate collections of cells on either side of the aorta appear sharply defined, but in most cases they are not truly encapsulated (fig. 11-4). There is a delicate microvasculature which subdivides the chromaffin cells into small nests and anastomosing short cords. These cells contrast sharply with the adjacent primitive neuroblasts, many of which will develop into ganglion cells (fig. 11-5). The fact that this chromaffin tissue complex resembled, but was not actually composed of true ganglia, prompted the designation *paraganglion* by Alfred Kohn in 1903 (17). These developing chromaffin cells have slightly larger nuclei which are pale staining, and there is an increased cytoplasmic volume with better defined borders. Paraganglia seen elsewhere in the abdomen or in other sites along the sympathetic axis (e.g., intrathoracic region) have a similar microscopic appearance (6). In the older fetus and young infant these paraganglia become better developed, with more mature chromaffin cells (fig. 11-6).

Intra-abdominal para-aortic paraganglia increase in size in humans up to 3 years of age; between 3 and 5 years they undergo degenerative changes with increased stroma (8). These changes are most marked in the organs of Zuckerkandl, with disintegration and involution

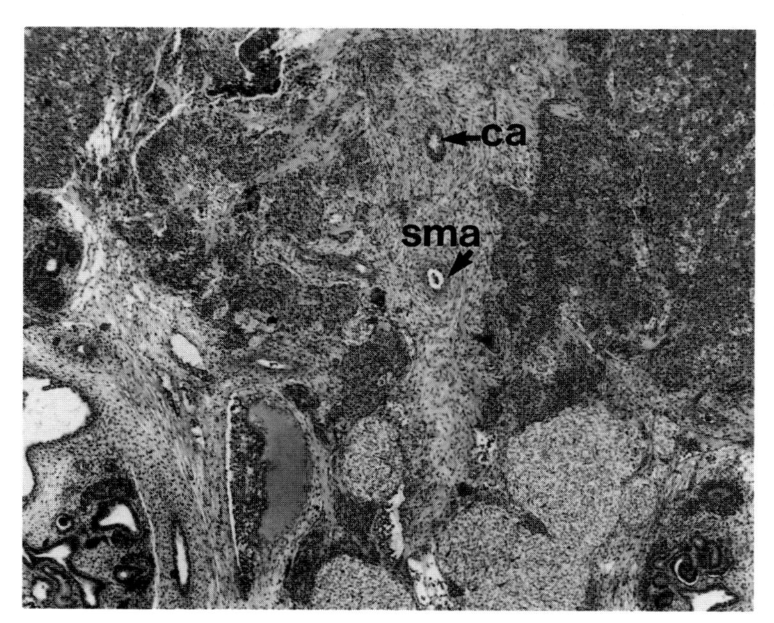

Figure 11-3
PARA-AORTIC PARAGANGLIA

Coronal section just anterior to the aorta in a human fetus shows elongate collections of paraganglia in a para-aortic location. Lower poles of kidneys are evident along with adrenal glands in relation to the large paravertebral and para-aortic sympathetic plexus. Seen are the celiac artery (ca) and superior mesenteric artery (sma) and below an oblique portion of the inferior mesenteric artery adventitia. (Fig. 1-5A from Lack EE, Kozakewich HP. Embryology, developmental anatomy, and selected aspects of non-neoplastic pathology. In: Lack EE, ed. Pathology of the adrenal glands. New York: Churchill Livingstone, 1990:1–74.)

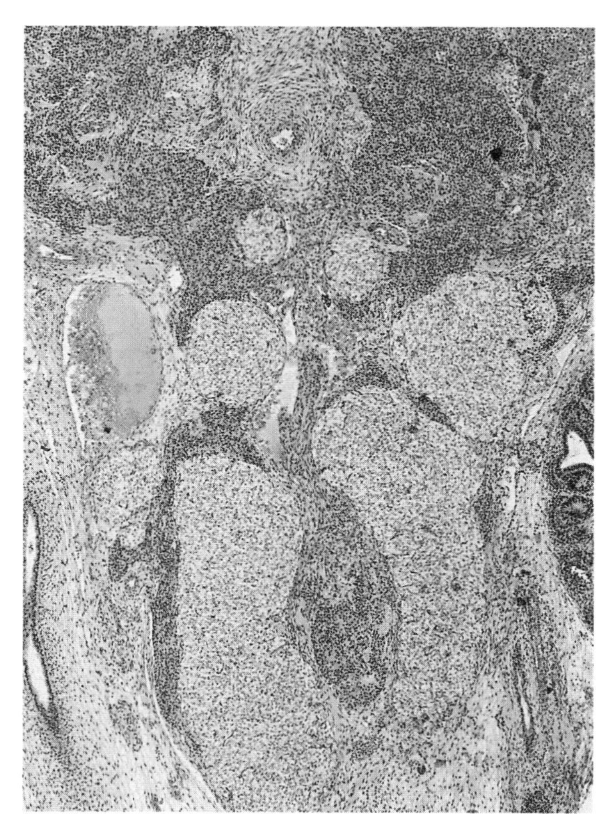

Figure 11-4
ORGANS OF ZUCKERKANDL

Closer view of organs of Zuckerkandl. Paraganglia are sharply circumscribed but not truly encapsulated.

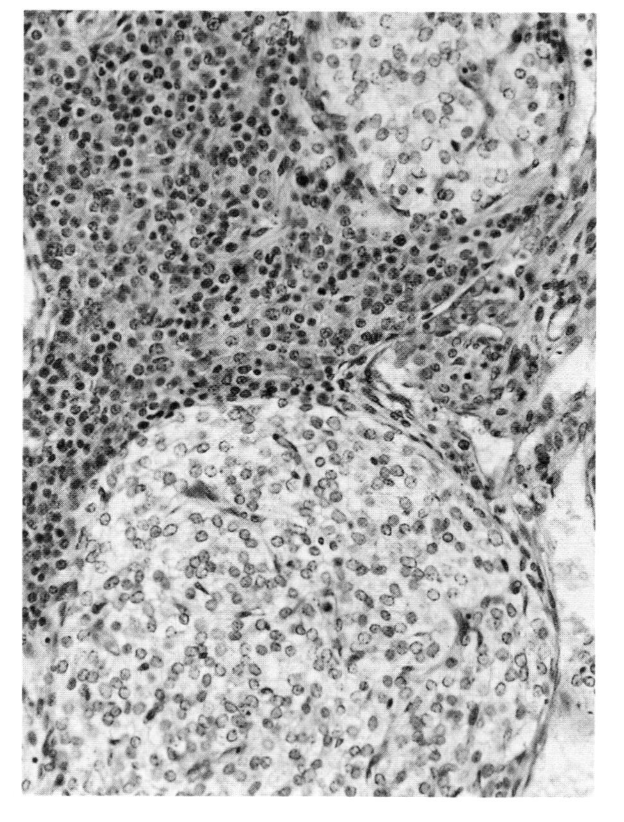

Figure 11-5
PARAGANGLION

The cells of this paraganglion in an 11-week-old fetus have pale cytoplasm with relatively indistinct borders. Nuclei are round to oval with dispersed chromatin. Contrast these cells with adjacent neuroblasts.

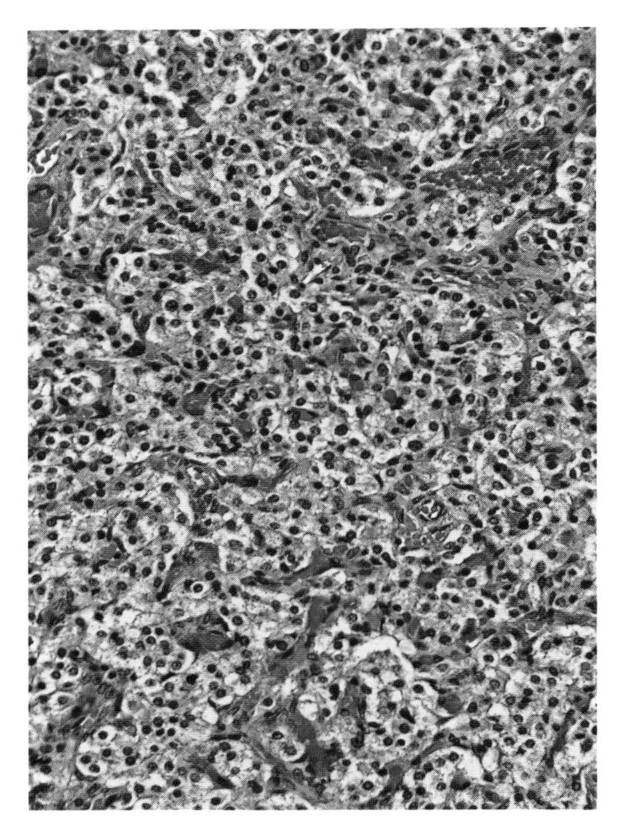

Figure 11-6
EXTRA-ADRENAL ABDOMINAL PARAGANGLION
This extra-adrenal abdominal paraganglion in a young child is composed of interanastomosing cords of cells separated by a rich microvasculature. Many cells have finely granular, light pink to amphophilic cytoplasm.

by 14 years of age (8). In adults, discrete microscopic collections of extra-adrenal chromaffin tissue persist (7,14). The microscopic appearance is virtually identical to that of the adrenal medulla (fig. 11-7A), and occasionally may be associated with ganglion cells (fig. 11-7B) or small myelinated nerve bundles (fig. 11-7C). The author has seen an intra-abdominal paraganglion in an adult with a small component present within the subcapsular sinusoid of an adjacent lymph node (fig. 11-8). Because of their catecholamine storage capacity, formaldehyde-induced fluorescence highlights small collections of extra-adrenal chromaffin cells (1,3,12,14).

Physiologic Function. The adrenal medullae attain structural maturity much later than the organs of Zuckerkandl (18,22). Extra-adrenal paraganglia are sparsely innervated (10), suggesting that chemical signals of some sort play a predominant role in stimulation (21). Norepinephrine is the predominant catecholamine in extra-adrenal chromaffin cells and in the fetal adrenal medulla (20,22). Since this amine is more potent as a pressor agent than epinephrine, it has been thought that the organs of Zuckerkandl in the fetus and newborn may help to maintain vascular tone; later this function gradually is taken over by the adrenal medullae and a more fully mature sympathetic nervous system (22). Abdominal chemoreceptors have been noted in the experimental animal in association with the vagus nerve (15,16), and the peripheral termination of vagal sensory and efferent fibers suggests that some of these paraganglia, including those in the adrenal medullae, may be involved in segmental reflex activity and more general homeostatic regulation (5). Hypoxia has been shown to cause a decrease in formaldehyde-induced fluorescence in extra-adrenal paraganglia in the human fetus (11) and release of norepinephrine in newborn rabbits exposed to severe asphyxia (2).

Immunohistochemical and Ultrastructural Features. Some of the enzymes involved in catecholamine synthesis have been identified in extra-adrenal collections of small, intensely fluorescent cells situated along blood vessels. Similar to neuroblasts of ganglia in the human fetus of 14 to 22 weeks' gestation, positive labeling was observed for tyrosine hydroxylase and dopamine beta-hydroxylase, but not for phenylethanolamine N-methyltransferase, which is consistent with the production of mainly norepinephrine (13). As expected, chromaffin cells of extra-adrenal paraganglia stain for neuroendocrine markers such as chromogranin A (fig. 11-9, left), and contain scattered sustentacular cells which are positive for S-100 protein (fig. 11-9, right). The ultrastructural features of paraganglia and adrenal medullae of the human fetus are covered in detail by Hervonen (10).

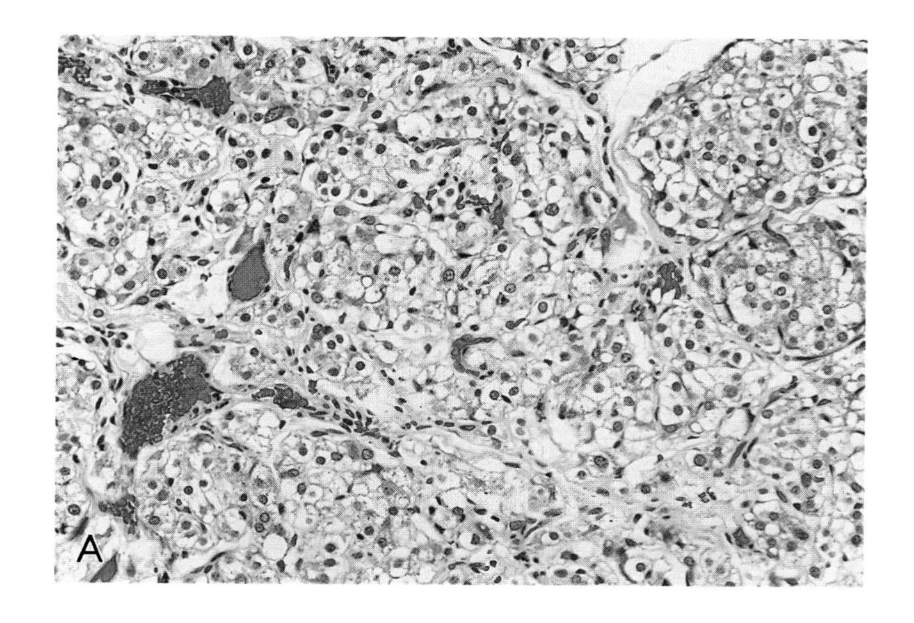

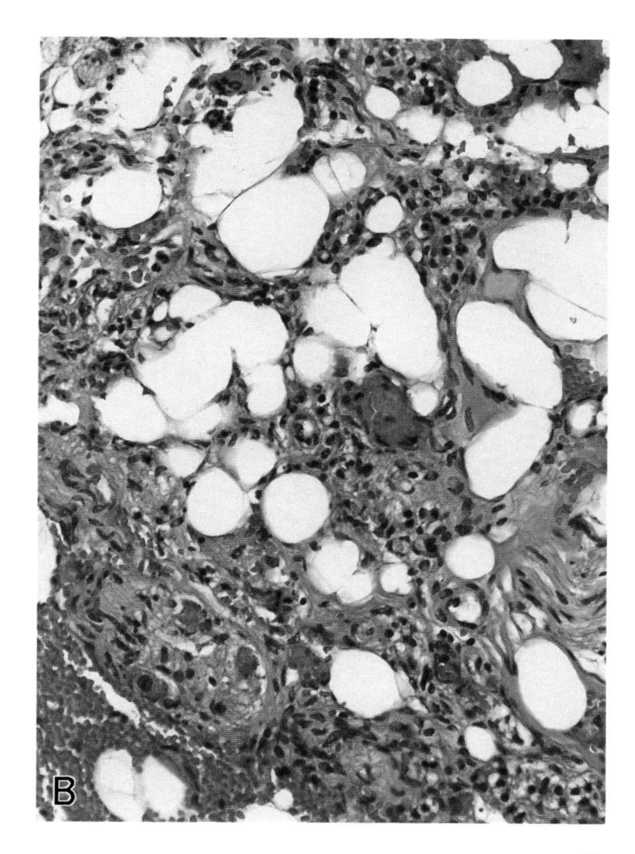

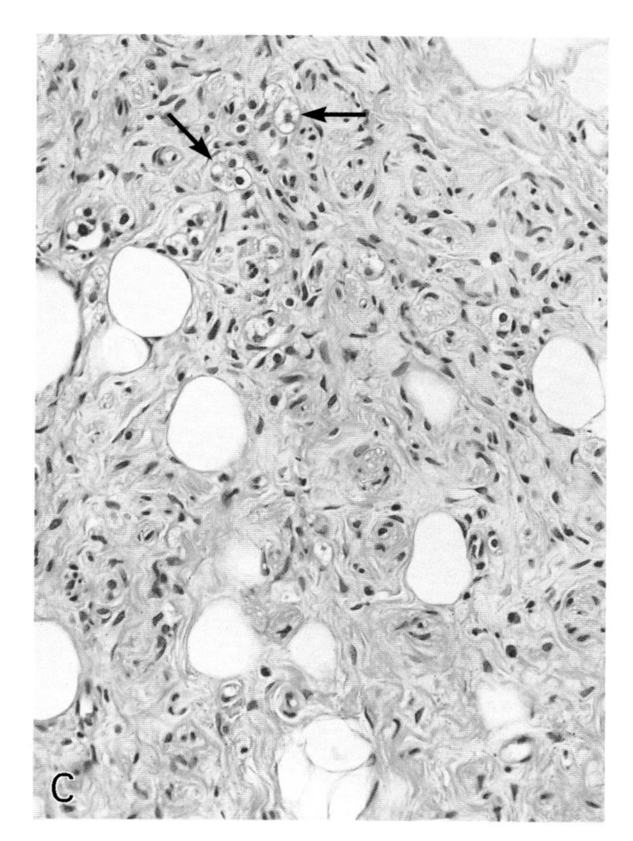

Figure 11-7
RETROPERITONEAL EXTRA-ADRENAL PARAGANGLIA IN ADULT PATIENTS

A: Aside from the lack of circumscription and intermingling with collections of fat cells (other areas), the tissue histomorphology of this extra-adrenal paraganglion closely resembles the adrenal medulla.

B: Small retroperitoneal paraganglion in an adult is associated with ganglion cells and a small component of neural tissue.

C: Small remnant of paraganglionic cells (straight arrows) are admixed with fibrous connective tissue, fat, and small nerves.

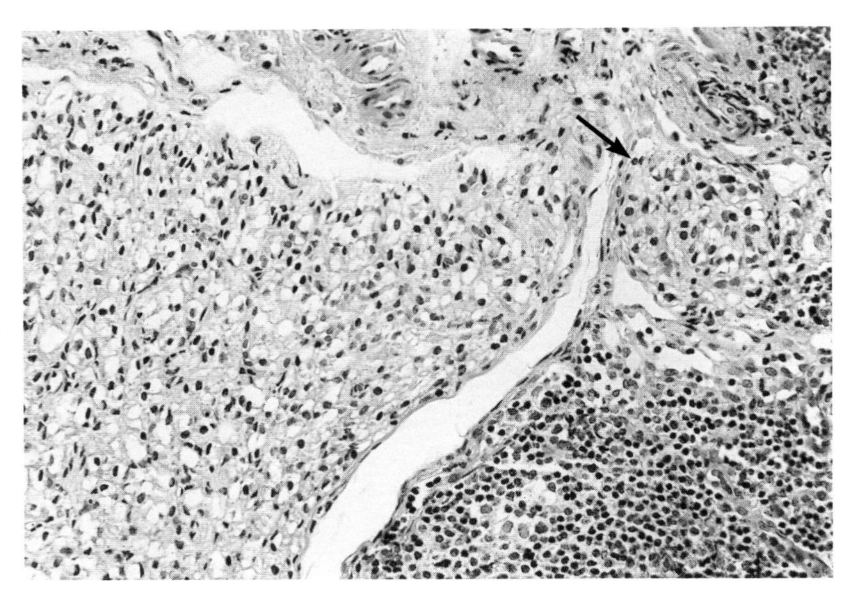

Figure 11-8
EXTRA-ADRENAL PARAGANGLION

This extra-adrenal paraganglion adjacent to a lymph node in an adult has a small component in the subcapsular sinusoid (arrow).

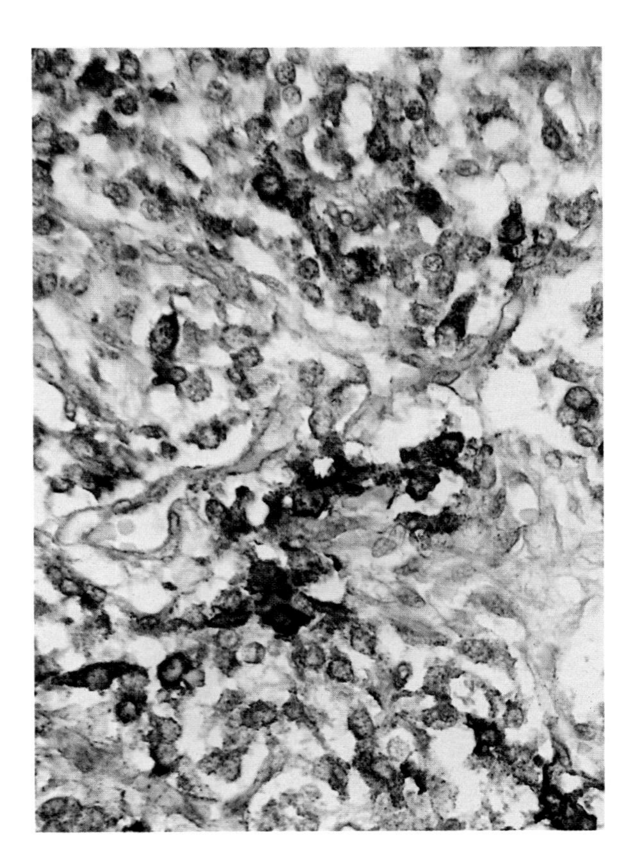

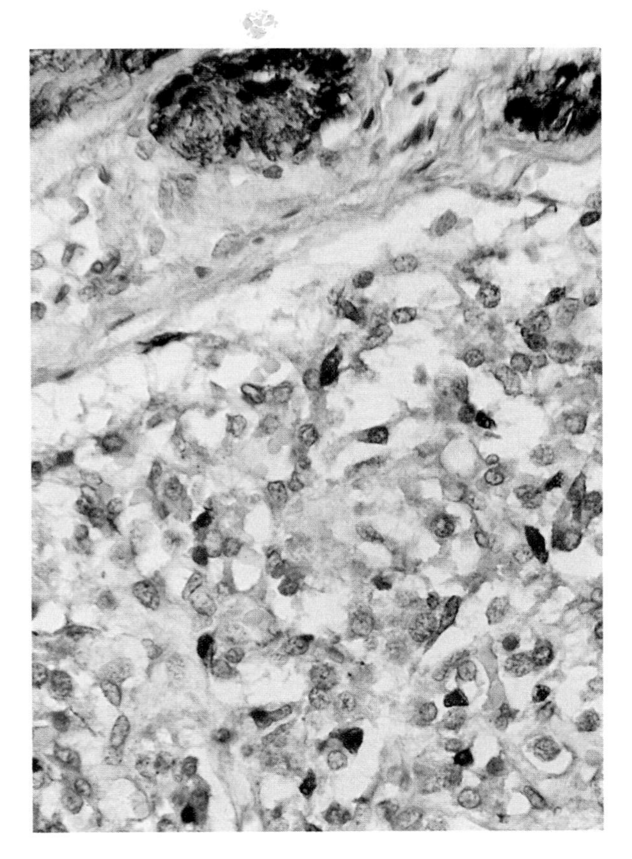

Figure 11-9
EXTRA-ADRENAL PARAGANGLION IN A CHILD

Left: Positive cytoplasmic immunostain for chromogranin A highlights clusters of paraganglion cells. (X350, Peroxidase-antiperoxidase stain)

Right: Immunostain for S-100 protein shows intense dark staining of ovoid to elongate nuclei of sustentacular cells. These are usually located near vascular channels. (X350, Peroxidase-antiperoxidase stain)

REFERENCES

1. Baljet B, Boekelaar AB, Groen GJ. Retroperitoneal paraganglia and the peripheral autonomic nervous system in the human fetus. Acta Morphol Neerl Scand 1985;23:137–49.
2. Brundin T. Studies on the preaortal paraganglia of newborn rabbits. Acta Physiol Scand 1966;290:1–54.
3. Chiba T. Monoamine fluorescence and electron microscopic studies on small intensely fluorescent (granule-containing) cells in human sympathetic ganglia. J Comp Neurol 1978;179:153–66.
4. Coupland RE. The natural history of the chromaffin cell. London: Longmans, 1965.
5. Coupland RE. The natural history of the chromaffin cell—twenty-five years on the beginning. Arch Histol Cytol 1989;52:331–41.
6. Coupland RE. Persistence of typical chromaffin cells in the human paravertebral sympathetic chain in the child and adult. Am J Anat 1979;129 (11a):196–7.
7. Coupland RE. The prenatal development of the abdominal para-aortic bodies in man. J Anat 1952;86:357–72.
8. Coupland RE. Postnatal fate of the abdominal para-aortic bodies in man. J Anat 1954;88:455–64.
9. Glenner GG, Grimley PM. Tumors of the extra-adrenal paraganglion system (including chemoreceptors), Atlas of Tumor Pathology, 2nd Series, Fascicle 9, Washington, D.C.: Armed Forces Institute of Pathology, 1974.
10. Hervonen A. Development of catecholamine-storing cells in human fetal paraganglia and adrenal medulla. A histochemical and electron microscopical study. Acta Physiol Scand 1971;368(suppl):1–94.
11. Hervonen A, Korkala O. The effect of hypoxia on the catecholamine content of human fetal abdominal paraganglia and adrenal medulla. Acta Obstet Gynecol Scand 1972;51:7–24.
12. Hervonen A, Partanen S, Vaalasti A, Partanen M, Kanerva L, Alho H: The distribution and endocrine nature of the abdominal paraganglia of adult man. Am J Anat 1978;153:563–72.
13. Hervonen A, Pickel VM, Joh TH, Reis DJ, Linnoila I, Miller RJ. Immunohistochemical localization of the catecholamine-synthesizing enzymes, substance P and enkephalin in the human fetal sympathetic ganglion. Cell Tissue Res 1981;214:33–42.
14. Hervonen A, Vaalasti A, Partanen M, Kanerva L, Vaalasti T. The paraganglia, a persisting endocrine system in man. Am J Anat 1976;146:207–10.
15. Hollinshead WH. Chemoreceptors in the abdomen. J Comp Neurol 1941;74:269–85.
16. Hollinshead WH. The function of the abdominal chemoreceptors of the rat and mouse. Am J Physiol 1946;147:654–60.
17. Kohn, A. Die paraganglien. Arch f Mikr Anat, Bd 1903:[62] S263–365.
18. Lack EE. Pathology of adrenal and extra-adrenal paraganglia. Major problems in pathology, Vol. 29. Philadelphia: WB Saunders, 1994.
19. Lack EE, Kozakewich HP. Embryology, developmental anatomy, and selected aspects of non-neoplastic pathology. In: Lack EE, ed. Pathology of the adrenal glands. New York: Churchill Livingstone, 1990:1–74.
20. Niemineva K, Pekkarinen A. Determination of adrenalin and noradrenalin in the human fetal adrenals and aortic bodies. Nature 1953;171:436–7.
21. Tischler AS. Paraganglia. In: Sternberg SS, ed. Histology for pathologists. New York: Raven Press, 1992:363–79.
22. West GB, Shepherd DM, Hunter RB, MacGregor AR. The function of the organs of Zuckerkandl. Clin Sci 1953;12:317–25.
23. Zuckerkandl E. The development of the chromaffin organs and the suprarenal glands. In: Kiebel F, Mall FP, eds. Manual of human embryology. Philadelphia: JB Lippincott, 1912:157–79.
24. Zuckerkandl E. Ueber nebenorgane des sympathicus im retroperitonaealraum des menschen. Verh Dtsch Anat Ges 1901;15:95–107.

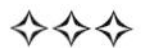

12

EXTRA-ADRENAL PARAGANGLIOMAS OF THE SYMPATHOADRENAL NEUROENDOCRINE SYSTEM

Extra-adrenal paragangliomas of the sympathoadrenal neuroendocrine system are located anywhere from the upper neck to the pelvic floor. According to Glenner and Grimley (2), the aorticosympathetic paraganglia are associated with segmental ganglia of the sympathetic chain while viscero-autonomic paraganglia are associated with viscera such as urinary bladder, gallbladder, and the intrathoracic area near the base of the heart. Results of a review by Fries and Chamberlin (1) of the distribution of 205 extra-adrenal paragangliomas are shown in Table 12-1. However, since only 5 to 10 percent of sporadic pheochromocytomas are extra-adrenal, the incidence figures shown in Table 12-1 decline considerably if adrenal medullary paragangliomas (pheochromocytomas) are included as a larger subset of sympathoadrenal paragangliomas (3). In a review by Melicow (4), 98 percent of 107 pheochromocytomas and extra-adrenal paragangliomas were intra-abdominal, only 2 percent were cervical or intrathoracic, and less than 1 percent arose in the urinary bladder.

EXTRA-ADRENAL INTRA-ABDOMINAL PARAGANGLIOMAS

Anatomic Distribution. Extra-adrenal paragangliomas of the abdomen are divided into three major groups (6). The largest group, superior para-aortic tumors (45 percent of cases), includes those located adjacent to the adrenal gland, in and around the hilum of the kidney, and the renal pedicle. Inferior para-aortic paragangliomas (30 percent of cases) arise below the inferior pole of the kidneys and extend down the aorta to include the iliac vessels; most extra-adrenal paragangliomas in this area arise from remnants of the organs of Zuckerkandl which persist into adult life (14). Some of these tumors have a midline or paramedian location anterior to the aorta or over the aortic bifurcation. The last group includes urinary bladder paragangliomas; these are considered separately because of clinical manifestations and what seems to be a somewhat better prognosis. Some have suggested that the anatomic localization of a tumor away from the aorta should essentially exclude a paraganglioma from the differential diagnosis (8), but important exceptions have been reported (14).

Clinical Features. Intra-abdominal extra-adrenal paragangliomas occur in virtually any age group, but most occur in the third to fifth decades of life (8,15,20,21). There is a roughly equal sex predilection, although there is a slight male predominance in some series (8,15,19,21). Signs and symptoms most likely due to excess catecholamine secretion have been reported in 25 to 86 percent of patients (8,15,21); in some asymptomatic patients the tumor is discovered at autopsy (7). Depending upon size and anatomic location, abdominal or flank pain may be a presenting complaint (15). Other unusual presentations include hydroureteronephrosis due to ureteral obstruction (9), gross hematuria due to invasion of the hilum of the kidney, obstructive jaundice due to compression of the common bile duct, and acute retroperitoneal hemorrhage (15). The rare patient may present with an osteolytic bony metastasis (16). Renovascular hypertension may result from unilateral compression of the renal artery without any evidence of excess catecholamine secretion (18). A rare case of a

Table 12-1

ANATOMIC DISTRIBUTION OF EXTRA-ADRENAL PARAGANGLIOMAS (Sympathoadrenal Neuroendocrine System)

Area	Incidence
Cervical	3%
Intrathoracic	12%
Intra-abdominal	85%
Superior para-aortic	45%
Inferior para-aortic	30%
Urinary bladder	10%

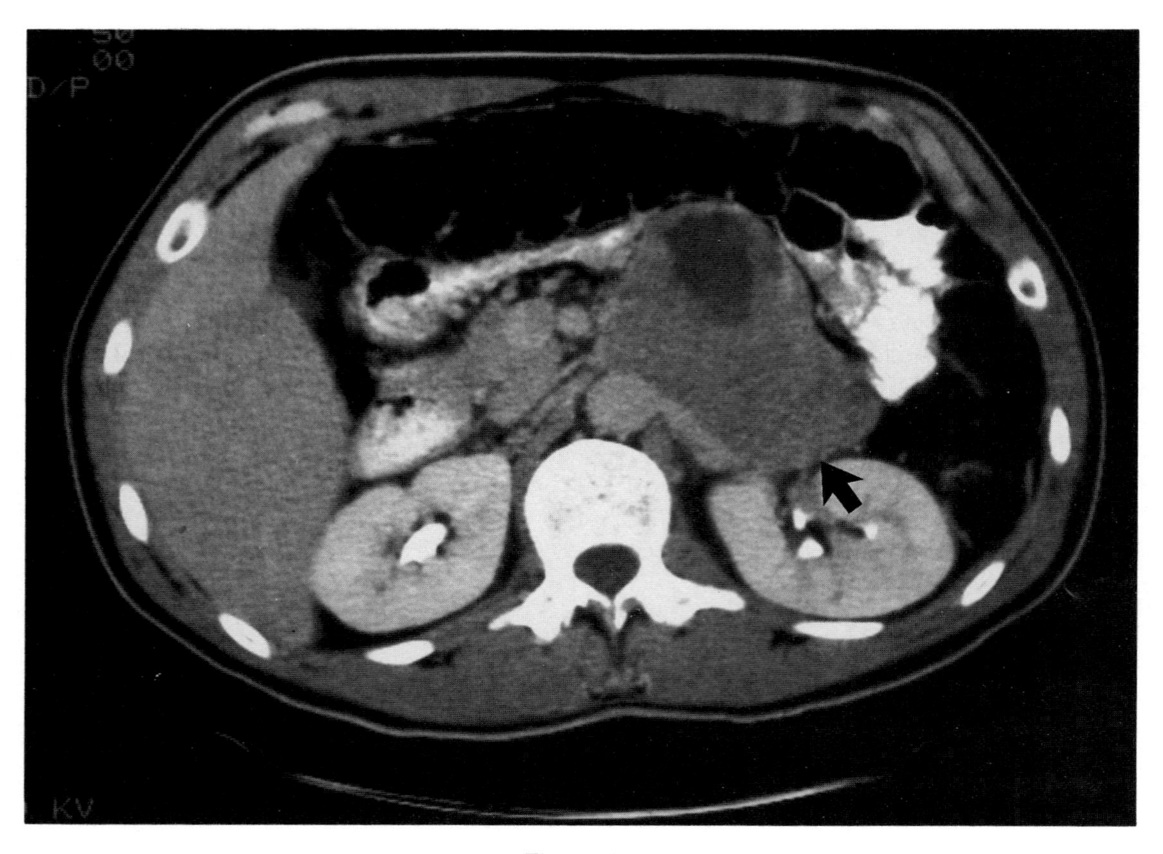

Figure 12-1
EXTRA-ADRENAL ABDOMINAL PARAGANGLIOMA
CT scan of the upper abdomen in a 28-year-old man who presented with symptoms suggesting pheochromocytoma shows a large preaortic and para-aortic paraganglioma (arrow). The paraganglioma is nonhomogeneous and grossly had areas of cystic degeneration. The ipsilateral adrenal gland was free of tumor.

malignant retroperitoneal paraganglioma was recently reported in a 12-year-old girl with evidence of Cushing's syndrome and virilization (12). Similar to pheochromocytomas, extra-adrenal paragangliomas may be localized by imaging modalities other than selective arteriography (fig. 12-1). On magnetic resonance imaging (MRI), the tumors usually have a hyperintense signal in T2-weighted images (fig. 12-2) (11).

Gross and Microscopic Findings. The tumors are usually solitary, particularly in adults, but in a review of nonfunctional, nonchromaffin paragangliomas two or more separate primary tumors were present in 5 of 21 patients (19). Occasional examples of paragangliomatosis have been reported, with multiple contiguous paragangliomas along the course of the sympathetic chain (8) or distributed from the neck to the pelvis (5,10). An unusual case of paragangliomatosis occurred in a teenager who had 21 separate tumors, and had evidence of additional paragangliomas (10). The average size of the tumors in two series was about 10 cm (fig. 12-3) (15,21), but there was a broad range in size of from 4 to 24 cm (21). The variety of gross morphologic features is similar to that of pheochromocytoma, although typically an adrenal remnant (entopic or ectopic) is not identified. Some tumors undergo marked cystic degeneration (fig. 12-4), and when the neoplasm shows extensive hemorrhage it can simulate a hematoma.

The most characteristic microscopic pattern is a trabecular arrangement with anastomosing cords of tumor cells (fig. 12-5). Some tumors may have a diffuse or alveolar (nesting) pattern (fig. 12-6). There is sufficient overlap in architecture

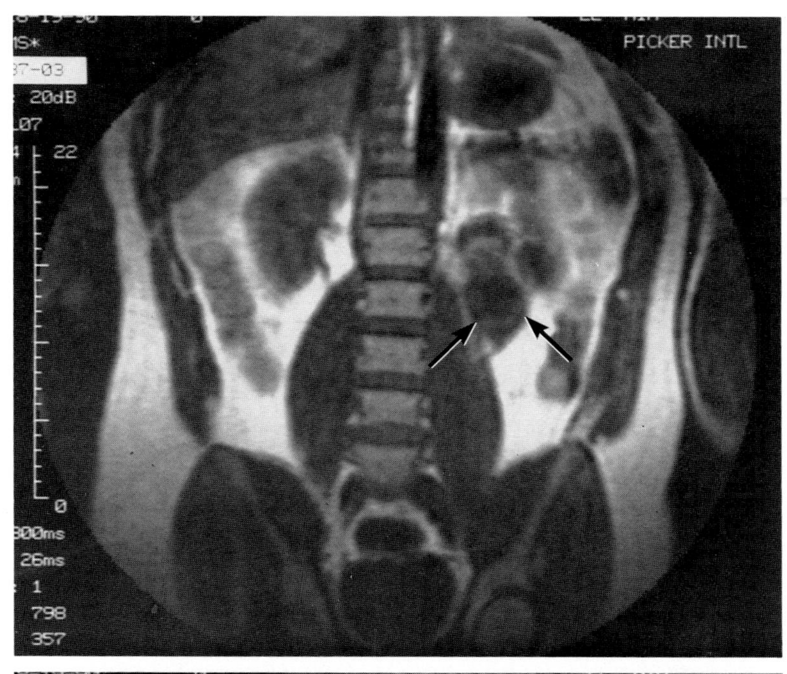

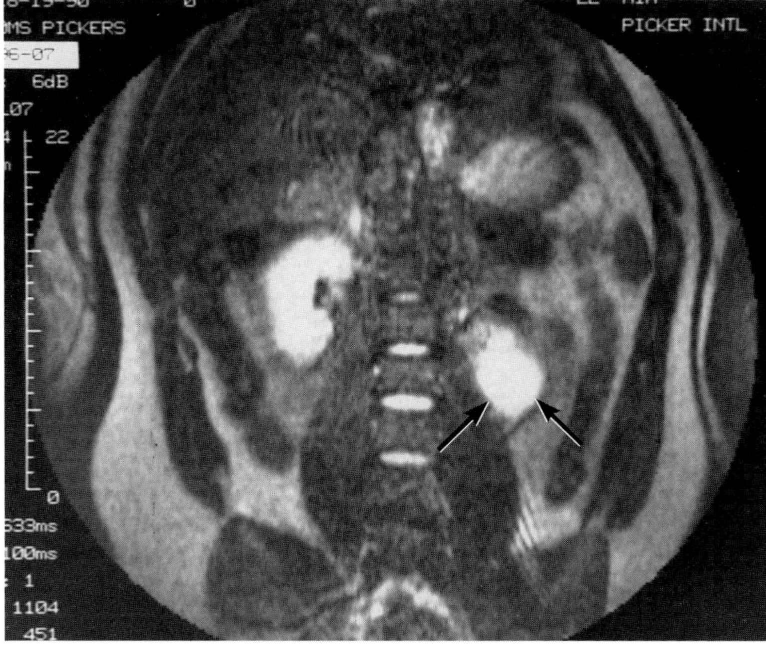

Figure 12-2
EXTRA-ADRENAL PARAGANGLIOMA

Top: This MRI shows a paraganglioma near the lower border of the kidney on the left side (arrows).

Bottom: There is an intense signal on a T2-weighted image (arrows). (Fig. 5-3A,B from Keiser HR, Doppman JL, Robertson CN, Linehan WM, Averbuch SD. Diagnosis, localization, and management of pheochromocytoma. In: Lack EE, ed. Pathology of the adrenal glands. New York: Churchill Livingstone, 1990:237–55.)

and cellular morphology that examination of isolated fields in any particular case may fail to reliably discriminate between an adrenal versus an extra-adrenal primary. Finding an attached adrenal remnant may be helpful, but some paragangliomas arise in an immediate periadrenal or juxta-adrenal location without intrinsic involvement of the gland. Preoperative localization studies or intraoperative findings at the time of laparotomy may distinguish the two (14).

Similar to pheochromocytomas, there may be a remarkable degree of nuclear pleomorphism and even occasional mitotic figures, but these and other histologic features, such as large size,

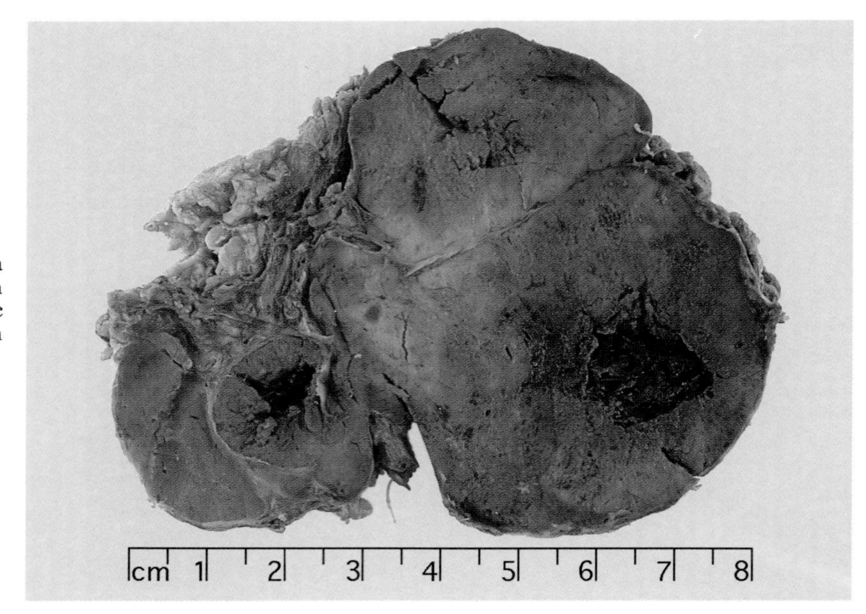

Figure 12-3
EXTRA-ADRENAL
ABDOMINAL PARAGANGLIOMA

In cross section, the paraganglioma seen in figure 12-1 is tan to dark brown with areas of hemorrhage and cystic degeneration. The tumor was 9.5 cm in diameter and weighed 208 g.

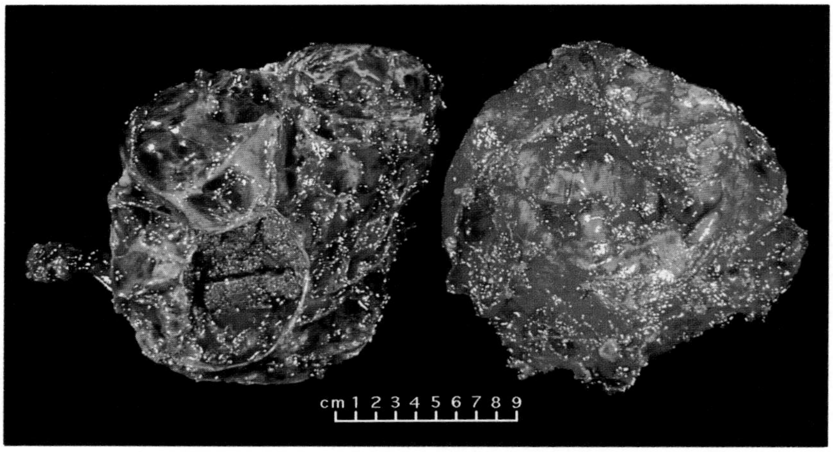

Figure 12-4
EXTRA-ADRENAL
ABDOMINAL PARAGANGLIOMA

This extra-adrenal abdominal paraganglioma resected from a 53-year-old man shows marked cystic degeneration on cross section. The tumor had been initially diagnosed as a hemangiopericytoma. It was 20 cm in diameter. The patient was alive and well 5 years later.

do not permit reliable classification of the paraganglioma as malignant (14). Intracytoplasmic hyaline globules can be found in some tumors, but the frequency in one study was lower (8.3 percent) (15) than the nearly one third incidence for pheochromocytoma (17). Prominent vascularity with abundance of plump endothelial cells may be mistaken for a primary vasoformative neoplasm (fig. 12-7). Occasionally, a few bundles of myelinated nerve are found within or immediately adjacent to the tumor; this may reflect a close relationship of extra-adrenal paraganglia with neural structures, and does not necessarily signify malignancy. An example of a composite extra-adrenal paraganglioma-ganglioneuroma has been reported which was clinically malignant (21). The author has seen a case of a heavily pigmented retroperitoneal extra-adrenal paraganglioma that contained abundant coarse granular pigment within the cytoplasm of most tumor cells, giving the tumor a jet black color (fig. 12-8). Ultrastructural study in this case showed numerous, relatively uniform ("epinephrine-type"), dense-core neurosecretory granules as well as electron-dense material consistent with neuromelanin, an electron-dense degradation

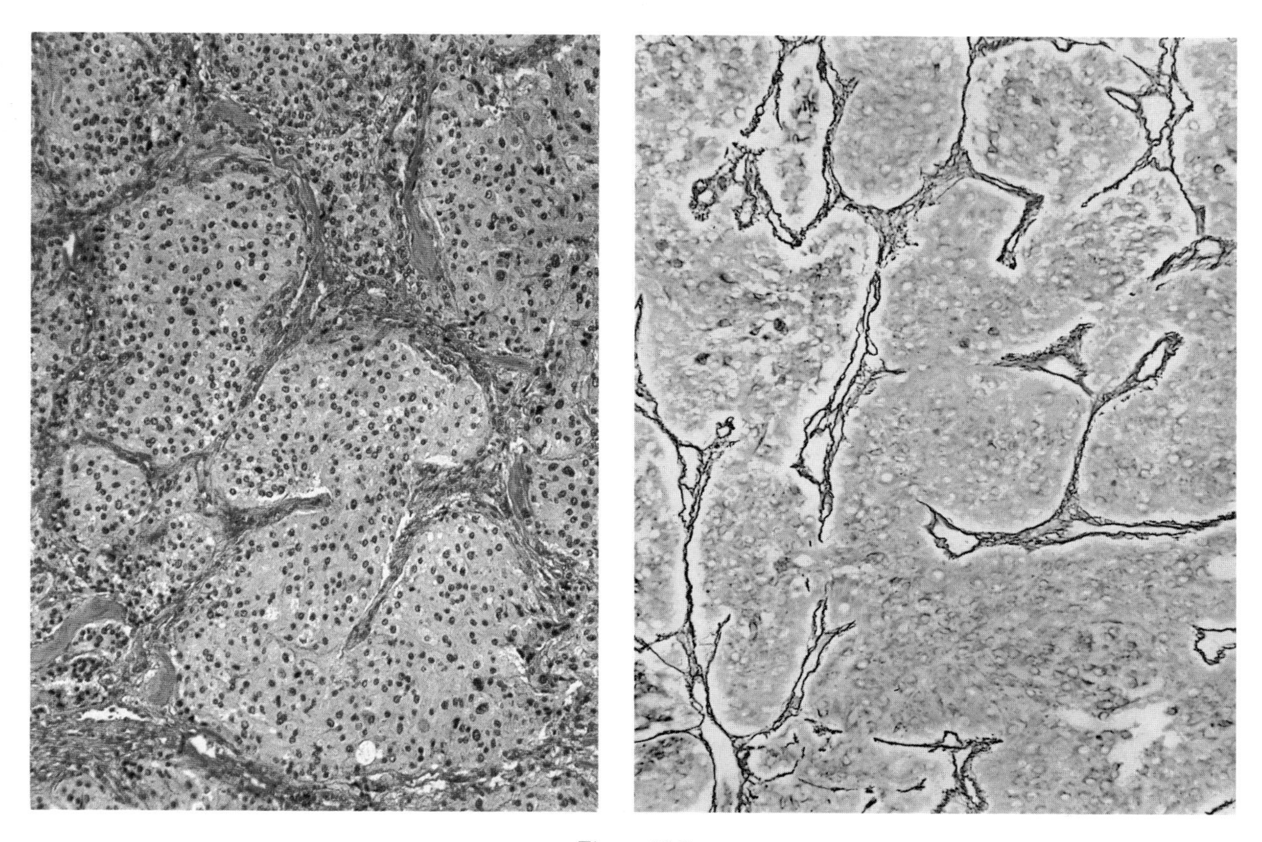

Figure 12-5
EXTRA-ADRENAL ABDOMINAL PARAGANGLIOMA
Left: An anastomosing trabecular pattern predominates in this field.
Right: Stain for reticulum greatly accentuates the interconnecting trabeculae with a delicate vascular pattern. (X200, Reticulum stain)

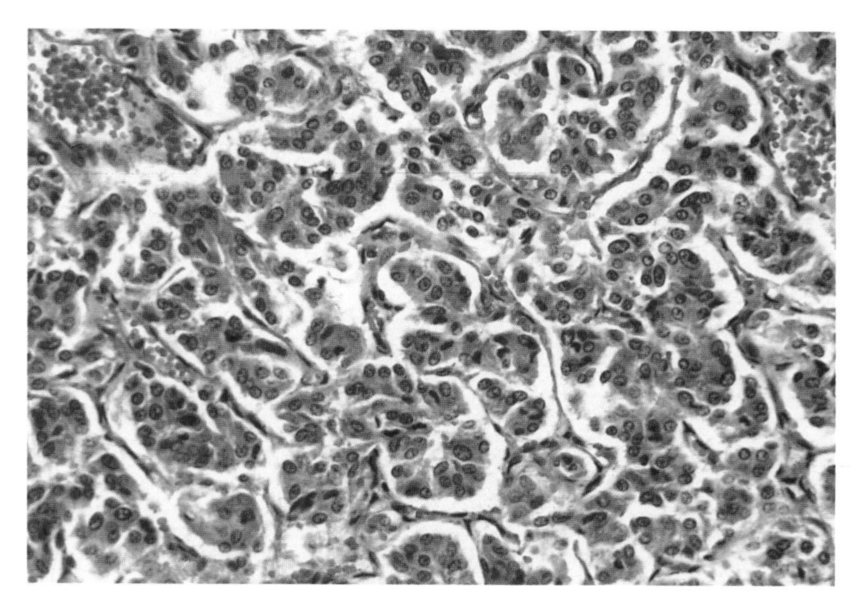

Figure 12-6
EXTRA-ADRENAL
ABDOMINAL PARAGANGLIOMA
There are small, relatively uniform nests of cells.

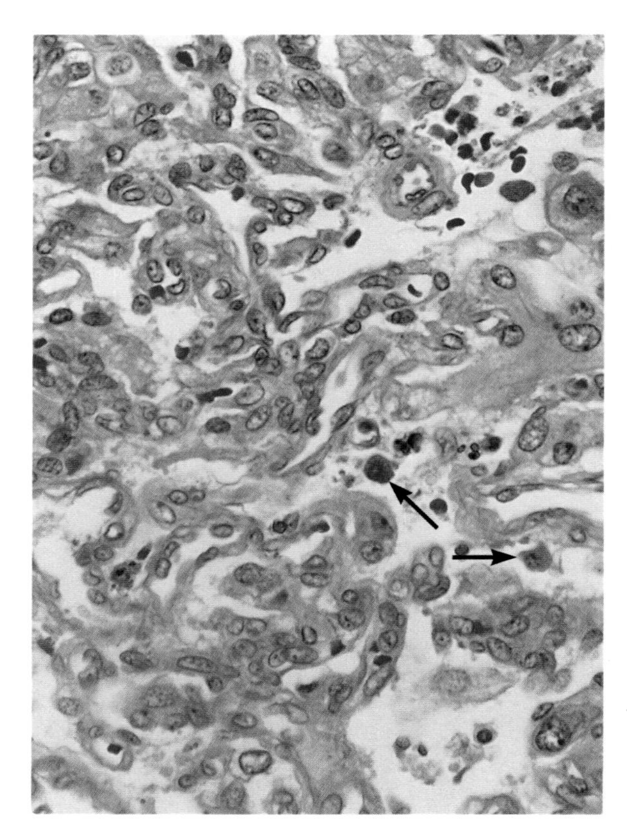

Figure 12-7
EXTRA-ADRENAL ABDOMINAL PARAGANGLIOMA
The prominent vascular pattern in this extra-adrenal abdominal paraganglioma can be misleading due to the component of plump endothelial cells. Note the scattered mast cells (arrows).

product of catecholamine metabolism (a lipofuscin-type secondary lysosome). No premelanosomes or melanosomes were identified.

Incidence of Malignancy. Intra-abdominal, extra-adrenal paragangliomas tend to be the most aggressive paragangliomas of the sympathoadrenal neuroendocrine system, compared with urinary bladder paragangliomas and probably paragangliomas in rare and exotic sites (there are too few cases to allow for a reliable prognostic profile for these rarer tumors) (14). The incidence of malignancy recorded in six large series is 14 percent (8), 24 percent (7), 29 percent (13), 33 percent (19), 42 percent (15), and 50 percent (21). The mode of spread (fig. 12-9) and pattern of metastasis are similar to that of pheochromocytoma, and sometimes prolonged follow-up is necessary before metastasis occurs. The 5-year survival rate in one series was 36 percent (21).

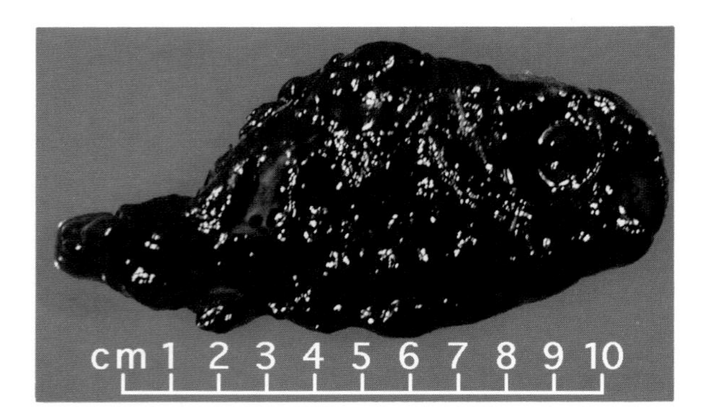

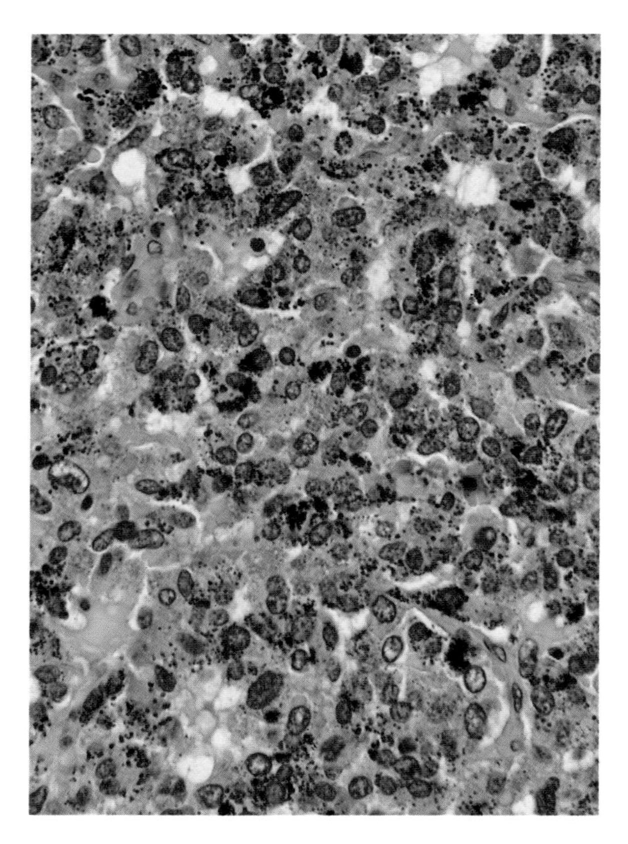

Figure 12-8
PIGMENTED (BLACK) EXTRA-ADRENAL PARAGANGLIOMA OF RETROPERITONEUM
Top: Tumor weighed 225 g and is jet black on cross section. Intact tumor measured 13 x 8 x 4.5 cm. (Courtesy of Dr. Hyunchul Kim, Des Moines, IA.)

Bottom: Tumor cells contain abundant granular pigment which on ultrastructural study was most consistent with neuromelanin or lipofuscin. There were no true melanosomes or premelanosomes identified. Tumor cells were positive for chromogranin A and synaptophysin and negative for S-100 protein and HMB-45. The pigment was positive with the Fontana-Masson silver stain and the staining reaction was abolished by bleaching procedure. Sustentacular cells were strongly S-100 protein positive.

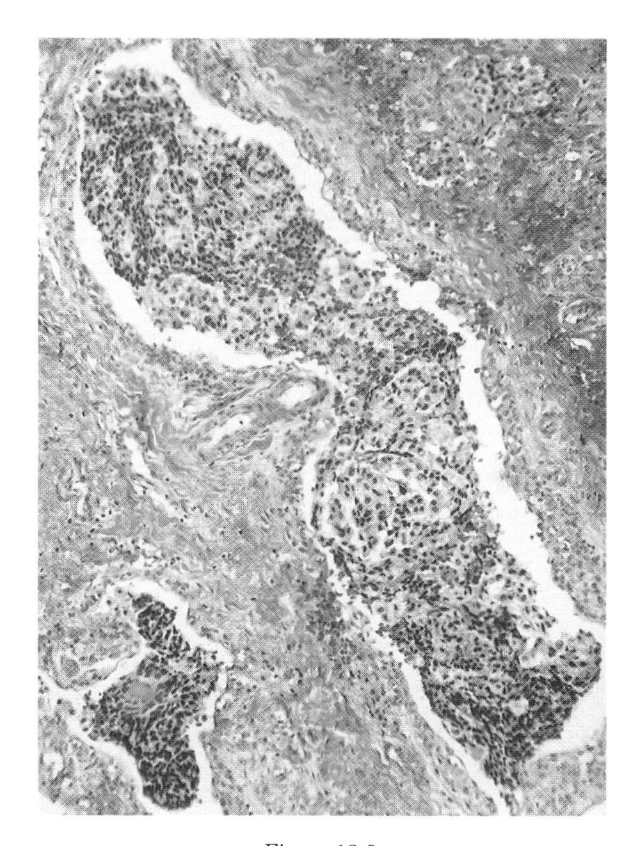

Figure 12-9
EXTRA-ADRENAL
ABDOMINAL PARAGANGLIOMA

This extra-adrenal abdominal paraganglioma probably arose from remnants of organs of Zuckerkandl. There are small foci of vascular invasion. The tumor proved to be clinically malignant.

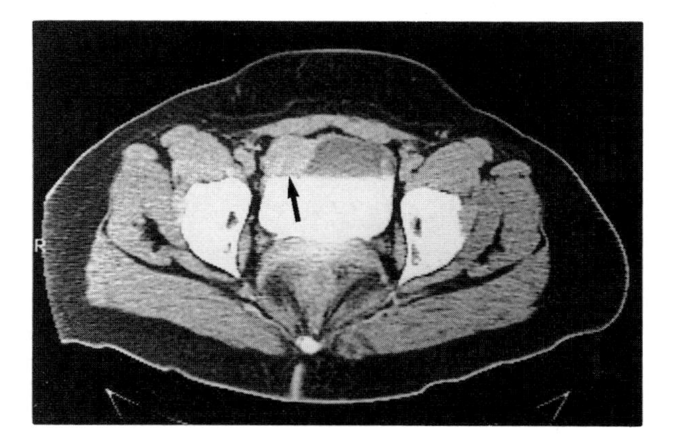

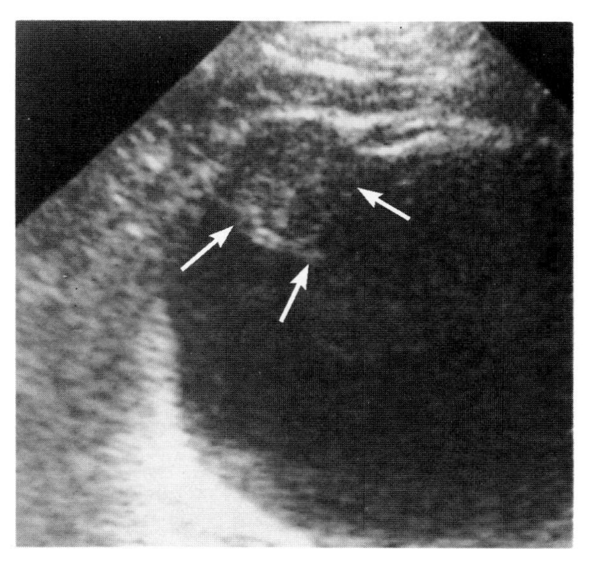

Figure 12-10
URINARY BLADDER PARAGANGLIOMA

Top: CT scan of a urinary bladder paraganglioma. The tumor is intramural in the right anterior aspect of the bladder (arrow). Water soluble contrast material layers out in the bladder posteriorly.

Bottom: Ultrasound showed a nonhomogeneous mass (arrows) involving the anterior wall of the urinary bladder. (Fig. 5-2A,B from Keiser HR, Doppman JL, Robertson CN, Linehan WM, Averbuch SD. Diagnosis, localization, and management of pheochromocytoma. In: Lack EE, ed. Pathology of the adrenal glands. New York: Churchill Livingstone, 1990:237–55.)

Urinary Bladder Paragangliomas

Clinical Features. Urinary bladder paragangliomas account for only 0.06 percent (28) to 0.5 percent (22) of all primary bladder tumors in adults. In the large series and literature review from the Armed Forces Institute of Pathology (AFIP) (28), there was a roughly equal sex predilection, and the average age at diagnosis was about 41 years (range, 11 to 78 years). The tumor is usually located in the trigone near the ureteral orifices, but can also arise in the dome and lateral walls. The clinical triad consists of paroxysmal (or sustained) hypertension, gross intermittent hematuria, and attacks, which may be precipitated by micturition, although this is not apparent in every case (28). Occasionally, tumors are multifocal in the bladder, are associated with extravesical paragangliomas (30), and occur in a familial setting (32). Cases have been associated with von Recklinghausen's disease (23), renal cell carcinoma (25), polycystic renal disease (26), and other conditions (27). Imaging studies may provide detailed information regarding location of the tumor (fig. 12-10).

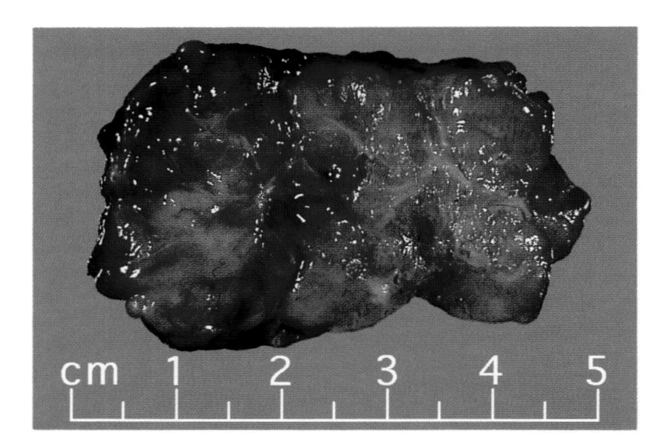

Figure 12-11
URINARY BLADDER PARAGANGLIOMA
This urinary bladder paraganglioma was removed by segmental resection of the bladder wall. The patient had intermittent symptoms of excess catecholamine secretion.

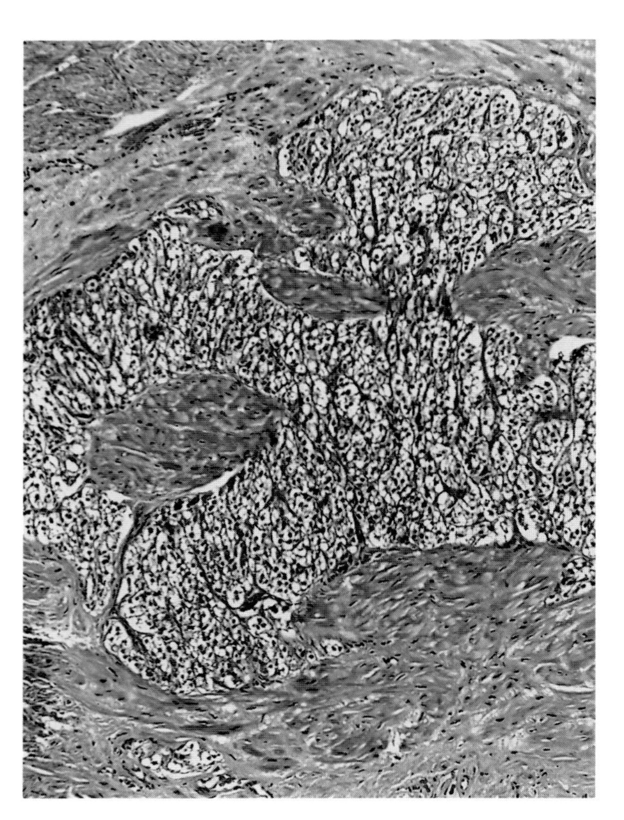

Figure 12-12
NON-NEOPLASTIC PARAGANGLION
This normal non-neoplastic paraganglion near the base of the bladder was an incidental finding in tissue obtained during transurethral resection for benign prostatic hyperplasia. Note the close relation with smooth muscle bundles.

Gross and Microscopic Findings. Urinary bladder paragangliomas tend to be relatively small, with an average diameter of 1.9 cm in one study, but can be much larger (fig. 12-11). The tumor may project into the bladder lumen. Several of the smaller tumors in the bladder submucosa (28,31) may represent a non-neoplastic paraganglion. Indeed, a normal paraganglion at the base of the bladder interdigitating with smooth muscle can be confused with a paraganglioma (fig. 12-12). Urinary bladder paragangliomas arise from small nests of paraganglia which have presumably migrated to various parts of the vesicle and bladder base during early embryonic development (27).

Microscopically, urinary bladder paragangliomas usually present little difficulty in diagnosis (fig. 12-13), but problems in interpretation may arise when there is ulceration, crush artifact, or suboptimal tissue fixation and processing (fig. 12-14, left). Some tumors may be misinterpreted as transitional cell carcinoma (29) or even granular cell tumor (myoblastoma) (28). Most urinary bladder paragangliomas are not well circumscribed microscopically, and may interdigitate with bundles of smooth muscle (fig. 12-14, right), an appearance that simulates invasion but is not considered to be reliable evidence of malignancy (27).

Biologic Behavior. In the review from the AFIP, metastases were noted in 3 of 58 cases (5 percent) (28). In a recent review of 87 urinary bladder paragangliomas, regional lymph node metastases were noted in 12 cases (13.8 percent), but distant metastases occurred in only 2 cases (2.3 percent) (24). Multicentric paragangliomas (vesical and extravesical) should not be overinterpreted as malignant (27).

Unusual Abdominal and Pelvic Sites of Paragangliomas

Paragangliomas have been reported in a number of unusual sites, sometimes where normal paraganglia have yet to be described (45), including various sites in the genitourinary tract such as kidney (33,39,46,51), urethra (34–37), prostate gland (40,47,49), and spermatic cord (41). Normal paraganglia have been described in the human prostate gland (50,53) as well as urinary bladder (45). In a recent study of radical prostatectomy specimens, periprostatic paraganglia (median size, 0.9 mm) were identified in about 8

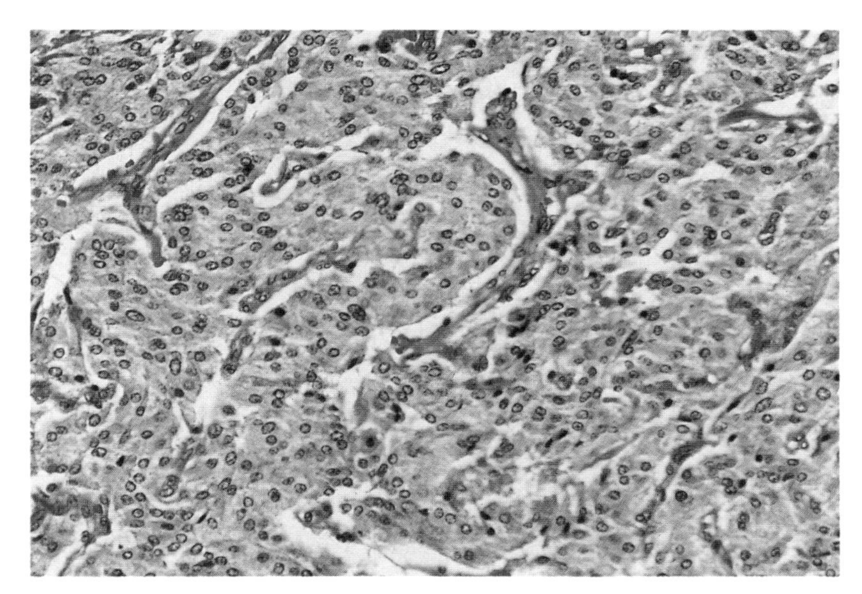

Figure 12-13
URINARY BLADDER PARAGANGLIOMA

Urinary bladder paraganglioma with a predominant anastomosing trabecular pattern. A nesting or alveolar arrangement of cells was also apparent in other areas.

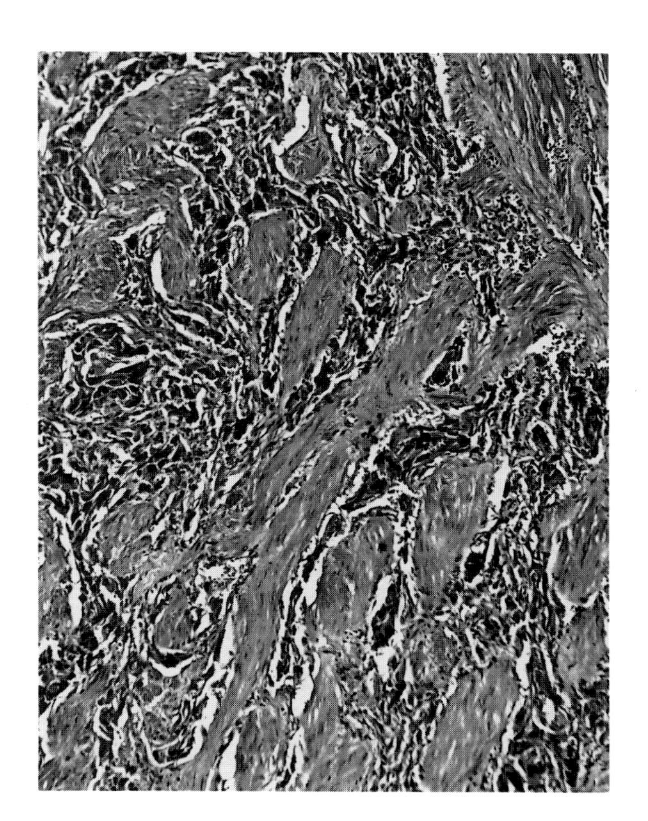

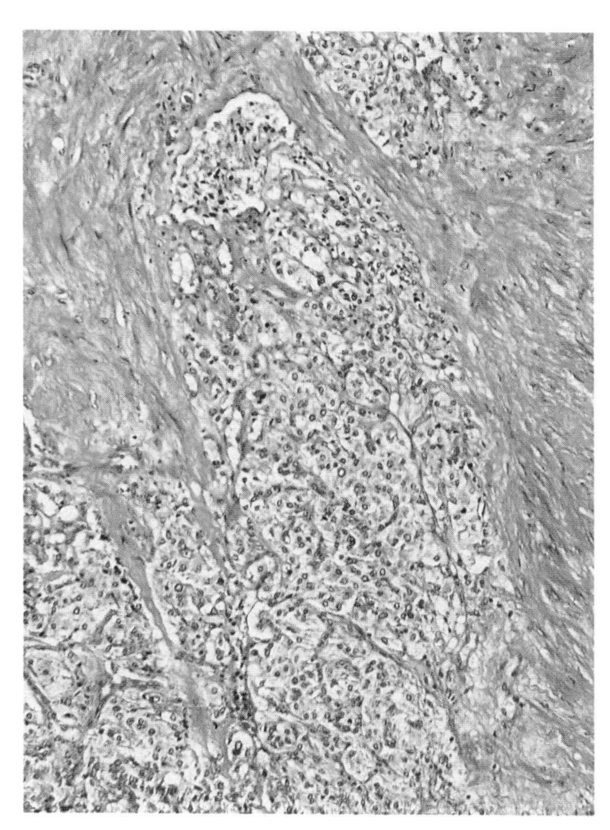

Figure 12-14
URINARY BLADDER PARAGANGLIOMA

Left: There is some crush artifact with strands of dark-staining tumor cells separating fibromuscular connective tissue.

Right: In another case, bundles of smooth muscle of bladder wall are separated by tumor, which has a predominantly nesting or alveolar pattern.

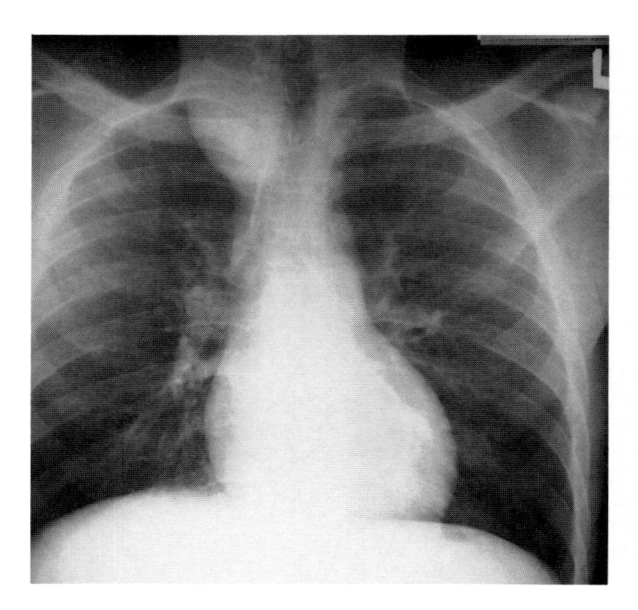

Figure 12-15
MALIGNANT PARAVERTEBRAL PARAGANGLIOMA
Posteroanterior chest roentgenogram in a 50-year-old man who presented initially with an osteolytic metastasis to right hip showed a primary paravertebral paraganglioma in the costovertebral sulcus in upper thorax on right side. (Figs. 12-15 through 12-18 are from the same case.) (Fig. 1 from Gallivan MV, Chun B, Rowden G, Lack EE. Intrathoracic paravertebral malignant paraganglioma. Arch Pathol Lab Med 1980;104:46–51.)

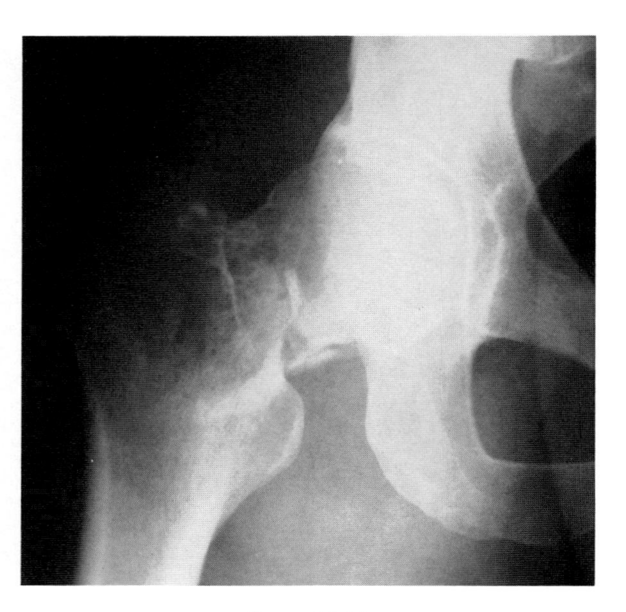

Figure 12-16
OSTEOLYTIC METASTASIS OF INTRATHORACIC PARAVERTEBRAL PARAGANGLIOMA
Intertrochanteric pathologic fracture of the right hip was the initial presentation, and later the patient was found to have a paravertebral intrathoracic paraganglioma. (Fig. 12-15A from Lack EE. Pathology of adrenal and extra-adrenal paraganglia. Major problems in pathology, Vol 29. Philadelphia: WB Saunders Co, 1994:283.)

percent of specimens; they were 1 to 3 mm, lateral and slightly posterior to the prostatic capsule, and often associated with neurovascular bundles (50). There have been several reports of gallbladder paragangliomas (43,48,54) and normal paraganglia within the subserosa, often close to blood vessels or nerves (42,44,52,54). Other exotic sites include uterus, ovary, vagina, vulva, and hepatobiliary tree (45) including liver parenchyma (38).

INTRATHORACIC PARAVERTEBRAL PARAGANGLIOMAS

Clinical Features. Intrathoracic paravertebral paragangliomas arise in areas closely related to the sympathetic axis (fig. 12-15), and in one review the tumors were usually located in the midthoracic region (55). About half of the tumors are functional, with excess catecholamine secretion. Some of the tumors arising in or near the base of the heart (i.e., aorticopulmonary paragangliomas) are also functionally active, thus suggesting a closer alignment with the sympathoadrenal neuroendocrine system; these tumors are considered separately. There is a predilection for males in the review by Gallivan et al. (55) with the average age at diagnosis of 29 years. Some cases have been reported in the pediatric age group (56). Rarely, Horner's syndrome is noted, and in exceptional cases an osteolytic metastasis may be the initial presentation (fig. 12-16). Tumors with a "dumbbell" configuration have been described (55); in one case, the tumor located away from the costovertebral sulcus simulated a primary rib tumor (59). Familial cases have occurred, and in some cases there may be paragangliomas in other sites, including neck and abdomen (55).

Gross and Microscopic Findings. The average size and weight of tumors in one review was 5.7 cm and 40 g, respectively; the largest tumor was 13 cm in diameter (55). Most tumors are detected in the right hemithorax (fig. 12-15). The gross appearance of an intrathoracic paravertebral paraganglioma is shown in figure 12-17. The histologic features are usually diagnostic,

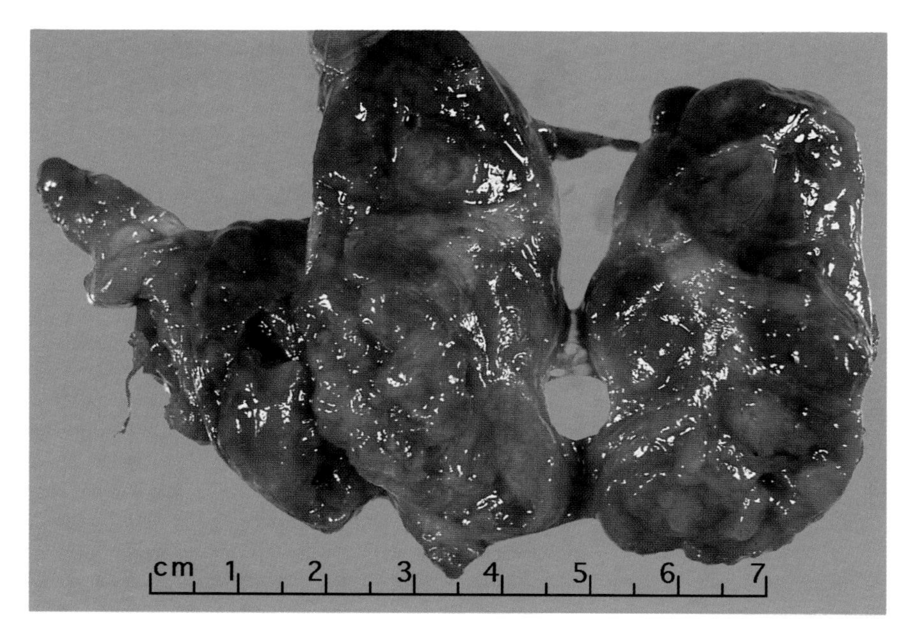

Figure 12-17
INTRATHORACIC PARAVERTEBRAL PARAGANGLIOMA

The tumor appeared well circumscribed and measured 6.5 cm in diameter. On cross section, the tumor is meaty tan-brown and deeply hemorrhagic in some areas. The tumor was extrapleural, overlying the heads of the first, second, and third ribs on the sympathetic chain. The patient died about 16 months later with multiple bony metastases as well as metastases to lung and liver.

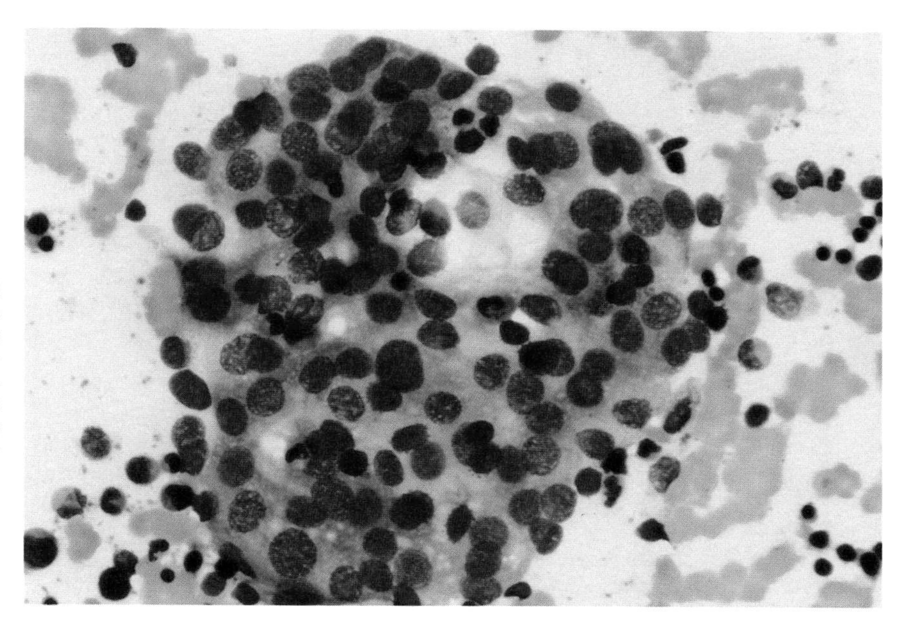

Figure 12-18
METASTATIC INTRATHORACIC PARAVERTEBRAL PARAGANGLIOMA

Intrathoracic paravertebral paraganglioma metastatic to iliac crest. Bone marrow aspirate of iliac crest showed relatively cohesive clusters of malignant cells which are difficult to classify accurately without further information or special stains to demonstrate neuroendocrine features. (X4 00, Wright-Giemsa stain)

although problems can arise in a limited biopsy of a primary tumor or when presentation is unusual, such as osseous metastasis in which the iliac crest bone marrow biopsy shows clusters of malignant cells which may be difficult to accurately classify (fig. 12-18) (55). On rare occasion, when tumor cells cling to delicate vascular channels with admixed hemorrhage, a paraganglioma may have a pseudopapillary or angiomatous appearance (fig. 12-19, left). Special stains can accentuate this pattern and provide valuable diagnostic information (fig. 12-19, right) (57).

Biologic Behavior. An initial review reported that 7 percent of intrathoracic paravertebral paragangliomas are clinically malignant (55), but in a recent report, 7 of 48 cases were malignant (13 percent) (58). There may be a greater tendency to report malignant paragangliomas arising in rare and exotic locations, thus overestimating the true incidence of malignant behavior.

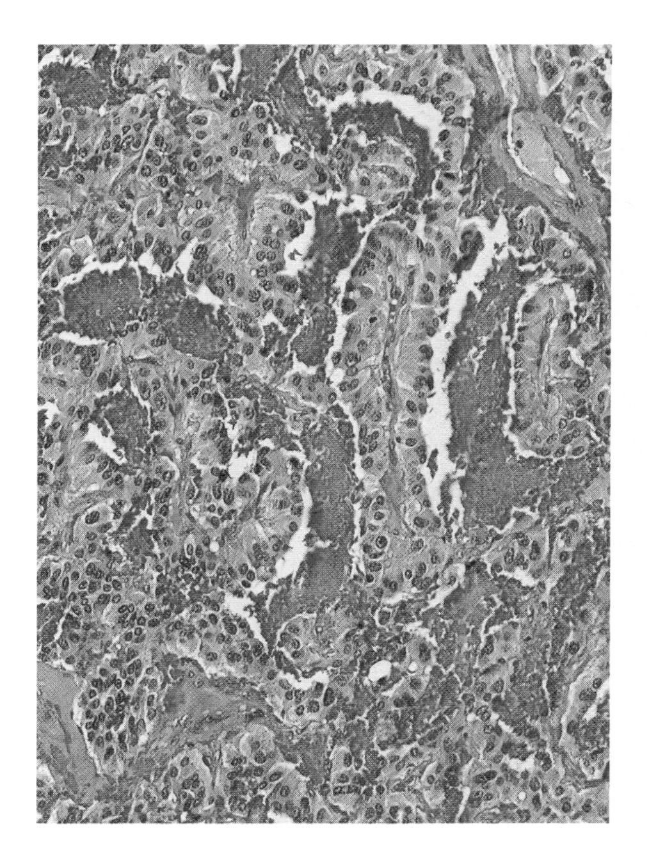

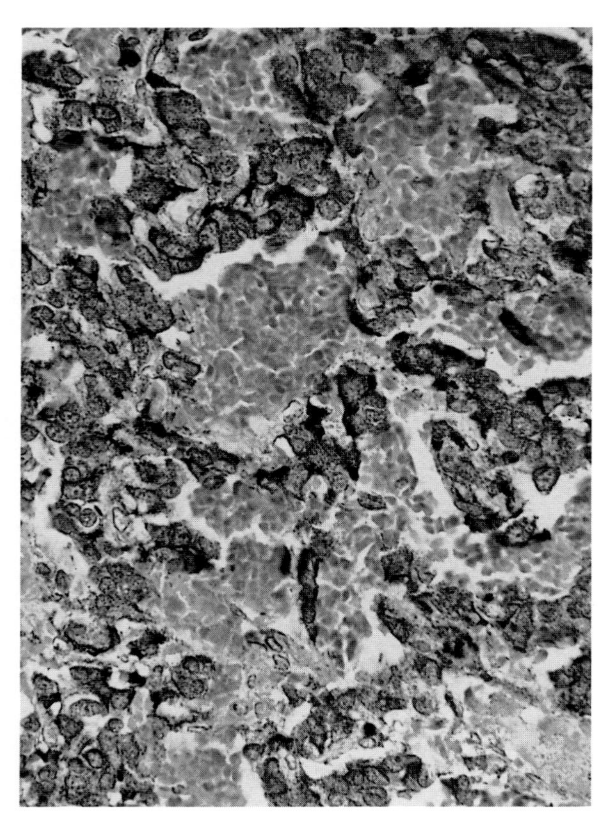

Figure 12-19
INTRATHORACIC PARAVERTEBRAL PARAGANGLIOMA
Left: There is a pseudopapillary pattern, with tumor cells clinging to vascular septa. Hemorrhage separated cell clusters.
Right: Stain for cytoplasmic argyrophilia highlights tumor cells separated by hemorrhage. (X200, Grimelius stain)

CERVICAL PARAVERTEBRAL PARAGANGLIOMAS

These tumors are very rare: in a review by Fries and Chamberlin (62) only five cases were identified. Only a few cases have been reported in the pediatric age group, and these may be associated with pheochromocytomas (60,63). At least two cases have been reported as carotid body type tumors, although anatomic localization supports an origin from the sympathoadrenal neuroendocrine system (61,64). Too few cases have been reported to allow for reliable prognostic assessment (65).

UNUSUAL NEOPLASMS

Gangliocytic Paraganglioma

This rare tumor was first described by Dahl et al. (67) as a duodenal ganglioneuroma. It was considered to be more closely related to a nonchromaffin paraganglioma (72), and was subsequently designated as gangliocytic paraganglioma (68). About 95 percent arise in the second portion of the duodenum (66,69–71), although occasionally in other sites such as jejunum (66, 70) and pylorus (66). The tumor may have areas resembling an endocrine tumor, but on close scrutiny this resemblance is superficial.

Paraganglioma of Cauda Equina

Paragangliomas of the cauda equina region are rare neoplasms which are usually intradural and limited to the filum terminale (73,76–78,80, 82–84); they occasionally involve conus medullaris, caudal nerve roots, and the thoracic region (81). Occasionally the tumor is epidural (73,81,83). Data from the Mayo Clinic (31 cases) show a slight

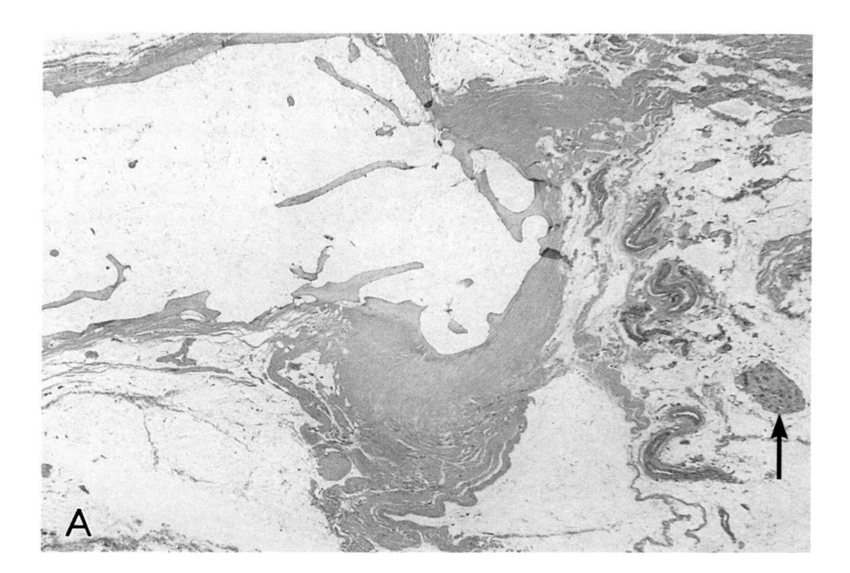

Figure 12-20
NORMAL GLOMUS COCCYGEUM

A: Sagittal section through coccyx from an adult at autopsy shows a glomus coccygeum (arrow) measuring 2 to 3 mm in size.

B: Glomus coccygeum is a well-circumscribed vascular structure with small vessels surrounded by a mantle of epithelioid cells, similar to cutaneous glomera.

C: Glomus coccygeum is not related to paraganglia. This normal anatomic structure near the tip of coccyx should not be confused with a neoplasm.

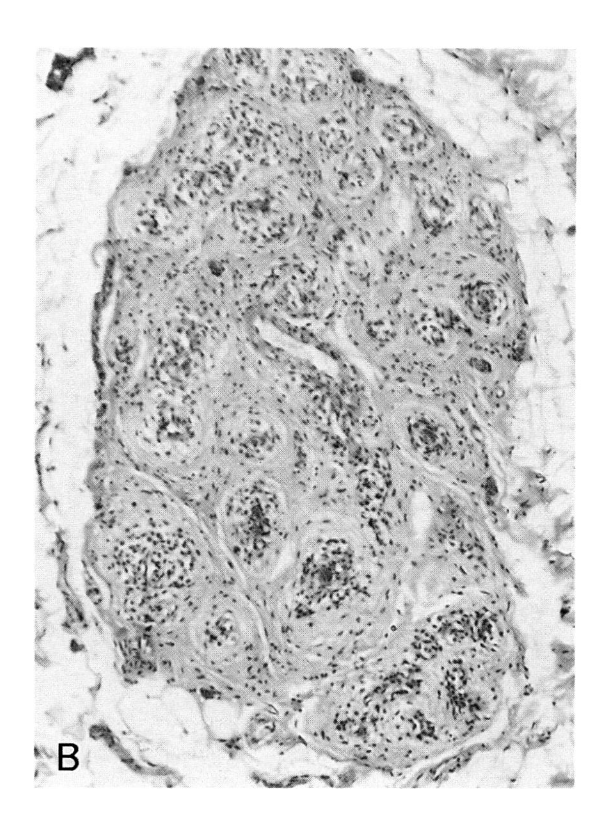

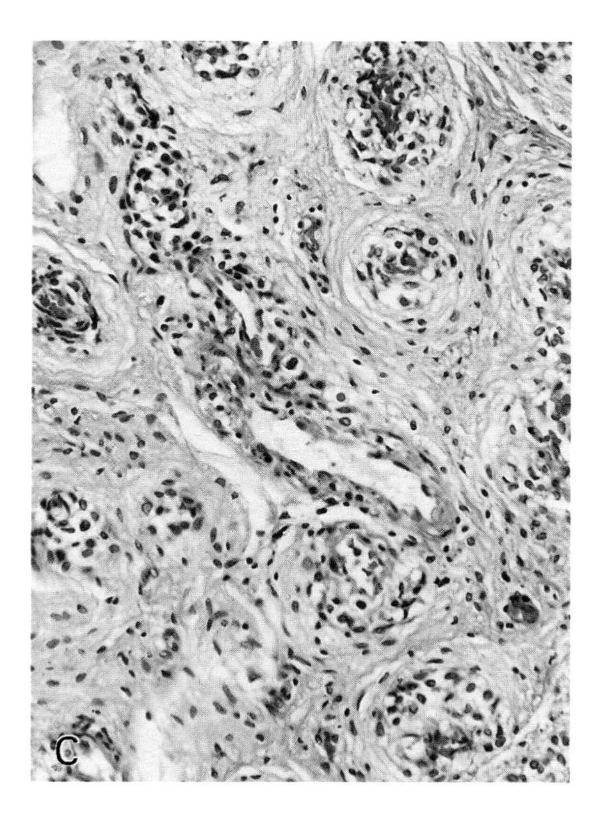

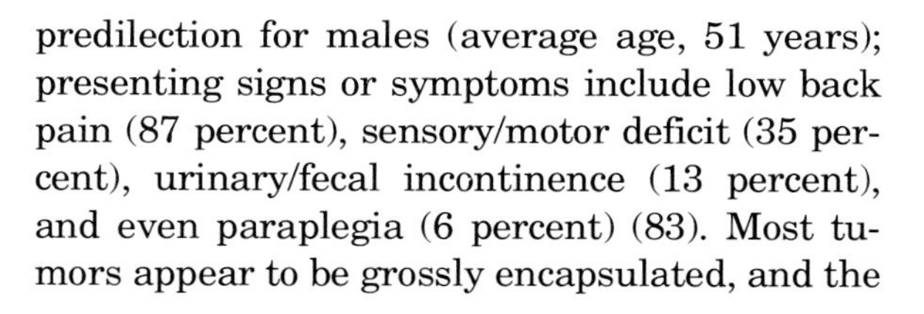

predilection for males (average age, 51 years); presenting signs or symptoms include low back pain (87 percent), sensory/motor deficit (35 percent), urinary/fecal incontinence (13 percent), and even paraplegia (6 percent) (83). Most tumors appear to be grossly encapsulated, and the histologic appearance is reported to resemble that of paragangliomas in other sites (83), although the full range of morphology is probably not known. Occasional cases have been reported with neuronal or ganglion cells (75,79), and ependymal differentiation has been described (74).

GLOMUS COCCYGEUM

The glomus coccygeum, first noted by Luschka (88,89), is a small, ovoid structure located near the tip of the coccyx and measuring only a few millimeters in diameter (fig. 12-20A). It receives its blood supply from the median sacral artery, and is innervated by the pelvic sympathetic plexus. It is composed of nests of epithelioid cells surrounding small vascular channels (fig. 12-20 B,C). The function of this normal anatomic structure is not yet established, and its importance to the pathologist is to know of its existence and not to mistake it for a neoplasm (85–87).

REFERENCES

1. Fries JG, Chamberlin JA. Extra-adrenal pheochromocytoma: literature review and report of a cervical pheochromocytoma. Surgery 1968;63:268–79.
2. Glenner GG, Grimley PM. Tumors of the extra-adrenal paraganglion system (including chemoreceptors). Atlas of Tumor Pathology, 2nd Series, Fascicle 9. Washington, D.C.: Armed Forces Institute of Pathology, 1974.
3. Lack EE. Pathology of adrenal and extra-adrenal paraganglia. Major problems in pathology, Vol 29. Philadelphia: WB Saunders, 1994.
4. Melicow MM. One hundred cases of pheochromocytoma (107 tumors) at the Columbia-Presbyterian Medical Center, 1926-1976: a clinicopathologic analysis. Cancer 1977;40:1987–2004.

Extra-Adrenal Intra-Abdominal Paragangliomas

5. Farhi F, Dikman SH, Lawson W, Cobin RH, Zak FG. Paragangliomatosis associated with multiple endocrine adenomas. Arch Pathol Lab Med 1976;100:495–8.
6. Fries JG, Chamberlin JA. Extra-adrenal pheochromocytoma: literature review and report of a cervical pheochromocytoma. Surgery 1968;63:268–79.
7. Glenn F, Gray GF. Functional tumors of the organ of Zuckerkandl. Ann Surg 1976;183:578–86.
8. Hayes WS, Davidson AJ, Grimley PM, Hartman DS. Extra-adrenal retroperitoneal paraganglioma: clinical, pathologic and CT findings. AJR Am J Roentgenol 1990;155:1247–50.
9. Immergut MA, Boldus R, Köllin CP, Rohlf P. The management of ectopic pheochromocytoma producing ureteral obstruction. J Urol 1970;104:337–41.
10. Karosov RS, Sheps SG, Carney JA, van Heerden JA, DeAuattro V. Paragangliomatosis with numerous catecholamine-producing tumors. Mayo Clin Proc 1982;57:590–5.
11. Keiser HR, Doppman JL, Robertson CN, Linehan WM, Averbuch SD. Diagnosis, localization, and management of pheochromocytoma. In Lack EE, ed. Pathology of the adrenal glands. New York: Churchill Livingstone, 1990:237–55.
12. Kitahara M, Mori T, Seki H, et al. Malignant paraganglioma presenting as Cushing's syndrome with virilism in childhood. Production of cortisol, androgens, and adrenocorticotrophic hormone by the tumor. Cancer 1993;72:3340–5.
13. Kryger-Baggesen N, Kjaergaard J, Sehested M. Nonchromaffin paraganglioma of the retroperitoneum. J Urol 1985;134:536–8.
14. Lack EE. Pathology of adrenal and extra-adrenal paraganglia. Major problems in pathology, Vol 29. Philadelphia: WB Saunders, 1994.
15. Lack EE, Cubilla AL, Woodruff JM, Lieberman PH. Extra-adrenal paragangliomas of the retroperitoneum. A clinicopathologic study of 12 tumors. Am J Surg Pathol 1980;4:109–20.
16. McCarthy EF, Bonfiglio M, Lawton W. A solitary functioning osseous metastasis from a malignant pheochromocytoma of the organ of Zuckerkandl. Cancer 1977;40:3092–6.
17. Medeiros LJ, Wolf BC, Balogh K, Federman M. Adrenal pheochromocytoma: a clinicopathologic review of 60 cases. Hum Pathol 1985;16:580–9.
18. Mundis RJ, Bisel HF, Sheps SG, Sheedy PF II, Gaffey TA, Sterioff S. Malignant nonfunctioning paraganglioma of the retroperitoneum producing renovascular hypertension. Mayo Clin Proc 1982;57:661–4.
19. Olson JR, Abell MR. Nonfunctional nonchromaffin paragangliomas of the retroperitoneum. Cancer 1969;23:1358–67.
20. Samaan NA, Hickey RC. Pheochromocytoma. Semin Oncol 1987;14:297–305.
21. Sclafani LM, Woodruff JM, Brennan MF. Extra-adrenal retroperitoneal paragangliomas: natural history and response to treatment. Surgery 1990;108:1124–30.

Urinary Bladder Paraganglioma

22. Albores-Saavedra J, Maldonado ME, Ibarra J, Rodriguez HA. Pheochromocytoma of the urinary bladder. Cancer 1969;23:1110–8.
23. Burton EM, Schellhammer PF, Weaver DL, Woolfitt RA Paraganglioma of urinary bladder in patient with neurofibromatosis. Urology 1986;27:550–2.
24. Davaris P, Petraki K, Arvanitis D, Papacharalammpous N, Morakis A, Zorzos, S. Urinary bladder paraganglioma (U.B.P.). Path Res Pract 1986;181:101–5.
25. DeKlerk DP, Catalona WJ, Nime FA, Freeman C. Malignant pheochromocytoma of the bladder: the late development of renal cell carcinoma. J Urol 1975; 113:864–8.

26. Jurascheck F, Egloff H, Buemi A, Laedlein-Greilsammer D. Paraganglioma of urinary bladder. Urology 1983;22:659–63.
27. Lack EE. Pathology of adrenal and extra-adrenal paraganglia. Major problems in pathology, Vol 29. Philadelphia: WB Saunders, 1994.
28. Leestma JE, Price EB Jr. Paraganglioma of the urinary bladder. Cancer 1971;28:1063–72.
29. Lieberman PH. Consultation case—paraganglioma in the neck of the bladder. Am J Surg Pathol 1977;1:83–4.
30. Lotz PR, Bogdasarian RS, Thompson NW, Seeger JF, Cho KJ. Paragangliomas of the head, neck, urinary bladder, and pelvis in a hypertensive woman. AJR Am J Roentgenol 1979;132:1001–4.
31. Scott WW, Eversole SL. Pheochromocytoma of the urinary bladder. J Urol 1960;83:656–64.
32. Spring DB, Palubinskas AJ. Familial pheochromocytoma: a rare case of hydronephrosis and hydroureter in two generations. Br J Radiol 1977;50:596–9.

Unusual Sites of Paragangliomas

33. Alcini E, Destito A, De Giovanni L, D'Addessi A, Wiel Marin A. Un raro caso di paraganglioma renale min. Minerva Urol 1981;33:191–4.
34. Altavilla G, Cavazzini L, Russo R. Secreting benign paraganglioma of the prostatic urethra. Tumori 1983;69:79–82.
35. Badalament RA, Kenworthy P, Pellegrini A, Drago JR. Paraganglioma of urethra. Urology 1991;38:76–8.
36. Bryant KR, Thompson IM, Ortiz R, Spence CR. Urethral paraganglioma presenting as a urethral polyp. J Urol 1983;130:571–2.
37. Cholhan HJ, Cagler H, Kremzier JE. Suburethral paraganglioma. Obstet Gynecol 1991;78:555–8.
38. Craig JR, Peters RL, Edmondson HA. Tumors of the liver and intrahepatic bile ducts. Atlas of Tumor Pathology, 2nd Series, Fascicle 26. Washington, D.C.: Armed Forces Institute of Pathology, 1989.
39. Dembitzer F, Greenebaum E. Fine needle aspiration of renal paraganglioma: an unusual location for a rare tumor [Abstract]. Mod Pathol 1993;6:29A(149).
40. Dennis PJ, Lewandowski AE, Rohner TJ Jr, Weidner WA, Mamourian AC, Stern DR. Pheochromocytoma of the prostate: an unusual location. J Urol 1989;141:130–2.
41. Dharkar D, Kraft JR. Paraganglioma of the spermatic cord. An incidental finding. J Urol Pathol 1994;2:89–93.
42. Fine G, Raju UB. Paraganglia in the human gallbladder. Arch Pathol Lab Med 1980;104:265–8.
43. Freschi M, Sassi I. Paraganglioma della colecisti. Pathologica 1990;82:459–63.
44. Kuo T, Anderson CB, Rosai J. Normal paraganglia in the human gallbladder. Arch Pathol 1974;97:46–7.
45. Lack EE. Pathology of adrenal and extra-adrenal paraganglia. Major problems in pathology, Vol 29. Philadelphia: WB Saunders, 1994.
46. Lagace R, Tremblay M. Non-chromaffin paraganglioma of the kidney with distant metastases. Can Med Assoc J 1968;99:1095–8.
47. Mehta M, Nadel NS, Lonni Y, Ali I. Malignant paraganglioma of the prostate and retroperitoneum. J Urol 1979;121:376–8.
48. Miller TA, Weber TR, Appelman HD. Paraganglioma of the gallbladder. Arch Surg 1972;105:637–9.
49. Nielsen VM, Skovgaard N, Kvist N. Pheochromocytoma of the prostate. Br J Urol 1987;59:478–9.
50. Ostrowski ML, Wheeler TM. Paraganglia of the prostate. Location, frequency, and differentiation from prostatic adenocarcinoma. Am J Surg Pathol 1994;18:412–20.
51. Pengelly CD. Pheochromocytoma within the renal capsule. Br Med J 1959;2:477–8.
52. Raju UB, Fine G. Ultrastructure of the gallbladder paraganglia. Arch Pathol Lab Med 1980;104:379–83.
53. Rode J, Bentley A, Parkinson C. Paraganglial cells of urinary bladder and prostate: potential diagnostic problem. J Clin Pathol 1990;43:13–6.
54. Wolff M. Paraganglioma of the gallbladder. Arch Surg 1973;107:493.

Intrathoracic Paravertebral Paraganglioma

55. Gallivan MV, Chun B, Rowden G, Lack EE. Intrathoracic paravertebral malignant paraganglioma. Arch Pathol Lab Med 1980;104:46–51.
56. Hodgkinson DJ, Telander RL, Sheps SG, Gilchrist GS, Crowe JK. Extra-adrenal intrathoracic functioning paraganglioma (pheochromocytoma) in childhood. Mayo Clin Proc 1980;55:271–76.
57. Lack EE. Pathology of adrenal and extra-adrenal paraganglia. Major problems in pathology, Vol 29. Philadelphia: WB Saunders, 1994.
58. Odze R, Bégin LR. Malignant paraganglioma of the posterior mediastinum. A case report and review of the literature. Cancer 1990;65:564–9.
59. Smalley JJ, Gallagher WB, Nichols CP. Paraganglioma simulating primary rib tumor. Arch Surg 1977;112:323–5.

Cervical Paravertebral Paraganglioma

60. Cone TE Jr. Recurrent pheochromocytoma: report of a case in a previously treated child. Pediatrics 1958;21:994–9.
61. Crowell WT, Grizzle WE, Siegel AL. Functional carotid paragangliomas. Biochemical, ultrastructural and histochemical correlation with clinical symptoms. Arch Pathol Lab Med 1982;106:599–603.
62. Fries JG, Chamberlin JA. Extra-adrenal pheochromocytoma: literature review and report of a cervical pheochromocytoma. Surgery 1968;63:268–79.
63. Gibbs MK, Carney JA, Hayles AB, Telander RL. Simultaneous adrenal and cervical pheochromocytomas in childhood. Ann Surg 1977;185:273–8.
64. Glenner GG, Crout JR, Roberts WC. A functional carotid-body-like tumor secreting levarterenol. Arch Pathol 1962;73:230–40.
65. Lack EE. Pathology of adrenal and extra-adrenal paraganglia. Major problems in pathology, Vol 29. Philadelphia: WB Saunders, 1994.

Gangliocytic Paraganglioma

66. Burke AP, Helwig EB. Gangliocytic paraganglioma. Am J Clin Pathol 1989;92:1–9.
67. Dahl EV, Waugh JM, Dahlin DC. Gastrointestinal ganglioneuromas. Brief review with report of a duodenal ganglioneuroma. Am J Pathol 1957;33:953–65.
68. Kepes JJ, Zacharias DL. Gangliocytic paragangliomas of the duodenum. A report of two cases with light and electron microscopic examination. Cancer 1971;27:61–70.
69. Perrone T, Sibley RK, Rosai J. Duodenal gangliocytic paraganglioma. An immunohistochemical and ultrastructural study with a hypothesis concerning its origin. Am J Surg Pathol 1985;9:31–41.
70. Reed RJ, Daroca PJ Jr, Harkin JC. Gangliocytic paraganglioma. Am J Surg Pathol 1977;1:207–16.
71. Scheithauer BW, Nora FE, Lechago J, et al. Duodenal gangliocytic paraganglioma. Clinicopathologic and immunocytochemical study of 11 cases. Am J Clin Pathol 1986;86:559–65.
72. Taylor HB, Helwig EB. Benign nonchromaffin paragangliomas of the duodenum. Virchow Arch [A] 1962;335:356–66.

Paraganglioma of Cauda Equina

73. Böker DK, Wassmann H, Solymosi L. Paragangliomas of the spinal canal. Surg Neurol 1983;19:461–8.
74. Caccamo DV, Ho KL, Garcia JH. Canda equina tumor with ependymal and paraganglionic differentiation. Hum Pathol 1992;23:835–8.
75. Djindjian M, Ayache P, Brugières P, Malpert D, Baudrimont M, Poirier J. Giant gangliocytic paraganglioma of the filum terminale. Case report. J Neurosurg 1990;73:459–61.
76. Hirose T, Sana T, Mori K, et al. Paraganglioma of the cauda equina: an ultrastructural and immunohistochemical study of two cases. Ultrastruct Pathol 1988;12:235–43.
77. Horoupian DS, Kerson LA, Saiontz H, Valsamis M. Paraganglioma of cauda equina. Clinicopathologic and ultrastructural studies of an unusual case. Cancer 1974;33:1337–48.
78. Kamalian N, Abbassioun K, Amirjamshidt A, Shams-Shahrabadi M. Paraganglioma of the filum terminale internum. Report of a case and review of the literature. J Neurol 1987;235:56–9.
79. Llena JF, Wisoff HS, Hirano A. Gangliocytic paraganglioma in canda equina region, with biochemical and neuropathological studies. Case report. J Neurosurg 1982;56:280–2.
80. Raftopoulos C, Flament-Durand J, Brucher JM, Stroobandt G, Chaskis C, Brotchi J. Paraganglioma of the cauda equina. Report of 2 cases and review of 59 cases from the literature. Clin Neurol Neurosurg 1990;92–3:263–70.
81. Shuangshoti S, Suwanwela N, Suwanwela C. Combined paraganglioma and glioma of conus medullaris and cauda equina. J Surg Oncol 1984;25:162–7.
82. Soffer DO, Pittaluga S, Caine Y, Feinsod M. Paraganglioma of cauda equina. A report of a case and review of the literature. Cancer 1983;51:1907–10.
83. Sonneland PR, Scheithauer BW, Lechago J, Crawford BG, Onofrio BM. Paraganglioma of the cauda equina region. Clinicopathologic study of 31 cases with special reference to immunocytology and ultrastructure. Cancer 1986;58:1720–35.
84. Taxy JB. Paraganglioma of the cauda equina. Report of a rare tumor. Cancer 1983;51:1904–6.

Glomus Coccygeum

85. Albrecht S, Zbieranowski I. Incidental glomus coccygeum. When a normal structure looks like a tumor. Am J Surg Pathol 1990;14:922–4.
86. Bell RS, Goodman SD, Fornasier VL. Coccygeal glomus tumors: a case of mistaken identity? J Bone Joint Surg 1982;64A:595–7.
87. Duncan L, Halverson J, DeSchryver-Kecskemeti K. Glomus tumor of the coccyx. A curable cause of coccydynia. Arch Pathol Lab Med 1991;115:78–80.
88. Luschka H. Die steissdrüse des menschen. Arch Pathol Anat 1860;18:106–15.
89. Luschka H. Ueber die drüsenartige natur des sogen annten ganglion intercaroticum. Arch Anat, Physiol, u Wissensch Med Jahrg 1862:405–14.

13
ULTRASTRUCTURAL AND OTHER FEATURES OF SYMPATHOADRENAL PARAGANGLIOMAS

Ultrastructural Findings. Examination of 1-μm sections from sympathoadrenal paragangliomas may reveal cells with different cytoplasmic staining characteristics; there may be a "light" and "dark" cell population as well as some variation in number and distribution of dense-core secretory granules (fig. 13-1). Pseudoacini, intracytoplasmic rounded vacuolar spaces of various size, may be numerous. Ultrastructural views of sympathoadrenal paragangliomas may show complex interdigitation of cytoplasmic processes (fig. 13-2). Endothelial cells and pericytes can be found and, occasionally, cells consistent with sustentacular cells; identification of the latter cell population is most readily done by immunostaining for S-100 protein.

The nuclei of paraganglioma cells are round to ovoid, often with some margination of chromatin against the nuclear membrane. The nucleolus may be prominent, depending upon the plane of section. The nuclei of some cells show nuclear folds with deep irregular extension or intrusion

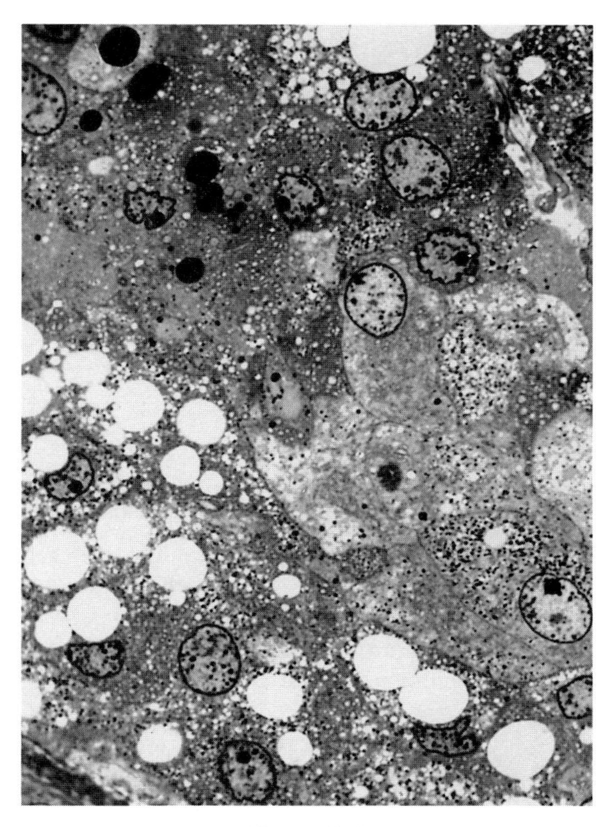

Figure 13-1
PHEOCHROMOCYTOMA

Pheochromocytoma with a variation in overall density of cytoplasm, with "light" and "dark" cells. Most of the dark granules represent neurosecretory granules. Prominent intracytoplasmic vacuoles (pseudoacini, see figure 13-8) are seen. (X1,000, Toluidine blue stain)

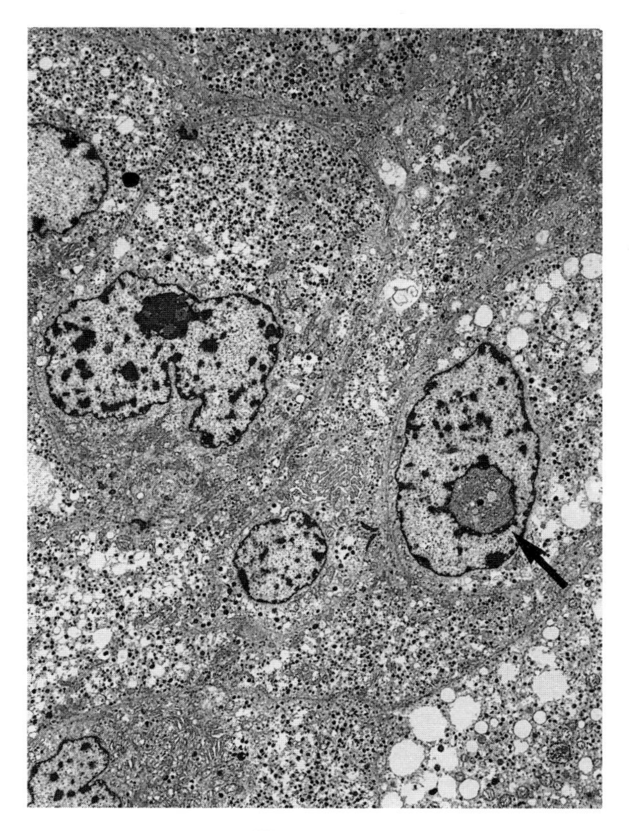

Figure 13-2
PHEOCHROMOCYTOMA

Some tumor cells have complex intertwining of cell processes. The dense-core neurosecretory granules vary in density. The nucleus on the left has an irregular contour while the nucleus on the right has small nuclear pseudoinclusion (arrow). (X2,500)

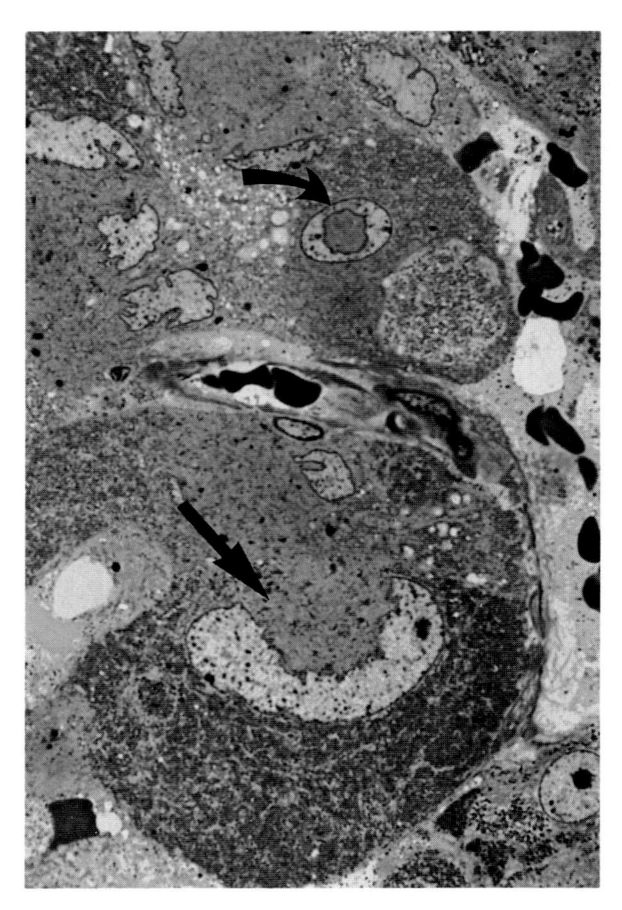

Figure 13-3
PHEOCHROMOCYTOMA
This 1-μm thick section of pheochromocytoma shows a deeply notched nucleus at the bottom (straight arrows) and nuclear pseudoinclusion at the top (curved arrow). (X1,000, Toluidine blue stain)

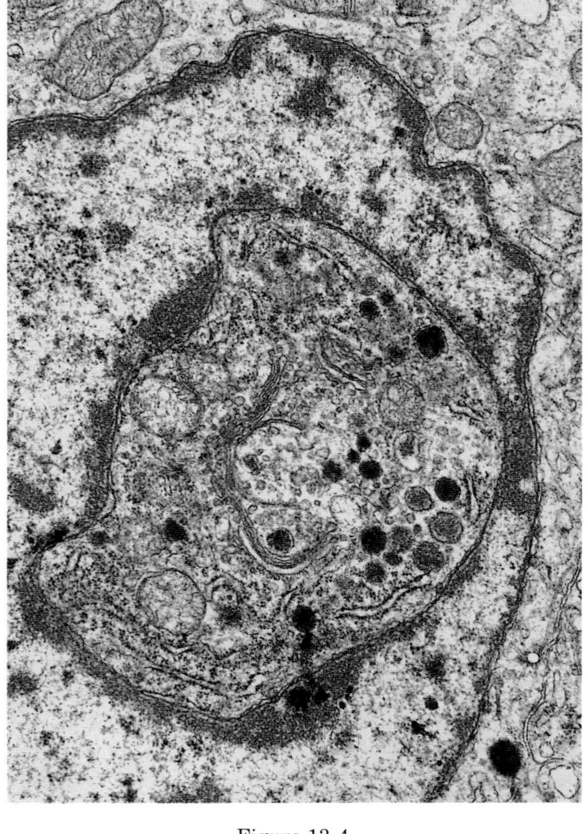

Figure 13-4
PHEOCHROMOCYTOMA
There are sparse numbers of dense-core neurosecretory granules, with increased density of organelles in the nuclear pseudoinclusion including rough endoplasmic reticulum and Golgi complex. (X42,000).

of cell cytoplasm forming a nuclear pseudoinclusion (3). A nuclear pseudoinclusion is viewed in profile in figure 13-3, and en face in figure 13-2 where it is surrounded by a continuous nuclear membrane. The density of cellular organelles within the intranuclear extension of cytoplasm may vary and result in differences in staining, and there may be empty spaces at the light microscopic level which ultrastructurally represent dilated cisternae of endoplasmic reticulum or nonspecific vacuolar change.

There may be a variation in density of cellular organelles from cell to cell or within a single cell (19). There are usually scattered profiles of rough endoplasmic reticulum, and there may be occasional lipofuscin. Intercellular junctions are sparse and simple in configuration. There are no true desmosomal attachments with insertion of intermediate filaments. The hallmark of these paragangliomas is the presence of dense-core neurosecretory granules (fig. 13-4), but when sparse they may be difficult to distinguish from small primary lysosomes. Often, the dense-core secretory granules vary in morphology (fig. 13-5). Tannenbaum (17) correlated the ultrastructural morphology of dense-core neurosecretory granules in 14 pheochromocytomas with norepinephrine and epinephrine content. In the tumors that contained predominantly epinephrine, the neurosecretory granules were of uniform type while

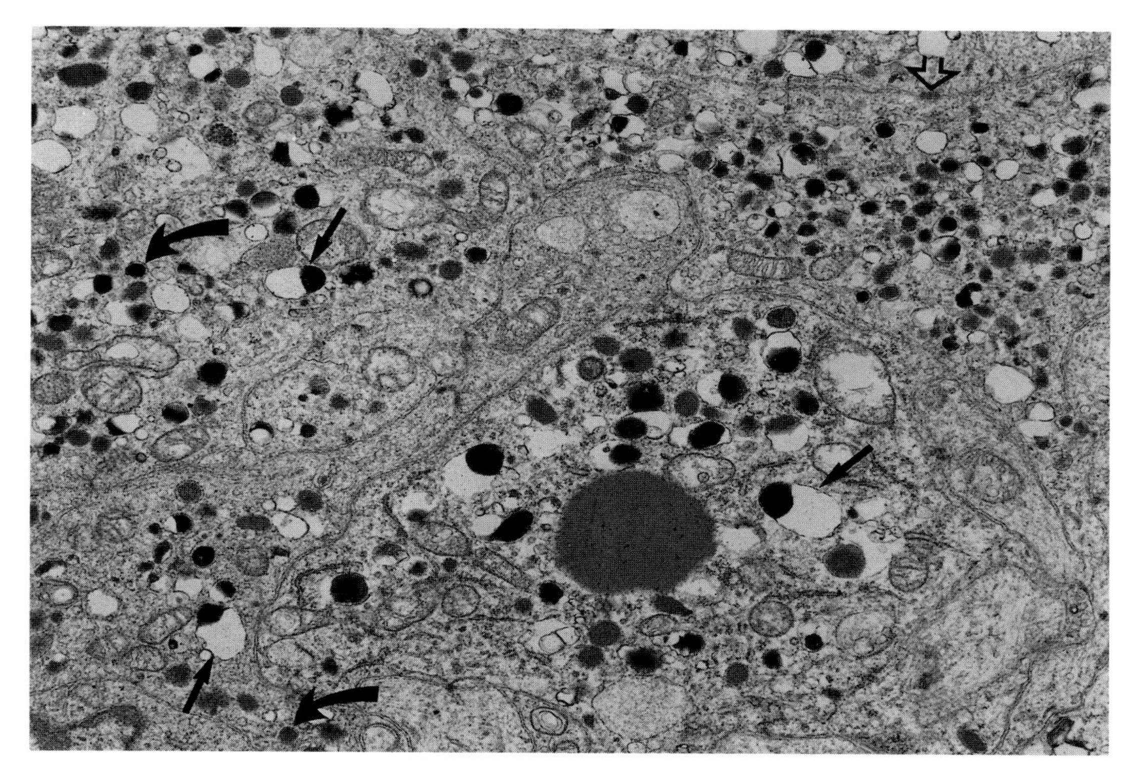

Figure 13-5
PHEOCHROMOCYTOMA
There is a range in morphology of dense-core neurosecretory granules. Some have an eccentric halo ("norepinephrine-type" granules, straight arrows) while others are more uniform ("epinephrine-type" granules, curved arrows). Note also the few profiles of rough endoplasmic reticulum as well as the simple cell junction (upper right, open arrow). (X18,000)

in the norepinephrine-containing tumors, they had a distinctive and entirely different appearance, with a prominent eccentric electron-lucent space (or halo) adjacent to the electron-dense core. Granule morphology can vary, however, and correlation with content of any particular hormone or neuropeptide is not reliable. Some granules may be found in close association with a Golgi complex (fig. 13-6); occasionally, intact neurosecretory granules with an investing membrane have been observed outside the cytoplasm of tumor cells, even within the vascular lumen (8,11,17), but given the normal sequence of events in fusion and exocytosis of dense-core granules this may be an artifact (11).

In one study, homogenates of normal adrenal medulla revealed an epinephrine level of 4.05 mg/g and norepinephrine level of 0.70 mg/g; ultrastructurally, 95 percent of neurosecretory granules were "epinephrine type" and 5 percent "norepinephrine type," a ratio of 20 to 1, which is very different from most pheochromocytomas (17). There also appears to be a correlation between the concentration of catecholamines and the density of neurosecretory granules (1). The average diameter varies from about 127 to 270 nm (17). An ultrastructural study reported 20 of 27 pheochromocytomas had a predominance of neurosecretory granules of type 1 morphology (typical of norepinephrine), while 20 of 23 extra-adrenal paragangliomas had granules with type 2 morphology (typical of epinephrine type); on the basis of the differences in granule morphology the pheochromocytomas were not considered synonymous with extra-adrenal paragangliomas (5).

Biochemical analysis has shown that extra-adrenal paragangliomas contain predominantly norepinephrine. A recent immunohistochemical study showed that 6 of 10 pheochromocytomas were positive for phenylethanolamine N-methyl

Table 13-1

IMMUNOHISTOCHEMICAL EXPRESSION OF NEURON-SPECIFIC ENOLASE AND 10 NEUROPEPTIDES IN 99 SYMPATHOADRENAL PARAGANGLIOMAS*

	Percent Positive
Neuron-specific enolase	100
[Leu^5]-enkephalin	76
[Met^5]-enkephalin	75
Somatostatin	67
Bovine pancreatic polypeptide	51
Vasoactive intestinal peptide	43
Substance P	31
ACTH	28
Calcitonin	23
Bombesin	15
Neurotensin	12

*From Linnoila RI, et al. Hum Pathol 1988;19:41–50.

Immunohistochemical Findings. *Neuroendocrine Markers and S-100 Protein Immunoreactivity.* A wide variety of regulatory peptides and hormones can be localized immunohistochemically in pheochromocytomas and extra-adrenal paragangliomas (Table 13-1) (23,25). All 99 sympathoadrenal paragangliomas studied at the National Cancer Institute (NCI) (25) were positive for neuron-specific enolase (NSE) (fig. 13-9, left), but similar immunoreactivity can be found in a large variety of other tumors. Staining for NSE and other neuroendocrine markers can also be seen in nuclear pseudoinclusions (fig. 13-9, right). Chromogranin A is a member of a family of acidic secretory proteins found in the matrix of dense-core granules; related proteins include chromogranin B and secretogranin II (21). Chromogranin A constitutes a large component of the soluble protein in secretory vesicles (31), and is a very good marker for neuroendocrine tumors such as sympathoadrenal paragangliomas (fig. 13-10). Chromogranin B and secretogranin II are additional markers for neuroendocrine neoplasms (27). Another useful marker is synaptophysin, an integral membrane glycoprotein of secretory vesicles (fig. 13-11);

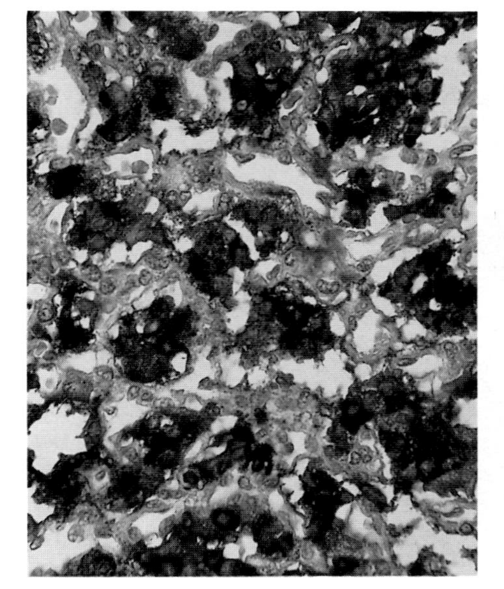

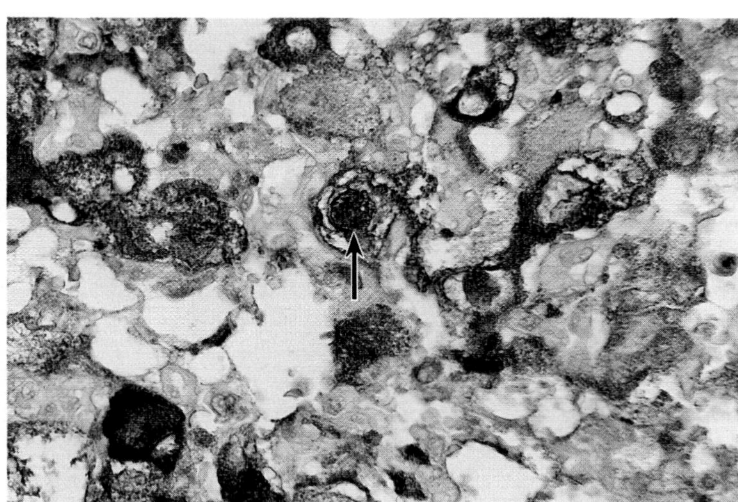

Figure 13-9

EXTRA-ADRENAL PARAGANGLIOMA OF ABDOMEN

Left: Extra-adrenal intra-abdominal paraganglioma probably arising from remnant(s) of organs of Zuckerkandl. The tumor showed diffuse, strong immunostaining for neuron-specific enolase. (X220, Peroxidase-antiperoxidase stain)

Right: Nuclear pseudoinclusion stains positively for neuron-specific enolase (arrow). (X400, Peroxidase-antiperoxidase stain)

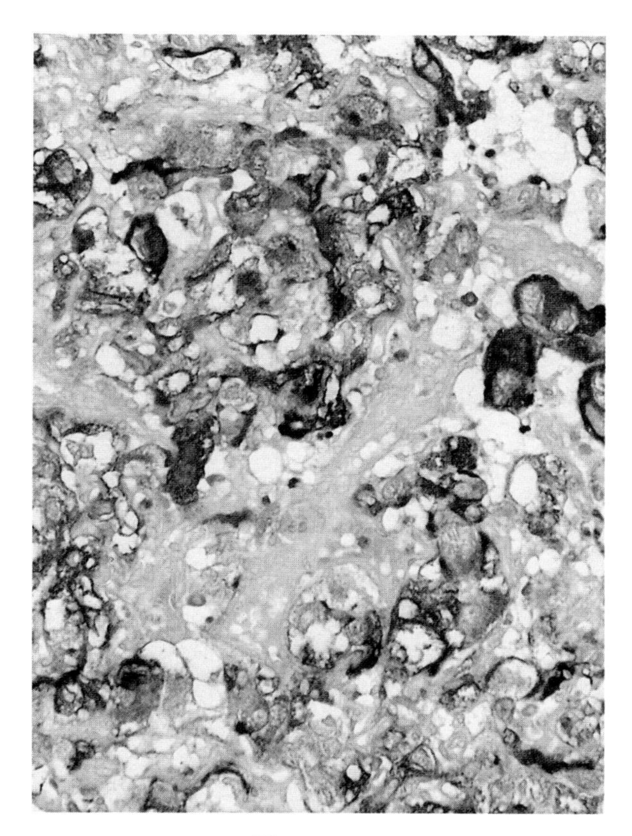

Figure 13-10
COMPOSITE PHEOCHROMOCYTOMA
Composite pheochromocytoma showing strong immunopositivity for chromogranin A. (X220, Peroxidase-antiperoxidase stain)

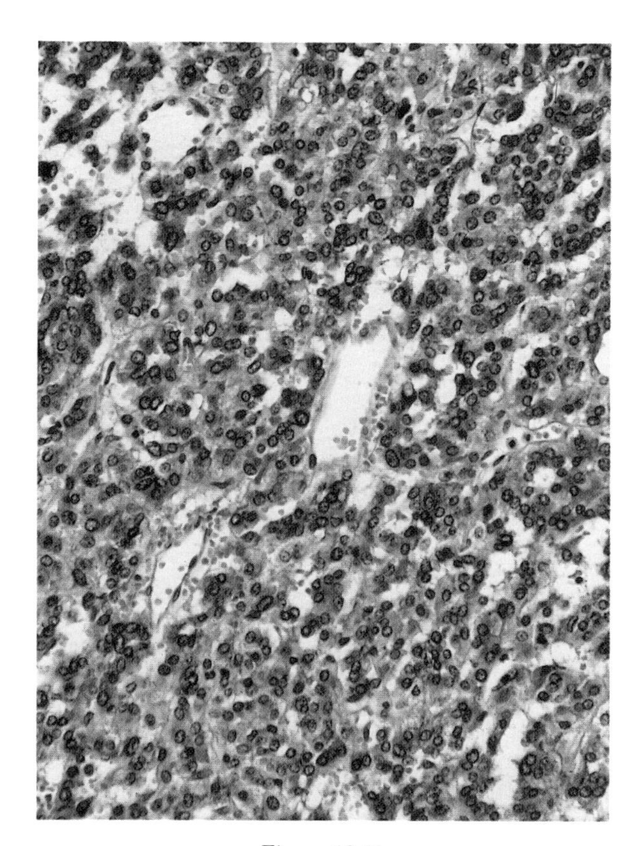

Figure 13-11
PHEOCHROMOCYTOMA
Extra-adrenal intra-abdominal paraganglioma shows positive immunostaining for synaptophysin. (X200, Peroxidase-antiperoxidase stain)

however, adrenal cortical neoplasms, both benign and malignant, can be immunoreactive (26,28) which may be a source of confusion and even lead to misdiagnosis (see fig. 5-30). The antilymphocyte antibody Leu-7 (HNK-1) (30), protein gene product (PGP) 9.5 (22,29), and cytochrome b561 (24) also have been used as neuroendocrine markers. Immunoreactivity for Leu-enkephalin has been reported in about 50 percent (20) to 75 percent (25) of pheochromocytomas and extra-adrenal paragangliomas. The most sensitive method for identifying sustentacular cells is by immunostaining for S-100 protein, a protein that decorates the nucleus and cytoplasm of elongate, stellate, or dendritic cells at the periphery of cords and clusters of tumor cells (fig. 13-12).

Associated Endocrine Syndromes and Other Features. Aside from these neuroendocrine markers, sympathoadrenal paragangliomas are capable of expressing a broad array of neuropeptides and hormones (Table 13-1). Immunostaining for [Leu^5]-enkephalin and [Met^5]-enkephalin was seen in three fourths of tumors studied at the NCI (fig. 13-13) (43). In one study, diffuse adrenal medullary hyperplasia consistently showed Leu-enkephalin–like immunoreactivity, whereas 50 percent of hyperplastic nodules, pheochromocytomas, and extra-adrenal paragangliomas were positive (33). Usually, however, there is no endocrine syndrome or other manifestation ascribed to any particular neuropeptide or hormone with the exception of catecholamines (41,42). In the study at the NCI, 28 percent of sympathoadrenal paragangliomas immunostained for ACTH; however, pheochromocytomas have rarely been the cause of Cushing's syndrome due to ectopic ACTH production (32, 35,37,46,48,51,54). Cushing's syndrome due to

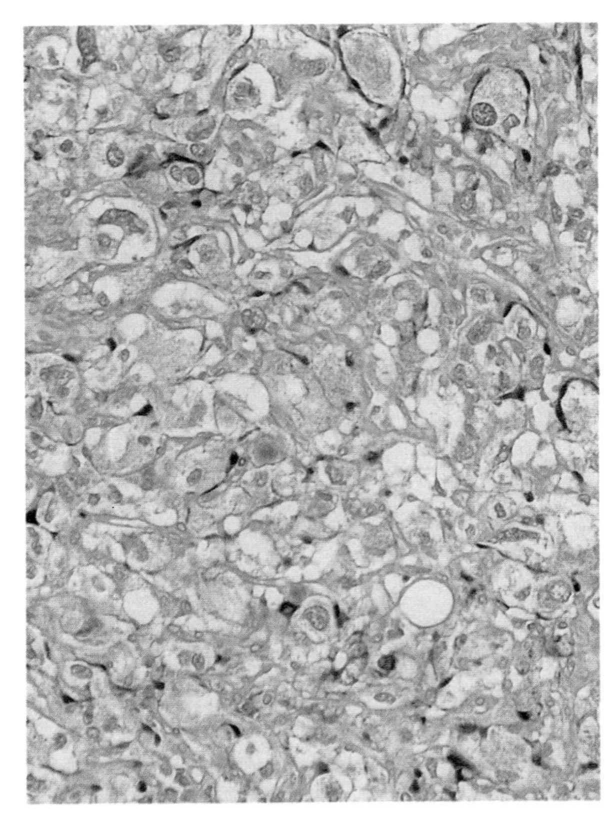

Figure 13-12
PHEOCHROMOCYTOMA
Stain for S-100 protein stain is positive in both nuclei and cytoplasm of stellate to dendritic sustentacular cells which are located at the edge of cords and clusters of neoplastic chromaffin cells. (X200, Peroxidase-antiperoxidase stain)

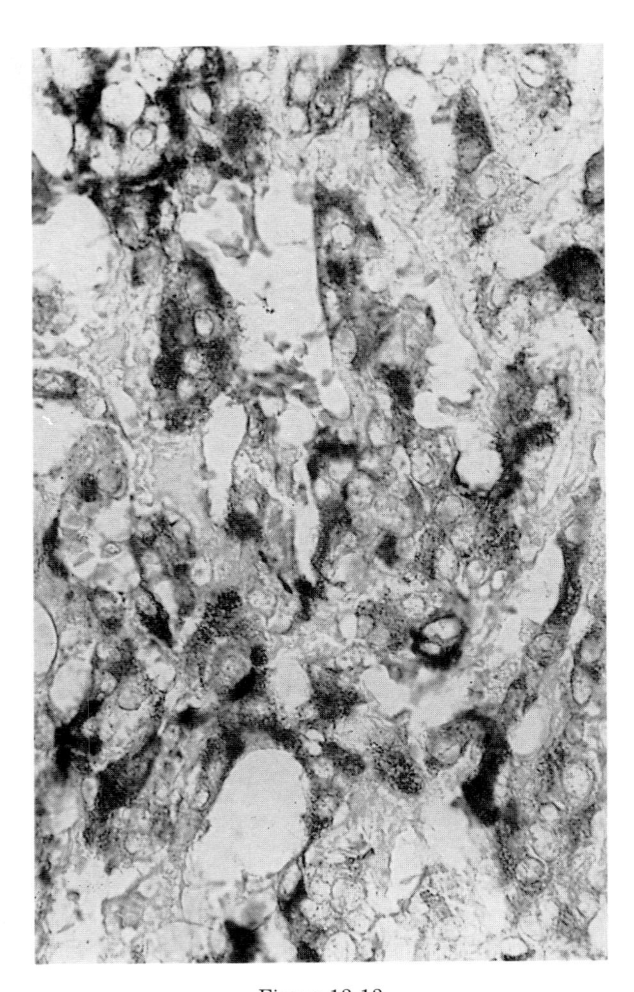

Figure 13-13
PHEOCHROMOCYTOMA
Pheochromocytoma showing positive immunostain for met-enkephalin. (X350, Peroxidase-antiperoxidase stain)

ectopic production of corticotropin-releasing factor by a pheochromocytoma has been reported (40). ACTH-like immunoreactivity has also been observed in the normal adrenal medulla (43,44). A review of endocrinologic data associated with ectopic ACTH production by pheochromocytomas indicated that indices of steroid production were markedly elevated in the presence of only modest plasma levels of ACTH, which might be explained by the close proximity of the pheochromocytoma to adrenal cortical sites of ACTH stimulation (37). Evaluation of a patient with Cushing's syndrome and an adrenal mass should include the possibility of an ACTH-producing pheochromocytoma (42).

A watery diarrhea syndrome, also referred to as the Verner-Morrison syndrome (58) or WDHA (watery diarrhea, hypokalemia, achlorhydria) syndrome, has been reported in association with pheochromocytoma (34,45,49) and composite pheochromocytoma (47,57), and has been attributed to release of vasoactive intestinal peptide (VIP). In the study at the NCI, 43 percent of sympathoadrenal paragangliomas stained for VIP, yet none of the patients had the watery diarrhea syndrome; few if any of the tumors showed any ganglionic or neuronal features (41, 43). Conversely, a number of tumors do show neuronal or ganglionic features as well as immunoreactivity for VIP, yet there is no associated diarrheal syndrome (fig. 13-14). Hypercalcemia has also been reported in association with pheochromocytoma (36,38,52,53,55,59), and in some

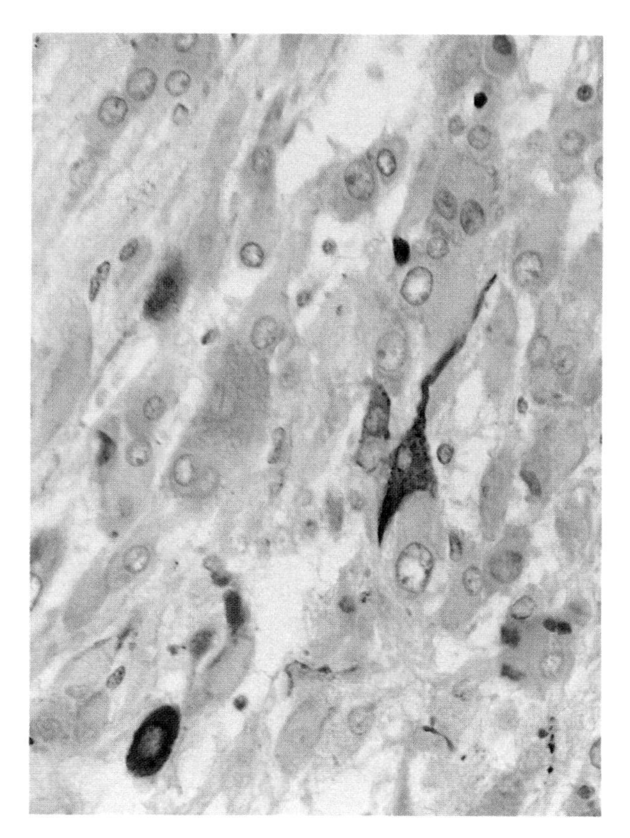

Figure 13-14
COMPOSITE PHEOCHROMOCYTOMA
Some tumor cells with neural features show intense immunoreactivity for vasoactive intestinal peptide. Areas elsewhere in the tumor resembled ganglioneuroblastoma. (X350, Peroxidase-antiperoxidase stain)

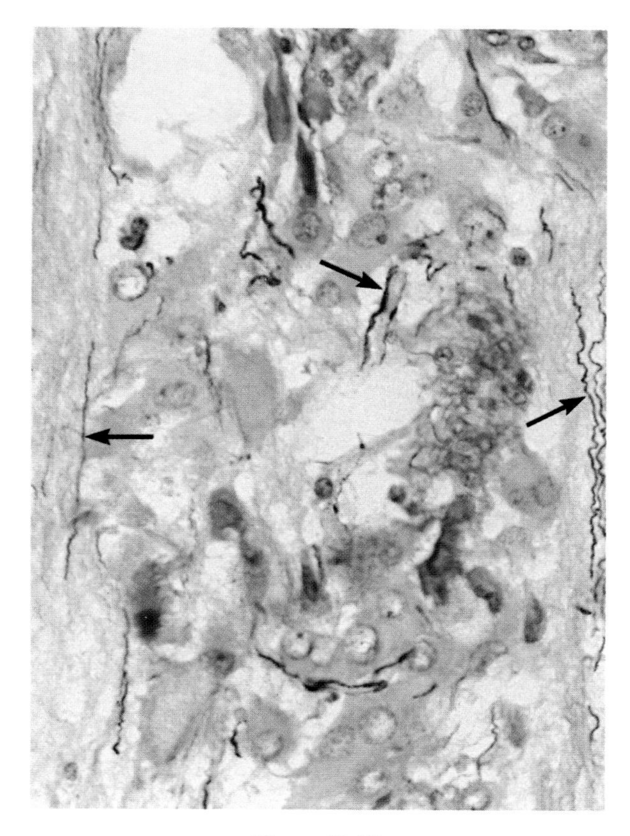

Figure 13-15
COMPOSITE PHEOCHROMOCYTOMA
Positive immunostaining for neurofilament protein is seen mainly in small neuritic processes (arrows); other areas resembled ganglioneuroblastoma. (X350, Peroxidase-antiperoxidase stain)

cases was attributed to production of a parathormone-like substance (53,55) or calcitonin (38, 59). Other unusual features associated with pheochromocytoma include polycythemia due to erythropoietin production (60), diarrhea, and steatorrhea (39) possibly due in one case to somatostatin production (56). Secretion of growth hormone-releasing factor has also been described (50).

Other Immunoreactive Substances. Other immunoreactive substances which have been reported in pheochromocytoma (or adrenal medulla) include galanin (61,69), renin (63), atrial natriuretic polypeptide (65), angiotensin-converting enzyme (67), insulin-like growth factor (64), and epidermal growth factor receptors (66). Positive immunostaining for J1-beta-tubulin, microtubule-associated protein 2 (MAP-2) (62), and neural cell adhesion molecule (N-CAM) has been reported (68). Pheochromocytoma joins the slowly growing number of tumors, in addition to malignant melanoma, that may be immunoreactive for HMB-45 (70).

Intermediate Filament Profile. Neurofilament (NF) proteins have been demonstrated in a high proportion of sympathoadrenal paragangliomas (fig. 13-15) (73,75–80). In the normal adrenal medulla, positive immunostaining for NF proteins has been localized in nerve axons, some ganglion cells, and chromaffin cells (80). In general, immunostaining for vimentin is usually restricted to vascular and connective tissue structures, but staining may be more widespread (71). Vimentin positivity has been reported in pheochromocytoma (73,75). Staining for cytokeratin has also been reported in pheochromocytoma (75), and similar staining has been observed in occasional

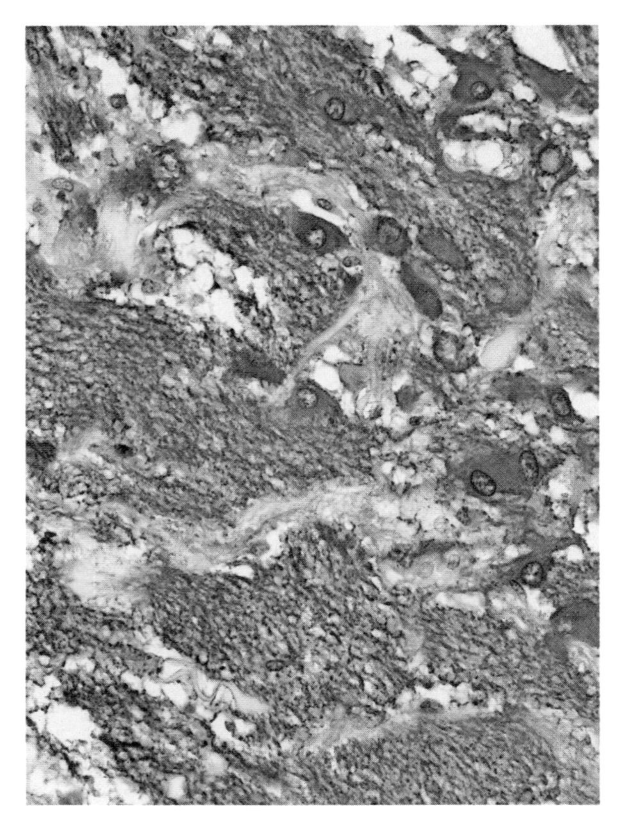

Figure 13-16
COMPOSITE PHEOCHROMOCYTOMA
Composite pheochromocytoma with dense mats of fibrillary matrix resembling neuropil. Scattered tumor cells as well as fibrillary matrix are strongly positive for neuron specific enolase (NSE). (X200, Peroxidase-antiperoxidase stain)

paragangliomas of the head and neck region using monoclonal antibodies AE1/AE3 and CAM 5.2 (74). The rat pheochromocytoma cell line (PC12) expresses markers for cytokeratin (72), and these cells, as well as tumor cells of human sympathoadrenal paraganglioma, appear capable of coexpressing both epithelial and neuronal immunomarkers. Globules in some pheochromocytomas have been positive for vimentin and glial fibrillary acidic protein (GFAP), and occasional staining has been demonstrated in cells of pheochromocytoma (73) or composite pheochromocytoma, where in addition the neurofibrillary matrix is positive for NSE (fig. 13-16).

Relation of Immunohistochemistry to Prognosis of Sympathoadrenal Paragangliomas. Some investigators report a paucity or absence of S-100 protein–positive (sustentacular) cells in clinically aggressive or metastasizing pheochromocytomas and extra-adrenal paragangliomas (81, 84,85,89,90); a recent study confirmed that clinically malignant tumors tend to have a reduced number of S-100 protein–positive cells, however, the presence or absence of this sustentacular cell population is not an absolutely reliable method for predicting biologic behavior (87). In a recent study of 64 sympathoadrenal paragangliomas (20 clinically malignant, 44 classified as clinically benign), 37 of the 44 benign tumors contained S-100 protein–positive cells (14 scored as 1+, 13 as 2+, 10 as 3+) and 7 tumors were negative; there was no S-100 protein in 12 of 20 malignant tumors (60 percent), but in 8 tumors there was a similar spectrum of reactivity (2 scored as 1+, 3 as 2+, 3 as 3+) (87). Clinically malignant sympathoadrenal paragangliomas express significantly fewer neuropeptides compared with benign tumors, although the spectrum of immunostaining is similar (Table 13-2). In one study, clinically benign tumors expressed an average of five neuropeptides compared with two for the malignant tumors (88). A few studies report abnormalities in neuropeptide Y and NSE expression or secretion (82,83,86). Further investigation is needed to identify truly reliable immunomarkers useful in predicting biologic behavior in these neoplasms.

In Situ Hybridization and Other Techniques. In situ hybridization shows great potential as a molecular probe in diagnosis, offering the pathologist the opportunity to combine molecular and morphologic methodologies (91–95). Detection of mRNA indicates actual production of the gene product by the cell in question rather than secondary absorption and the technique does not require expression of the gene product because DNA or mRNA gene substance can be detected directly (92). The polymerase chain reaction (PCR) also has potential application in endocrine pathology for studying oncogene amplification as well as identification and analysis of mutations in DNA (96).

Cytologic Findings. Cytologic results of fine-needle aspiration (FNA) of pheochromocytomas and extra-adrenal paragangliomas have been reported (97–99,102,104–108), including a case of composite pheochromocytoma-ganglioneuroma (103). However, problems occur with cytologic interpretation, especially when malignancy is diagnosed based solely on cytologic atypia, which can

Table 13-2

SIMULTANEOUS EXPRESSION OF MULTIPLE NEUROPEPTIDES IN BENIGN AND MALIGNANT SYMPATHOADRENAL PARAGANGLIOMAS

						Number of Neuropeptides*						
	0	**1**	**2**	**3**	**4**	**5**	**6**	**7**	**8**	**9**	**10**	**Index****
Benign Tumors	2	2	4	8	9	11	12	5	3	0	0	5
Malignant Tumors	4	3	5	7	2	1	2	0	1	0	0	2

*The presence of the 10 neuropeptides was assessed in two or more blocks of each tumor by immunohistochemistry.
**The average number of neuropeptides per tumor.

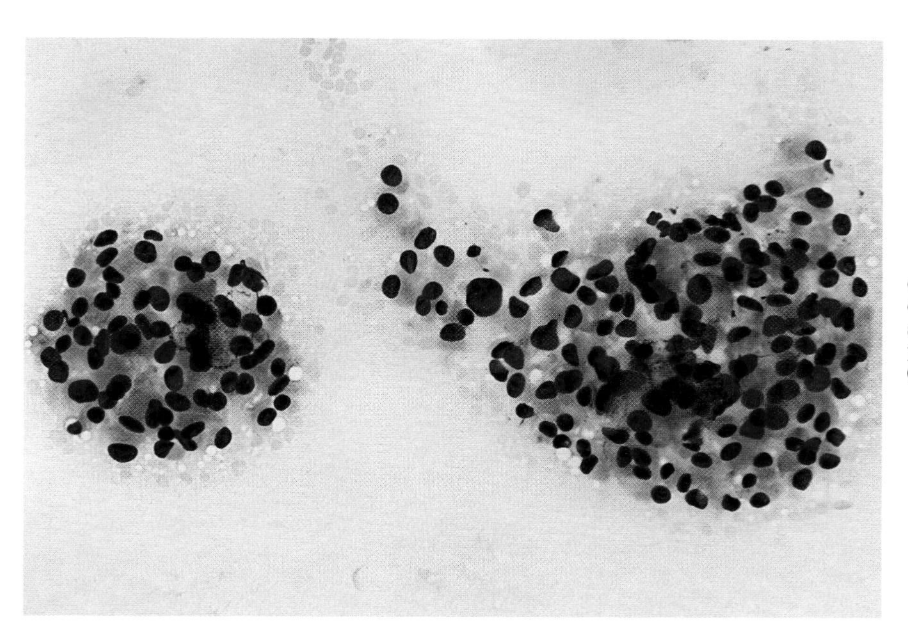

Figure 13-17
PHEOCHROMOCYTOMA
Touch imprint of a pheochromocytoma showing clusters of epithelioid cells with darkly stained nuclei. The tumor had a predominantly alveolar pattern. (X200, Diff Quik stain)

be rather marked in these tumors, similar to head and neck paragangliomas (99,102,105, 106). Potentially fatal consequences have been reported with the use of FNA in these tumors including marked alteration in blood pressure (97,102,104), sometimes complicated by uncontrollable intra-abdominal hemorrhage (104). Caution is necessary when knowingly aspirating a suspected catecholamine-producing paraganglioma (100,101). FNA of pheochromocytomas has been reported to show binucleated or multinucleated cells and prominent intranuclear pseudoinclusions. Precise anatomic localization and close correlation with clinical and endocrinologic data may provide some important advantage in cytologic interpretation, recognizing of course other endocrine tumors that can mimic a paraganglioma such as a pancreatic islet cell tumor (101). Smear/imprint preparations of surgically resected tumors may provide the opportunity to gain familiarity with the cytologic features of these rare tumors (figs. 13-17, 3-18).

Role of Quantitative DNA Analysis in Prognosis. There have been several studies of the DNA content of pheochromocytomas using flow cytometry and static image analysis of tissue sections (109–113,115,118–122) or cytology specimens (114) in order to predict biologic behavior, but there have been conflicting interpretations (117). Koss et al. (116) discuss some of the pitfalls in techniques and histogram interpretation, and caution that for most cancers studied

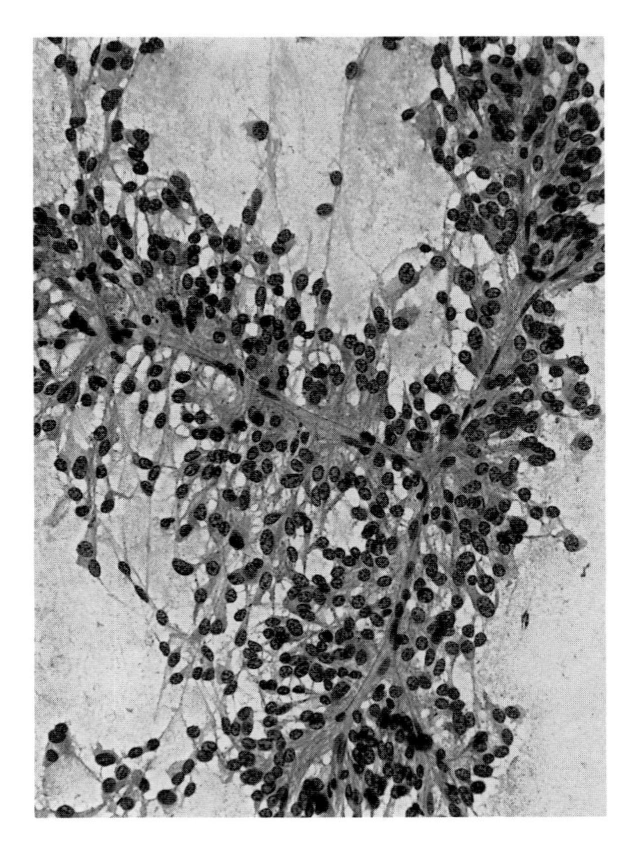

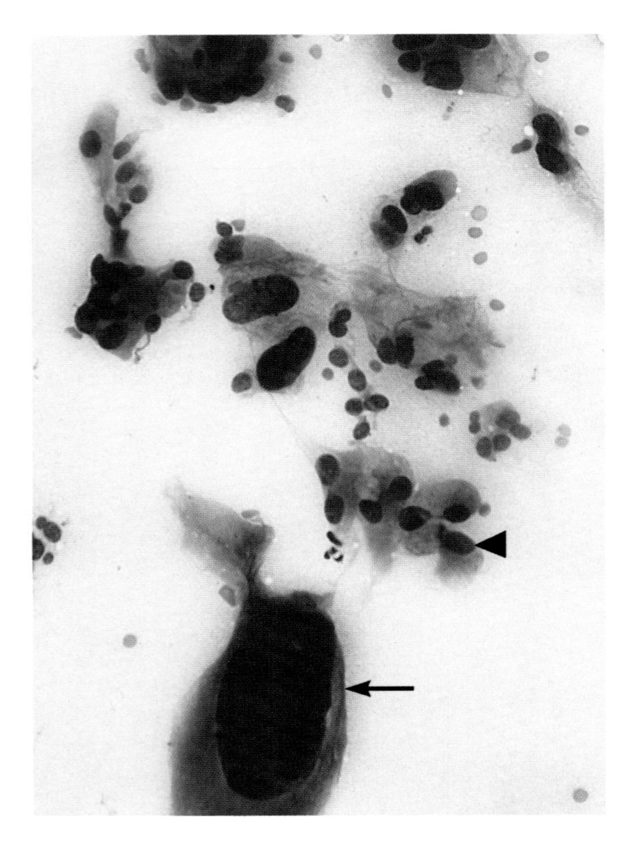

Figure 13-18
PHEOCHROMOCYTOMA

Left: Smear/imprint shows a delicate branching vessel with surrounding mantles of partially disrupted tumor cells. Note the relatively uniform nuclear morphology.

Right: Smear/imprint of a pheochromocytoma showing greatly enlarged hyperchromatic nuclei (arrow). Compare these with the smaller nuclei of adjacent tumor cells (arrowhead). The tumor proved to be clinically benign.

to date information regarding DNA quantitation remains incomplete. Two successive series of DNA flow cytometric analyses from the Mayo Clinic suggest that DNA ploidy patterns offer independent prognostic value for patients with sympathoadrenal paragangliomas (fig. 13-19): all 12 patients who died of tumor-related disease had abnormal DNA ploidy, whereas none of the 64 patients with DNA diploid tumors died (113, 120). These findings are in contrast to other studies using flow cytometry and DNA cytophotometry (fig. 13-20) which indicate that on a statistical basis DNA quantitation does not reliably discriminate between clinically benign and malignant sympathoadrenal paragangliomas (109–111,114,118,121,122). A recent study documented DNA tetraploidy or aneuploidy in 16 of 72 clinically benign adrenal and extra-adrenal paragangliomas (122). Indeed, the surgical pathologist dealing with endocrine tumors in general encounters a significant number of cases with aberrations in nuclear size and shape along with hyperchromasia in which long-term clinical follow-up indicates a benign course (117).

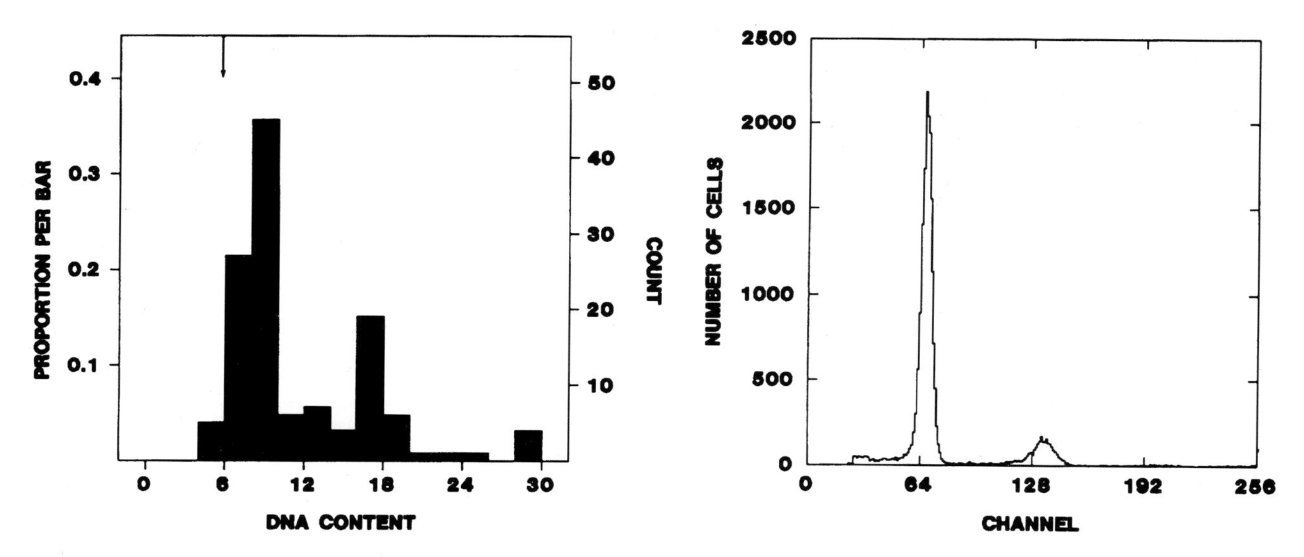

Figure 13-19

CLINICALLY MALIGNANT EXTRA-ADRENAL ABDOMINAL PARAGANGLIOMA

Left: Static image analysis of DNA content shows aneuploid peaks.

Right: Flow cytometric analysis of DNA content in same case shows concordance for peak number and placement, although image analysis suggests the presence of a tetraploid subpopulation of cells not evident by flow analysis.

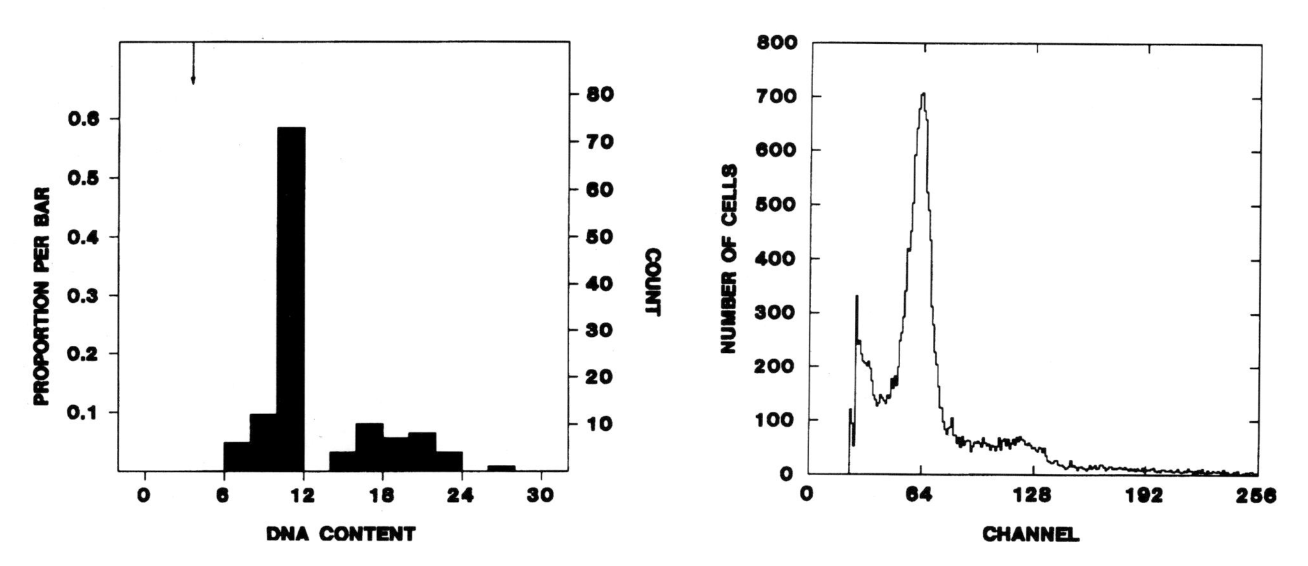

Figure 13-20

CLINICALLY BENIGN PHEOCHROMOCYTOMA

Left: Aneuploidy is evident on static image analysis DNA histogram.

Right: Flow cytometric analysis of DNA content in same case. There is better discrimination of aneuploidy by image analysis (left) when the diploid flow peak is obscured due to paucity of diploid cells or prevalence of debris.

REFERENCES

Ultrastructural Findings

1. Brown WJ, Barajas L, Waisman J, DeQuattro V. Ultrastructural and biochemical correlates of adrenal and extra-adrenal pheochromocytoma. Cancer 1972;29:744–59.
2. Damjanov I, Chang AE, Blechner JN, Foster J. Ultrastructure of malignant paraganglioma of organ of Zuckerkandl. Urology 1978;11:414–7.
3. DeLellis RA, Suchow E, Wolfe HJ. Ultrastructure of nuclear inclusions in pheochromocytoma and paraganglioma. Hum Pathol 1980;11:205–7.
4. Glenner GG, Grimley PM. Tumors of the extra-adrenal paraganglion system (including chemoreceptors). Atlas of Tumor Pathology, 2nd Series, Fascicle 9. Washington, D.C.: Armed Forces Institute of Pathology, 1974.
5. Gómez RR, Osborne BM, Ordoñez NG, Mackay B. Pheochromocytoma. Ultrastruct Pathol 1991;15:557–62.
6. Gordon RE, Taff ML, Schwartz IS, Kleinerman J. Malignant retroperitoneal paraganglioma: unusual light and electron microscopic findings. Mt Sinai J Med 1983;50:507–13.
7. Izumiyama N, Asami E, Itoh Y, Ohtsubo K. Alzheimer's neurofibrillary tangles and paired helical filaments in the pheochromocytoma cells of the adrenal medulla—electron microscopic and immunoelectron microscopic observations. Acta Neuropathol (Berl) 1990;81:213–6.
8. Kay S. Hyperplasia and neoplasia of the adrenal gland. Pathol Annu 1976;11:103–39.
9. Kimura N, Miura Y, Nagatsu I, Nagura H. Catecholamine synthesizing enzymes in 70 cases of functioning and nonfunctioning pheochromocytoma and extra-adrenal paraganglioma. Virchows Arch [A] 1992;421:25–32.
10. Kyriacou K, Shipkey FH, Loewen R. Crystalloid structures in retroperitoneal paragangliomas: a light and electron microscopic study. Ultrastruct Pathol 1991;15:57–67.
11. Lack EE. Pathology of adrenal and extra-adrenal paraganglia. Major problems in pathology, Vol 29. Philadelphia: WB Saunders, 1994.
12. Lloyd RV, Sisson JC, Shapiro B, Verhofstad AA. Immunohistochemical localization of epinephrine, norepinephrine, catecholamine-synthesizing enzymes, and chromogranin in neuroendocrine cells and tumors. Am J Pathol 1986;125:45–54.
13. Meideros LJ, Wolf BC, Balogh K, Federman M. Adrenal pheochromocytoma: a clinicopathologic review of 60 cases. Hum Pathol 1985;16:580–9.
14. Mendelsohn G, Olson JL. Pheochromocytoma [Letter]. Hum Pathol 1978;9:607–8.
15. Osamura RY, Yasuda O, Kawai K, et al. Immunohistochemical localization of catecholamine-synthesizing enzymes in human pheochromocytomas. Endocr Pathol 1990;1:102–8.
16. Pollock WJ, Lim JY, McClellan SL. An adrenal gland tumor in a 24-year-old woman. Ultrastruct Pathol 1986;10:369–76.
17. Tannenbaum M. Ultrastructural pathology of adrenal medullary tumors. Pathol Annu 1970;5:145–71.
18. Wilson RA, Ibanez ML. A comparative study of 14 cases of familial and nonfamilial pheochromocytoma. Hum Pathol 1978;9:181–8.
19. Yokoyama M, Takayasu H. An electron microscopic study of the human adrenal medulla and pheochromocytoma. Urol Int 1969;24:79–95.

Immunohistochemical Findings

20. DeLellis RA, Tischler AS, Lee AK, Blount M, Wolfe HJ. Leu-enkephalin-like immunoreactivity in proliferative lesions of the human adrenal medulla and extra-adrenal paraganglia. Am J Surg Pathol 1983;7:29–37.
21. Eiden LE, Huttner WB, Mallet J, O'Connor DT, Winkler H, Zanini A. A nomenclature proposal for the chromogranin/secretogranin proteins. Neuroscience 1987;21:1019–21.
22. Hamid Q, Varndell IM, Ibrahim NB, Mingazzini P, Polak JM. Extra-adrenal paragangliomas. An immunocytochemical and ultrastructural report. Cancer 1987;60:1776–81.
23. Lack EE. Pathology of adrenal and extra-adrenal paraganglia. Major problems in pathology, Vol 29. Philadelphia: WB Saunders, 1994.
24. Lee I, Gong G, Yu E, Wiedenmann B, Franke WW. Cytochrome b561: molecular marker of a subset of neuroendocrine cells and neoplasms. Mod Pathol 1993;6:39A(209).
25. Linnoila RI, Lack EE, Steinberg SM, Keiser HR. Decreased expression of neuropeptides in malignant paragangliomas: an immunohistochemical study. Hum Pathol 1988;19:41–50.
26. Miettinen M. Neuroendocrine differentiation in adrenocortical carcinoma. New immunohistochemical findings supported by electron microscopy. Lab Invest 1992;66:169–74.
27. Schmid KW, Schröder S, Dockhorn-Dworniczak B, et al. Immunohistochemical demonstration of chromogranin A, chromogranin B, and secretogranin II in extra-adrenal paragangliomas. Mod Pathol 1994;7:347–53.
28. Schröder S, Padberg BC, Achilles E, Holl K, Dralle H, Klöppel G. Immunocytochemistry in adrenocortical tumors: a clinicomorphological study of 72 neoplasms. Virchows Arch [A] 1992;420:65–70.
29. Thompson RJ, Doran JF, Jackson P, Dhillon AP, Rode J. PGP 9.5 a new marker for vertebrate neurons and neuroendocrine cells. Brain Res 1983;278:224–8.
30. Tischler AS, Mobtaker H, Mann K, et al. Anti-lymphocyte antibody leu-7 (HNK-1) recognizes a constituent of neuroendocrine granule matrix. J Histochem Cytochem 1986;34:1213–6.
31. Winkler H, Apps DK, Fischer-Colbrie R. The molecular function of adrenal chromaffin granules: established facts and unresolved topics. Neurosci 1986;18:261–90.

Associated Endocrine Syndromes and Other Features

32. Beaser RS, Guay AT, Lee AK, Silverman ML, Flint LD. An adrenocorticotropic hormone-producing pheochromocytoma: diagnostic and immunohistochemical studies. J Urol 1986;135:10–3.
33. DeLellis RA, Tischler AS, Lee AK, Blount M, Wolfe HJ. Leu-enkephalin-like immunoreactivity in proliferative lesions of the human adrenal medulla and extra-adrenal paraganglia. Am J Surg Pathol 1983;7:29–37.
34. Fisher BM, MacPhee GJ, Davies DL, McPherson SG, Brown IL, Goldberg A. A case of watery diarrhoea syndrome due to an adrenal phaeochromocytoma secreting vasoactive intestinal polypeptide with coincidental autoimmune thyroid disease. Acta Endocrinol (Copenh) 1987;114:340–4.
35. Forman BH, Marban E, Kayne RD, et al. Ectopic ACTH syndrome due to pheochromocytoma. Yale J Biol Med 1979;82:181–9.
36. Garbini A, Mainardi M, Grimi M, Repaci G, Nanni G, Bragherio G. Pheochromocytoma and hypercalcemia due to ectopic production of parathyroid hormone. NY State J Med 1986;86:25–7.
37. Grizzle WE, Tolbert L, Pittman CS, Siegel AL, Aldrete JS. Corticotropin production by tumors of the autonomic nervous system. Arch Pathol Lab Med 1984;108:545–50.
38. Heath H III, Edis AJ. Pheochromocytoma associated with hypercalcemia and ectopic secretion of calcitonin. Ann Intern Med 1979;91:208–10.
39. Interlandi JW, Hundley RF, Kasselberg AG, Orth DN, Salmon WD Jr, Sullivan JN. Hypercortisolism, diarrhea with steatorrhea and massive proteinuria due to pheochromocytoma. South Med J 1985;78:879–83.
40. Jessop DS, Cunnah D, Millar JG, et al. A phaeochromocytoma presenting with Cushing's syndrome associated with increased concentrations of circulating corticotrophin-releasing factor. J Endocr 1987;113:133–8.
41. Lack EE. Adrenal medullary hyperplasia and pheochromocytoma. In: Lack EE, ed. Pathology of the adrenal glands. New York: Churchill Livingstone, 1990:173–235.
42. Lack EE. Pathology of adrenal and extra-adrenal paraganglia. Major problems in pathology, Vol 29. Philadelphia: WB Saunders, 1994.
43. Linnoila RI, Lack EE, Steinberg SM, Keiser HR. Decreased expression of neuropeptides in malignant paragangliomas: an immunohistochemical study. Hum Pathol 1988;19:41–50.
44. Lloyd RV, Shapiro B, Sisson JC, Kalff V, Thompson NW, Beierwaltes WA. An immunohistochemical study of pheochromocytomas. Arch Pathol Lab Med 1984;108:541–4.
45. Matta MK, Prorok JJ, Trimpi HD, Sheets JA, Stasik JJ Jr, Khubchandani IT. WDHA syndrome caused by pheochromocytoma: report of a case. Dis Colon Rect 1978;21:297–301.
46. Meloni CR, Tucci J, Canary JJ, Kyle LH. Cushing's syndrome due to bilateral adrenocortical hyperplasia caused by a benign adrenal medullary tumor. J Clin Endocrinol Metab 1966;26:1192–200.
47. Mendelsohn G, Eggleston JC, Olson JL, Said SI, Baylin SB. Vasoactive intestinal peptide and its relationship to ganglion cell differentiation in neuroblastic tumors. Lab Invest 1979;31:144–9.
48. Perry RR, Nieman LK, Cutler GB Jr, et al. Primary adrenal causes of Cushing's syndrome. Diagnosis and surgical management Ann Surg 1989;210:59–68.
49. Sackel SG, Manson JE, Harawi SJ, Burakoff R. Watery diarrhea syndrome due to an adrenal pheochromocytoma secreting vasoactive intestinal polypeptide. Dig Dis Sci 1985;30:1201–7.
50. Sano T, Saito H, Yamasaki R, et al. Production and secretion of immunoreactive growth hormone-releasing factor by pheochromocytoma. Cancer 1986;57:1788–93.
51. Schteingart DE, Conn JW, Orth DN, Harrison TS, Fox JE, Bookstein JJ. Secretion of ACTH and beta-MSH by an adrenal medullary paraganglioma. J Clin Endocrinol Metab 1972;34:676–83.
52. Shanberg AM, Baghdassarian R, Tansey LA, Bacon D, Greenberg P, Perley M. Pheochromocytoma with hypercalcemia: case report and review of literature. J Urol 1985;133:258–9.
53. Shimbo, S, Nakano, Y. A case of malignant pheochromocytoma producing parathyroid hormone-like substance. Calcif Tissue Res 1974;15:155–6.
54. Spark RF, Connolly PB, Gluckin DS, White R, Sacks B, Landsberg L. ACTH secretion from a functioning pheochromocytoma. N Engl J Med 1979;301:416–8.
55. Swinton NW Jr, Clerkin EP, Flint LD. Hypercalcemia and familial pheochromocytoma. Correction after adrenalectomy. Ann Intern Med 1972;76:455–7.
56. Thesleff P, Benoni C, Mårtensson H, Nilsson Å, Sundler F, Åkesson B. A mixed endocrine adrenal tumour causing steatorrhea. Gut 1987;28:1298–301.
57. Trump DL, Livingstone JN, Baylin SB. Watery diarrhea syndrome in an adult with ganglioneuroma-pheochromocytoma: identification of vasoactive intestinal peptide, calcitonin and catecholamines and assessment of their biologic activity. Cancer 1977;40:1526–33.
58. Verner JV, Morrison AB. Islet cell tumor and a syndrome of refractory watery diarrhea and hypokalemia. Am J Med 1958;25:374–80.
59. White MC, Hickson BR. Multiple paragangliomata secreting catecholamines and calcitonin with intermittent hypercalcaemia. J Royal Soc Med 1979;72:532–8.
60. Young JD Jr, Qureshi AS, Connor TB, Wiswell JG. Problem lesions in adrenal surgery. J Urol 1969;101:233–40.

Other Immunoreactive Substances

61. Bauer FE, Hacker GW, Terenghi G, Adrian TE, Polak JM. Localization and molecular forms of galanin in human adrenals: elevated levels in pheochromocytomas. J Clin Endocrinol Metab 1986;63:1372–8.
62. Franquemont DW, Mills SE, Lack EE. Immunohistochemical detection of neuroblastomatous foci in composite adrenal pheochromocytoma-neuroblastoma. Am J Clin Pathol 1994;102:163–70.

63. Fried G, Wikström LM, Höög A, et al. Mutiple neuropeptide immunoreactivities in a renin producing human paraganglioma. Cancer 1994;74:142–51.
64. Haselbacher GK, Irminger JC, Ziegler WH, Humbel RE. Insulin-like growth factor II in human adrenal pheochromocytomas and Wilms' tumors: expression at the mRNA and protein level. Proc Natl Acad Sci 1987;84:1104–6.
65. Inagaki S, Kubota Y, Kito S, Kangawa K, Matsuo H. Immunoreactive atrial natriuretic polypeptides in the adrenal medulla and sympathetic ganglia. Regul Peptides 1986;15:249–60.
66. Kamio T, Shigematsu K, Sou H, Kawai K, Tsuchiyama H. Immunohistochemical expression of epidermal growth factor receptor in human adrenocortical carcinoma. Hum Pathol 1990;21:277–82.
67. Laliberte F, Laliberte MF, Alhenc-Gelas F, Chevillard C. Cellular and subcellular immunohistochemical localization of angiotensin-converting enzyme in the rat adrenal gland. Lab Invest 1987;56:364–71.
68. Miettinen M, Cupo W. Neural cell adhesion molecule distribution in soft tissue tumors. Hum Pathol 1993;24:62–6.
69. Sano T, Vrontakis ME, Kovacs K, Asa SL, Friesen HG. Galanin immunoreactivity in neuroendocrine tumors. Arch Pathol Lab Med 1991;115:926–9.
70. Unger PD, Hoffman K, Thung SN, Pertsemlides D, Wolfe D, Keneko M. HMB-45 reactivity in adrenal pheochromocytomas. Arch Pathol Lab Med 1992;116:151–3.

Intermediate Filament Profile

71. Azumi N, Battifora H. The distribution of vimentin and keratin in epithelial and nonepithelial neoplasms. A comprehensive immunohistochemical study on formalin- and alcohol-fixed tumors. Am J Clin Pathol 1987;88:286–96.
72. Franke WW, Grund C, Achtstätter T. Coexpression of cytokeratins and neurofilament proteins in permanent cell line: cultural rat PC12 cells combine neuronal and epithelial features. J Cell Biol 1986;103:1933–43.
73. Franquemont DW, Mills SE, Lack EE. Immunohistochemical detection of neuroblastomatous foci in composite adrenal pheochromocytoma-neuroblastoma. Am J Clin Pathol 1994;102:163–70.
74. Johnson TL, Zarbo RJ, Lloyd RV, Crissman JD. Paragangliomas of the head and neck: immunohistochemical neuroendocrine and intermediate filament typing. Mod Pathol 1988;1:216–23.
75. Kimura N, Nakazato Y, Nagura H, Sasano N. Expression of intermediate filaments in neuroendocrine tumors. Arch Pathol Lab Med 1990;114:506–10.
76. Lehto VP, Virtanen I, Miettinen M, Dahl D, Kahri A. Neurofilaments in adrenal and extra-adrenal pheochromocytoma. Demonstration using immunofluorescence microscopy. Arch Pathol Lab Med 1983;107:492–4.
77. Miettinen M. Synaptophysin and neurofilament proteins as markers for neuroendocrine tumors. Arch Pathol Lab Med 1987;111:813–8.
78. Miettinen M, Lehto VP, Dahl D, Virtanen I. Immunofluorescence microscopic evaluation of the intermediate filament expression of the adrenal cortex and medulla and their tumors. Am J Pathol 1985;118:360–6.
79. Shah IA, Schlageter MO, Netto D. Immunoreactivity of neurofilament proteins in neuroendocrine neoplasms. Mod Pathol 1991;4:215–9.
80. Trojanowski JQ, Lee VM. Expression of neurofilament antigens by normal and neoplastic human adrenal chromaffin cells. N Engl J Med 1985;313:101–4.

Relation of Immunohistochemistry to Prognosis

81. Bernardello F, Zamboni G, Pea M, et al. Retroperitoneal paragangliomas: correlation between S-100 positive cells and prognosis. Mod Pathol 1994;7:51A.
82. Grouzmann E, Gicquel C, Plouin PF, Schlumberger M, Comoy E, Bohuon C. Neuropeptide Y and neuron-specific enolase levels in benign and malignant pheochromocytomas. Cancer 1990;66:1833–5.
83. Helman LJ, Cohen PS, Averbuch SD, Cooper MJ, Keiser HR, Israel MA. Neuropeptide Y expression distinguishes malignant from benign pheochromocytoma. J Clin Oncol 1989;7:1720–5.
84. Kliewer KE, Cochran AJ. A review of the histology, ultrastructure, immunohistology, and molecular biology of extra-adrenal paragangliomas. Arch Pathol Lab Med 1989;113:1209–18.
85. Kliewer KE, Wen DR, Cancilla PA, Cochran AJ. Paragangliomas: assessment of prognosis by histologic, immunohistochemical, and ultrastructural techniques. Hum Pathol 1989;20:29–39.
86. Kuvshinoff BW, Nussbaum MS, Richards AF, Bloustein P, McFadden DW. Neuropeptide Y secretion from a malignant extra-adrenal retroperitoneal paraganglioma. Cancer 1992;70:2350–3.
87. Linnoila RI, Becker RL Jr, Steinberg SM, Keiser HR, Lack EE. The role of S-100 protein containing cells in the prognosis of sympathoadrenal paragangliomas. Mod Pathol 1993;6:39A(210).
88. Linnoila RI, Lack EE, Steinberg SM, Keiser HR. Decreased expression of neuropeptides in malignant paragangliomas: an immunohistochemical study. Hum Pathol 1988;19:41–50.
89. Lloyd RV, Blaivas M, Wilson BS. Distribution of chromogranin and S-100 protein in normal and abnormal adrenal medullary tissues. Arch Pathol Lab Med 1985;109:633–5.
90. Unger P, Hoffman K, Pertsemlidis D, Thung S, Wolfe D, Kaneko M. S-100 protein-positive sustentacular cells in malignant and locally aggressive adrenal pheochromocytomas. Arch Pathol Lab Med 1991;115:484–7.

In Situ Hybridization and Other Techniques

91. DeLellis RA. In situ hybridization techniques for the analysis of gene expression: applications in tumor pathology. Hum Pathol 1994;25:580–5.
92. Lloyd RV. Introduction to molecular endocrine pathology. Endocr Pathol 1993;4:64–72.
93. Lloyd RV. Molecular probes and endocrine diseases. Am J Surg Pathol 1990;14:34–44.
94. Lloyd RV, Jin L, Kulig E, Fields K. Molecular approaches for the analysis of chromogranins and secretogranins. Diagn Mol Pathol 1992;1:2–15.
95. Long AA, Mueller J, Andre-Schwartz J, Barrett KJ, Schwartz R, Wolfe H. High specificity in-situ hybridization: methods and application. Diagn Mol Pathol 1992;1:45–57.
96. Templeton NS. The polymerase chain reaction. History, methods and applications. Diagn Mol Pathol 1992;1:58–72.

Cytologic Findings and Fine-Needle Aspiration

97. Casola G, Nicolet V, von Sonnenberg E. Unsuspected pheochromocytoma and risk of blood-pressure alterations during percutaneous adrenal biopsy. Radiology 1986;159:733–5.
98. González-Cámpora R, Otal-Salaverri C, Panea-Flores P, Lerma-Puertas E, Galera-Davidson H. Fine needle aspiration cytology of paraganglionic tumors. Acta Cytol 1988;32:386–90.
99. Heaston DK, Handel DB, Ashton PR, Korobkin M. Narrow gauge needle aspiration of solid adrenal masses. AJR Am J Roentgenol 1982;138:1143–8.
100. Lack EE. Adrenal medullary hyperplasia and pheochromocytoma. In: Lack EE, ed. Pathology of the adrenal glands. New York: Churchill Livingstone, 1990:173–235.
101. Lack EE. Pathology of adrenal and extra-adrenal paraganglia. Major problems in pathology, Vol 29. Philadelphia: WB Saunders, 1994.
102. Lambert MA, Hirschowitz L, Russell RC. Fine needle aspiration biopsy: a cautionary tale. Br J Surg 1985;72:364.
103. Layfield LJ, Glasgow BJ, Du Puis MH, Bhuta S. Aspiration cytology and immunohistochemistry of a pheochromocytoma-ganglioneuroma of the adrenal gland. Acta Cytologica 1987;31:33–9.
104. McCorkell SJ, Niles NL. Fine-needle aspiration of catecholamine-producing adrenal masses: a possibly fatal mistake. AJR Am J Roentgenol 1985;145:113–4.
105. Montali G, Solbiati L, Bossi MC, De Pra L, Di Donna A, Ravetto C. Sonographically guided fine-needle aspiration biopsy of adrenal masses. AJR Am J Roentgenol 1984;143:1081–4.
106. Nguyen GK. Cytopathologic aspects of adrenal pheochromocytoma in a fine needle aspiration biopsy. A case report. Acta Cytologica 1982;26:354–8.
107. Rupp M, Ehya H. Fine needle aspiration cytology of retroperitoneal paraganglioma with lipofuscin pigmentation. Acta Cytol 1990;34:84–8.
108. Wadih GE, Nance KV, Silverman JF. Fine-needle aspiration cytology of the adrenal gland. Fifty biopsies in 48 patients. Arch Pathol Lab Med 1991;116:841–6.

Quantitative DNA Analysis

109. Amberson JB, Vaughan ED Jr, Gray GF, Naus GJ. Flow cytometric differentiation of nuclear DNA content in benign adrenal pheochromocytomas. Urology 1987;30:102–4.
110. González-Cámpora R, Cano SD, Lerma-Puertas E, et al. Paragangliomas. Static cytometric studies of nuclear DNA patterns. Cancer 1993;71:820–4.
111. Grignon DJ, Ro JY, Mackay B, et al. Paraganglioma of the urinary bladder: immunohistochemical, ultrastructural, and DNA flow cytometric studies. Hum Pathol 1991;22:1162–9.
112. Hoffman K, Gil J, Barba J, et al. Morphometric analysis of benign and malignant adrenal pheochromocytomas. Arch Pathol Lab Med 1993;117:244–7.
113. Hosaka Y, Rainwater LM, Grant CS, Farrow GM, van Heerden JA, Lieber MM. Pheochromocytoma: nuclear deoxyribonucleic acid patterns studied by flow cytometry. Surgery 1986;100:1003–10.
114. Kimura N, Watanabe M, Ookuma T, et al. DNA ploidy of pheochromocytoma on cytology specimen by image analysis. Endocr Pathol 1994;5:178–82.
115. Klein FA, Kay S, Ratliff JA, White FK, Newsome HH. Flow cytometric determinations of ploidy and proliferation patterns of adrenal neoplasms: an adjunct to histological classifications. J Urol 1985;134:862–6.
116. Koss LG, Czerniak B, Herz F, Wersto RP. Flow cytometric measurements of DNA and other cell components in human tumors. A critical appraisal. Hum Pathol 1989;20:528–48.
117. Lack EE. Pathology of adrenal and extra-adrenal paraganglia. Major problems in pathology, Vol 29. Philadelphia: WB Saunders, 1994.
118. Lewis PD. A cytophotometric study of benign and malignant pheochromocytomas. Virchows Arch [Cell Pathol] 1971;9:371–6.
119. Linnoila RI, Becker RL Jr, Steinberg SM, Keiser HR, Lack EE. The role of S-100 protein containing cells in the prognosis of sympathoadrenal paragangliomas [Abstract]. Mod Pathol 1993;6:39A.
120. Nativ O, Grant CS, Sheps SG, et al. The clinical significance of nuclear DNA ploidy pattern in 184 patients with pheochromocytoma. Cancer 1992;69:2683–7.
121. Padberg BC, Garbe E, Achilles E, Dralle H, Bressel M, Schröder S. Adrenomedullary hyperplasia and pheochromocytoma. DNA photometric findings in 47 cases. Virchows Archiv [A] 1990;416:443–6.
122. Pang LC, Tsao KC. Flow cytometric DNA analysis for the determination of malignant potential in adrenal and extra-adrenal pheochromocytomas or paragangliomas. Arch Pathol Lab Med 1993;117:1142–7.

14
PARAGANGLIA OF THE HEAD AND NECK REGION

Extra-adrenal paraganglia have a centripetal and roughly symmetric distribution on either side of the midline, extending from the middle ear region and base of the skull to the pelvic floor. All of these endocrine cells are assumed to have common embryogenesis from the neural crest, similar to chromaffin cells of adrenal medulla and chief cells of the carotid body (25). As noted earlier, the sympathoadrenal neuroendocrine system has a different anatomic distribution and mediates rapid adaptations to changes in the environment by a combination of neural (norepinephrine release from postganglionic sympathetic neurons) and hormonal effects, with the latter due to secretion of catecholamines (mainly epinephrine) from the adrenal medullae. Paraganglia of the head and neck region are more closely aligned with the parasympathetic nervous system, and often have an intimate association with vascular and neural structures (fig. 14-1). Many of these paraganglia have a branchiomeric distribution which parallels, in large part, the location of branchial arch mesodermal structures such as carotid artery and great vessels near the base of the heart; this anatomic distribution suggests an atavistic relation to the gill arches of aquatic species which are vital to respiratory function. The strategic location of some of these head and neck paraganglia makes them likely candidates for having a chemoreceptor role in reflex changes in respiratory and cardiovascular activities in response to alterations in the composition of arterial blood.

Based upon early reports of a positive chromaffin reaction (although notably weaker in the carotid body) and presumed neural connections with the sympathetic nervous system, Kohn (19) regarded the carotid bodies as paraganglia similar to the adrenal medullae. Some have questioned the propriety of the term paraganglia for carotid bodies, and by extrapolation, for similar endocrine structures in the head and neck region that are nonchromaffin and have a chemosensory role (22). Nonetheless, the term has become widely accepted, although it undoubtedly embraces a wider group of neuroendocrine cells than was originally envisioned by Kohn. Although paraganglia of the head and neck region are structurally and functionally distinct from those of the sympathoadrenal neuroendocrine system, there is some overlap in morphology, and similarity in the immunohistochemical phenotype of normal endocrine cells and the paragangliomas arising from them.

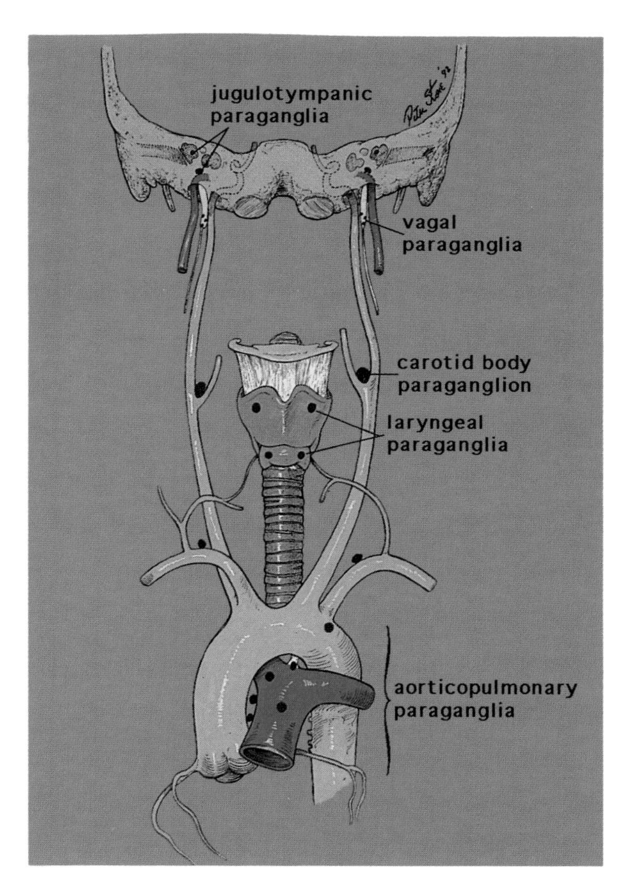

Figure 14-1
ANATOMIC DISTRIBUTION OF PARAGANGLIA IN HEAD AND NECK REGION

The anatomic distribution of most paraganglia in the head and neck region, including those located near the base of heart and great vessels, is shown. Carotid bodies comprise the largest compact collection of paraganglia in this anatomic distribution. Note the close relationship of paraganglia to vascular and neural structures some of which are embryologically associated with branchial arches. Paragangliomas can arise in sites where normal paraganglia have not yet been adequately characterized (e.g., orbit).

PARAGANGLIA AS PART OF A DIFFUSE NEUROENDOCRINE SYSTEM

Paraganglia are members of a very complex and intriguing family of endocrine cells that have a wide anatomic distribution and varied regulatory functions. The APUD (amine precursor uptake and decarboxylation) cell concept was introduced by Pearse (29) in an attempt to bond a vast array of endocrine cells having shared metabolic characteristics as well as presumed common embryogenesis from the neural crest. The term *APUDoma* soon became a popular reference to a variety of endocrine tumors. Although no longer in wide use, this concept was an important stimulus for scientific investigation, particularly in the areas of immunology and molecular biology (22). The term neurocristopathy was proposed by Bolande (7) for a disparate group of endocrine neoplasms and disorders with common embryogenesis but remarkably diverse clinical and pathologic features.

Feyrter (12) recognized certain endocrine cells of the gastrointestinal tract that were presumed to have an influence on neighboring cells (paracrine function), and later postulated that similar endocrine cells of the bronchial mucosa might give rise to carcinoid tumors; this endocrine unit in the gastrointestinal tract was conceptualized as a "diffuse endocrine epithelial organ." The designation *neuroendocrine* has now become popular since it emphasizes the close functional relationship between the nervous system (e.g., neurons and ganglion cells) and endocrine cells (10). This diffuse or dispersed neuroendocrine system has evolved as a general unifying concept without focusing on a common path of embryogenesis or shared cytochemical features. A wide variety of hormones, amines, and regulatory peptides have been identified in endocrine cells of normal paraganglia in the head and neck region as well as their respective paragangliomas. Some of these substances are capable of eliciting a more conventional endocrine effect (e.g., the rare paraganglioma with excess catecholamine secretion), while others mediate a regulatory function on adjacent cells (paracrine action) or an autoregulatory role on the same cells secreting the product (autocrine effect).

The literature dealing with paraganglia is immense, particularly relating to carotid bodies

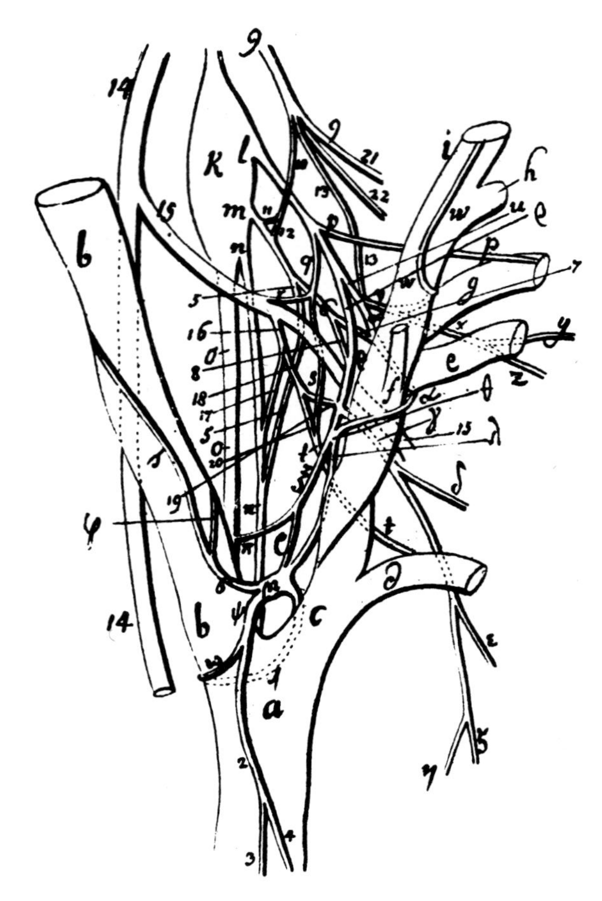

Figure 14-2
CAROTID BODY

Carotid body appears as a small quadrangular structure at the carotid bifurcation, with rich neural connections. The carotid body was originally referred to as "ganglion parvum" or "ganglion minutum." (Illustrated by Neubauer, 1772 [28].)

which have been most accessible to study because of their macroscopic size and relatively constant anatomic location. Investigation of these and other paraganglia in humans has been limited to either autopsy material or, occasionally, tissue obtained during surgery such as therapeutic glomectomy specimens. The first published account of the human carotid body is attributed to Taube, a pupil of Albrecht von Haller, who in 1743 delivered a dissertation on the "ganglion minutum" (15). The carotid body was illustrated by Neubauer in 1772 (28) who portrayed it as a small quadrangular structure in the carotid bifurcation (fig. 14-2). A detailed account of the early history of the carotid body can be found in the work by Adams (2). Svitzer (33) in his anatomic illustrations suggested that

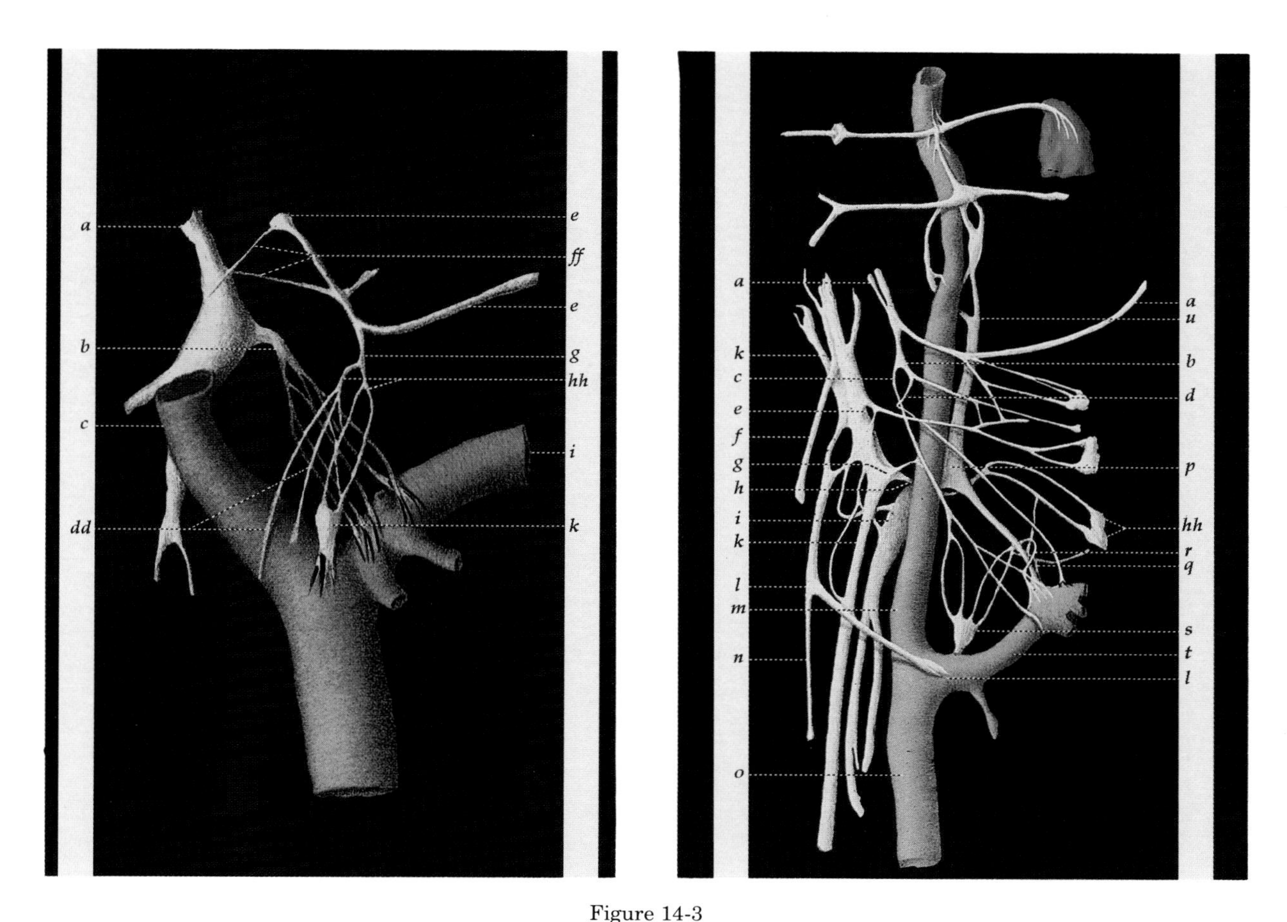

Figure 14-3
CAROTID BODY
Left, right: A carotid body with its neural connections was illustrated in greater detail by Svitzer in 1863 (33).

the carotid body might be innervated solely by the glossopharyngeal nerve without significant sympathetic innervation (fig. 14-3).

For nearly 175 years since the discovery of the carotid body, its physiological function remained a mystery. DeCastro (8) established the predominantly glossopharyngeal innervation of the carotid body in 1926, and in a subsequent study proposed a novel chemoreceptor function for this structure by sensing (or "tasting") alterations in blood. Figure 14-4 shows the neural connections and vascular supply in the experimental animal (9). Conclusive physiologic evidence of chemoreceptor function was provided by Heymans et al. (17) who demonstrated reflex changes in respiration and cardiovascular activity in response to alterations in arterial PaO2, PaCO2, pH, and other agents. The Nobel Prize in physiology and medicine was awarded to this group in 1938 (35).

Other investigators confirmed the chemoreceptor role of carotid bodies as well as small collections of paraganglia located near the base of the heart (11), collectively referred to as aorticopulmonary paraganglia.

PHYSIOLOGIC FUNCTION IN EXPERIMENTAL ANIMALS

Space constraints do little justice to the vast literature on the physiology of chemoreceptors, particularly carotid bodies, in animals. The peripheral arterial chemoreceptors are responsible for the immediate increase in breathing produced by hypoxia (5). Chemoreceptor discharge along the carotid sinus nerve (nerve of Hering), a branch of the ninth cranial nerve, is stimulated by a decrease in PaO_2, increase in $PaCO_2$, and lowered pH. Other excitatory factors include an

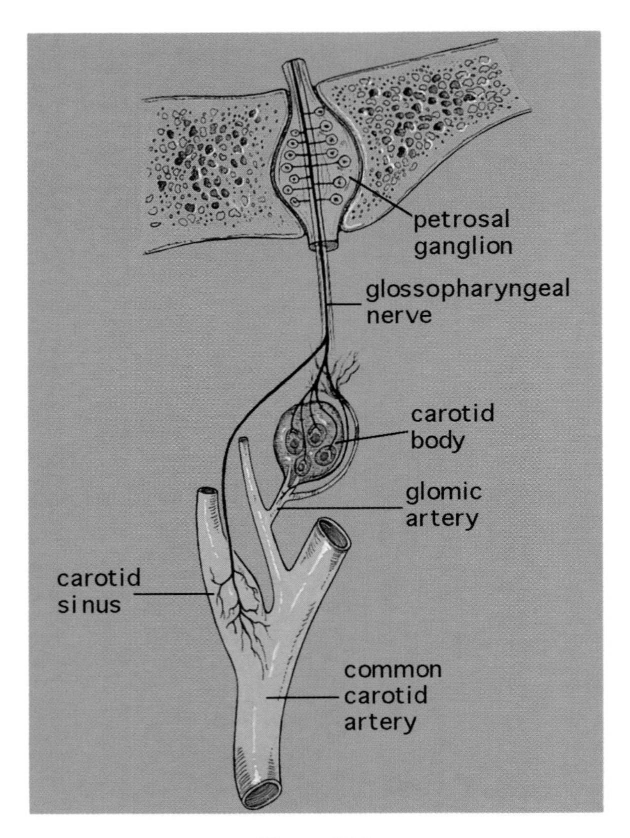

Figure 14-4
NEURAL AND VASCULAR SUPPLY
OF CAT CAROTID BODY

Afferent fibers of the glossopharyngeal nerve innervate the baroreceptor apparatus on the left and the carotid body, which also receives its blood supply from the "glomic artery." An arteriovenous anastomosis is also shown. Note that afferent fibers terminate on or within the cell body of chief cells. (Fig. 10 from DeCastro F. Sur la structure de la synapse dans les chemorecepteurs: leur mechanisme d'excitation et role dans la circulation sanguine locale. Acta Physiol Scand 1951;22:14–43.)

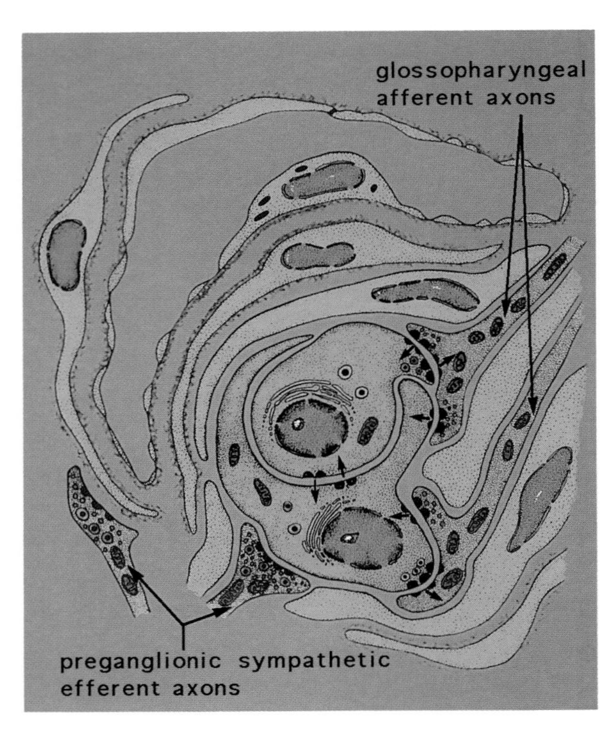

Figure 14-5
NEURAL CONNECTIONS IN THE
RAT CAROTID BODY

Schematic diagram of the spatial relation of carotid body chief cells and afferent terminals of the ninth cranial nerve in the rat. The chief cells are both presynaptic and postsynaptic to glossopharyngeal nerve fibers and the direction of synaptic discharge is indicated by arrows. Note the reciprocal synapses between adjacent chief cells. Sustentacular cells envelop chief cells and neural processes. Pericytes and endothelial cells are also present, with the latter having cytoplasmic fenestrations. Note also the efferent sympathetic fibers. Based upon this model, an antidromic generation of nerve impulses from central terminals of chemoreceptor neurons might contribute to the efferent activity in the glossopharyngeal nerve even though this nerve is primarily sensory.

increase in temperature or osmotic pressure and a variety of chemical substances. Some agents appear to have a stimulatory effect in some animals while being inhibitory in others. Despite the immense research effort, the precise mode of chemosensation or transduction in the carotid body is still not entirely clear. There appears little doubt that chemoreceptor activity involves interaction between nerve endings and chief (glomus type 1) cells. In rats, the chief cell has been regarded as an inhibitory interneuron secreting dopamine which modulates impulse generation along the afferent nerve terminals (fig. 14-5) (27); in this experimental animal the chief cells are both presynaptic and postsynaptic to the nerve terminals, and have reciprocal synapses, features that have not been well characterized for the human carotid body chief cell. Currently, most investigators favor the chief cell as the primary chemosensor or transducer, and some feel that the most likely candidate for a pO_2 sensor is the respiratory chain in mitochondria of chief cells (1,6). Aorticopulmonary paraganglia have a more pronounced effect on the cardiovascular system, depending upon the animal species studied, but the precise mechanism of chemoreception and transduction is unclear. A chemoreceptor function has also been suggested for vagal paraganglia, perhaps mediated through the ganglion nodosum, with reflex changes such as apnea, bradycardia, hypotension, and vomiting (18,22). Laryngeal and endoneurial paraganglia are in an ideal location for regulation of laryngeal airway resistance during hypoxia, but their precise physiologic role is undefined at present (22). A chemoreceptor role has not been established for histologically similar paraganglia elsewhere in the head and neck region.

PHYSIOLOGIC FUNCTION OF CHEMORECEPTORS IN HUMANS

Knowledge about the physiologic role of peripheral arterial chemoreceptors in humans is essentially limited to carotid body paraganglia. Much of the evidence for a chemoreceptor role is based upon the study of ventilatory dynamics in patients who have undergone bilateral glomectomy in an attempt to ameliorate symptoms of obstructive pulmonary disease (e.g., asthma), an operation which has recently been viewed with considerable skepticism regarding its efficacy. Carotid bodies contribute to the sensation of breathlessness which results in a break from breathholding, and following glomectomy there may be a diminution in exercise hyperpnea as well as a decrease in minute ventilation (22). A relationship with essential hypertension and cluster headaches has also been reported (22). Other important lines of evidence supporting a chemoreceptor role in humans are the hypertrophy and hyperplasia of carotid body paraganglia in individuals dwelling at high altitudes (3,30), and those at sea level with chronic hypoxemia or systemic hypertension (16,20–23, 32), and the increased incidence of carotid body paragangliomas ("chemodectomas") at high altitude (22,30). It has been postulated that an attenuated sensitivity of carotid bodies with prolonged hypoxia may play a role in the deterioration of the patient with chronic obstructive pulmonary disease (4).

NOMENCLATURE OF PARAGANGLIOMAS

It is preferable to designate paragangliomas based upon the primary anatomic site of origin. Glenner and Grimley (14) in the second series Fascicle, Tumors of the Extra-Adrenal Paraganglion System, recognized several interrelated "families" of paraganglia and corresponding paragangliomas based upon anatomic distribution, innervation, and microscopic anatomy; these families included branchiomeric, intravagal, aorticosympathetic, and viscero-autonomic paraganglia and corresponding paragangliomas. Adrenal medullary paraganglioma (commonly designated pheochromocytoma) was considered separately. Classification of paragangliomas based upon the chromaffin or nonchromaffin status of the tumor has significant limitations because fresh tissue must be promptly fixed in the appropriate dichromate solution (or exposed to other oxidizing agents), correlation with endocrine function is not always reliable, and a negative reaction does not ensure the absence of catecholamines. The paragangliomas covered in this section, however, are characteristically chromaffin negative. Carotid body paraganglia have been shown to contain catecholamines, mainly dopamine, along with lower levels of norepinephrine and only a trace amount of epinephrine (13, 23,24,36). Acetylcholine has also been identified. Enzymes involved in catecholamine biosynthesis, such as tyrosine hydroxylase and dopamine beta-hydroxylase, have been localized in chief cells (34), while phenylethanolamine N-methyl transferase (PNMT) is presumed to be present, but in low concentrations since the epinephrine level is so low (13). A negative chromaffin reaction might be attributed to the absence or low level of epinephrine which is responsible for the dark brown color (31). Although norepinephrine has been localized in some head and neck paragangliomas, along with the expected enzymes involved in synthesis of this catecholamine, PNMT and its end product epinephrine are identified mainly in cardiac paragangliomas (26). Cardiac paragangliomas are frequently associated with excess catecholamine secretion, as are pheochromocytomas, causing one to speculate whether some of these paraganglia, and their respective tumors, are more closely aligned with the sympathoadrenal neuroendocrine system. Glenner and Grimley (14) recognized five families of para ganglia and their corresponding tumors; the branchiomeric and intravagal groups account for most of those depicted in figure 14-1.

REFERENCES

1. Acker H. Importance of oxygen supply in the carotid body for chemoreception. Biomed Biochim Acta 1987;46:885–98.
2. Adams WE. The comparative morphology of the carotid body and carotid sinus. Springfield, IL: Charles C. Thomas, 1958.
3. Arias-Stella J, Valcarcel J. Chief cell hyperplasia in the human carotid body at high altitudes: physiologic and pathologic significance. Hum Pathol 1976;7:361–73.
4. Bee D, Howard P. The carotid body: a review of its anatomy, physiology and clinical importance. Monaldi Arch Chest Dis 1993;48(1):48–53.
5. Berger AJ, Mitchell RA, Severinghaus JW. Regulation of respiration (first of three parts). N Engl J Med 1977;297:92–7.
6. Biscoe TJ, Duchen MR. Cellular basis of transduction in carotid chemoreceptors. Am J Physiol 1990; 258:L271–8.
7. Bolande RP. The neurocristopathies. A unifying concept of disease arising in neural crest development. Hum Pathol 1974;5:409–29.
8. DeCastro F. Sur la structure et l'innervation du sinus carotidien de l'homme et des mammifères. Nouveaux faits sur l'innervation et la fonction du glomus caroticum. Études anatomiques et physiologiques. Trab Lab Invest Biol Univ Madr 1928;25:331–80.
9. DeCastro F. Sur la structure de la synapse dans les chemorecepteurs: leur mechanisme d'excitation et role dans la circulation sanguine locale. Acta Physiol Scand 1951;22:14–43.
10. DeLellis RA, Dayal Y. Neuroendocrine system. In: Sternberg SS, ed. Histology for pathologists. New York: Raven Press, 1992:347–62.
11. Dripps RD Jr, Comroe JH Jr. The clinical significance of the carotid and aortic bodies. Am J Med Sci 1944;208:681–94.
12. Feyrter F. Über die these von den peripheren endokrinen drusen. Wien Innere Med Grenzgeb 1946;10:9–36.
13. Fidone SJ, Gonzalez C, Yoshizaki K. Putative neurotransmitters in the carotid body: the case for dopamine. Fed Proc 1980;39:2636–40.
14. Glenner GG, Grimley PM. Tumors of the extra-adrenal paraganglion system (including chemoreceptors). Atlas of Tumor Pathology, 2nd Series, Fascicle 9. Washington, D.C.: Armed Forces Institute of Pathology, 1974.
15. Haller A. Disputationes anatomicae selectae de vera nervi intercostalis origine. Praeside D. Alberto Haller. Gottingae: A Vandenhoeck, Vol II, 1747:939–51.
16. Heath D, Edwards C, Harris P. Post-mortem size and structure of the human carotid body. Its relation to pulmonary disease and cardiac hypertrophy. Thorax 1970;25:129–40.
17. Heymans C, Bouckhaert JJ, Dautrebande L. Sinus carotidien et reflexes respiratoires. II. Influences respiratoires reflexes de l'acidose, de l'alkalose, de l'anhydride carbonique, de l'ion hydrogene et de l'anoxéme. Sinus carotidien et echanges respiratoires dans les poumons et au dela des poumons. Arch Int Pharmacodyn Ther 1930;39:400–50.
18. Jacobs L, Comroe JH Jr. Reflex apnea, bradycardia, and hypotension produced by serotonin and phenyldiguanide acting on the nodose ganglia of the cat. Circ Res 1971;29:145–55.
19. Kohn A. Die paraganglien. Arch fur Mikr Anat 1903;62:263–365.
20. Lack EE. Carotid body hypertrophy in patients with cystic fibrosis and cyanotic congenital heart disease. Hum Pathol 1977;8:39–51.
21. Lack EE. Hyperplasia of vagal and carotid body paraganglia in patients with chronic hypoxemia. Am J Pathol 1978;91:497–516.
22. Lack EE. Pathology of adrenal and extra-adrenal paraganglia. Major problems in pathology, Vol 29. Philadelphia: WB Saunders, 1994.
23. Lack EE, Perez-Atayde AR, Young JB. Carotid body hyperplasia in cystic fibrosis and cyanotic heart disease. A combined morphometric, ultrastructural and biochemical study. Am J Pathol 1985;119:301–14.
24. Lack EE, Perez-Atayde AR, Young JB. Carotid bodies in sudden infant death syndrome: a combined light microscopic, ultrastructural and biochemical study. Ped Pathol 1986;6:335–50.
25. LeDouarin N. The neural crest. Cambridge: Cambridge University Press, 1982.
26. Lloyd RV, Sisson JC, Shapiro B, Verhofstad AA. Immunohistochemical localization of epinephrine, norepinephrine, catecholamine-synthesizing enzymes, and chromogranin in neuroendocrine cells and tumors. Am J Pathol 1986;125:45–54.
27. McDonald DM. Regulation of chemoreceptor sensitivity in the carotid body: the role of presynaptic sensory nerves. Fed Proc 1980;39:2627–35.
28. Neubauer JE. Descriptio anatomica nervorum cardiacorum. Sectio prima de nervo intercostali cervicali, dextri imprimis lateris. Frankfurt and Leipzig: Fleischer, 1772.
29. Pearse AG. The cytochemistry and ultrastructure of polypeptide hormone-producing cells of the APUD series and the embryologic, physiologic and pathologic implications of the concept. J Histochem Cytochem 1969;17:303–13.
30. Saldana MJ, Salem LE, Travezan R. High altitude hypoxia and chemodectomas. Hum Pathol 1973;4:251–63.
31. Sherwin RP. Histopathology of pheochromocytoma. Cancer 1959;12:861–77.
32. Smith P, Jago R, Heath D. Anatomical variation and quantitative histology of the normal and enlarged carotid body. J Pathol 1982;137:287–304.
33. Svitzer E. Einige untersuchungen über das ganglion intercaroticum. Copenhagen: Thiele, 1863.
34. Wang ZZ, Stensaas LJ, Dinger B, Fidone SJ. Co-existence of tyrosine hydroxylase and dopamine beta-hydroxylase immunoreactivity in glomus cells of the cat carotid body. J Auton Nerv Syst 1991;32:259–64.
35. Zak FG, Lawson W. The paraganglionic chemoreceptor system: physiology, pathology and clinical medicine. New York: Springer-Verlag, 1982.
36. Zapata P, Hess A, Bliss EL, Eyzaguirre C. Chemical, electron microscopic and physiological observations on the role of catecholamines in the carotid body. Brain Res 1969;14:473–96.

15
CAROTID BODY PARAGANGLIA

NORMAL ANATOMY OF CAROTID BODY PARAGANGLIA

Gross Morphology. Carotid body paraganglia are distinguished by their location, macroscopic dimensions, compactness, and multilobular architecture; aside from these features the fundamental microanatomy is virtually identical to that of other paraganglia of the head and neck region. Carotid bodies are round to ovoid or flattened structures which are pale tan to pink and situated on both sides of the neck in close relation to the medial aspect of the common carotid artery bifurcation (fig. 15-1). Occasionally the carotid body is located along the internal or external carotid artery branch or even adjacent to the uppermost part of the common carotid artery, a location that can explain the rare angiographic appearance of a carotid body paraganglioma without significant splaying apart of the carotid artery branches (14). Carotid body paraganglia are located within adventitia without being directly connected to the media of the adjacent artery. Their average dimensions are 3.3 x 2.2 x 1.7 mm in adults (3), but they are often considerably smaller in infants. Occasionally the carotid body appears bilobed (fig. 15-1) or even trilobed (16). A fibrovascular pedicle (ligament of Mayer) may be seen carrying one or more small glomic arteries which supply the lower pole of the carotid body (4,10), as well as small myelinated nerve bundles (fig. 15-2) (12). The average combined weight of carotid bodies in patients under age 50 years (fig. 15-3) is normally a little over 12 mg, but this depends upon the effort taken to remove excess connective tissue, preferably with the aid of a dissecting microscope (14,16). The weight of bilateral carotid bodies is similar (3,13,15,16,22).

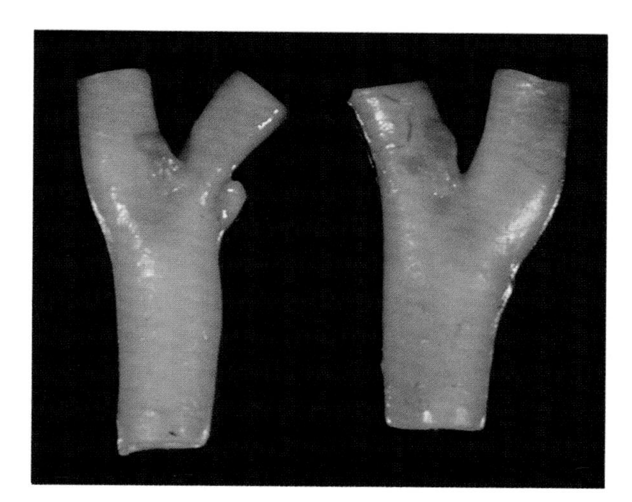

Figure 15-1
BILATERAL CAROTID BODIES

Bilateral carotid bodies from a 12-year-old boy who died of metastatic malignant melanoma. Combined weight of both carotid bodies was 13.3 mg, and both are located on the medial aspect of the carotid bifurcation. Carotid body on right is bilobed. (Fig. 2 from Lack EE. Paragangliomas. In: Sternberg SS, ed. Diagnostic surgical pathology. 2nd ed. New York: Raven Press, 1994:600.)

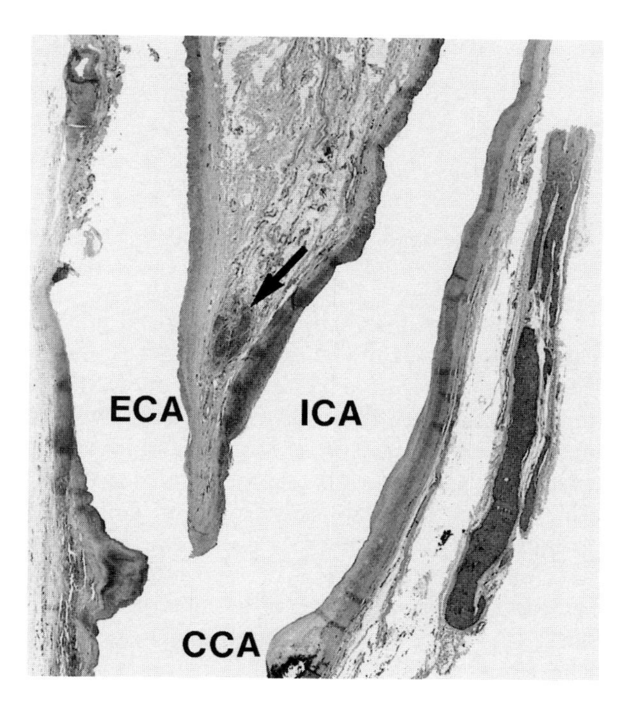

Figure 15-2
CAROTID BODY PARAGANGLION

Common carotid artery (CCA) with external (ECA) and internal (ICA) carotid artery branches from an adult patient at autopsy. Note the carotid body paraganglion in the adventitial connective tissue of the carotid bifurcation (arrow). Dilation of the proximal ICA represents carotid sinus which has baroreceptor function. Profiles of small glomic arteries are present in fibrous connective tissue near the inferior pole of the carotid body.

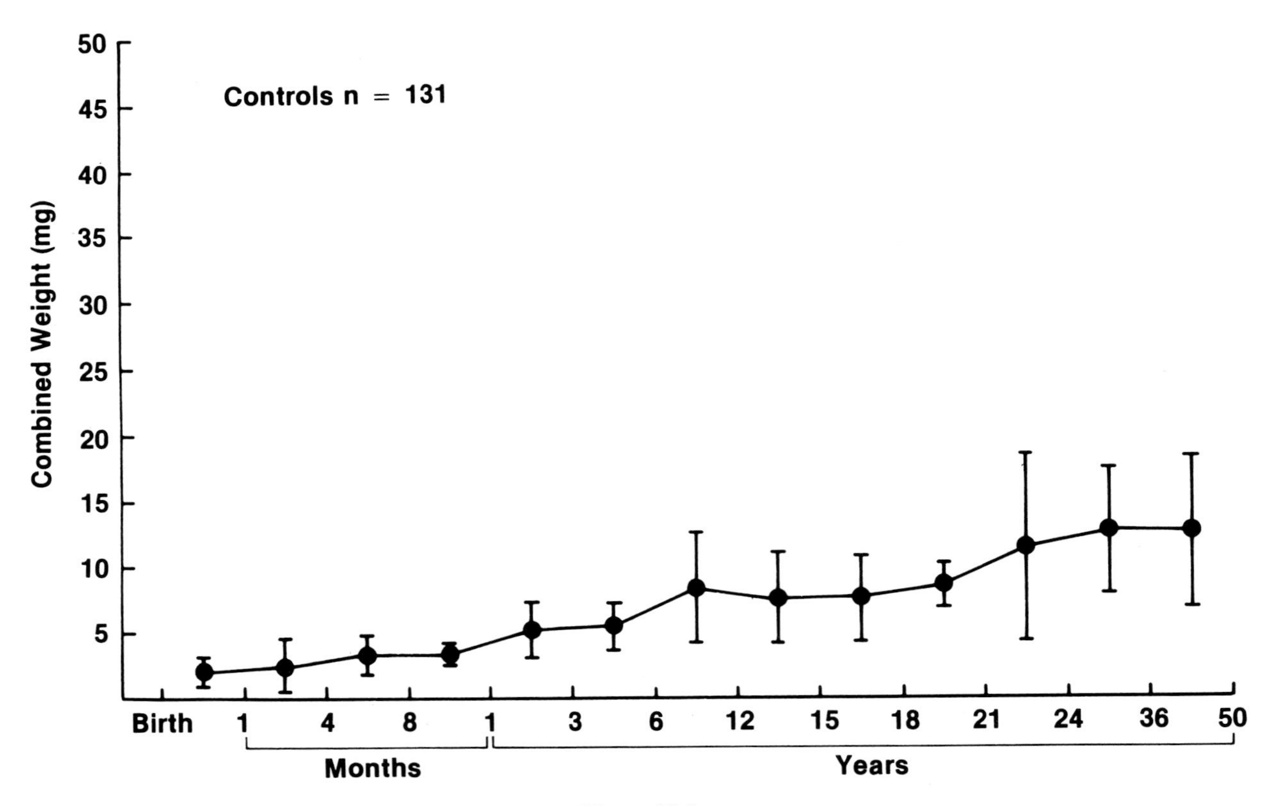

Figure 15-3
AVERAGE COMBINED WEIGHTS OF CAROTID BODIES
Average combined weight of both carotid bodies is plotted according to arbitrary age intervals up to 50 years of age. The average combined weights in adults is a little over 12 mg. The control population (n=131) had no evidence of chronic hypoxemia or systemic hypertension. Vertical bars represent one standard deviation.

Microscopic Anatomy. The carotid body is composed of multiple lobules which are rounded, ovoid, or angular, and may appear partially molded to each other (fig. 15-4). The average number of lobules in cross section usually varies from 11 to 14 for various age intervals into adult life (16). Similar to individual or combined weights of carotid bodies, there is an increase with age in area of the entire structure in cross section or area occupied by lobules (arbitrarily designated functional parenchyma) (fig. 15-5). There are two basic types of cells: chief (or glomus type 1) cells and sustentacular (glomus type 2) cells. There is good experimental evidence for a neural crest origin of carotid body chief cells (19), and presumably, chief cells of other paraganglia in the head and neck region share a similar line of embryogenesis. Chief cells are arranged in round to elongated nests, and often have an eccentric, dark-staining nucleus with granular eosinophilic or amphophilic cytoplasm (fig. 15-6). Three types of chief cells have been recognized: "light" cells, "dark" cells, and pyknotic cells (subsequently referred to as progenitor cells [6]), but there is some question as to whether the nuclear changes are related to postmortem autolysis (18). At present there is no known functional significance that can be ascribed to these different types of chief cells (14).

Sustentacular cells have pale, indistinct cytoplasm with an elongated or crescentic nucleus; they are located at the periphery of clusters of chief cells (fig. 15-6). Ultrastructurally, these cells have been reported to resemble Schwann cells, enough so, in fact, that distinction between the two is not always possible (11). As one might anticipate, doing reliable differential cell counts of chief, sustentacular, and other cells can be very difficult (14). The sustentacular cells can be demonstrated by staining for S-100 protein (fig. 15-7),

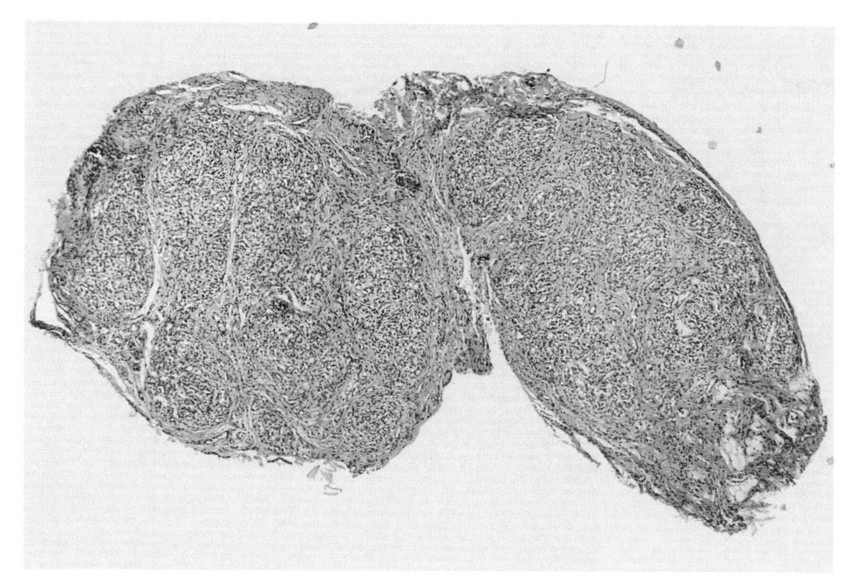

Figure 15-4
CAROTID BODY PARAGANGLIA
Both carotid bodies are from a 38-year-old patient. Note the ovoid shape with multiple lobules. These carotid bodies are well-circumscribed but not truly encapsulated. (X25, Hematoxylin and eosin stain)

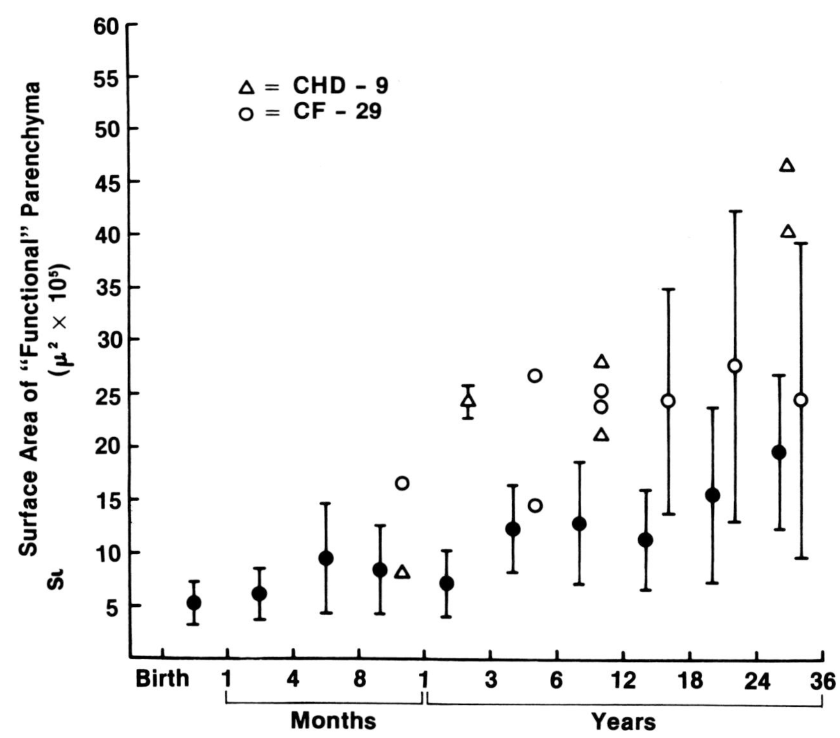

Figure 15-5
AREA OCCUPIED BY LOBULES
This area occupied by lobules has arbitrarily been designated "functional parenchyma" and is plotted according to arbitrary age intervals. Note the gradual increase with age similar to carotid body weight. Vertical bar represents one standard deviation. (Fig. 10 from Lack EE, Perez-Atayde AR, Young JB. Carotid body hyperplasia in cystic fibrosis and cyanotic heart disease. A combined morphometric, ultrastructural, and biochemical study. Am J Pathol 1985;119:301–14.) (CHD = cyanotic heart disease; CF = cystic fibrosis.)

but given the rich innervation of the carotid body, some of these immunopositive cells are likely to be Schwann cells. The nesting pattern of chief cells can be accentuated by staining for cytoplasmic argyrophilia (fig. 15-8, left) or chromogranin A (fig. 15-8, right). Carotid body paraganglia contain catecholamines of which dopamine is present in greatest concentration, followed by norepinephrine (15,16,23). Enzymes involved in epinephrine synthesis (e.g., tyrosine hydroxylase) have been localized immunocytochemically in chief cells (24) along with a variety of neuropeptides

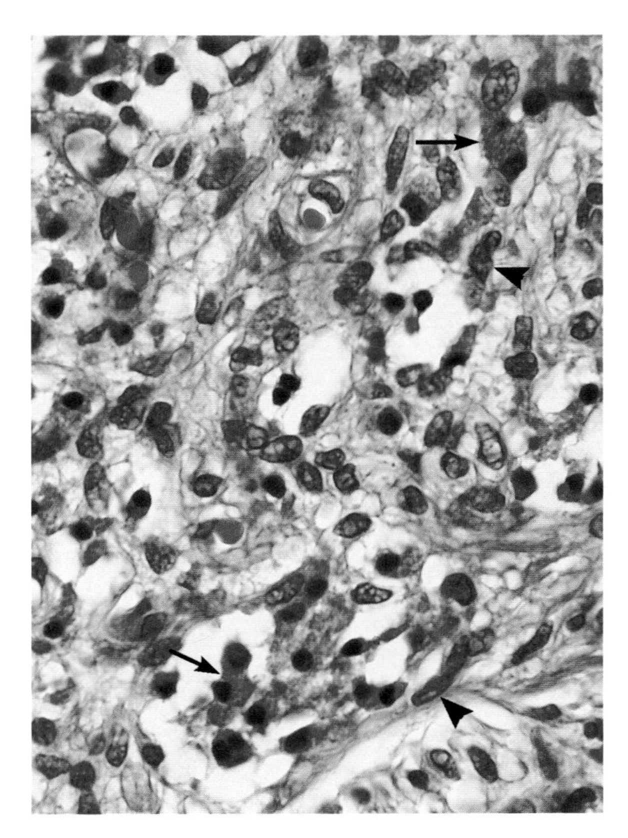

Figure 15-6
CAROTID BODY PARAGANGLION
FROM NEWBORN INFANT

There are clusters of chief cells with dark staining nuclei and eosinophilic, somewhat granular cytoplasm (arrows). Sustentacular cells are in close association with chief cells and have ovoid to elongate, pale-staining nuclei (arrowheads).

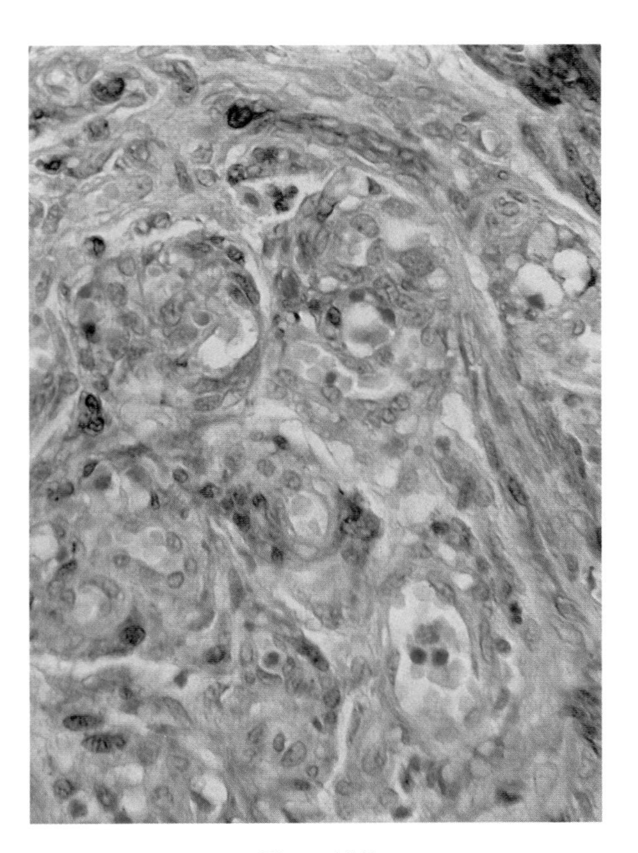

Figure 15-7
SUSTENTACULAR CELLS
POSITIVE FOR S-100 PROTEIN

These cells, positive for S-100 protein, show staining of both nucleus and cytoplasm and are situated at the periphery of chief cell nests and cords. (X200, Peroxidase-antiperoxidase stain)

(6,7,14,21). A variety of histologic changes have been described in carotid bodies such as decrease in lobule size and fibrosis with aging (9,17), chronic carotid glomitis (5), vascular telangiectasia (probably agonal due to passive congestion), and Schwann cell proliferation which may be focal or diffuse in distribution (14). Ganglion cells have only rarely been reported within interlobular connective tissue of the carotid body (20).

Ultrastructural Anatomy. There have been relatively few ultrastructural studies done on human carotid body and other head and neck paraganglia, and only selected references are cited (1,2,8,11,12,15,16); because of advanced autolysis in postmortem material there are certain limitations in performing optimal electron microscopy (14). Ultrastructural study of glomectomy specimens obtained surgically from patients with underlying pulmonary disease might provide more optimal morphology, but the endocrine tissue in this setting may not be entirely normal (14). Survey views show the complexity of carotid body paraganglia, as well as other paraganglia in the head and neck region (fig. 15-9) (12). Chief cells often show a mosaic interdigitation of cell cytoplasm, sometimes with partial encirclement of one cell by another, the so-called cell-embracing which can also be found in the corresponding paraganglioma (14). Light and dark cells have been identified, with the latter often having numerous dense-core neurosecretory granules (fig. 15-10). Neurosecretory granules usually have a uniform electron-dense core with a narrow symmetric halo between the

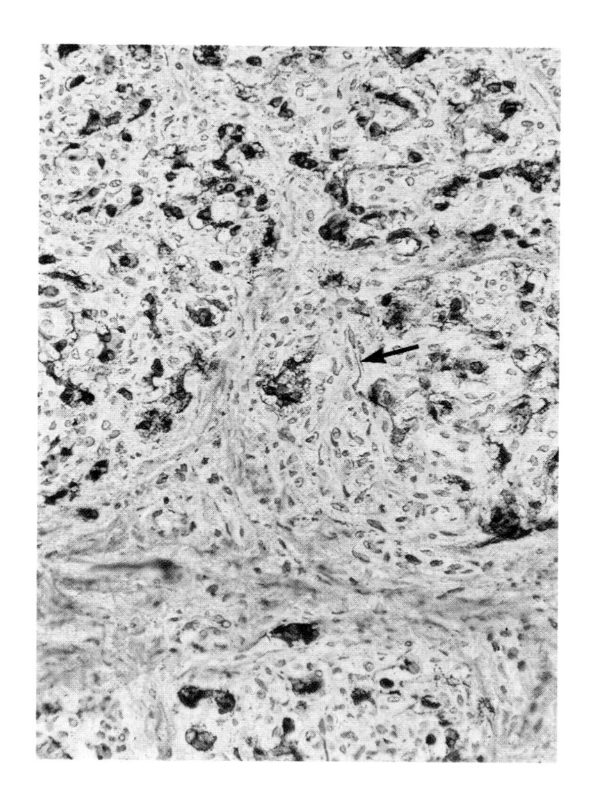

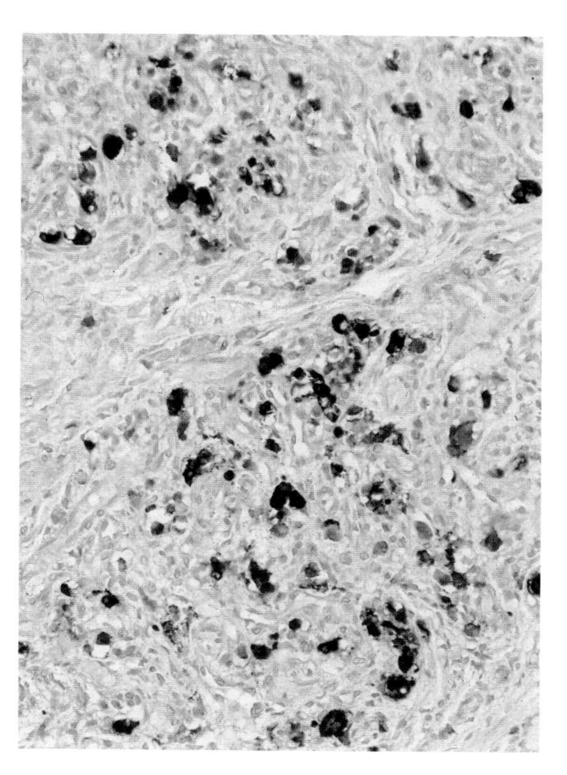

Figure 15-8
NORMAL CAROTID BODY PARAGANGLION

Left: Normal carotid body from an adult showing cytoplasmic argyrophilia of chief cell cytoplasm. The staining reaction within the multiple lobules reveals the distinct clusters and short cords of chief cells. Axonal or dendritic neural processes are also well delineated (arrow) between and within lobules. (X120, Bodian axon stain)

Right: Normal carotid body from a young adult. Distinct clusters of chief cells are seen within several lobules and show strong immunostaining for chromogranin A. (X140, Peroxidase-antiperoxidase stain)

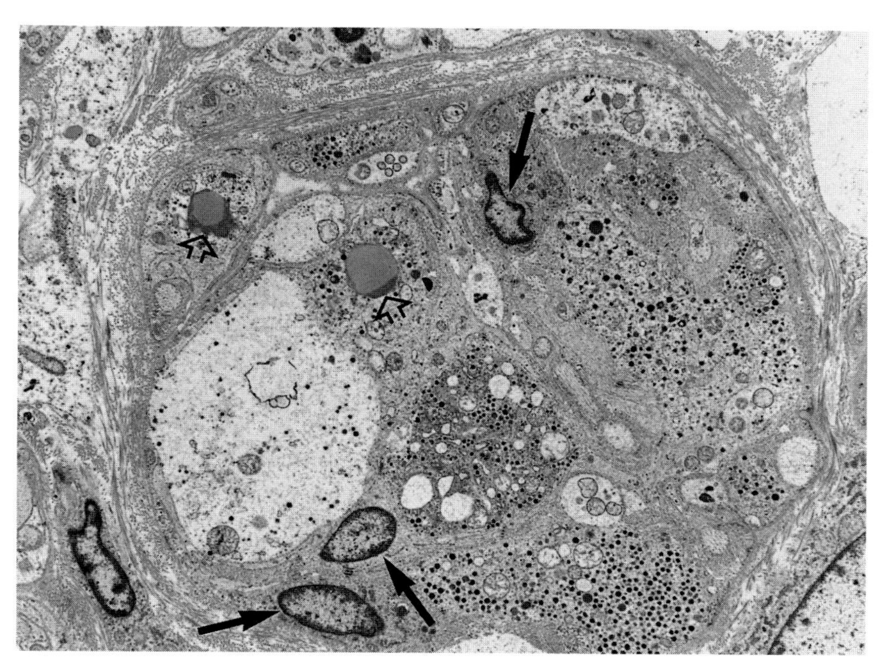

Figure 15-9
ADULT CAROTID BODY OBTAINED AT AUTOPSY

Clusters of chief cells within a carotid body lobule. There is an admixture of both "light" and "dark" chief cells, with the latter having increased number and higher density of dense-core neurosecretory granules. Sustentacular cells (straight arrows) are located at the periphery and have thin, complex cytoplasmic extensions which partially envelop the chief cells. Lipofuscin is indicated by open arrows. (X2,000)

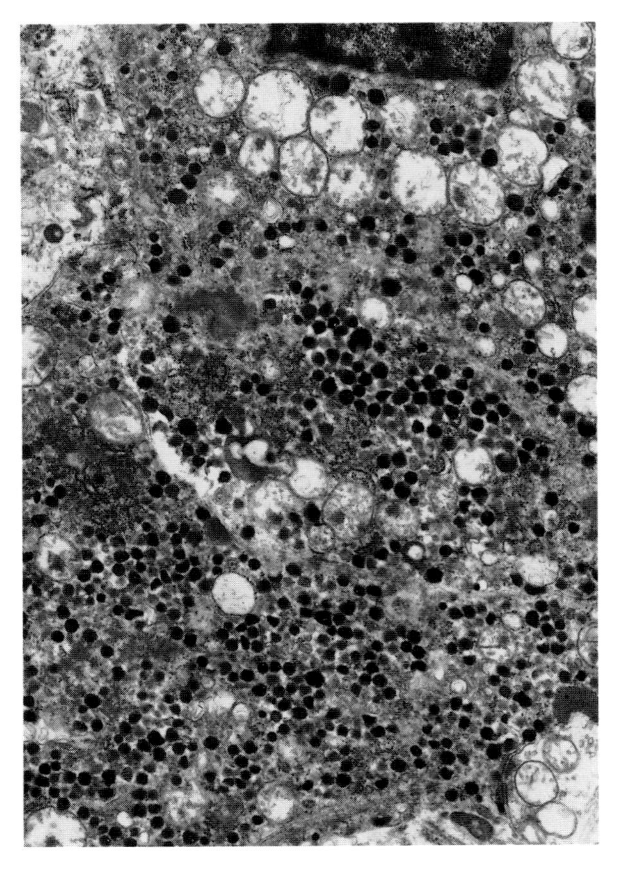

Figure 15-10
CAROTID BODY FROM A VICTIM OF SUDDEN INFANT DEATH SYNDROME

The chief cells contain numerous dense-core neurosecretory granules. There was no evidence of significant depletion of granules compared with carotid bodies from an age-related group without SIDS. (X11,600) (Fig. 2-19 from Lack EE. Pathology of adrenal and extra-adrenal paraganglia. In: Major problems in pathology, Vol 29. Philadelphia: WB Saunders Co, Philadelphia, 1994:28.)

limiting membrane. Granule diameters usually range from 100 to 200 nm; in a study of the fetal carotid body the average diameter of neurosecretory granules was 110 nm (12). Some chief cells contain electron-dense material associated with lipid droplets, typical for lipofuscin (14).

Sustentacular cells have sparse cellular organelles with small amounts of rough endoplasmic reticulum and bundles of thin (actin-like) filaments. Sustentacular cells in close proximity to chief cells usually have long, tapering cytoplasmic processes, occasionally forming simple mesaxons with axonal processes; Schwann cells are readily distinguished from sustentacular cells when the myelin sheath is well developed. According to Jago et al. (11) the only reliable feature that distinguishes sustentacular cells is the extension of the cell processes which envelop chief cells. Other types of cells in carotid body and other head and neck paraganglia include abundant endothelial cells, pericytes, and occasional mast cells. Efferent-type synaptic junctions have been noted in the human fetus; some are probably sympathetic due to very small dense-core granules (8); in the study by Grimley and Glenner (2), afferent-type terminals were not identified, although there is compelling experimental data to presume their existence in humans.

HYPERPLASIA OF CAROTID BODY PARAGANGLIA

Definition. Carotid body hyperplasia represents an increase in number of chief (glomus type 1) cells, often accompanied by proliferation of other cell types such as sustentacular (glomus type 2) cells. Cellular proliferation may result in carotid body hypertrophy, which is usually bilateral and roughly symmetrical.

General Remarks. Hyperplasia (diffuse or nodular) of adrenal medullae with consequent hypertrophy has been covered in chapter 9, particularly in the setting of multiple endocrine neoplasia (MEN) syndromes type IIa and IIb in which the pathologic changes clearly antedate the development of pheochromocytomas. The gross and microscopic counterparts in paraganglia of the head and neck region, particularly carotid bodies, are much smaller, and the underlying or associated abnormalities for the most part appear to be basically physiologic (42). Although carotid body and other types of paragangliomas may have familial occurrence with varied Mendelian inheritance patterns (43), many pathologic abnormalities are reported in individuals dwelling at high altitudes (25,27,28,31,39,47–49), where a 10-fold increased incidence of "chemodectomas" has been reported (49). A relationship between chronic hypoxemia and carotid body enlargement (sometimes resembling "chemodectomas") has been noted in bovines at high altitude (26). Carotid body hypertrophy and hyperplasia has also been reported under normobaric conditions in individuals with chronic obstructive pulmonary disease and systemic hypertension (29,32,33,35,37,38,41,46,

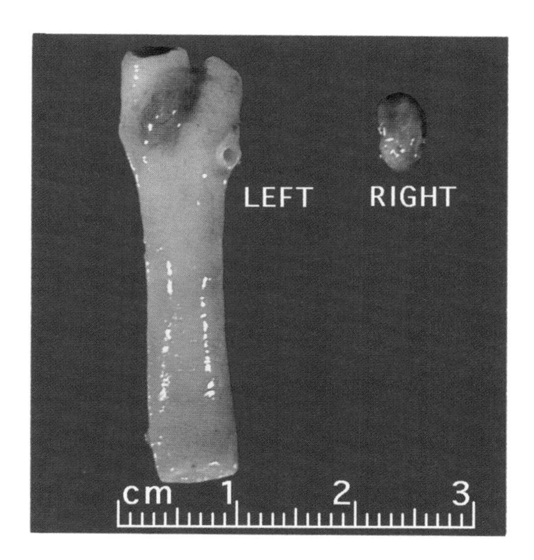

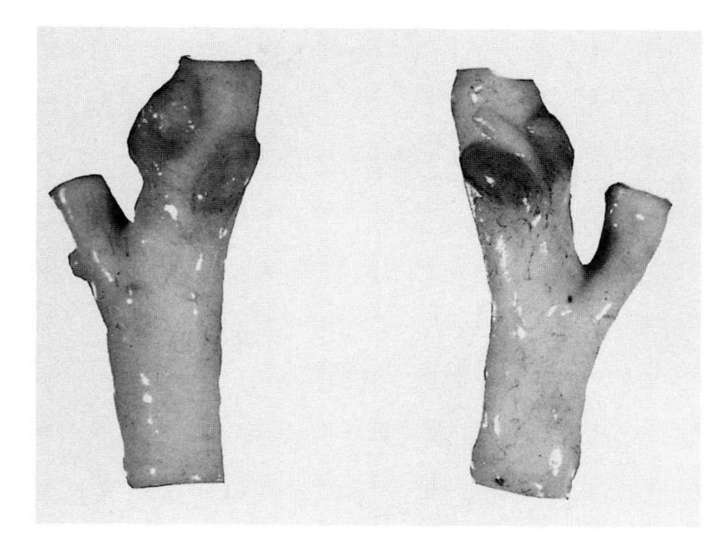

Figure 15-11
HYPERPLASTIC CAROTID BODY PARAGANGLIA

Left: An enlarged hyperplastic carotid body from a 21-year-old woman with cystic fibrosis is located on the medial aspect of the carotid bifurcation. Both carotid bodies were dark compared with normal, and had a combined weight of 70.0 mg.

Right: Enlarged hyperplastic carotid bodies from a 24-year-old woman with cystic fibrosis had a combined weight of 80.3 mg. Both are bilobed and situated along the medial aspect of the internal carotid arteries. The bilobed carotid body on one side has a small vessel emerging from internal carotid artery. (Modified from fig. 4 from Lack EE. Carotid body hypertrophy in patients with cystic fibrosis and cyanotic congenital heart disease. Hum Pathol 1977;8:39–51.)

50), as well as in patients with chronic hypoxemia due to cystic fibrosis and cyanotic heart disease (40,44). Hyperplasia of vagal (41,43) and aorticopulmonary paraganglia (43) has been described, thus supporting a chemoreceptor role for these paraganglia. Chemodectoma-like tumors have been described in relatively stationary cod fish dwelling in more or less polluted waters, but the etiology of these tumors is unclear (45).

Gross Morphology. The hyperplastic carotid body is enlarged, ovoid, often dark in color (fig. 15-11, left), and occasionally bilobed (fig. 15-11, right). Three criteria have been proposed for the diagnosis of carotid body hyperplasia: 1) combined carotid body weight over 30 mg; 2) mean diameter of lobules greater than 565 μm; and 3) a more than 47 percent increase in the differential count of elongated cells over chief cells (50). Individual or combined weight of carotid bodies should be correlated with an age-related control population because there is variation in weight and surface area with age (40,43,44).

Microscopic Anatomy. With carotid body hypertrophy and hyperplasia there is an increase in total cross sectional surface area as well as area occupied by lobules, and in some cases there may be an increase in the number of lobules (fig. 15-12). Hyperplasia of lobules may be accompanied by an attenuation in intervening fibrovascular connective tissue, resulting in what appears to be confluence of lobules (43). There tends to be a roughly proportional increase in chief cells as well as sustentacular cells (fig. 15-13); there may also be variation in size, shape, and intensity of nuclear staining of chief cells (43). Depletion of naturally fluorescing biogenic amines has been reported at high altitudes (27); as a corollary to this observation, there may be greatly diminished staining for cytoplasmic argyrophilia (fig. 15-14, left) and chromogranin A immunoreactivity (fig. 15-14, right) compared with controls (43). In adult and elderly patients, some investigators have noted a significant proliferation of elongated cells, mainly sustentacular cells, with a concentric or "onion skin" configuration and apparent compression of central cores of chief cells (fig. 15-15) (50). Proliferation of dark cells has also been described (34). It is difficult to envision how this type of hyperplasia can progress to the histologic appearance of the chief cell hyperplasia and "chemodectomas"

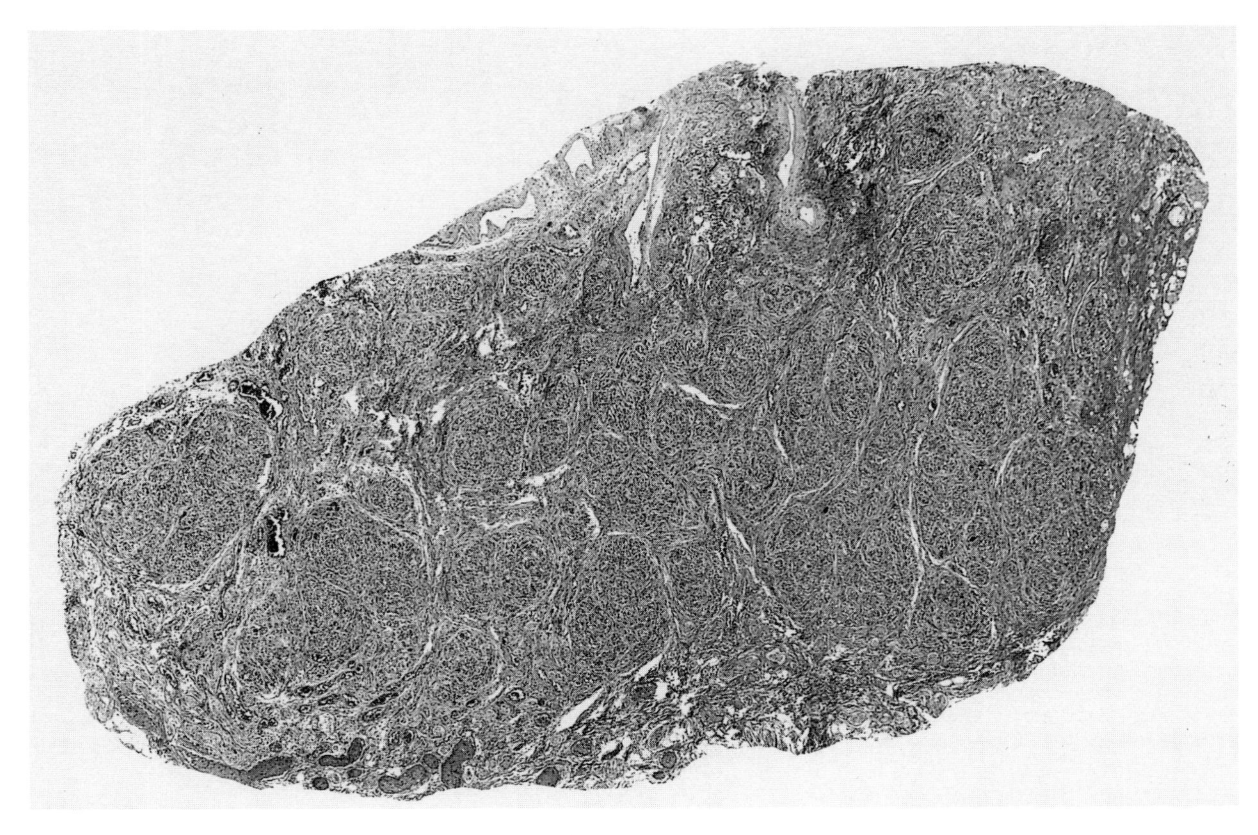

Figure 15-12
HYPERPLASTIC CAROTID BODY PARAGANGLION

Enlarged hyperplastic carotid body from a 21-year-old woman with cystic fibrosis (see figure 15-11, left). This carotid body contains increased numbers of lobules compared with control carotid bodies. Some appear to become confluent. Compare the size with normal carotid bodies in figure 15-4 which were photographed at a slightly higher magnification. (X20, Hematoxylin and eosin)

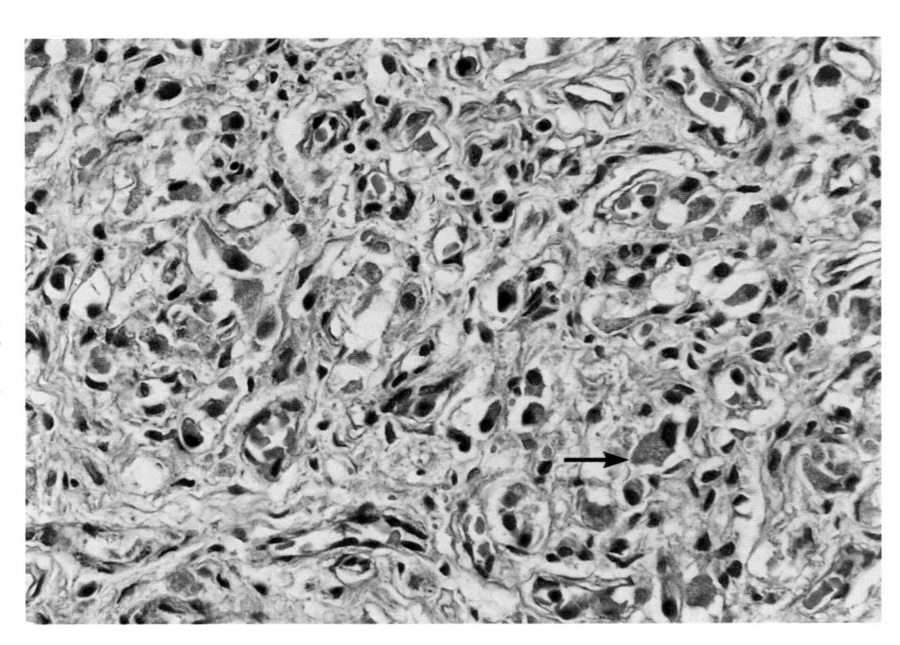

Figure 15-13
HYPERPLASTIC
CAROTID BODY

Enlarged hyperplastic carotid body from a young adult with cystic fibrosis. Lobules are increased in size and appear to merge. Most chief cell nuclei are hyperchromatic and some are enlarged slightly. Some chief cells had small cytoplasmic vacuoles (arrow).

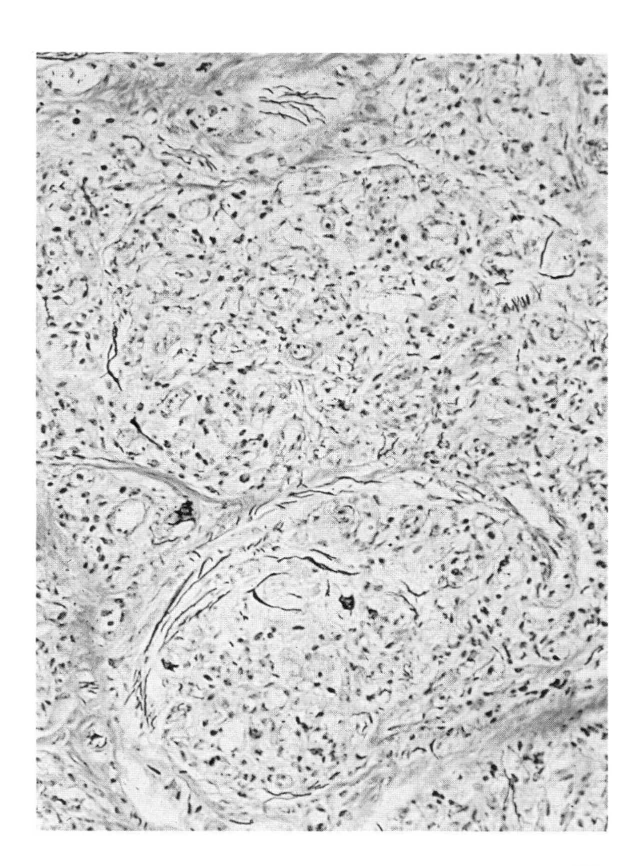

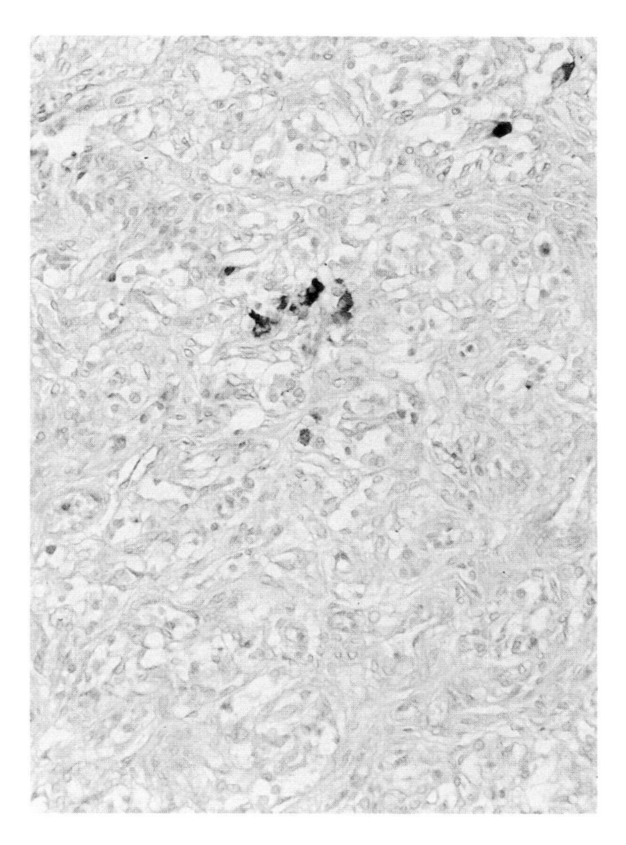

Figure 15-14
CAROTID BODY HYPERTROPHY AND HYPERPLASIA

Left: Carotid body hypertrophy and hyperplasia in a young adult with cystic fibrosis. The carotid body lobules show a marked decrease in argyrophilia of chief cell cytoplasm, yet neural processes stain well. Compare with the normal carotid body in figure 15-8, left. (X120, Bodian axon stain)

Right: Hyperplastic carotid body from a different patient with cystic fibrosis. There is a marked decrease in immunostaining of chief cells for chromogranin A compared with figure 15-8, right. (X120, Peroxidase-antiperoxidase stain)

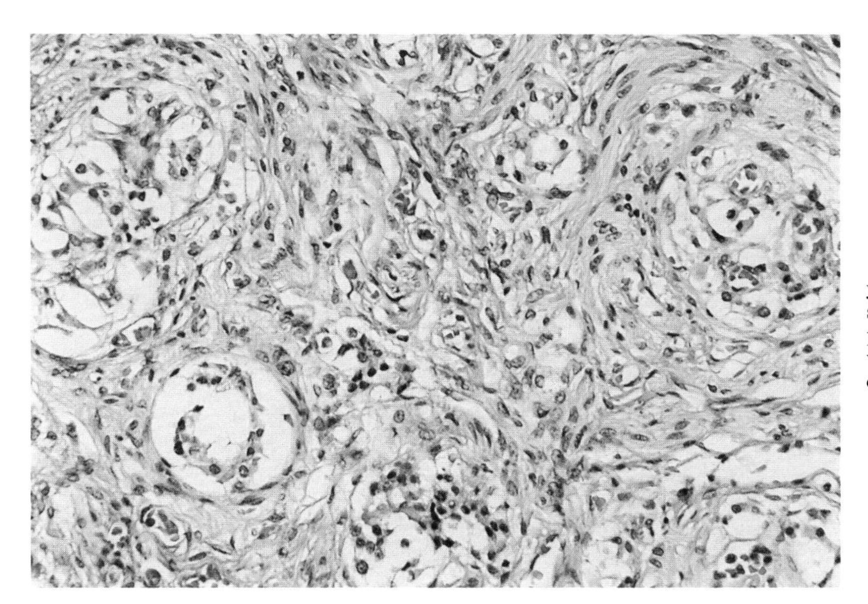

Figure 15-15
HYPERPLASTIC CAROTID BODY

Hyperplastic carotid body from a 54-year-old woman with severe chronic obstructive pulmonary disease. Note the prominent spindle cell component within the lobules surrounding clusters of chief cells.

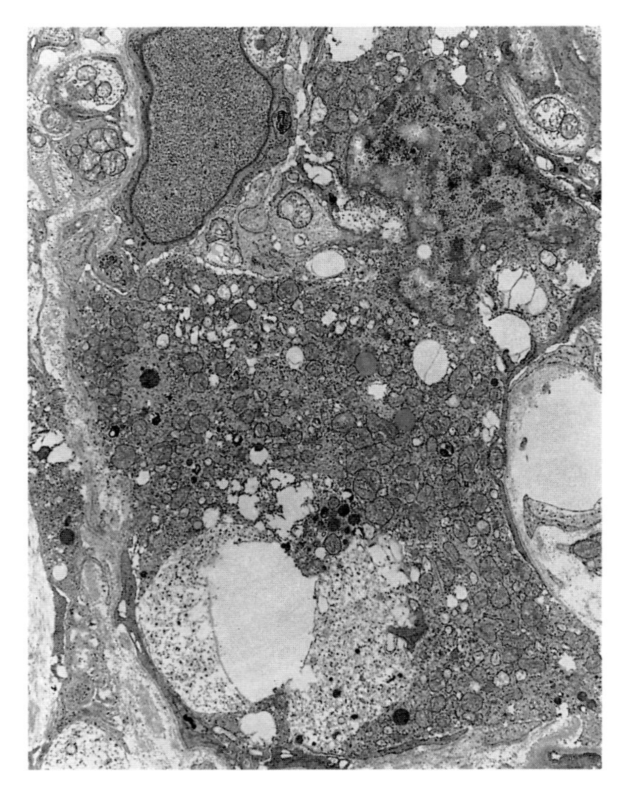

Figure 15-16
HYPERPLASTIC CAROTID BODY
Enlarged hyperplastic carotid body obtained at autopsy from a young adult with cystic fibrosis. Chief cells showed severe depletion of dense-core neurosecretory granules. (X6,500)

which have been illustrated in humans (27,49) and bovines at high altitude (26).

Ultrastructural Anatomy. In a recent study of carotid bodies from eight patients with cystic fibrosis, each showed a moderate to marked decrease in the number of dense-core neurosecretory granules (fig. 15-16) which were either patchy or diffuse throughout the lobules studied (44). In another study, proliferation of sustentacular cells was reported in a patient with carotid body hyperplasia while chief cells were not considered to be abnormal (36). Proliferation of nerve axons has also been described (30,36).

RISK FOR DEVELOPMENT OF "CHEMODECTOMA" UNDER NORMOBARIC CONDITIONS

There are only anecdotal accounts of carotid body paragangliomas occurring under normobaric conditions in humans with chronic obstructive pulmonary disease (52), systemic hypertension (53), and cyanotic heart disease (56), including a patient with a malignant paraganglioma in another location (51). In general, however, there is currently no convincing evidence of any significant risk of developing a paraganglioma of peripheral arterial chemoreceptors, such as carotid bodies, in patients who have these conditions (54,55).

REFERENCES

Normal Anatomy of Carotid Body Paraganglia

1. Böck P, Stockinger L, Vyslonzil E. Die feinstruktur des glomus caroticum beim menschen. Z Zellforsch Mikrosk Anat 1970;105:543–68.
2. Grimley PM, Glenner GG. Ultrastructure of the human carotid body. A perspective on the mode of chemoreception. Circulation 1968;37:648–65.
3. Heath D, Edwards C, Harris P. Post-mortem size and structure of the human carotid body. Thorax 1970;25:129–40.
4. Heath D, Jago R, Smith P. The vasculature of the carotid body. Cardiovasc Res 1983;17:33–42.
5. Heath D, Khan Q. Focal chronic thyroiditis and chronic carotid glomitis. J Pathol 1989;159:29–34.
6. Heath D, Khan Q, Smith P. Histopathology of the carotid bodies in neonates and infants. Histopathology 1990;17:511–20.
7. Heath D, Quinzanini M, Rodella A, Albertini A, Ferrari R, Harris P. Immunoreactivity to various peptides in the human carotid body. Res Commun Chem Pharmacol 1988;62:289–93.
8. Hervonen A, Korkala O. Fine structure of the carotid body of the midterm human fetus. Z Anat Entwicklungsmach Gesch 1972;138:135–44.
9. Hurst G, Heath D, Smith P. Histological changes associated with ageing of the human carotid body. J Pathol 1985;147:181–7.
10. Jago R, Heath D, Smith P. Structure of the glomic arteries. J Pathol 1982;138:205–18.
11. Jago R, Smith P, Heath D. Electron microscopy of carotid body hyperplasia. Arch Pathol Lab Med 1984;108:717–22.
12. Kjaergaard J. Anatomy of the carotid glomus, and carotid glomus-like bodies (non-chromaffin paraganglia). With electron microscopy and comparison of human fetal carotid, aorticopulmonary, subclavian, tympanojugular, and vagal glomera. Copenhagen: FADL's Forlag, 1973.

13. Lack EE. Carotid body hypertrophy in patients with cystic fibrosis and cyanotic congenital heart disease. Hum Pathol 1977;8:39–51.
14. Lack EE. Pathology of adrenal and extra-adrenal paraganglia. Major problems in pathology, Vol 29. Philadelphia: WB Saunders, 1994.
15. Lack EE, Perez-Atayde AR, Young JB. Carotid bodies in sudden infant death syndrome: a combined light microscopic, ultrastructural, and biochemical study. Pediatr Pathol 1986;6:335–50.
16. Lack EE, Perez-Atayde AR, Young JB. Carotid body hyperplasia in cystic fibrosis and cyanotic heart disease. A combined morphometric, ultrastructural, and biochemical study. Am J Pathol 1985;119:301–14.
17. Lowe P, Heath D, Smith P. Relation between histological age-changes in the carotid body and atherosclerosis in the carotid arteries. J Laryngol Otol 1987;101:1271–5.
18. Pallot DJ, Seker M, Abramovici A. Post-mortem changes in the normal rat carotid body: possible implications for human histopathology. Virchows Arch [A] 1992:420:31–5.
19. Pearse AG, Polak JM, Rost FW, Fontaine J, Le Lievre C, Le Douarin N. Demonstration of the neural crest origin of type I (APUD) cells in the avian carotid body, using a cytochemical marker system. Histochemie 1973;34:191–203.
20. Pryse-Davies J, Dawson IM, Westbury G. Some morphologic, histochemical, and chemical observations on chemodectomas and the normal carotid body, including a study of the chromaffin reaction and possible ganglion cell elements. Cancer 1964;17:185–202.
21. Smith P, Gosney J, Heath D, Burnett H. The occurrence and distribution of certain polypeptides within the human carotid body. Cell Tissue Res 1990;261:565–71.
22. Smith P, Jago R, Heath D. Anatomical variation and quantitative histology of the normal and enlarged carotid body. J Pathol 1982;137:287–304.
23. Steele RH, Hinterberger H. Catecholamines and 5-hydroxytryptamine in the carotid body in vascular, respiratory and other diseases. J Lab Clin Med 1972;80:63–70.
24. Tischler AS. Paraganglia. In: Sternberg SS, ed. Histology for pathologists, New York: Raven Press, 1992:363–79.

Hypertrophy and Hyperplasia of Carotid Body Paraganglia

25. Arias-Stella J. Human carotid body at high altitude [Abstract]. Am J Pathol 1969;55:82a.
26. Arias-Stella J, Bustos F. Chronic hypoxia and chemodectomas in bovines at high altitudes. Arch Pathol Lab Med 1976;100:636–9.
27. Arias-Stella J, Valcarcel J. Chief cell hyperplasia in the human carotid body at high altitudes: physiologic and pathologic significance. Hum Pathol 1976;7:361–73.
28. De La Vega J, Takano J. Tumores del corpusculo carotideo en el hombre de las grandes alturas. Presented at the Ninth Latin-American Congress of Pathology, Merida, Yucatan, Mexico, November 25–30, 1973.
29. Edwards C, Heath D, Harris P. The carotid body in emphysema and left vertricular hypertrophy. J Pathol 1971;104:1–13.
30. Fitch R, Smith P, Heath D. Nerve axons in carotid body hyperplasia. A quantitative study. Arch Pathol Lab Med 1985;109:234–7.
31. Gaylis H, Davidge-Pitts K, Pantanowitz D. Carotid body tumors. A review of 52 cases. S Afr Med J 1987;72:493–6.
32. Habeck JO. Morphological findings at the carotid bodies of humans suffering from different types of systemic hypertension or severe lung diseases. Anat Anz 1986;162:17–27.
33. Heath D, Edwards C, Harris P. Post-mortem size and structure of the human carotid body. Thorax 1970;25:129–40.
34. Heath D, Smith P, Jago R. Dark cell proliferation in carotid body hyperplasia. J Pathol 1984;142:39–49.
35. Heath D, Smith P, Jago R. Hyperplasia of the carotid body. J Pathol 1982;138:115–27.
36. Jago R, Smith P, Heath D. Electron microscopy of carotid body hyperplasia. Arch Pathol Lab Med 1984;108:717–22.
37. Janzer RC, Schneider J. The influence of chronically hypoxemic states on human carotid body structure and cardiac hypertrophy. Virchows Arch [A] 1977;376:75–87.
38. Kluge P. Vascularization and morphology of carotid bodies in patients with essential hypertension. Acta Physiol Pol 1985;36:76–82.
39. Krause-Senties L. Tumores del cuerpo carotideo. Arch Invest Med 1971;2:25–30.
40. Lack EE. Carotid body hypertrophy in patients with cystic fibrosis and cyanotic congenital heart disease. Hum Pathol 1977;8:39–51.
41. Lack EE. Hyperplasia of vagal and carotid body paraganglia in patients with chronic hypoxemia. Am J Pathol 1978;91:497–516.
42. Lack EE. Paragangliomas. In: Sternberg SS, ed. Diagnostic surgical pathology, 2nd ed. New York: Raven Press, 1994:599–621.
43. Lack EE. Pathology of adrenal and extra-adrenal paraganglia. Major problems in pathology, Vol 29. Philadelphia: WB Saunders, 1994.
44. Lack EE, Perez-Atayde AR, Young JB. Carotid body hyperplasia in cystic fibrosis and cyanotic heart disease. A combined morphometric, ultrastructural, and biochemical study. Am J Pathol 1985;119:301–14.
45. Lange E, Johannessen JV. Histochemical and ultrastructural studies of chemodectoma-like tumors in the cod (Gadus morrhua L.). Lab Invest 1977;37:96–104.
46. Lange F. Vergröberung des glomus caroticum bei allen formen der hypertonie. Dtsch Med Wschr, Stuttgart 1962;87:13–6.
47. Pacheco-Ojeda L, Darango E, Rodriguez C, Vivar N. Carotid body tumors at high altitudes: Quito, Ecuador, 1987. World J Surg 1988;12:856–60.
48. Rodriguez-Cuevas H, Lau I, Rodriguez HP. High altitude paragangliomas, diagnostic and therapeutic considerations. Cancer 1986;57:672–76.
49. Saldana MJ, Salem LE, Travezan R. High altitude hypoxia and chemodectomas. Hum Pathol 1973;4:251–63.
50. Smith P, Jago R, Heath D. Anatomical variation and quantitative histology of the normal and enlarged carotid body. J Pathol 1982;137:287–304.

"Chemodectomas" Under Normobaric Conditions

51. Bockelman HW, Arya S, Gilbert EF. Cyanotic congenital heart disease with malignant paraganglioma. Cancer 1982;50:2513–7.
52. Chedid A, Jao W. Hereditary tumors of the carotid bodies and chronic obstructive pulmonary disease. Cancer 1974;33:1635–41.
53. Heath D, Smith P, Jago R. Hyperplasia of the carotid body. J Pathol 1982;138:115–27.
54. Lack EE. Paragangliomas. In: Sternberg SS, ed. Diagnostic surgical pathology, 2nd ed. New York: Raven Press, 1994:599–621.
55. Lack EE. Pathology of adrenal and extra-adrenal paraganglia. Major problems in pathology, Vol 29. Philadelphia: WB Saunders, 1994.
56. Nissenblatt MJ. Cyanotic heart disease: low altitude risk for carotid body tumor? J Hop Med J 1978;142:12–21.

16
CAROTID BODY PARAGANGLIOMA

Definition. Carotid body paraganglioma (CBP) is an endocrine neoplasm arising from the chief cells of carotid body paraganglia. It is also referred to as a *chemodectoma.*

General Remarks. Paragangliomas in the head and neck region are termed according to the anatomic site of origin. Five families of paraganglia (and the respective paragangliomas) were described by Glenner and Grimley (2): branchiomeric, intravagal, aorticosympathetic, visceral-autonomic, and adrenal; the branchiomeric and intravagal are the main groups recognized in the head and neck region. CBP is the prototypic tumor of the head and neck paraganglion system, analogous to pheochromocytoma (adrenal medullary paraganglioma) of the sympathoadrenal neuroendocrine system (4,5). The term chemodectoma (chemeia: infusion; deschesthai: to receive; oma: tumor) was introduced by Mulligan in 1950 (9), but some have objected to its use for a neoplasm such as CBP since none of these tumors have been shown to have any chemoreceptor function (5), and based upon morphologic features, a chemoreceptor role would not even be anticipated.

The first CBP was reported by Marchand in 1891 (6), and from the illustration of the resected tumor and carotid vessels (fig. 16-1), it is not surprising that the patient died of complications several days after surgery. Four other patients with CBP were reported from Vienna by Paltauf in the same year (10). These early cases underscore the potential peril to the patient in attempting complete surgical resection because of vascular and neurologic complications; indeed, one is reminded of the intraoperative challenge by the statement of Mathews in 1915 (7): "This rare tumor presents unusual difficulties to the surgeon, and should one encounter it without having suspected the diagnosis, the experience will not soon be forgotten." This poignant phrase is reinforced by intraoperative photographs of a patient undergoing resection of a CBP complicated by excessive bleeding during surgery (fig. 16-2). Scudder in 1903 (11) is credited with the first description of a CBP surgically resected in the United States; the tumor was classified as a variety of angiosarcoma known as perithelioma. Middleton in 1897 (8) gave the first description of a CBP which was most likely bilateral. Historically, CBPs were at one time referred to as "potato tumors" (1), although this designation had been used for fungating tumors of the neck, most of which were probably malignant lymphomas (3).

Clinical Features. The sex incidence in most series is roughly equal, although some report a slight predilection for females. The average age of presentation is usually in the fifth decade of life (21–24), but CBPs have even been reported in the first year of life (15). Studies of CBPs at

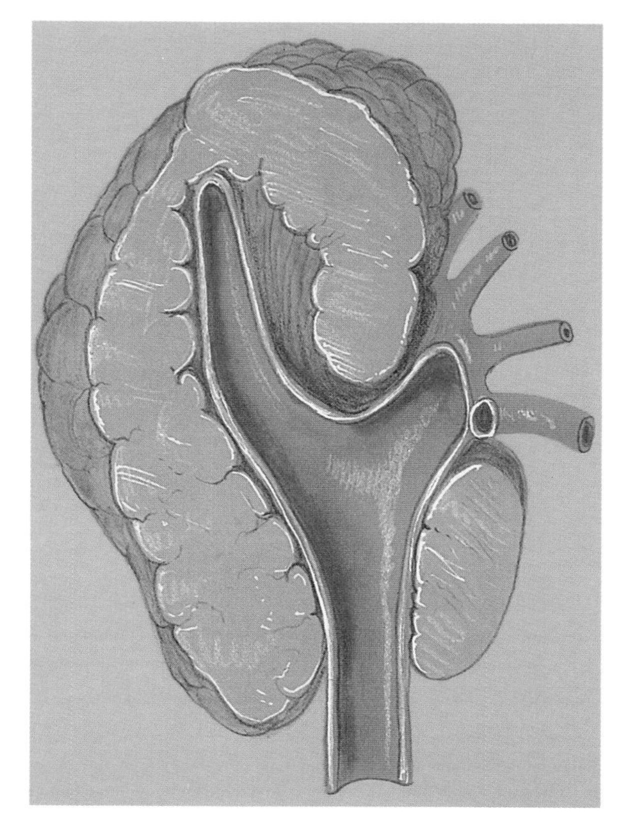

Figure 16-1
CAROTID BODY PARAGANGLIOMA
Cross section of carotid vessels and large carotid body paraganglioma (CBP). Modification of original illustration of CBP from work by Marchand in 1891.

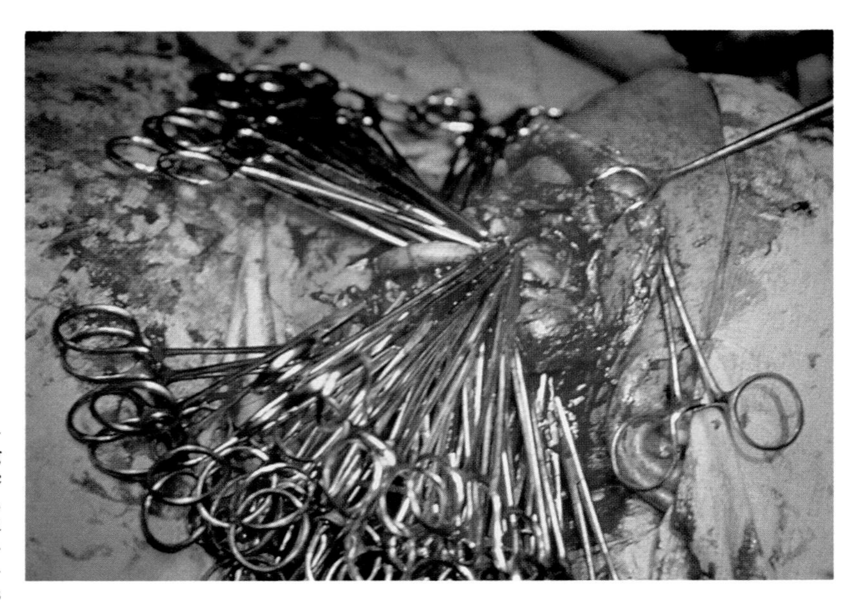

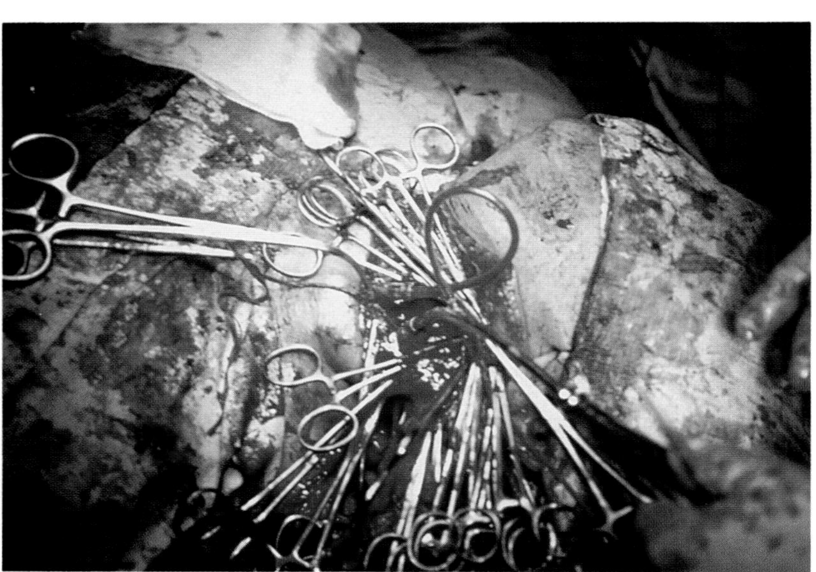

Figure 16-2
CAROTID BODY
PARAGANGLIOMA

Top: A 30-year-old man noted a painless neck mass on the left side during the past year. A high pitched systolic bruit was noted over the carotid vessels, and the carotid arteriogram showed a hypervascular tumor diagnostic of a carotid body paraganglioma. During surgical resection 2,000 ml of blood was lost. The number of hemostats in the field is ample testimony to the difficulty in controlling the bleeding.

Bottom: A vascular shunt was inserted between the common carotid artery and internal branch to permit resection of tumor from bifurcation. (Courtesy of Dr. Hollon W. Farr, New York, NY.)

high altitude have noted a marked predilection for females. The most common presentation is a painless, slow-growing neck mass near the angle of the mandible (16,22,24,27,29,34), with little to no mobility in the vertical plane (fig. 16-3) (22). Only rarely is the mass painful or tender. Fluctuation in size is also uncommon, but it has been reported in one case in association with upper respiratory tract infections (23,24). There may be signs or symptoms of cranial nerve palsy, usually involving a combination of the 7th, 10th, and 12th cranial nerves (24,26,29). Horner's syndrome is occasionally seen due to involvement of the cervical sympathetic chain (22). The rate of postoperative cranial nerve dysfunction observed at the Mayo Clinic remained relatively unchanged over a 50-year period (the rate in the most recent 10 years was 40 percent) (19). The average duration of symptoms usually ranges from 5 (23,24) to nearly 7 years (34), but is sometimes as much as 20 years or more (22–24). Farr (14) has estimated a growth rate of about 5 mm per year or about 2 cm in 5 years. Carotid sinus syndrome with bradycardia and syncopal

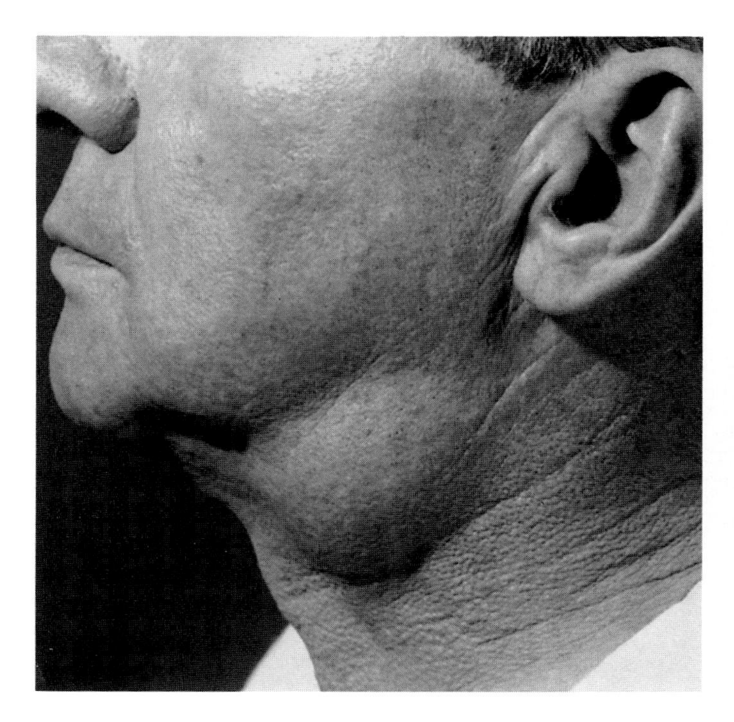
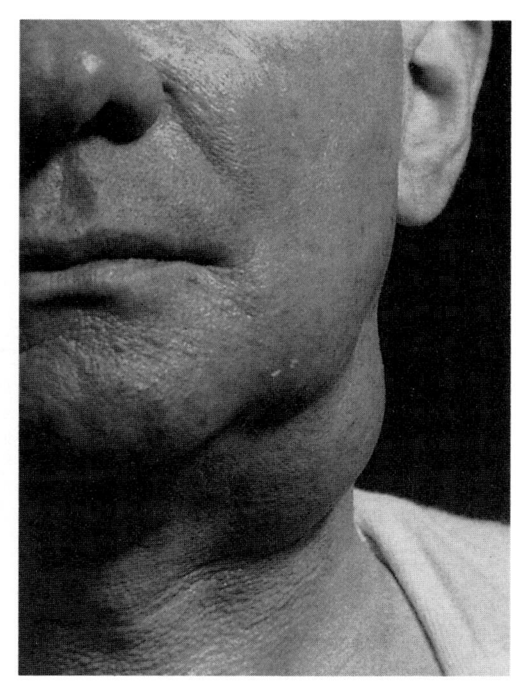

Figure 16-3
CAROTID BODY PARAGANGLIOMA

Left: A 57-year-old man noted a soft nontender mass in the left neck 14 years ago which had been slowly enlarging. During the past several months, the mass had become slightly painful and tender on pressure.

Right: The mass measured 5 cm in diameter, and was thought to be a branchogenic cyst. Several aspiration biopsies yielded only blood. The patient developed a hematoma, about twice the size of the original tumor, and this feature, coupled with the large amount of blood aspirated, raised the clinical suspicion of a CBP. (Fig. 3-7 from Lack EE. Pathology of adrenal and extra-adrenal paraganglia. Major problems in pathology, Vol 29. Philadelphia: WB Saunders Co, 1994:47.)

episodes is occasional (24,31,37). A patient with bilateral CBPs presented with transient ischemic attacks (33). Unusual functionally active CBPs and vagal and jugulotympanic paragangliomas with excess catecholamine secretion have been reported (17,20,36). In a review of the world literature, Zak and Lawson (38) identified 20 cases of functional paragangliomas of the head and neck region. Some of these reports should be interpreted with caution since some tumors arise along the cervical sympathetic chain (12,18) and are therefore sympathoadrenal paragangliomas. Clinically, the differential diagnosis includes a variety of entities such as salivary gland enlargement, lymphadenopathy, branchial cleft cyst, and even carotid aneurysm (22,24). On physical examination, a thrill or bruit is occasionally noted with CBP (and some other head or neck paragangliomas), but it is not a common finding. Medial protrusion by a carotid body or vagal paraganglioma may simulate tonsillar enlargement or an oropharyngeal mass (fig. 16-4) (22,24).

Preoperative Localization Studies. Preoperative selective angiography is useful for delineating tumor location, defining the blood supply, demonstrating other paragangliomas (13), and providing a route for selective embolization if this is considered prior to surgery. Preoperative embolization has been used to reduce blood loss during surgery (32,35), but it is not without complications (25,30). Characteristically with CBP, there is lateral displacement of the carotid bifurcation and both carotid artery branches (fig. 16-5A); the lateral view shows a widening of the bifurcation with “lyre-like” splaying apart of both branches (fig. 16-5B,C). A schematic view of the relation of CBP to the carotid bifurcation is seen in figure 16-5D. On rare occasion, a CBP may be located medial to the bifurcation without significant

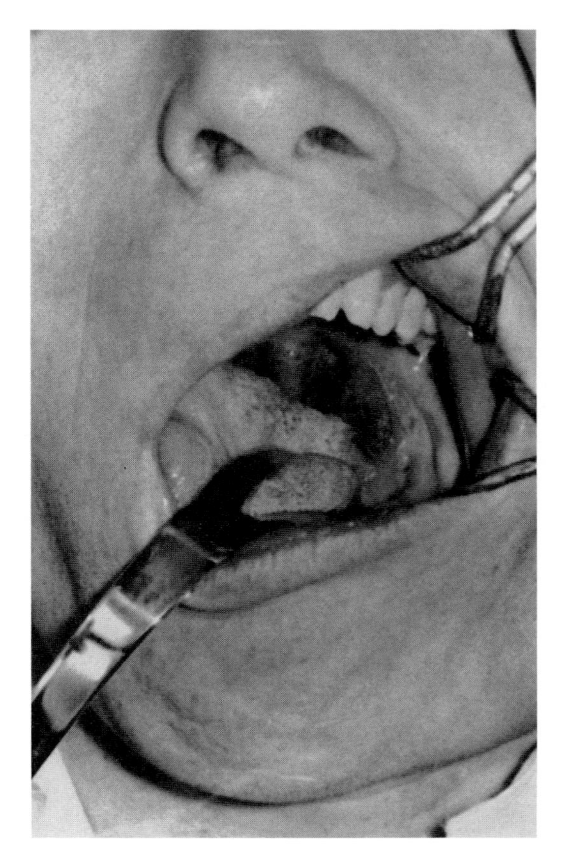

Figure 16-4
CAROTID BODY PARAGANGLIOMA
A 31-year-old man presented in 1942 with a 3-year history of a painless neck mass associated with dysphagia. The CBP caused medial protrusion of the soft palate and pharynx. The patient died on the fourth postoperative day due to complications from ligation of major carotid vessels.

widening of the carotid branches (fig. 16-6). Magnetic resonance imaging (MRI) is also useful in tumor localization and diagnosis (28). Multiplanar imaging, good tissue contrast, and clear anatomic detail display the CBP in relation to the carotid vessels (fig. 16-7). Computed tomography (CT) also provides valuable information.

Familial and Multicentric Paragangliomas. In the familial setting about one third of patients with CBPs have bilateral tumors (fig. 16-8), either synchronous or metachronous, and multicentric paragangliomas may develop at other sites in the head and neck region (fig. 16-9). Some studies of family pedigrees indicate an autosomal dominant mode of inheritance with variable penetrance and expression (39,45,47,48). In some series the sex ratio is equal (39) while in others there is a predilection for females (40,42, 46). Occasional tumors are transmitted almost exclusively along the paternal line, and a genomic imprinting hypothesis has been proposed (50). Patients with familial CBP may be diagnosed at a slightly younger age than those with sporadic tumors (45), and the tumors may develop in childhood (44). In a review of the familial occurrence of head and neck paragangliomas, 78 percent were CBPs, 16 percent jugular paragangliomas, and 4.5 percent vagal paragangliomas (49). Sympathoadrenal paragangliomas can also occur in association with familial paragangliomas of the head and neck region (42). Hereditary deficiencies of clotting factors VII and X have been reported in patients with familial CBP (41). Multicentric or bilateral paragangliomas can also occur in a nonfamilial or sporadic fashion (42,43); bilateral tumors occur in 4 to 8 percent of patients with CBP (39,45).

Association with Other Endocrine Disorders. CBPs have occurred in association with the triad of gastric epithelioid leiomyosarcoma, pulmonary chondroma, and functioning extra-adrenal paraganglioma (53–55); papillary thyroid carcinoma (51,57); hyperparathyroidism (58); and unusual endocrine disorders, raising the possibility of a new pattern of multiple endocrine neoplasia (52,56).

Pathology. In general it is not possible to distinguish CBP from other head and neck paragangliomas on purely morphologic grounds, although some gross or microscopic features permit distinction, such as residual ganglion nodosum at the periphery of a vagal paraganglioma or the small irregular fragments of a jugulotympanic paraganglioma, with or without bone involvement (65). Details of CBP morphology are covered in this chapter and paragangliomas at other sites in the head and neck region will emphasize special characteristics or amplify a broader range of morphology.

Gross Findings. CBPs are often sharply demarcated, and occasionally give the impression of true encapsulation, but careful histologic study often shows an expansile border with what is best regarded as a fibrous pseudocapsule. The average size in the Memorial Hospital series was 3.8 cm (range, 1.9 to 8.5 cm) (66). In a study of CBPs in patients born and living at high altitude the average dimensions were 3.9 x 2.8 x 2.6 cm;

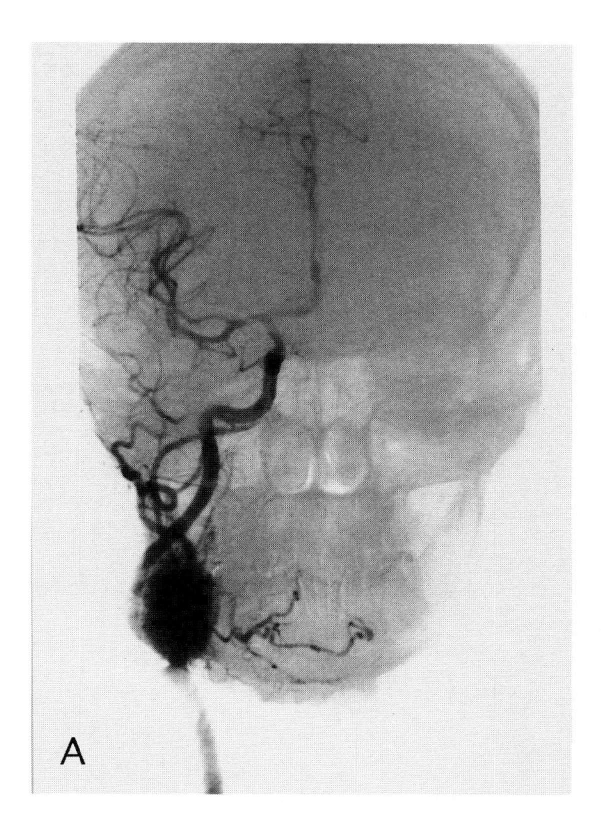

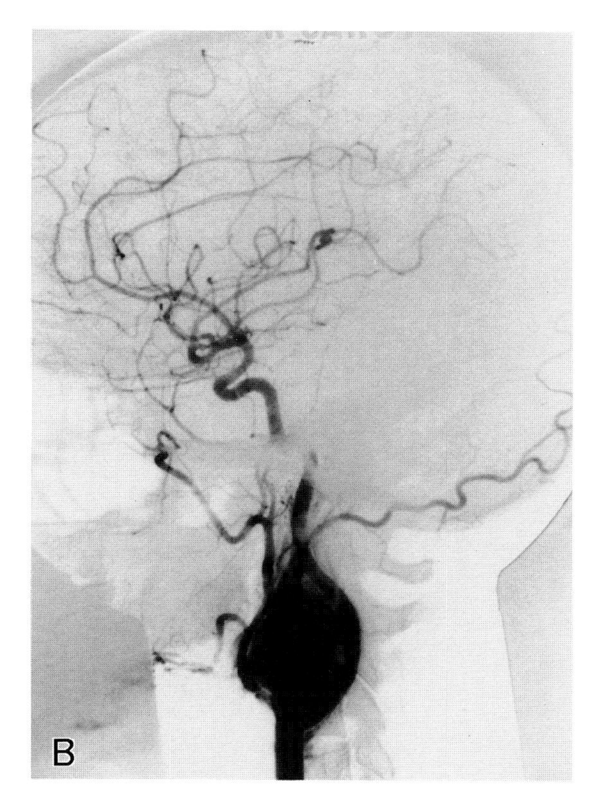

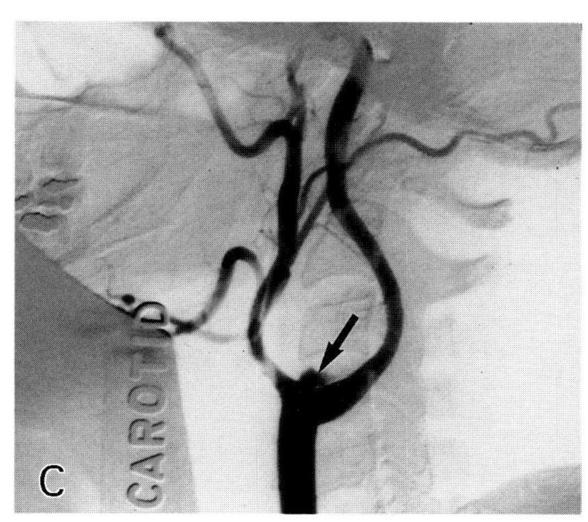

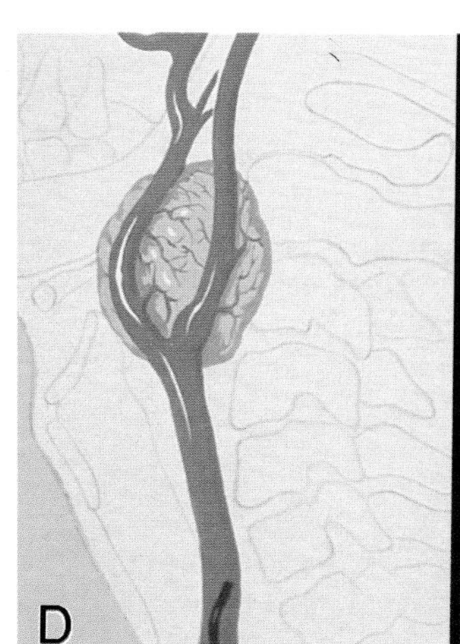

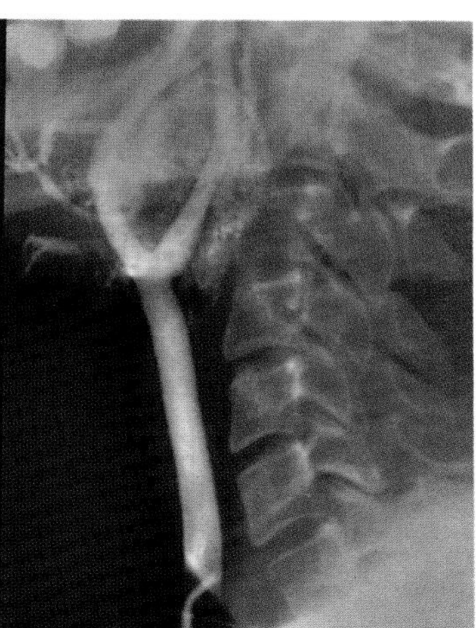

Figure 16-5
CAROTID BODY PARAGANGLIOMA

A: A 40-year-old woman had a right neck mass of about 5-months' duration. Selective right carotid angiogram in the anterior-posterior plane shows a hypervascular mass with some lateral displacement of the common carotid artery and bifurcation. Digital subtraction enhances contrast with bony densities.

B: Lateral view with digital subtraction showed a mass in the carotid bifurcation which measured 3.5 cm in diameter.

C: Lateral view after selective embolization. Note the "lyre-like" configuration of the carotid bifurcation. A small vascular stump at the base of the bifurcation (arrow) represents the ascending pharyngeal artery which had been selectively embolized. The patient had a similar CBP removed from the left neck over a decade earlier, and had a family history of similar tumors. (Fig. 3-9 from Lack EE. Pathology of adrenal and extra-adrenal paraganglia. Major problems in pathology, Vol 29. Philadelphia: WB Saunders Co., 1994:48.)

D: Schematic diagram of CBP and its relation to the carotid artery bifurcation.

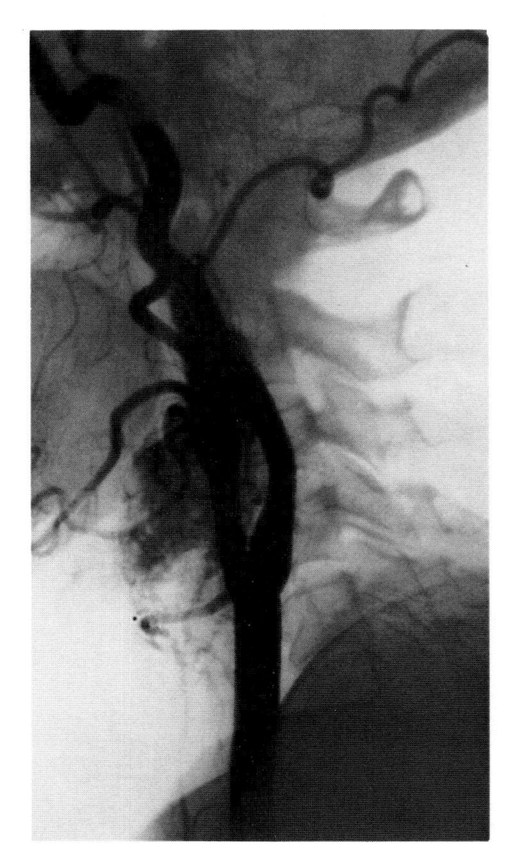

Figure 16-6
CAROTID BODY PARAGANGLIOMA
A 54-year-old woman presented with a painless right neck mass measuring 4.5 x 3.5 cm. Lateral view of the CBP shows no significant widening of the carotid bifurcation, which is very unusual. The tumor was located medial to the carotid bifurcation (see figure 16-7). (Fig. 3-10B from Lack EE. Pathology of adrenal and extra-adrenal paraganglia. Major problems in pathology, Vol 29. Philadelphia: WB Saunders Co., 1994:49.)

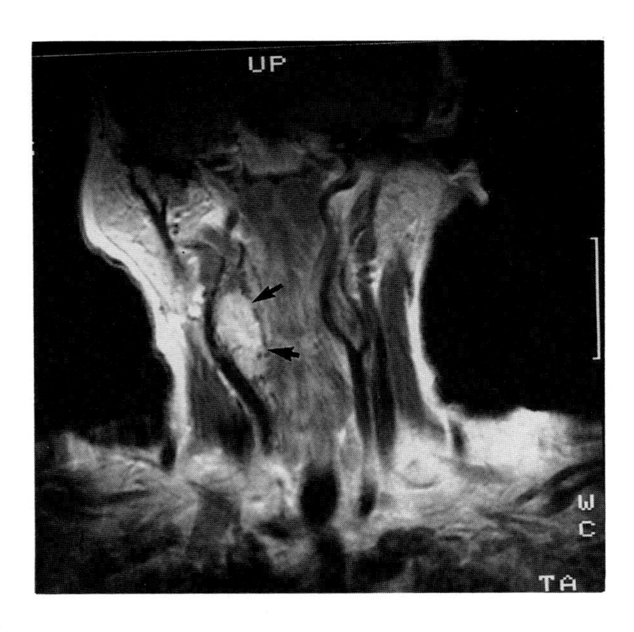

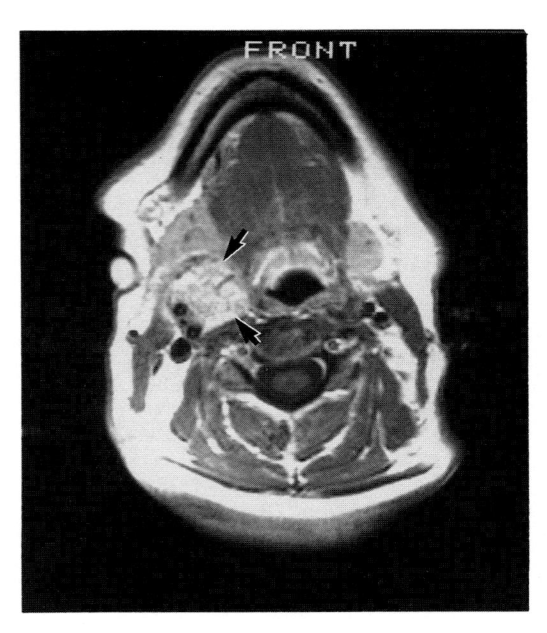

Figure 16-7
CAROTID BODY PARAGANGLIOMA
Top: MRI in coronal plane shows well-demarcated cervical mass (arrows) with bright image after gadolinium contrast administration. Note lateral displacement of carotid vessels. (Fig. 3-11B from Lack EE. Pathology of adrenal and extra-adrenal paraganglia Major problems in pathology, Vol 29. Philadelphia: WB Saunders Co., 1994:50.)

Bottom: MRI in transverse plane after gadolinium contrast administration. Carotid body paraganglioma was located medial to carotid vessels and bifurcation (see figure 16-6). (Fig. 3-11C from Lack EE. Pathology of adrenal and extra-adrenal paraganglia. Major problems in pathology, Vol 29. Philadelphia: WB Saunders Co., 1994:51.)

some of the smaller tumors weighed 369 to 550 mg (75). On external examination there may be indentation of the surface of the CBP made by one or both carotid vessels. CBPs usually have a meaty to light tan appearance (fig. 16-10), but with much mechanical manipulation during surgery, the tumor may become quite congested or frankly hemorrhagic (fig. 16-11). Close inspection of the cut surface may reveal punctate, linear, or curvilinear profiles of vessels which may be retracted slightly beneath the surface (65). Areas of tumor necrosis are rare, unless of course the tumor has been successfully embolized prior to surgery (fig. 16-12). In a recent study there was no significant difference between surface areas

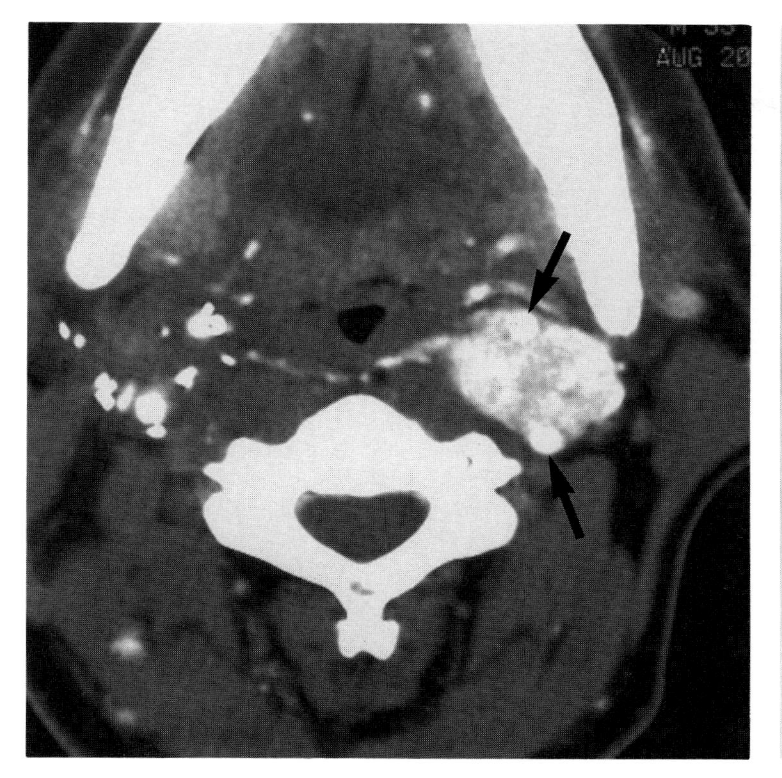

Figure 16-8
CAROTID BODY PARAGANGLIOMA
Familial CBP in a patient with a strong history of similar tumors in related family members. CT scan with intravenous contrast shows a bright image of the CBP along with both carotid vessels which indent the tumor (arrows). Note the surgical clips in the opposite neck where a CBP had been previously resected.

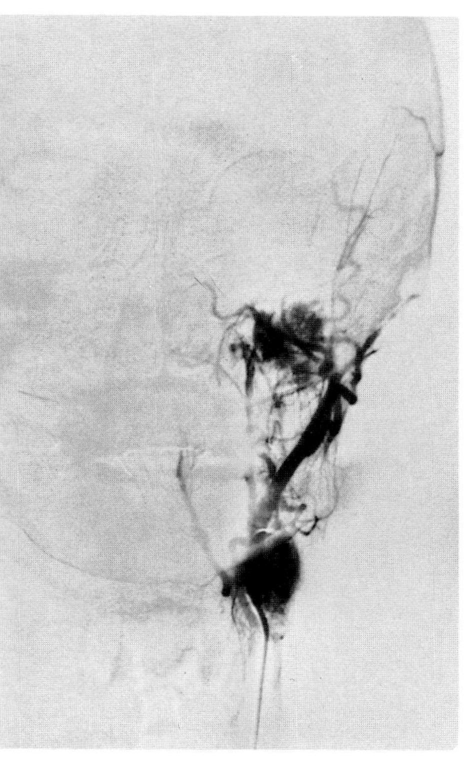

Figure 16-9
CAROTID BODY PARAGANGLIOMA
A 15-year-old girl had a family history of head and neck paragangliomas. Carotid arteriogram on the left side shows a CBP which measured 2 cm in diameter and a jugulotympanic paraganglioma.

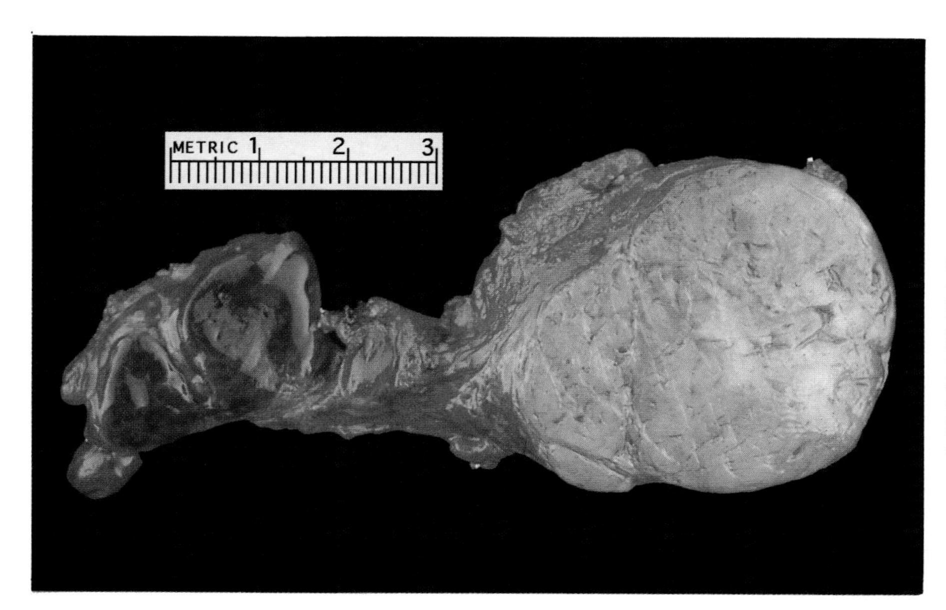

Figure 16-10
CAROTID BODY PARAGANGLIOMA
Cross section of CBP resected from an adult patient with a familial history of similar tumors. Grooves on either side represent impressions left by internal and external carotid artery branches. Deeply congested lymph nodes attached to the specimen were negative for tumor.

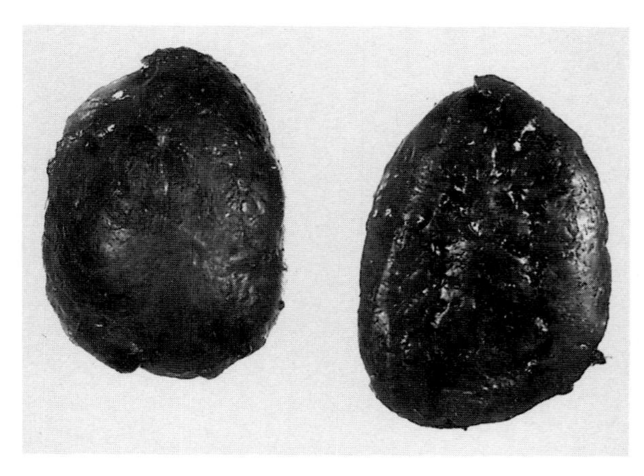

Figure 16-11
CAROTID BODY PARAGANGLIOMA
The bisected CBP is deeply congested and hemorrhagic on cross section (right side). The external aspect of the tumor (left side) is relatively smooth.

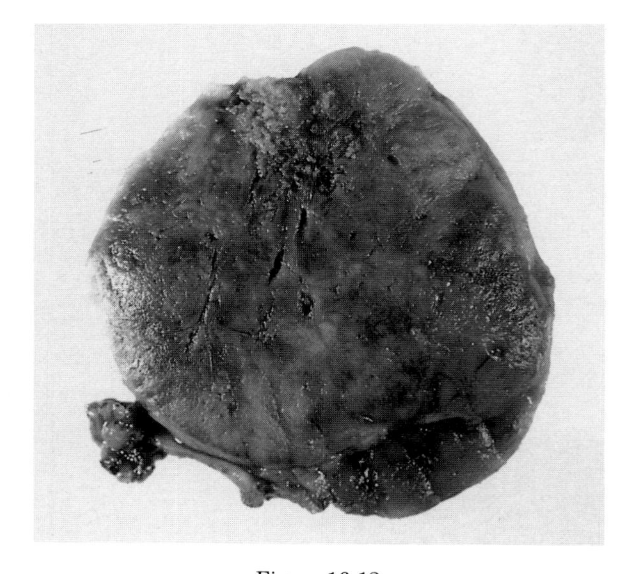

Figure 16-12
CAROTID BODY PARAGANGLIOMA
CBP on cross section has irregular areas of pallor and congestion. The tumor had been embolized via the ascending pharyngeal artery, resulting in confluent areas of tumor necrosis.

of embolized versus nonembolized CBP, although the intraoperative blood loss was lower in embolized tumors (average, 372 ml versus 609 ml) (67). Occasionally, there are areas of sclerosis or cystic change (fig. 16-13). On rare occasion, a CBP invades the lumen of the carotid artery or causes total carotid artery occlusion (74,77).

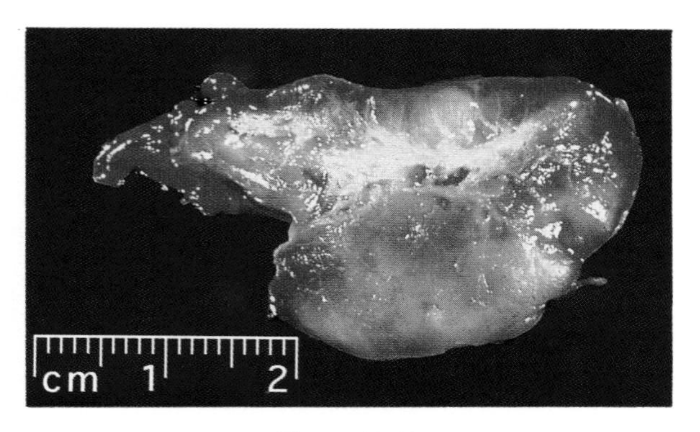

Figure 16-13
CAROTID BODY PARAGANGLIOMA
CBP resected from a young man shows areas of sclerosis with mild cystic degeneration.

Three groups of CBP have been identified (fig. 16-14) (76). Group I tumors (26 percent of cases) do not adhere significantly to adventitia and are relatively small (calculated median volume of tumor, 7 cm^3) (figs. 16-15, 16-16); group II (46.5 percent of cases) are more adherent to the adventitia of vessel wall and partially surround one or both carotid vessels (median volume, 11 cm^3); and group III tumors (27.6 percent of cases) intimately adhere to the entire circumference of the bifurcation (median volume, 22 cm^3) (71). Correlation of increasing size of CBP with each consecutive group has been reported (63).

Microscopic Findings. *Architectural and Other Features.* On low-power magnification, CBPs are often well demarcated, with a well-developed fibrous pseudocapsule (fig. 16-17). Examination of the periphery of the tumor may reveal areas where the fibrous pseudocapsule is deficient, but this should not be regarded as true capsular invasion (fig. 16-18). The tumor may intimately involve the adventitia of one or both carotid artery branches, and complete resection may necessitate vascular grafting. There may not be a discernible plane of dissection from the vessel wall (fig. 16-19). The most characteristic pattern in CBPs (and other head and neck paragangliomas) is a relatively uniform nesting arrangement of cells or formation of "zellballen" (fig. 16-20, left), a pattern that can be greatly accentuated in reticulin-stained sections (fig. 16-20, right). Three basic histologic patterns were recognized by LeCompte (68,69): usual, adenoma-like, and angioma-like. Sometimes there

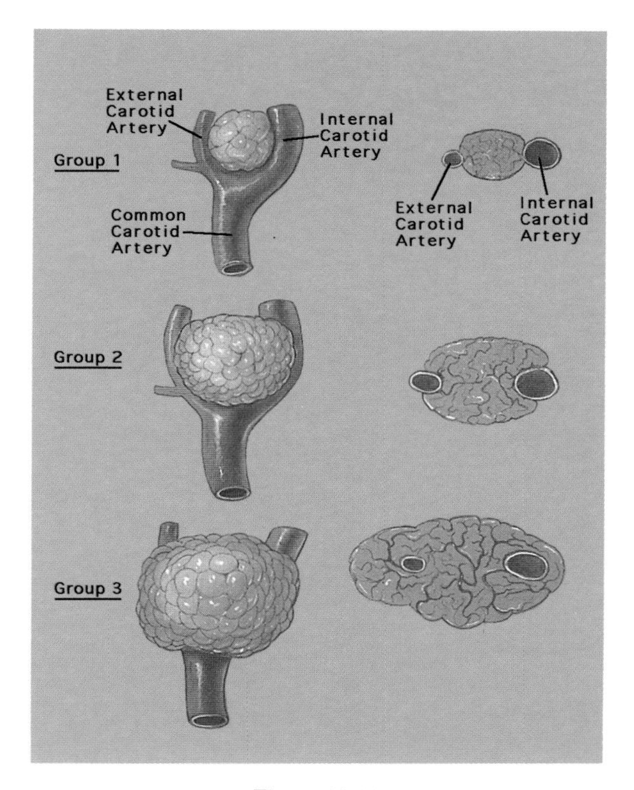

Figure 16-14
CAROTID BODY PARAGANGLIOMA
Three groups of CBP are schematically represented. The tumors get progressively bigger, and in group III it encircles the carotid bifurcation and carotid vessels.

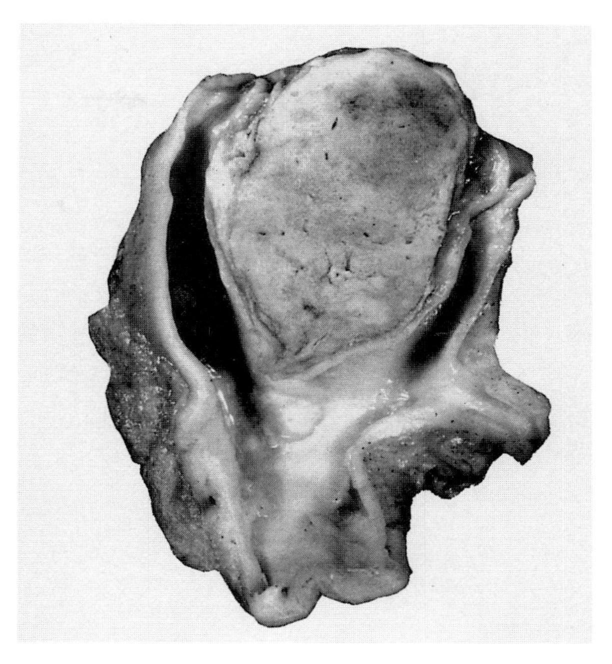

Figure 16-15
CAROTID BODY PARAGANGLIOMA
CBP obtained at autopsy from the left neck of a 52-year-old man who had a CBP on the opposite side for nearly a decade. During surgical resection of the right CBP, the common carotid artery was ligated, and the patient developed a left-sided hemiplegia which soon proved fatal. There was no family history of other head and neck paragangliomas.

is artifactual separation of nests of tumor cells from vascular stroma, probably related to shrinkage during fixation (fig. 16-21). Clusters of neoplastic chief cells may vary in size and shape. Occasionally, the zellballen focally become quite large and seem to compress adjacent areas within the tumor (fig. 16-22); extremely large nests of tumor cells may have a central area of degeneration or necrosis (fig. 16-23).

Some CBPs have areas of hemorrhage which, if marked, can separate individual clusters of neoplastic chief cells, giving a somewhat misleading picture (fig. 16-24). In sections taken through the periphery of the tumor or fibrous pseudocapsule small remnants of normal carotid body may be seen, a feature that shows that the neoplastic process only affected a portion of the carotid body (fig. 16-25). When the neoplasm has been embolized to decrease vascularity it may result in geographic areas of necrosis, but this is

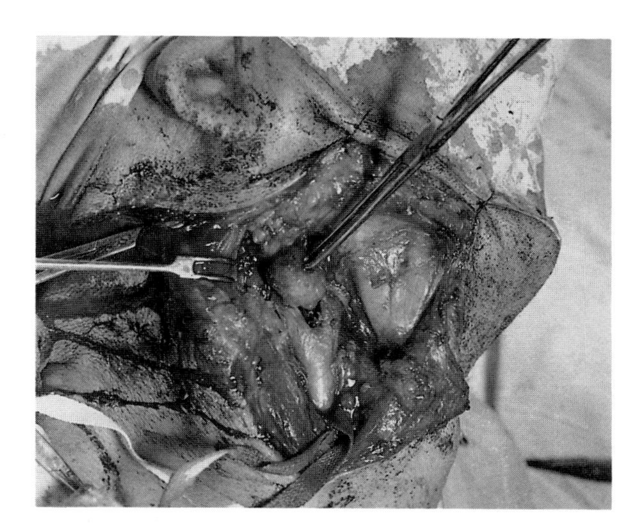

Figure 16-16
CAROTID BODY PARAGANGLIOMA
A 63-year-old man had a firm nontender mass of the right neck which was felt clinically to be enlarged jugular lymph nodes. The CBP measured 2.2 x 1.2 cm. The tumor has been mobilized from the carotid bifurcation by dissection through the adventitial plane. Preoperative needle aspiration biopsy had yielded only blood.

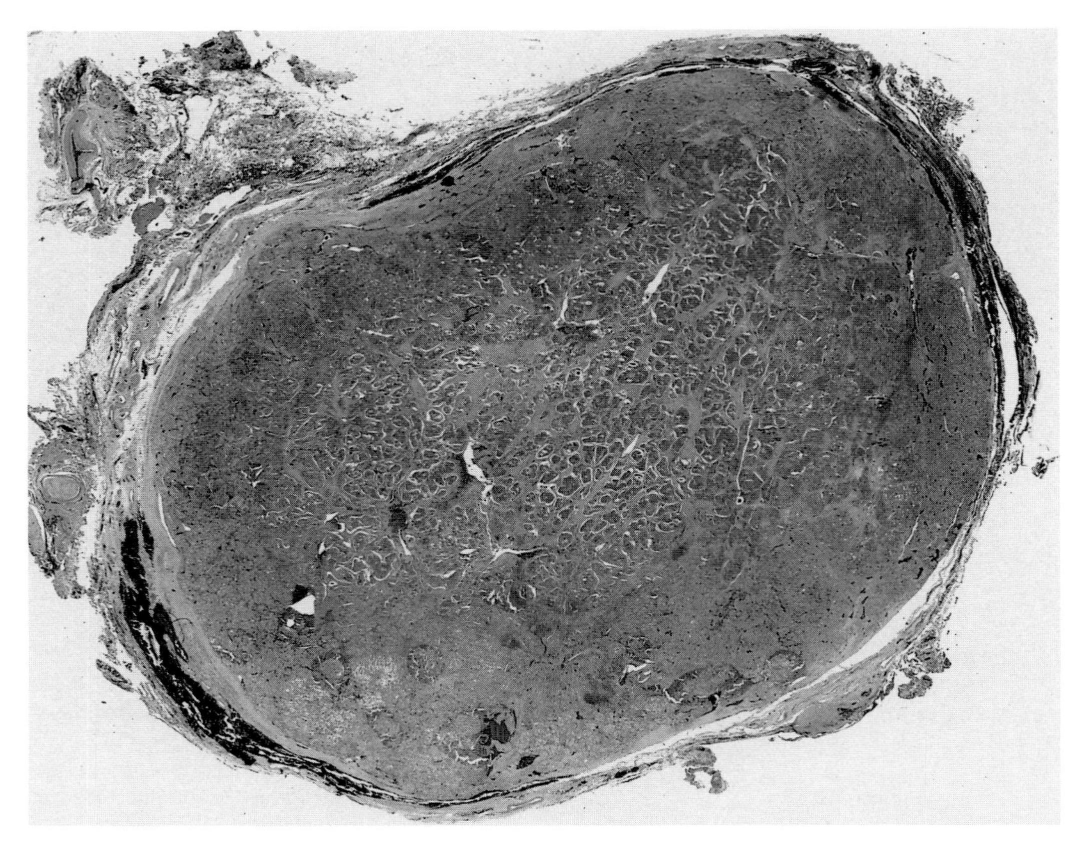

Figure 16-17
CAROTID BODY PARAGANGLIOMA

This CBP is sharply circumscribed with a fibrous pseudocapsule. Central portions of the tumor contained larger clusters of tumor cells ("zellballen") with some showing central degeneration and necrosis. The patient had bilateral CBPs and was alive and well 10 years after resection of the second tumor.

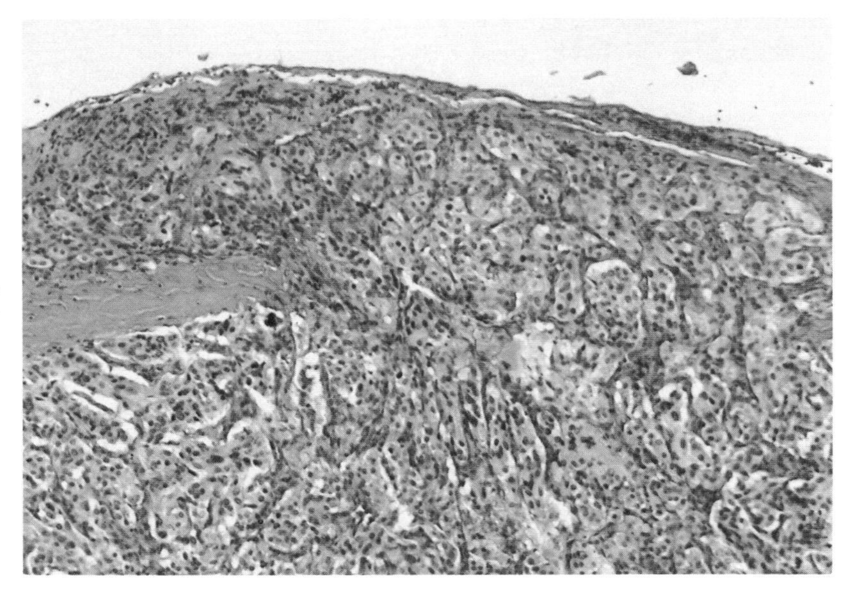

Figure 16-18
CAROTID BODY PARAGANGLIOMA

Clinically benign CBP shows discontinuity in the fibrous pseudocapsule, a feature that mimics true capsular invasion.

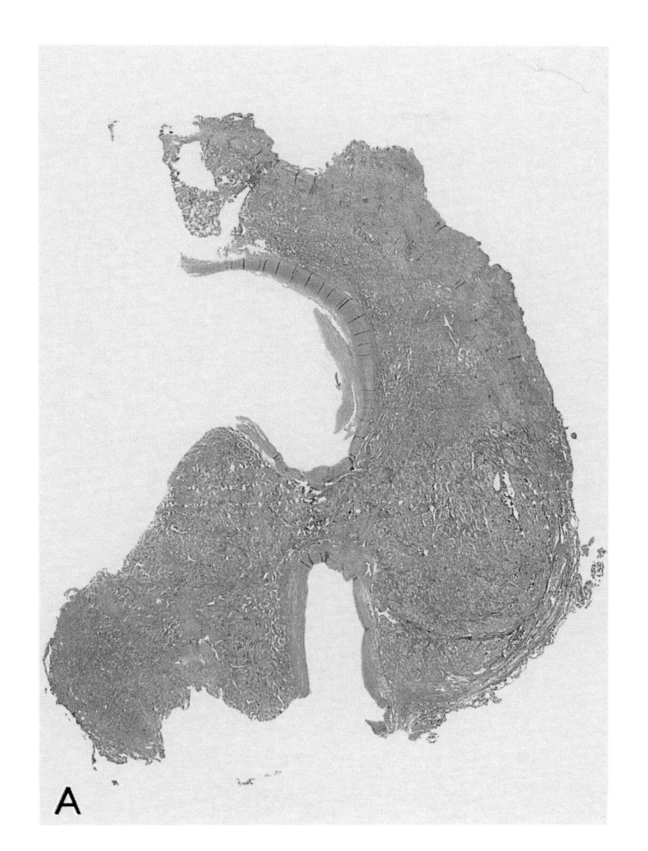

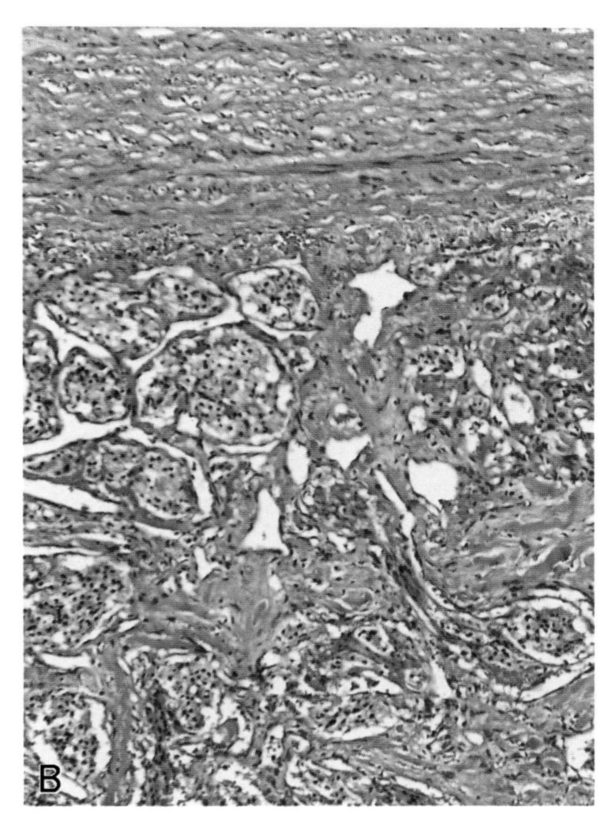

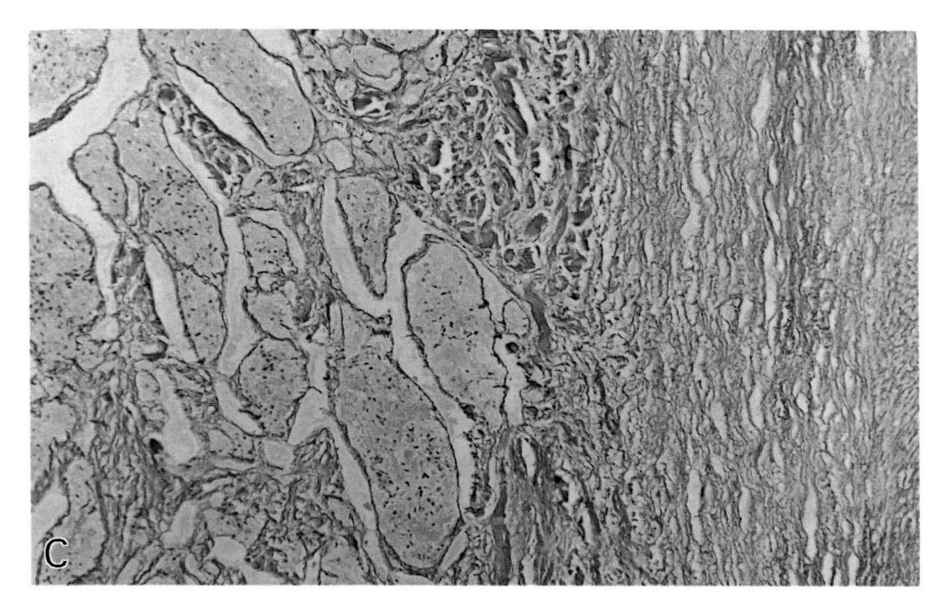

Figure 16-19
CAROTID BODY PARAGANGLIOMA

A: This CBP almost completely encircled the carotid bifurcation and both internal and external carotid branches (group III tumor). The tumor was firmly adherent to vessels, with no definable plane of dissection.

B: CBP is densely adherent to the vessel wall, but does not invade the media.

C: Stain for reticulum shows dense condensation of connective tissue adjacent to the media of the vessel wall. (X120, Reticulum stain)

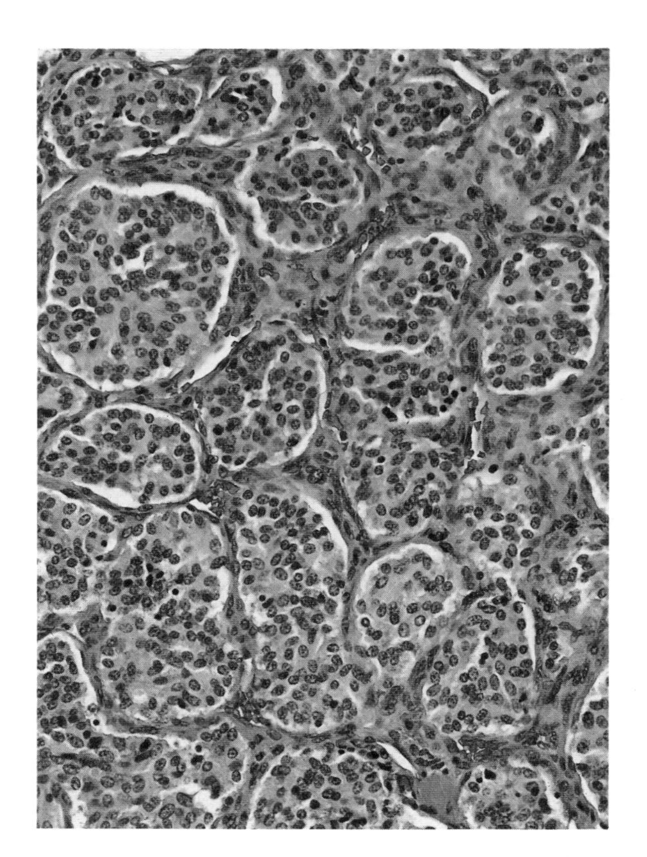

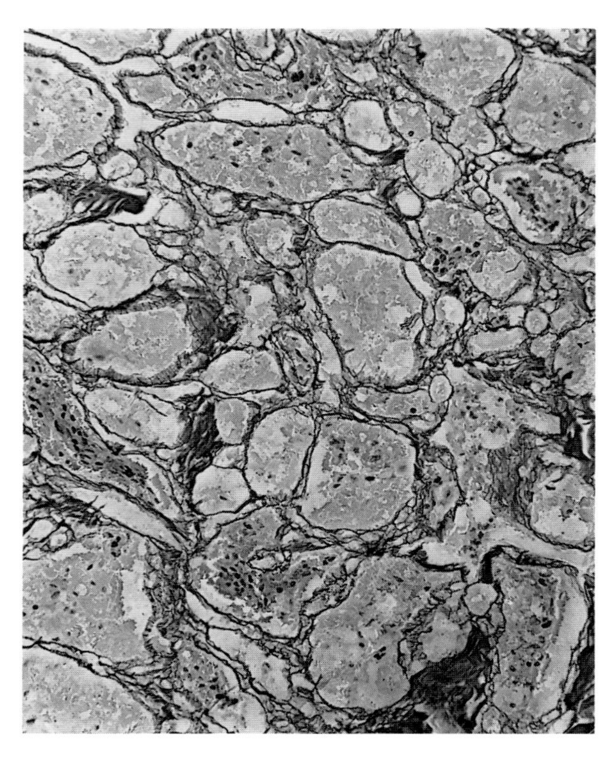

Figure 16-20
CAROTID BODY PARAGANGLIOMA
Left: CBP with distinct nests ("zellballen") of tumor cells.
Right: Stain for reticulum greatly accentuates the nesting pattern. (X120, Reticulum stain)

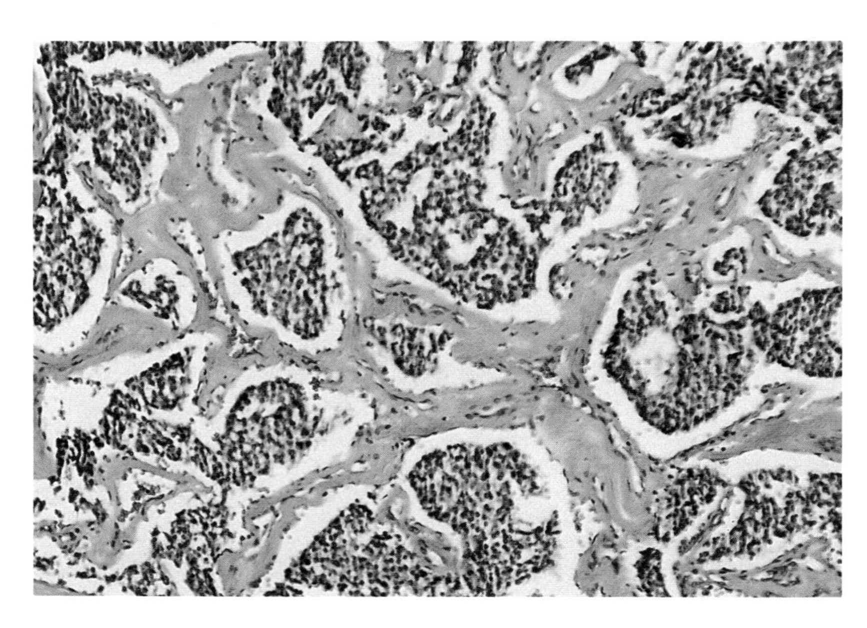

Figure 16-21
CAROTID BODY PARAGANGLIOMA
Clusters of tumor cells show some retraction from the fibrovascular stroma.

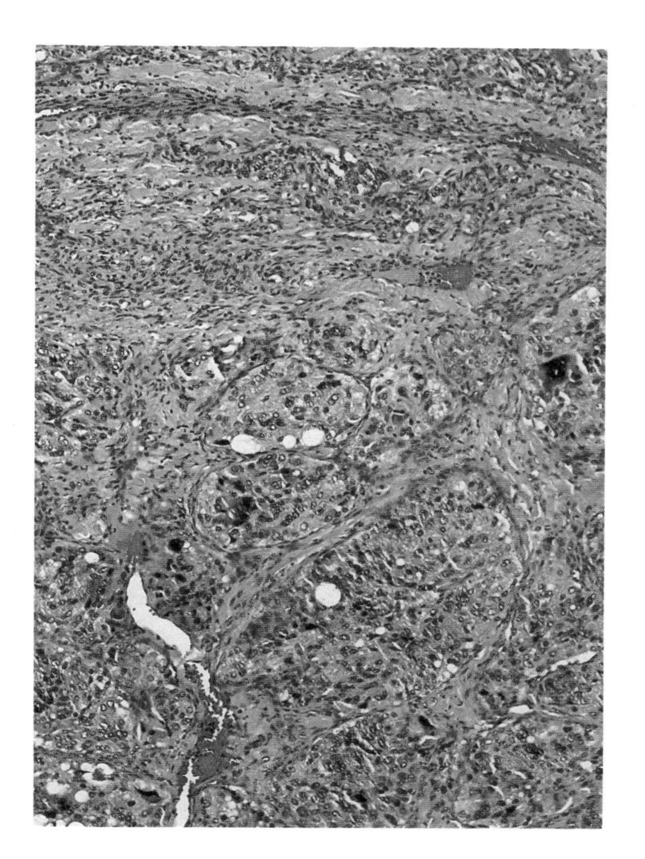

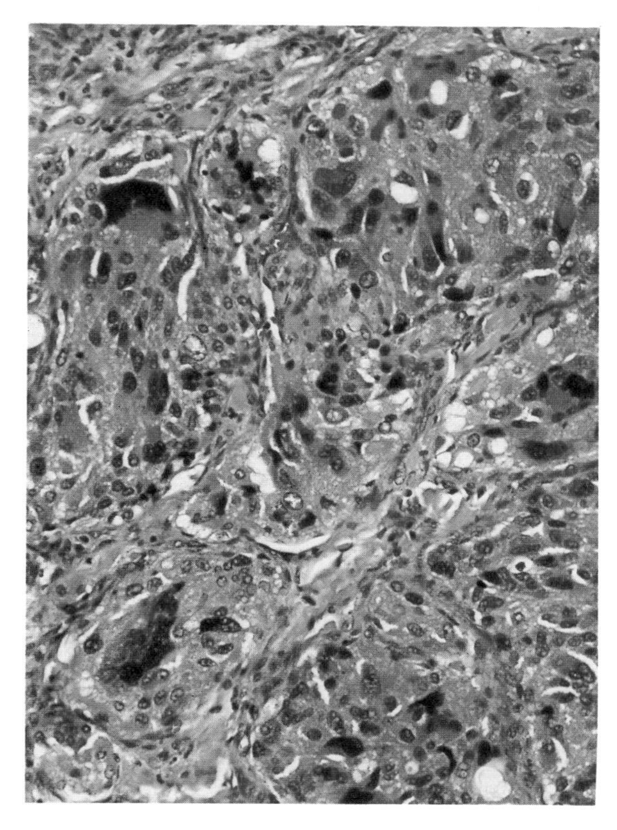

Figure 16-22
CAROTID BODY PARAGANGLIOMA

Left: Area within the CBP shown in figure 16-17 shows marked enlargement of "zellballen." Contrast the size and irregular shape of these clusters of neoplastic chief cells with the adjacent tumor at top of field.

Right: Enlarged hyperchromatic nuclei are seen in this field. Some "zellballen" also had areas of central necrosis.

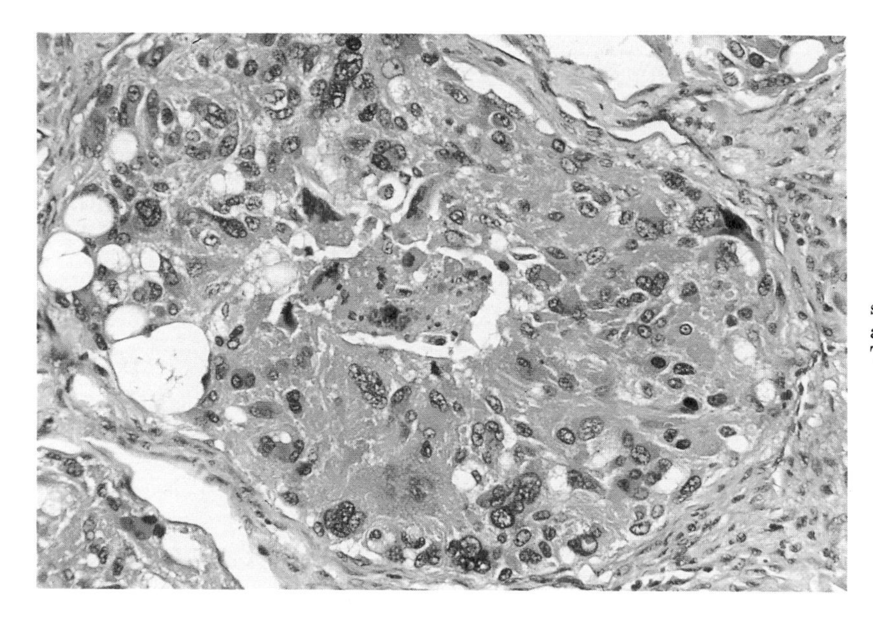

Figure 16-23
CAROTID BODY PARAGANGLIOMA

A few greatly enlarged "zellballen," some with central areas of degeneration and necrosis, were seen in this CBP. The tumor was clinically benign.

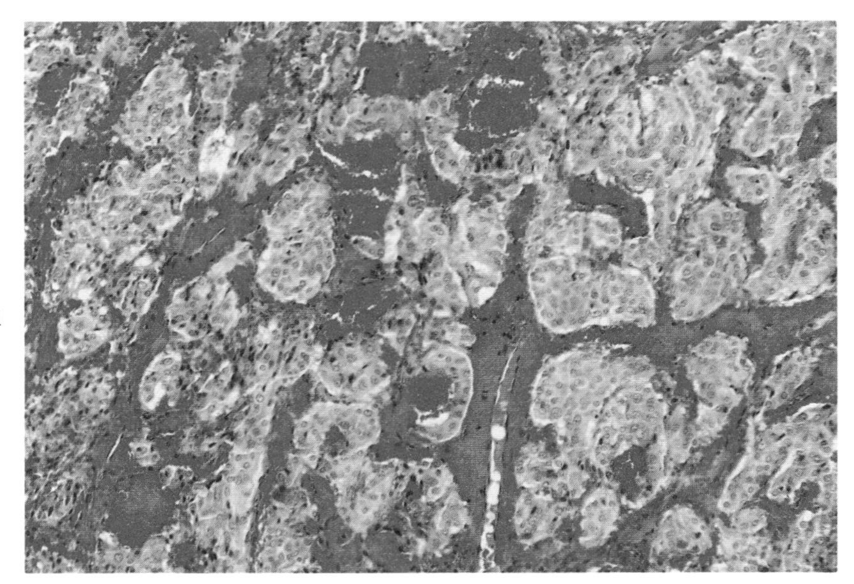

Figure 16-24
CAROTID BODY PARAGANGLIOMA
Nests of tumor cells are separated by hemorrhage.

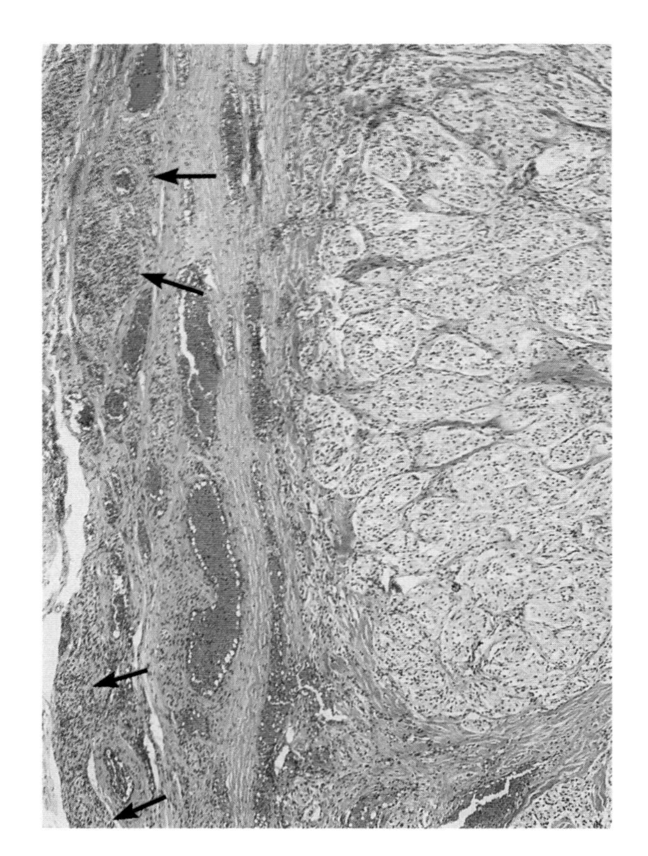

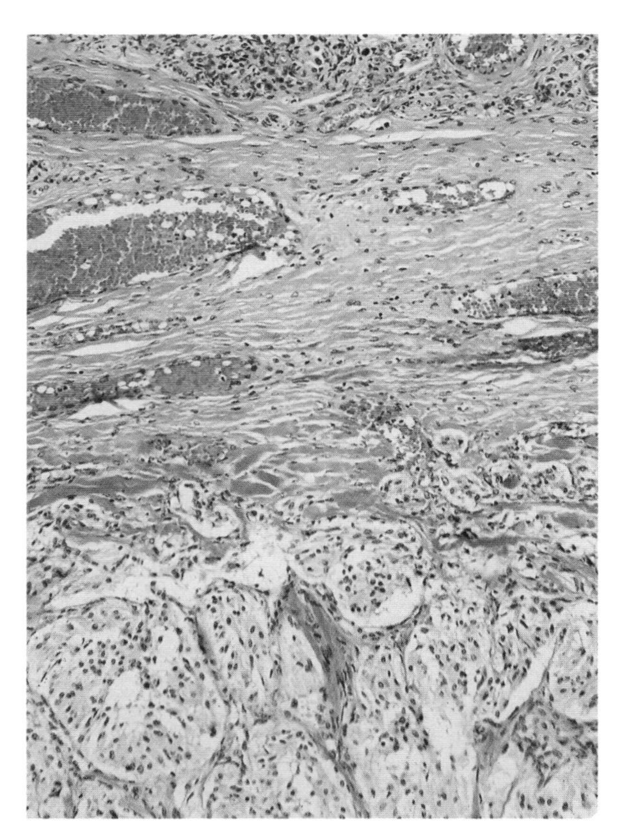

Figure 16-25
CAROTID BODY PARAGANGLIOMA
Left: Residual lobules of non-neoplastic carotid body paraganglion are present within the fibrous pseudocapsule (arrows).
Right: Portions of residual non-neoplastic carotid body within the fibrous pseudocapsule (very top of field).

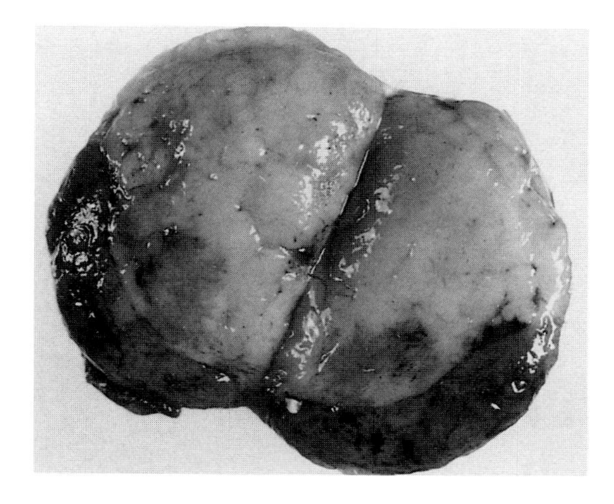

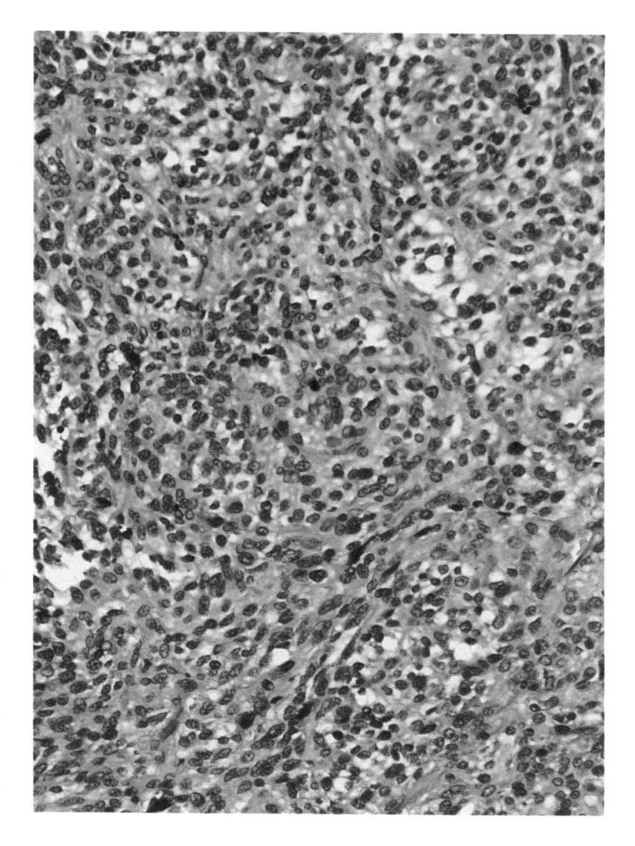

Figure 16-26
CAROTID BODY PARAGANGLIOMA

Above: Bivalved CBP was resected from the right neck of a 62-year-old woman and measured 3.0 x 2.5 x 2.5 cm. The tumor was yellowish gray and focally hemorrhagic. (Fig. 5 from Lack EE, Cubilla AL, Woodruff JM. Paragangliomas of the head and neck region. A pathologic study of tumors from 71 patients. Hum Pathol 1979;10:191–218.)

Right: Spindle cell or pseudosarcomatous pattern was apparent in much of the tumor, but a more characteristic nesting pattern was also present in other areas. The late Dr. F.W. Stewart commented that "if one can guess that one (CBP) will prove malignant, this one would be," but the patient was alive and well 16 years later.

not always the case. A most unusual pattern is a spindle cell or pseudosarcomatous arrangement of cells (65,66). The author has encountered only one example of CBP with this pattern (fig. 16-26), but the neoplasm had more characteristic features in additional sections.

Cellular Features. CBPs have a higher cell density of neoplastic chief cells compared with chief cells in non-neoplastic carotid body paraganglia (70). Neoplastic chief cells usually have ample, finely granular, eosinophilic cytoplasm; cell borders may be indistinct or at times well defined with polygonal or angular contours. Some tumor cells have such abundant, deeply eosinophilic cytoplasm that the neoplasm appears oncocytic (fig. 16-27); this has been attributed to the presence of numerous mitochondria (61). Nuclei may be round to oval and stain uniformly or there may be conspicuous nuclear pleomorphism and hyperchromasia (fig. 16-28), but this feature by itself is not a reliable indication of malignancy. Nuclear pseudoinclusions, similar to those of sympathoadrenal paragangliomas, are sometimes seen. A vacuolar change in the cytoplasm of tumor cells may be found in the occasional CBP as well as other paragangliomas, and these spaces have been referred to as pseudoacini (fig. 16-29) (64); they are also found in some sympathoadrenal paragangliomas.

Sustentacular cells account for 1 to 5 percent of cells in paragangliomas (59). These cells are almost impossible to identify in routinely stained sections, and they may be difficult to identify even ultrastructurally (65). A finding that is rare (72) and observed only twice by the author, is the presence of ganglion cells within a CBP; this phenomena can not be adequately explained by secondary incorporation of ganglia (fig. 16-30). It could be a manifestation of composite neural and endocrine differentiation in vivo similar to composite pheochromocytomas; in the study by Costero (62) some of the surviving tumor cells grown in tissue culture spontaneously developed long neuritic cell processes.

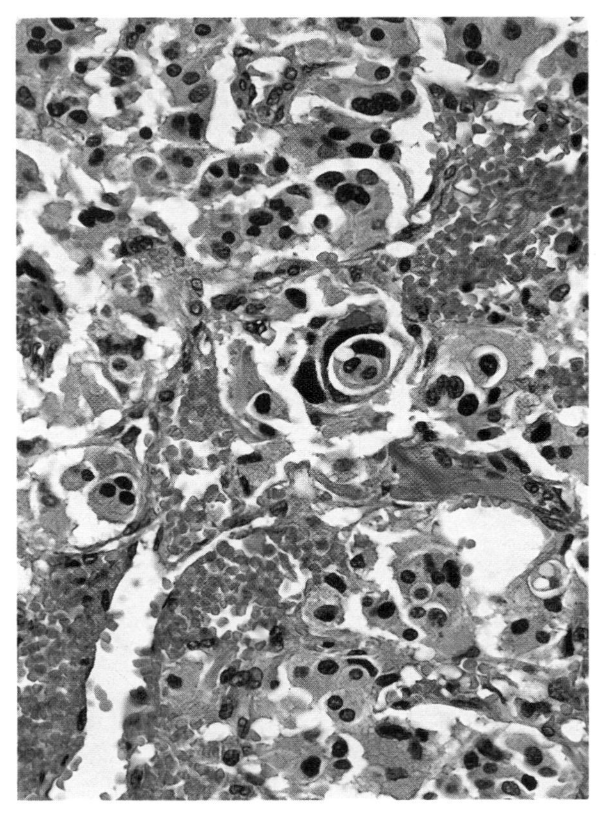

Figure 16-27
CAROTID BODY PARAGANGLIOMA
WITH ONCOCYTIC FEATURES

Most nuclei are hyperchromatic, with a few showing mild pleomorphism. Some tumor cells encircle other cells, an appearance referred to as "cell embracing."

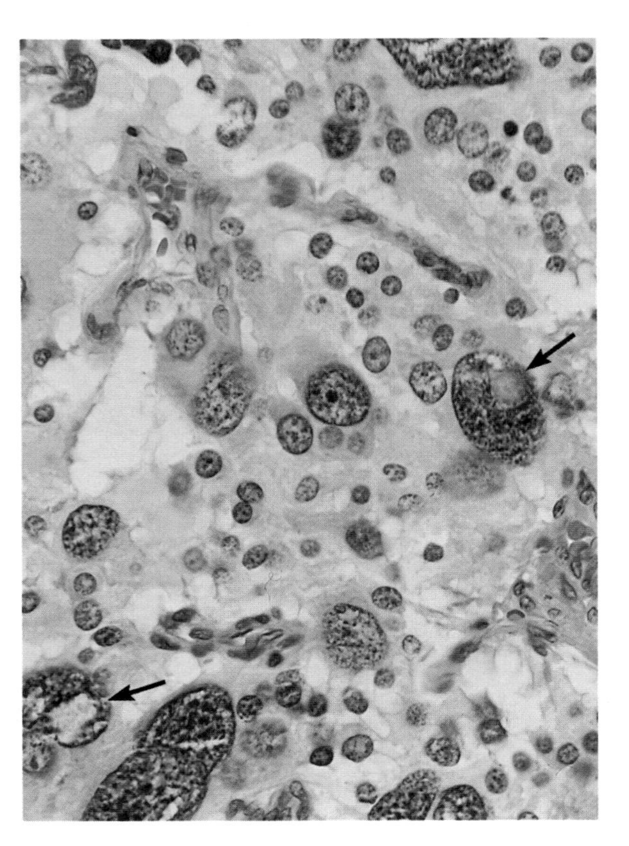

Figure 16-28
CAROTID BODY PARAGANGLIOMA

Marked nuclear pleomorphism and hyperchromasia as well as a nuclear "pseudoinclusion" (arrows) are seen in this CBP.

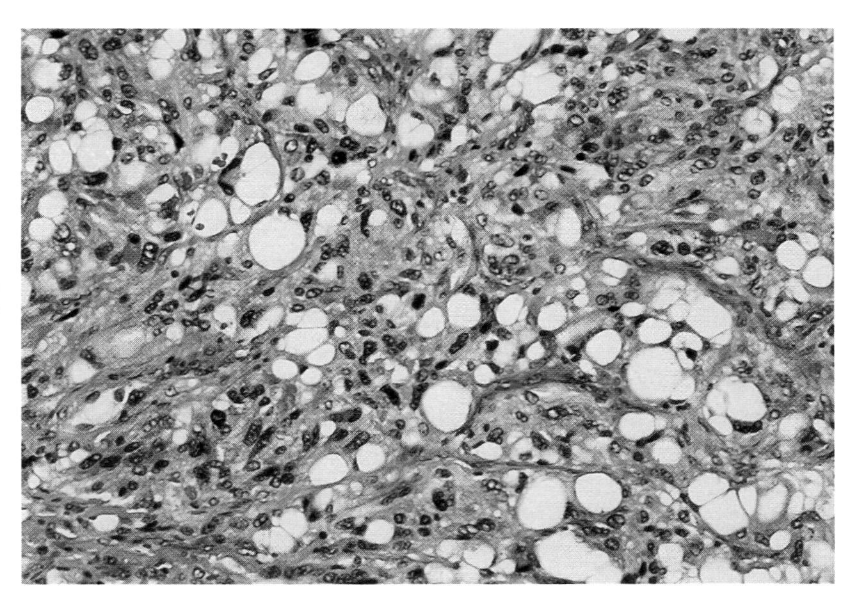

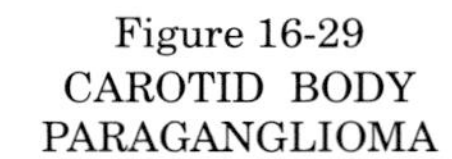

Figure 16-29
CAROTID BODY
PARAGANGLIOMA

Nests of neoplastic chief cells have a striking amount of vacuolar spaces. These have been referred to as "pseudoacini."

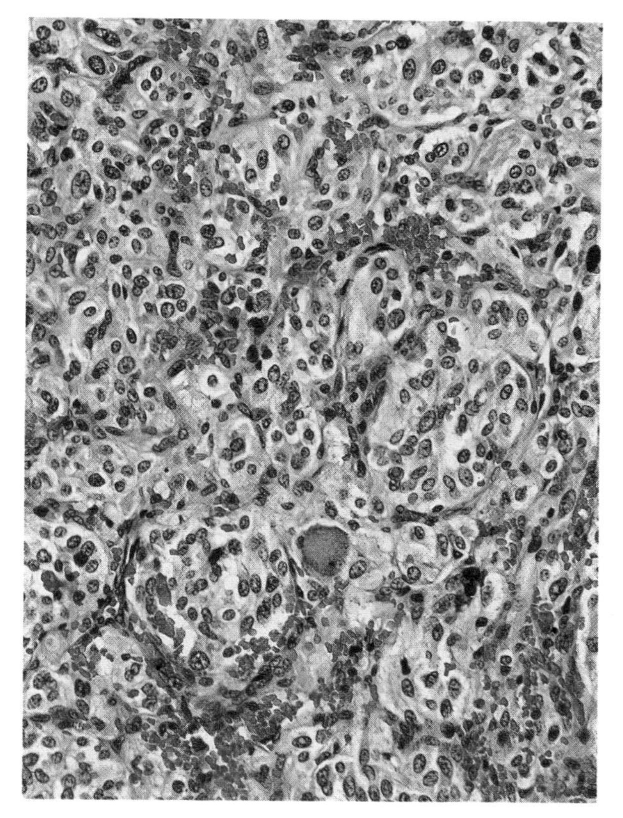

Figure 16-30
CAROTID BODY PARAGANGLIOMA
This CBP contained a few scattered cells with cytomorphology typical for ganglion cells (lower half of field).

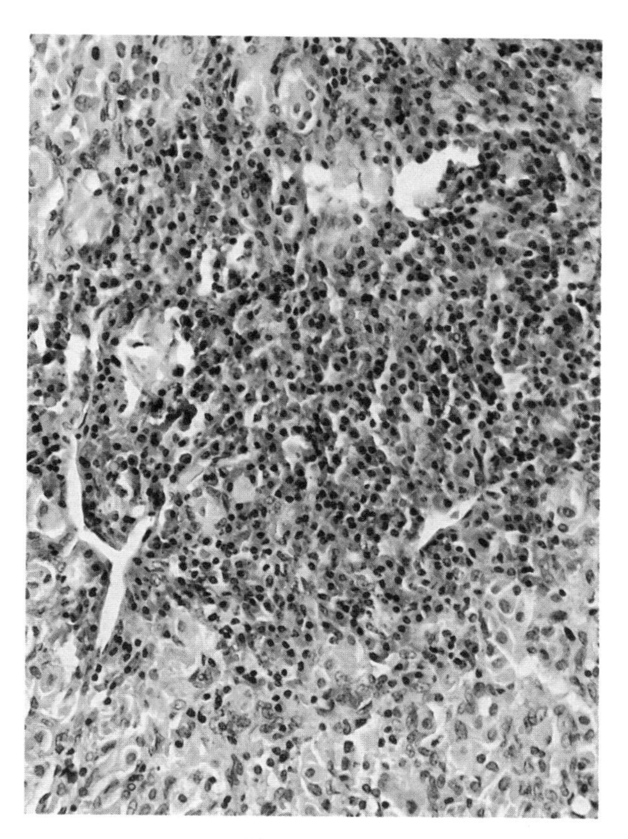

Figure 16-31
CAROTID BODY PARAGANGLIOMA
The patient complained of intermittent swelling of a neck mass in association with upper respiratory tract infections. The CBP contained abundant lymphocytes and plasma cells with a few lymphoid follicles with reactive germinal centers.

Another unusual histologic feature is significant chronic inflammation. Small perivascular collections of inflammatory cells may be present, particularly near the fibrous pseudocapsule, but their presence within the tumor and causing architectural distortion is rare. One patient in the Memorial Hospital series complained of intermittent swelling of a lateral cervical mass in association with upper respiratory tract infections, and on histologic study the CBP was initially confused with a metastatic Hurthle cell carcinoma of thyroid to a cervical lymph node (fig. 16-31) (66). While some observers have regarded CBPs as representing hyperplasia rather than neoplasia (62,73), the histopathology strongly supports a true neoplasm.

Stromal Features. Alterations in the stromal connective tissue and vascular framework of CBPs and other paragangliomas may be extensive, and at times may partially obscure the diagnosis. Fibrosis may be a conspicuous feature in some cases, and can cause compression and distortion of nests of tumor cells (fig. 16-32). There may be evidence of old hemorrhage with hemosiderin deposition, and on rare occasion fibrosiderotic nodules (Gamna-Gandy bodies) (66). Foci of metaplastic bone have also occasionally been reported (66). Alteration in vascular structures can add to diagnostic difficulties (65). There may be areas of sinusoidal sclerosis, for example, which may cause significant architectural distortion (fig. 16-33). Occasionally, there are arcades of dilated vessels which might be confused with a vascular neoplasm such as hemangiopericytoma or hemangioendothelioma (fig. 16-34). Stromal amyloid deposits have been noted

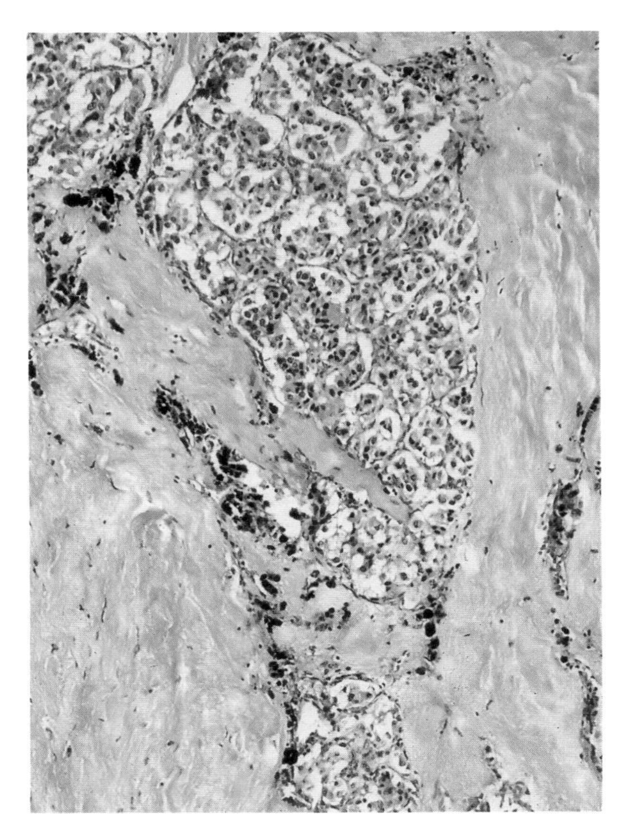

Figure 16-32
CAROTID BODY PARAGANGLIOMA
Multiple areas of marked fibrosis are seen. Hemosiderin deposits were also present.

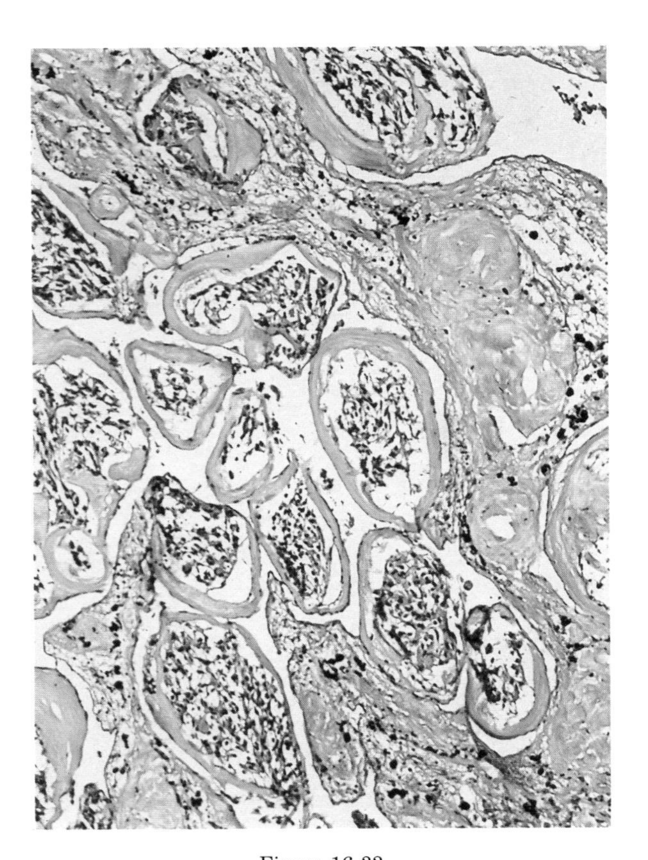

Figure 16-33
CAROTID BODY PARAGANGLIOMA
Sinusoidal sclerosis compresses nests of neoplastic chief cells. The dark granular material in the interstitium of the lower portion of field represents hemosiderin.

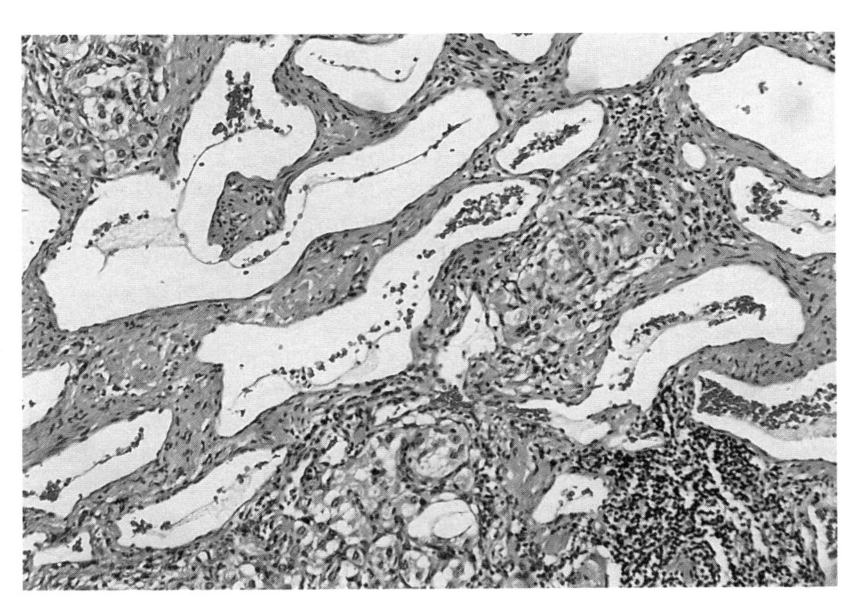

Figure 16-34
CAROTID BODY PARAGANGLIOMA
This CBP has an irregular vascular pattern which might be mistaken for a vasoformative neoplasm. Note the small lymphoid aggregate in the right corner near the tumor periphery.

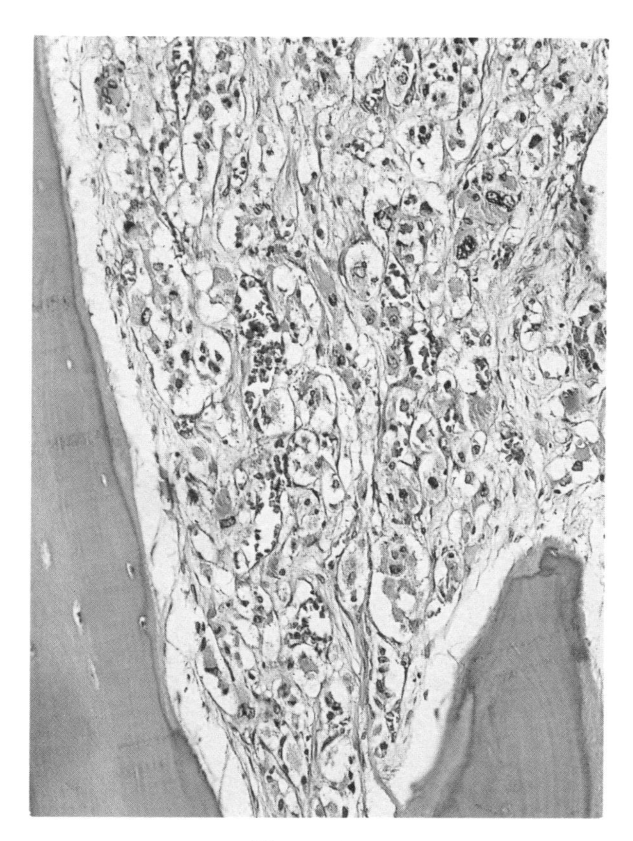

Figure 16-35
METASTATIC CAROTID BODY
PARAGANGLIOMA TO BONE
Patient had several osteolytic bony metastases.

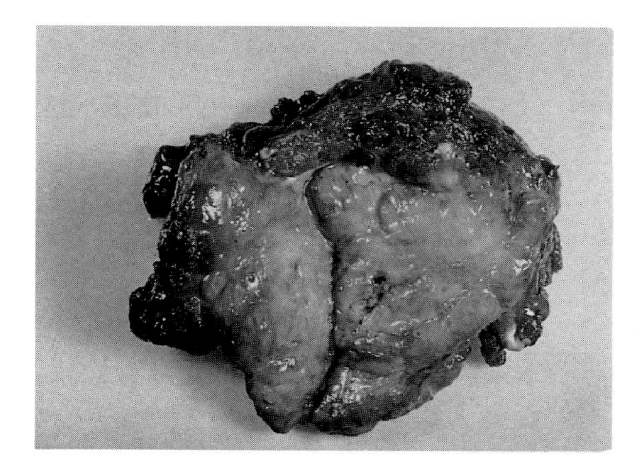

Figure 16-36
CLINICALLY MALIGNANT
CAROTID BODY PARAGANGLIOMA
The bisected tumor was adherent to skeletal muscle and fat in the right neck, and recurred locally with extension up to the base of the skull. The patient died almost 3 years later with clinically apparent cervical lymph node metastases.

in two CBPs on ultrastructural study, but no illustrations were provided (60).

Treatment and Prognosis. As with paragangliomas in general, complete surgical resection is the treatment of choice if it can be done safely; paragangliomas involving the base of the skull may require adjuvant therapy. Carotid body and other head and neck paragangliomas are seldom malignant. In an early study of CBPs, 50 percent of the tumors were considered malignant based upon histologic findings such as mitotic activity, capsular invasion, and cellular pleomorphism (79). Documentation of malignancy usually depends upon demonstration of metastasis to regional lymph nodes, liver, lung, or bone (fig. 16-35). Rarely, a patient presents with miliary infiltrates in lung (89). Aggressive local growth with large size, encirclement of carotid vessels, incorporation of nerves, or invasion near the base of the skull (fig. 16-36) may also suggest malignancy, although undoubted evidence is provided by metastases. Multicentric paragangliomas must be distinguished from true metastases. The incidence of metastasizing CBPs ranges from 6.4 percent (88) to 12.5 percent (90). Some series report a higher incidence of malignancy (18 percent [78] and 23 percent [82]), or categorically classify all CBPs as malignant (86), but this is an overestimate of the malignant potential of this tumor. Prolonged follow-up may be necessary since the neoplasm may metastasize after a long interval (84). Data from the Mayo Clinic over two long periods of treatment indicate a 2 percent rate of malignancy (83,87); a relatively low incidence of malignancy was also reported by Padberg et al. (2.7 percent) (85). There are no individual or group of histopathologic findings which can reliably predict metastases (80). Data from Memorial Hospital suggest that confluent necrosis, vascular invasion, and increased mitotic activity may be adverse prognostic findings, but these features were not considered to be conclusive (81).

REFERENCES

Introduction and Historical Perspective

1. Gilford H, Davis KL. "Potato" tumours of the neck and their origin as endotheliomata of carotid body, with account of three cases. Practioner (London), 1904;73:729–39.
2. Glenner GG, Grimley PM. Tumors of the extra-adrenal paraganglion system (including chemoreceptors). Atlas of Tumor Pathology, 2nd Series, Fascicle 9. Washington, D.C.: Armed Forces Institute of Pathology, 1974.
3. Hutchinson J. Sarcomatous tumours under the upper part of the stermomastoid (potato-like tumours). Illust Med News, Lond 1888–9;1:50.
4. Lack EE. Adrenal medullary hyperplasia and pheochromocytoma. In: Lack EE, ed. Pathology of the adrenal glands. New York: Churchill Livingstone, 1990:173–235.
5. Lack EE. Pathology of adrenal and extra-adrenal paraganglia. Major problems in pathology, Vol 29. Philadelphia: WB Saunders, 1994.
6. Marchand F. Beiträge zur kenntniss der normalen und pathologischen anatomie der glandula carotica und der nebennieren. Festschr für Rudolf Virchow 1891;1:535–81.
7. Mathews FS. Surgery of the neck. In: Johnson AB, ed. Operative therapeusis. Vol 3. New York: Appleton-Century-Crofts, 1915:315.
8. Middleton WD. Some curiosities in surgical pathology. Trans Iowa State Med Soc 1897;15:94–6.
9. Mulligan RM. Chemodectoma in the dog. Am J Pathol 1950;26:680–1.
10. Paltauf R. Ueber geschwülste der glandula carotica nebst einem beitrage zur histologie und entwickelungsgeschichte derselben. Ziegler's Beitr z path Anat u alleg Path, Jena 1891–1892;11:260–301.
11. Scudder CL. Tumor of the intercarotid body. A report of one case, together with all cases in the literature. Am J Med Sci 1903;126:384–9.

Clinical Features of Carotid Body Paragangliomas and Preoperative Localization

12. Crowell WT, Grizzle WE, Siegel AL. Functional carotid paragangliomas. Biochemical, ultrastructural, and histochemical correlation with clinical symptoms. Arch Pathol Lab Med 1982;106:599–603.
13. Duncan AW, Lack EE, Deck MF. Radiological evaluation of paragangliomas of the head and neck. Radiology 1979;132:95–105.
14. Farr HW. Carotid body tumors. A thirty year experience at Memorial Hospital. Am J Surg 1967;114:614–9.
15. Fletcher WE, Arnold JH. Carotid body tumors: review of the literature and report of unusual case. Am J Surg 1954;87:617–9.
16. Gaylis H, Davidge-Pitts K, Pantanowitz D. Carotid body tumours. A review of 52 cases. S Afr Med J 1987;72:493–6.
17. Glasscock ME, Schwaber MK, Nissen AJ, Jackson CG, Smith PG. Diagnosis and management of catecholamine secreting glomus tumors. Laryngoscope 1984;94:1008–15.
18. Glenner GG, Crout JR, Roberts WC. A functional carotid-body-like tumor secreting levarterenol. Arch Pathol 1962;73:230–40.
19. Hallett JW Jr, Nora JD, Hollier LH, Cherry KJ Jr, Pairolero PC. Trends in neurovascular complications of surgical management of carotid body and cervical paragangliomas: a fifty-year experience with 153 tumors. J Vasc Surg 1988;7:284–91.
20. Hamberger CA, Hamberger CB, Wersäll J, Wägermark J. Malignant catecholamine-producing tumor of the carotid body. Acta Path et Microbiol Scandinav 1967;69:489–92.
21. Lack EE. Paragangliomas. In: Sternberg SS, ed. Diagnostic surgical pathology, 2nd ed. New York: Raven Press, 1994:599–621.
22. Lack EE. Pathology of adrenal and extra-adrenal paraganglia. Major problems in pathology, Vol 29. Philadelphia: WB Saunders, 1994.
23. Lack EE, Cubilla AL, Woodruff JM. Paragangliomas of the head and neck region. A pathologic study of tumors from 71 patients. Hum Pathol 1979;10:191–218.
24. Lack EE, Cubilla AL, Woodruff JM, Farr HW. Paragangliomas of the head and neck region. A clinical study of 69 patients. Cancer 1977;39:397–409.
25. LaMuraglia GM, Fabian RL, Brewster DC, et al. The current surgical management of carotid body paragangliomas. J Vasc Surg 1992;15:1038–45.
26. Nora JD, Hallett JW Jr, O'Brien, PC, Naessens JM, Cherry KJ Jr, Pairolero PC. Surgical resection of carotid body tumors: long-term survival, recurrence, and metastasis. Mayo Clin Proc 1988;63:348–52.
27. Oberman HA, Holtz F, Sheffer LA, Magielski JE. Chemodectomas (nonchromaffin paragangliomas) of the head and neck. A clinicopathologic study. Cancer 1968;21:838–51.
28. Olsen WL, Dillon WP, Kelly WM, Norman D, Brant-Zawadzki M, Newton TH. MR imaging of paragangliomas. Am J Roentgenol 1987;148:201–4.
29. Padberg FT Jr, Cady B, Persson AV. Carotid body tumor. The Lahey Clinic experience. Am J Surg 1983;145:526–8.
30. Pandya S, Nagpal R, Desai A, Purohit A. Death following external carotid artery embolization for a functioning glomus jugulare chemodectoma. Case report. J Neurosurg 1978;48:1030–4.
31. Patel AK, Yap VU, Fields J, Thomsen JH. Carotid sinus syncope induced by malignant tumors in the neck. Emergence of vasodepressor manifestations following pacemaker therapy. Arch Intern Med 1979;139:1281–4.
32. Robison JG, Shagets FW, Beckett WC Jr, Spies JB. A multidisciplinary approach to reducing morbidity and operative blood loss during resection of carotid body tumor. Surg Gynecol Obstet 1989;168:166–70.
33. Sanchez AC, de Seijas EV, Matesanz JM, Trapero VL. Carotid body tumor: unusual cause of transient ischemic attacks. Stroke 1988;19:102–3.
34. Shamblin WR, ReMine WH, Sheps SG, Harrison EG Jr. Carotid body tumor (chemodectoma). Clinicopathologic analysis of ninety cases. Am J Surg 1971;122:732–9.

35. Smith RF, Shelty PC, Reddy DJ. Surgical treatment of carotid paragangliomas presenting unusual technical difficulties. The value of preoperative embolization. J Vasc Surg 1988;7:631–7.
36. White MC, Hickson BR. Multiple paragangliomata secreting catecholamines and calcitonin with intermittent hypercalcaemia. J Roy Soc Med 1979;72:532–8.
37. You-xian F, Qun S. Surgical treatment of carotid body tumors. Review of 63 cases. Chinese Med J 1982;95:417–22.
38. Zak FG, Lawson W. The paraganglionic chemoreceptor system: physiology, pathology, and clinical medicine. New York: Springer-Verlag, 1982.

Familial and Multicentric Paragangliomas

39. Grufferman S, Gillman MW, Pasternak LR, Peterson CL, Young WG. Familial carotid body tumors: case report and epidemiologic review. Cancer 1980;46:2116–22.
40. Jensen JC, Choyke PL, Rosenfeld M, et al. A report of familial carotid body tumors and multiple extra-adrenal pheochromocytomas. J Urol 1991;145:1040–2.
41. Kroll AJ, Alexander B, Cochios F, Pechet L. Hereditary deficiencies of clotting factors VII and X associated with carotid body tumors. N Engl J Med 1964;270:6–13.
42. Lack EE. Pathology of adrenal and extra-adrenal paraganglia. Major problems in pathology, Vol 29. Philadelphia: WB Saunders, 1994.
43. Lattes R, McDonald JJ, Sproul E. Nonchromaffin paraganglioma of carotid body and orbit. Report of a case. Ann Surg 1954;139:382–4.
44. Ophir D. Familial multicentric paragangliomas in a child. J Laryngol Otol 1991;105:376–80.
45. Parry DM, Li FP, Strong LC, et al. Carotid body tumors in humans: genetics and epidemiology. JNCI 1982;68:573–8.
46. Pratt LW. Familial carotid body tumors. Arch Otolaryngol 1973;97:334–6.
47. Sobol SM, Dailey JC. Familial multiple cervical paragangliomas: report of a kindred and review of the literature. Otololaryngol Head Neck Surg 1990;102:382–90.
48. van Baars FM, Cremers CW, van den Broek P, Veldman JE. Familial nonchromaffin paragangliomas (glomus tumors). Clinical and genetic aspects. Acta Otolaryngol 1981;91:589–93.
49. van Baars FM, van den Broek P, Cremers C, Veldman J. Familial non-chromaffin paragangliomas (glomus tumors): clinical aspects. Laryngoscope 1981;91:988–96.
50. Van der May AG, Maaswinkel-Mooy PD, Cornelisse CJ, Schmidt PH, van de Kamp JJ. Genetic imprinting in hereditary glomus tumors: evidence for new genetic theory. Lancet 1989;2:1291–4.

Association with Other Endocrine Disorders

51. Albores-Saavedra J, Durán ME. Association of thyroid carcinoma and chemodectoma. Am J Surg 1968;116:887–90.
52. Berg B, Biörklund A, Grimelius L, et al. A new pattern of multiple endocrine adenomatosis: chemodectoma, bronchial carcinoid, GH-producing pituitary adenoma, and hyperplasia of the parathyroid glands, and antral and duodenal gastrin cells. Acta Med Scand 1976;200:321–6.
53. Carney JA. The triad of gastric epithelioid leiomyosarcoma, functioning extra-adrenal paraganglioma, and pulmonary chondroma. Cancer 1979;43:374–82.
54. Carney JA. The triad of gastric epithelioid leiomyosarcoma, pulmonary chondroma, and functioning extra-adrenal paraganglioma: a five year review. Medicine 1983;62:159–69.
55. Carney JA, Sheps SG, Go VL, Gordon H. The triad of gastric leiomyosarcoma, functioning extra-adrenal paraganglioma and pulmonary chondroma. N Engl J Med 1977;296:1517–8.
56. Larraza-Hernandez O, Albores-Saavedra J, Benavides G, Krause LG, Perez-Merizaldi JC, Ginzo A. Multiple endocrine neoplasia. Pituitary adenoma, multicentric papillary thyroid carcinoma, bilateral carotid body paraganglioma, parathyroid hyperplasia, gastric leiomyoma, and systemic amyloidosis. Am J Clin Pathol 1982;78:527–32.
57. Parry DM, Li FP, Strong LC, et al. Carotid body tumors in humans: genetics and epidemiology. JNCI 1982;68:573–8.
58. Steely WM, Davies RS, Brigham RA. Carotid body tumor and hyperparathyroidism. A case report and review of the literature. Amer Surg 1987;53:337–8.

Pathology of Carotid Body Paragangliomas

59. Capella C, Riva C, Cornaggia M, Chiaravalli AM, Frigerio B. Histopathology, cytology and cytochemistry of pheochromocytomas and paragangliomas including chemodectomas. Path Res Pract 1988;183:176–87.
60. Capella C, Solcia E. Optical and electron microscopical study of cytoplasmic granules in human carotid body, carotid body tumors and glomus jugulare tumors. Virchows Arch [Cell Pathol] 1971;7:37–53.
61. Chang A, Harawi SJ. Oncocytes, oncocytosis and oncocytic tumors. Pathol Annu 1992;27:263–304.
62. Costero I. Recent advances in the knowledge concerning chemodectomas. Lab Invest 1963;12:270–84.
63. Davidge-Pitts KJ, Pantanowitz D. Carotid body tumors. Surg Ann 1984;16:203–27.
64. Glenner GG, Grimley PM. Tumors of the extra-adrenal paraganglion system (including chemoreceptors). Atlas of Tumor Pathology, 2nd Series, Fascicle 9. Washington, D.C.: Armed Forces Institute of Pathology, 1974.
65. Lack EE. Pathology of adrenal and extra-adrenal paraganglia. Major problems in pathology, Vol 29. Philadelphia: WB Saunders, 1994.

66. Lack EE, Cubilla AL, Woodruff JM. Paragangliomas of the head and neck region. A pathologic study of tumors from 71 patients. Hum Pathol 1979;10:191–218.
67. LaMuraglia GM, Fabian RL, Brewster DC, et al. The current surgical management of carotid body paragangliomas. J Vasc Surg 1992;15:1038–45.
68. Le Compte PM. Tumors of the carotid body. Am J Pathol 1948:24:305–16.
69. Le Compte PM. Tumors of the carotid body and related structures (chemoreceptor system). Atlas of Tumor Pathology, 1st Series, Fascicle 16. Washington, D.C.: Armed Forces Institute of Pathology, 1951.
70. Mauri MF, Mingazzini P, Sisti S, Montironi R, Scarpelli M. Histomorphometric and morphologic studies of the carotid body and aortic paragangliomas. Appl Pathol 1989;7:310–7.
71. Nora JD, Hallett JW Jr, O'Brien PC, Naessens JM, Cherry KJ Jr, Pairolero PC. Surgical resection of carotid body tumors: long-term survival, recurrence, and metastasis. Mayo Clin Proc 1988;63:348–52.
72. Pryse-Davies J, Dawson IM, Westbury G. Some morphologic, histochemical, and chemical observations on chemodectomas and the normal carotid body, including a study of the chromaffin reaction and possible ganglion cell elements. Cancer 1964;17:185–202.
73. Rodriguez-Cuevas H, Lau I, Rodriguez HP. High-altitude paragangliomas diagnostic and therapeutic considerations. Cancer 1986;57:672–6.
74. Sacher M, Som PM, Lanzieri CF, Biller HF. Total internal carotid artery occlusion by a benign carotid body tumor: a rare occurrence. J Comput Assist Tomogr 1985;9:213–7.
75. Saldana MJ, Salem LE, Travezan R. High altitude hypoxia and chemodectomas. Hum Pathol 1973;4:251–63.
76. Shamblin WR, ReMine WH, Sheps SG, Harrison EG Jr. Carotid body tumor (chemodectoma). Clinicopathologic analysis of ninety cases. Am J Surg 1971;122:732–9.
77. Warshawski SJ, de Souza FM. The carotid body tumor. J Otolaryngol 1989;18:306–10.

Biologic Behavior of Carotid Body Paragangliomas

78. Gaylis H, Davidge-Pitts K, Pantanowitz D. Carotid body tumours. A review of 52 cases. S Afr Med J 1987;72:493–6.
79. Harrington SW, Clagett OT, Dockerty MB. Tumors of the carotid body. Clinical and pathologic considerations of twenty tumors affecting nineteen patients (one bilateral). Ann Surg 1941;114:820–33.
80. Lack EE. Pathology of adrenal and extra-adrenal paraganglia. Major problems in pathology, Vol 29. Philadelphia: WB Saunders, 1994.
81. Lack EE, Cubilla AL, Woodruff JM. Paragangliomas of the head and neck region. A pathologic study of tumors from 71 patients. Hum Pathol 1979;10:191–218.
82. Martin CE, Rosenfeld L, McSwain B. Carotid body tumors: a 16-year follow-up of seven malignant cases. South Med J 1973;66:1236–43.
83. Nora JD, Hallett JW Jr, O'Brien PC, Naessens JM, Cherry KJ Jr, Pairolero PC. Surgical resection of carotid body tumors: long-term survival, recurrence, and metastasis. Mayo Clin Proc 1988;63:348–52.
84. North CA, Zinreich ES, Christensen WN, North RB. Multiple spinal metastases from paraganglioma. Cancer 1990;66:2224–8.
85. Padberg FT Jr, Cady B, Persson AV. Carotid body tumor. The Lahey Clinic experience. Am J Surg 1983;145:526–8.
86. Pantanowitz D, Davidge-Pitts K, Gaylis H, Hale MJ. Are carotid body tumours malignant? S Afr J Surg 1990;28:97–9.
87. Shamblin WR, ReMine WH, Sheps SG, Harrison EG Jr. Carotid body tumor (chemodectoma). Clinicopathologic analysis of ninety cases. Am J Surg 1971;122:732–9.
88. Staats EF, Brown RL, Smith RR. Carotid body tumors, benign and malignant. Laryngoscope 1966;76:907–15.
89. Tu H, Bottomley RH. Malignant chemodectoma presenting as a miliary infiltrate. Cancer 1974;33:244–9.
90. Zbaren P, Lehmann W. Carotid body paraganglioma with metastases. Laryngoscope 1985;95:450–4.

◇◇◇

17
JUGULOTYMPANIC PARAGANGLIOMA

The first description of a "carotid body tumor," located in the middle ear and mastoid, was by Rosenwasser in 1945 (10), but it was Otani (10,11) who actually made the pathologic diagnosis. The tumor was considered to arise from the minute paraganglia located near the base of the skull. Several other carotid body–like tumors of the middle ear and base of skull were reported over the next few years (3,7,8,13), including the first case associated with a carotid body paraganglioma (3).

JUGULOTYMPANIC PARAGANGLIA

In 1941 Guild (1) described microscopic structures resembling the carotid body that were located in adventitia of the dome of the jugular bulb beneath the bony floor of the middle ear or along the ramus tympanicus of the glossopharyngeal nerve. In a subsequent study in 1953 (2), Guild examined 88 temporal bones from 44 individuals, and identified 248 collections of paraganglia: 135 in close association with the tympanic branch of the ninth cranial nerve (nerve of Jacobson) and 113 near the auricular branch of the tenth cranial nerve (nerve of Arnold) (fig. 17-1). He believed that previous reports by Krause (5) and Valentin (12), did not validly document the "glomus jugulare." This minor historical dispute aside, the study published in 1953 provided valuable anatomic data regarding number, size, and distribution of the paraganglia in humans (2). An average of 2.82 paraganglia were identified in each temporal bone (range, 0 to 12), but this was probably a low estimate: 7 of 82 temporal bones contained more than six paraganglia. A little over half of the paraganglia were present in adventitia of the dome of the jugular bulb and along the nerves of Jacobson and Arnold, and 25 percent were within mucosa of the cochlear promontory in association with the tympanic plexus of the nerve of Jacobson (fig. 17-1, bottom).

The microanatomy of jugulotympanic paraganglia is virtually identical to carotid body paraganglia except for smaller size and lack of multilobelation (fig. 17-2) (6). Most are ovoid or flattened and measure 0.5 mm or less in diameter (2). A chemoreceptor role has been postulated in response to changes in gas composition of the middle ear, but inconsistency of anatomic localization in a recent study has cast some doubt on this proposal (9). Results of ultrastructural study of jugulotympanic paraganglia in the human fetus were essentially identical to those of carotid body paraganglia (4).

CLINICAL FEATURES OF JUGULOTYMPANIC PARAGANGLIOMA

Definition. Jugular and tympanic paragangliomas arise from anatomically dispersed paraganglia near the base of the skull and middle ear.

Clinical Features. Jugulotympanic paragangliomas (JTPs) usually occur in adult patients in the fifth to sixth decade of life (14,17), but have been diagnosed even in early childhood (18,19). A distinct predilection for female patients has been reported: in one large series the female to male ratio was 6 to 1 (198 females, 33 males), with an average age of 55 years at diagnosis (17). At the Mayo Clinic, 55 patients (43 females, 12 males) were evaluated for a tympanic paraganglioma (TP) at an average age of 52 years (range, 22 to 81 years) (25). There is no apparent bias in laterality: JTPs have a roughly equal distribution on either side.

TYMPANIC PARAGANGLIOMA

Tympanic paragangliomas (TPs) are usually located along the course of Jacobson's nerve in the middle ear cavity. They are often associated with tinnitus or aural pulsations, and may cause conduction-type hearing loss due to involvement of middle ear ossicles (24). Other manifestations include ear fullness or pain, otorrhea, vertigo/dizziness, and symptoms of chronic otitis media. Facial palsy has also been noted in a small number of patients. A TP can be quite small on the promontory of the middle ear (fig. 17-3), or when it becomes large, it can fill the middle ear cavity, engulf the middle ear ossicles, bulge or protrude through the tympanic membrane, and present as an aural polyp in the external ear canal. Biopsy of such a lesion can result in brisk, copious bleeding. TP can

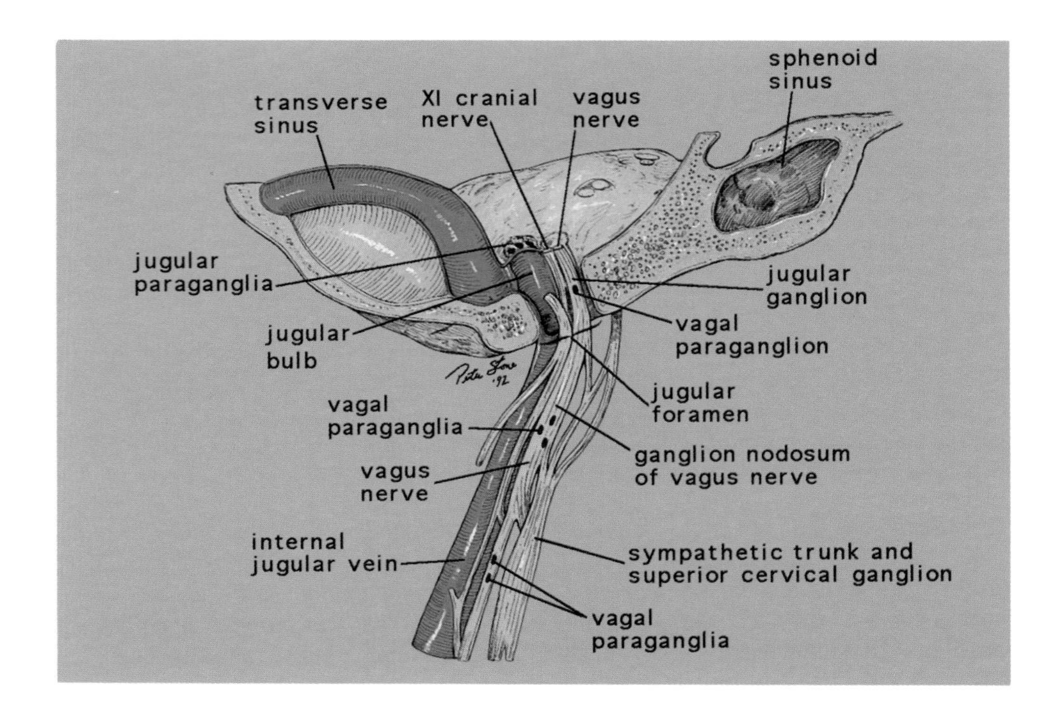

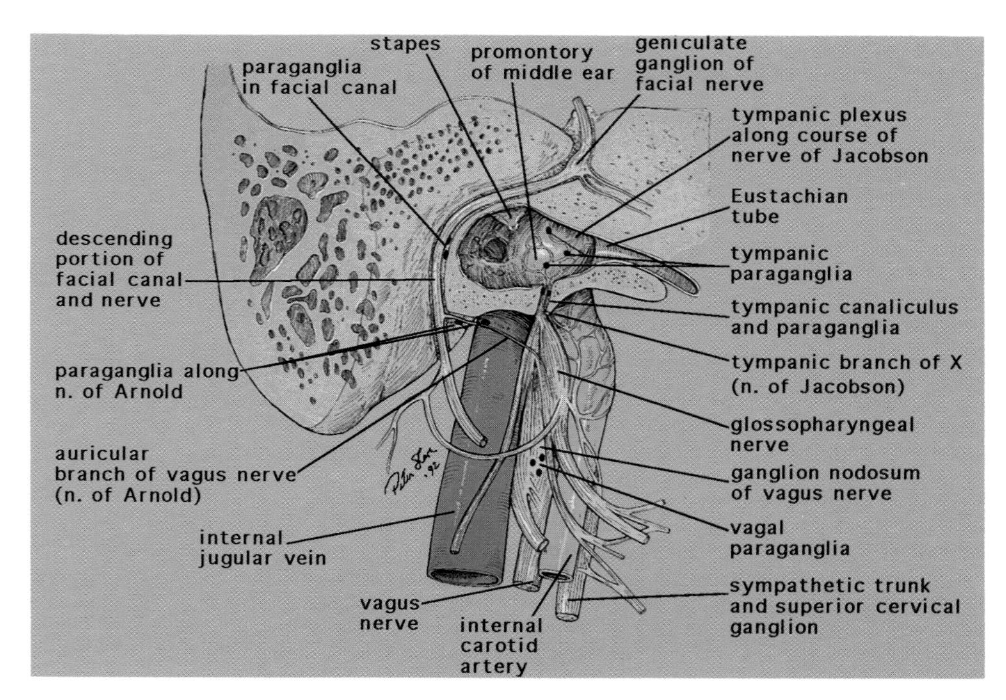

Figure 17-1
JUGULOTYMPANIC PARAGANGLIA

Top: Diagram showing plane of section through base of skull and lateral temporal bone. Jugulotympanic paraganglia are present within the adventitia near the jugular bulb. Note also the vagal paraganglia in relation to the ganglion nodosum of the vagus nerve and the vagal paraganglion higher up, in or near a superior jugular ganglion.

Bottom: A different plane of section through the base of the skull shows paraganglia within the facial canal, middle ear over promontory, and along nerves of Arnold and Jacobson. Note also the vagal paraganglia in close association with the ganglion nodosum of the vagus nerve.

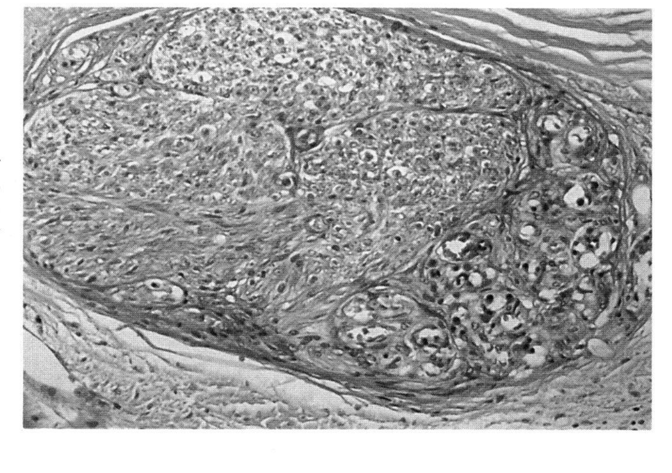

Figure 17-2
SMALL JUGULOTYMPANIC PARAGANGLION

This small paraganglion is located paraneurally along the nerve of Jacobson. The cytoarchitecture is identical to that of a portion of carotid body lobule. Chief cells have eccentric, dark-staining nuclei. Courtesy of Dr. Karoly Balogh, Boston, MA.)

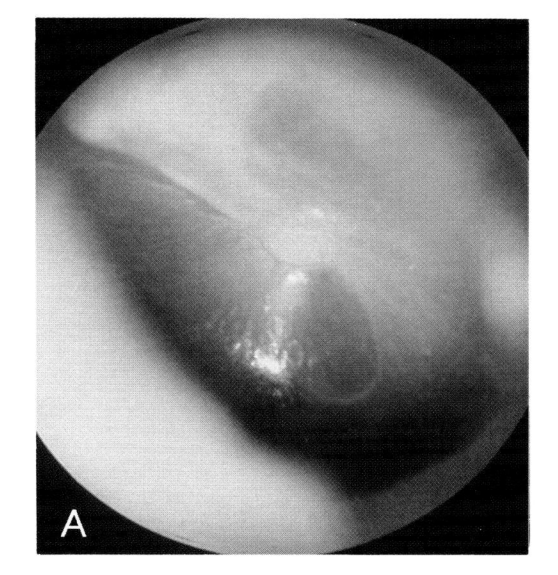

Figure 17-3
TYMPANIC PARAGANGLIOMA

A: Tympanic paraganglioma appears as a small, deeply congested lesion on the cochlear promontory of the middle ear. The tumor is apparent through intact tympanic membrane. (Courtesy of Dr. W. R. Wilson, Washington, DC.)

B: Schematic diagram of the anatomic relation of the tympanic paraganglioma shown in A.

C: Small tympanic paraganglioma was removed by transmeatal approach from the cochlear promontory of the middle ear.

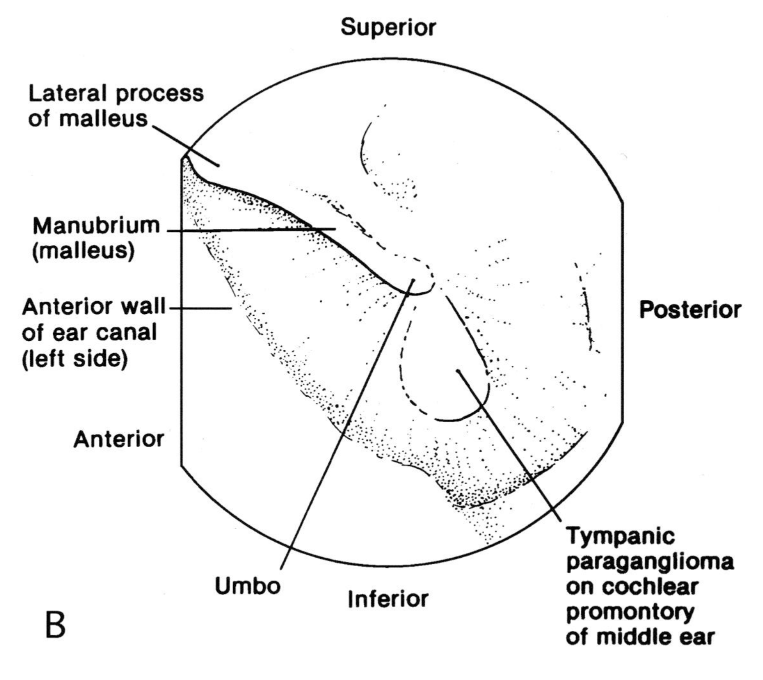

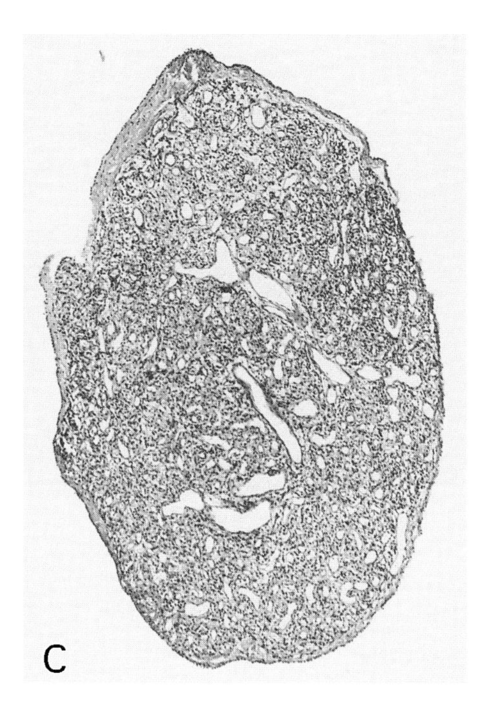

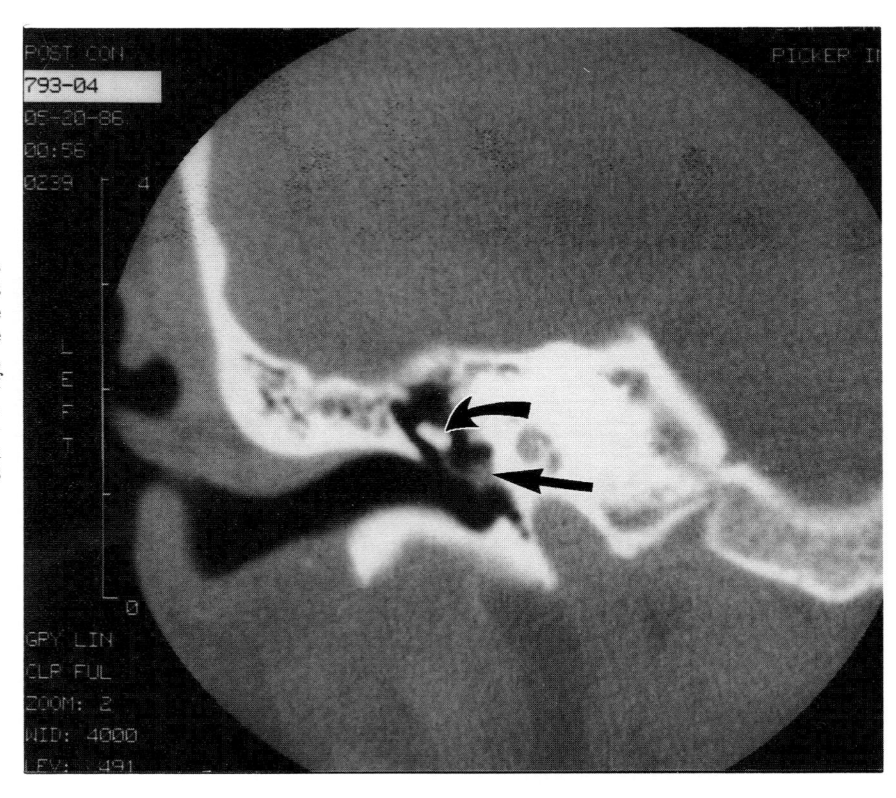

Figure 17-4
TYMPANIC PARAGANGLIOMA

Coronal plane of CT scan shows a tympanic paraganglioma (straight arrow) on the promontory of middle ear. Other structures in this plane include malleus (curved arrow), semicircular canal, and basal turn of the cochlea. (Fig. 4-5 from Lack EE. Pathology of adrenal and extra-adrenal paraganglia. Major problems in pathology, Vol 29. Philadelphia: WB Saunders Co, 1994:81.)

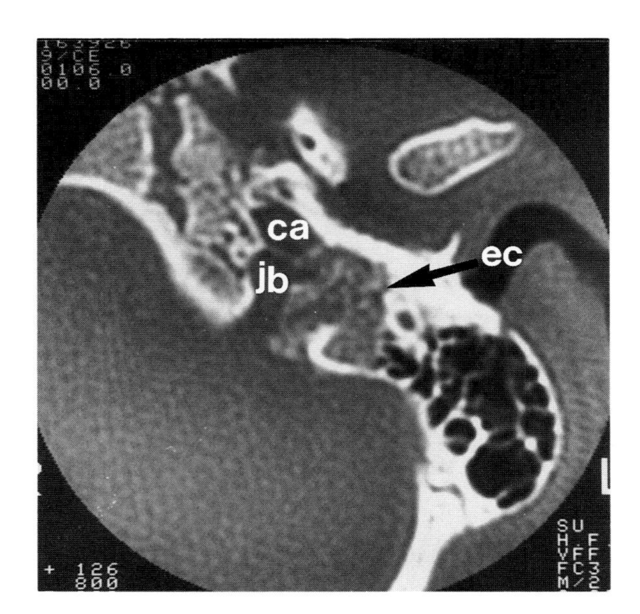

Figure 17-5
JUGULAR PARAGANGLIOMA

CT scan in horizontal (axial) plane shows a JP (arrow) on the left side in a 15-year-old girl with a family history of head and neck paragangliomas. Patient also had an ipsilateral carotid body paraganglioma. Jugular bulb (jb), internal carotid artery (ca), and external ear canal (ec) are indicated.

also extend into the orifice of the eustachian tube or aditus ad antrum (24). The lesion can be visualized using high resolution computed tomographic (CT) scans (fig. 17-4) (28). Magnetic resonance imaging (MRI) also provides high resolution, but it is less sensitive in identifying bone erosion or destruction. Direct visualization of the middle ear mass or bulging tympanic membrane typically shows a red, pink, or bluish lesion. Problems associated with hemorrhage are clearly conveyed in a report of surgery on a young girl with a JTP: "... the most vivid vascular experience we have ever encountered requiring 6 hours and 17 bottles of blood" (27).

JUGULAR PARAGANGLIOMA

Jugular paragangliomas (JPs) involve the lateral temporal bone at the base of the skull (fig. 17-5). They may grow within the petrous bone, sometimes extending intracranially and simulating a cerebellopontine angle tumor or a mass in the middle cranial fossa (24). The tumor may have a dumbbell configuration, grow through the jugular foramen, and occasionally occlude the superior part of the internal jugular vein and

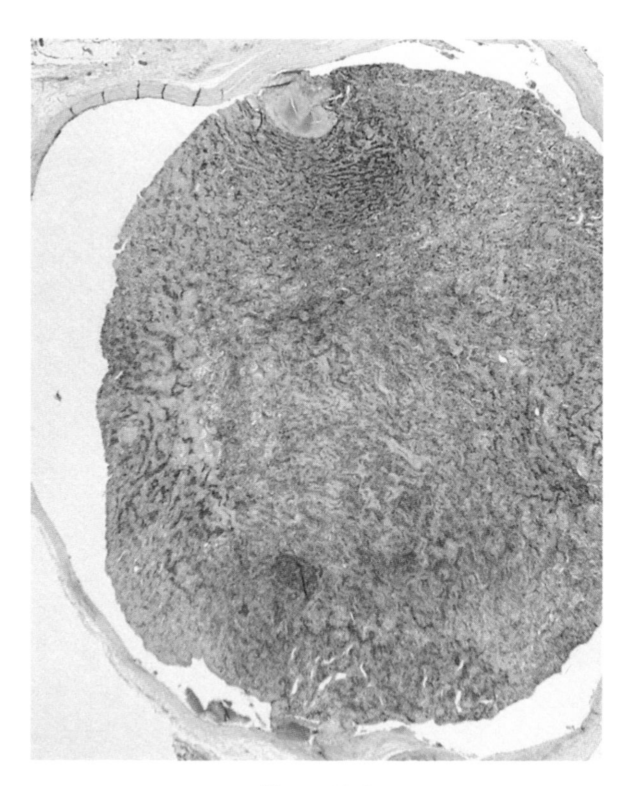

Figure 17-6
JUGULAR PARAGANGLIOMA
This jugular paraganglioma grew within the lumen of the internal jugular vein. In this plane of section the tumor appears "free floating," but more rostrally there was a broad-based attachment to the wall of the vessel.

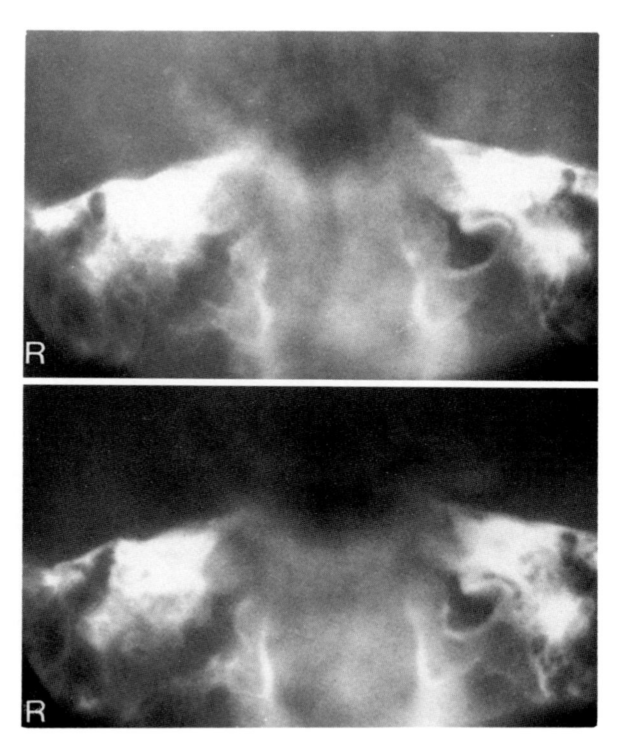

Figure 17-7
JUGULAR PARAGANGLIOMA
Tomogram of base of skull of a woman with a JP on the right side. The patient also had a history of multiple familial paragangliomas of the head and neck region. (Fig. 5 from Duncan AW, Lack EE, Deck MF. Radiological evaluation of paragangliomas of the head and neck. Radiology 1979;132:99–105.)

bulb. The tumor may extend as a sausage-like projection into the lumen of the internal jugular vein (fig. 17-6). Theoretical complications include contiguous extension into the right heart and fatal embolization at the time of surgery or even during the course of radiation treatment (24). In one case the tumor caused extensive bone destruction at the base of the skull, and extended in a continuous fashion into the internal jugular vein, superior vena cava, and on into the right atrium; the surgically resected tumor was 15 cm in length and 3 cm in diameter when it was transected near the base of the skull (20). A retrograde venous jugulogram can document intravenous growth by the tumor (22). The jugular foramen syndrome may occur with paresis due to compression of cranial nerves 9, 10, 11, and 12 in various combinations (24).

Ragged erosion of the jugular fossa or foramen is important radiographic evidence of a JP (fig. 17-7), but erosion should not be confused with simple asymmetry in size and shape of the jugular foramen which can occur under normal conditions (21,28). JPs can also erode the thin bony plate overlying the dome of the jugular fossa, and present as an aural or middle ear polyp (fig. 17-8). The tumor has also been reported to cause parotid swelling, and mimic an acinic cell neoplasm on pathologic examination of the parotidectomy specimen (16). Upper cervical growth can also cause medial deviation of nasopharyngeal soft tissue (29). Small biopsy specimens of JP might also be misinterpreted as meningioma, and in one case the tumor radiographically simulated a meningioma, with extension medially to the area of the foramen magnum and extensive calcification (26). Based upon extent and location of some of these paragangliomas of the skull base it may not be possible to neatly designate the tumor as tympanic or jugular, hence the composite designation

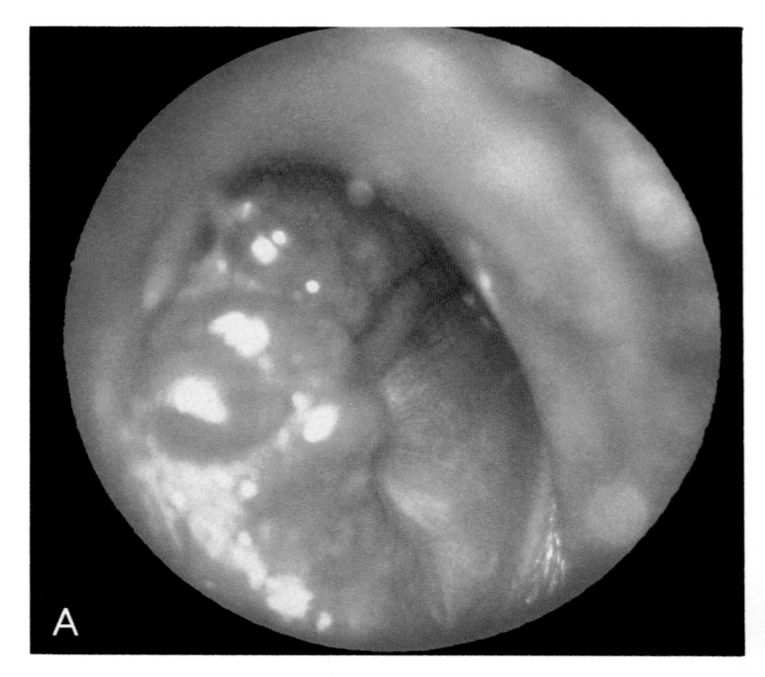

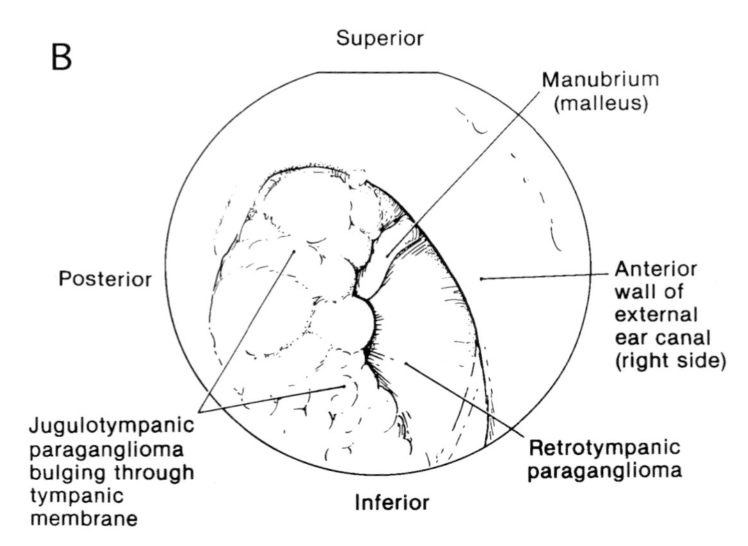

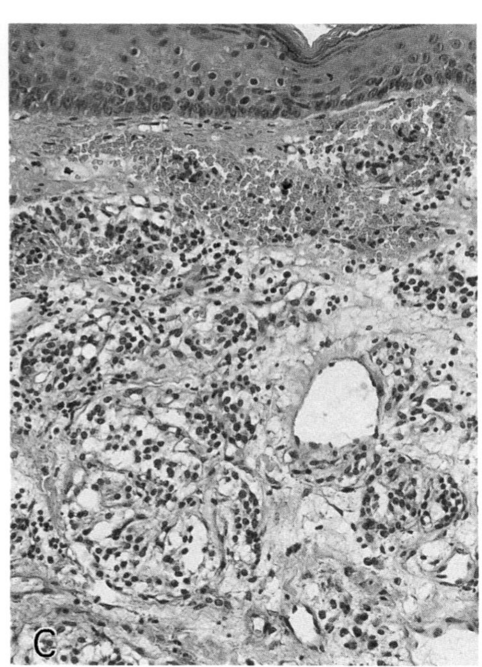

Figure 17-8
JUGULAR PARAGANGLIOMA

A: JP appears as a lobulated, deeply congested mass bulging out the tympanic membrane. The tumor has completely filled the middle ear cavity. (Courtesy of Dr. A. Julianna Gulya, Washington, DC.)

B: Diagram depicting anatomic regions of the JP.

C: The paraganglioma protrudes behind the tympanic membrane. There is a well-developed organoid arrangement of neoplastic chief cells.

jugulotympanic paraganglioma (JTP) (24). Some vagal paragangliomas are difficult to distinguish from JTPs because of the close spatial relationship of the ganglion nodosum and jugular foramen and the fact that vagal paraganglia sometimes occur rostral to this ganglion, or even within the jugular ganglion of the vagus nerve (15). Due to the complexities of these paragangliomas of the skull base, and some controversy regarding optimal treatment regimens, several clinical classification schemes (e.g., the McCabe-Fletcher classification [30] and the Glasscock-Jackson classification [23,25]) have been proposed in an attempt to promote consistency in communication, and permit a more standardized analysis of treatment results.

OTHER INTRACRANIAL PARAGANGLIOMAS

Rare intrasellar (31) and parasellar (33) paragangliomas have been reported. One patient had several extra-adrenal paragangliomas; one that arose near the clivus and upper cervical spine had increased catecholamine secretion (32). A paraganglioma was reported in the region of the pineal gland (34), but the histopathology in this case was somewhat atypical. Expanding the concept of tumors of "glomic" tissue, Zak (35) referred to tumors arising from aberrant cranial "glomera" over the cerebral convexity, in the ventricular lumen, and in other locations, and questioned whether some meningiomas and hemangioblastomas were of glomic origin. This concept has not been accepted, since these tumors have specific histopathology distinct from paragangliomas.

HORMONAL MANIFESTATIONS

Rare examples of functionally active or catecholamine-producing paragangliomas of the skull base or infratemporal fossa (39,41,42,44–47) and wide fluctuations in systemic blood pressure during surgical removal of JTPs (38,42) have prompted some observers to advise that "gentle handling" of all large glomus jugulare tumors is imperative (38). A JTP was reported with the carcinoid syndrome, but there was no biochemical documentation (43). Norepinephrine (37,40) and dopamine (36) have been detected in several cases of JTP.

PATHOLOGY OF JUGULOTYMPANIC PARAGANGLIOMA

Gross Findings. Surgically resected specimens of JTP are often small or fragmentary. A tumor that appears significant in size under the operating microscope and has caused significant symptoms for the patient may be actually quite small after transmeatal tumor resection (see fig. 17-3C) (50). Massive JTPs with petrosal extension and intracranial impingement with fatal consequences are rare. Selective tumor embolization and radiation therapy may also limit the gross characterization of JTP. The rare intravenous extensions may be more significant in terms of gross pathology.

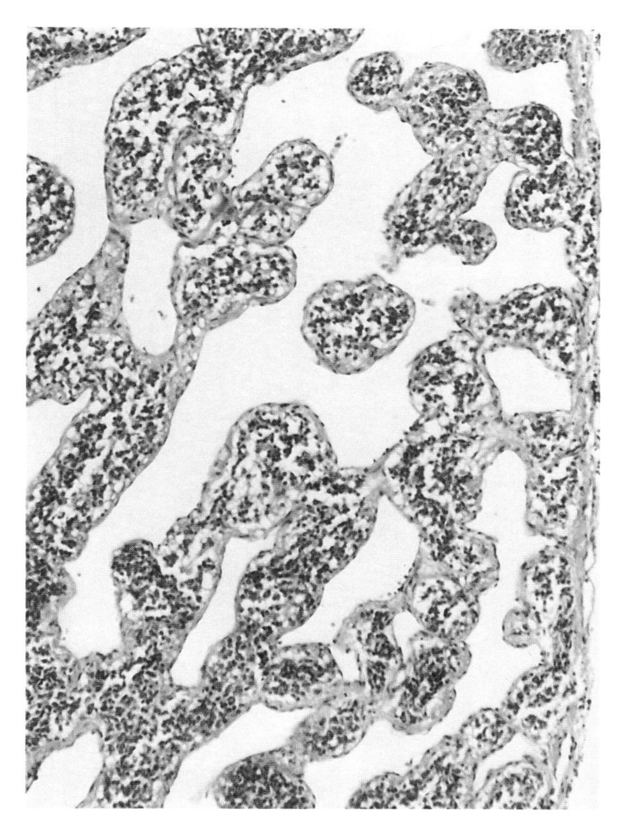

Figure 17-9
JUGULOTYMPANIC PARAGANGLIOMA
Anastomosing arcades of relatively small tumor cells were focally evident in this JTP. Vascular channels appear devoid of blood which is artifactual due to mechanical manipulation of tumor during surgery.

Microscopic Findings. Microscopically, JTPs are similar to paragangliomas at other sites in the head and neck region, although sometimes there are features that allow prediction of anatomic location with relative assurance. Examples include the circumscribed small tumor removed from the cochlear promontory on transmeatal approach (see fig. 17-3), or a portion of attached tympanic membrane or middle ear mucosa. JTPs are more vascular (49), cell nests are less uniform and frequently smaller, and the chief cell nuclei are smaller compared with other paragangliomas (figs. 17-9, 17-10) (52). A remarkable feature of some JTPs (and also some vagal paragangliomas) is the degree of sclerosis present (fig. 17-11) (50). In a recent review of a large number of head and neck paragangliomas, stromal sclerosis was most marked in JTPs and vagal

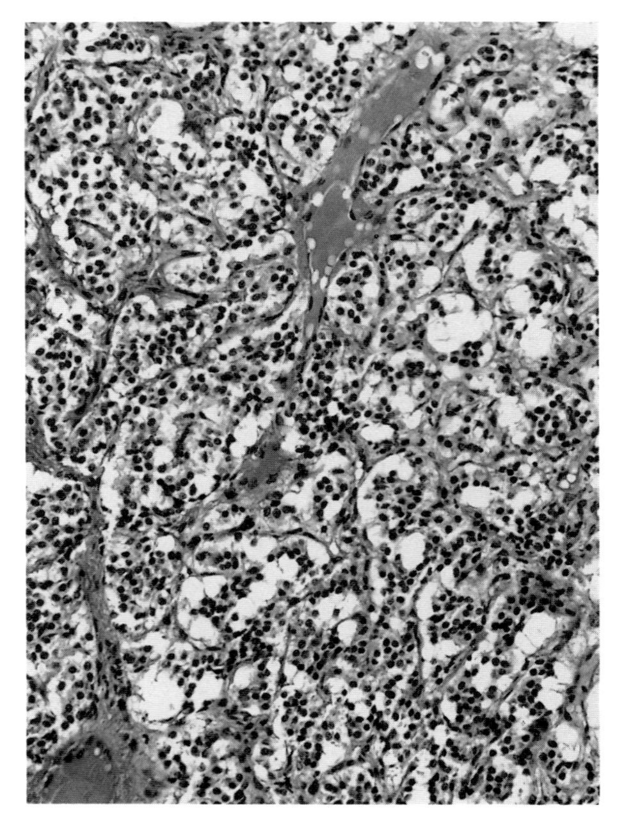

Figure 17-10
JUGULOTYMPANIC PARAGANGLIOMA

Other areas of the same tumor show a more organoid or nesting pattern, with formation of small "zellballen." The tumor cells have uniform, small, hyperchromatic nuclei.

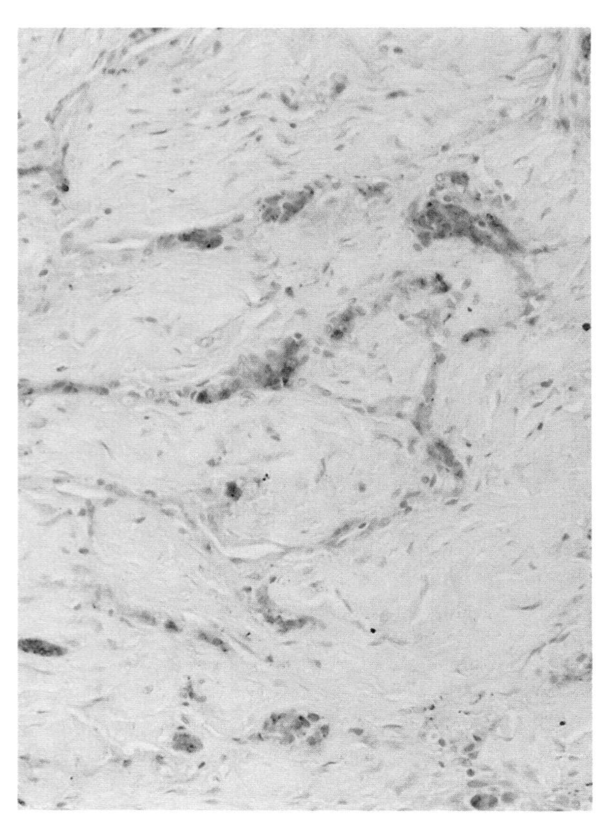

Figure 17-11
JUGULOTYMPANIC PARAGANGLIOMA

There are areas of marked sclerosis. The stain for chromogranin immunoreactivity highlights thin cords of compressed tumor cells. (X200, Streptavidin alkaline phosphatase method)

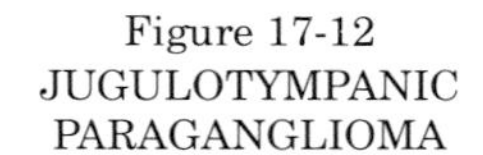

Figure 17-12
JUGULOTYMPANIC
PARAGANGLIOMA

JTP invades the bony structures at the base of the skull, with evidence of some bone remodeling. This represents local invasion and not a metastasis.

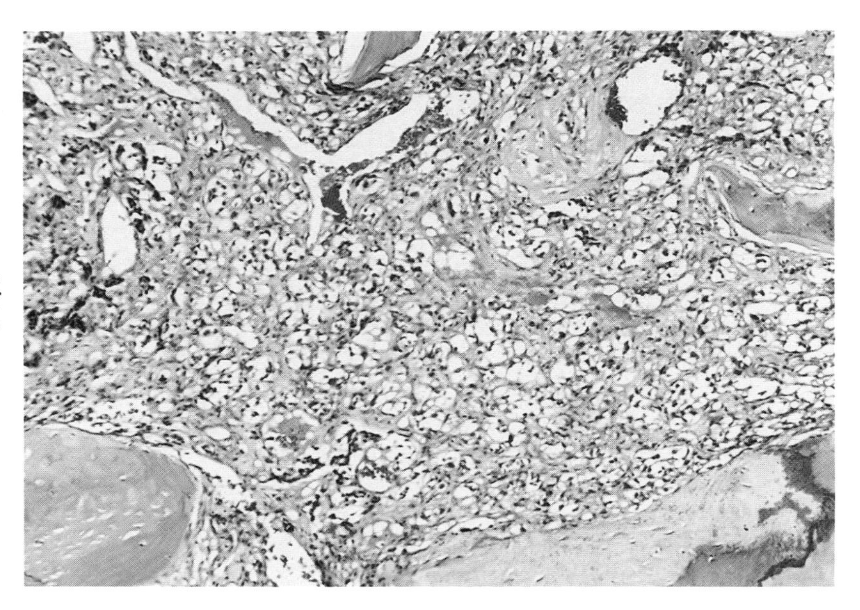

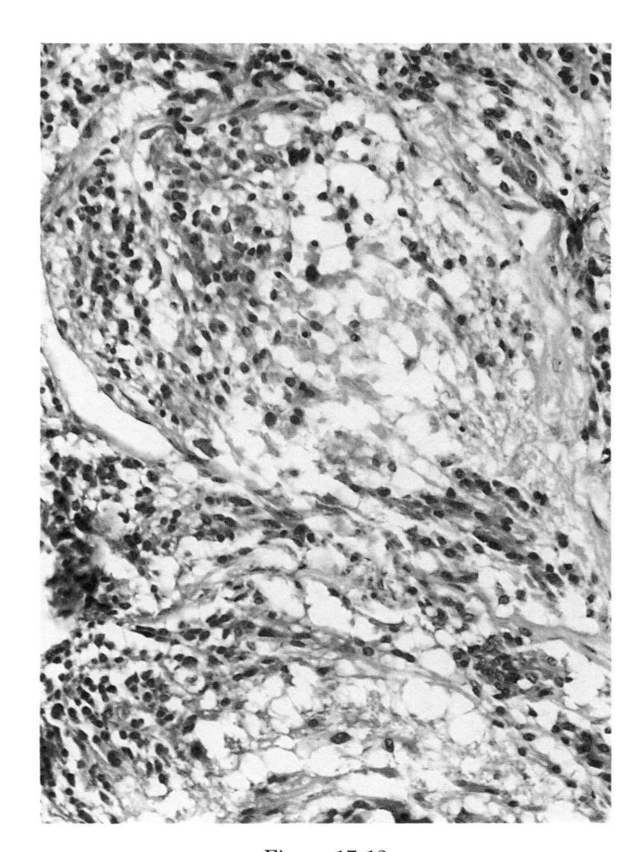

Figure 17-13
JUGULOTYMPANIC PARAGANGLIOMA
Areas of tumor were composed of small "neuroblast-like" cells associated with a distinct fibrillary matrix resembling neuropil. Other areas showed a pattern typical for a paraganglioma.

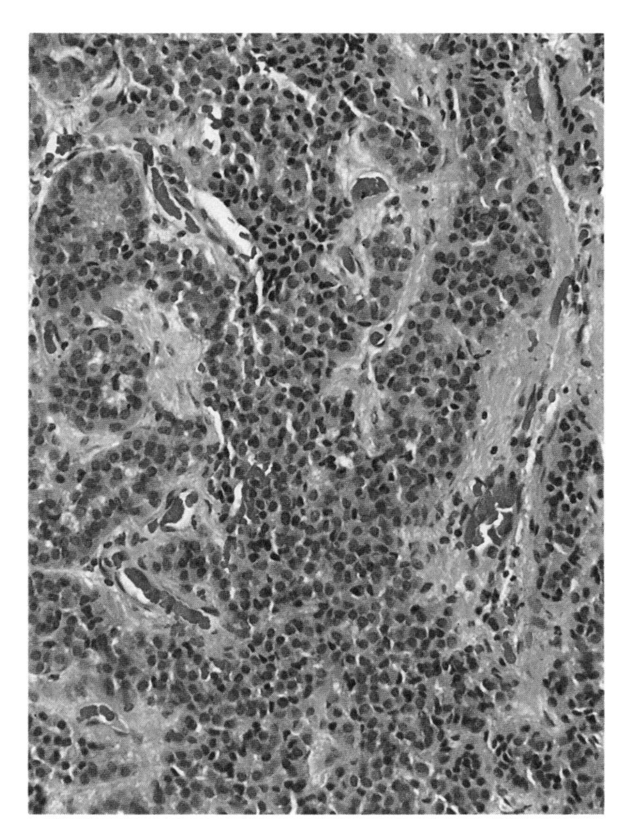

Figure 17-14
ADENOMATOUS NEOPLASM
OR ADENOMA OF MIDDLE EAR
Adenomatous neoplasm of the middle ear or middle ear adenoma from a woman with conductive-type hearing loss. The tumor is composed of uniform cells organized into interconnecting trabeculae. Mucicarminophilic material was present in gland-like spaces in some areas of tumor.

paragangliomas (48). Due to location at the skull base with access to bony recesses and foramina, JTPs can involve adjacent bone, with pressure erosion and marked bony destruction (fig. 17-12) (50). Occasionally there is extensive calcification (51). The rare small cell, almost neuroblastic component replete with a fibrillary matrix resembling neuropil (fig. 17-13) (50), may represent a divergent path of differentiation, analogous to composite pheochromocytomas (see chapter 10).

Differential Diagnosis. An important neoplasm to consider in the differential diagnosis is a middle ear adenoma or adenomatous neoplasm (60), an indolent tumor which arises in the middle ear and often causes conductive-type hearing loss (54,59). These tumors may have a neuroendocrine component as shown by immunohistochemistry and electron microscopy and may be confused with paraganglioma (60). The tumor is usually associated with an intact tympanic membrane, and is composed of remarkably uniform cuboidal or cylindrical cells often in thin anastomosing cords or trabeculae (figs. 17-14, 17-15). This neoplasm is usually not as vascular as a paraganglioma. The histogenesis is apparently from epithelium lining the middle ear (60). Other tumors in the differential diagnosis include meningioma (fig. 17-16) (55,56) (or meningeal hemangiopericytoma [58]), metastatic renal cell carcinoma (53), and several non-neoplastic entities such as lateral aberrant internal carotid artery (or aneurysmal intrapetrosal internal carotid artery) which can present in the middle ear as a "blue" retrotympanic lesion (57), and aberrant jugular bulb due to anatomic extension into the middle ear (61,62).

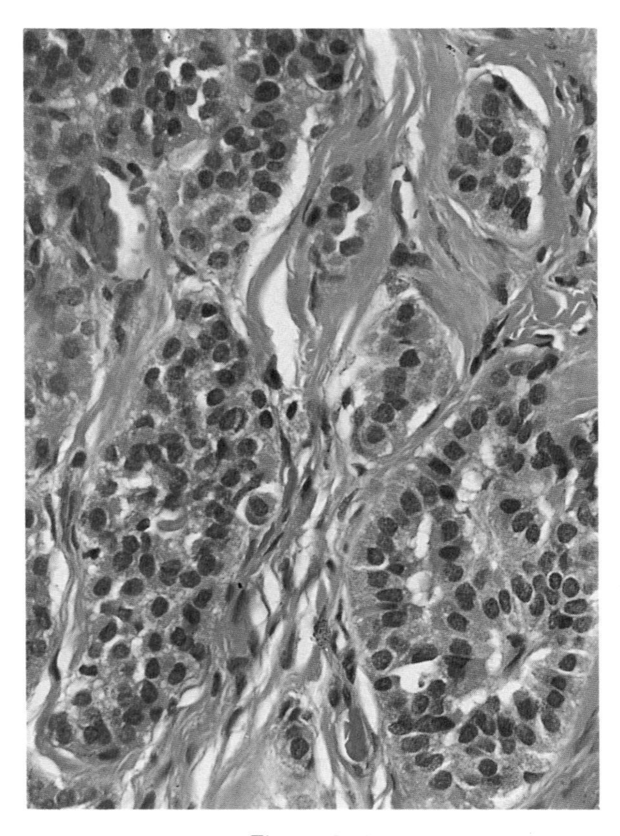

Figure 17-15
ADENOMATOUS NEOPLASM
OR ADENOMA OF MIDDLE EAR
Nuclei of tumor cells are round to oval and relatively uniform. No mitotic figures could be identified.

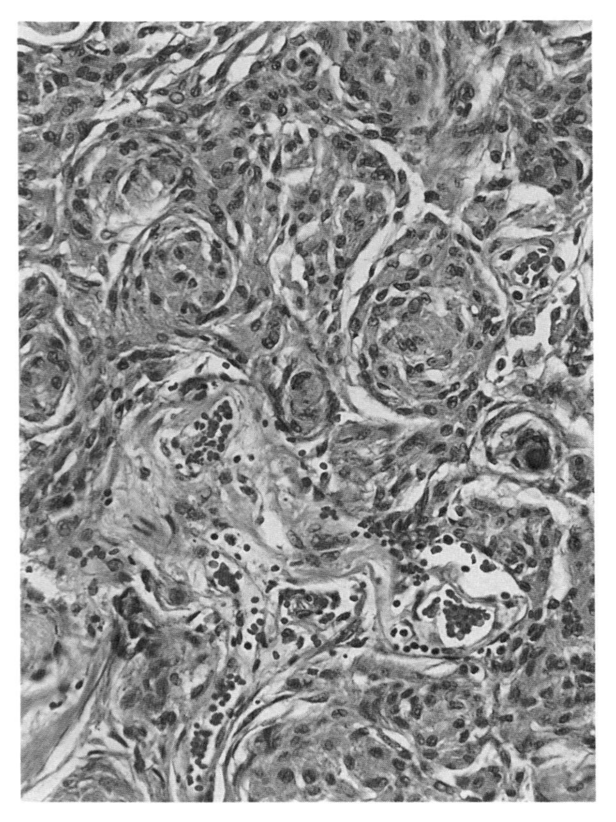

Figure 17-16
MENINGIOMA
Meningioma showing tight clusters of cells. This tumor may occasionally enter into differential diagnosis of a paraganglioma.

BIOLOGIC BEHAVIOR AND TREATMENT OF JUGULOTYMPANIC PARAGANGLIOMA

Biologic Behavior. JTPs can be locally aggressive neoplasms, with bony destruction and intracranial extension, and they may recur (or persist) locally (64). They extend in a centrifugal pattern, following multiple pathways simultaneously, with growth along paths of least resistance offered by bony fissures, air cells, vascular channels, and neural foramina (67). Regional or distant metastases are very uncommon: in the literature review by Alford and Guilford (63), only 1.9 percent of tumors metastasized; others estimate 3 percent of tumors to be clinically malignant (70). The true incidence of malignancy, however, may be even lower since there is a greater tendency to report clinically malignant tumors. None of the patients reported by Larson et al. (65) with tympanic paragangliomas had a clinically malignant tumor with metastases. A most unusual mode of spread is extension through the dura, with seeding and dissemination within the subarachnoid space via the cerebrospinal fluid (69).

Treatment. Because of inherent problems in safe, complete resection of some JTPs, much has been written about the relative efficacy of radiation treatment, with or without surgery. In a recent literature review, local control rates were similar for surgery alone (86 percent), radiation before and after surgery (90 percent), and radiation alone (93 percent), but there was a higher incidence of treatment-related morbidity following surgical resection of JTPs (68). In some studies radiation may not entirely obliterate the tumor (66).

REFERENCES

Jugulotympanic Paraganglia

1. Guild SR. A hitherto unrecognized structure, the glomus jugularis, in man. Anat Rec 1941;79:29.
2. Guild SR. The glomus jugulare, a nonchromaffin paraganglion in man. Ann Otol Rhinol Laryngol 1953;62:1045–71.
3. Kipkie GF. Simultaneous chromaffin tumors of the carotid body and the glomus jugularis. Arch Path 1947;44:113–8.
4. Kjaergaard J. Anatomy of the carotid glomus-like bodies (nonchromaffin paraganglia): with electron microscopy and comparison of human foetal carotid, aorticopulmonary, subclavian, tympanojugular, and vagal glomera. Copenhagen: FADL's Forlag, 1973:76–92.
5. Krause W. Die glandula tympanica des menschen. Centralbl Med Wissenschaften 1878;16:737–9.
6. Lack EE. Pathology of adrenal and extra-adrenal paraganglia. Major problems in pathology, Vol 29. Philadelphia: WB Saunders, 1994.
7. Lattes R, Waltner JG. Nonchromaffin paraganglioma of the middle ear. Carotid body-like tumor: glomus jugulare tumor. Cancer 1949;2:447–68.
8. LeCompte PM, Sommers SC, Lathrop FD. Tumor of carotid body type arising in the middle ear. Arch Path 1947;44:78–81.
9. Rockley TJ, Hawke M. The glomus tympanicum: a middle ear chemoreceptor? J Otolaryngol 1989;18:370–3.
10. Rosenwasser H. Carotid body tumor of the middle ear and mastoid. Arch Otolaryngol 1945;41:64–7.
11. Rosenwasser H. Glomus jugulare tumors. II. Pathology. Arch Otolaryngol 1968;88:27–40.
12. Valentin G. Ueber eine gangliöse anschwellung in der Jacobsonschen anastomose des menschen. Arch Anat Physiol Wissensch Med 1840:287–90.
13. Winship T, Klopp CT: Glomus-jugularis tumors. Cancer 1948;1:441–8.

Clinical Features of Jugulotympanic Paraganglioma

14. Alford BR, Guilford FR. A comprehensive study of tumors of the glomus jugulare. Laryngoscope 1962;72:765–87.
15. Birrell JH. The jugular body and its tumors. Aust N Z J Surg 1955;24:195–206.
16. Brandrick JT, Das Gupta AR, Singh R. Jugulotympanic paraganglioma (glomus jugulare tumour) presenting as a parotid neoplasm (a case report and review of the literature). J Laryngol Otol 1988;102:741–4.
17. Brown JS. Glomus jugulare tumors revisited: a ten-year statistical follow-up of 231 cases. Laryngoscope 1985;95:284–8.
18. Busby DR, Hepp VE. Glomus tympanicum tumor in infancy. Arch Otolaryngol Head Neck Surg 1974;99:377–8.
19. Choa DI, Colman BH. Paraganglioma of the temporal bone in infancy. A congenital lesion? Arch Otolaryngol Head Neck Surg 1987;113:421–4.
20. Chretien PB, Engleman K, Hoye RC, Geelhoed GW. Surgical management of intravascular glomus jugulare tumor. Am J Surg 1971;122:740–3.
21. Duncan AW, Lack EE, Deck MF. Radiological evaluation of paragangliomas of the head and neck. Radiology 1979;132:99–105.
22. Gejrot T, Laurén T. Retrograde jugularography in diagnosis of glomus tumours in the jugular region. Acta Otolaryngol (Stockholm) 1964;58:191–207.
23. Jackson CG, Glasscock ME III, Harris PF. Glomus tumors. Diagnosis, classification, and management of large lesions. Arch Otolaryngol 1982;108:401–6.
24. Lack EE. Pathology of adrenal and extra-adrenal paraganglia. Major problems in pathology, Vol 29. Philadelphia: WB Saunders, 1994.
25. Larson TC III, Reese DF, Baker HL Jr, McDonald TJ. Glomus tympanicum chemodectomas: radiographic and clinical characteristics. Radiology 1987;163:801–6.
26. Moody DM, Ghatak NR, Kelly DL Jr. Extensive calcification in a tumor of the glomus jugulare. Neuroradiology 1976;12:131–5.
27. Parkinson D. Intracranial pheochromocytomas (active glomus jugulare). Case report. J Neurosurg 1969;31:94–100.
28. Phelps PD, Stansbie JM. Glomus jugulare or tympanicum? The role of CT and MR imaging with gadolinium DTPA. J Laryngol Otol 1988;102:766–76.
29. Stewart JP, Ogilvie RF, Sammon JD. Tumours of the glomus jugulare and paraganglion juxtavagale of the ganglion nodosum. J Laringol Otol 1956;70:196–239.
30. Wang ML, Hussey DH, Doornbos JF, Vigliotti AP, Wen BC. Chemodectoma of the temporal bone: a comparison of surgical and radiotherapeutic results. Int J Radiation Oncology Biol Phys 1988;14:643–8.

Other Intracranial Paragangliomas

31. Bilbao JM, Horvath E, Kovacs K, Singer W, Hudson AR. Intrasellar paraganglioma associated with hypopituitarism. Arch Pathol Lab Med 1978;102:95–8.
32. Nelson MD, Kendall BE. Intracranial catecholamine-secreting paragangliomas. Neuroradiology 1987;29:277–82.
33. Prabhaker S, Sawhney IM, Chopra JS, Kak VK, Banerjee AK. Hemibase syndrome: an unusual presentation of intracranial paraganglioma. Surg Neurol 1984;22:39–42.
34. Smith WT, Hughes B, Ermocilla R. Chemodectoma of the pineal region, with observations on the pineal body and chemoreceptor tissue. J Pathol Bacteriol 1966;92:69–72.
35. Zak FG. An expanded concept of tumors of glomic tissue. NY State J Med 1954;54:1153–65.

Hormonal Manifestations

36. Azzarelli B, Fetten S, Muller J, Miyamoto R, Purvin V. Dopamine in paragangliomas of the glomus jugulare. Laryngoscope 1988;98:573–8.
37. Balogh K Jr, Drasköczy PR, Caulfield JB. Norepinephrine in tumors of the jugular glomus. Am J Pathol 1966;48:40a.
38. Brown JS. Glomus jugulare tumors revisited: a ten-year statistical follow-up of 231 cases. Laryngoscope 1985;95:284–8.
39. Cantrell RW, Kaplan MJ, Atuk NO, Winn HR, Jahrsdoerfer RA. Catecholamine-secreting infratemporal fossa paraganglioma. Ann Otol Rhinol Laryngol 1984;93:583–8.
40. DeLellis RA, Roth JA. Norepinephrine in a glomus jugulare tumor. Histochemical demonstration. Arch Path 1971;92:73–5.
41. Duke WW, Boshell BR, Stores P, Carr TH. A norepinephrine secreting glomus jugulare tumor presenting as a pheochromocytoma. Ann Intern Med 1946;60:1040–7.
42. Farrior J. Surgical management of glomus tumors: endocrine-active tumors of the skull base. South Med J 1988;81:1121–6.
43. Farrior JB III, Hyams VJ, Benke RH, Farrior JB. Carcinoid apudoma arising in a glomus jugulare tumor: review of endocrine activity in glomus jugulare tumors. Laryngoscope 1980;90:110–9.
44. Matishak MZ, Symon L, Cheeseman A, Pamphlett R. Catecholamine-secreting paragangliomas of the base of the skull. Report of two cases. J Neurosurg 1987;66:604–8.
45. Nelson MD, Kendall BE. Intracranial catecholamine-secreting paragangliomas. Neuroradiology 1987;29:277–82.
46. Parkinson D. Intracranial pheochromocytomas (active glomus jugulare). Case report. J Neurosurg 1969;31:94–100.
47. Terracol J, Guerrier Y. Les tumeurs du glomus jugulaire. Montpellier Med 1951;41–2:289–340.

Pathology of Jugulotympanic Paraganglioma

48. Bitterman P, Sherman M, Lack EE. Paragangliomas of the head and neck region: clinicopathologic and immunohistochemical evaluation of 88 cases. Patologia 1992;25:493A.
49. Glenner GG, Grimley PM. Tumors of the extra-adrenal paraganglion system (including chemoreceptors). Atlas of Tumor Pathology, 2nd Series, Fascicle 9. Washington, D.C.: Armed Forces Institute of Pathology, 1974.
50. Lack EE. Pathology of adrenal and extra-adrenal paraganglia. Major problems in pathology, Vol 29. Philadelphia: WB Saunders, 1994.
51. Moody DM, Ghatak NR, Kelly DL Jr. Extensive calcification in a tumor of the glomus jugulare. Neuroradiology 1976;12:131–5.
52. Oberman HA, Holtz F, Sheffer LA, Magielski JE. Chemodectomas (nonchromaffin paragangliomas) of the head and neck. A clinicopathologic study. Cancer 1968;21:838–51.

Differential Diagnosis of Jugulotympanic Paraganglioma

53. Boileau MA, Grotta JC, Borit A, et al. Metastatic renal cell carcinoma simulating glomus jugulare tumor. J Surg Oncol 1987;35:201–3.
54. Derlacki EL, Barney PL. Adenomatous tumors of the middle ear and mastoid. Laryngoscope 1976;86:1123–35.
55. Fleury P, Caron JP, Basset JM, et al. Méningíomes de l'orielle simulant une tumeur glomique. Deux nouveaux cas. Ann Oto-Laryng 1982;99:199–202.
56. Ford CN, Kurtycz DF, Brandenburg JH, Hafez GR. Significance of apparent intratympanic meningiomas. Laryngoscope 1983;93:1397–404.
57. Goldman NC, Singleton GT, Holly EA. Aberrant internal carotid artery presenting as a mass in the middle ear. Arch Otolaryngol 1971;94:269–73.
58. Guthrie BL, Ebersold MJ, Scheithauer BW, Shaw EG. Meningeal hemangiopericytoma: histological features, treatment, and long-term follow-up of 44 cases. Neurosurgery 1989;25:514–22.
59. Hyams VJ, Michaels L. Benign adenomatous neoplasm (adenoma) of the middle ear. Clin Otolaryngol 1976;1:17–26.
60. Lack EE. Pathology of adrenal and extra-adrenal paraganglia. Major problems in pathology, Vol 29. Philadelphia: WB Saunders, 1994.
61. Rauch SD, Xu WZ, Nadol JB Jr. High jugular bulb: implications for posterior fossa neurotologic and cranial base surgery. Ann Otol Rhinol Laryngol 1993;102:100–7.
62. West JM, Bandy BC, Jafer BW. Aberrant jugular bulb in the middle ear cavity. Arch Otolaryngol 1974;100:370–2.

Biologic Behavior and Treatment of Jugulotympanic Paraganglioma

63. Alford BR, Guilford FR. A comprehensive study of tumors of the glomus jugulare. Laryngoscope 1962;72:765–87.
64. Lack EE. Pathology of adrenal and extra-adrenal paraganglia. Major problems in pathology, Vol 29. Philadelphia: WB Saunders, 1994.
65. Larson TC III, Reese DF, Baker HL Jr, McDonald TJ. Glomus tympanicum chemodectomas: radiographic and clinical characteristics. Radiology 1987;163:801–6.
66. Spector GJ, Compagno J, Perez CA, Maisel RH, Ogura JH. Glomus jugulare tumors: effects of radiotherapy. Cancer 1975;35:1316–21.
67. Spector GJ, Sobol S, Thawley SE, et al. Panal discussion: glomus jugulare tumors of the temporal bone: patterns of invasion in the temporal bone. Laryngoscope 1979;89:1628–39.
68. Springate SC, Haraf D, Weichselbaum RR. Temporal bone chemodectomas: comparing surgery and radiation therapy. Oncology (Williston Park) 1991;5:131–7.
69. Welsh LW, Welsh JJ, Huck GF Jr. Glomus jugulare tumor. Disseminated form in the central nervous system. Arch Otolaryngol 1976;102:507–10.
70. Zak FG, Lawson W. The paraganglionic chemoreceptor system: physiology, pathology, and clinical medicine. New York: Springer-Verlag, 1982:372–5.

18
VAGAL PARAGANGLIOMA

VAGAL PARAGANGLIA

Anatomy of the Rostral Vagus Nerve. The vagus nerve is a mixed sensory and motor nerve which exits the medulla as fila radicularia. It consists of 10 to 18 small nerve bundles which converge to form the larger vagal trunk (fig. 18-1). The ganglion nodosum is a fusiform expansion of the nerve, measuring about 1.5 cm in length in adults; it contains cell bodies of visceral afferent fibers from pharynx, larynx, and trachea as well as intrathoracic and intra-abdominal viscera (7). The superior or jugular ganglion of the vagus nerve contains cell bodies of somatic efferent nerve fibers. The vagus nerve also has special visceral efferent fibers to the voluntary musculature of the upper aerodigestive tract, and has an important role in regulation and control of respiratory, cardiovascular, and gastrointestinal function. Among sensory ganglia, those of the vagus nerve are seemingly unique in containing paraganglionic tissue (7).

Distribution and Normal Microanatomy of Vagal Paraganglia. The terms vagal body and vagal body paraganglia collectively refer to the multiple, spatially dispersed paraganglia usually found at or just below the lower border of the ganglion nodosum (fig. 18-2). Muratori (9) described vagal paraganglia in birds in 1932, and White (11) identified them in humans in 1935 within the rostral vagus nerve in juxtaposition to ganglion cells. Because these paraganglia do not form a single compact structure, the term vagal body is technically a misnomer. These paraganglia are microscopic structures that have virtually the same microanatomy as subunits of the carotid body (fig. 18-3). The varied anatomic locations of paraganglia adjacent to or within the substance of nerve bundles of the vagus nerve may help to explain some of the characteristic clinicopathologic features of vagal paragangliomas and the problems inherent in complete surgical resection. Paraganglia have also been identified higher in the vagus nerve, in or near the jugular ganglion (1), and vagal paragangliomas arising in this more rostral location may have radiographic and clinical features suggesting a jugular paraganglioma (7). Paraganglia have also been identified well below the inferior pole of the nodose ganglion (8,10), even in laryngeal nerves (2,10); in the experimental animal paraganglia have been found associated with the abdominal portion of the vagus nerve and even in the hilum of the liver (3).

In a study in humans using a step sectioning technique (5), an average of seven separate paraganglia were found on the left side of the vagus nerve and six on the right. They are usually ovoid

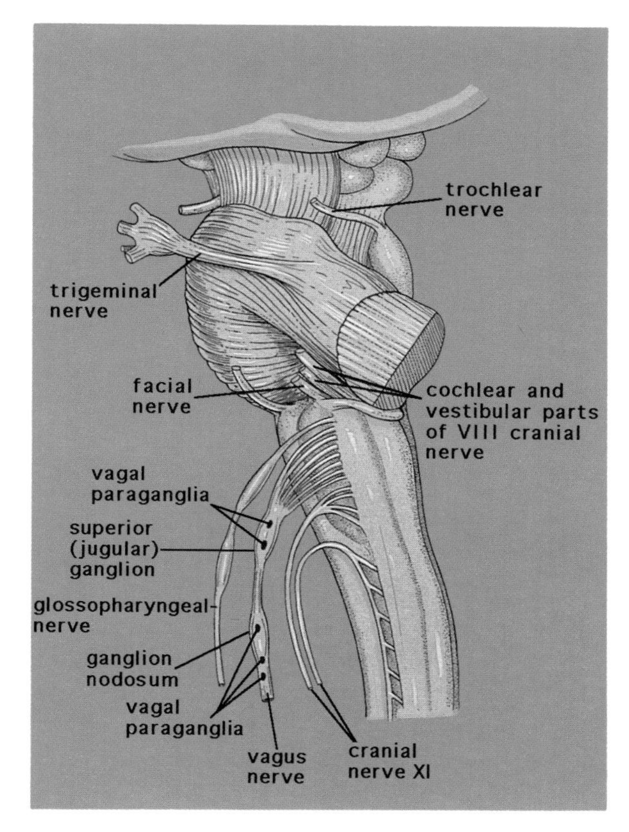

Figure 18-1
VAGUS NERVE

Lateral view of brain stem and upper cervical spinal cord. The trunk of the vagus nerve is formed after confluence of fila radicularia. The position of the superior (jugular) ganglion and ganglion nodosum (inferior ganglion) are indicated. Vagal paraganglia are usually found at or near the lower border of the nodose ganglion.

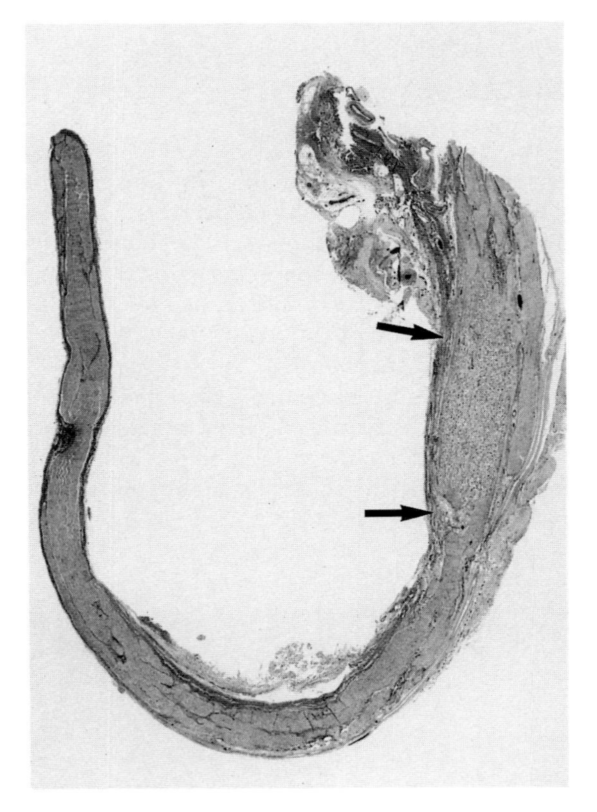

Figure 18-2
VAGUS NERVE
Rostral portion of the vagus nerve from an infant in the first year of life. The ganglion nodosum is seen as a fusiform expansion of nerve between the arrows. Vagal paraganglia are usually located near the lower border of the ganglion. (Fig. 5-1 from Lack EE. Pathology of adrenal and extra-adrenal paraganglia. Major problems in pathology, Vol 29. Philadelphia: WB Saunders Co, 1994:96.)

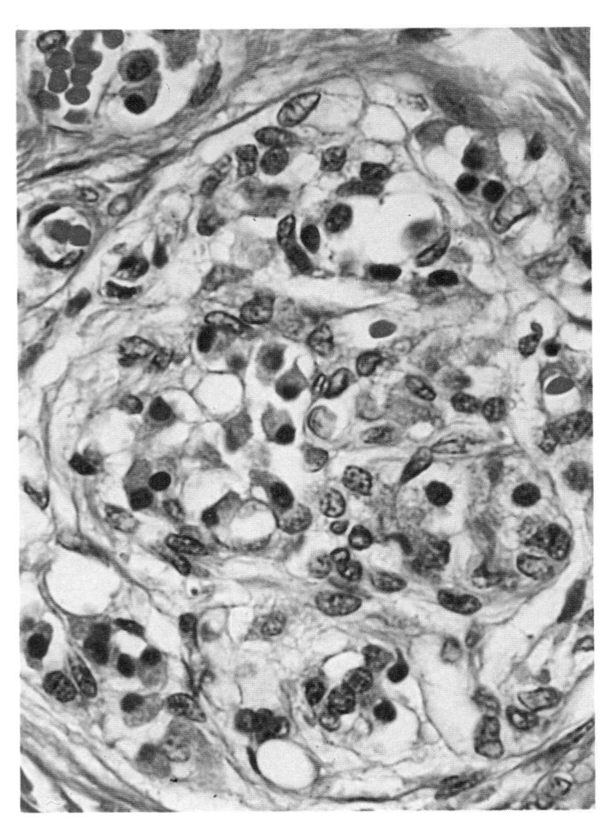

Figure 18-3
VAGAL PARAGANGLION
Vagal paraganglion is present within the interstitium of the vagus nerve, with small bundles of myelinated nerve adjacent to it. The paraganglion is identical to the lobular subunit of the carotid body. Clusters of chief cells are seen along with a few sustentacular cells.

structures with average dimensions in adults of about 160 x 350 μm, but tend to be smaller in young children (6). Vagal paraganglia are located within interstitial connective tissue of the nerve (fig. 18-3), within large nerve trunks just beneath the perineurium (fig. 18-4A), partially surrounding small nerve bundles within the vagus nerve (fig. 18-4B), or occasionally, immediately adjacent to ganglion cells of the ganglion nodosum (fig. 18-4C). Rarely, an intravascular protrusion of a vagal paraganglion is covered by an intact continuous layer of endothelial cells (fig. 18-5). An ultrastructural study of vagal paraganglia in the human fetus showed morphologic features indistinguishable from the carotid body (4).

Hyperplasia of Vagal Paraganglia. Hyperplasia of vagal paraganglia has been reported in some patients with chronic hypoxemia due to chronic obstructive pulmonary disease (5), cystic fibrosis (fig. 18-6), and cyanotic heart disease (fig. 18-7). This hyperplasia tends to parallel similar changes in carotid body paraganglia, but the findings are not always concordant (7). Hyperplasia provides additional support for a chemoreceptor role for vagal paraganglia, but there are essentially no data available which indicate a relationship between hyperplasia and the development of a paraganglioma, even at high altitude (7). A brief discussion of possible physiologic functions of vagal paraganglia is provided elsewhere (7).

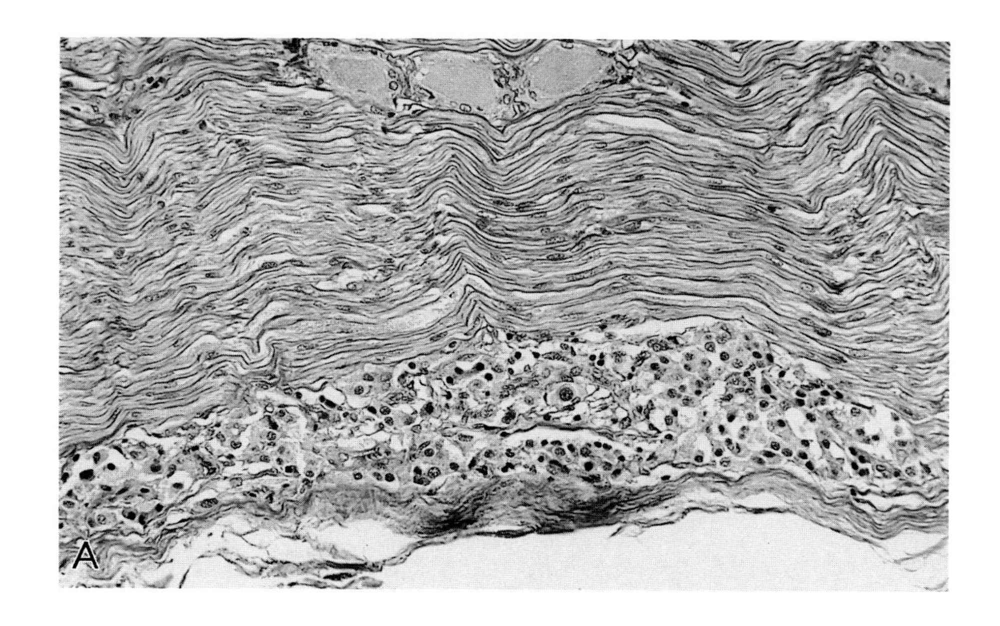

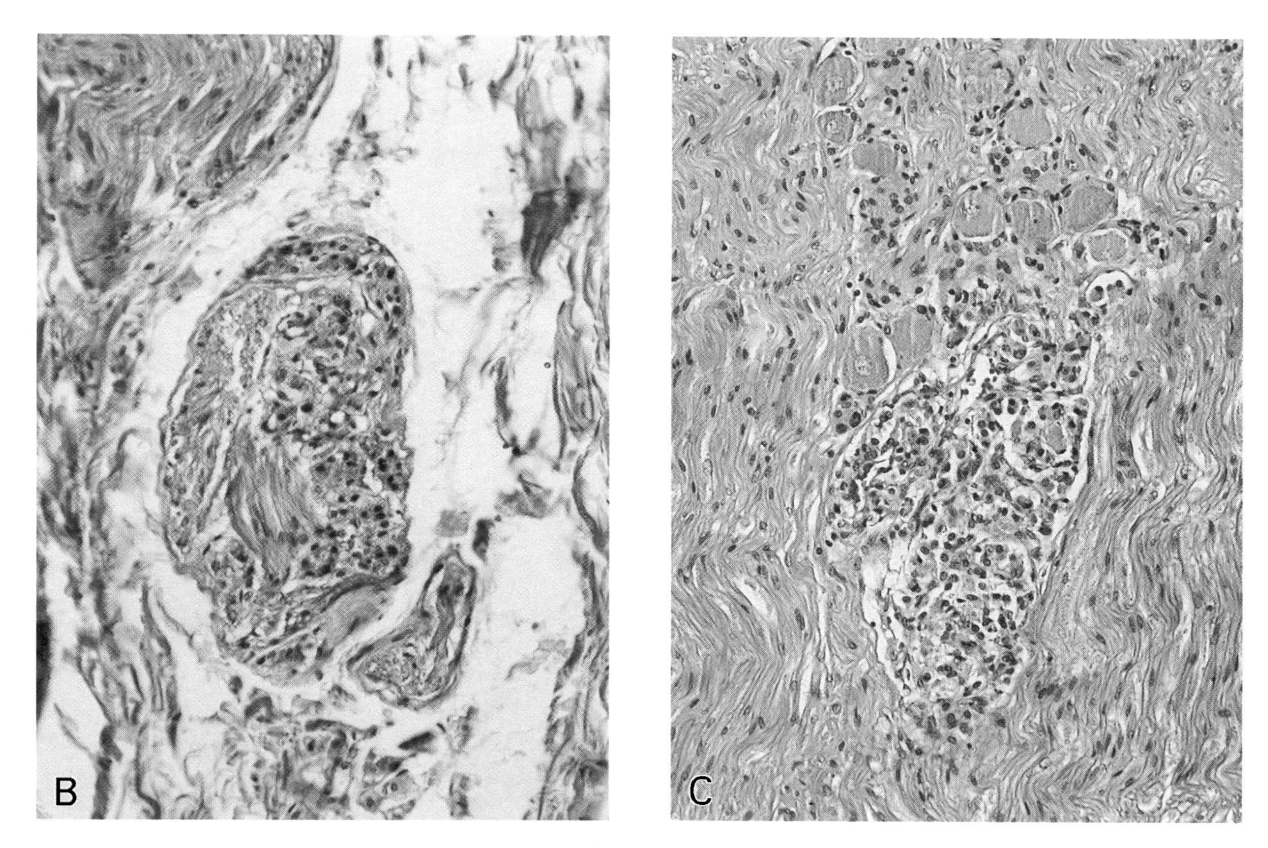

Figure 18-4
VAGAL PARAGANGLIA

A: Vagal paraganglion has an elongate profile beneath the perineurium of the vagus nerve.
B: A small vagal paraganglion partially surrounds a myelinated nerve bundle seen in cross section.
C: This vagal paraganglion is located at the lower border of the nodose ganglion immediately adjacent to ganglion cells.

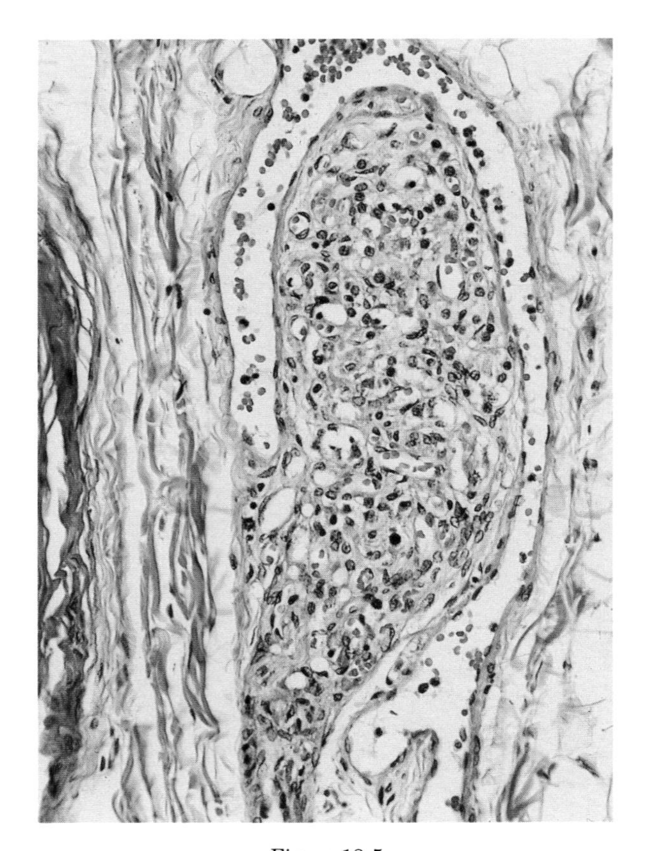

Figure 18-5
INTRAVASCULAR POLYPOID PROTRUSION
BY NORMAL VAGAL PARAGANGLION

The intraluminal surface is covered by a continuous layer of endothelial cells.

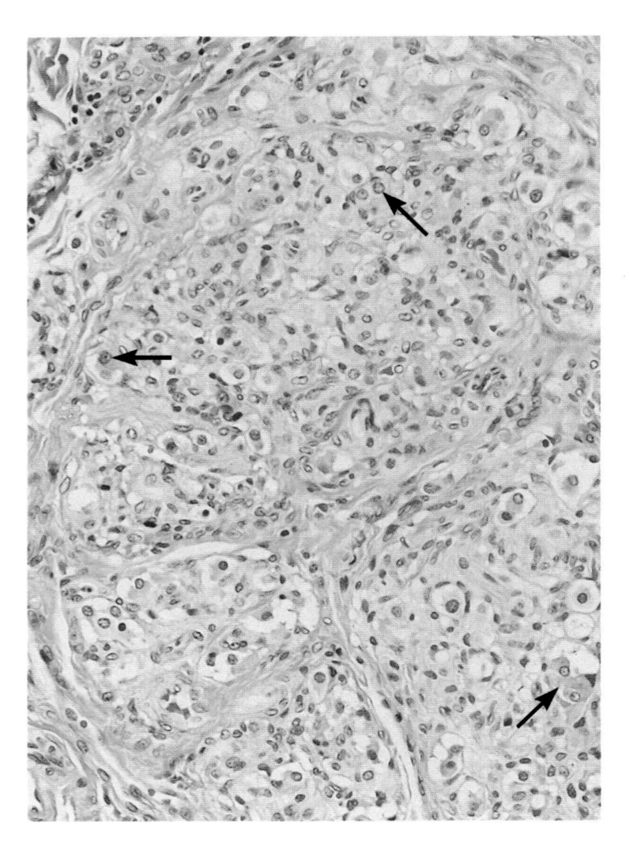

Figure 18-6
ENLARGED HYPERPLASTIC VAGAL PARAGANGLION

Enlarged hyperplastic vagal paraganglion in a young adult with cystic fibrosis. Note the enlarged hyperplastic chief cells (arrows).

Figure 18-7
HYPERPLASIA OF
VAGAL PARAGANGLION

Hyperplasia of vagal paraganglion in a young patient with digital clubbing and cyanosis due to congenital heart disease. The patient had a simple left ventricle with transposition of the great vessels. The paraganglion shown here was enlarged, cellular, and measured 320 x 1,100 μm. Note the enlarged hyperplastic chief cells which predominate throughout field

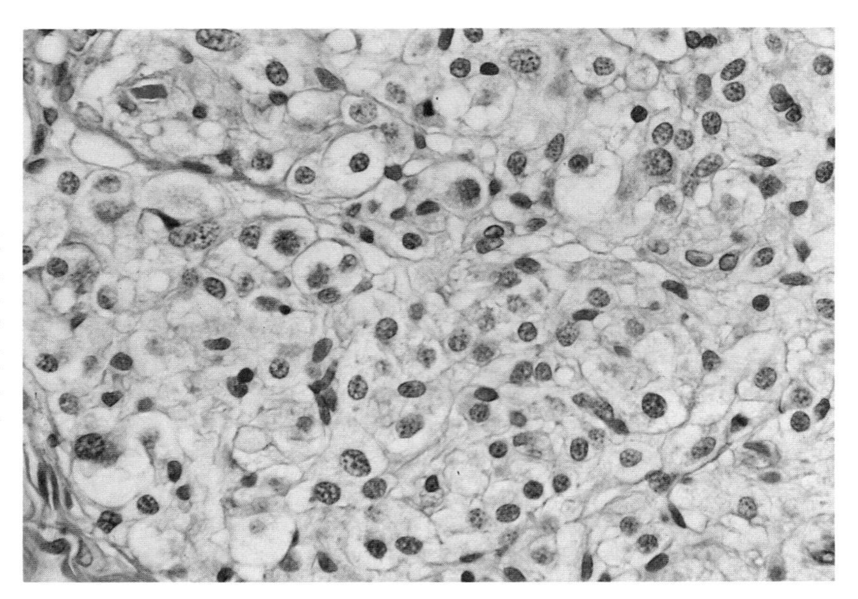

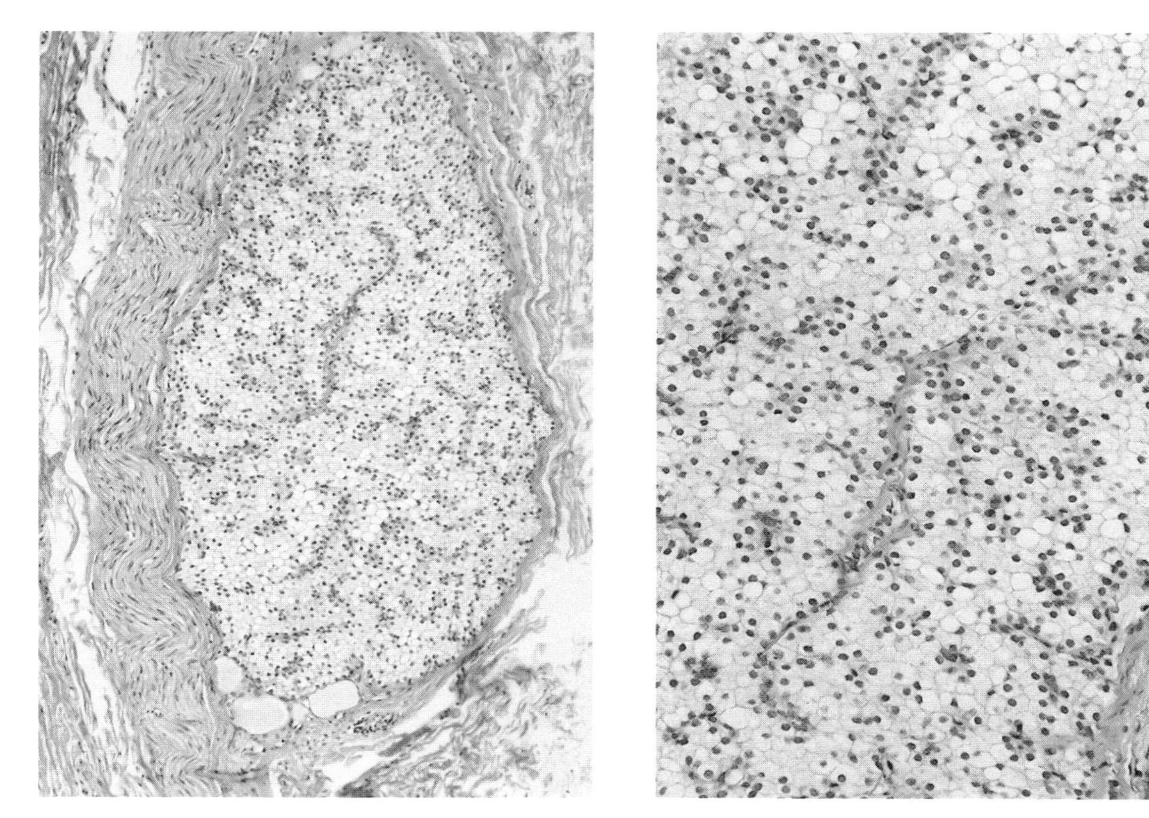

Figure 18-8
ECTOPIC PARATHYROID TISSUE

Left: The ectopic parathyroid tissue is located beneath the perineurium of the rostral portion of the vagus nerve. The tissue is subdivided by small, branching vascular channels.

Right: Higher magnification shows uniform round nuclei and distinct cell borders. Small cytoplasmic vacuoles are present, probably due to lipid accumulation.

PARATHYROID TISSUE WITHIN THE VAGUS NERVE

A small collection of uniform cells resembling parathyroid chief cells can sometimes be seen in sections of the rostral vagus nerve (fig. 18-8) (13–15). Ectopic parathyroid tissue has been reported in the cervical vagus nerve in 4 percent of adults (14) and 6 percent of children in the first year of life (15). These collections of cells vary in size: some are small enough to evade detection on casual inspection (fig. 18-9). They may simulate a vagal paraganglion, but their cytologic uniformity, distinct cell borders, and pale-staining or clear cytoplasm permits distinction. The cells may contain abundant intracytoplasmic glycogen (fig. 18-10, left) (14), and stain for chromogranin and parathormone (fig. 18-10, right) (15). Rare examples of aberrant parathyroid adenoma with primary hyperparathyroidism have been reported within the cervical vagus nerve (12,17,18). Ectopic parathyroid tissue has also been noted within a cervical ganglion (probably related to the vagus nerve) in a patient undergoing surgery for papillary thyroid carcinoma (16).

VAGAL PARAGANGLIOMA

Definition. This paraganglioma arises from dispersed paraganglia located within or immediately adjacent to the vagus nerve, especially the most rostral portion of the nerve in relation to the ganglion nodosum. The tumor is also referred to as *vagal body paraganglioma.*

Clinical Features. Vagal paraganglioma (VP) is the third most frequent paraganglioma of the head and neck region. There is a distinct predilection for female patients, usually in the

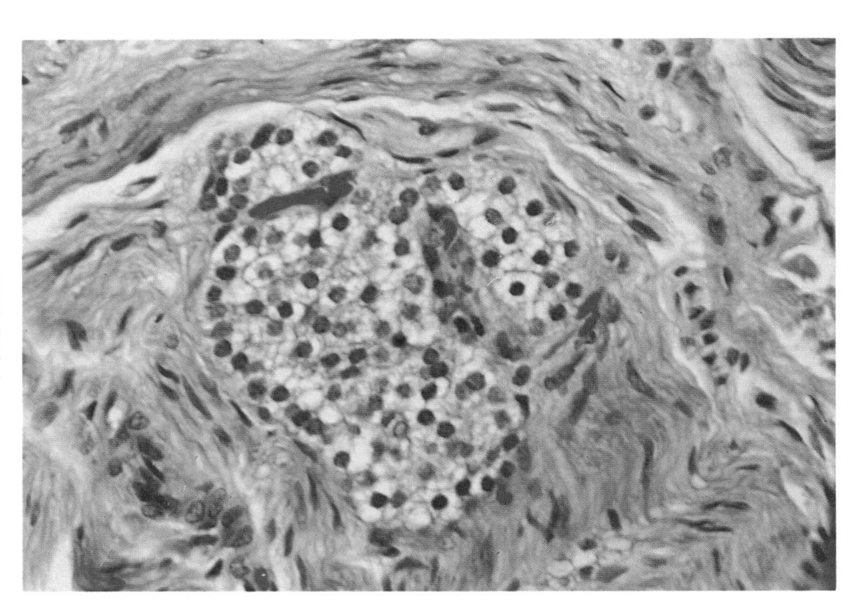

Figure 18-9
INTRAVAGAL PARATHYROID CHIEF CELLS

A small collection of parathyroid chief cells is present within a myelinated nerve bundle of the vagus nerve. The cells have relatively clear cytoplasm with distinct cell borders and small uniform nuclei.

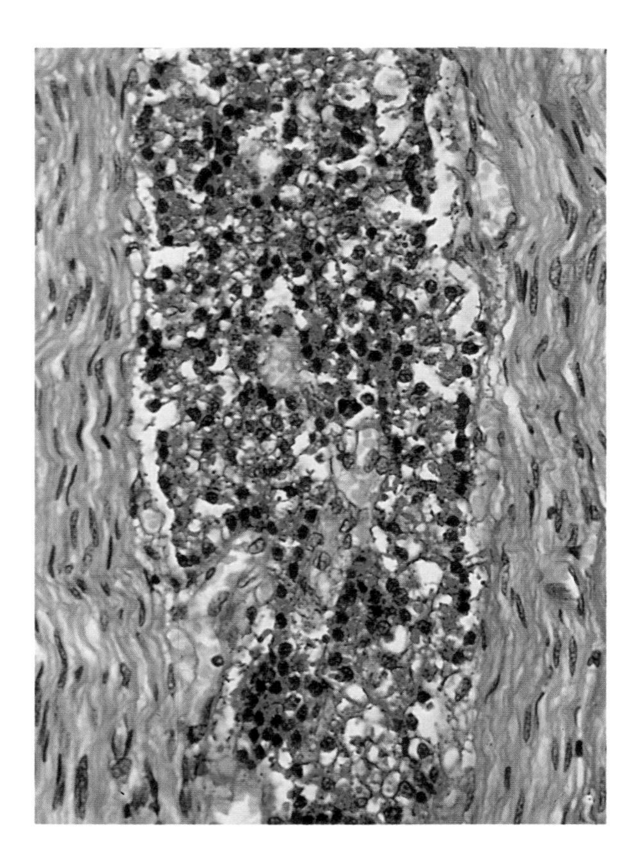

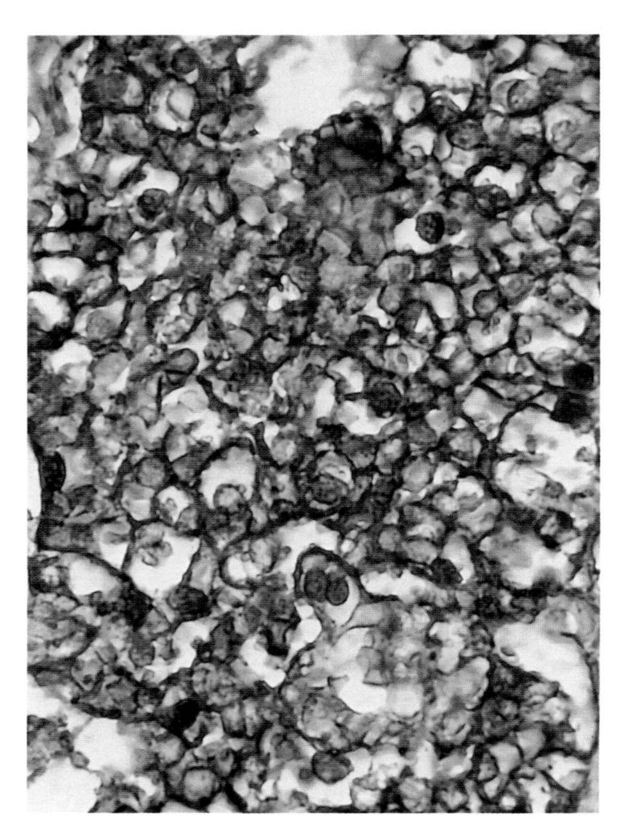

Figure 18-10
INTRAVAGAL PARATHYROID CHIEF CELLS

Left: These parathyroid chief cells within the vagus nerve are strongly PAS positive. The reaction was entirely ablated by pretreatment with diastase, indicating the presence of glycogen. (X250, Periodic-acid–Schiff stain)

Right: This collection of intravagal parathyroid chief cells immunostains strongly for parathormone. (X400, Peroxidase-antiperoxidase stain)

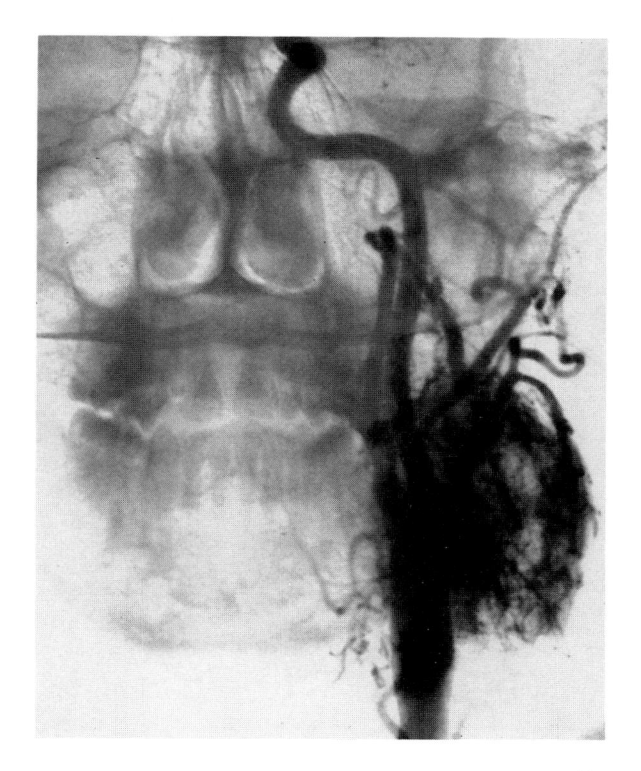

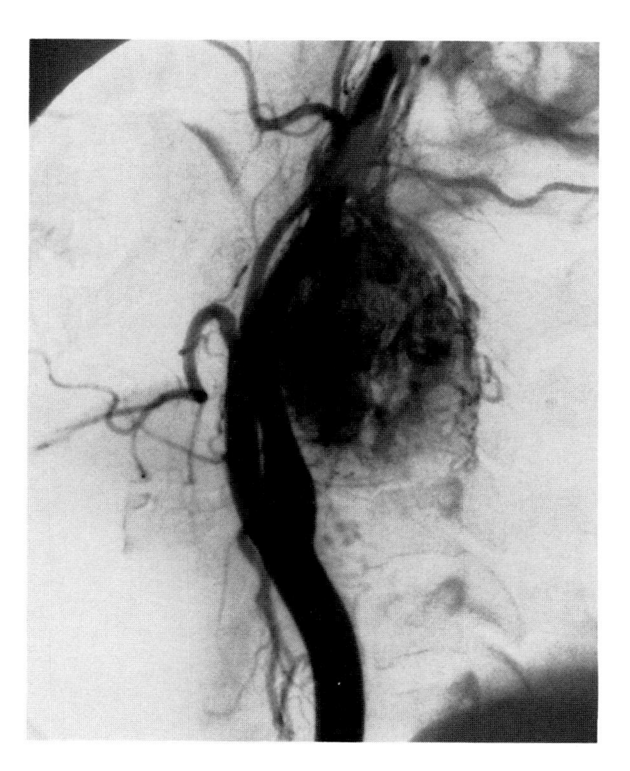

Figure 18-11
VAGAL PARAGANGLIOMA

Left: Vagal paraganglioma in a 29-year-old patient who presented with a 3-year history of a painless, slow-growing mass in the left neck associated with dysphagia. Selective carotid arteriogram in the anteroposterior projection shows a distinct tumor blush near the angle of mandible without lateral displacement of the carotid vessels.

Right: Lateral view of same vagal paraganglioma shows anterior bowing of both internal and external carotid artery branches without direct involvement of the carotid bifurcation. (Fig. 5-11B from Lack EE. Pathology of adrenal and extra-adrenal paraganglia. Major problems in pathology, Vol 29. Philadelphia: WB Saunders Co, 1994:105.) (Figures 18-11 and 18-13 are from the same case.)

fourth and fifth decades of life (25,27,28,30,34). The patient may present with a painless, slowly growing neck mass, and there may be medial deviation of tonsillar or oropharyngeal tissue. There may be a variety of cranial nerve palsies, mostly involving the vagus nerve, with ipsilateral vocal cord dysfunction, hoarseness, or dysphagia (28); local expansion by a VP can cause compression of other nerves in the jugular foramen with paresis of the ninth, eleventh, and twelfth cranial nerves in various combination (32). An occasional patient may have an ipsilateral Horner's syndrome. A rare VP may have a dumbbell configuration with extension up into the jugular foramen (20), or arise above the level of the nodose ganglion (35). Functionally active VPs have occasionally been reported, with resultant signs and symptoms of excess catecholamine secretion (21,23,26,33,37,38). Intraoperative traction on the vagus nerve can be complicated by cardiac arrest, probably related to bradycardia (39).

On selective arteriography, VPs typically cause anterior displacement of the carotid vessels without direct involvement of the bifurcation (figs. 18-11, 18-12) (22); in lateral views, therefore, there is no "lyre-like" widening of the common carotid artery bifurcation as expected with a carotid body paraganglioma. Other effective means of tumor localization are computed tomography (CT) (fig. 18-13) and magnetic resonance imaging (MRI). VPs may be associated with other paragangliomas and occur in a familial setting (28).

Gross Findings. VPs may have a fusiform or globular configuration and abut directly onto the base of the skull. When the tumor grows directly within the vagus nerve and nerve bundles splay over much or all of the surface of the paraganglioma (fig. 18-14), it may be impossible to simply "shell

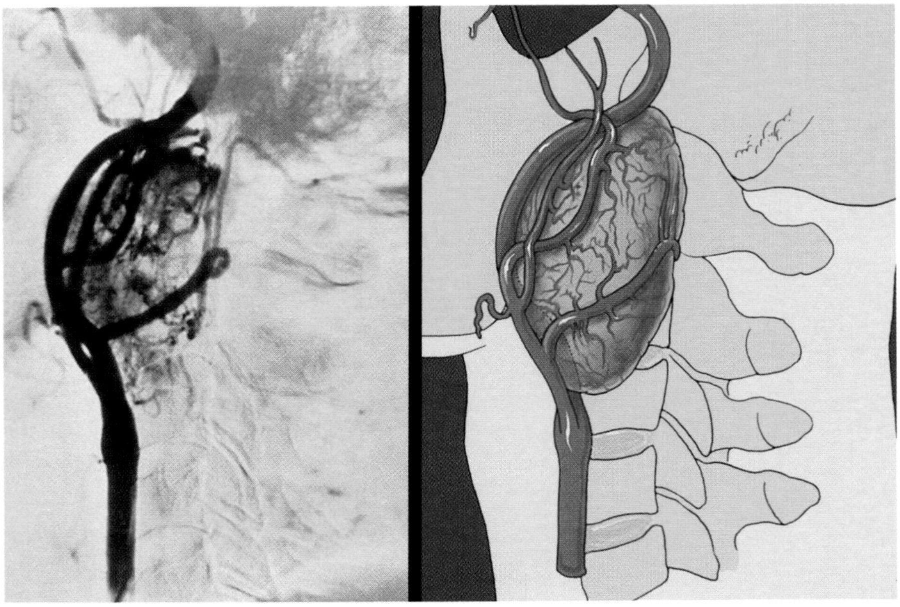

Figure 18-12
VAGAL PARAGANGLIOMA
Schematic diagram illustrating the relationship of a vagal paraganglioma to the carotid vessels. The tumor does not directly involve the carotid bifurcation and is located more cephalad than carotid body paragangliomas.

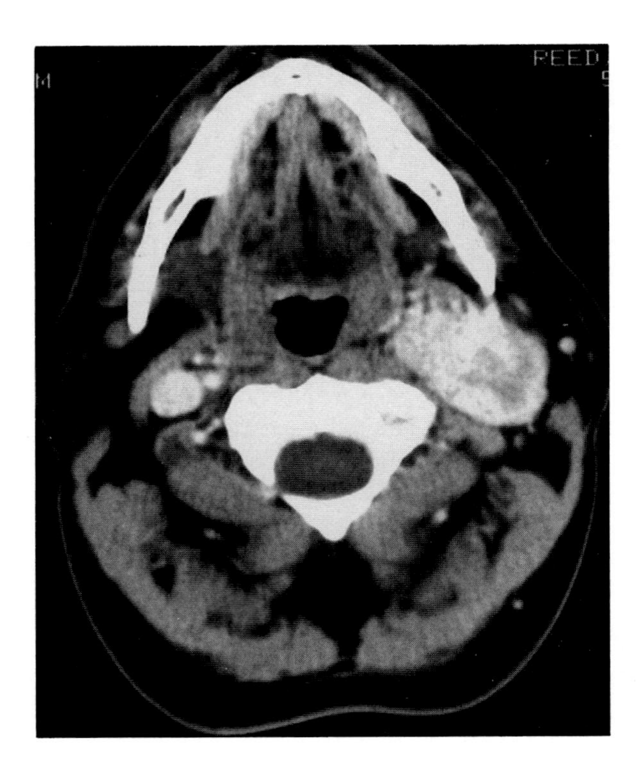

Figure 18-13
VAGAL PARAGANGLIOMA
Vagal paraganglioma of left neck on CT scan. The tumor appears as a bright ovoid mass which can not be distinguished from the carotid artery and internal jugular vein with intravenous contrast.

out" the tumor at surgery. In some cases, however, the tumor causes lateral displacement of the vagus nerve, thus permitting preservation of much of the nerve (28). On gross inspection, the cut surface of VP is similar to other head and neck paragangliomas, although these neoplasms may be quite sclerotic, similar to jugulotympanic paragangliomas (28). Gross identification of a stump of resected vagus nerve helps identify the anatomic site of origin (fig. 18-15).

Microscopic Findings. The organoid arrangement of tumor cells is similar to that of other head and neck paragangliomas; the pattern seen in figure 18-16, left, emphasizes the disparity in size of "zellballen," and staining for reticulum may highlight this (fig. 18-16, right). Microscopic sections may reveal a close relationship with a large ganglion (fig. 18-17), helping in the localization of the VP. Multiple myelinated nerve bundles may be seen in sections taken from the periphery of the tumor (fig. 18-18); these represent components of the vagus nerve. Other head and neck paragangliomas may have nerve bundles at the periphery of the tumor (e.g., carotid body tumors) or actually incorporate them within the substance of the tumor. Because of the anatomic location of vagal paraganglia within myelinated nerve bundles of the vagus nerve, there is occasional close paraneural, or

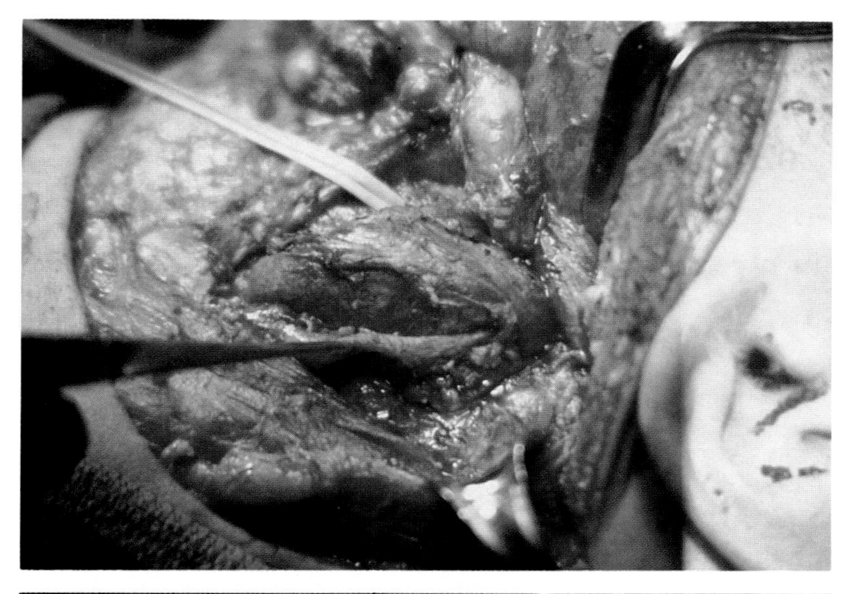

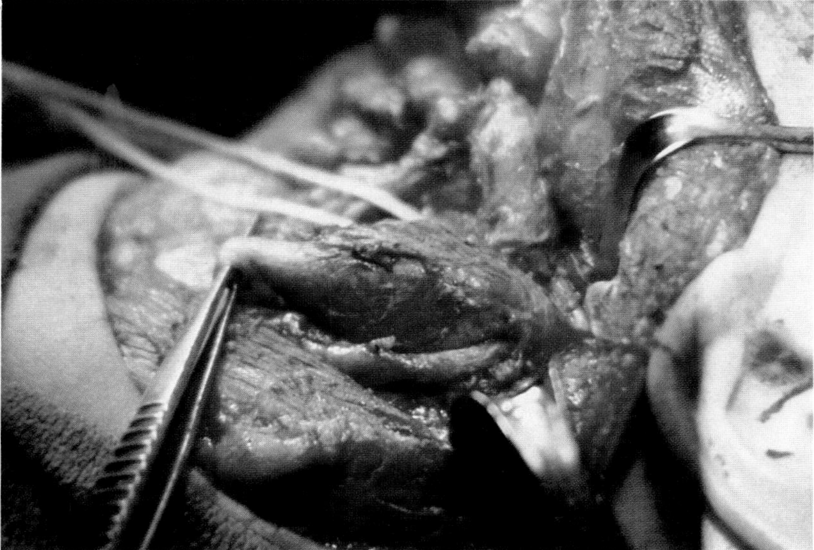

Figure 18-14
VAGAL PARAGANGLIOMA
OF LEFT NECK

Top: Tumor is apparent as a fusiform expansion of the vagus nerve and extended up to the base of the skull.

Bottom: The forcep in the left portion of field is elevating the trunk of vagus nerve at the lower aspect of tumor. Bundles of vagus nerve were splayed over surface of tumor, and were densely adherent to the fibrous pseudocapsule. (Courtesy of Dr. Roy B. Sessions, Washington, DC.)

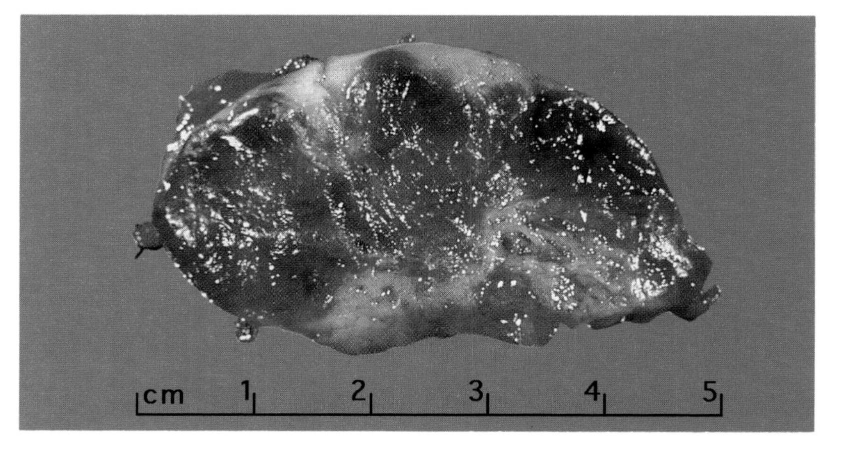

Figure 18-15
VAGAL PARAGANGLIOMA

Vagal paraganglioma from a 69-year-old woman is deeply congested, with some areas of sclerosis evident on cross section. A portion of the resected vagus nerve is attached to the tumor on the right side. The left portion of the tumor extended up to base of skull near the jugular foramen.

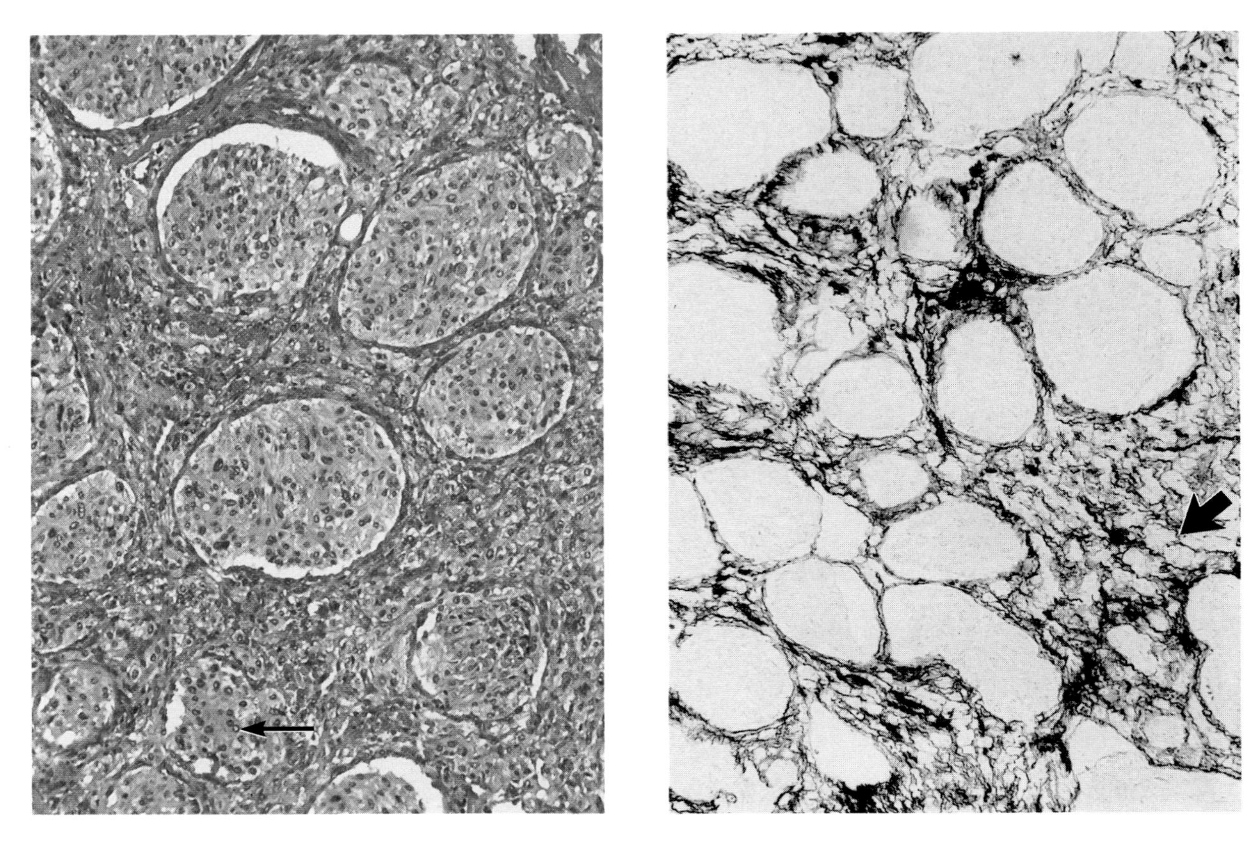

Figure 18-16
VAGAL PARAGANGLIOMA

Left: Vagal paraganglioma shows "zellballen" of varying size, with some being quite small and difficult to identify. Note the nuclear "pseudoinclusions" (arrow).

Right: Stain for reticulum highlights the round to ovoid zellballen. Some are quite small (arrow). (X200, Reticulum stain)

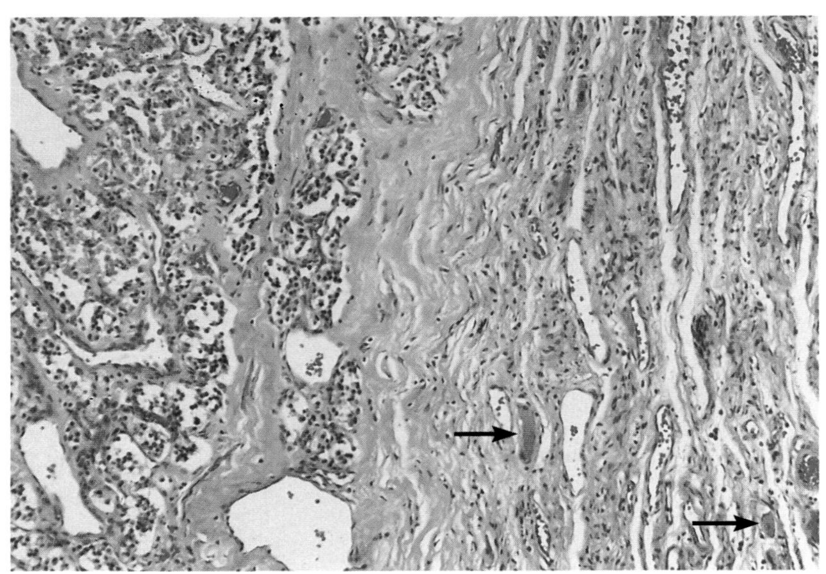

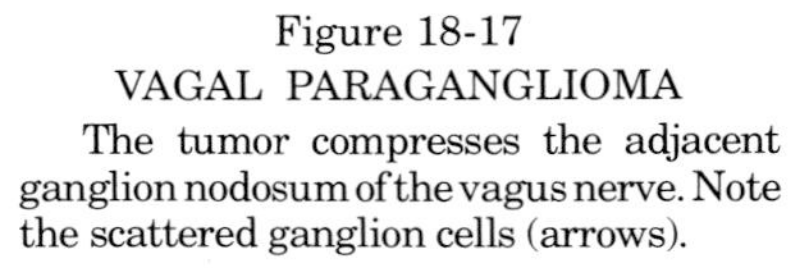

Figure 18-17
VAGAL PARAGANGLIOMA

The tumor compresses the adjacent ganglion nodosum of the vagus nerve. Note the scattered ganglion cells (arrows).

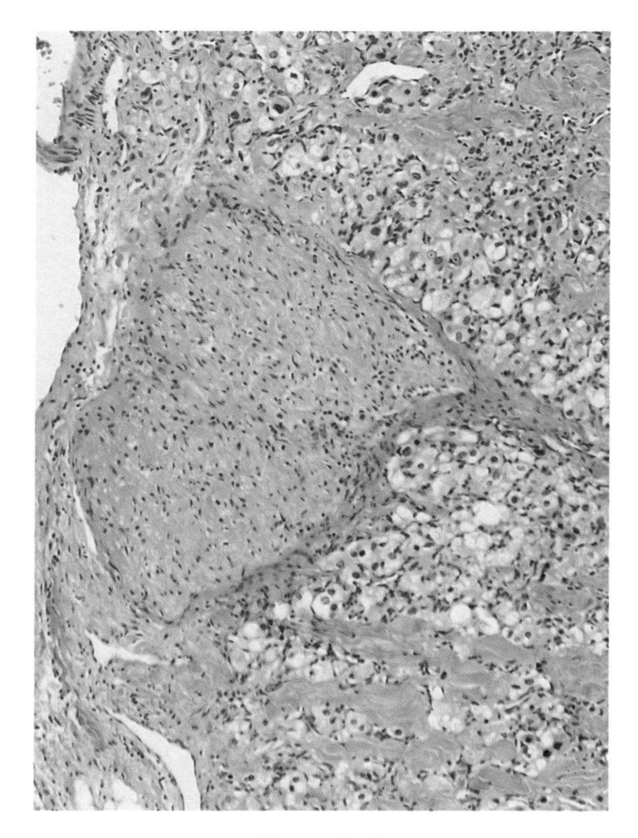

Figure 18-18
VAGAL PARAGANGLIOMA
Sections taken through the periphery of the tumor showed several bundles of myelinated nerve. Some are compressed and distorted.

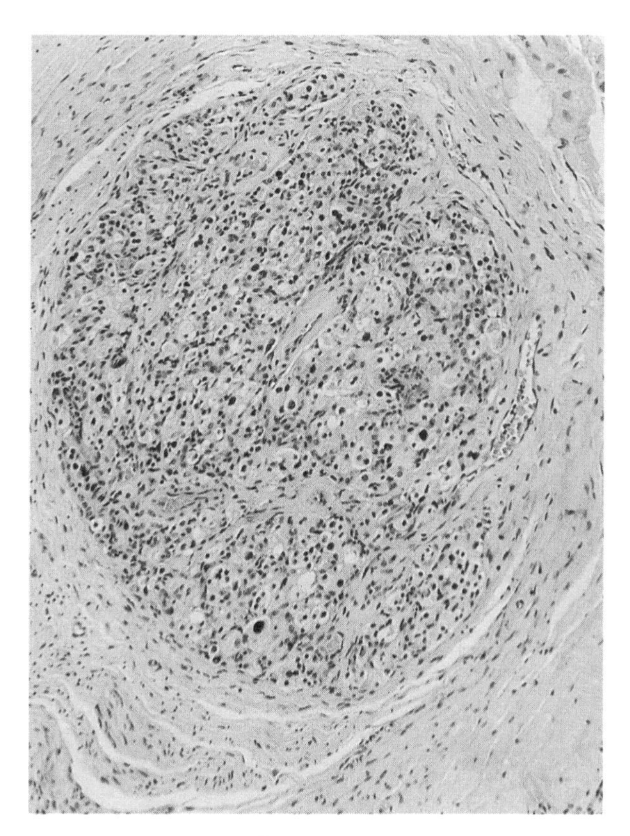

Figure 18-19
VAGAL PARAGANGLIOMA
There is a focus of intraneural growth along with some sclerosis. The tumor proved to be clinically benign.

even intraneural (fig. 18-19), growth by neoplastic chief cells (29). This does not necessarily indicate malignancy. Stromal changes such as sclerosis may be prominent in some tumors while interstitial edema with prominent vascularity (fig. 18-20) may cause difficulty in accurate diagnosis.

The first VP was reported by Stout in 1935 (36) in a 52-year-old woman; the tumor cells were reported to contain brown pigment, presumably melanin. The same case was reported again by Lattes in 1950 (31), and the tumor proved to be clinically benign after a 19-year follow-up, despite the fact that in the original article intravascular plugs of tumor were shown side by side in vein and artery (36). Occasional foci may suggest angioinvasion by a VP (or other head and neck paraganglioma), but it is unclear whether that illustrated in figure 18-21 is true vascular invasion or merely intravascular protrusion similar to figure 18-5.

Treatment and Biologic Behavior. The optimal treatment for VP is complete surgical resection. Complications may result from intraoperative hemorrhage or postoperative sequelae of sacrifice of the tenth cranial (or other) nerves. Adjuvant therapy may provide some palliation. Although some have felt that VPs are hyperplastic rather than truly neoplastic (19), these tumors are considered to be authentic neoplasms (28). The actual or true incidence of malignant behavior of VP may be slightly inflated because of the increased tendency to report individual cases of a rare tumor which prove to be malignant. Heinrich et al. (24) identified 151 cases of VP reported in the English language literature: 10.6 percent were malignant (15 cases), of which 73 percent metastasized to one or more cervical lymph nodes (fig. 18-22); distant metastases to sites such as lung and bone occurred in 4 of 15 cases.

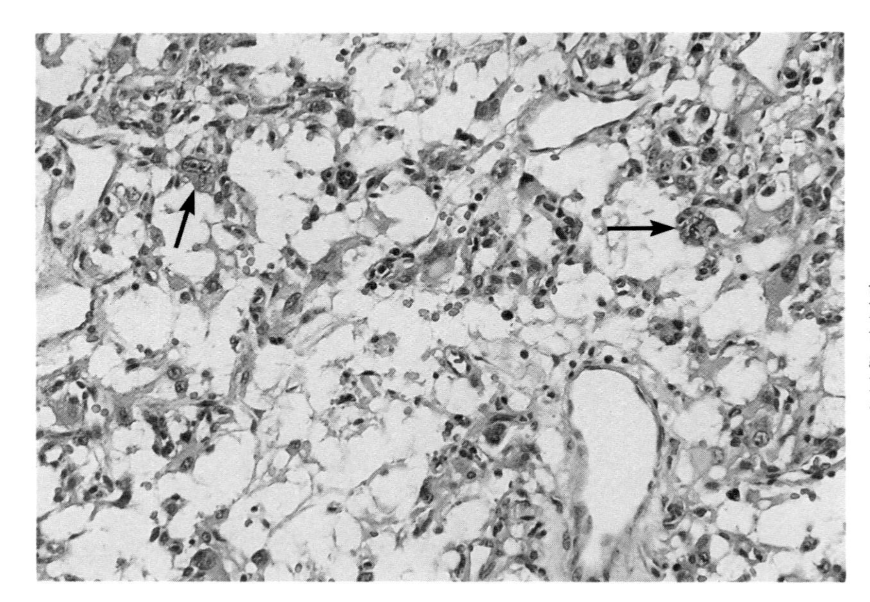

Figure 18-20
VAGAL PARAGANGLIOMA

Prominent vascularity and interstitial edema separate tumor cells. Some have enlarged nuclei (arrows). The tumor was diagnosed as a hemangioendothelioma of the vagus nerve; the patient was alive and well 10 years after surgical resection.

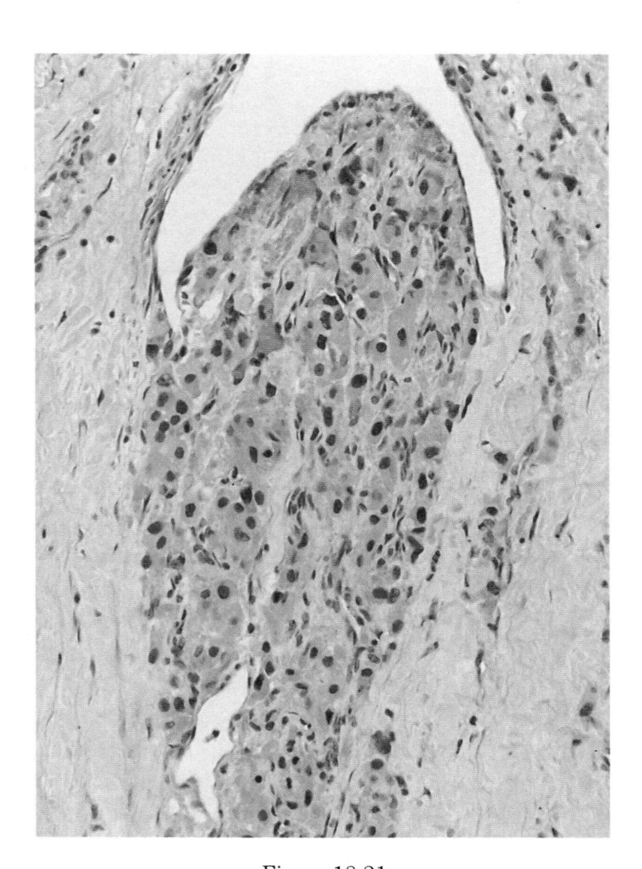

Figure 18-21
VAGAL PARAGANGLIOMA

Few areas of intravascular extension (or protrusion) were present. The tumor was benign after a follow-up of nearly 6 years.

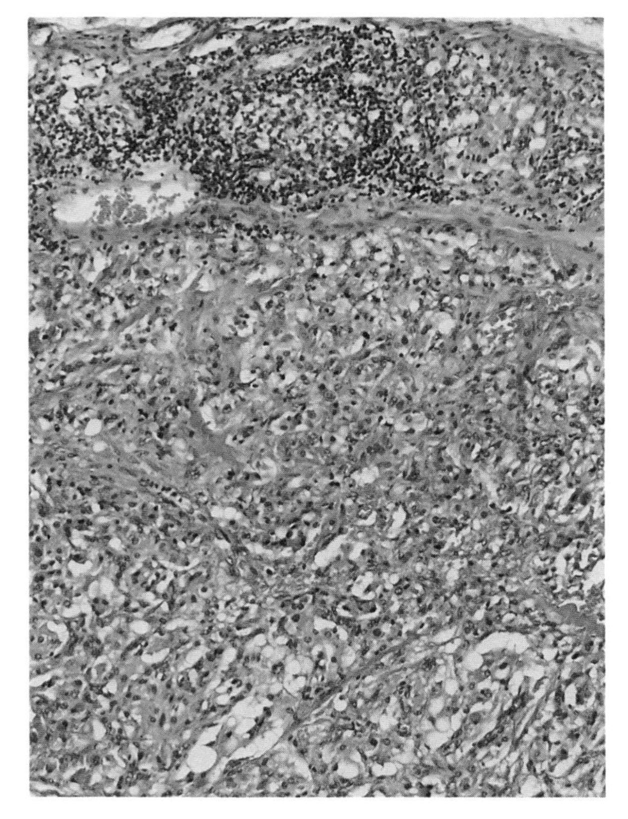

Figure 18-22
VAGAL PARAGANGLIOMA

This malignant vagal paraganglioma in a 49-year-old female metastasized to a regional cervical lymph node.

REFERENCES

Vagal Paraganglia

1. Birrell JH. Jugular body and its tumour. Aust N Z J Surg 1955;24:195–206.
2. Dahlqvist A, Carlsöö B, Hellstöm S. Paraganglia of the human recurrent laryngeal nerve. Am J Otolaryngol 1986;7:366–9.
3. Goormaghtigh N. On the existence of abdominal vagal paraganglia in the adult mouse. J Anat 1936;71:77–90.
4. Kjaergaard J. Anatomy of the carotid glomus and carotid glomus-like bodies (nonchromaffin paraganglia). With electron microscopy and comparison of human foetal carotid, aorticopulmonary, subclavian, tympanojugular, and vagal glomera. Copenhagen: FADL's Forlag, 1973.
5. Lack EE. Hyperplasia of vagal and carotid body paraganglia in patients with chronic hypoxemia. Am J Pathol 1978;91:497–516.
6. Lack EE. Microanatomy of vagal body paraganglia in infancy including victims of sudden infant death syndrome. Ped Pathol 1989;9:373–86.
7. Lack EE. Pathology of adrenal and extra-adrenal paraganglia. In: Major problems in pathology, Vol 29. Philadelphia: WB Saunders, 1994.
8. Marcuse RM, Chamberlin JA. Multicentric paragangliomas. Case report with demonstration of intravagal paraganglionic tissue at a previously undescribed level. Cancer 1956;9:288–92.
9. Muratori G. Contributo all' innervazione del tessuto paragangliare annesso al sistema del vago (glomo carotico, paragangli estravagali, ed intravagali) e all' innervazione del seno carotideo. Anat Anz 1932;75:115–23.
10. Plenat F, Leroux P, Floquet J, Floquet A. Intra and juxtavagal paraganglia: a topographical, histochemical, and ultrastructural study in the human. Anat Rec 1988;221:743–53.
11. White EG. Die struktur des glomus caroticum, seine pathologie und physiologie und seine beziehung zum nervensystem. Beitr Path Anat 1935;96:177–227.

Parathyroid Tissue Within the Vagus Nerve

12. Doppman JL, Shawker TH, Fraker DL, et al. Parathyroid adenoma within the vagus nerve. AJR Am J Roentgenol 1994;163:943–5.
13. Gilmour JR. Some developmental abnormalities of the thymus and parathyroids. J Pathol Bacteriol 1941;52:213–8.
14. Lack EE. Hyperplasia of vagal and carotid body paraganglia in patients with chronic hypoxemia. Am J Pathol 1978;91:497–516.
15. Lack EE, Delay S, Linnoila RI. Ectopic parathyroid tissue within the vagus nerve. Incidence and possible clinical significance. Arch Pathol Lab Med 1988;112:304–6.
16. Michal M. Ectopic parathyroid within a neck paraganglion. Histopathology 1993;22:85–7.
17. Reiling RB, Cady B, Clerkin EP. Aberrant parathyroid adenoma within vagus nerve. Lahey Clin Bull 1972;21:158–62.
18. Takimoto T, Okabe Y, Ito M, Umeda R. Intravagal parathyroid adenoma. J Laryngol Otol 1989;103:704–6.

Vagal Paraganglioma

19. Birrell JH. The vagal body and its tumour. Aust N Z J Surg 1953–4;23:48–54.
20. Black FO, Myers EN, Parnes SM. Surgical management of vagal chemodectomas. Laryngoscope 1977;87:1259–69.
21. Chen E, DeSanto LW, Gaffey TA. Intravagal paraganglioma: report of a case and review of the literature. Ear Nose Throat J 1985;64:54–62.
22. Duncan AW, Lack EE, Deck MF. Radiological evaluation of paragangliomas of the head and neck. Radiology 1979;132:95–105.
23. Green JD Jr, Olsen KD, DeSanto LW, Scheithauer BW. Neoplasms of the vagus nerve. Laryngoscope 1988;98: 648–54.
24. Heinrich MC, Harris AE, Bell WR. Metastatic intravagal paraganglioma. Case report and review of the literature. Am J Med 1985;78:1017–24.
25. Johnson WS, Beahrs OH, Harrison EG Jr. Chemodectoma of the glomus intravagale (vagal-body tumor). Am J Surg 1962;104:812–20.
26. Karusseit VO, Lodder JV. Functioning vagal body tumour. Br J Surg 1987;74:1184.
27. Kissel P, Floquet J, André JM, Picard L, Frisch R. Les chémodectomes du vague. Hypothèses pathogéniques à partir d'une revue du cent cas. Rev Neural (Paris) 1976;132:391–404.
28. Lack EE. Pathology of adrenal and extra-adrenal paraganglia. Major problems in pathology, Vol 29. Philadelphia: WB Saunders, 1994.
29. Lack EE, Cubilla AL, Woodruff JM. Paragangliomas of the head and neck region. A pathologic study of tumors from 71 patients. Hum Pathol 1979;10:191–218.
30. Lack EE, Cubilla AL, Woodruff JM, Farr HW. Paragangliomas of the head and neck region: a clinical study of 69 patients. Cancer 1977;39:397–409.
31. Lattes R. Nonchromaffin paraganglioma of ganglion nodosum, carotid body, and aortic-arch bodies. Cancer 1950;3:667–94.
32. Lawson W. Glomus bodies and tumors. NY State J Med 1980;80:1567–75.
33. Levit SA, Sheps SG, Espinosa RE, ReMine WH, Harrison EG Jr. Catecholamine-secreting paraganglioma of glomus-jugulare region resembling pheochromocytoma. N Engl J Med 1969;281:805–11.
34. Murphy TE, Huvos AG, Frazell EL. Chemodectomas of the glomus intravagale: vagal body tumors, nonchromaffin paragangliomas of the nodose ganglion of the vagus nerve. Ann Surg 1970;172:246–55.
35. Perez PE, Harrison EG Jr, ReMine WH. Vagal-body tumor (chemodectoma of the glomus intravagale). N Engl J Med 1960;263:1116–21.
36. Stout AP. Malignant tumors of peripheral nerves. Am J Cancer 1935;25:1–36.
37. Sundaram M, Cope V. Paragangliomas in the neck. Br J Surg 1976;63:182–5.
38. Tannir NM, Cortas N, Allam C. A functioning catecholamine-secreting vagal body tumor. A case report and review of the literature. Cancer 1983;52:932–5.
39. Wong GT, Stokes BA, Khangure MS, Apsimon HT, Sterrett GF. Glomus intravagale tumour: aspects of management. Aust NZ J Surg 1987;57:199–204.

19
LARYNGEAL PARAGANGLIOMA

LARYNGEAL PARAGANGLIA

Laryngeal paraganglia are microscopic structures that have a variable anatomic distribution in relation to the cricoid and thyroid cartilages (6,9). They have been divided into a superior and inferior group (fig. 19-1) (8); the size and location of the superior laryngeal paraganglia are more constant (5). A midline paraganglion has been designated as the anterior laryngeal glomus (6). Laryngeal paraganglia can sometimes be found immediately adjacent to the thyroid gland or as an ovoid structure within the capsule of the gland (10). They have also been described within the recurrent laryngeal nerve (3). Laryngeal paraganglia seem to be radioresistant since there are no detectable structural changes following therapeutic doses of radiation (10). Their basic histology is virtually identical to that of paraganglia elsewhere in the head and neck region (fig. 19-2) (7).

The precise physiologic role of laryngeal paraganglia is not known. The larynx has been characterized as a respirator effector organ capable of regulating respiratory flow of air, particularly during expiration (2). Fine motor control of the vocal cords modulates changes in airway resistance during the respiratory cycle; vagal innervation appears to be important in keeping laryngeal resistance low in conditions with hypoxia, and may help to prevent partial airway obstruction and thereby blunt the ventilatory work load (1). Some have postulated that endoneurial paraganglia might function as chemoreceptors, and that the chemosensory input to the central nervous system during hypoxia may represent a summation of stimuli from a variety of chemoreceptor sites (4).

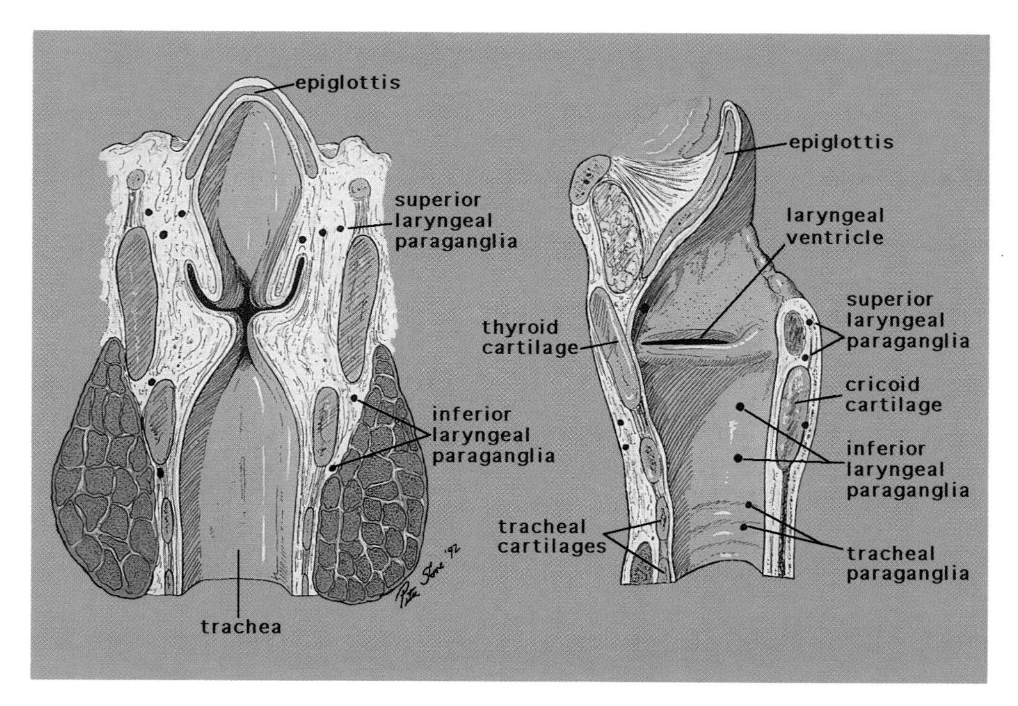

Figure 19-1
DISTRIBUTION OF HUMAN LARYNGEAL AND TRACHEAL PARAGANGLIA
Most paraganglia are paired structures located in superior and inferior locations in the lateral larynx.

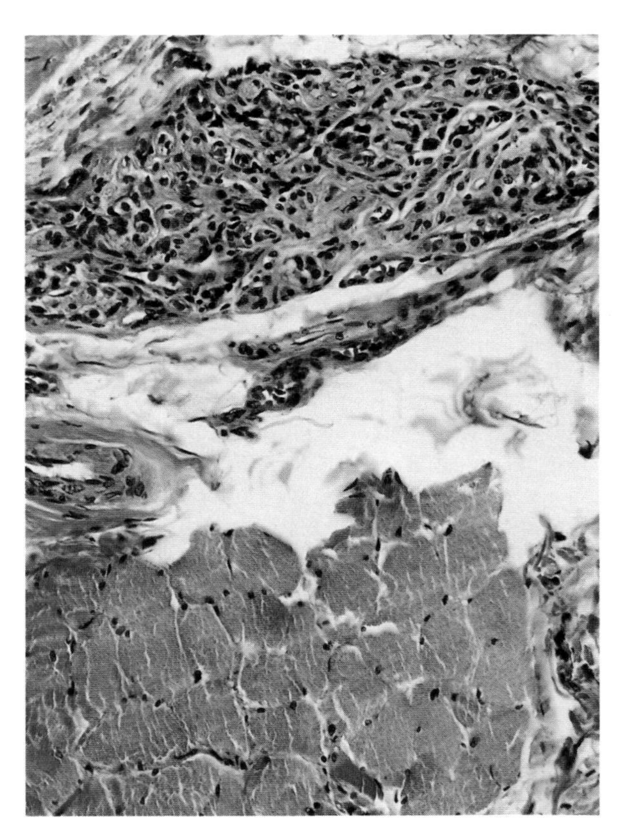

Figure 19-2
NORMAL LARYNGEAL PARAGANGLION
The normal laryngeal paraganglion is ovoid, and is morphologically identical to a lobule of carotid body.

LARYNGEAL PARAGANGLIOMA

Definition. This is a paraganglioma arising from dispersed paraganglia located near the larynx.

Clinical Features. Most laryngeal paragangliomas (LPs) present as a submucosal mass in the supraglottic larynx which may impinge on the glottic airway (fig. 19-3). The usual presenting complaint is hoarseness; other signs and symptoms include dysphagia, dyspnea, stridor, dysphonia, hemoptysis, and a cervical mass (15, 21). Throat pain has been a prominent symptom in some cases (27). In a critical review of the literature on LPs, Barnes (13) identified 81 cases, of which 34 were considered acceptable for analysis. There was a predilection for females (25 females, 9 males), average age at diagnosis of 47 years (range, 14 to 80 years), and average duration of symptoms of 26 months. Only 15 percent of LPs were primary in the subglottis and 3

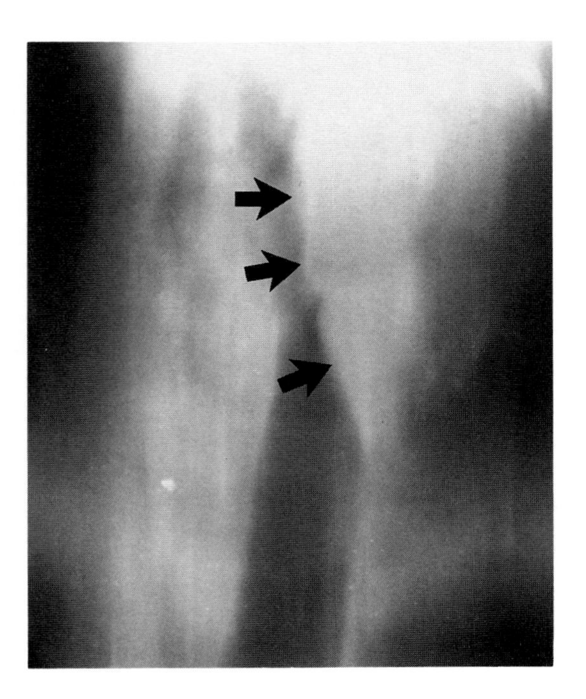

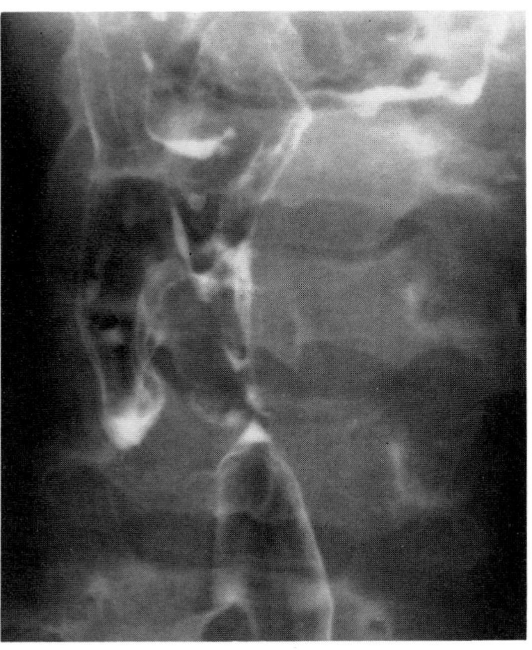

Figure 19-3
LARYNGEAL PARAGANGLIOMA
Top: A 26-year-old woman presented with progressive hoarseness of 5 months' duration. A tomogram of the larynx shows impingement on glottic airway by a soft tissue mass (arrows).

Bottom: Laryngogram shows mass effect with smooth overlying mucosa. The tumor originated in the area of the left piriform sinus and measured 4 x 6 cm. (Fig. 1A,B from Gallivan MV, Chun B, Rowden G, Lack EE. Laryngeal paraganglioma. Case report with ultrastructural analysis and literature review. Am J Surg Pathol 1979;3:85–92.)

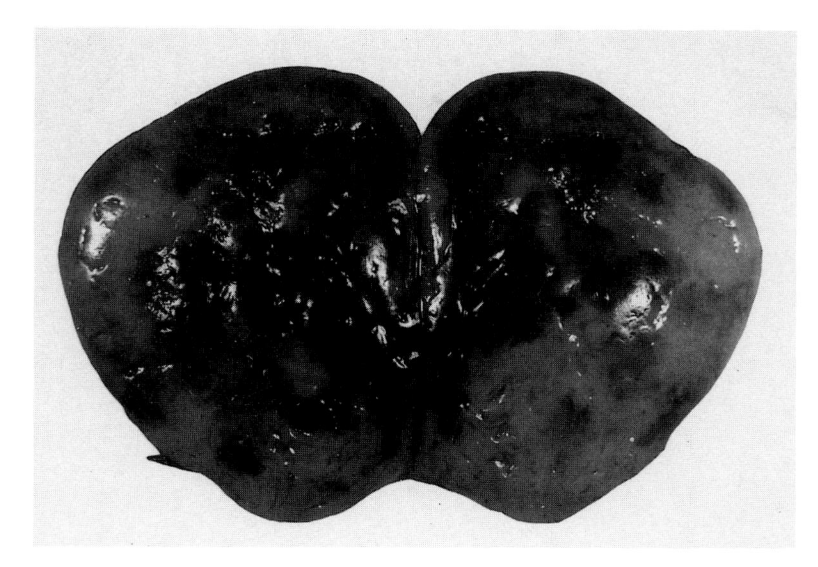

Figure 19-4
LARYNGEAL PARAGANGLIOMA
Bisected laryngeal paraganglioma from a 57-year-old woman who presented with a 3-year history of hoarseness and dysphagia. Preoperative diagnosis was a laryngeal chondroma. The patient was alive and well 15 years later. (Modified from fig. 7 from Lack EE, Cubilla AL, Woodruff JM. Paragangliomas of the head and neck region: a pathologic study of tumors from 71 patients. Hum Pathol 1979;10:191–218.)

percent in the glottis. One LP may have been hormonally active since the patient experienced hypertension and tachycardia, but there was no biochemical documentation of excess catecholamine secretion (22).

Pathologic Findings. The average size of LPs in the review by Barnes (13) was 2.5 cm (range, 0.5 to 6 cm). Most arose in the right side of the larynx. A dumbell-shaped LP extended into the larynx and prelaryngeal space adjacent to the thyroid gland (16). There may be multicentric paragangliomas in other sites (18), but several of these cases were excluded in the review by Barnes (including a tracheal paraganglioma): cases were also excluded if the tumor had not been illustrated or the illustrations were not considered confirmatory of the diagnosis (11,14, 17,25,28–30). LPs are described as a red or blue-red submucosal mass, and on cross section may have a meaty to tan appearance, with areas of congestion and hemorrhage (fig. 19-4).

The histologic appearance is usually typically that of a paraganglioma, but the unusual location or a prominent vascular pattern with plump endothelial cells can cause problems in interpretation (fig. 19-5). Accurate diagnosis is also hindered by technical alterations induced by a limited biopsy specimen or crush artifact. Barnes found few mitotic figures. Frank invasion into adjoining soft tissues is uncommon and should raise the possibility of another type of laryngeal neuroendocrine neoplasm with more aggressive behavior (20).

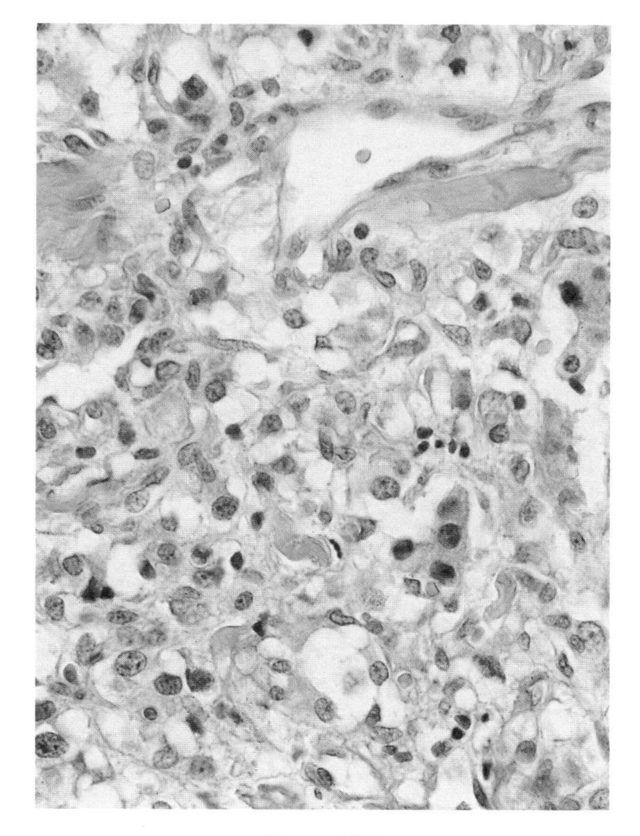

Figure 19-5
LARYNGEAL PARAGANGLIOMA
This tumor initially had been misinterpreted as a hemangioendothelioma because of the marked vasculature.

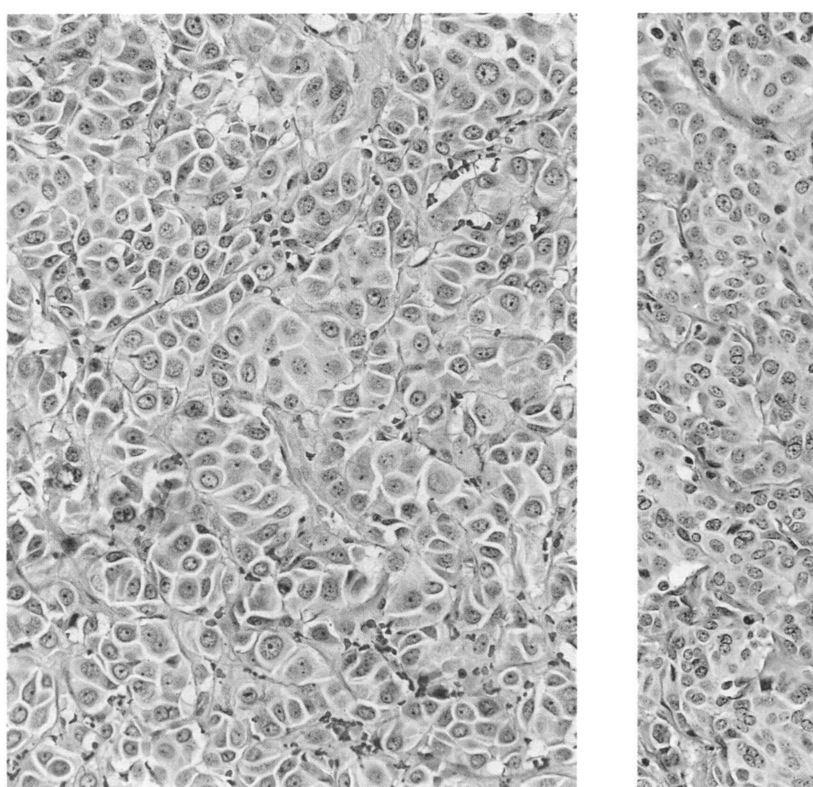
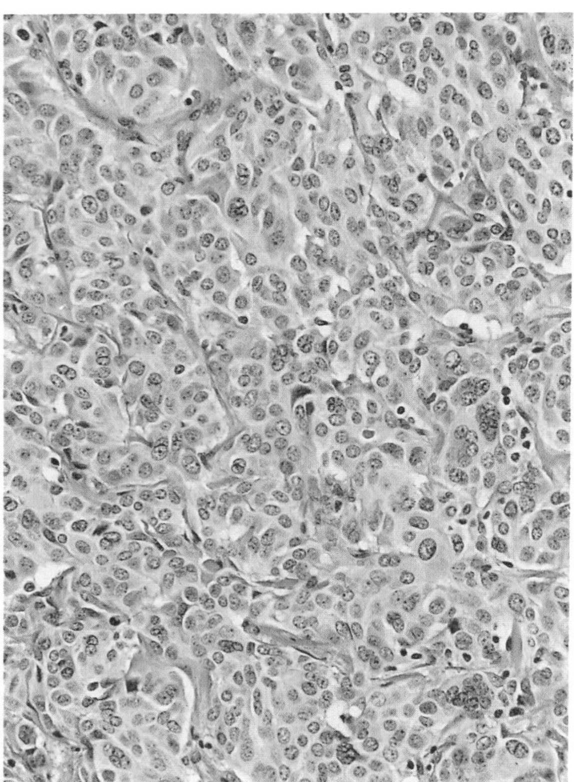

Figure 19-6
LARYNGEAL ATYPICAL CARCINOID

Left: A 66-year-old female had a 1-cm tumor in the submucosa of the supraglottic larynx. There is a nested and trabecular arrangement of cells with ample, granular eosinophilic cytoplasm.

Right : Same laryngeal atypical carcinoid tumor with a vague organoid pattern which can cause confusion with laryngeal paraganglioma. (Figs. 19-6 and 19-7 are from the same case.)

Biologic Behavior. Gallivan et al. (15) found that 25 percent of laryngeal tumors reported as LP were clinically malignant. This incidence was considered to be "spuriously high" since some of the cases reported as LP were actually atypical laryngeal carcinoid tumors (13,19,23,24). Based upon the world literature review by Barnes (13), local recurrence of LP was noted in 5 of 30 patients (17 percent); only one was malignant (3 percent) and metastasized to the lumbar spine 16 years after diagnosis of the primary tumor (12,26). These data indicate that LPs have a significantly lower incidence of malignancy than previously reported (20).

Differential Diagnosis. The differential diagnosis includes a variety of tumors such as malignant melanoma, either primary (39) or metastatic to the larynx (31,34), and hemangiopericytoma (40), but the primary neoplasm that has caused the greatest diagnostic confusion with LP is the laryngeal atypical carcinoid tumor (LAC) (43) which has also been referred to as large cell (38,44) or moderately differentiated neuroendocrine carcinoma (32,42). The average size of LAC in the review by Woodruff and Senie (43) was 1.6 cm. An organoid or trabecular pattern in a LAC can be readily confused with an LP (fig. 19-6) (37), and similar to LP, neuroendocrine neoplasms of the larynx can express markers such as chromogranin (fig. 19-7, left), protein gene product 9.5, and neuron-specific enolase (35). The LAC, however, is typically positive for epithelial markers such as cytokeratin (fig. 19-7, right) (35,42,43) and carcinoembryonic antigen (35). Positive staining for S-100 protein was found in 20 percent of LACs in the study by

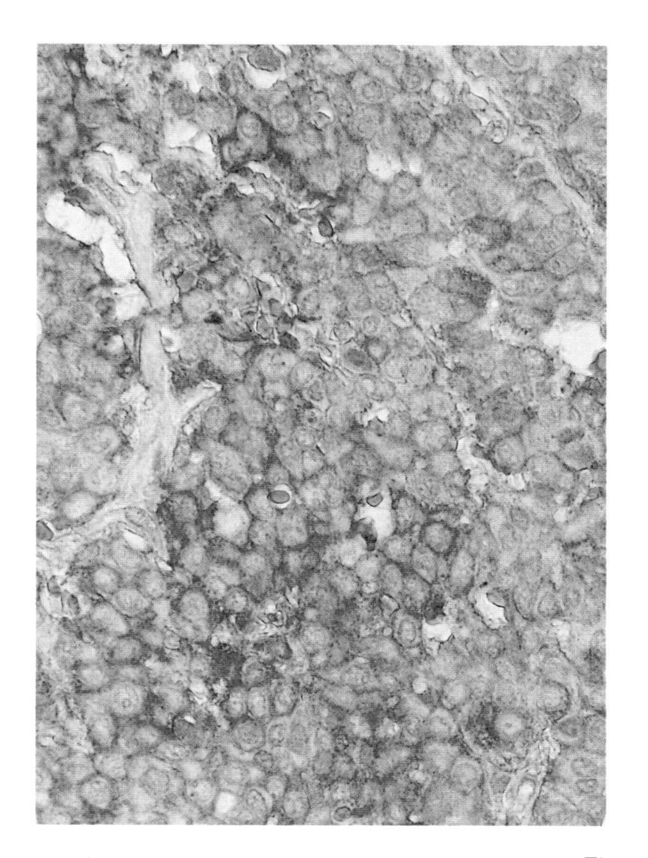

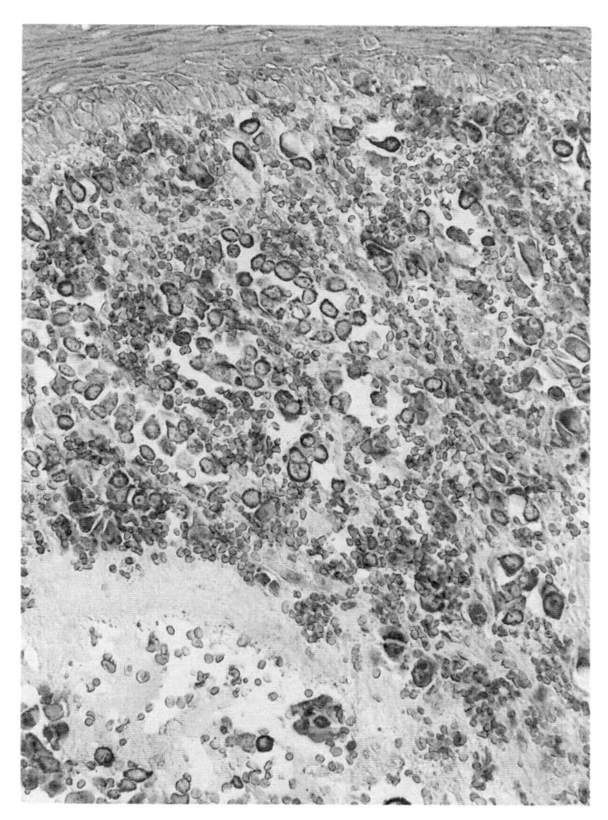

Figure 19-7
LARYNGEAL ATYPICAL CARCINOID
Left: Laryngeal atypical carcinoid shows positive immunostaining for chromogranin. (X200, Peroxidase-antiperoxidase stain)
Right: Same case with diffuse cytoplasmic immunoreactivity for cytokeratin. (X100, Peroxidase-antiperoxidase stain)

Wenig et al. (42), while in LPs, S-100 protein-positive cells are sustentacular cells and are distributed at the periphery of clusters of neoplastic chief cells (37). In a comprehensive review of LACs, the survival at 5 years was 48 percent and at 10 years 30 percent; a poorer survival rate was noted for patients having tumors over 1 cm in diameter and tumors involving skin and subcutaneous tissue (43). There has been some attempt at standardization of nomenclature of neuroendocrine neoplasms of the upper respiratory tract: the currently accepted three groups are laryngeal carcinoid, laryngeal atypical carcinoid (LAC), and small cell carcinoma (33,36,41).

REFERENCES

Anatomy and Physiology of Laryngeal Paraganglia

1. Bartlett D. Effects of vagal afferents on laryngeal responses to hypercapnia and hypoxia. Respir Physiol 1980;42:189–98.
2. Bartlett D Jr, Remmers JE, Gautier H. Laryngeal regulation of respiratory airflow. Resp Physiol 1973;18:194–204.
3. Dahlqvist A, Carlsöö B, Hellström S. Paraganglia of the human recurrent laryngeal nerve. Am J Otolaryngol 1986;7:366–9.
4. Dahlqvist A, Pequignot JM, Hellström S. Catecholamines of endoneurial laryngeal paraganglia in the rat. Acta Physiol Scand 1986;127:257–61.
5. Jansen HH, Netty-Marbell AO. Die parasympathischen paraganglien des menschlichen kehlkopfes. Zbl Allg Path 1967;110:246–50.
6. Kleinsasser O. Das glomus laryngicum inferior. Ein bisher unbekanntes, nichtchromaffines. Paraganglion vom Bau der sog. Carotisdrüse im menschlichen kehlkopf. Archiv Ohren-Nasen-und Kehlkopfheilk 1964;184:214–24.

7. Lack EE. Pathology of adrenal and extra-adrenal paraganglia. Major problems in pathology, Vol 29. Philadelphia: WB Saunders, 1994.
8. Lawson W, Zak FG. The glomus bodies (paraganglia) of the human larynx. Laryngoscope 1974;84:98–111.
9. Watzka M. Über die paraganglion in der plica ventricularis des menschlichen kehlkopfes. Dtsch Med Forsch 1963;1:19–20.
10. Zak FG, Lawson W. Glomic (paraganglionic) tissue in the larynx and capsule of the thyroid gland. Mt Sinai J Med 1972;39:82–90.

Laryngeal Paraganglioma

11. Ali S, Aird DW, Bihari J. Pain-inducing laryngeal paragangliomas (non-chromaffin). J Laryngol Otol 1983;97:181–8.
12. Azevedo-Gamas A, Gloor F. Un cas très rare de tumeur du larynx. Diagnostic anatomo-pathologique inattendu. Ann Otolaryngol (Paris) 1968;85:329–35.
13. Barnes L. Paraganglioma of the larynx. A critical review of the literature. ORL J Otorhinolaryngol Relat Spec 1991;53:220–34.
14. Crowther JA, Colman BH. Chemodectoma of the larynx. J Otolaryngol Otol 1987;101:1095–8.
15. Gallivan MV, Chun B, Rowden G, Lack EE. Laryngeal paraganglioma. Case report with ultrastructural analysis and literature review. Am J Surg Pathol 1979;3:85–92.
16. Googe PB, Ferry JA, Bhan AK, Dickersin GR, Pilch BZ, Goodman M. A comparison of paraganglioma, carcinoid tumor, and small-cell carcinoma of the larynx. Arch Pathol Lab Med 1988;112:809–15.
17. Hanna GS, Ali MH. Chemodectoma of the larynx. J Laryngol Otol 1986;100:1081–7.
18. Hartmann E. Chemodectoma laryngis. Acta Otolaryngol 1960;51:528–32.
19. Justrabo E, Michiels R, Calmettes C, et al. An uncommon apudoma: a functional chemodectoma of the larynx. Report of a case and review of the literature. Acta Otolaryngol 1980;89:135–43.
20. Lack EE. Pathology of adrenal and extra-adrenal paraganglia. Major problems in pathology, Vol 29. Philadelphia: WB Saunders, 1994.
21. Lack EE, Cubilla AL, Woodruff JM. Paragangliomas of the head and neck region: a pathologic study of tumors from 71 patients. Hum Pathol 1979;10:191–218.
22. Laudadio P. Chemodectoma (paraganglioma noncromaffine) del glomo laringeo superiore. Otolaringol Ital 1971;39:19–31.
23. Marks PV, Brookes GB. Malignant paraganglioma of the larynx. J Laryngol Otol 1983;97:1183–8.
24. Milroy CM, Rode J, Moss E. Laryngeal paragangliomas and neuroendocrine carcinomas. Histopathology 1991;18:201–9.
25. Ohsawa M, Kurita Y, Horie A, Kurita KI. Malignant chemodectoma (paraganglioma) of the larynx. A case report with electron microscopy and biochemical assay. Acta Pathol Jpn 1983;33:1279–88.
26. Rüfenacht H, Mihatsch MJ, Jundt K, Gächter A, Tanner K, Heitz PU. Gastric epithelioid leiomyomas, pulmonary chondroma, non-functioning metastasizing extra-adrenal paraganglioma and myxoma: a variant of Carney's triad. Report of a patient. Klin Wochenschr 1985;63:282–4.
27. Stanley RJ, Weiland LH, Neel HB III. Pain-inducing laryngeal paraganglioma: report of the ninth case and review of the literature. Otolaryngol Head Neck Surg 1986;95:107–12.
28. Stearns MP. Chemodectoma of the larynx. J Laryngol Otol 1982;96:1181–5.
29. van Vroonhoven TJ, Peutz WH, Tjan TG. Presurgical devascularization of a laryngeal paraganglioma. Arch Otolaryngol 1982;108:600–2.
30. Wetmore RF, Tronzo RD, Lane RJ, Lowry LD. Nonfunctional paraganglioma of the larynx: clinical and pathological considerations. Cancer 1981;48:2717–23.

Differential Diagnosis of Laryngeal Paragangliomas

31. Batsakis JG, Luna MA, Byers RM. Metastases to the larynx. Head Neck Surg 1985;7:458–60.
32. Dictor M, Tennvall J, Åkerman M. Moderately differentiated neuroendocrine carcinoma (atypical carcinoid) of the supraglottic larynx. Arch Pathol Lab med 1992;116:253–7.
33. El-Naggar A. Laryngeal neuroendocrine carcinoma. Victims of semantics. Arch Pathol Lab Med 1992;116:237–8.
34. Ferlito A, Caruso G, Recher G. Secondary laryngeal tumors. Report of seven cases with review of the literature. Arch Otolaryngol Head Neck Surg 1988;114:635–9.
35. Ferlito A, Friedmann I. Contribution of immunohistochemistry in the diagnosis of neuroendocrine neoplasms of the larynx. ORL J Otorhinolaryngol Relat Spec 1991;53:235–44.
36. Ferlito A, Rosai J. Terminology and classification of neuroendocrine neoplasms of the larynx. ORL J Otorhinolaryngol Relat Spec 1991;53:185–7.
37. Lack EE. Pathology of adrenal and extra-adrenal paraganglia. Major problems in pathology, Vol 29. Philadelphia: WB Saunders, 1994.
38. Milroy CM, Rode J, Moss E. Laryngeal paragangliomas and neuroendocrine carcinomas. Histopathology 1991;18:201–9.
39. Reuter VE, Woodruff JM. Melanoma of the larynx. Laryngoscope 1986;94:389–93.
40. Schwartz MR, Donovan DT. Hemangiopericytoma of the larynx: a case report and review of the literature. Otolaryngol Head Neck Surg 1987;96:369–72.
41. Shanmugaratnam K, Sobin LH, Barnes L, et al. Histological typing of tumors of the upper respiratory tract and ear. Berlin: Springer-Verlag, 1991.
42. Wenig BM, Hyams VJ, Heffner DK. Moderately differentiated neuroendocrine carcinoma of the larynx. A clinicopathologic study of 54 cases. Cancer 1988;62:2658–76.
43. Woodruff JM, Senie RT. Atypical carcinoid tumor of the larynx. A critical review of the literature. ORL J Otorhinolaryngol Relat Spec 1991;53:194–209.
44. Woodruff JM, Shah JP, Huvos AG, Gerold FP, Erlandson RA. Neuroendocrine carcinomas of the larynx. Am J Surg Pathol 1985;9:771–90.

20
AORTICOPULMONARY PARAGANGLIOMA

AORTICOPULMONARY PARAGANGLIA

Since the beginning of this century there have been descriptions of paraganglia in various sites near the base of the heart and great vessels; early descriptions by Wiesel (14), Busacchi (4), Penitschka (13), and others (12) leave little doubt that these microscopic structures have a varied anatomic distribution. They may be very difficult to recognize in histologic sections unless systematically searched for. In the study by Blessing (2), several thousand serial sections from the supracardiac region in an infant revealed 56 separate paraganglia (fig. 20-1). Paraganglia in this area are collectively referred to as aorticopulmonary paraganglia. Boyd (3) subdivided aorticopulmonary paraganglia into three groups at the base of the heart, while in an extensive study by Becker (1) four groups were recognized, including those located along the course of the left coronary artery in adventitia of the pulmonary trunk.

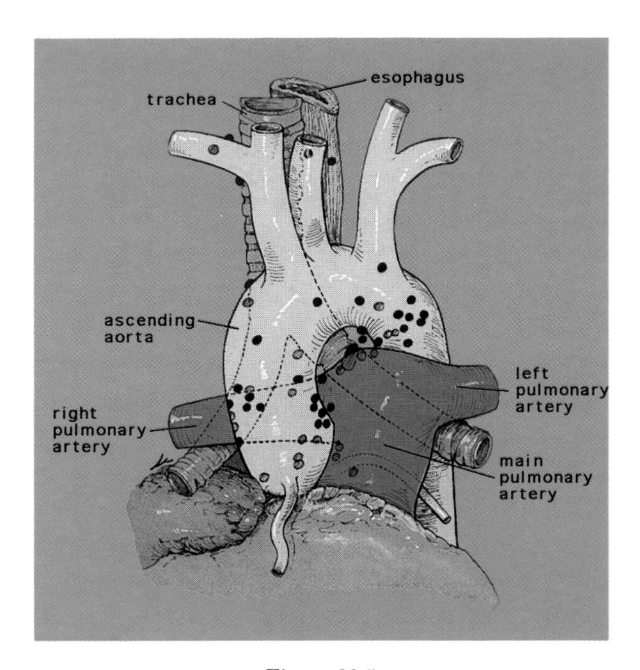

Figure 20-1
ANATOMIC DISTRIBUTION OF
AORTICOPULMONARY PARAGANGLIA

Cross-hatched dots indicate distribution in the dorsal aspect, while solid black dots show location in the ventral aspect. Some paraganglia are located on the superior aspect of the aortic arch and more cephalad near the subclavian artery. (Modified from fig. 1 from Blessing MH. Über glomuszellen im suprakardialraum. Klin Wochenschr 1963;41:1025–6.)

Since some (or all) aorticopulmonary paraganglia have a chemoreceptor function, the nature of the vascular supply is important. Although there was some controversy in early studies (6), and some consider the blood supply to be partially derived from the pulmonary artery trunk (11), several studies have convincingly demonstrated that the arterial supply is systemic and originates from the left coronary artery via the intertruncal branch (1,7) or the aorta (1). Aorticopulmonary paraganglia are also found in or near the interatrial septum (5,8), as well as along the proximal course of the left coronary artery (8); the subgroup of tumors designated cardiac paragangliomas may originate from some of these paraganglia.

Aorticopulmonary paraganglia are microscopic structures which are histologically identical to the lobular subunits of carotid bodies. These paraganglia may be closely associated with small vascular units (fig. 20-2, left) or myelinated nerve bundles (fig. 20-2, right). The precise dimensions and histologic appearance of these paraganglia do not correlate with age or any specific disease process. In one study, the maximum size of paraganglia in the fetus and newborn was 140 to 250 µm (1); in another study, 14 fetal paraganglia were identified ranging in size from 45 to 180 µm (10). In the latter study, it was estimated that collectively the aorticopulmonary paraganglia make up a total volume about one third that of the carotid body; the ultrastructural appearance is similar to other head and neck paraganglia. Hyperplasia of aorticopulmonary paraganglia has been observed in some patients with cystic fibrosis (12). The largest paraganglion measured 1,360 by 1,800 µm. Hyperplasia is evidenced basically by an increase in size, sometimes with multilobulation; chief cells may be prominent (fig. 20-3). It

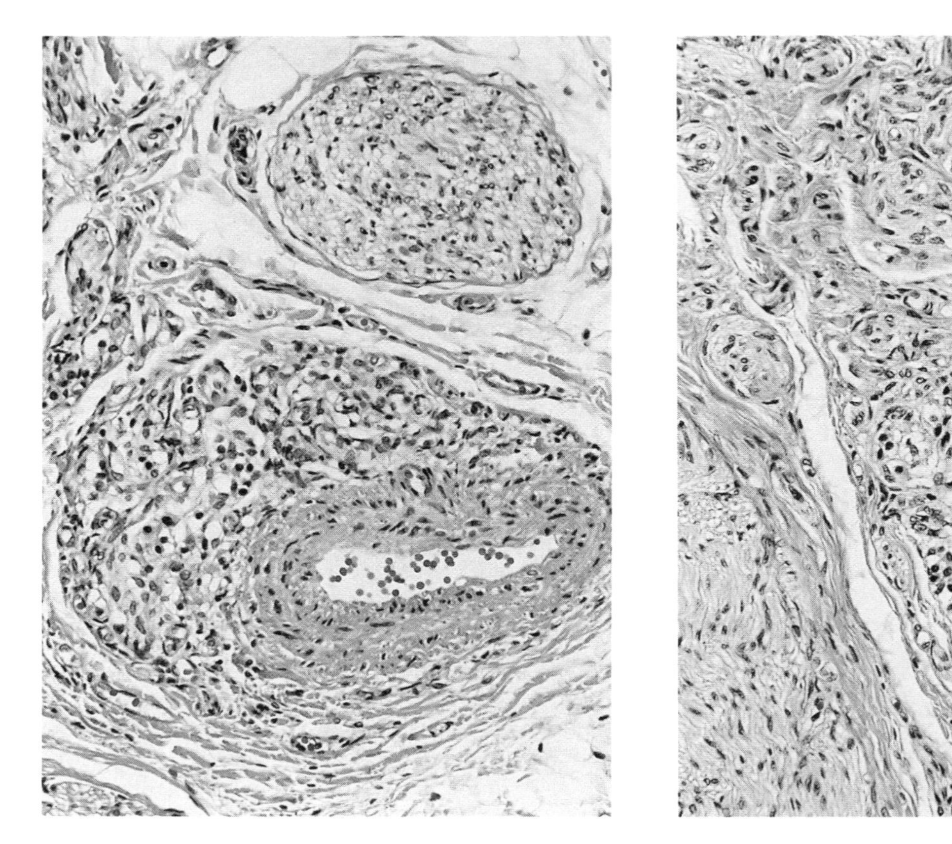

Figure 20-2
AORTICOPULMONARY PARAGANGLIA

Left: Aorticopulmonary paraganglion is identical to the lobular subunit of the carotid body. Note the small vascular channel in the lower field. Chief cells are arranged in small clusters and many have dark-staining nuclei.

Right: Small lobules of aorticopulmonary paraganglion are located adjacent to myelinated nerve bundles. Note the ganglion cell (arrow).

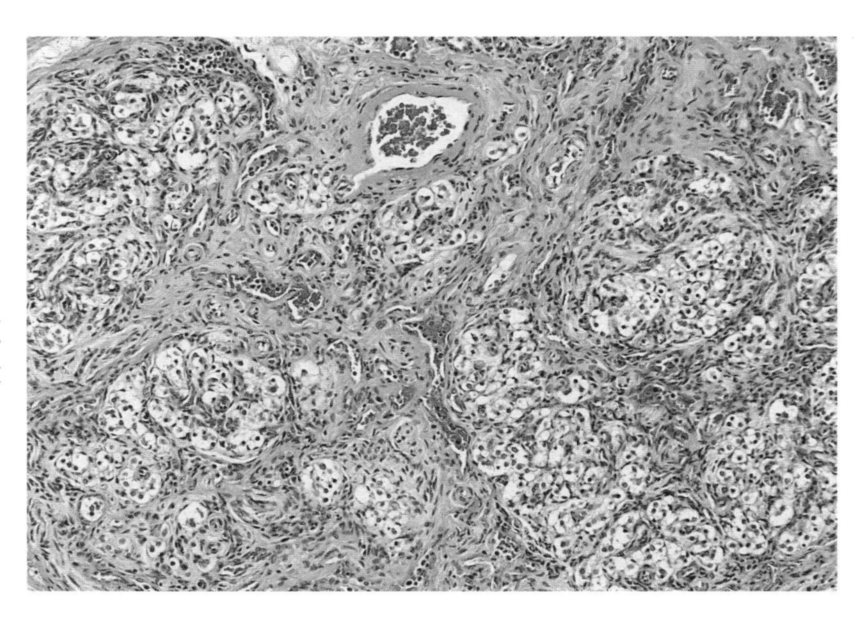

Figure 20-3
HYPERPLASTIC AORTICOPULMONARY PARAGANGLION

A portion of a hyperplastic aorticopulmonary paraganglion in an 18-year-old man with cystic fibrosis. Carotid bodies were also enlarged. Note the accentuated lobular architecture and prominent array of chief cells.

would be interesting to systematically study these and other extracarotid paraganglia in the head and neck region in individuals residing at high altitude or in individuals with altered physiologic function resulting in chronic hypoxemia (12). Morphologic alterations of some aorticopulmonary paraganglia have been reported in victims of sudden unexpected death, and it has been suggested on theoretical grounds that these alterations could lead to disturbance of cardiac rhythm, conduction, or repolarization (9).

AORTICOPULMONARY PARAGANGLIOMA

Definition. This is a paraganglioma arising from paraganglia near the base of the heart and great vessels.

General Remarks. Aorticopulmonary paragangliomas (APPs) arise from paraganglia which may be intracardial, usually at the level of the atria; intrapericardial but extracardiac; or in more diverse sites above or below the aortic arch as indicated in figure 20-1 (23). The collective group of APPs can be subdivided into cardiac and extracardiac paragangliomas. These tumors account for about 1 percent of all primary mediastinal neoplasms (15). The term APP is not used for paragangliomas located in the paravertebral sulcus paralleling the sympathetic chain.

Clinical Features. *Cardiac Paragangliomas.* Over 20 cases of primary cardiac paraganglioma (CP) have been reported, some more than once (16–32). This subset of APP may require special techniques for surgical management, such as cardiopulmonary bypass with cardioplegia and coronary artery reconstruction; human cardiac explantation and autotransplantation has even been attempted following resection of a large atrial paraganglioma (17,21). CPs arise within the pericardium and involve some intrinsic aspect of the heart. In a review by Johnson et al. (22), females were affected more often, and the average age at diagnosis was 45 years. Some of the presenting signs or symptoms include cardiomegaly, retrosternal pain, hemoptysis, palpitations, and murmur (23). A few patients have symptoms of ischemic heart disease (19,25). Occlusion of the left anterior descending coronary artery has been reported, probably due to extrinsic compression by a CP (24).

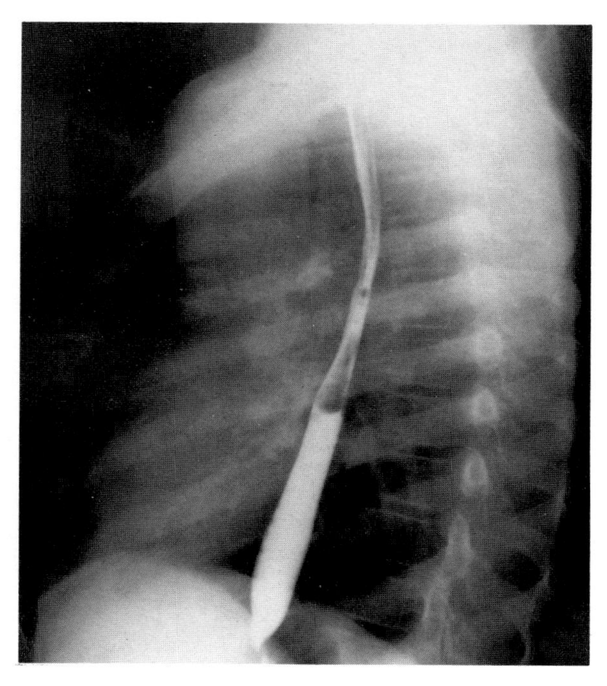

Figure 20-4
AORTICOPULMONARY PARAGANGLIOMA
Chest radiograph with barium esophagogram of an 11-year-old girl with an aorticopulmonary paraganglioma. A middle mediastinal mass impinging on the esophagus was initially interpreted as a vascular structure. (Figures 20-4 and 20-5 are from the same case.)

About half of the reported CPs have been associated with signs or symptoms of excess catecholamine secretion; these tumors (and the associated paraganglia) may be related to sympathoadrenal paragangliomas (23). Several patients have undergone failed abdominal exploration for suspected pheochromocytoma (16,20, 32). CPs can involve the walls of the atria, interatrial septum or groove, and the aorticopulmonary sulcus, and have been described within the pericardium overlying the right or left ventricle toward the base of the heart. Some CPs are not detectable by routine tomography or computed tomography (CT) (20), and ^{131}I-metaiodobenzylguanidine (MIBG) scintigraphy is used to show localized iodine uptake in the cardiac region (26,29,30).

Extracardiac Paragangliomas. A greater number of extracardiac paragangliomas (ECPs) have been reported, that is, paragangliomas outside the pericardial cavity in the area of the base of the heart and great vessels (figs. 20-4, 20-5), than cardiac paragangliomas (35,38,40–46,48).

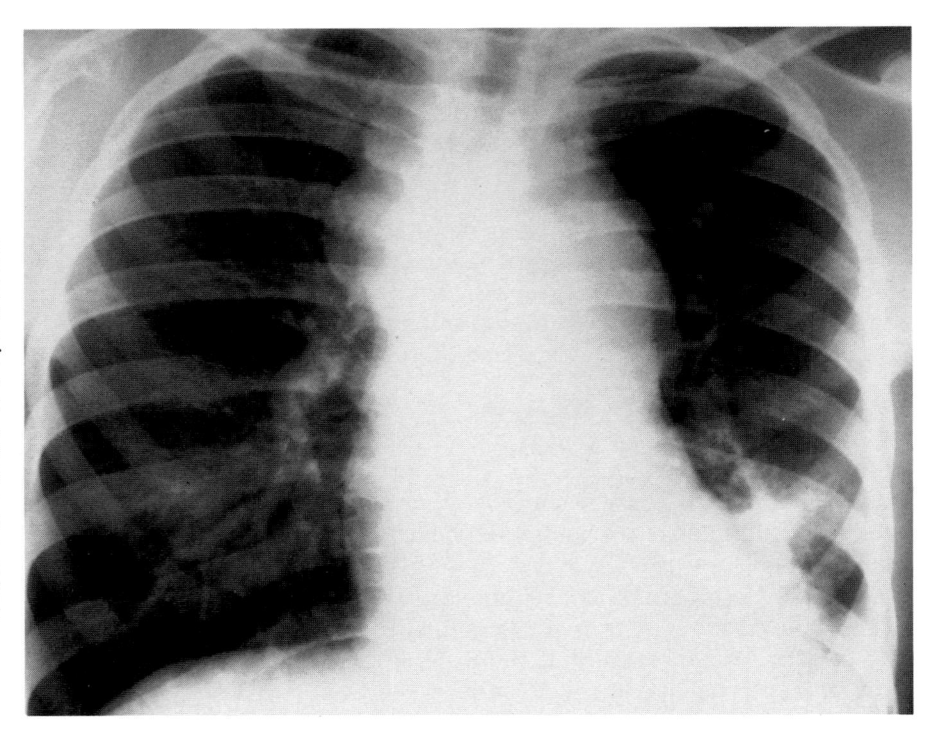

Figure 20-5
AORTICOPULMONARY PARAGANGLIOMA

Anteroposterior radiograph of the chest 4 years later with enlargement of the mediastinal mass. Left lower lobe infiltrate most likely represents pneumonitis secondary to compression of the main-stem bronchus. The patient had complained of recent cough with sputum production. There was no evidence of excess catecholamine secretion. (Fig. 2 from Lack EE, Stillinger RA, Colvin DB, Groves RM, Burnette DG. Aortico-pulmonary paraganglioma. Report of a case with ultrastructural study and review of the literature. Cancer 1979;43:269–78.)

ECPs were first reported in 1950 (42,44). A female predominance is apparent with an age distribution similar to that of CPs (40). In a recent study of 16 mediastinal paragangliomas there was slight male predominance, but most of the tumors were located in the posterior mediastinum (45), raising the possibility that some were in fact paravertebral paragangliomas of the sympathoadrenal neuroendocrine system. Hoarseness, dysphagia, cough, and chest pain are common manifestations, and occasionally patients present with superior vena cava syndrome (41).

Occasionally, ECPs and CPs are associated with paragangliomas in other sites (36,37) including pheochromocytoma (50) or extra-adrenal abdominal paraganglioma (49), and some patients may have a family history of similar tumors (36). A number of APPs have been reported in association with the triad of gastric epithelioid leiomyosarcoma, functioning extra-adrenal paraganglioma, and pulmonary chondroma (33).

Gross Findings. APPs range considerably in size, from 1.2 (42) to 17 cm, but are usually 5 to 7 cm in diameter (40,41). They may be round to ovoid and sharply demarcated, or may be flattened and expansile with indistinct borders and tenacious attachment to vital structures, making complete surgical removal difficult (40). Because of their location, APPs may encircle or partially envelop large vascular channels or encase or displace neural structures (40). Unless the pericardium is opened, some CPs escape detection if they are flattened and easily compressed. An occasional tumor may have a polyploid configuration with protrusion into the atrium.

Microscopic Findings. With adequate tissue sampling the diagnosis of APP can be readily made based upon the organoid clustering of neoplastic cells forming "zellballen" (fig. 20-6), but with small biopsy specimens the diagnosis may be difficult, particularly if there is crush artifact. A sustentacular cell population can be demonstrated in APPs and other paragangliomas by staining for S-100 protein. Intracytoplasmic hyaline globules are rare in these and other head and neck paragangliomas. An unusual spindle cell pattern was reported recently (45). The presence of apparent "infiltration" of cardiac connective tissue or muscle is not considered a reliable indicator of malignancy (39). A variety of other neoplasms enter into the differential diagnosis of APP, and several of these are discussed elsewhere (40).

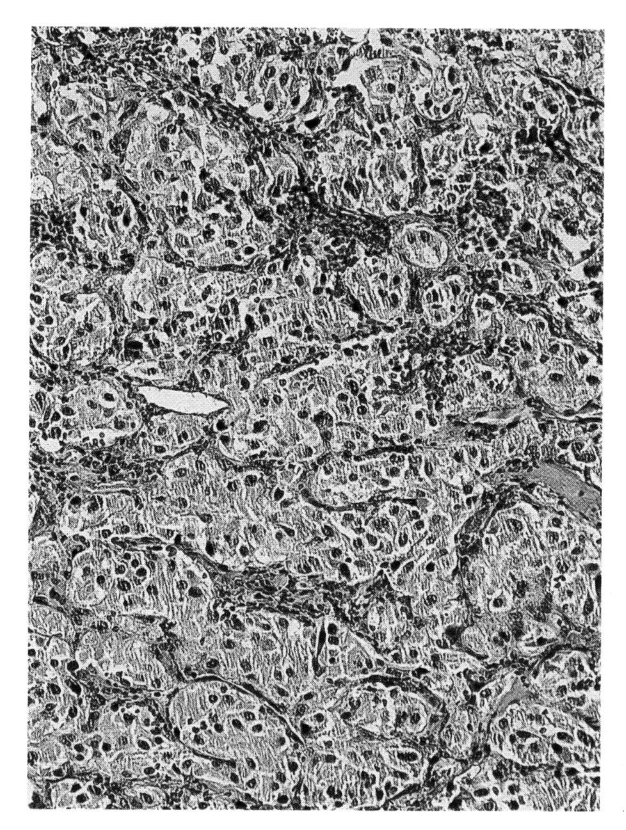

Figure 20-6
AORTICOPULMONARY PARAGANGLIOMA
Biopsy of an aorticopulmonary paraganglioma shows a nesting pattern of tumor cells with relatively abundant granular cytoplasm. Small nests and short cords of tumor cells were highlighted by reticulin stain.

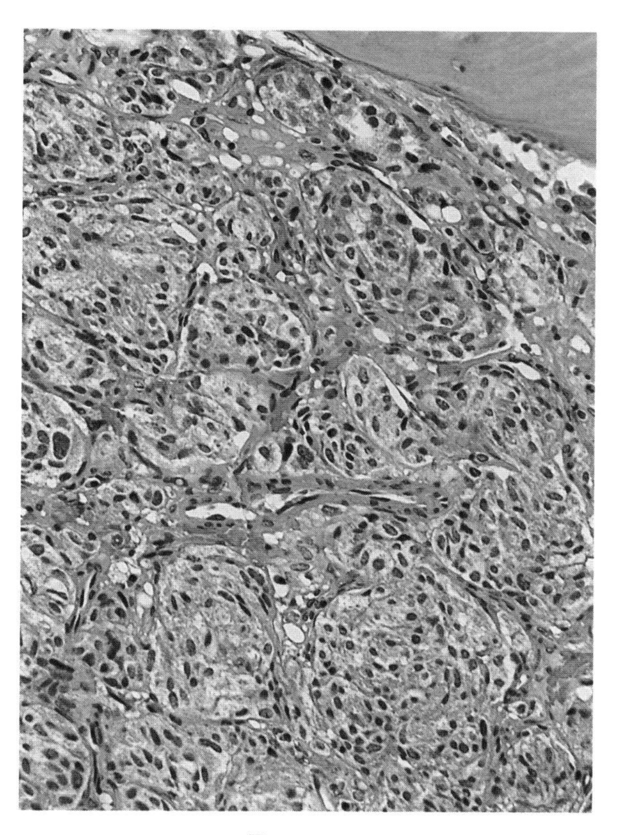

Figure 20-7
AORTICOPULMONARY PARAGANGLIOMA
Metastatic aorticopulmonary paraganglioma arising near the root of the lung. The skeletal metastasis has a well-developed nesting ("zellballen") pattern.

Biologic Behavior. The incidence of malignancy of APPs with metastasis has been estimated at 13 percent (41) to 20 percent (51) of cases (fig. 20-7); however, the rarity of these tumors, particularly the malignant ones, may make them more likely to be reported and hence result in an overestimation of the true malignant potential. An even greater problem, however, is the relatively high rate of unresectability due to dense adherence to or direct involvement of vital structures (40). Only 60 percent of patients with APPs have had complete surgical resection (51); this figure varies with APP size and precise anatomic location. Surgical resection may necessitate cardiopulmonary bypass with removal of portions of heart involved by tumor, and fatalities have occurred intraoperatively due to excess bleeding (34,47).

THE ENDOCRINE LUNG AND PULMONARY CHEMORECEPTORS: INNERVATED CLUSTERS OF PULMONARY NEUROENDOCRINE CELLS

Pulmonary neuroendocrine (NE) cells are solitary or arranged in small, discrete collections referred to as neuroepithelial bodies (NEBs). These form ovoid to triangular corpuscles intercalated within respiratory mucosa (56), and in experimental animals have been shown to be innervated by sensory nerve fibers of the vagus nerve (58). The corpuscular cell appears presynaptic to the nerve ending, thus permitting discharge of nerve impulses to the central nervous system (57). It has been proposed that innervated clusters of NE cells (i.e., NEBs) may function as pulmonary airway chemoreceptors sensitive to hypoxia (55). It is clear from recent experimental data, coupled with results of a symposium on pulmonary NE cells in health and disease (60), that the bronchopulmonary tree has physiologic functions and is not merely an airway conduit. Structural changes, including hyperplasia of pulmonary NE cells, have been reported in experimental animals (61), and in humans living at high altitude (59) and with chronic bronchitis, emphysema (54), and pulmonary hypertension (53). A recent study of high altitude dwellers and lowlanders found no significant differences in structure, number, content, or distribution of pulmonary NE cells, but the number of cases was small and subtle changes might not achieve statistical significance (62). Presently, there does not appear to be sufficient data from human studies to draw any valid conclusions on the effects of high altitude on pulmonary NE cells (52).

PULMONARY PARAGANGLIA

There are very few references to pulmonary paraganglia in the literature, and they are difficult to document in humans (64). In a study by Blessing and Hora (63) involving over 5,000 serial sections of a newborn human lung, 68 separate pulmonary paraganglia were identified (fig. 20-8). These paraganglia were in close proximity to blood vessels and nerves, and were often located near the pulmonary artery, especially in areas of branching. Based upon most of the illustrations, these appear to be genuine paraganglia, and the authors considered them to be chemoreceptors involved in regulating respirations and pulmonary blood flow. It is important to note that these paraganglia were not identified within the interstitium of alveolar walls or in conducting airway epithelium.

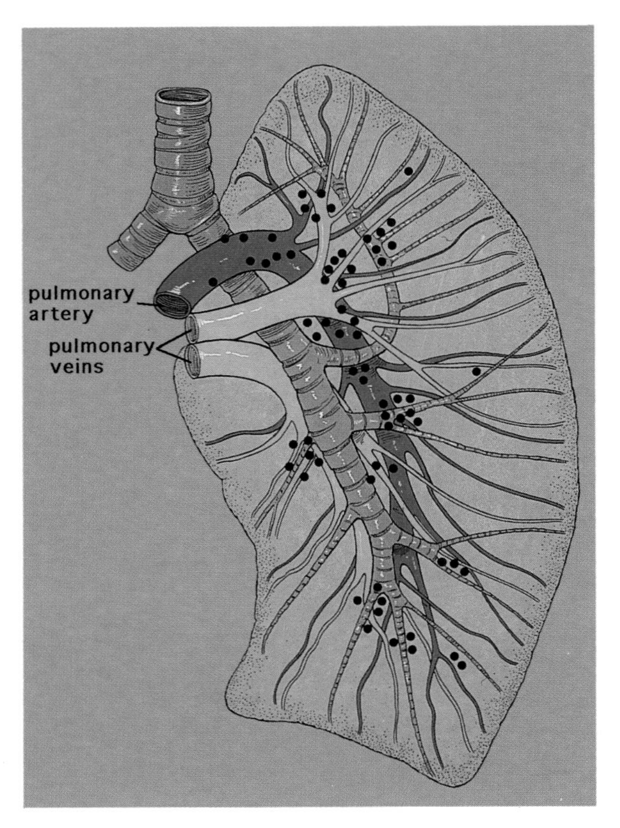

Figure 20-8
PULMONARY PARAGANGLIA
Distribution of pulmonary paraganglia in human fetal lung. Most have a centripetal location in relation to vessels and nerves. (Modified from fig. 1 from Blessing MH, Hora BI. Glomera in der lunge des menschen. Z Zellforsch Mikrosk Anat 1968;87:567–70.)

PULMONARY PARAGANGLIOMA

Clinical and Pathologic Findings. If the occurrence of normal paraganglia within the lung in association with blood vessels and nerves is accepted, then it follows that pulmonary paragangliomas exist as well, and indeed a number of such tumors have been reported in the literature (65–71,73–78). The author has not personally seen a case of primary pulmonary paraganglioma. A meaningful review of the clinical and pathologic features of these tumors is not possible because: 1) some reports lack detailed illustrations of pathology; 2) the tumors are difficult (if not impossible) to distinguish from some bronchial carcinoid tumors (fig. 20-9); and 3) distinction from metastatic paraganglioma to lung is difficult (72). Some of the reported pulmonary paragangliomas appear to have the typical architectural patterns seen in paragangliomas elsewhere in the head and neck region (66,69,73).

Differential Diagnosis. *Bronchial Carcinoid Tumors.* As stated above, pulmonary paragangliomas may be difficult to distinguish from bronchial carcinoid tumors. There are a number of morphologic features seen in bronchial carcinoid tumors that are not typical for a paraganglioma, but distinguishing the two may be more of an academic exercise since bronchial

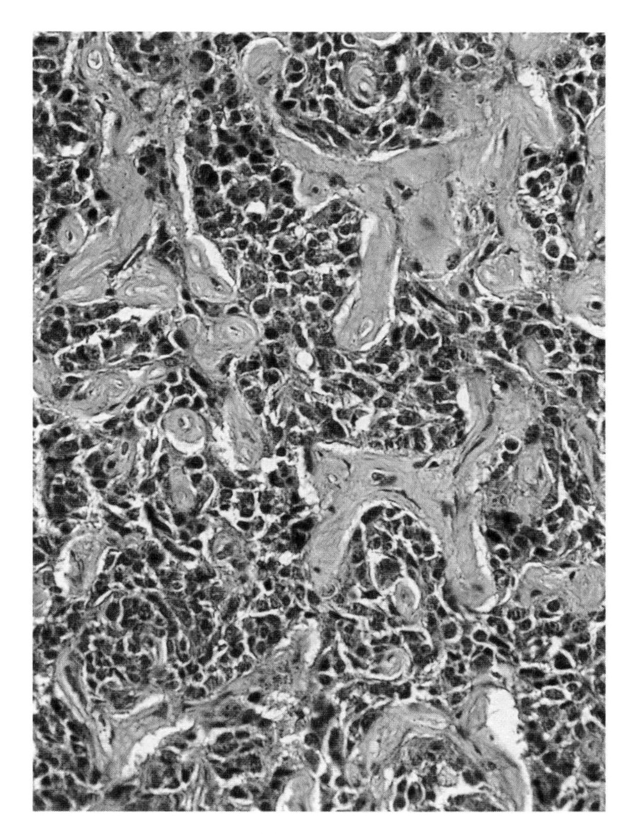

Figure 20-9
BRONCHIAL CARCINOID TUMOR
MIMICKING PARAGANGLIOMA
Bronchial carcinoid tumor with areas showing a nesting arrangement of cells with fibrosis mimicking a paraganglioma. Some cells have nuclei with dispersed or stippled chromatin.

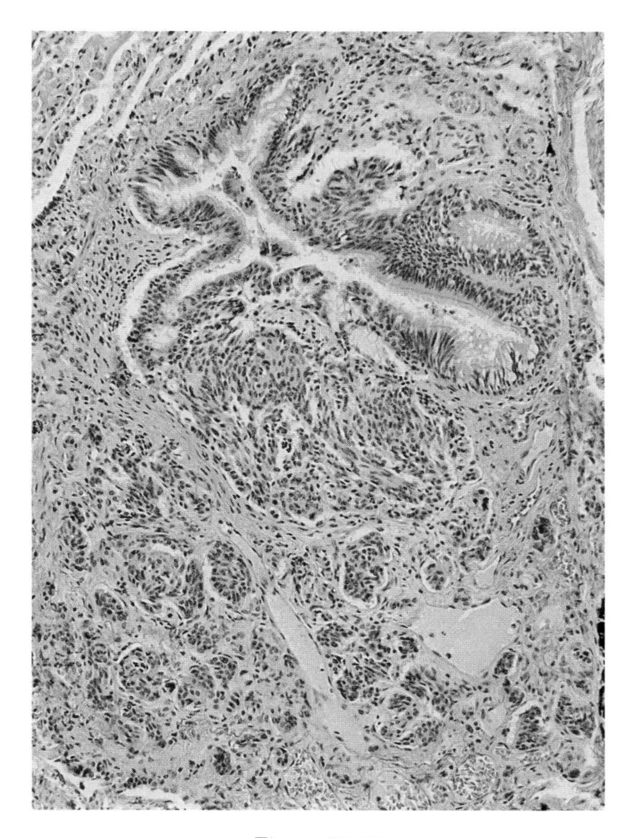

Figure 20-10
MULTIPLE CARCINOID TUMORLETS
Multiple carcinoid tumorlets were found incidentally in a lobectomy specimen from a patient with bronchiectasis. Lesions abut the epithelial lining of the terminal bronchiole and nests of spindle to ovoid cells are separated by collagenous stroma.

carcinoid tumors and most paragangliomas of the head and neck region have relatively limited malignant potential (72).

Carcinoid Tumorlets. Another lesion that may be part of the differential diagnosis of a primary pulmonary paraganglioma is carcinoid tumorlet. These are usually peripheral in the lung and microscopic or only a few millimeters in diameter (figs. 20-10, 2-11). Carcinoid tumorlets are often related to bronchial or bronchiolar epithelium which may progress to luminal obliteration or extend to involve adjacent lung parenchyma, with proliferation of connective tissue including elastosis (80). The organoid clustering of cells faintly resembles a paraganglioma, but close sectioning reveals continuity of one nest with another (83). Neurosecretory-type granules have been demonstrated by electron microscopy (79,80,82,83). Carcinoid tumorlets are usually incidental findings, sometimes in lung parenchyma involved by bronchiectasis or other inflammatory processes, and are of no consequence to the patient. Metastases to regional hilar lymph nodes occur occasionally (81): 2 of 85 cases originally reported by Whitwell in 1955 metastasized (84).

Minute Meningothelial-Like Nodules. Minute meningothelial-like nodules were described by Korn et al. in 1960 (93), and were regarded as minute pulmonary tumors resembling chemodectomas. They have been reported in 1 of 60 (91) to 1 of 300 autopsies (93), and there appears to be an increased frequency in lungs from patients with cardiac failure, chronic bronchitis, emphysma (86,93) and thromboemboli (95). A number of

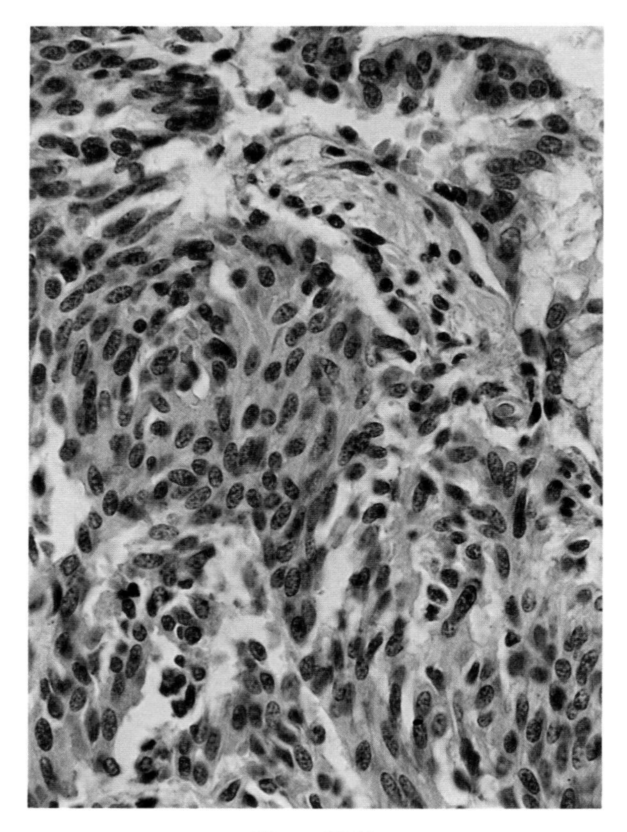

Figure 20-11
MULTIPLE CARCINOID TUMORLETS
Carcinoid tumorlet has oval to elongated nuclei with a lightly stippled nuclear chromatin pattern.

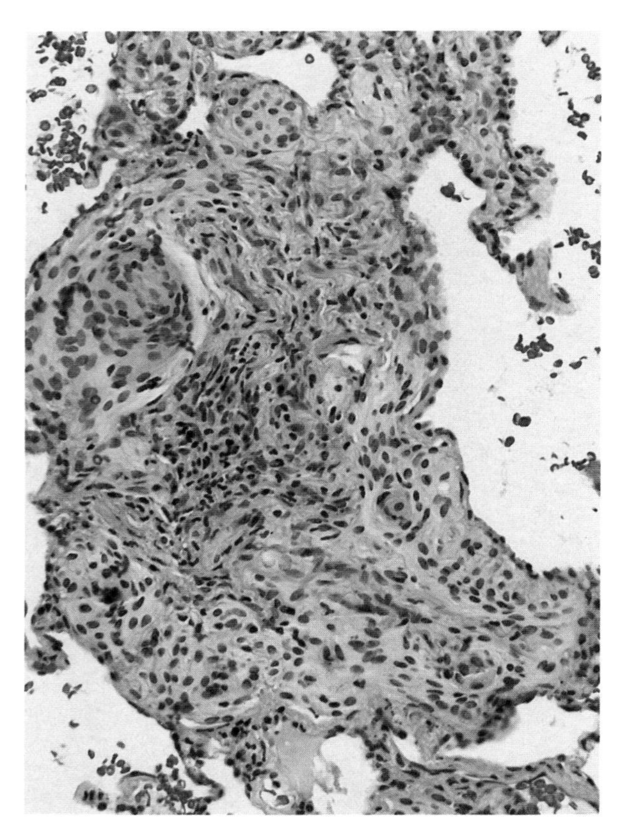

Figure 20-12
MINUTE MENINGOTHELIAL-LIKE NODULE
The lesion formerly referred to as pulmonary "chemodectoma" is composed of nests of oval uniform cells which expand interstitium of alveolar septa.

other investigators have regarded minute meningothelial-like nodules as pulmonary chemoreceptors or chemodectomas analogous to the carotid body (85,89,92,95,97). Some even report an intensely positive argentaffin reaction consistent with hyperplasia of endocrine-type chemoreceptor tissue (85), although a subsequent ultrastructural study provided different conclusions and suggested a pleural origin (87). There is no relationship to paraganglia or paraganglioma. Other ultrastructural studies have confirmed the nonendocrine nature of these cells and a strong resemblance to meningothelial cells (94,96). Minute meningothelial-like nodule often appears as a 1- to 3-mm, tan-yellow lesion which may be detected on gross examination and is characteristically located in the interstitium with expansion of alveolar septa (fig. 20-12). The cells have bland oval nuclei, often with a small dot-like nucleolus, and pale eosinophilic cytoplasm with indistinct borders. The cells may be arranged in nests or "zellballen" (93). The existence of minute meningothelial-like nodules may help to explain the rare occurrence of primary pulmonary meningiomas (88,90).

REFERENCES

Distribution and Anatomy of Aorticopulmonary Paraganglia

1. Becker AE. The glomera in the region of the heart and great vessels. A microscopic-anatomical and histochemical study. MD thesis, Laboratory of Pathological Anatomy of the University of Amsterdam, 1966.
2. Blessing MH. Über glomuszellen im suprakardialraum. Klin Wochenschr 1963;41:1025–6.
3. Boyd JD. The inferior aortico-pulmonary glomus. Brit Med Bull 1961;17:127–31.
4. Busacchi P. I corpi cromaffini del cuore umano. Arch Ital Anat Embriol 1912-1913;11:352–76.
5. Dail WG Jr, Palmer GC. Localization and correlation of catecholamine-containing cells with adenyl cyclase and phosphodiesterase activities in the human fetal heart. Anat Rec 1973;177:265–88.
6. Edwards C, Heath D. Microanatomy of glomic tissue of the pulmonary trunk. Thorax 1969;24:209–17.
7. Edwards C, Heath D. Site and blood supply of the intertruncal glomera. Cardiovasc Res 1970;4:502–8.
8. Gobbi H, Barbosa AJ, Teixeira VP, Almeida HO. Immunocytochemical identification of neuroendocrine markers in human cardiac paraganglion-like structures. Histochemistry 1991;95:337–40.
9. James TN. Degenerative lesions of a coronary chemoreceptor and nearby neural elements in the hearts of victims of sudden death. J Am Coll Cardiol 1986;8:12A–21A.
10. Kjaergaard J. Anatomy of the carotid glomus and carotid glomus-like bodies (nonchromaffin paraganglia) with electron microscopy and comparison of human foetal carotid, aorticopulmonary, subclavian, tympanojugular, and vagal glomera. Copenhagen: FADL's Forlag, 1973.
11. Krahl VE. The glomus pulmonale: its location and microscopic anatomy. In: De Reuck AU, O'Connor M, eds. Ciba foundation symposium on pulmonary structure and function. Boston: Little Brown and Co, 1962:53–76.
12. Lack EE. Pathology of adrenal and extra-adrenal paraganglia. Major problems in pathology, Vol 29. Philadelphia: WB Saunders, 1994.
13. Penitschka W. Paraganglion aorticum supracardiale. Z Mikros Anat Forsch 1931;24:24–37.
14. Wiesel J. Über erkrankungen der koronararterien im verlaufe akuter infektionskrankheiten. Wien Klin Wochenschr 1906;19:723–5.

Aorticopulmonary Paragangliomas: Cardiac Paraganglioma

15. Benjamin SP, McCormack LJ, Effler DB, Groves LK. Primary tumors of the mediastinum. Chest 1972;62:297)6303.
16. Besterman E, Bromley LL, Peart WS. An intrapericardial phaeochromocytoma. Br Heart J 1974;36:318–20.
17. Cooley DA, Reardon MJ, Frazier OH, Angelini P. Human cardiac explantation and autotransplantation: application in a patient with a large cardiac pheochromocytoma. Tex Heart Inst J 1985;12:171–6.
18. Del Fante FM, Watkins E Jr. Chemodectoma of the heart in a patient with multiple chemodectomas and familial history. Lahey Clin Found Bull 1967;16:224–9.
19. Dunn GD, Brown MJ, Sapsford RN, et al. Functioning middle mediastinal paraganglioma (phaeochromocytoma) associated with intercarotid paragangliomas. Lancet 1986;1:1061–4.
20. Hodgson SF, Sheps SG, Subramanian R, Lie JT, Carney JA. Catecholamine-secreting paraganglioma of the interatrial septum. Am J Med 1984;77:157–61.
21. Hui G, McAllister HA. Left atrial paraganglioma: report of a case and review of the literature. Am Heart J 1987;113:1230–34.
22. Johnson TL, Lloyd RV, Shapiro B, et al. Cardiac paragangliomas. A clinicopathologic and immunohistochemical study of four cases. Am J Surg Pathol 1985;9:827–34.
23. Lack EE. Pathology of adrenal and extra-adrenal paraganglia. Major problems in pathology, Vol 29. Philadelphia: WB Saunders, 1994.
24. Levi B, Cain AS, Dorzab WE. Coronary paraganglioma. Clin Cardiol 1982;5:505–10.
25. Orenstein HH, Green GE, Kancherla PL. Aortocoronary paraganglioma. Anatomic relationship of left coronary artery to paraganglia of aorta. NY State J Med 1984;84:33–6.
26. Orringer MB, Sisson JC, Glazer G, et al. Surgical treatment of cardiac pheochromocytomas. J Thorac Cardiovasc Surg 1984;89:753–7.
27. Saad MF, Frazier OH, Hickey RC, Samaan NA. Intrapericardial pheochromocytoma. Am J Med 1983;75:371–6.
28. Shapiro B, Kalff V, Glazer G, Thompson N, Beierwaltes W. The location of middle mediastinal pheochromocytomas. J Thorac Cardiovasc Surg 1984;87:814–20.
29. Sheps SG, Brown ML. Localization of mediastinal paragangliomas (pheochromocytoma). Chest 1985;87:807–9.
30. Swensen, SJ, Brown, ML, Sheps, SG, et al. Use of 131I MIBG scintigraphy in the evaluation of suspected pheochromoctyoma. Mayo Clin Proc 1985;60:299–304.
31. Voci V, Olson H, Beilin L. A malignant primary cardiac pheochromocytoma. Surg Rounds 1982;5:88–90.
32. Wilson AC, Bennett RC, Niall JF, Clarebrough JK, Doyle AE, Louis WJ. An unusual case of intrathoracic pheochromocytoma. Aust N Z J Surg 1974;44:27–32.

Extracardiac Paraganglioma

33. Carney JA. The triad of gastric epithelioid leiomyosarcoma, pulmonary chondroma, and functioning extra-adrenal paraganglioma: a five-year review. Medicine (Baltimore) 1983;62:159–69.
34. Cooley DA, Reardon MJ, Frazier OH, Angelini P. Human cardiac explantation and autotransplantation: application in a patient with a large cardiac pheochromocytoma. Tex Heart Inst J 1985;12:171–6.
35. Cueto-Garcia L, Shub C, Sheps SG, Puga FJ. Two-dimensional echocardiographic detection of mediastinal pheochromocytoma. Chest 1985;87:834–6.

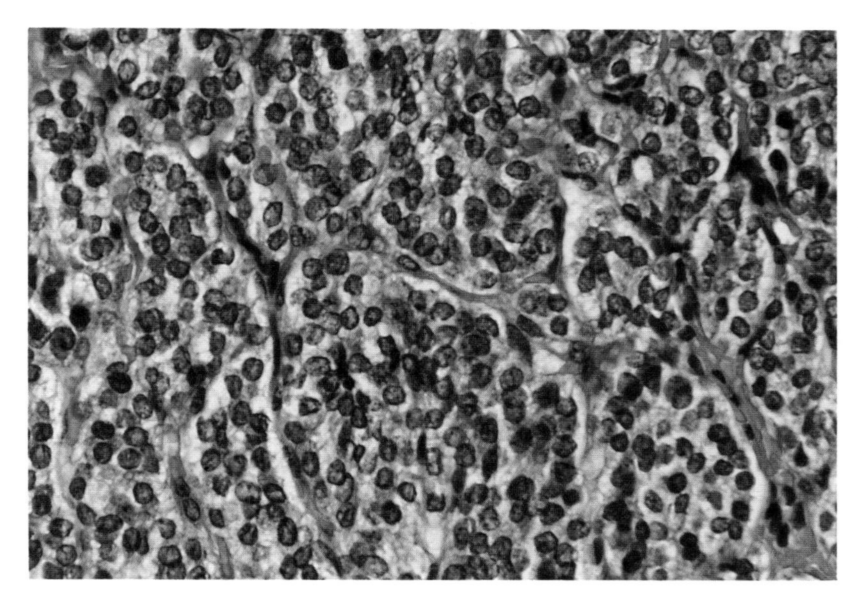

Figure 21-3
CARCINOID TUMOR
This biopsy of an orbital tumor was initially interpreted as a nonchromaffin paraganglioma, but is considered most likely a carcinoid tumor. The patient had no evidence of a primary tumor elsewhere. Ultrastructural study showed dense-core neurosecretory-type granules.

PARAGANGLIOMAS OF NASAL CAVITY AND NASOPHARYNX

Rare paragangliomas have been reported primary in the nasopharynx and nasal cavity (30, 31,33–35,37–39,41–45) as well as soft palate (32) and pterygopalatine fossa (40). A few paragangliomas reported in the nasopharynx were presumed to originate in the area of the ganglion nodosum and hence may be vagal paragangliomas (36). Most patients are female, and the range in age at diagnosis is wide. In most cases the tumor is a polypoid or exophytic mass ranging in size from 1.5 to 4 cm (36). Profuse bleeding had been noted either spontaneously or during attempted surgery. Normal paraganglia do not correlate with the varied anatomic locations of nasal and nasopharyngeal paragangliomas (36). One nasal paraganglioma recurred several times over a 4-year period (37,38), and was diagnosed by the late Dr. F. Foote (36) as a "carotid body-type tumor" (fig. 21-4).

PRIMARY THYROID PARAGANGLIOMA

There have been a small number of paragangliomas originating within thyroid parenchyma (48,50,53,55,59,61,62) or immediately adjacent to the gland (46,58). Zak and Lawson (65) documented paraganglionic tissue over or within the thyroid capsule, but there is no documentation of paraganglia actually within the substance of the gland (59). In one case the thyroid paraganglioma was associated with bilateral carotid body paragangliomas (55), while in another case there was a papillary thyroid carcinoma and a parathyroid adenoma (50). Thyroid paraganglioma can be mistaken for medullary thyroid carcinoma, but the classic nesting pattern (fig. 21-5, 21-6) and absence of amyloid stroma are two helpful features in making the distinction. Immunohistochemical staining for chromogranin is usually positive in both tumors (fig. 21-7), but the demonstration of sustentacular cells at the periphery of clusters of chief cells is a characteristic feature of thyroid paraganglioma (fig. 21-8). A recent case of medullary thyroid carcinoma was reported with S-100 protein-positive sustentacular-like cells which might make distinction from paraganglioma more problematic (52). The tumor illustrated in figures 21-5 and 21-6 was negative for thyrocalcitonin, carcinoembryonic antigen, and cytokeratin. Of thyroid paragangliomas reported to date, one was locally invasive (62) and another recurred locally and had invasive features (59).

Another thyroid lesion that might mimic a primary thyroid paraganglioma is hyalinizing trabecular adenoma (HTA) (49,54,57,60,64). Bronner et al. (47) refer to this lesion of the thyroid, which may have histologic features resembling paraganglioma, as "paraganglioma-like

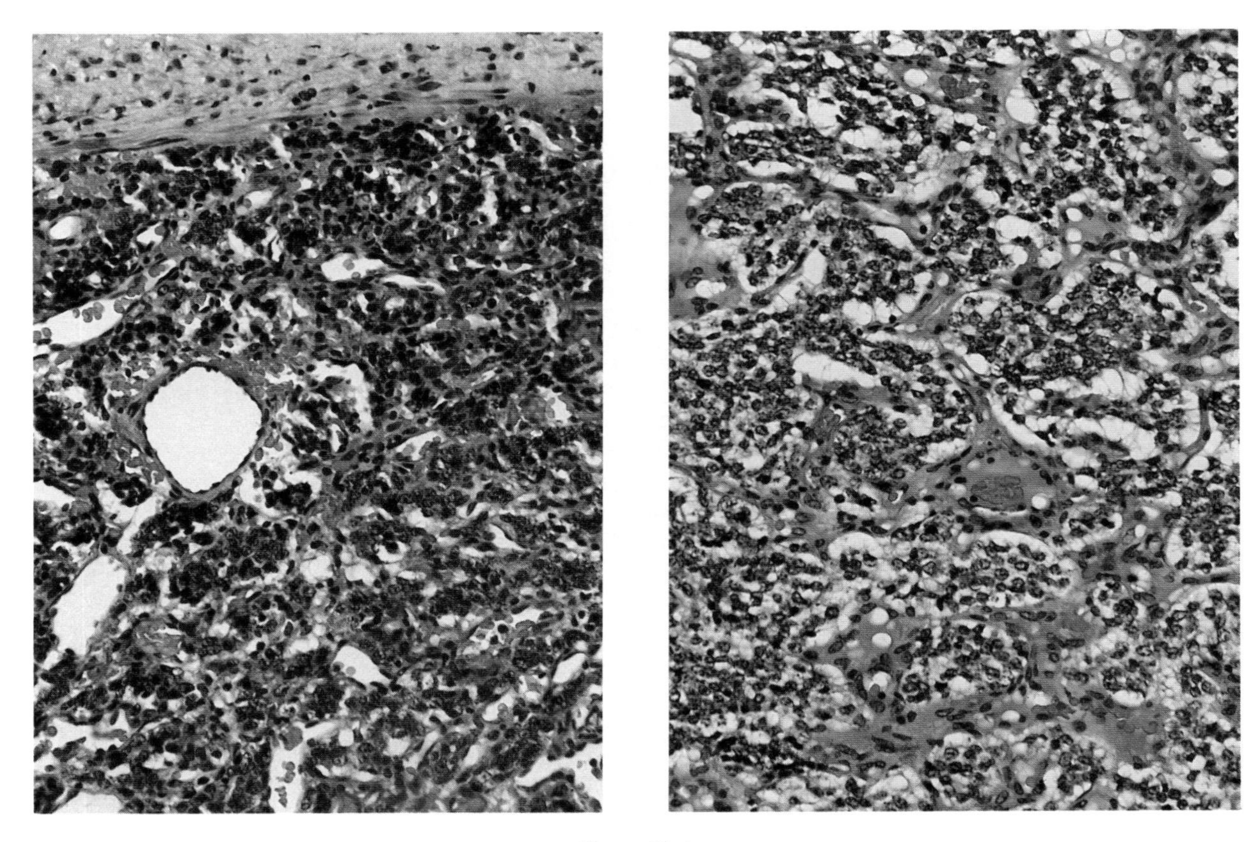

Figure 21-4
PRIMARY NASAL PARAGANGLIOMA

Left: Primary nasal paraganglioma had recurred locally on three occasions and at final surgery appeared as a polypoid mass attached to the cribriform plate. Respiratory-type mucosa was present over a portion of tumor.

Right: A prominent nesting pattern with "zellballen" is seen. Most of the intervening vascular spaces appear devoid of blood.

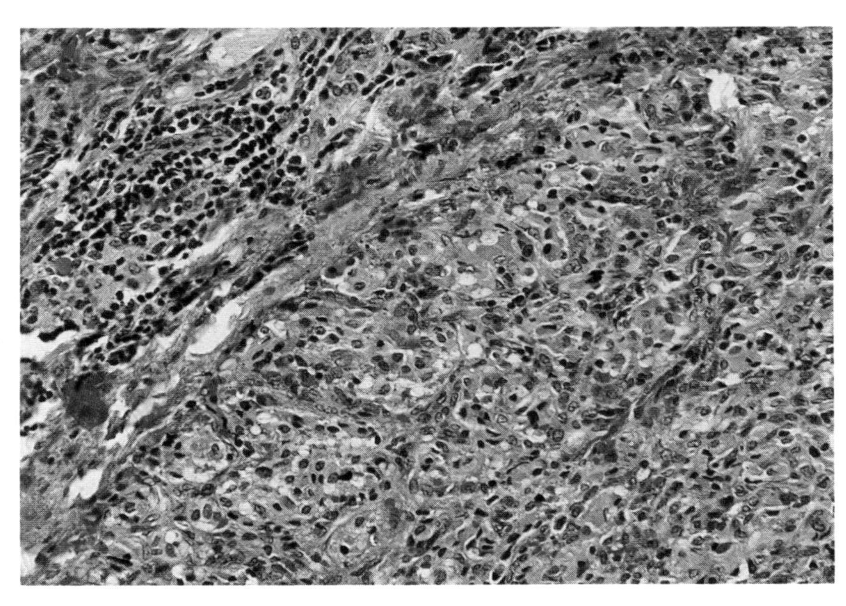

Figure 21-5
PRIMARY THYROID PARAGANGLIOMA

This primary thyroid paraganglioma in a 56-year-old woman was originally regarded as a medullary thyroid carcinoma. The tumor has fine interlacing fibrous stroma with distinct nests of neoplastic epithelioid chief cells. Residual inflamed thyroid is present at top left. (Figures 21-5–21-8 are from the same case.)

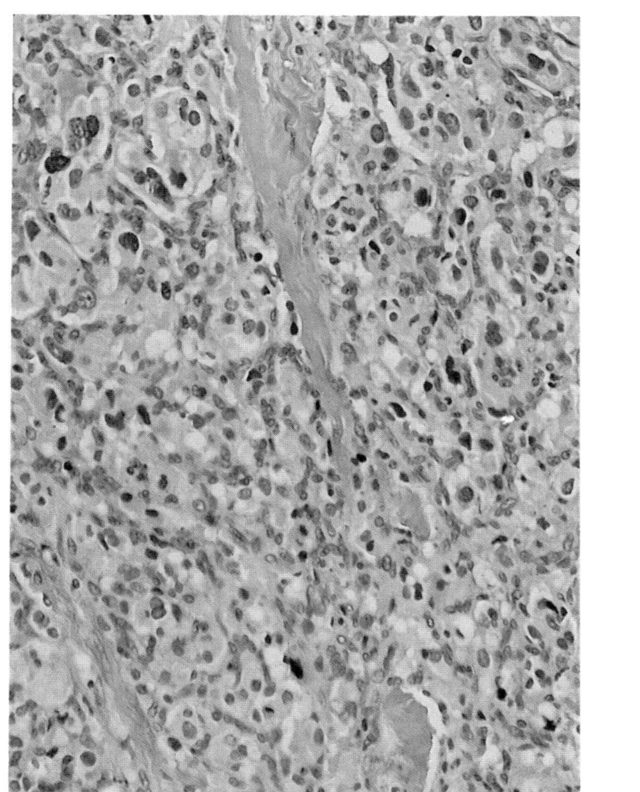

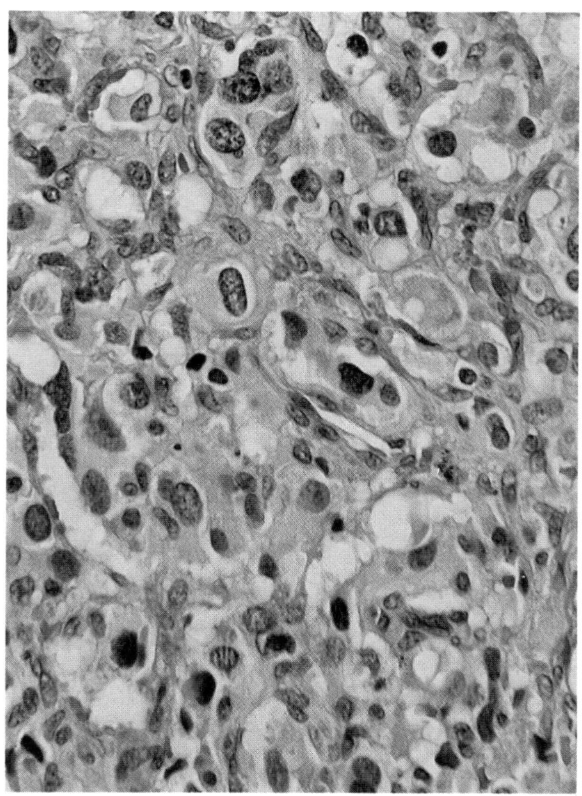

Figure 21-6
PRIMARY THYROID PARAGANGLIOMA
Left: Primary thyroid paraganglioma is composed of organoid clusters of cells with prominent microvasculature.
Right: Features are indistinguishable from paragangliomas elsewhere in the head and neck region.

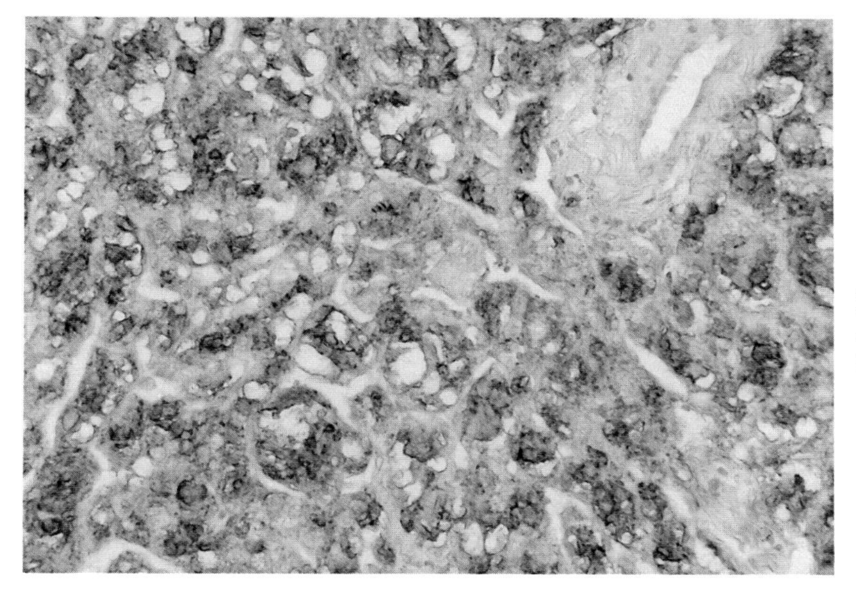

Figure 21-7
PRIMARY THYROID PARAGANGLIOMA
Recurrent primary thyroid paraganglioma contains numerous cells which are strongly immunoreactive for chromogranin. (X200, Peroxidase-antiperoxidase stain)

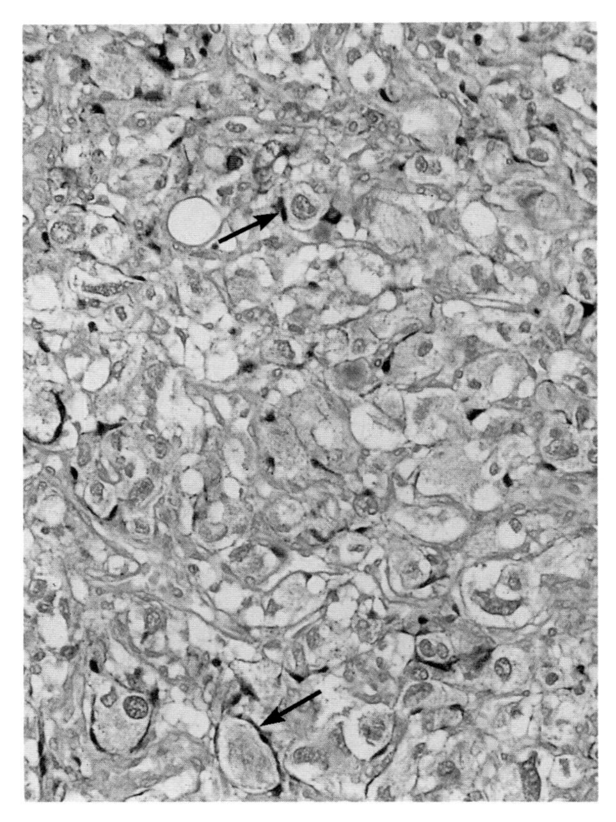

Figure 21-8
PRIMARY THYROID PARAGANGLIOMA
Immunostain for S-100 protein shows numerous slender to dendritic sustentacular cells (both nucleus and cytoplasm are immunoreactive) at the periphery of clusters of neoplastic chief cells (arrows). (X200, Peroxidase-antiperoxidase stain)

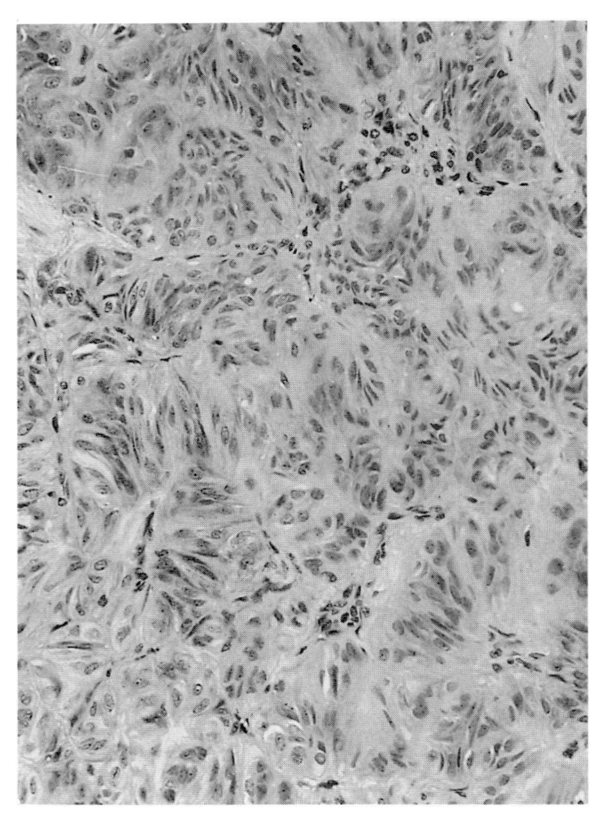

Figure 21-9
ADENOMATOUS NODULE RESEMBLING HTA
Adenomatous nodule in a young female had an area resembling hyalinizing trabecular adenoma or paraganglioma-like adenoma of the thyroid .

adenoma of the thyroid." The specificity of these lesions might be questioned since a HTA-like pattern has been reported in adenomatous nodules (fig. 21-9) (59), lymphocytic thyroiditis, and a thyroid adenoma (51), and some have identified malignant features in HTA (63). HTA of thyroid may be regarded as a reasonably distinct variant of thyroid adenoma when it occurs as a solitary, well-circumscribed or encapsulated mass. An encapsulated variant of medullary thyroid carcinoma has been described which also resembles the HTA (paraganglioma-like adenoma) of the thyroid (56).

PARAGANGLIOMAS IN OTHER LOCATIONS

Paragangliomas have been reported in exotic sites such as face (69), external ear (71), tongue (70), and cheek (66), anatomic sites in which normal paraganglionic tissue is not documented. Paraganglioma of trachea has also been reported (67), and if the tumor arises superiorly near the thyroid or cricoid cartilage it could originate from paraganglia normally residing there (68).

REFERENCES

Orbital Paraganglioma

1. Archer KF, Hurwitz JJ, Balogh JM, Fernandes BJ. Orbital nonchromaffin paraganglioma. A case report and review of the literature. Ophthalmology 1989;96:1659–66.
2. Botár J, Pribék L. Corpuscle paraganglionnaire dans l'orbite. Ann D'Anat Path 1935;12:227–8.
3. Deutsch AR, Duckworth JK. Nonchromaffin paraganglioma of the orbit. Am J Opthalmol 1969;68:659–63.
4. Fisher ER, Hazard JB. Nonchromaffin paraganglioma of the orbit. Cancer 1952;5:521–4.
5. Lack EE. Pathology of adrenal and extra-adrenal paraganglia. Major problems in pathology, Vol 29. Philadelphia: WB Saunders, 1994.
6. Lattes R, McDonald JJ, Sproul E. Non-chromaffin paraganglioma of carotid body and orbit. Ann Surg 1954;139:382–4.
7. Mawas J. Sur un organe épithélial non décrit, le paraganglion infra-orbitaire. Compt Rend Acad d Sci 1936;202:977–8.
8. Paulus W, Jellinger K, Brenner H. Melanotic paraganglioma of the orbit: a case report. Acta Neuropathol (Berl) 1989;79:340–6.
9. Thacker WC, Duckworth JK. Chemodectoma of the orbit. Cancer 1969;23:1233–8.
10. Vara Thorbeck R, Morales Valentin OI, Ruiz Morales M. Non-chromaffin paraganglioma of the orbit. Case Report. Zentralbl Chir 1986;111:46–9.
11. Venkataramana NK, Sastry Kolluri VR, Raj Kumar DV, Vasedev Rao T, Das BS. Paraganglioma of the orbit with extension to the middle cranial fossa: case report. Neurosurgery 1989;24:762–4.
12. Zak FG, Lawson W. The paraganglionic chemoreceptor system: physiology, pathology, and clinical medicine. New York: Springer-Verlag, 1982:419–23.

Alveolar Soft-Part Sarcoma

13. Benfu W. Orbital chemodectoma. Clinical and pathologic analysis of 2 cases. Chinese Med J 1981;94:419–22.
14. Christopherson WM, Foote FW, Stewart FW. Alveolar soft-part sarcomas. Cancer 1952;5:100–11.
15. Enzinger FM, Weiss SW. Soft tissue tumors, 2nd ed. St Louis: CV Mosby, 1988:929–36.
16. Font RL, Jurco S III, Zimmerman LE. Alveolar soft-part sarcoma of the orbit: a clinicopathologic analysis of seventeen cases and a review of the literature. Hum Pathol 1982;13:569–79.
17. Lieberman PH, Brennan MF, Kimmel M, Erlandson RA, Garin-Chesa P, Flehinger BY. Alveolar soft part sarcoma. A clinico-pathologic study of half a century. Cancer 1989;63:1–13.
18. Lieberman PH, Foote FW Jr, Stewart FW, Berg JW. Alveolar soft part sarcoma. JAMA 1966;198:1047–51.
19. Nirankari MS, Greer CH, Chaddah MR. Malignant nonchromaffin paraganglioma in the orbit. Brit J Ophthalmol 1963;47:357–63.
20. Shipkey FH, Lieberman PH, Foote FW Jr, Stewart FW. Ultrastructure of alveolar soft part sarcoma. Cancer 1964;17:821–30.
21. Smetana HF, Scott WF Jr. Malignant tumors of nonchromaffin paraganglia. Milit Surg 1951;109:330–49.
22. Varghese S, Nair B, Joseph TA. Orbital malignant non-chromaffin paraganglioma. Alveolar soft part sarcoma. Brit J Ophthalmol 1968;52:713–5.

Carcinoid Tumors of the Eye and Orbit

23. Braffman BH, Bilaniuk LT, Eagle RC Jr, et al. MR imaging of carcinoid tumor metastatic to the orbit. J Computer Assist Tomogr 1987;11:891–4.
24. Duncan AW, Lack EE, Deck MF. Radiological evaluation of paragangliomas of the head and neck. Radiology 1979;132:99–105.
25. Lack EE, Cubilla AL, Woodruff JM. Paragangliomas of the head and neck region. A pathologic study of tumors from 71 patients. Hum Pathol 1979;10:191–218.
26. Lack EE, Cubilla AL, Woodruff JM, Farr HW. Paragangliomas of the head and neck region: a clinical study of 69 patients. Cancer 1977;39:397–409.
27. Riddle PJ, Font RL, Zimmerman LE. Carcinoid tumors of the eye and orbit: a clinicopathologic study of 15 cases, with histochemical and electron microscopic observations. Hum Pathol 1982;13:459–69.
28. Rush JA, Waller RR, Campbell RJ. Orbital carcinoid tumor metastatic from the colon. Am J Ophthalmol 1980;89:636–40.
29. Zimmerman LE, Stangl R, Riddle PJ. Primary carcinoid tumor of the orbit. A clinicopathologic study with histochemical and electron microscopic observations. Arch Ophthalmol 1983;101:1395–8.

Paragangliomas of Nasal Cavity and Nasopharynx

30. Apple D, Kreines K. Cushing's syndrome due to ectopic ACTH production by a nasal paraganglioma. Am J Med Sci 1982;283:32–5.
31. Chambers EF, Norman D, Dedo HH, Ferrell LD. Primary nasopharyngeal chemodectoma. Neuroradiology 1982;23:285–8.
32. Dasgupta G, Deodhare SG. Chemodectoma of the soft palate. Internat Surg 1967;62:366–7.
33. Govasi DK, Mohidekar AT. Chemodectoma of the nose and sphenoid sinus. J Laryngol Otol 1978;92:813–6.
34. Himelfarb MZ, Ostrzega NL, Samuel J, Shanon E. Paraganglioma of the nasal cavity. Laryngoscope 1983;93:350–2.

35. Holmes KM. Chemodectoma of the nasopharynx. Eye Ear Nose Throat Mon 1976;55:152–5.
36. Lack EE. Pathology of adrenal and extra-adrenal paraganglia. Major problems in pathology, Vol 29. Philadelphia: WB Saunders, 1994.
37. Lack EE, Cubilla AL, Woodruff JM. Paragangliomas of the head and neck region. A pathologic study of tumors from 71 patients. Hum Pathol 1979;10:191–218.
38. Lack EE, Cubilla AL, Woodruff JM, Farr HW. Paragangliomas of the head and neck region: a clinical study of 69 patients. Cancer 1977;39:397–409.
39. Moran TE. Nonchromaffin paraganglioma of the nasal cavity. Laryngoscope 1962;72:201–6.
40. Otokida K, Ohira A, Kamimura A, et al. Cervical catecholamine-secreting paraganglioma in the pterygopalatine fossa. Tohoku J Exp Med 1987;153:347–54.
41. Parisier SC, Sinclair GM. Glomus tumor of the nasal cavity. Laryngoscope 1968;78:2013–24.
42. Schuller DE, Lucas JG. Nasopharyngeal paraganglioma. Report of a case and review of the literature. Arch Otolaryngol 1982;108:667–70.
43. Scoppa J, Tonkin JP. Non-chromaffin paraganglioma of the nasopharynx. J Laryngol Otol 1975;89:653–6.
44. Smith JC, Kohut RI, Million RR. Chemodectomas of the nasopharynx. An unusual case associated with unilateral ocular proptosis. Laryngoscope 1973;83:330–5.
45. Watson DJ. Nasal paraganglioma. J Laryngol Otol 1988;102:526–9.

Primary Thyroid Paraganglioma

46. Banner B, Morecki R, Eviatar A. Chemodectoma in the mid-thyroid region. J Otolaryngol 1979;8:271–3.
47. Bronner M, LiVolsi VA, Jennings T. Plat: paraganglioma-like adenomas of the thyroid. Surg Pathol 1988;1:383–9.
48. Buss DH, Marshall RB, Baird FG, Myers RT. Paraganglioma of the thyroid gland. Am J Surg Pathol 1980; 4:589–93.
49. Carney JA, Ryan J, Goellner JR. Hyalinizing trabecular adenoma of the thyroid gland. Am J Surg Pathol 1987;11:583–91.
50. Cayot F, Bastien H, Justrabo E, et al. Paragangliomes multiples du cou avec localization thyroidienne. Cancer papillaire thyroïdien et adénome parathyroïdien associés. Sem Hop Paris 1982;58:2004–7.
51. Chetty R, Beydoun R, LiVolsi V. Paraganglioma-like nodular proliferations in chronic lymphocytic thyroiditis. Mod Pathol 1993;6:38A(203).
52. Collina G, Maiorana A, Fano RA, Cesinaro AM, Trentini GP. Medullary carcinoma of the thyroid gland with sustentacular cell-like cells in a patient with multiple endocrine neoplasia type IIA. Report of a case with ultrastructural and immunohistochemical studies. Arch Pathol Lab Med 1994;118:1041–4.
53. de Vries EJ, Watson CG. Paraganglioma of the thyroid. Head Neck 1989;11:462–5.
54. Goellner JR, Carney JA. Cytologic features of fine-needle aspirates of hyalinizing trabecular adenoma of the thyroid. Am J Clin Pathol 1989;91:115–9.
55. Haegert DG, Wang NS, Farrer PA, Seemayer TA, Thelmo W. Non-chromaffin paragangliomatosis manifesting as a cold thyroid nodule. Am J Clin Pathol 1974;61:561–70.
56. Huss LJ, Mendelsohn G. Medullary carcinoma of the thyroid gland: an encapsulated variant resembling the hyalinizing trabecular (paraganglioma-like) adenoma of thyroid. Mod Pathol 1990;3:581–5.
57. Katoh R, Jasani B, Williams ED. Hyalinizing trabecular adenoma of the thyroid. A report of three cases with immunohistochemical and ultrastructural studies. Histopathology 1989;15:211–24.
58. Kay S, Montague JW, Dodd RW. Nonchromaffin paraganglioma (chemodectoma) of thyroid region. Cancer 1975:36:582–5.
59. Lack EE. Pathology of adrenal and extra-adrenal paraganglia. Major problems in pathology, Vol 29. Philadelphia: WB Saunders, 1994.
60. LiVolsi VA. Surgical pathology of the thyroid. In: Bennington JL, (consulting ed). Major problems in pathology, Vol 22. Philadelphia: WB Saunders, 1990:338.
61. Massaioli N, Balbo G, Fausone G, Negro D. Paraganglioma branchiomerico endotiroideo (non cromaffine). Minerva Chir 1979;34:867–74.
62. Mitsudo SM, Grajower MM, Balbi H, Silver C. Malignant paraganglioma of the thyroid gland. Arch Pathol Lab Med 1987;111:378–80.
63. Sambade C, Franssila KO, Cameselle-Teijeiro J, Nesland JM, Sobrinho-Simões M. Hyalinizing trabecular adenoma. A misnomer for a peculiar tumor of the thyroid gland. Endocr Pathol 1991;2:83–91.
64. Sambade C, Sarabando F, Nesland JM, Sobrinho-Simões M. Hyalinizing trabecular adenoma of the thyroid. Ultrastr Pathol 1989;13:275–80.
65. Zak FG, Lawson W. Glomic (paraganglionic) tissue in the larynx and capsule of the thyroid gland. Mt. Sinai J Med 1972;39:82–90.

Paragangliomas in Other Locations

66. DeLozier HL. Chemodectoma of the cheek. A case report. Ann Otol Rhinol Laryngol 1983;92:109–12.
67. Horree WA. An unusual primary tumour of the trachea (chemodectoma). Pract Oto-, Rhino, Laryngol 1963;25:125–6.
68. Lack, EE. Pathology of adrenal and extra-adrenal paraganglia. Major problems in pathology, Vol 29. Philadelphia: WB Saunders, 1994.
69. Milroy HJ. Chemodectoma (non-chromaffin paraganglioma) of the face. Brit J Surg 1969;56:510–2.
70. Scopelliti G, Camera A, Barbato U. Chemodectoma della lingua: criteri diagnostico-differenziali ed istogenetici. Ann Stomatol 1970;19:819–34.
71. Volchek GB, Bolotnaia RD. Chemodectoma of the auricular concha. Vestnik Otorinolaryngol 1970;32:103–4.

22
ULTRASTRUCTURAL AND OTHER FEATURES OF PARAGANGLIOMAS OF HEAD AND NECK REGION

General Features. Paragangliomas of the head and neck region (including non-neoplastic paraganglia such as carotid bodies) are typically nonchromaffin (3), and except for cardiac paragangliomas are unreactive for phenylethanolamine N-methyltransferase (PNMT) (5). The excess catecholamine secretion seen with some of these tumors suggests a closer alignment with paragangliomas of the sympathoadrenal neuroendocrine system. For diagnostic purposes it is not essential to document the presence of catecholamines within head and neck paragangliomas. The demonstration of cytoplasmic argyrophilia using a variety of staining procedures is occasionally useful in diagnosis (fig. 22-1) (1,2,6), and has been shown by electron microscopy to be associated with endocrine granules (7). Positive cytoplasmic argyrophilia was observed focally or diffusely in virtually all paragangliomas studied at Memorial Hospital in which paraffin blocks were available (4). The tumors are typically argentaffin negative. Sophisticated and specific immunohistochemical markers and various molecular probes can establish a diagnosis if routine morphology is equivocal.

Ultrastructural Findings. The ultrastructure of various paragangliomas from different sites in the head and neck region is quite similar, and it is not possible to distinguish one particular tumor from another based upon fine structural characteristics (8–16,18–21,23–29). Examination of 1-mm thick sections provides some insight into the different types of cells found in these paragangliomas: neoplastic chief cells greatly outnumber other cell types, which is out of proportion compared with normal (17,22) or hyperplastic paraganglia (fig. 22-2). Reliable identification of sustentacular cells is very difficult in routine or thin sections, and they may be difficult to recognize on ultrastructural study as well. The easiest way of detecting these cells is by immunohistochemical staining for S-100 protein (or occasionally glial fibrillary acidic protein [GFAP]).

Ultrastructurally, paragangliomas are not as complicated as normal or hyperplastic paraganglia: the clusters of neoplastic chief cells appear sharply demarcated, and may be subtended by thin, continuous or discontinuous extensions of sustentacular cell cytoplasm (fig. 22-3). Nuclei of chief cells may have irregular folds and indentations, and when marked this may result in formation of nuclear pseudoinclusions as seen with sympathoadrenal paragangliomas. It is advantageous when identifying cell types other than neoplastic chief cells to examine profiles of vascular channels and then proceed into nests of neoplastic chief cells (fig. 22-4). Endothelial cells

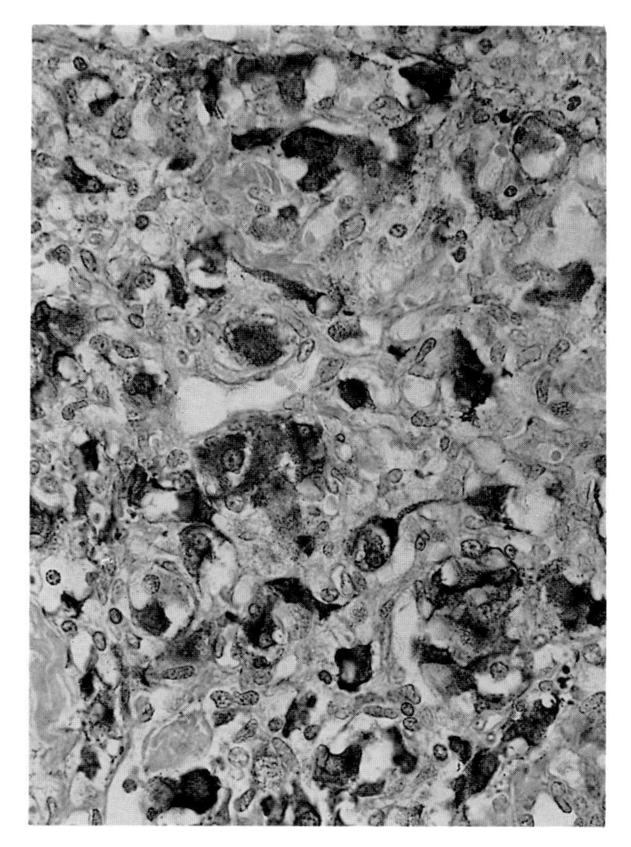

Figure 22-1
LARYNGEAL PARAGANGLIOMA
Grimelius stain for cytoplasmic argyrophilia stains numerous neoplastic chief cells. Many have a myriad of pinpoint black granules. (X200, Grimelius stain)

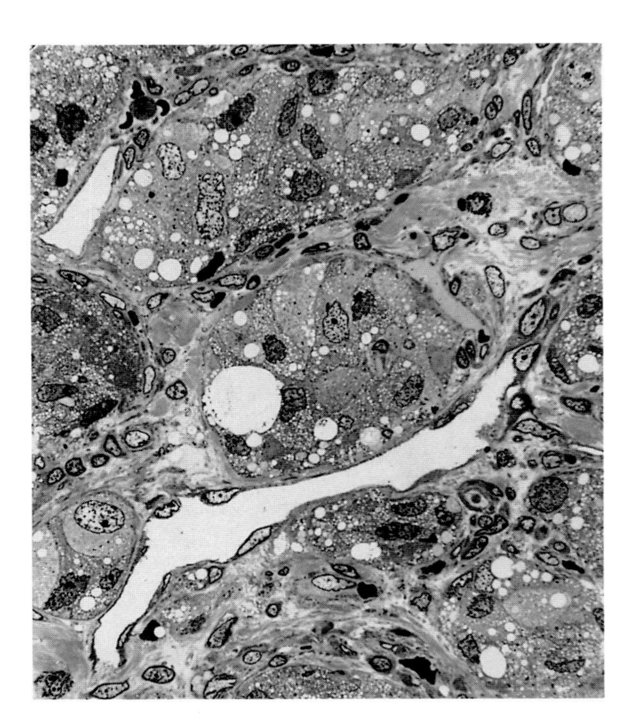

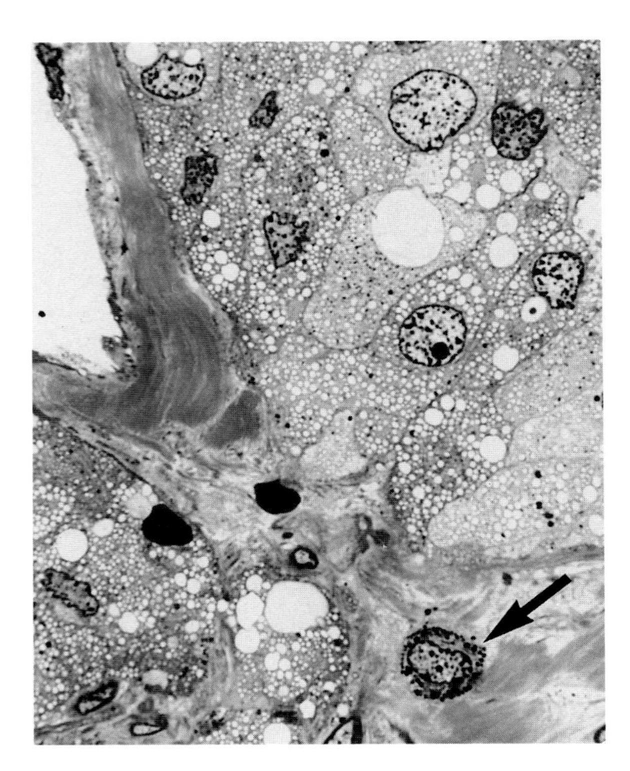

Figure 22-2
CAROTID BODY PARAGANGLIOMA

Left: The neoplastic chief cells have a discrete nesting pattern. Some have medium to large cytoplasmic vacuoles, so-called pseudoacini. (X400, Toluidine blue stain)

Right: Neoplastic chief cells contain sparse, dark-staining granules, most of which represent neurosecretory granules. Note the mast cell in the interstitium (arrow). (X1000, Toluidine blue stain)

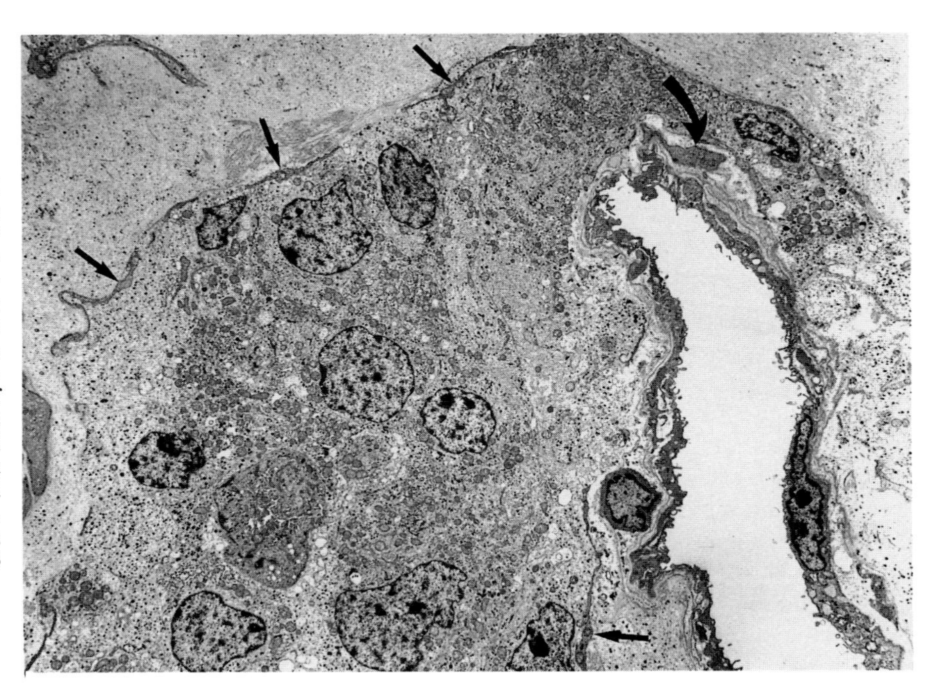

Figure 22-3
CAROTID BODY
PARAGANGLIOMA

Survey view shows rounded to ovoid nuclei of neoplastic chief cells, some with irregular contour, and an occasional nucleolus. Note the slender, discontinuous wisps of cytoplasm around the outer aspect of a cluster of tumor cells (straight arrows). This represents sustentacular cells. A portion of pericyte cytoplasm is evident near an endothelial cell (curved arrow). (X2,000) (Fig. 9-3 from Lack EE. Pathology of adrenal and extra-adrenal paraganglia. Major problems in pathology, Vol 29. Philadelphia: WB Saunders Co, 1994:168.)

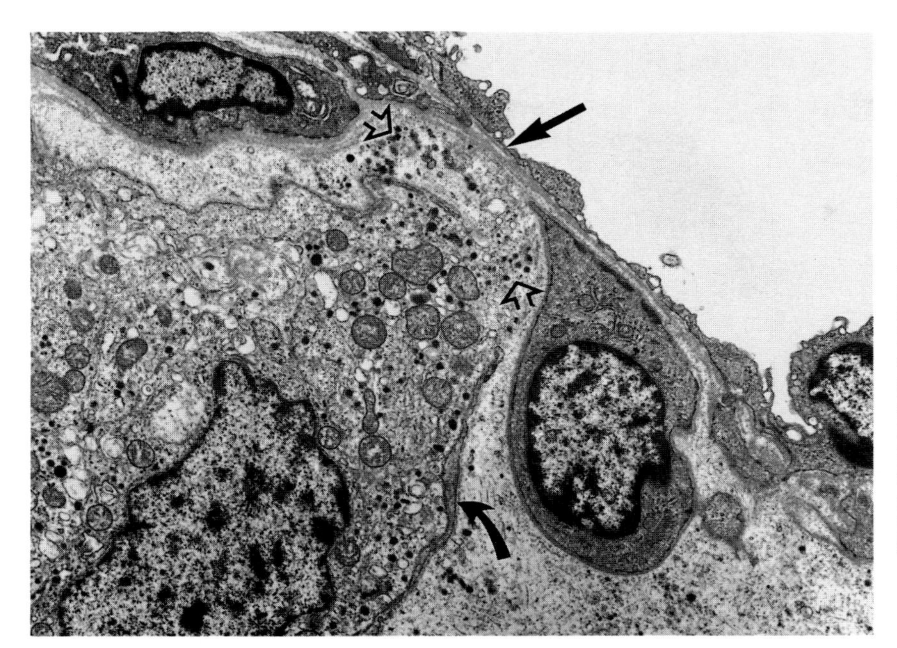

Figure 22-4
CAROTID BODY
PARAGANGLIOMA

Attenuated endothelial lining of a vascular channel is seen, with few cytoplasmic fenestrations (straight arrow). Several pericytes are present with plasmalemmal densities, few pinocytotic vesicles, and a layer of continuous basement membrane. Note the slender extension of a sustentacular cell (curved arrow) and the presence of dense-core neurosecretory granules free in the interstitium (open arrows). This may be artifactual due to mechanical disruption of cytoplasm. (X6,000) (Fig. 9-8 from Lack EE. Pathology of adrenal and extra-adrenal paraganglia. Major problems in pathology, Vol 29. Philadelphia: WB Saunders Co. 1994:172.)

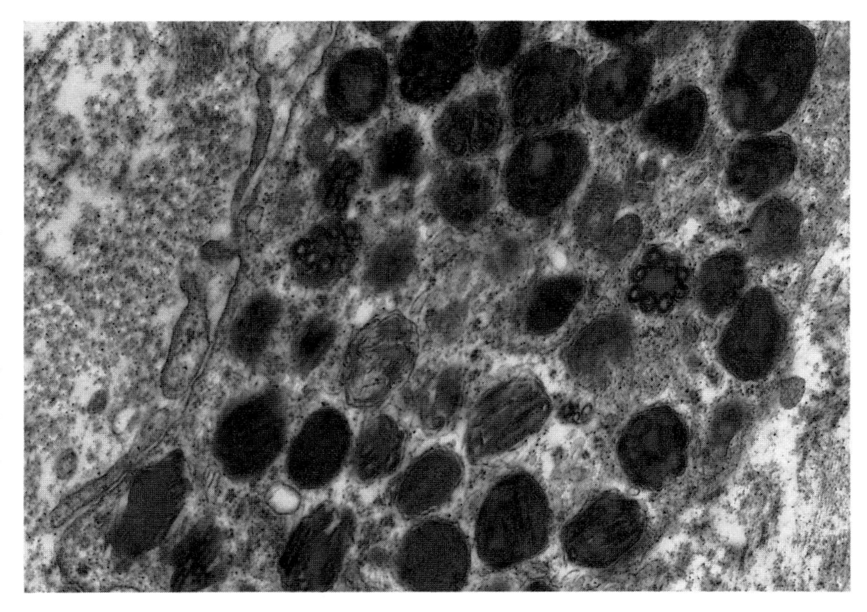

Figure 22-5
CAROTID BODY
PARAGANGLIOMA

A mast cell is seen within the interstitium near the vascular channel in a carotid body paraganglioma. The cytoplasm contains numerous electron-dense structures which have scroll-like, lamellar, or curvilinear profiles. Because of the large size and heterogeneity, the mast cell granules should not be confused with neurosecretory granules. (X22,500) (Fig. 9-11 from Lack EE. Pathology of adrenal and extra-adrenal paraganglia. Major problems in pathology, Vol 29. Philadelphia: WB Saunders Co., 1994:173.)

are ubiquitous, and may have small cytoplasmic fenestrations. Pericytes are also present proximal to endothelial cells. Examination of the interstitium adjacent to vascular spaces may reveal occasional mast cells, and the heterogeneous, scroll-like, lamellar or curvilinear granules should not be confused with neurosecretory-type granules of chief cells (fig. 22-5). Interstitial collagen may be a prominent feature. Amyloid deposits have been reported, but not illustrated (11).

The variation in the overall electron density of the cytoplasm of neoplastic chief cells gives the impression of two polar cell populations of "light" and "dark" cells (23). This has been ascribed to a variation in the density of hyaloplasm (8,15), or disparity in compactness or density of cellular organelles such as mitochondria and even neurosecretory granules (fig. 22-6) (16,22). Forms transitional in cellular density have also been described. There does not appear to be any biologic

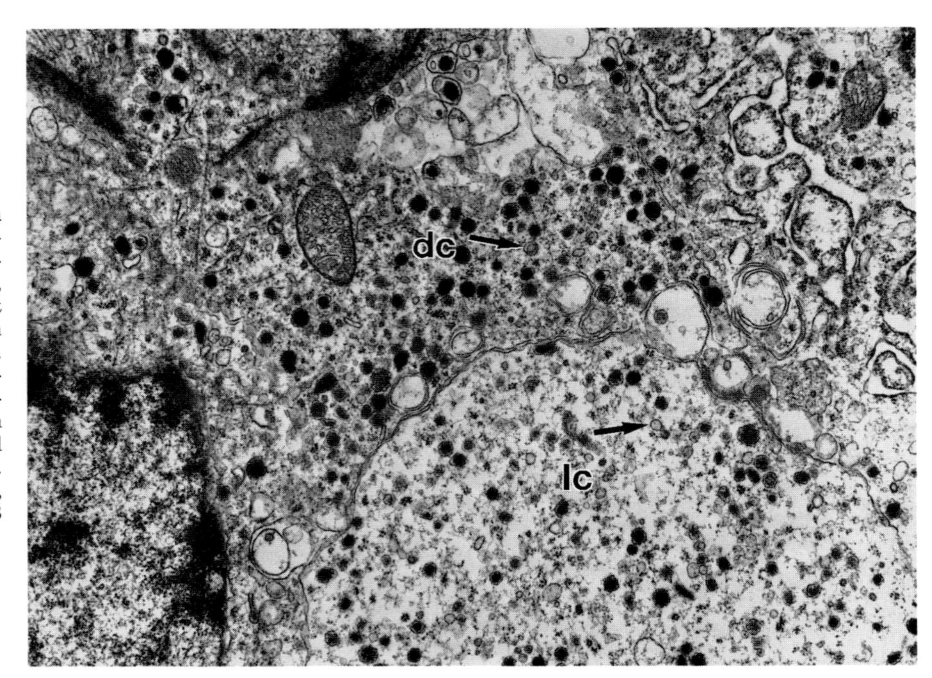

Figure 22-6
CAROTID BODY
PARAGANGLIOMA

The "dark" cell (dc) has a slightly greater density of cellular organelles, including dense-core neurosecretory granules, compared with the adjacent "light" cell (lc). The cells contain a few empty vesicles (arrows). Profiles of dilated rough endoplasmic reticulum are also present. (X20,000) (Fig. 9-4 from Lack EE. Pathology of adrenal and extra-adrenal paraganglia. Major problems in pathology, Vol 29. Philadelphia: WB Saunders Co, 1994:169.)

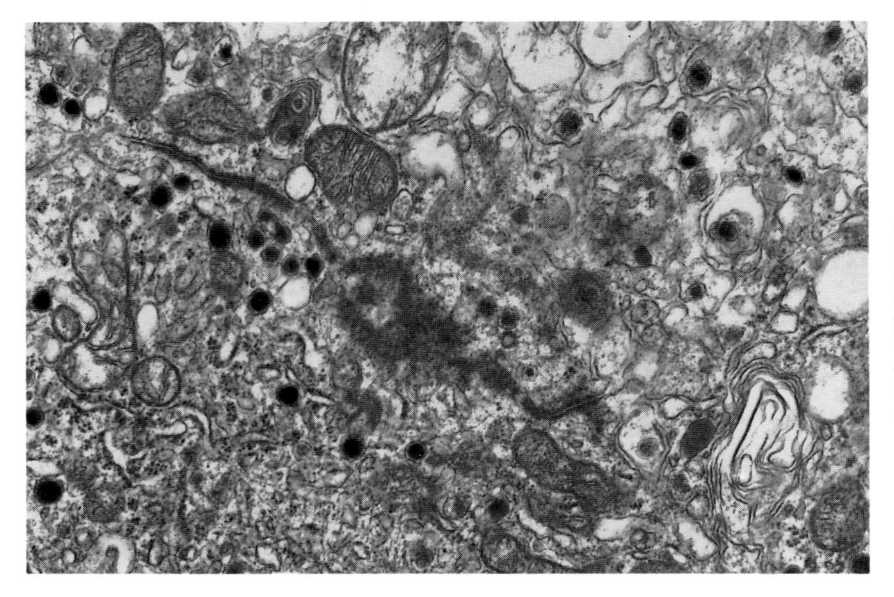

Figure 22-7
CAROTID BODY
PARAGANGLIOMA

Simple belt-like intercellular attachments are present between two neoplastic chief cells. Note both smooth and rough endoplasmic reticulum along with some free polyribosomes. (X30,000) (Fig. 9-7 from Lack EE. Pathology of adrenal and extra-adrenal paraganglia. Major problems in pathology, Vol 29. Philadelphia: WB Saunders Co, 1994:171.)

significance attached to this cellular variation at the ultrastructural level (23). There may be irregular profiles of rough and smooth endoplasmic reticulum, and some appear slightly dilated. Free polyribosomes are also seen. Some cells have simple intercellular junctions without formation of true desmosomal attachments (fig. 22-7), but usually these are rare.

The diagnostic feature of the neoplastic chief cells is the presence of dense-core neurosecretory-type granules; however, the distribution and density of these granules can vary considerably. Some secretory vesicles appear empty since tangential sectioning or vagaries in fixation may give an inaccurate impression (23). Most neurosecretory-type granules are relatively uniform in

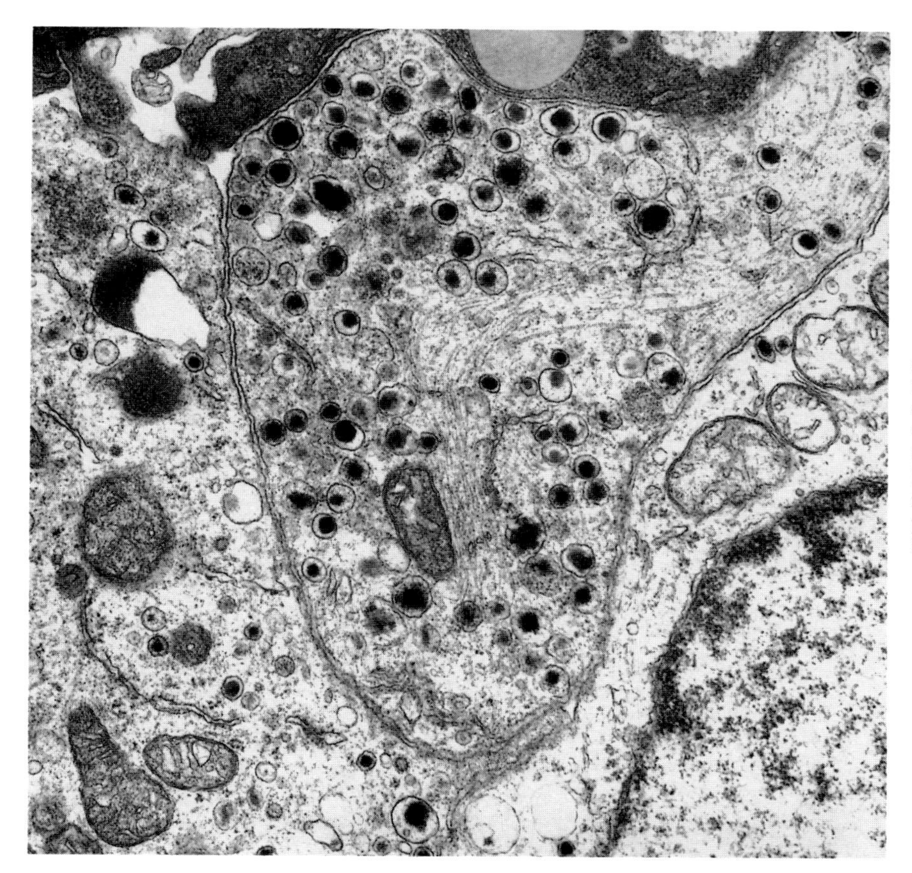

Figure 22-8
CAROTID BODY
PARAGANGLIOMA

Some dense-core neurosecretory granules have a symmetric halo beneath the limiting membrane while other granules have a wider halo which is somewhat asymmetric. (X21,250) (Fig. 9-5 from Lack EE. Pathology of adrenal and extra-adrenal paraganglia. Major problems in pathology, Vol 29. Philadelphia: WB Saunders Co., 1994:170.)

size and shape, depending upon the precise plane of section, and most are in the size range of 70 to 200 nm (23). Some granules have a wide, asymmetric halo between the limiting membrane which may simulate "norepinephrine-type" granules (fig. 22-8), but correlation of granule morphology with content of particular catecholamine or neuropeptide is unreliable (23). There may be some variability in granule morphology, with an elongate or "sausage" shape (23). Close association of neurosecretory-type granules with a Golgi complex may also be seen. Occasionally, dense-core granules are observed in an extracellular location (see figure 22-4), and some investigators have speculated that this represents release of catecholamines during surgical manipulation of the tumor (19). A synaptic connection between nerve fibers and neoplastic chief cells is not a feature of true paragangliomas (23). An extraordinary case of a jugulotympanic paraganglioma (JTP) was reported: membrane-bound, rhomboid crystals nearly identical to those seen in alveolar soft-part sarcoma were seen and a similar mode of origin from smaller dense-core granules was postulated (18).

Immunohistochemical Findings. The immunohistochemical profile of paragangliomas displays a diversity similar to that of sympathoadrenal paragangliomas (Table 22-1) (30,36,44). In the diagnostic interpretation of these immunohistochemical stains, artifacts and technical problems may occur, and caution should be exercised when contradicting an opinion based upon sound clinical information and experienced evaluation of morphology (31). There are a number of good, reliable immunomarkers for neuroendocrine differentiation. Staining for neuron-specific enolase is uniformly positive under optimal conditions (fig. 22-9), but the lack of specificity limits its diagnostic value (32,40). An immunoprofile using a selected battery of stains may yield more specific results with monoclonal antibodies directed against chromogranin A (fig. 22-10) (34), related substances such as chromogranin B, or

Table 22-1

IMMUNOPROFILE FOR CAROTID BODY (N=11) AND JUGULOTYMPANIC (N=7) PARAGANGLIOMAS*

Markers	No. Positive
Neuron-specific enolase (NSE)	18/18
Serotonin	13/18
Leu-enkephalin	10/18
Gastrin	7/18
Substance P	7/18
Vasoactive intestinal peptide	7/18
Somatostatin	5/18
Bombesin	2/18
Alpha-MSH	2/18
Calcitonin	2/18
Adrenocorticotrophic hormone (ACTH)	0/18
Glucagon	0/18
Human chorionic gonadotrophin (HCG)	0/18
Insulin	0/18
Vasopressin	0/18

*Table 1 from Warren WH, Lee I, Gould VE, Memoli VA, Jao W. Paragangliomas of the head and neck: ultrastructural and immunohistochemical analysis. Ultrastr Pathol 1985;8:336.

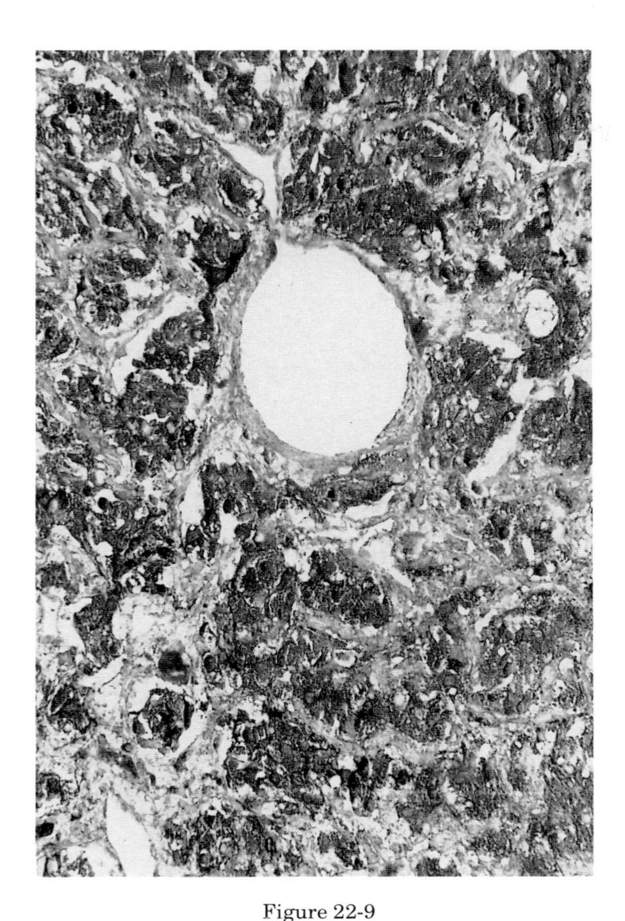

Figure 22-9
VAGAL PARAGANGLIOMA

Immunoreactivity for neuron-specific enolase is diffusely strong within the cytoplasm of tumor cells. (X100, Peroxidase-antiperoxidase stain)

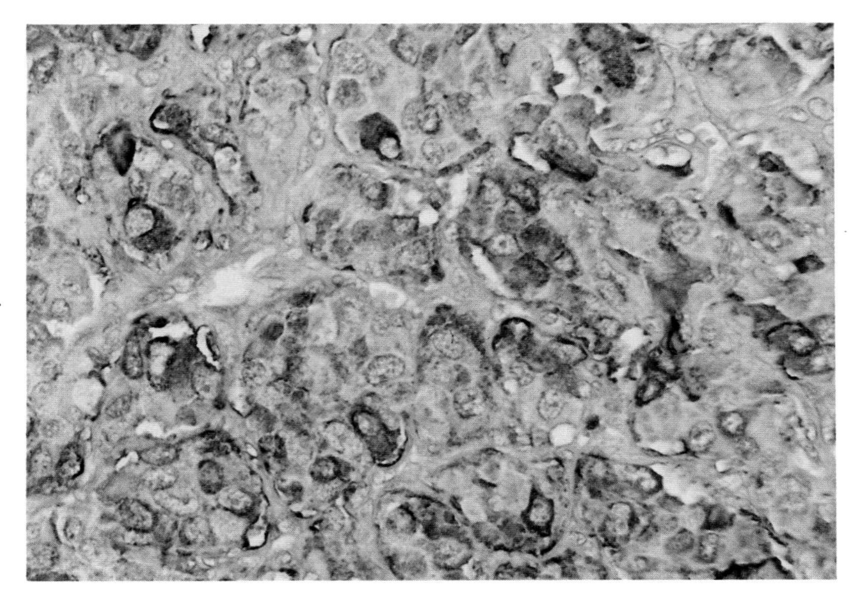

Figure 22-10
VAGAL PARAGANGLIOMA

Most tumor cells show strong immunostaining for chromogranin A. Some cells were only weakly positive, suggesting a paucity or low density of neurosecretory granules. (X100, Peroxidase-antiperoxidase stain)

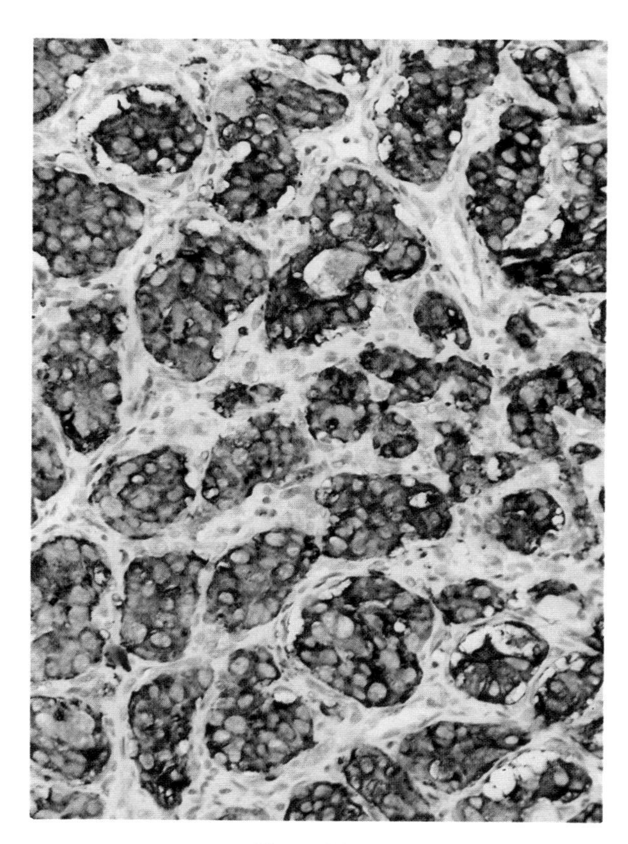

Figure 22-11
CAROTID BODY PARAGANGLIOMA
Nests of neoplastic chief cells are vividly accentuated by strong immunoreactivity for synaptophysin. (X100, Peroxidase-antiperoxidase stain)

Table 22-2

NEUROENDOCRINE MARKERS AND INTERMEDIATE FILAMENT TYPING FOR CAROTID BODY (N=9) AND JUGULOTYMPANIC (N=20) PARAGANGLIOMAS*

Neuroendocrine Markers	No. Positive
Neuron-specific enolase (NSE)	29/29
Chromogranin A	26/29
Synaptophysin	28/29
Serotonin	25/29
S-100 protein	29/29
substentacular vs. chief cells (100%) (24%)	
Intermediate Filaments	
Cytokeratin	3/29
Neurofilament	0/29
Desmin	0/29
Vimentin	rarely + in chief cells
Glial fibrillary acidic protein (GFAP)	0/29

*Data from reference 33.

synaptophysin, an integral and specific component of the membranes of presynaptic vesicles (fig. 22-11). Given the localization of chromogranin A in the matrix of granules and not in the investing membranes, staining may be granular, and differences in intensity or distribution of staining (under optimal conditions) may reflect a variation in content or density of neurosecretory-type granules (36). Molecular probes may detect mRNA for the chromogranin and secretogranin family of acidic proteins in endocrine tumors which have a paucity of neurosecretory granules (37). Results of immunostaining for various neuroendocrine markers from a study by Johnson et al. (33) involving 29 head and neck paragangliomas are shown in Table 22-2. A recent study using specific antibodies against chromogranin A and B and secretogranin II revealed divergent staining patterns in parasympathetic paragangliomas (i.e., carotid body paraganglioma [CBP] and JTP) versus sympathetic (extra-adrenal) paragangliomas, probably reflecting the different histogenesis of these tumors. The parasympathetic tumors expressed both chromogranin B and secretogranin II in most neoplastic chief cells of all 14 tumors while chromogranin A reactivity was strong in only 2 tumors and weak to absent in the rest; 12 of 12 sympathetic paragangliomas showed immunoreactivity for chromogranin A and 11 of 12 for chromogranin B while secretogranin II was found in less than half of the cases (41). Immunoreactivity of endocrine cells with the antilymphocyte antibody Leu-7 (HNK-1) has also been reported (43).

Results of intermediate filament typing have been reported (33,39). Some tumors stain for neurofilament protein (38,39). Vimentin staining is occasionally noted in chief and sustentacular cells (33), but positive results are most notable in endothelial cells in which the stain highlights the

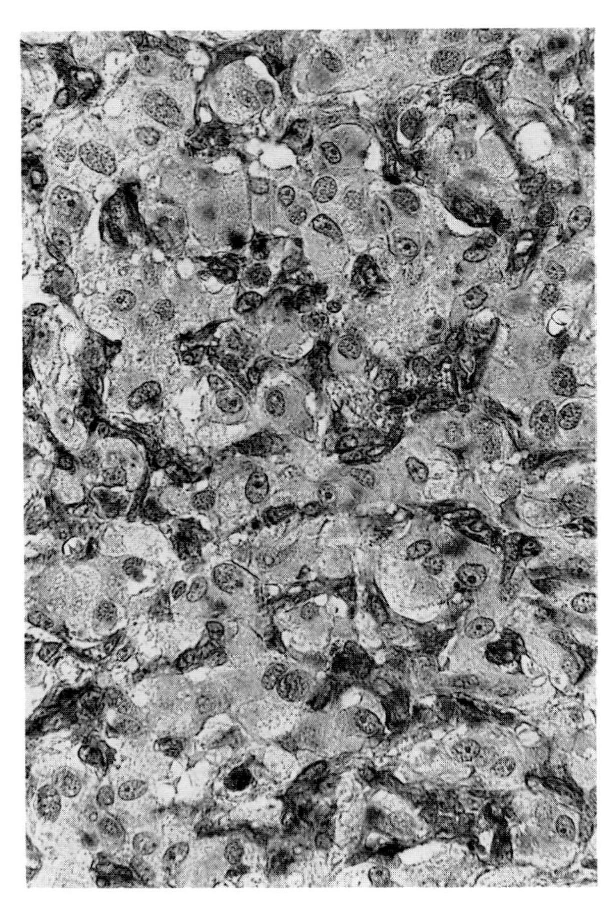

Figure 22-12
CAROTID BODY PARAGANGLIOMA
Immunostaining for vimentin highlights the intricate endothelial network of the tumor. (X200, Peroxidase-antiperoxidase stain)

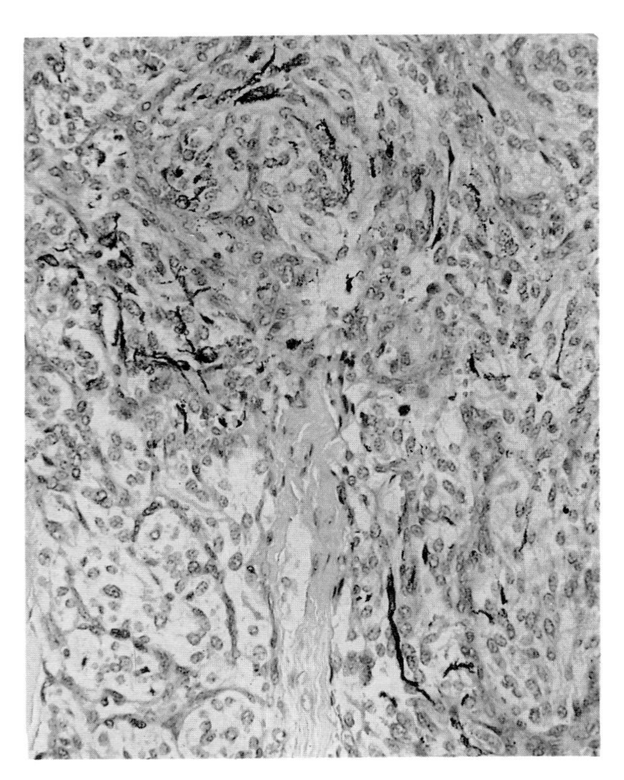

Figure 22-13
CAROTID BODY PARAGANGLIOMA
Carotid body paraganglioma immunostained for cytokeratin (AE1/AE3 monoclonal antibodies) shows staining of rare cells with dendritic or spindle cell configuration. Some ovoid cells could be neoplastic chief cells. (X100, Peroxidase-antiperoxidase stain)

organoid arrangement of neoplastic chief cells (fig. 22-12). Immunostaining for cytokeratin has been reported to be positive in a small number of JTPs and CBPs when a combination of monoclonal antibodies including CAM 5.2 is used (fig. 22-13); this may be a potential source of immunohistochemical misinterpretation unless a panel of markers is included (33). GFAP has been used as a marker for sustentacular cells (fig. 22-14), but results of staining are variable (33,35,38,42).

Based upon a number of studies, the identification of sustentacular cells is most reliably done by immunostaining for S-100 protein. These cells characteristically appear as elongate or dendritic cells at the periphery of neoplastic chief cells and may demonstrate nuclear positivity, cytoplasmic positivity, or both (fig. 22-15). Ultrastructurally, sustentacular cells closely "embrace" neoplastic chief cells with slender wisp-like extensions of cytoplasm (fig. 22-16); these cells have relatively sparse numbers of cellular organelles and lack neurosecretory-type granules. Some chief cells have also been reported to be immunoreactive for S-100 protein (33,38). The role of in situ hybridization and other molecular probes has been briefly referred to in chapter 13.

S-100 Protein–Positive Cells and Prognosis. Some investigators have reported a decrease in density of S-100 protein–positive sustentacular cells in malignant paragangliomas of the head and neck region (45,49–52). In a recent review, paragangliomas were assigned three grades (Table 22-3); JTPs (n=10) accounted for over 50 percent of all recurrent or locally aggressive tumors, and were reported to have strikingly few sustentacular cells regardless of behavior (51). In

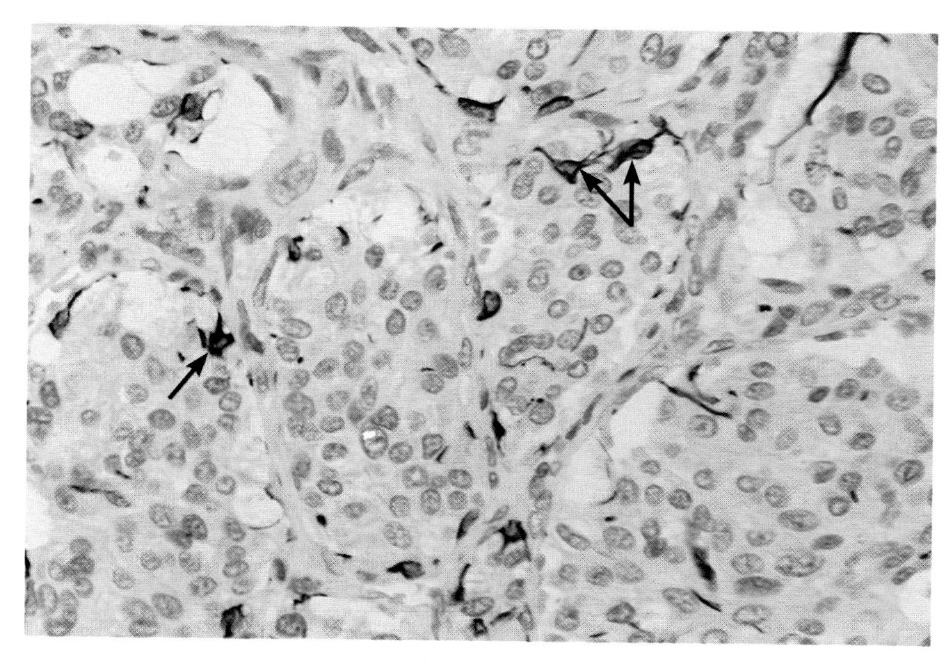

Figure 22-14
CAROTID BODY PARAGANGLIOMA
Immunostain for glial fibrillary acidic protein intensely stains the stellate to dendritic cells near the vascular channels (arrows), the characteristic distribution for sustentacular cells. (X200, Peroxidase-antiperoxidase stain)

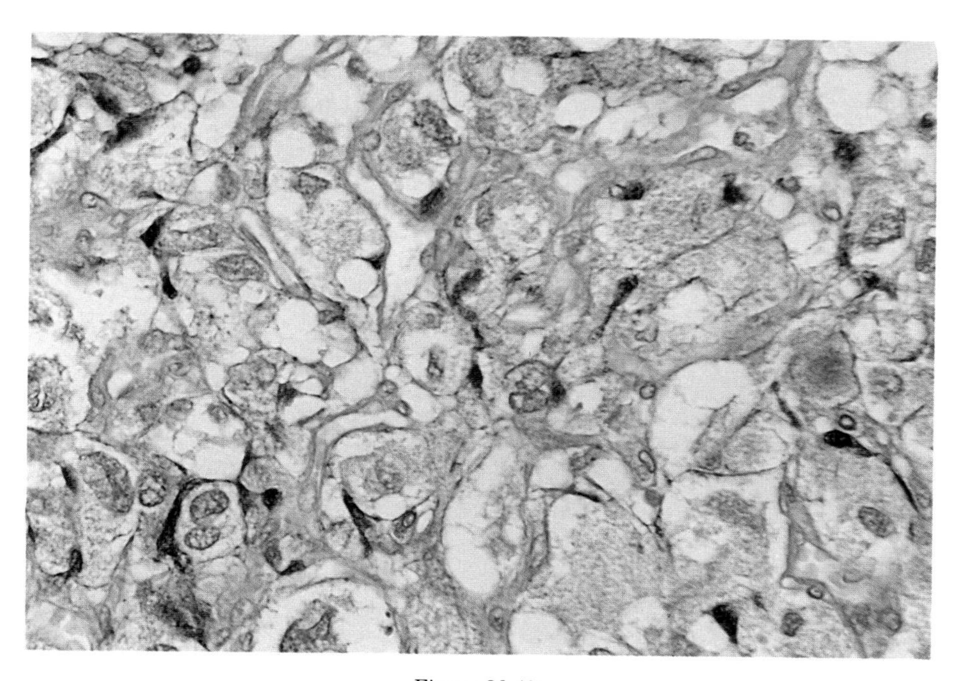

Figure 22-15
PRIMARY MALIGNANT THYROID PARAGANGLIOMA
Immunostaining for S-100 protein shows intense reactivity in numerous slender to curvilinear sustentacular cells closely applied to the microvasculature at the periphery of neoplastic chief cells. The tumor recurred locally, with extensive invasion of laryngotracheal structures. (X200, Peroxidase-antiperoxidase stain)

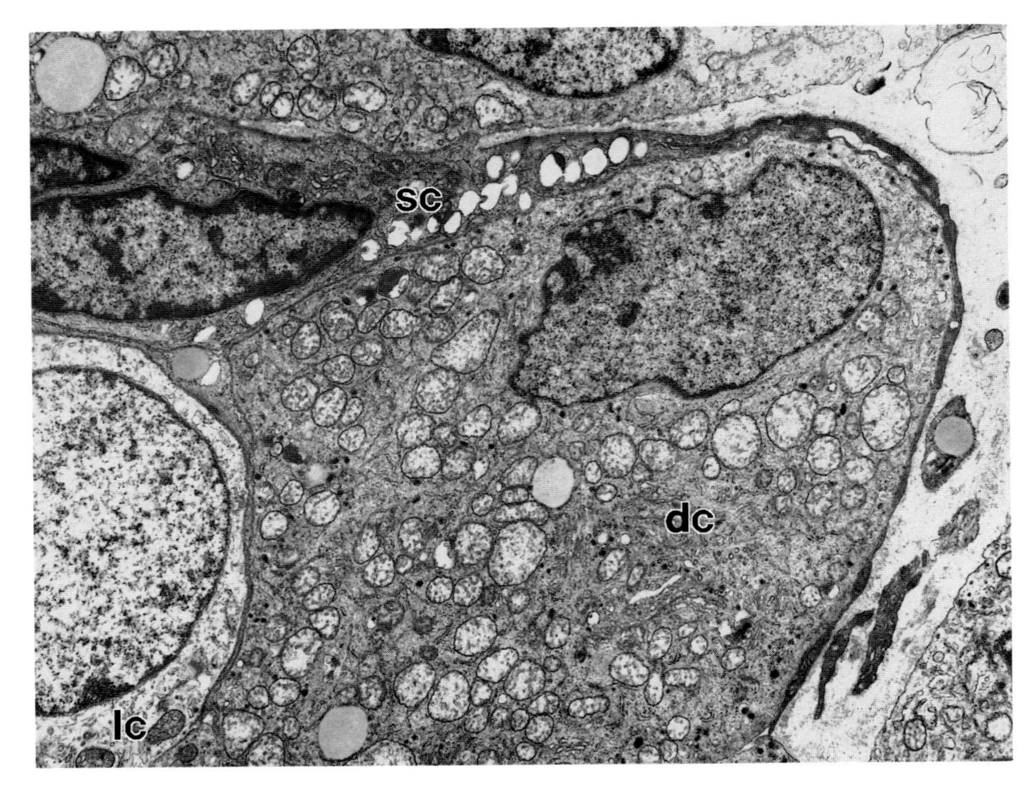

Figure 22-16
CAROTID BODY PARAGANGLIOMA
Nests of neoplastic "dark" (dc) and "light" (lc) chief cells are partially surrounded by cytoplasmic extensions of a sustentacular cell (sc). Both chief cells contain sparse neurosecretory granules, but the sustentacular cell contains none. (X8,000) (Fig. 9-9 from Lack EE. Pathology of adrenal and extra-adrenal paraganglia. Major problems in pathology, Vol 29. Philadelphia: WB Saunders Co, 1994:172.)

a recent study of over 50 head and neck paragangliomas, semiquantitative analysis of overall density of S-100 protein was not considered to be a reliable means of distinguishing clinically benign from malignant (i.e., metastasizing) paragangliomas (46), and a number of JTPs contained demonstrable sustentacular cells (fig. 22-17). A similar study of benign and malignant sympathoadrenal paragangliomas showed no statistically significant difference in density of S-100 protein–positive sustentacular cells, although there was a trend toward decreased density in malignant tumors (53). A malignant CBP had a high sustentacular cell density in both the primary tumor and the pulmonary metastasis (48).

A recent study showed that benign pheochromocytomas contain an increased density of HLA-DR–positive and S-100 protein–negative cells (double immunostaining technique), whereas relatively few such cells were seen in

Table 22-3

GRADING SCHEME PROPOSED FOR VARIOUS PARAGANGLIOMAS OF THE HEAD AND NECK REGION*

Paragangliomas (n=42; 37 patients)
- CBP - 46%; JTP - 27%; VP-1, LP-1, NP-1, other
  - Low Grade = benign, nonrecurrent (n=24)
  - Intermediate Grade = recurrent, locally aggressive (n=8)
  - High Grade = metastasizing (n=5)

Conclusions using panel of immunohistochemical stains
1) Useful in confirming diagnosis
2) Decline in relative proportion of type II (sustentacular) cells (S-100, GFAP) correlates with aggressive behavior/metastases

*Data from reference 51.

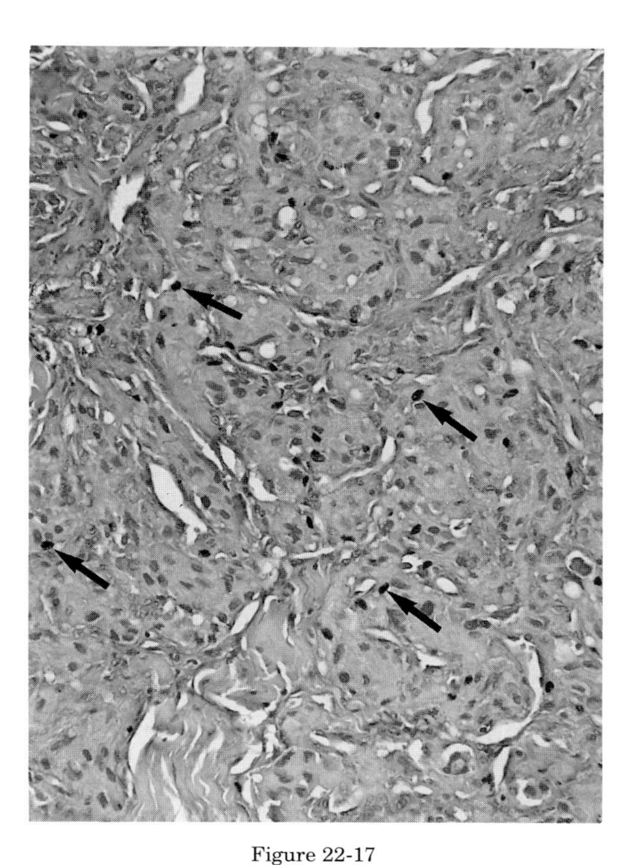

Figure 22-17
JUGULOTYMPANIC PARAGANGLIOMA
Jugulotympanic paraganglioma contained scattered sustentacular cells showing strong nuclear immunostaining for S-100 protein (arrows). (X100, Peroxidase-antiperoxidase stain)

tumors which were aggressive or metastasized; one clinically benign CBP also had a few dendritic cells (47). Another study reported positive immunostaining for tyrosine hydroxylase in two primary CBPs and one JTP, but cervical lymph node metastases in two cases were negative, suggesting an immature phenotype for the more aggressive component of the tumors (54).

Fine-Needle Aspiration and Cytologic Findings. It may be very difficult, or even impossible, to make a specific diagnosis of paraganglioma without heightened clinical suspicion, pertinent correlation with clinical history (e.g., positive family history of similar tumors), or precise anatomic localization. Without additional information, the variability in nuclear size and shape, and intensity of staining may easily lead to a mistaken diagnosis of malignancy (fig. 22-18A) or of an entirely different neoplasm, either benign or malignant (56,58,65,68,72). Fine-needle aspiration (FNA) has been used as a diagnostic technique for various head and neck paragangliomas. There are significantly different views on the efficacy or role of this technique in diagnosing CBP, a neoplasm which may simulate enlarged cervical lymph nodes (fig. 22-18B,C) (55,57,59,61–63). Some regard the procedure as a safe (58,71) and accurate means of diagnosing CBP (58); to enhance accuracy, skill in interpretation of aspirates is important, coupled with in-depth knowledge of surgical pathology. Still, one can not emphasize enough the importance of factors embodied in the first sentence of this paragraph.

Complications appear to be extremely rare with fine-needle biopsy, but include hemorrhage (see fig. 16-3), and thrombosis of the common carotid artery with cerebral embolism and death (56). In the Memorial Hospital review of 73 head and neck paragangliomas, 15 patients had undergone fine-needle aspiration and diagnosis was suggested in 6 (40 percent) (66,67). Needle aspiration of tumors has been performed at Memorial Hospital since 1926 (69); Stewart (73) studied smears of material from 2,500 tumors obtained by aspiration with an 18-gauge needle, but there was no specific reference to head and neck paragangliomas. One important clue to a paraganglioma on FNA is the aspiration of much blood (57). Aspirates often yield only a few clusters of tumor cells, and strands of cytoplasm may give a lattice-like appearance (71). Nuclei may appear "naked" or stripped of cytoplasm (60), and the presence of prominent nuclear vacuoles (nuclear pseudoinclusions) can simulate a papillary thyroid carcinoma (64). Rarely, tumor cells may envelop one another (cell embracing) (70). Immunohistochemical stains may aid in the diagnosis of aspirates or cell block preparations if a paraganglioma is suspected (65).

Quantitative Determination of DNA Content. Quantitation of DNA content in paragangliomas of the head and neck region has been done using flow cytometry or static image analysis of Feulgen-stained tissue sections (74–83). Several recent studies have shown that abnormal DNA content of CBPs and other paragangliomas is common, and that DNA ploidy is not reliable in determining malignant potential (75,77,80,83). Some malignant CBPs have even been reported to have normal diploid DNA (79).

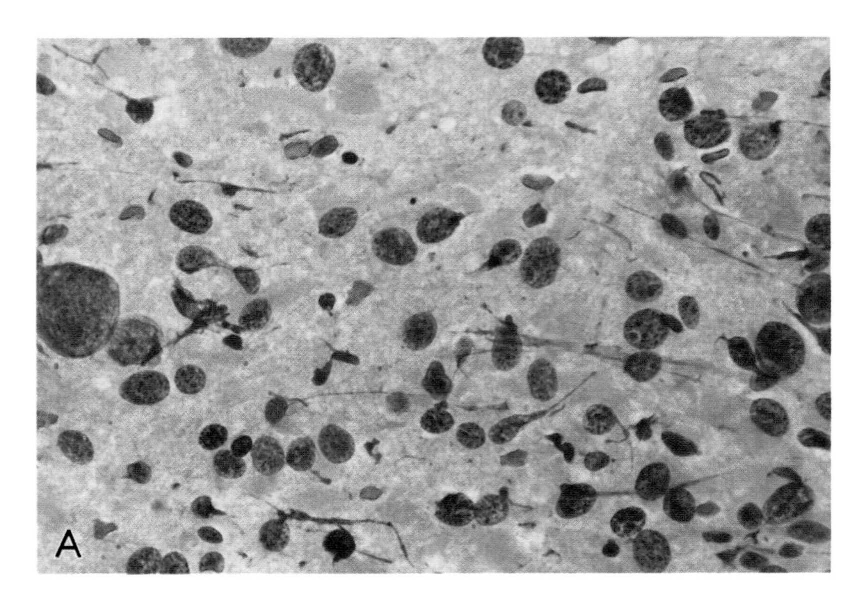

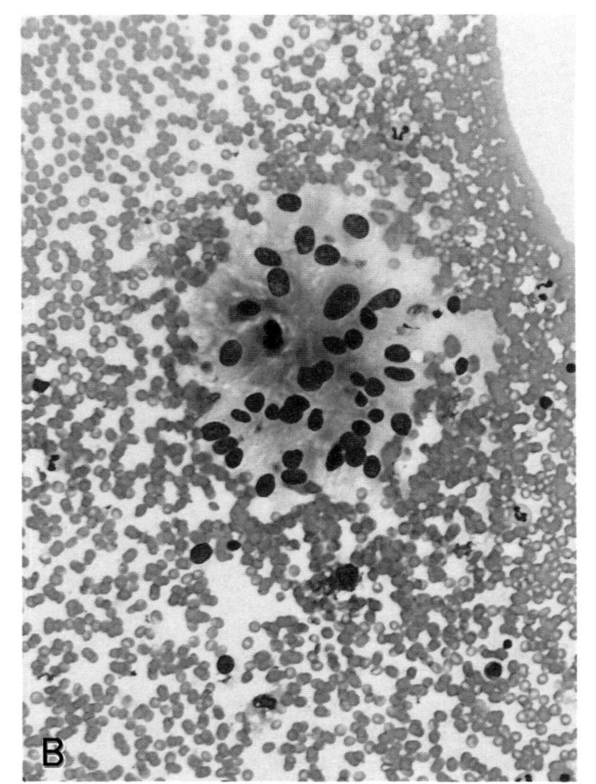

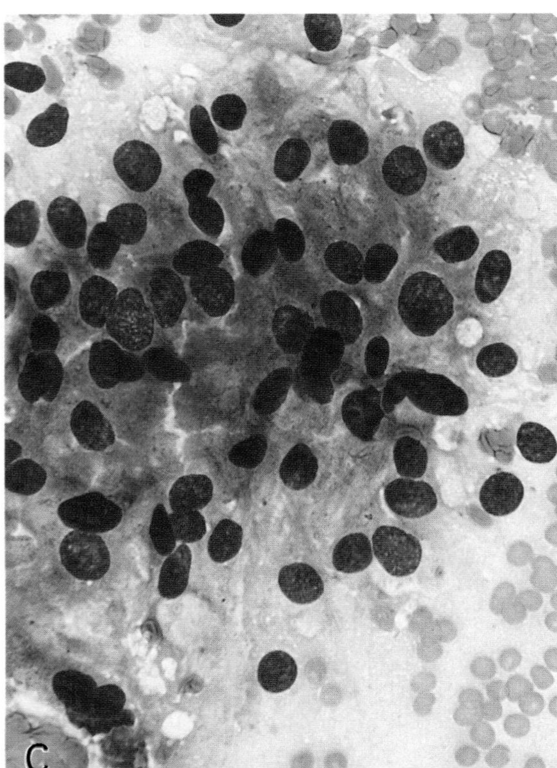

Figure 22-18
CAROTID BODY PARAGANGLIOMA

A: Smear/imprint of a surgically resected CBP. The variability in nuclear size might be confused with malignancy. (X400, Papanicolaou stain)

B: Fine-needle aspiration of a different CBP. A small cluster of loosely cohesive tumor cells is present within a bloody background. Small vacuolar spaces are present giving a lattice-like appearance. The nuclei are darkly stained, with a mild degree of irregularity in size and shape. (X200, Diff-Quik stain)

C: Same case as B showing a bloody background and greater degree of variation in nuclear size. A heightened clinical suspicion for paraganglioma along with correlation with clinical findings and anatomic localization are critical factors in making an accurate diagnosis. (X400, Diff-Quik stain)

In a large study of 99 paragangliomas from 77 patients (average duration of follow-up 10 years or more), aneuploidy was noted in 37 tumors (37 percent), none of which proved to be malignant (83). While DNA aneuploidy in hereditary and sporadic paragangliomas does not reliably predict malignant behavior, it does provide strong support that these paragangliomas are truly neoplastic (83). There also appears to be no relation between DNA ploidy and the location of the paraganglioma in the neck (83). Precautions in interpretation of DNA histograms must be observed, with rigorous adherence to standardized methods (85). Cytogenetic analysis of a head and neck paraganglioma has only rarely been reported. In a recent case of bilateral familial CBP, no evidence of numerical or structural alteration was seen (78). The oncogenes c-*myc*, *bcl*-2, and c-*jun* are abnormally expressed in some CBPs, suggesting that deregulation of these oncogenes may contribute to the genesis of some of these tumors (84).

REFERENCES

General Features

1. Churukian CJ, Schenk EA. A modification of Pascual's argyrophil method. J Histotechnol 1979;2:102–3.
2. Grimelius L. A silver nitrate stain for alpha 2 cells in human pancreatic islets. Acta Soc Med Upsala 1968;73:243–70.
3. Lack EE. Pathology of adrenal and extra-adrenal paraganglia. Major problems in pathology, Vol 29. Philadelphia: WB Saunders, 1994.
4. Lack EE, Cubilla AL, Woodruff JM. Paragangliomas of the head and neck region. A pathologic study of tumors from 71 patients. Hum Pathol 1979;10:191–218.
5. Lloyd RV, Sisson JC, Shapiro B, Verhofstad AA. Immunohistochemical localization of epinephrine, norepinephrine, catecholamine-synthesizing enzymes, and chromogranin in neuroendocrine cells and tumors. Am J Pathol 1986;125:45–54.
6. Pascual JS. A new method for easy demonstration of argyrophil cells. Stain Technol 1976;51:231–5.
7. Vassallo G, Capella C, Solcia E. Grimelius silver stain for endocrine cell granules, as shown by electron microscopy. Stain Technol 1971;46:7–13.

Ultrastructural Findings

8. Alpert LI, Bochetto JF. Carotid body tumor: ultrastructural observations. Cancer 1974;34:564–73.
9. Archer KF, Hurwitz JJ, Balogh JM, Fernandes BJ. Orbital nonchromaffin paraganglioma. A case report and review of the literature. Ophthalmology 1989;96:1659–66.
10. Barnes L. Paraganglioma of the larynx. A critical review of the literature. ORL J Otorhinolaryngol Relat Spec 1991;53:220–34.
11. Capella C, Solcia E. Optical and electron microscopical study of cytoplasmic granules in human carotid body, carotid body tumours and glomus jugulare tumours. Virchows Arch [Cell Pathol] 1971;7:37–53.
12. Chaudhry AP, Haar JG, Koul A, Nickerson PA. A nonfunctioning paraganglioma of vagus nerve. An ultrastructural study. Cancer 1979;43:1689–701.
13. Erlandson RA. Diagnostic transmission electron microscopy of tumors: with clinicopathological, immunohistochemical, and cytogenetic correlations. New York: Raven Press, 1994.
14. Gallivan MV, Chun B, Rowden G, Lack EE. Laryngeal paraganglioma. Case report with ultrastructural analysis and literature review. Am J Surg Pathol 1979;3:85–92.
15. Gonzalez-Angulo A, Feria-Velasco A, Corvera J, Yabur-Elias E. Ultrastructure of the glomus jugulare tumor. Arch Otolaryngol 1968;87:13–21.
16. Grimley PM, Glenner GG. Histology and ultrastructure of carotid body paragangliomas. Comparison with the normal gland. Cancer 1967;20:1473–88.
17. Grimley PM, Glenner GG. Ultrastructure of the human carotid body. A perspective on the mode of chemoreception. Circulation 1968;37:648–65.
18. Horváth KK, Ormos J, Ribári O. Crystals in a jugulotympanic paraganglioma. Ultrastr Pathol 1986;10:257–64.
19. Hui G, McAllister HA, Angelini P. Left atrial paraganglioma: report of a case and review of the literature. Am Heart J 1987;113:1230–4.
20. Johnson TL, Lloyd RV, Shapiro B, et al. Cardiac paragangliomas. A clinicopathologic and immunohistochemical study of four cases. Am J Surg Pathol 1985;9:827–34.
21. Kahn LB. Vagal body tumor (nonchromaffin paraganglioma, chemodectoma, and carotid body-like tumor) with cervical node metastasis and familial association. Ultrastructural study and review. Cancer 1976;38:2367–77.
22. Kjaergaard J. Anatomy of the carotid glomus and carotid glomus-like bodies (non-chromaffin paraganglia). With electron microscopy and comparison of human foetal carotid, aorticopulmonary, subclavian, tympanojugular, and vagal glomera. Copenhagen: FADL's Forlag, 1973.
23. Lack EE. Pathology of adrenal and extra-adrenal paraganglia. Major problems in pathology, Vol 29. Philadelphia: WB Saunders, 1994.

24. Lack EE, Cubilla AL, Woodruff JM. Paragangliomas of the head and neck region: a pathologic study of tumors from 71 patients. Hum Pathol 1979;10:191–218.
25. Lack EE, Stillinger RA, Colvin DB, Groves RM, Burnette DG. Aortico-pulmonary paraganglioma. Report of a case with ultrastructural study and review of the literature. Cancer 1979;43:269–78.
26. Smith KR, Gladney JH. The ultrastructure of a tumor of the glomus jugulare. Laryngoscope 1968;78:1999–2012.
27. Stiller D, Katenkamp D, Küttner K. Jugular body tumors: hyperplasias or true neoplasms? Light and electron microscopical investigations. Virchows Arch [A] 1975;365:163–77.
28. Thomsen J, Jorgensen MB. Electron microscopy as a supplement in the diagnosis of glomus jugulare tumors. J Laryngol Otol 1974;88:543–50.
29. Ueda N, Yoshida A, Fukunishi R, Fujita H, Yanagihara N. Nonchromaffin paraganglioma in the nose and paranasal sinuses. Acta Pathol Jpn 1985;35:489–95.

Immunohistochemical Findings

30. Capella C, Riva C, Cornaggia M, Chiaravalli AM, Frigerio B. Histopathology, cytology and cytochemistry of pheochromocytomas and paragangliomas including chemodectomas. Path Res Pract 1988;183:176–87.
31. Erlandson RA. Diagnostic immunohistochemistry of human tumors. An interim evaluation. Am J Surg Pathol 1984;8:615–24.
32. Haimoto H, Takahashi Y, Koshikawa T, Nagura H, Kato K. Immunohistochemical localization of gamma-enolase in normal human tissues other than nervous and neuroendocrine tissues. Lab Invest 1985;52:257–63.
33. Johnson TL, Zarbo RJ, Lloyd RV, Crissman JD. Paragangliomas of the head and neck: immunohistochemical neuroendocrine and intermediate filament typing. Mod Pathol 1988;1:216–23.
34. Kimura N, Sasano N, Yamada R, Satoh J. Immunohistochemical study of chromogranin in 100 cases of pheochromocytoma, carotid body tumour, medullary thyroid carcinoma and carcinoid tumour. Virchows Arch [A] 1988;413:33–8.
35. Korat O, Trojanowski JQ, LiVolsi VA, Merino MJ. Antigen expression in normal paraganglia and paragangliomas. Surg Pathol 1988;1:33–40.
36. Lack EE. Pathology of adrenal and extra-adrenal paraganglia. In: Major problems in pathology, Vol 29. Philadelphia: WB Saunders, 1994.
37. Lloyd RV, Jin L, Kulig E, Fields K. Molecular approaches for the analysis of chromogranins and secretogranins. Diagn Mol Pathol 1992;1:2–15.
38. Martinez-Madrigal F, Bosq J, Micheau CH, Nivet P, Luboinski B. Paragangliomas of the head and neck. Immunohistochemical analysis of 16 cases in comparison with neuro-endocrine carcinomas. Pathol Res Pract 1991;187:814–23.
39. Mukai M, Torikata C, Iri H, et al. Expression of neurofilament triplet proteins in human neural tumors. An immunohistochemical study of paraganglioma, ganglioneuroma, ganglioneuroblastoma, and neuroblastoma. Am J Pathol 1986;122:28–35.
40. Schmechel DE. Gamma-subunit of the glycolytic enzyme enolase: nonspecific or neuron-specific? Lab Invest 1985;52:239–42.
41. Schmid KW, Schröder S, Duckhorn-Dworniczak B, et al. Immunohistochemical demonstration of chromogranin A, chromogranin B, and secretogranin II in extra-adrenal paragangliomas. Mod Pathol 1994;7:347–53.
42. Schroder HD, Johannsen L. Demonstration of S-100 protein sustentacular cells of phaeochromocytomas and paragangliomas. Histopathology 1986;10:1023–33.
43. Tischler AS, Mobtaker H, Mann K, et al. Anti-lymphocyte antibody leu-7 (HNK-1) recognizes a constituent of neuroendocrine granule matrix. J Histochem Cytochem 1986;34:1213–6.
44. Warren WH, Lee I, Gould VE, Memoli VA, Jao W. Paragangliomas of the head and neck: ultrastructural and immunohistochemical analysis. Ultrastr Pathol 1985;8:333–43.

Relation of S-100 Protein–Positive Cells to Prognosis

45. Bhansali SA, Bojrab DI, Zarbo RJ. Malignant paragangliomas of the head and neck: clinical and immunohisto-chemical characterization. Otolaryngol Head Neck Surg 1991;104:132.
46. Bitterman P, Sherman M, Lack EE. Paragangliomas of the head and neck region: clinicopathologic and immunohistochemical evaluation of 88 cases. Patologia 1992;25:493A.
47. Furihata M, Ohtsuki Y. Immunohistochemical characterization of HLA-DR-antigen positive dendritic cells in phaeochromocytomas and paragangliomas as a prognostic marker. Virchows Archiv [A] 1991;418:33–9.
48. Granger JK, Houn HY. Head and neck paragangliomas: a clinicopathologic study with DNA flow cytometric analysis. Southern Med J 1990;83:1407–12.
49. Kliewer KE, Cochran AJ. A review of the histology, ultrastructure, immunohistology, and molecular biology of extra-adrenal paragangliomas. Arch Pathol Lab Med 1989;113:1209–18.
50. Kliewer KE, Cochran AJ, Wen DR, Cheng L, Cancilla PA. An immunohistochemical study of 37 paragangliomas. Med Sci Res 1987;15:87–8.
51. Kliewer KE, Wen DR, Cancilla PA, Cochran AJ. Paragangliomas: assessment of prognosis by histologic, immunohistochemical, and ultrastructural techniques. Hum Pathol 1989;20:29–39.
52. Korat O, Trojanowski JQ, LiVolsi VA, Merino MJ. Antigen expression in normal paraganglia and paragangliomas. Surg Pathol 1988;1:33–40.
53. Linnoila RI, Becker RL Jr, Steinberg SM, Kaiser HR, Lack EE. The role of S-100 protein containing cells in the prognosis of sympathoadrenal paragangliomas [Abstract]. Mod Pathol 1993;6:39A.
54. Takahashi H, Nakashima S, Kumanishi T, Ikuta F. Paragangliomas of the craniocervical region. An immunohistochemical study on tyrosine hydroxylase. Acta Neuropathol 1987;73:227–32.

Fine-Needle Aspiration and Cytologic Findings

55. Conley JJ. The carotid body tumor. Arch Laryngol 1965;81:187–93.
56. Engzell U, Franzén S, Zajicek J. Aspiration biopsy of tumors of the neck II. Cytologic findings in 13 cases of carotid body tumor. Acta Cytol 1971;15:25–30.
57. Farr HW. Carotid body tumors. A thirty year experience at Memorial Hospital. Am J Surg 1967;114:614–9.
58. Fleming MV, Oertel YC, Rodriguez ER, Fidler WJ. Fine-needle aspiration of six carotid body paragangliomas. Diagn Cytopathol 1993;9:510–5.
59. Frable WJ. Thin-needle aspiration biopsy. Major problems in pathology, Vol 14. Philadelphia: WB Saunders, 1983.
60. González-Cámpora R, Otal-Salaverri C, Panea-Flores P, Lerma-Puertas E, Galera-Davidson H. Fine needle aspiration cytology of paraganglionic tumors. Acta Cytol 1988;32:386–90.
61. Harrington SW, Clagett OT, Dockerty MB. Tumors of the carotid body. Clinical and pathologic considerations of twenty tumors affecting nineteen patients (one bilaterally). Ann Surg 1941;114:820–33.
62. Hodge KM, Byers RM, Peters LJ. Paragangliomas of the head and neck. Arch Otolaryngol Head Neck Surg 1988;114:872–7.
63. Irons GB, Weiland LH, Brown WL. Paragangliomas of the neck: clinical and pathological analysis of 116 cases. Surg Clin North Am 1977;57:575–83.
64. Jacobs DM, Waisman J. Cervical paraganglioma with intranuclear vacuoles in a fine needle aspirate. Acta Cytol 1987;31:29–32.
65. Lack EE. Pathology of adrenal and extra-adrenal paraganglia. Major problems in pathology, Vol 29. Philadelphia: WB Saunders, 1994.
66. Lack EE, Cubilla AL, Woodruff JM. Paragangliomas of the head and neck region. A pathologic study of tumors from 71 patients. Hum Pathol 1979;10:191–218.
67. Lack EE, Cubilla AL, Woodruff JM, Farr HW. Paragangliomas of the head and neck region: a clinical study of 69 patients. Cancer 1977;39:397–409.
68. MacComb WS. Carotid body tumors. Ann Surg 1948;127:269–77.
69. Martin HE, Ellis EB. Biopsy by needle puncture and aspiration. Ann Surg 1930;92:169–81.
70. Mincione GP, Urso C. Carotid body paraganglioma (chemodectoma): cytologic remarks. Pathologica 1989;81:179–83.
71. Qizilbash AH, Young JE. Guides to clinical aspiration biopsy. Head and neck. New York: Igaku-Shoin, 1988:279–89.
72. Soares MA, Apel RL, Bédard YC. Carotid body tumor mimicking adenocarcinoma on fine-needle aspiration. Endocr Pathol 1994;5:131–5.
73. Stewart FW. The diagnosis of tumors by aspiration. Am J Pathol 1933;9:801–12.

Quantitative Determination of DNA Content

74. Barnes L. Paraganglioma of the larynx. A critical review of the literature. ORL J Otorhinolaryngol Relat Spec 1991;53:220–34.
75. Barnes L, Taylor SR. Carotid body paragangliomas. A clinicopathologic and DNA analysis of 13 tumors. Arch Otolaryngol Head Neck Surg 1990;116:447–53.
76. Barnes L, Taylor SR. Vagal paragangliomas: a clinical, pathological and DNA assessment. Clin Otolaryngol 1991;16:376–82.
77. González-Cámpora R, Cano SD, Lerma-Puertas E, et al. Paragangliomas. Static cytometric studies of nuclear DNA patterns. Cancer 1993;71:820–4.
78. Granger JK, Houn HY. Bilateral familial carotid body paragangliomas. Report of a case with DNA flow cytometric and cytogenetic analyses. Arch Pathol Lab Med 1990;114:1272–5.
79. Granger JK, Houn HY. Head and neck paragangliomas: a clinicopathologic study with DNA flow cytometric analysis. Southern Med J 1990;83:1407–12.
80. Milroy CM, Williams RA, Charlton IG, Moss E, Rode J. Nuclear ploidy in neuroendocrine neoplasms of the larynx. ORL J Otorhinolaryngol Relat Spec 1991;53:245–9.
81. Sauter ER, Hollier LH, Bolton JS, Ochsner JL, Sardi A. Prognostic value of DNA flow cytometry in paragangliomas of the carotid body. J Surg Oncol 1991;46:151–3.
82. Sauter ER, Hollier LH, Farr GH Jr. The value of flow cytometric analysis in multicentric glomus tumors of the head and neck. Cancer 1992;69:1452–6.
83. van der Mey AG, Cornelisse CJ, Hermans J, Terpstra JL, Schmidt PH, Fleuren GJ. DNA flow cytometry of hereditary and sporadic paragangliomas (glomus tumours). Br J Cancer 1991;63:298–302
84. Wang DG, Barros D'Sa AA, Johnston CF, Buchanan KD. Oncogene expression in carotid body tumors. Cancer 1996;77:2581–7.
85. Wersto RP, Liblit RL, Koss LG. Flow cytometric DNA analysis of human solid tumors: a review of the interpretation of DNA histograms. Hum Pathol 1991;22:1085–98.

✧✧✧

23
NEUROBLASTOMA, GANGLIONEUROBLASTOMA, AND OTHER RELATED TUMORS

NEUROBLASTOMA AND GANGLIONEUROBLASTOMA

Definition. Neuroblastoma is a primitive neoplasm of neuroectodermal origin which arises in sites paralleling the distribution of the sympathetic nervous system. Ganglioneuroblastoma is a closely related neoplasm showing variable cyto-differentiation into ganglion cells which may or may not be accompanied by a spindle cell schwannian matrix.

Epidemiology. Neuroblastoma (NB) and ganglioneuroblastoma (GNB) are the fourth most common malignant tumors in childhood after leukemia, brain tumors, and malignant lymphoma (23,24). The incidence of NB in the United States is estimated to be 8.7 per million white population and GNB 1.8 per million, with a slightly lower incidence in blacks. About 85 percent of all cases of NB and GNB occur in the first 4 years of life, and there are no sex-related differences in incidence rates (24). Both NB and GNB make up 7.9 percent of the 9,308 childhood cancers followed by the Surveillance, Epidemiology, and End Results (SEER) program in children younger than age 15 years (19). In a series of 118 patients, 88 percent were 5 years of age or younger at diagnosis, with a median age of 21 months (fig. 23-1) (20). These tumors are uncommon in the second decade, and are rare in adult life, although NB and GNB have been reported at nearly every age (14).

NB has an unusual geographic distribution, with a low incidence in certain areas, particularly the "Burkitt lymphoma belt" of Africa (18). Familial occurrence of NB has been reported (6), and in some cases appears to have an autosomal dominant pattern of inheritance, but there are obvious difficulties in determining the incidence and penetrance of an inherited susceptibility for this neoplasm given its capacity for regression, maturation, and early death, and treatment

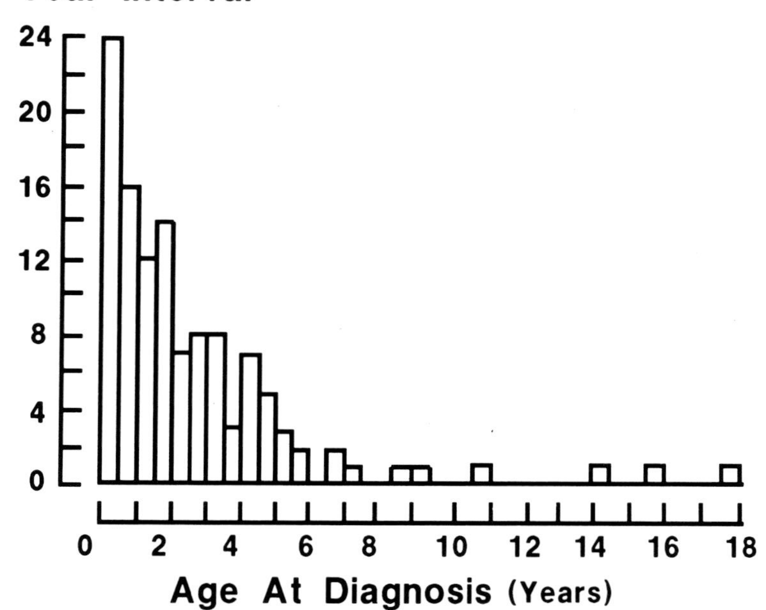

Figure 23-1
AGE DISTRIBUTION OF 118 PATIENTS WITH NEUROBLASTOMA

Median age at diagnosis was 21 months. (Fig. 1 from Rosen EM, Cassady JR, Frantz CN, Kretschmar C, Levey R, Sallan SE. Neuroblastoma: the Joint Center for Radiation Therapy/Dana-Farber Cancer Institute/Children's Hospital experience. J Clin Oncol 1984;2:719–32.)

Table 23-1

UNUSUAL MANIFESTATIONS OR ASSOCIATIONS WITH CHILDHOOD NEUROBLASTOMA*

Congenital neuroblastoma
Cutaneous metastases and "blueberry muffin" baby
Placental enlargement with hydrops fetalis
Neuroblastoma "leukemia"
Opsoclonus/myoclonus
Alopecia
Heterochromia iridis
Horner's syndrome
Watery diarrhea (vasoactive intestinal peptide [VIP] secretion)
Cushing's syndrome
Asymmetric crying facies
Central hypoventilation syndrome ("Ondine's curse")
Late recurrence and death
Familial neuroblastoma
Association with von Recklinghausen's disease

*Table 14-1 from Lack EE. Pathology of adrenal and extra-adrenal paraganglia. Major problems in pathology, Vol 29. Philadelphia: WB Saunders Co, 1994:318.

complications that preclude reproduction and prevent multigenerational pedigrees for evaluation (13). Some studies indicate essentially no risk of offspring of surviving patients with NB or GNB developing similar tumors (1). In a two-mutation model of cancer applied to NB and pheochromocytoma, nonhereditary cases have both events occurring in somatic cells and the tumor is characteristically solitary, whereas in hereditary cases the tumors may be multiple (11).

There are a variety of disorders or unusual manifestations associated with these tumors (Table 23-1) (14). A watery diarrhea syndrome has been reported with NB (2), GNB (4,7,9, 10,12,15), ganglioneuroma (5,12), and pheochromocytoma with (17,22) or without (14) composite features. This diarrheal syndrome has been reported in 6 percent of children with NB and GNB (20) and secretion of vasoactive intestinal peptide (VIP) has been implicated as an etiologic agent (2,5,7,9,10,15). Ganglion cell differentiation has been considered a prerequisite for VIP production, but as indicated for pheochromocytomas, this may not always be true. Adrenergic overactivity due to excess catecholamine release is uncommon with NB and GNB, and in one series only 4 percent of patients were hypertensive at the time of diagnosis (20). Opsoclonus/myoclonus ("dancing eyes, dancing feet") is present in about 2 to 7 percent of patients with NB and GNB, and has been associated with a favorable prognosis, but may present a diagnostic dilemma in a child without a palpable mass or abnormalities in excretion of catecholamines or their metabolites (3, 20). Heterochromia iridis is a rare but potentially important sign associated with cervical or mediastinal NB or GNB (8,16), and has even been reported in a patient with paravertebral neurilemoma (fig. 23-2); the heterochromia results from prenatal or postnatal interruption of sympathetic tracts that mediate pigmentation of the iris (21).

Mass Screening Programs for Neuroblastoma. Mass screening for NB began in Kyoto, Japan in 1974 (32), and other screening programs have been subsequently developed in other areas of Japan (29,31) as well as other countries (27,28). Mass screening in infancy, usually at 6 months of age, with a qualitative vanillylmandelic acid (VMA) spot test, has resulted in an increased annual detection rate of 93 per million compared with a baseline annual rate of 13.3 per million without screening (33). The prognosis for childhood NB detected by screening is favorable, since important factors are low clinical stage and early age at diagnosis (28). In a recent study, most children detected by screening were considered to be in a low-risk subgroup with potential for spontaneous tumor regression (25). Tumors not detected through screening but diagnosed clinically in children over 12 months of age are predominantly of unfavorable histology with poor outcome (34). Some have recommended additional screening of children over 12 months of age (26), since NBs missed in earlier screening have poor prognostic features (over 1 year of age and advanced stage) (27,30). More data are needed to tell whether preclinical detection will truly result in a decline in population-based mortality for NB.

Anatomic Distribution of Primary Tumors. The anatomic distribution of NB and GNB closely parallels that of the sympathetic nervous system with which they are so closely aligned (45). Data compiled from 10 reference sources by Jaffe (42) are shown in Table 23-2. The anatomic

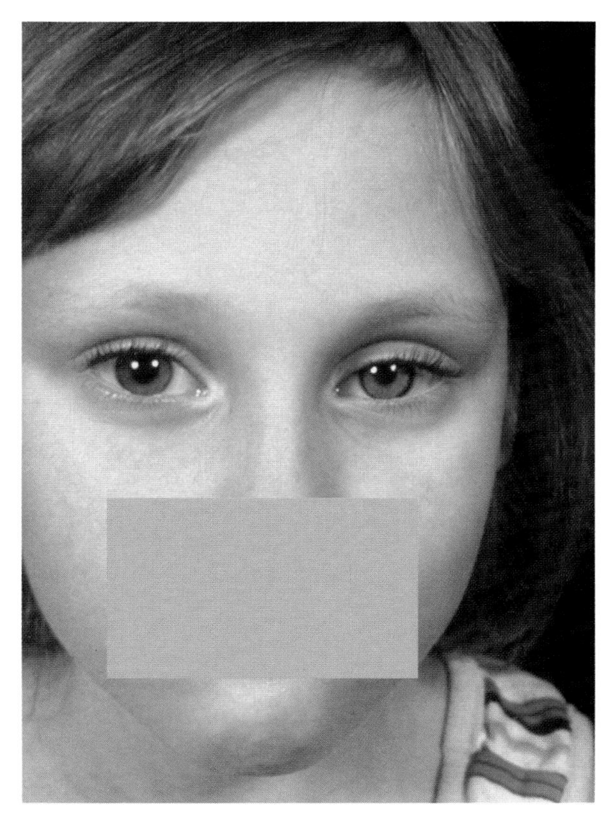

Figure 23-2
HETEROCHROMIA IRIDIS ASSOCIATED WITH PARAVERTEBRAL NEURILEMOMA

A 7-year-old girl had Horner's syndrome on the right side and heterochromia iridis. The patient had an upper thoracic paravertebral neurilemoma on the left side measuring 4 cm in diameter. Half of the right iris was brown, and the other half blue, while the left iris was uniformly blue throughout.

Table 23-2

INCIDENCE AND SURVIVAL DATA BASED UPON PRIMARY ANATOMIC SITE OF NEUROBLASTOMA*

Primary Site	Incidence (%)	Survival (%)
Head	2	33
Neck	5	15
Thorax	14	61
Abdomen	54	20
Adrenal	36	9
Nonadrenal	18	32
Pelvis	5	41
Other	10	21
Unknown	10	17

*Data from reference 42.

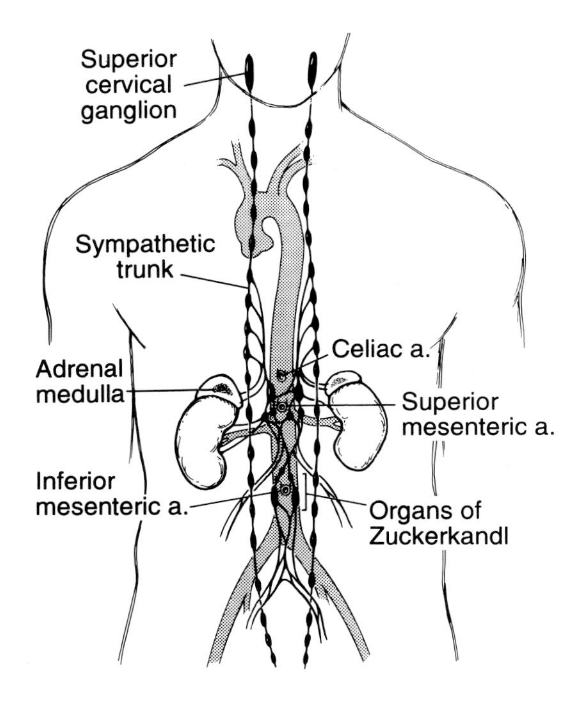

Site	Number	(%)		
Unknown	6	(5.1)		
Cervical	4	(3.4)		
Thoracic	24	(20.3)		
Abdomen	80	(67.8)		
Adrenal	--		45	(38.1)
Extra-adrenal	--		35	(29.7)
Pelvic	4	(3.4)		
All sites	**118**	**(100.0)**		

Figure 23-3
ANATOMIC DISTRIBUTION OF PRIMARY NEUROBLASTOMA AND GANGLIONEUROBLASTOMA IN 118 PATIENTS

Most tumors were intra-abdominal, arising in adrenal glands or upper abdomen. (Data from Rosen EM, Cassady JR, Frantz CN, Kretschmar C, Levey R, Sallan SE. Neuroblastoma: the Joint Center for Radiation Therapy/Dana-Farber Cancer Institute/Children's Hospital experience. J Clin Oncol 1984;2:719–32.)

distribution of NB and GNB in 118 patients is shown in figure 23-3 (48). Unusual anatomic sites of origin include orbit (37,43), intrarenal (49), and ovary (cystic teratoma) (47). An improved survival rate has been noted for patients with NB and GNB located in the neck, thorax (fig. 23-4) (39), and pelvis, but this may be attributed in large part to early stage disease and younger age at diagnosis (38). Thoracic NB has

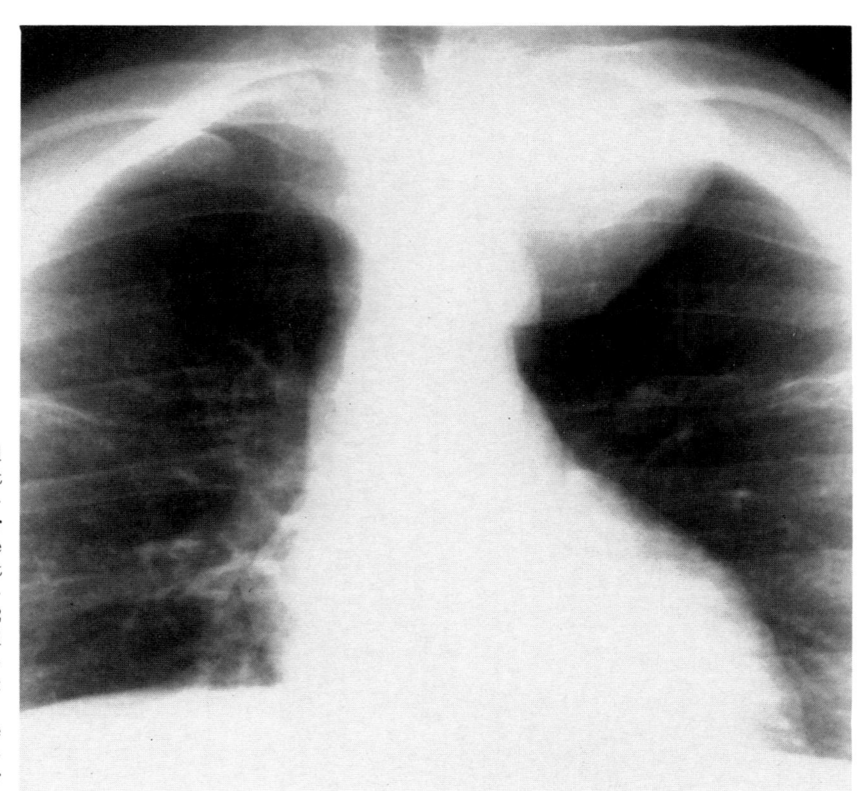

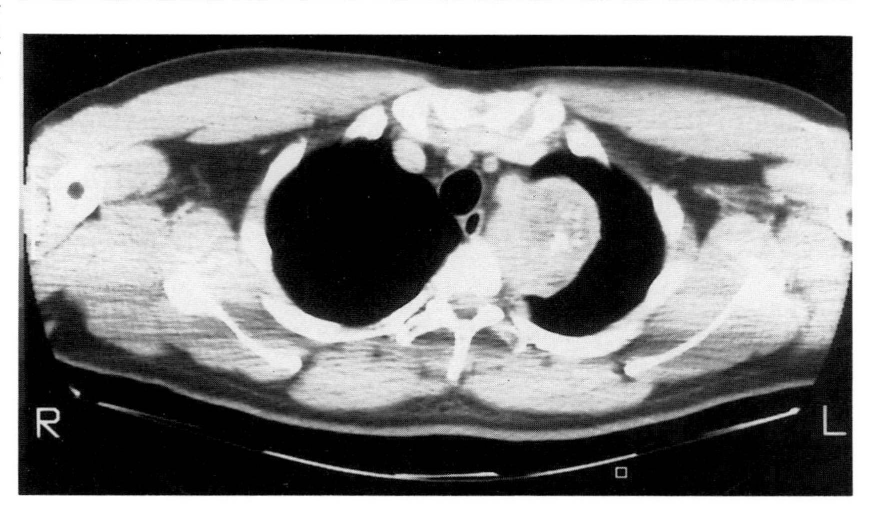

Figure 23-4
STROMA-POOR
NEUROBLASTOMA

Top: A 25-year-old man presented with a history of dry cough and on chest roentgenogram showed a large intrathoracic paravertebral mass. Tumor was a stroma-poor neuroblastoma in the Shimada classification with ≥5 percent differentiating elements and a low mitosis-karyorrhexis index (MKI). (Fig. 14-2 from Lack EE. Pathology of adrenal and extra-adrenal paraganglia. Major problems in pathology, Vol 29. Philadelphia: WB Saunders Co., 1994:319.)

Bottom: CT scan of the same case showed the tumor in the paravertebral sulcus on the left side. The tumor is nonhomogeneous and had spotty areas of dystrophic calcification. An earlier biopsy of a left supraclavicular lymph node showed metastatic neuroblastoma.

been reported to contain more complex gangliosides of the b series and few monosialogangliosides, suggesting a more differentiated cellular composition (50). Only about 2 to 3 percent of all primary NBs arise in the cervical area of the sympathetic chain (fig. 23-5) (40,42,48); they may encase the nodose ganglion of the vagus nerve (36) and occasionally cause Horner's syndrome (46).

There may be intraspinal extension of NB and GNB with compression of the spinal cord, and extradural intraspinal extension has also been reported with ganglioneuroma (35,41). King et al. (44) found intraspinal extension ("dumbbell" NB) in 10 percent of abdominal NBs, 28 percent of thoracic NBs (fig. 23-6), and one of four cervical NBs (25 percent).

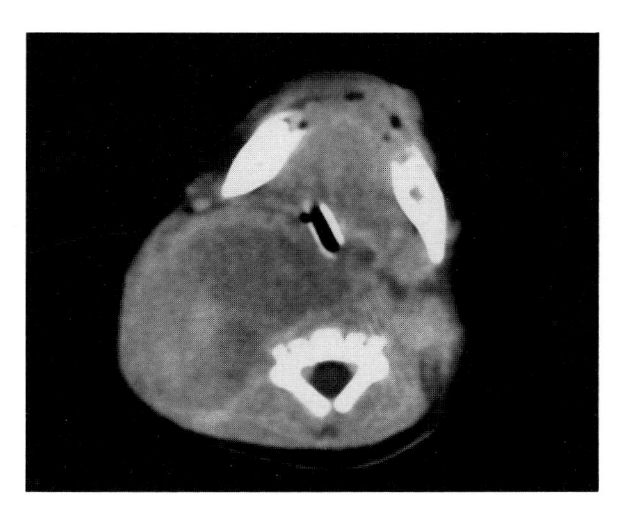

Figure 23-5
CONGENITAL CERVICAL NEUROBLASTOMA
Newborn female with a large congenital neuroblastoma in the right neck. The tumor was stroma-poor with a low mitosis-karyorrhexis index (MKI), a favorable subgroup in the Shimada classification. (Fig. 14-6 from Lack EE. Pathology of adrenal and extra-adrenal paraganglia. Major problems in pathology, Vol 29. Philadelphia: WB Saunders Co., 1994:320.)

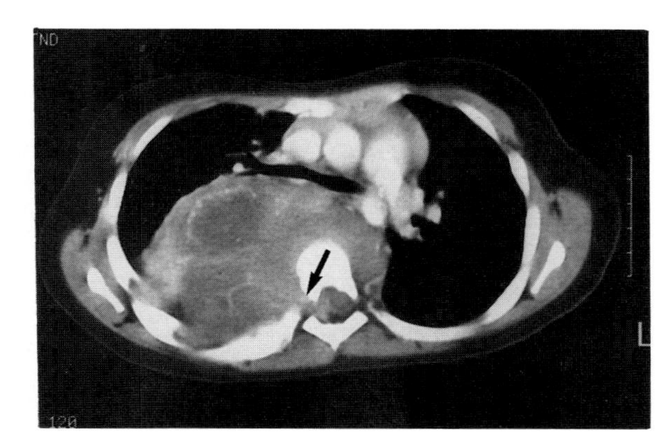

Figure 23-6
INTRATHORACIC GANGLIONEUROBLASTOMA
A large intrathoracic ganglioneuroblastoma in a 5-year-old girl partially destroyed the rib posteriorly and extended across the midline. Note the spotty areas of calcification within the tumor as well as erosion of the intervertebral foramen on the right side (arrow) due to intraspinal extradural extension by tumor.

Staging Systems. The staging system proposed by Evans et al. (56) has been very popular and continues to provide valuable information regarding prognosis, but other staging classifications have been proposed and comparative studies of many of them have been reported (51, 53,57). An international NB staging system, very similar to the original Evans classification, may avoid some disparities in staging criteria (Table 23-3). Based upon several clinical series, the relative proportion of patients at each stage at diagnosis is 6 to 8 percent at stage I, 9 to 24 percent at stage II, 9 to 23 percent at stage III (58,59,61), 48 to 52 percent at stage IV, and 8 to 12 percent at stage IV-S (S = special) (55,59–62). Between 60 and 70 percent of patients with NB and GNB have advanced stage or metastases at presentation (stages IV and IV-S), while 30 to 40 percent have more localized disease (stages I,II, and III) (54,58,61). The IV-S category includes patients with bone marrow involvement; although it is not limited to the age of 1 year, few patients are older than this (52).

In Situ Neuroblastoma. The concept of in situ NB was introduced by Beckwith and Perrin (64) for a small nodule of NB cells within the adrenal gland (fig. 23-7) which was histologically

Table 23-3

INTERNATIONAL STAGING SYSTEM FOR NEUROBLASTOMA*

Stage I:	Localized tumor confined to the area of origin; complete gross excision, with or without microscopic residual disease; identifiable ipsilateral and contralateral lymph nodes negative microscopically
Stage IIA:	Unilateral tumor with incomplete gross excision; identifiable ipsilateral and contralateral lymph nodes negative microscopically
Stage IIB:	Unilateral tumor with complete or incomplete gross excision; positive ipsilateral regional lymph nodes; identifiable contralateral lymph nodes negative microscopically
Stage III:	Tumor infiltrating across the midline with or without regional lymph node involvement; or, unilateral tumor with contralateral regional lymph node involvement; or, midline tumor with bilateral lymph nodes negative
Stage IV:	Dissemination of tumor to distant lymph nodes, bone, bone marrow, liver, and/or other organs (except as defined in stage IV-S)
Stage IV-S:	Localized primary tumor as defined for stage I or II with dissemination limited to liver, skin, and/or bone marrow

*Data from reference 52.

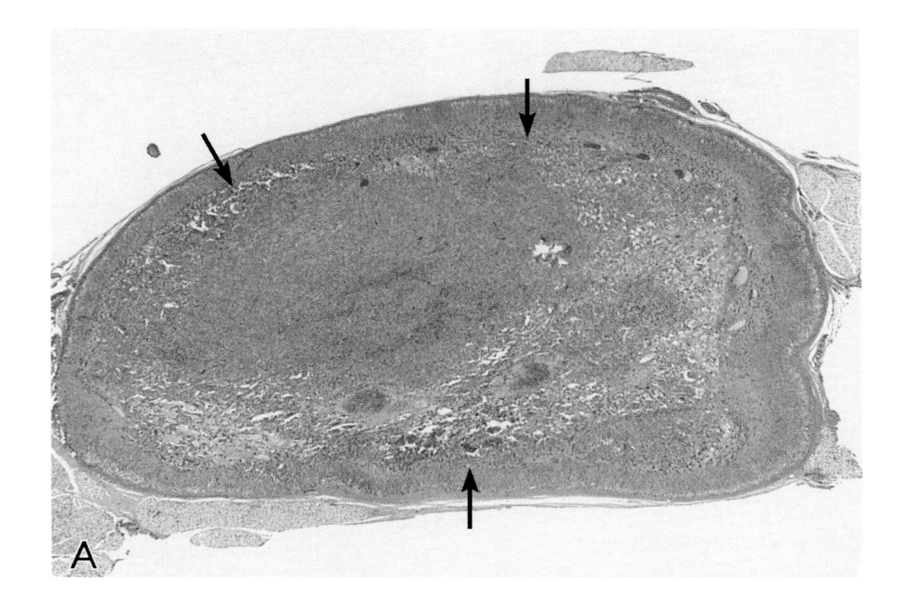

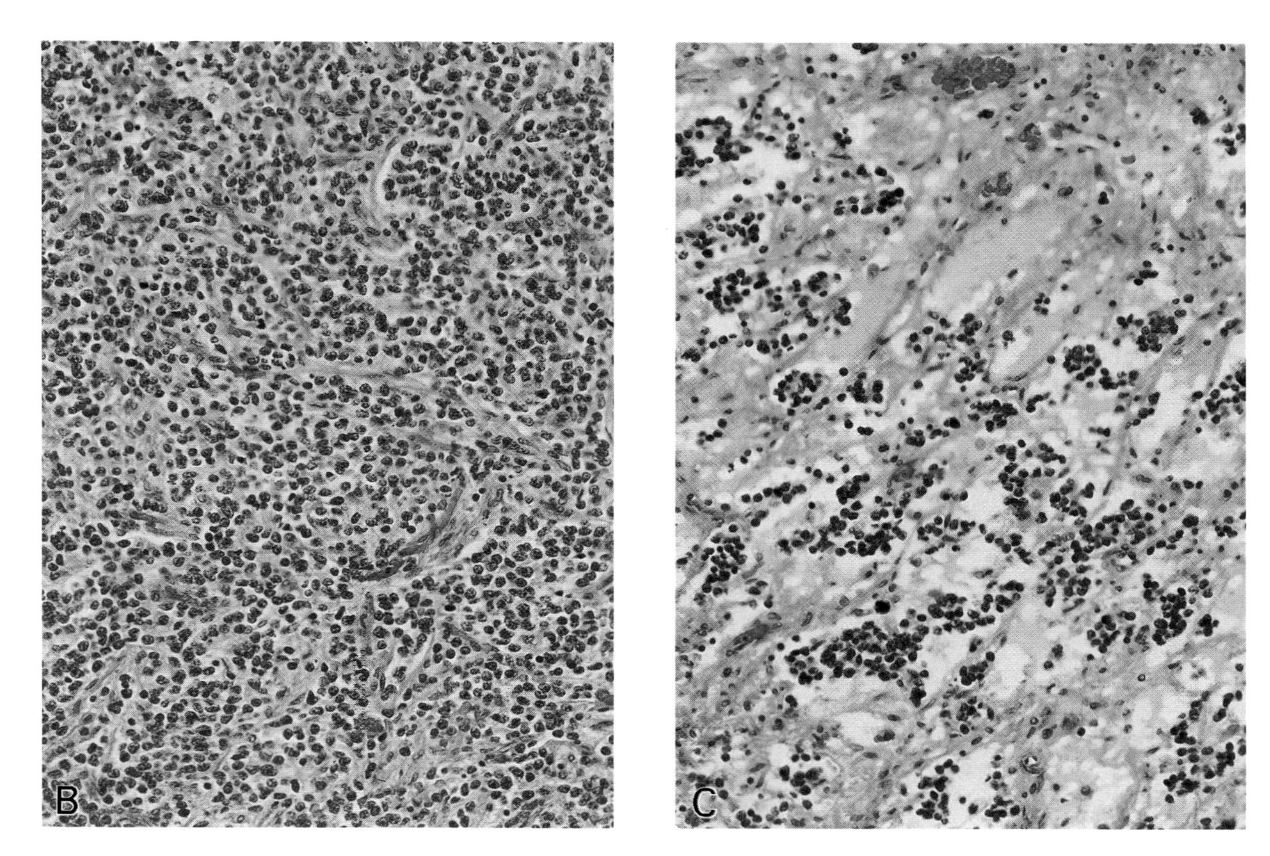

Figure 23-7
IN SITU NEUROBLASTOMA

A: Incidental in situ neuroblastoma in a 26-day-old girl who died of congenital heart disease. The tumor measured 6 mm in diameter. The junction with residual adult or definitive cortex is indicated by arrows.

B: This in situ neuroblastoma is composed of sheets of monotonous primitive cells.

C: Secondary degenerative features can sometimes be found, such as edema and microcystic change.

indistinguishable from childhood NB, but without evidence of tumor anywhere else. The size of the in situ NBs in their study ranged from 0.7 to 9.5 mm. In situ NB has been found anywhere from 1 in 39 (65) to 1 in 244 autopsies (64) on infants less than 3 months of age, a greater incidence than for clinically overt NB, suggesting that the lesion involutes or matures "spontaneously" or otherwise remains clinically occult (63). The increased frequency reported in the study by Guin et al. (65) was due to careful prospective evaluation of adrenal glands yielding 5 to 12 specimen blocks from each gland. Other possibilities include evolution into an adrenal cyst or a calcified scar (68). In situ NB has been associated with an adrenal cyst, very similar to cystic NB (69). The nodules of neuroblasts which are an integral part of normal development of the adrenal gland (see chapter 1) may be hard to distinguish from in situ NB (66,67,70).

Stage IV-S Neuroblastoma. Stage IV-S NB is a distinctive subgroup with distant metastases to liver (fig. 23-8), skin (fig. 23-9), or bone marrow without evidence of bone metastases

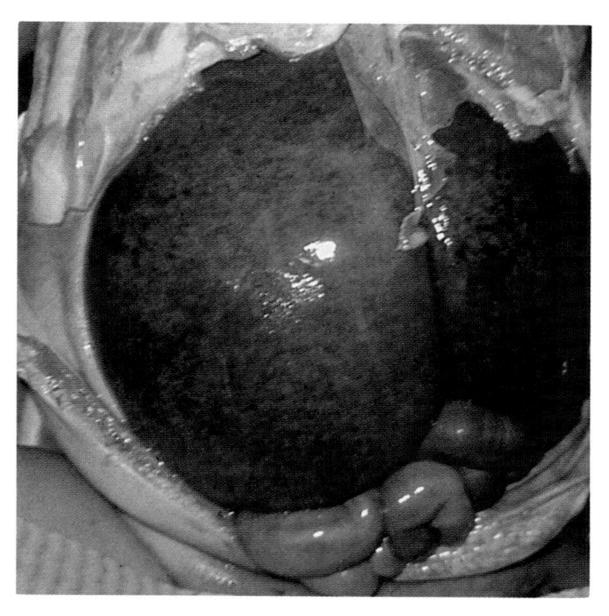

Figure 23-8
STAGE IV-S NEUROBLASTOMA
An infant with stage IV-S neuroblastoma massively involving the liver at autopsy. Marked hepatomegaly such as this due to metastatic neuroblastoma can compromise function of vital organs and result in death.

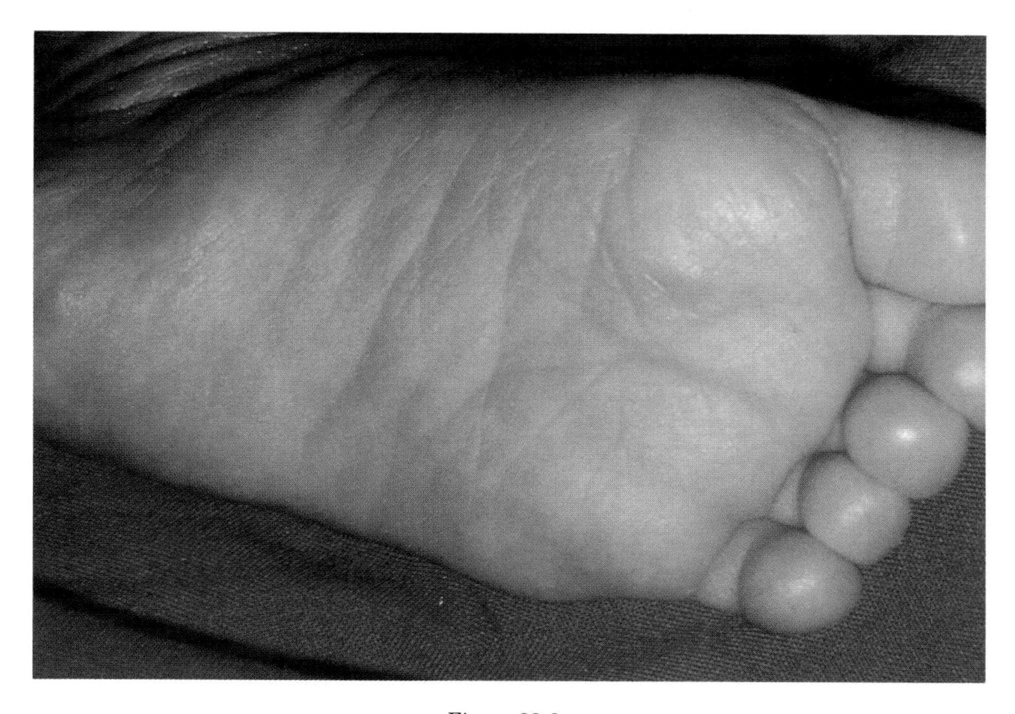

Figure 23-9
STAGE IV-S NEUROBLASTOMA
Stage IV-S neuroblastoma with multiple cutaneous metastases presenting as mobile blue-gray nodules. This appearance has led to the fanciful description "blueberry muffin" baby.

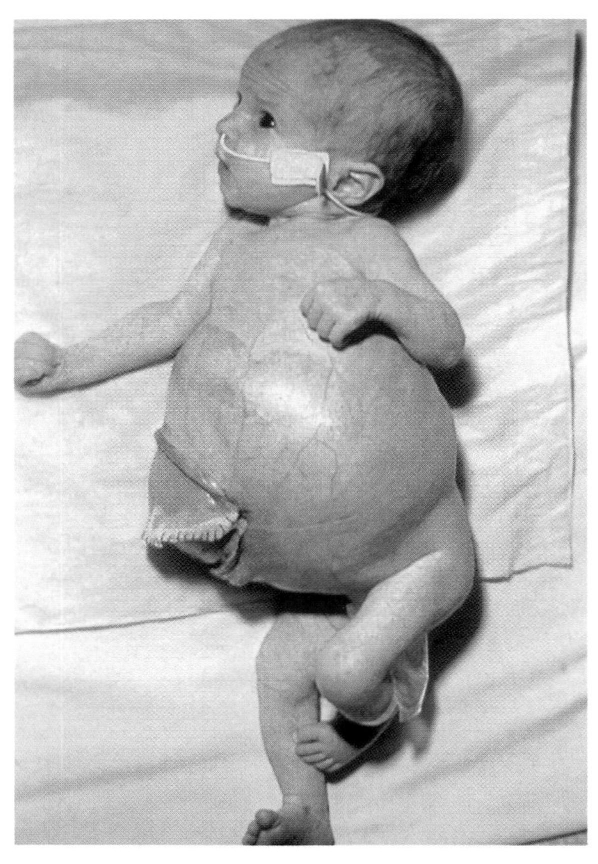

Figure 23-10
STAGE IV-S NEUROBLASTOMA
This infant has massive hepatomegaly due to metastatic neuroblastoma. Intra-abdominal pressure is partially relieved by a silastic pouch.

(see Table 23-3) (72,73,82). There is usually a small intra-abdominal adrenal primary, but in 10 percent of cases no primary tumor can be identified (72). Stage IV-S NB usually occurs in infants, with a median age of about 3 months (78), but is occasionally found in those over the age of 1 year. The prognosis is good, with survival rates of 80 to 87 percent (72,73,81) despite an immense tumor burden. Spontaneous regression has been documented, and some have proposed that stage IV-S NB represents hyperplastic nodules of nonmalignant neural tissue bearing a mutation that interferes with normal development, and a second "hit" or further event transforms the lesions into malignant neoplasms such as malignant schwannoma or NB (77). No significant cytogenetic abnormalities have been described (71), and the patients usually lack the adverse prognostic findings associated with stage IV NB (76) or the high frequency of N-*myc* oncogene amplification (74,75), although exceptions have been noted (79).

In 1901 Pepper (80) described six infants who were noted in the first 6 weeks of life to have abdominal distension and massive liver enlargement due to "congenital sarcoma of the liver and suprarenal," which proved fatal 10 days to 16 weeks later. These patients probably had the "high-risk" type of stage IV-S NB with massive enlarging hepatomegaly and secondary complications such as compromise of cardiac, respiratory, and renal function (81). Low-dose radiotherapy or chemotherapy may be of benefit in stage IV-S disease; surgical procedures such as formation of a silastic pouch relieve intra-abdominal pressure (fig. 23-10) (73,81). The designation IV-P (P = Pepper) has been proposed for this high-risk group (81).

Gross Findings. The gross morphology of NB and GNB can vary considerably from a relatively circumscribed ovoid mass to a massive multilobulated tumor measuring 10 cm or larger (99). A very small adrenal primary may give the impression of "encapsulation" (fig. 23-11), but part of the perceived capsule may be that of the adrenal capsule proper. Some tumors are massive (fig. 23-12), and entirely eclipse the associated adrenal gland, making it difficult or impossible to determine the precise anatomic site of origin (fig. 23-13). The tumor usually presents as a solitary, unicentric mass or contiguous aggregation of large nodules of tumor; bilateral adrenal NB or GNB or multicentric nondisseminated tumors are unusual (91,97,100). Several examples of NB extending into the inferior vena cava have been reported, including one extending into the right atrium (88). The color and consistency of tumors in cross section may vary depending upon the extent of hemorrhage or necrosis, and the amount and distribution of the stromal component, be it the fibrillary component resembling neuropil or a cellular, schwannian matrix (fig. 23-14). In some tumors the composition may be strikingly different, with one portion well differentiated (e.g., ganglioneuroma) and one or more areas of NB; such tumors were referred to as *composite GNB* by Stout (84,104), and are included under the stroma-rich nodular grouping in the classification described by Shimada et al. (103).

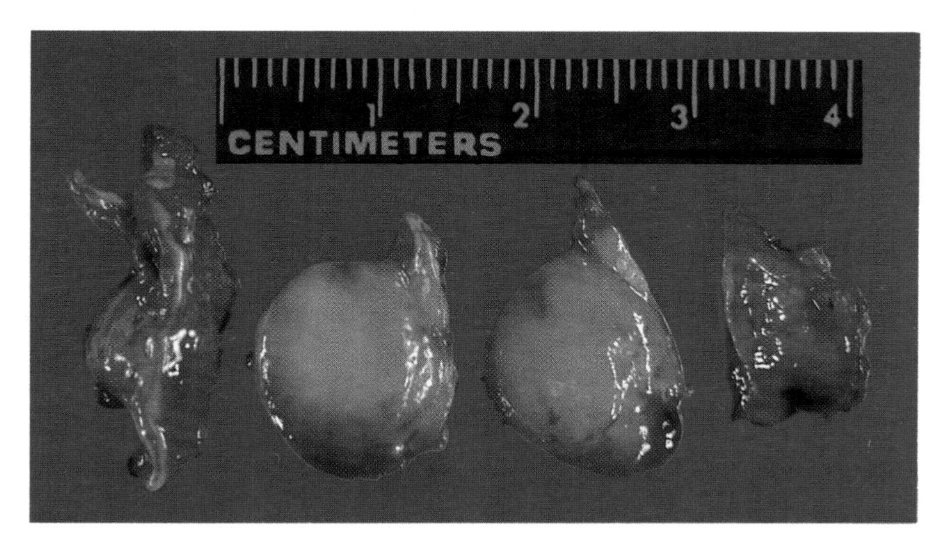

Figure 23-11
ADRENAL GANGLIONEUROBLASTOMA
Small adrenal ganglioneuroblastoma from a 3-year-old boy with stage IV neuroblastoma. The tumor is well-circumscribed and gray-white.

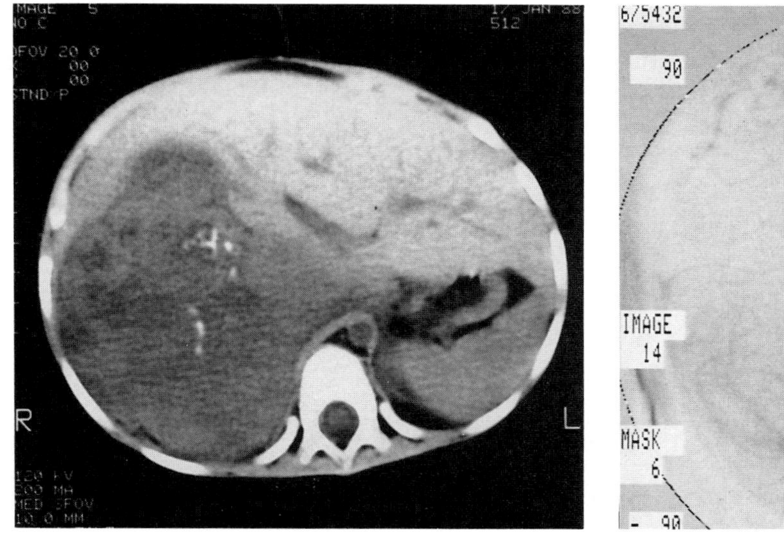

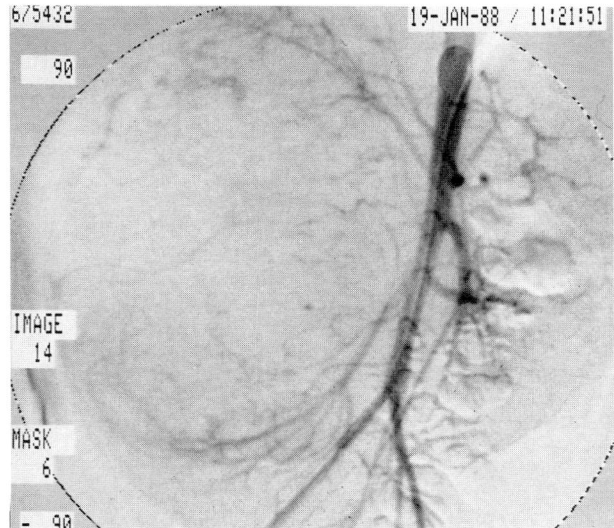

Figure 23-12
ABDOMINAL NEUROBLASTOMA
Left: Abdominal CT scan from a 2-year-old girl with a large neuroblastoma in right hemiabdomen with extension across the midline and some displacement of the aorta. Note also irregular calcifications within the tumor. (Fig. 14-14A,B from Lack EE. Pathology of adrenal and extra-adrenal paraganglia. Major problems in pathology, Vol 29. Philadelphia: WB Saunders Co., 1994:327.)
Right: Aortogram from the same case showing tenting and stretching of vessels by a large abdominal neuroblastoma.

On close inspection, bulging lobules of tumor may be deeply congested or hemorrhagic with a soft, almost encephaloid consistency (fig. 23-15). Cystic degeneration can be seen in some tumors, and on rare occasion a NB can rupture leading to retroperitoneal hemorrhage and shock (85, 102). Calcification may be apparent on gross inspection as punctate, opaque foci; as a conspicuous feature that can be readily appreciated on gross examination (fig. 23-16A,B); or as a gritty sensation. A specimen radiograph may vividly demonstrate the calcifications (fig. 23-16C).

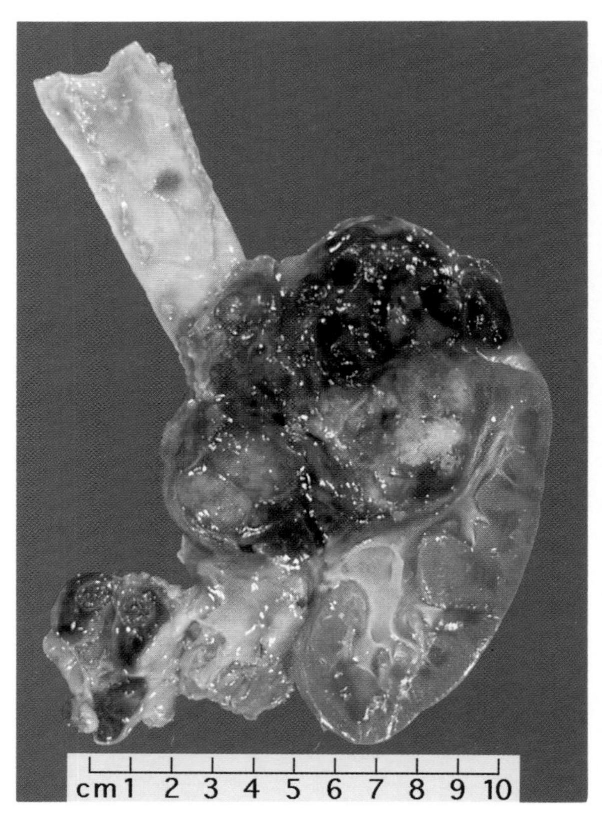

Figure 23-13
HEMORRHAGIC NEUROBLASTOMA

Cross section of a large hemorrhagic neuroblastoma of the left adrenal gland. The tumor replaced the entire adrenal gland and invaded the renal parenchyma. Note the coarse lobulations on cross section, with bulging nodules showing irregular areas of hemorrhage. The tumor had a soft, almost encephaloid, texture.

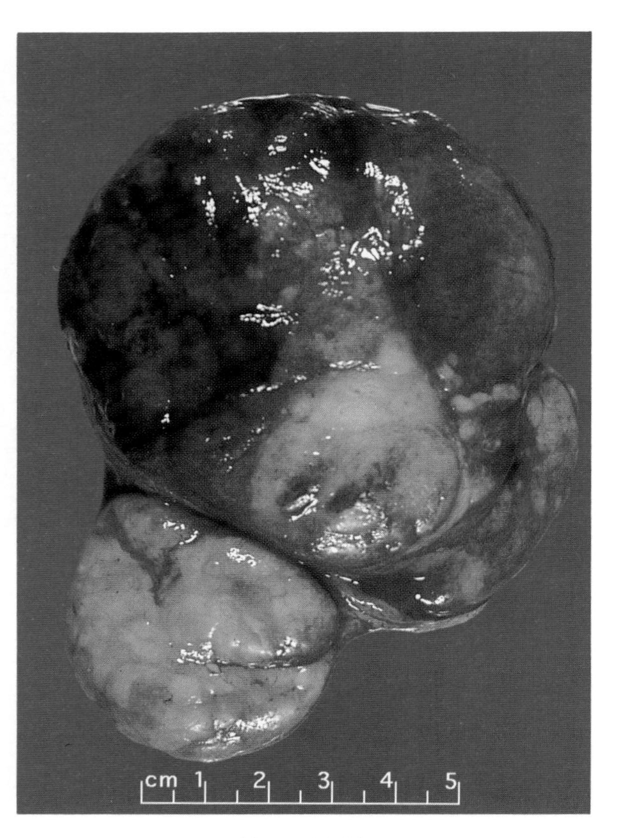

Figure 23-14
GANGLIONEUROBLASTOMA

This ganglioneuroblastoma on cross section shows a variation from hemorrhagic, bulging, irregular lobules to more pale, homogeneous foci. The tumor was stroma-poor by the Shimada classification.

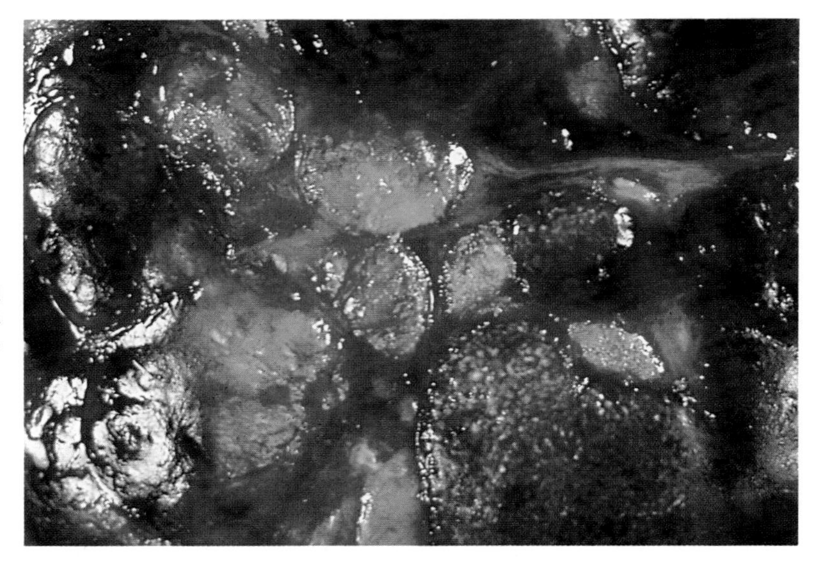

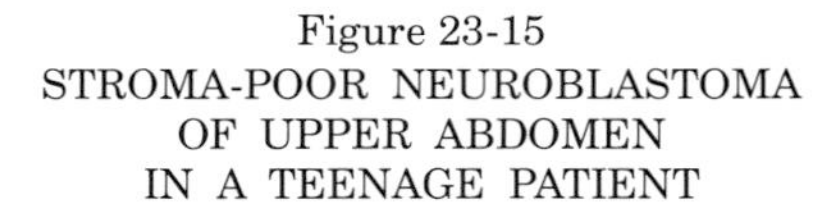

Figure 23-15
STROMA-POOR NEUROBLASTOMA
OF UPPER ABDOMEN
IN A TEENAGE PATIENT

Bulging nodules of tumor are congested and hemorrhagic with punctate yellowish areas representing dystrophic calcification.

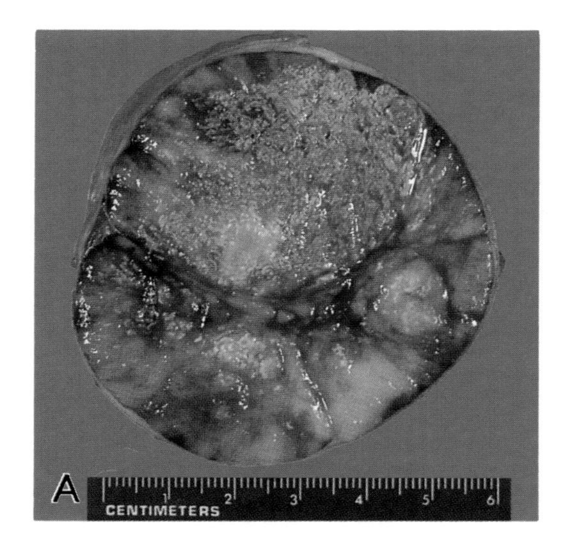

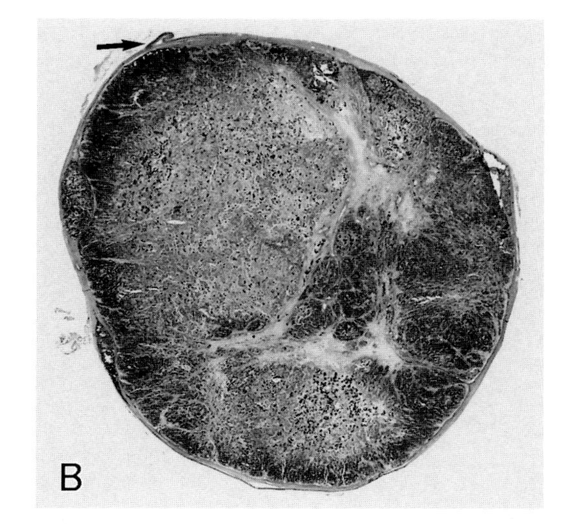

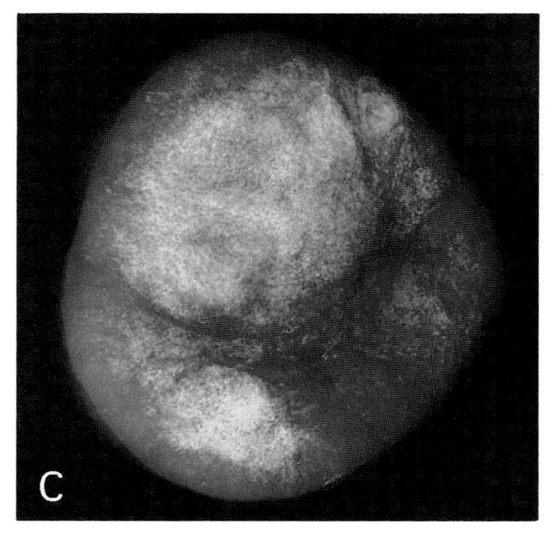

Figure 23-16
ADRENAL NEUROBLASTOMA

A: Cross section of a 174 g adrenal neuroblastoma from a 5-month-old boy. There is extensive calcification.

B: Low-power view of a histologic section of the same tumor shows punctate dark-staining areas corresponding to dystrophic calcifications. The adrenal remnant is at the top (arrow).

C: Specimen radiograph shows extensive foci of dystrophic calcification. (Figures B and C are figs. 7-6B, C from Lack EE, Kozakewich HP. Adrenal neuroblastoma, ganglioneuroblastoma, and related tumors. In: Lack EE, ed. Pathology of the adrenal glands. New York: Churchill Livingstone, 1990:282.)

Microscopic Findings. *Architectural Pattern.* NBs and GNBs often have a lobular growth pattern with delicate, often incomplete fibrovascular septa (fig. 23-17) (99,103). Sometimes there are areas with a more diffuse or solid pattern. A distinct organoid pattern has been recently described in which a thin fibrovascular meshwork isolates regular nests of NB cells; this is reported to be an indicator of good prognosis in younger children (92). Immunostaining for S-100 protein shows a prominent spindle cell component suggesting a close relationship between NB and Schwann cells. There is a continuum of microscopic morphology between undifferentiated NB (fig. 23-18) and GNB (83): at one end of the spectrum is the prototypical small "blue cell" tumor of childhood with a range of patterns which merge imperceptibly with GNB (fig. 23-19); at the other end are tumors which are so highly differentiated (in part or throughout) that they resemble ganglioneuroma (fig. 23-20). Most clinical series of childhood NBs include all neoplasms which fall within this wide spectrum (98,99). The correct diagnosis may be difficult, particularly with undifferentiated NBs, tumors that have been poorly fixed, or in biopsy specimens with crush artifact.

Cytomorphology. One of the most characteristic features of NB is the formation of Homer Wright rosettes (fig. 23-21) (106), although well-formed rosettes are often difficult to identify. The rosettes are circular, ovoid, or angular zones of

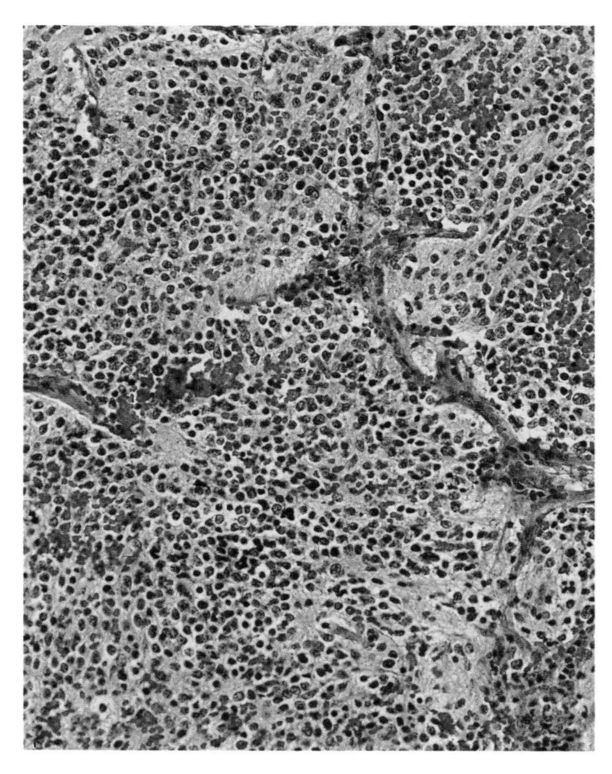

Figure 23-17
NEUROBLASTOMA
This neuroblastoma has a lobular architecture, but is not as well developed and organoid as pheochromocytomas or extra-adrenal paragangliomas.

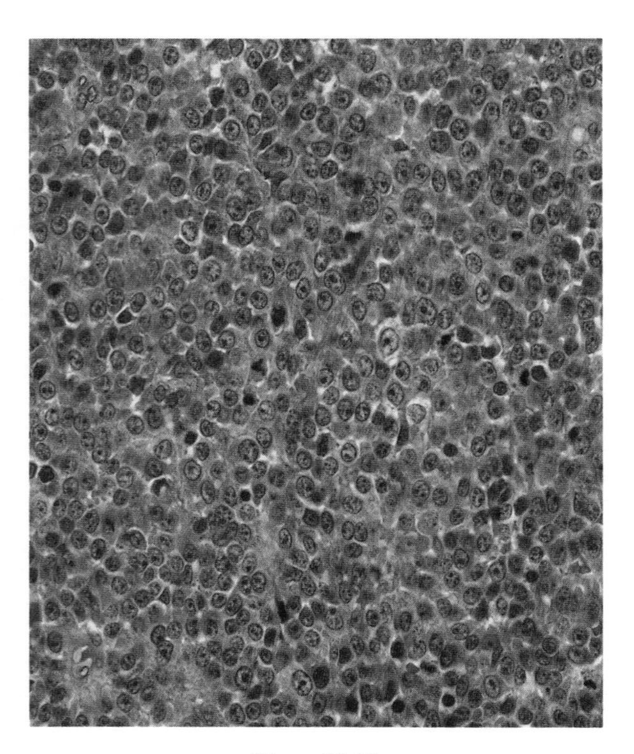

Figure 23-18
UNDIFFERENTIATED NEUROBLASTOMA
Closely packed, poorly differentiated neuroblasts form solid sheets. Patterns such as this may cause confusion with other childhood neoplasms such as malignant lymphoma. Many nuclei have a single, small nucleolus. The tumor had been fixed in B-5 fixative.

pale-staining, fibrillar material flanked circumferentially by tumor cells. The fibrillar matrix represents a tangled skein of neuritic cell processes. Sometimes a small vascular channel or collagenous tissue within the fibrillar zone is seen which is sometimes referred to as a pseudorosette. Homer Wright rosettes contrast sharply with the Flexner-Wintersteiner rosettes seen in retinoblastoma (fig. 23-22). Occasionally, Homer Wright rosettes have a prominent rhythmic or palisaded arrangement (fig. 23-23).

Nuclei of typical NBs are round or ovoid, often with dispersed nuclear chromatin, giving a stippled appearance or one likened to "salt and pepper" (fig. 23-24). Rarely, eosinophilic inclusions within nuclei have been reported (94). Anaplasia has been noted in some NBs with a striking degree of cellular and nuclear pleomorphism (fig. 23-25), which is different from the large maturing cells with ganglionic differentiation (87). Although anaplasia, as rigidly defined in Wilms' tumor (nephroblastoma), has important prognostic implications, at least before the use of more intensive chemotherapy (107), it appears doubtful that anaplasia in NB can be tested as a prognostic factor until more effective treatment is available (89). One study reported no statistically significant differences in survival with regard to anaplasia, and stage III and IV NB (86). Foci of spindle-shaped neuroblasts have also been reported (94), and may resemble those of rhabdomyosarcoma. Nuclei of most NBs are usually larger than nuclei of mature lymphocytes. Aggregates of lymphocytes may be seen in NB, GNB, and ganglioneuroma, and should not be confused with small primitive neuroblasts; if confusion arises, immunostaining for lymphoid markers should quickly resolve the issue (fig. 23-26A,B). Rarely, the lymphocytic and plasma cell infiltrate can be so intense that there may be some obliteration of the primary tumor (fig. 23-26C) (94).

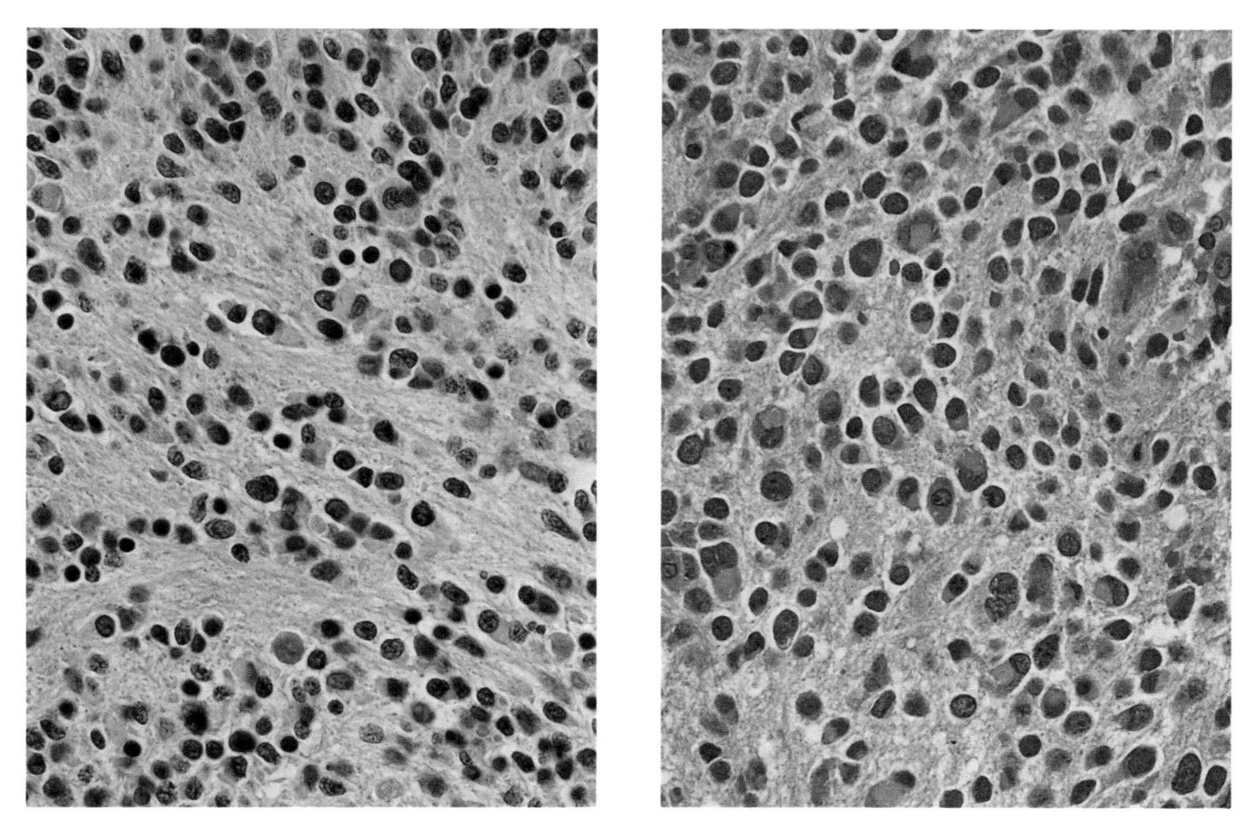

Figure 23-19
NEUROBLASTOMA AND GANGLIONEUROBLASTOMA

Left: Tumor cells of neuroblastoma are separated by pale pink fibrillar material representing neuritic cell processes. The tumor was largely undifferentiated, with only rare cells showing early ganglion cell differentiation.

Right: An area of ganglioneuroblastoma showing abundant, relatively immature ganglion cells.

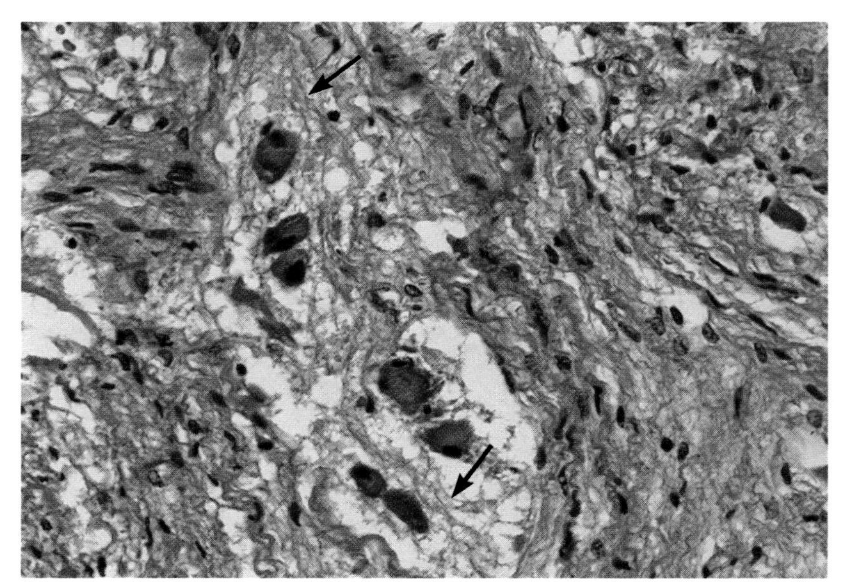

Figure 23-20
GANGLIONEUROBLASTOMA

A high level of ganglion cell differentiation was apparent along with a prominent schwannian spindle cell stroma, but the tumor is still incompletely differentiated as evidenced by fibrillary matrix (arrows).

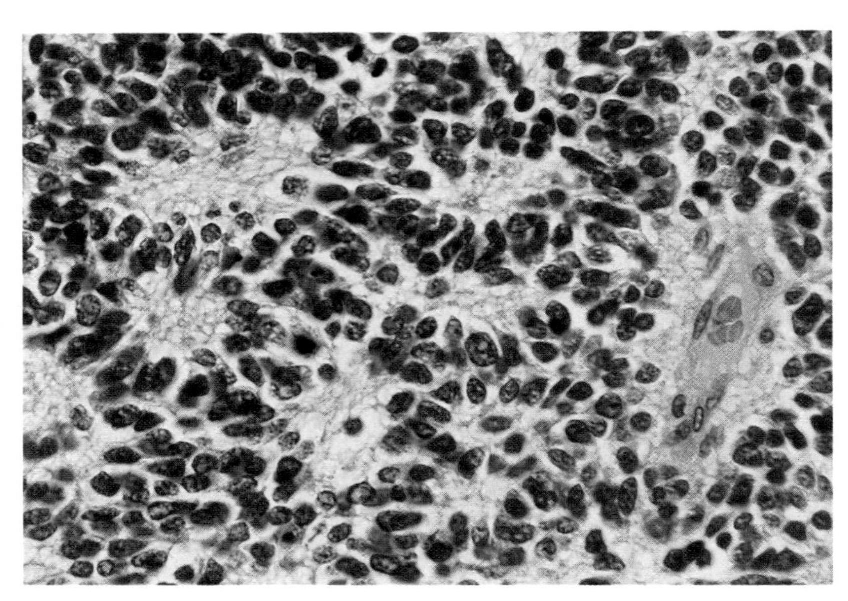

Figure 23-21
HOMER WRIGHT ROSETTES
IN A NEUROBLASTOMA

These Homer Wright rosettes appear as pale zones with fibrillar matrix corresponding to neuritic cell processes.

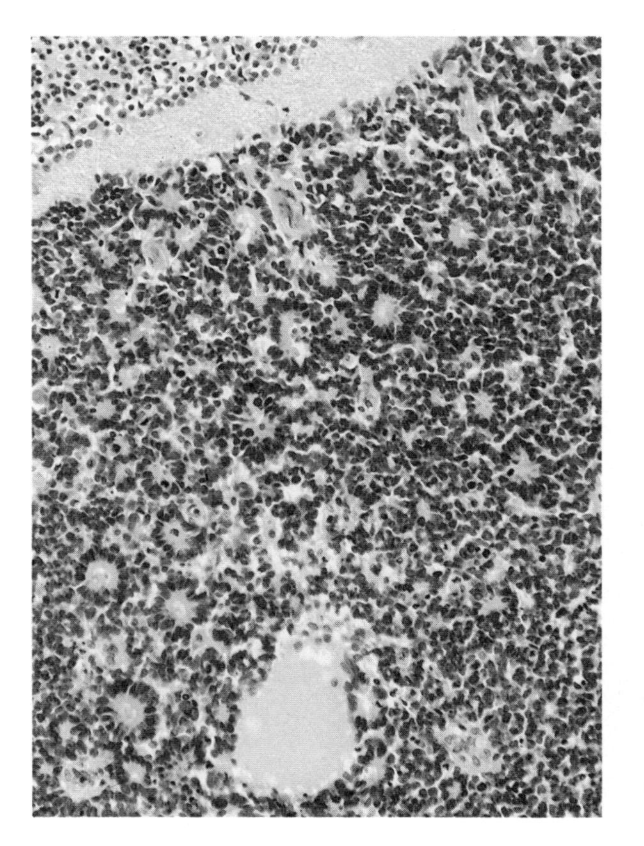

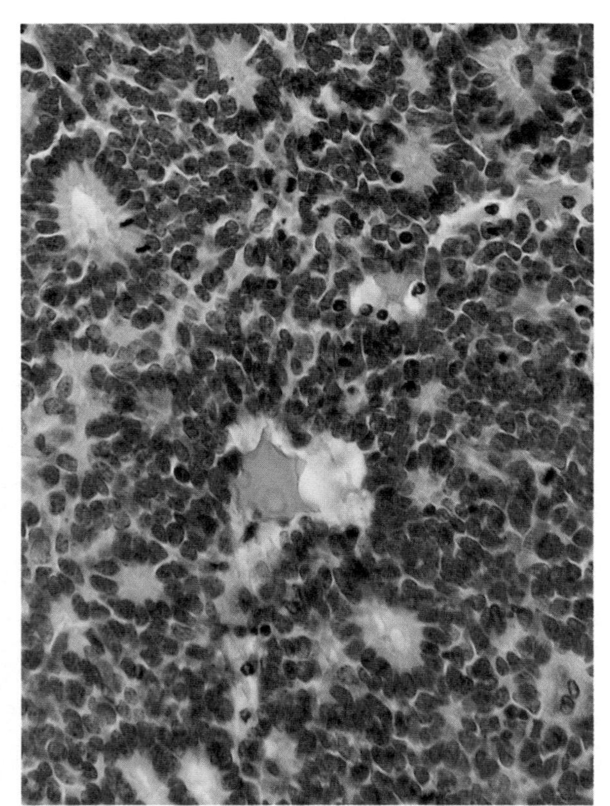

Figure 23-22
RETINOBLASTOMA

Left and right: This retinoblastoma has characteristic Flexner-Wintersteiner rosettes with circular alignment of short columnar cells around a central lumen.

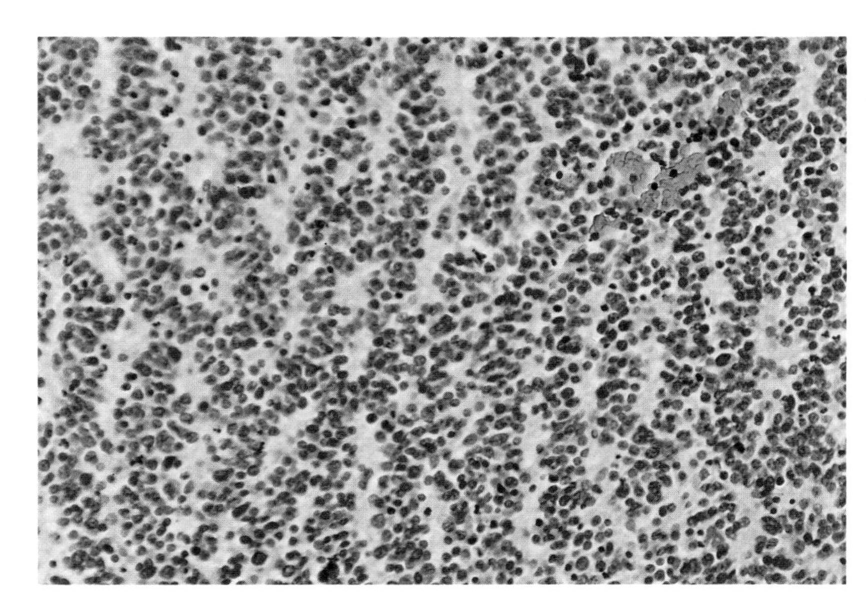

Figure 23-23
NEUROBLASTOMA
There is unusual palisading of Homer Wright rosettes in an almost parallel array.

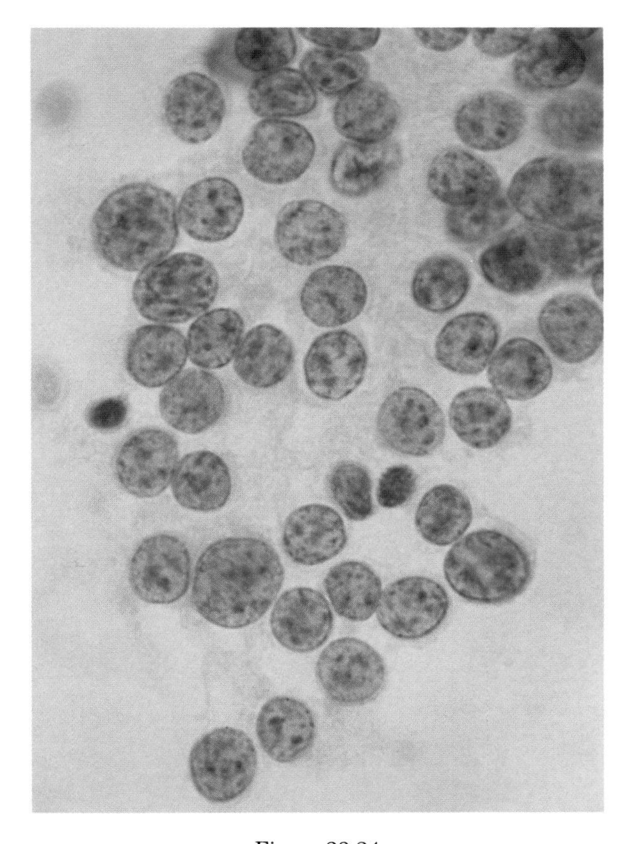

Figure 23-24
TOUCH IMPRINT OF NEUROBLASTOMA
Nuclei are round to oval, variable in size, and have a stippled chromatin pattern. Some cells have shaggy strands of pale cytoplasm.

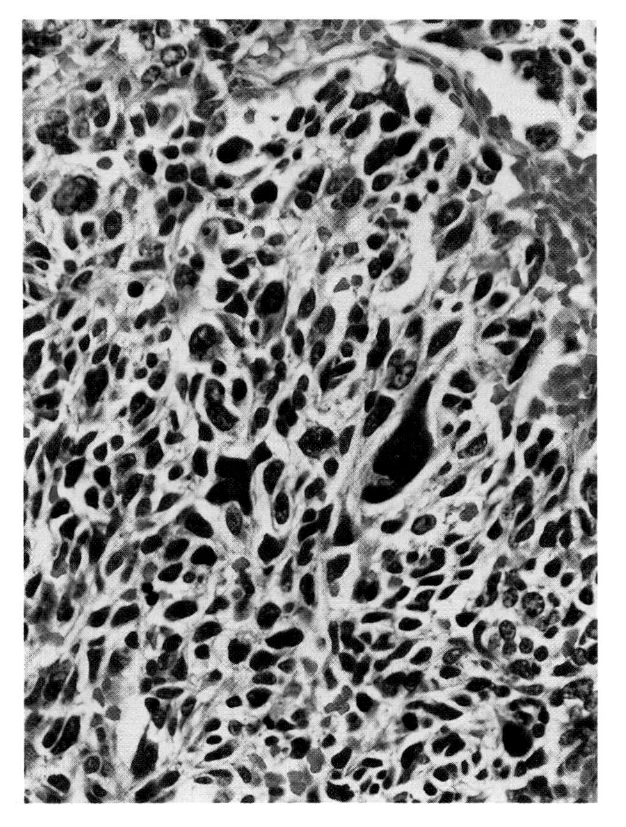

Figure 23-25
ANAPLASTIC NEUROBLASTOMA
Cells have pleomorphic, hyperchromatic nuclei.

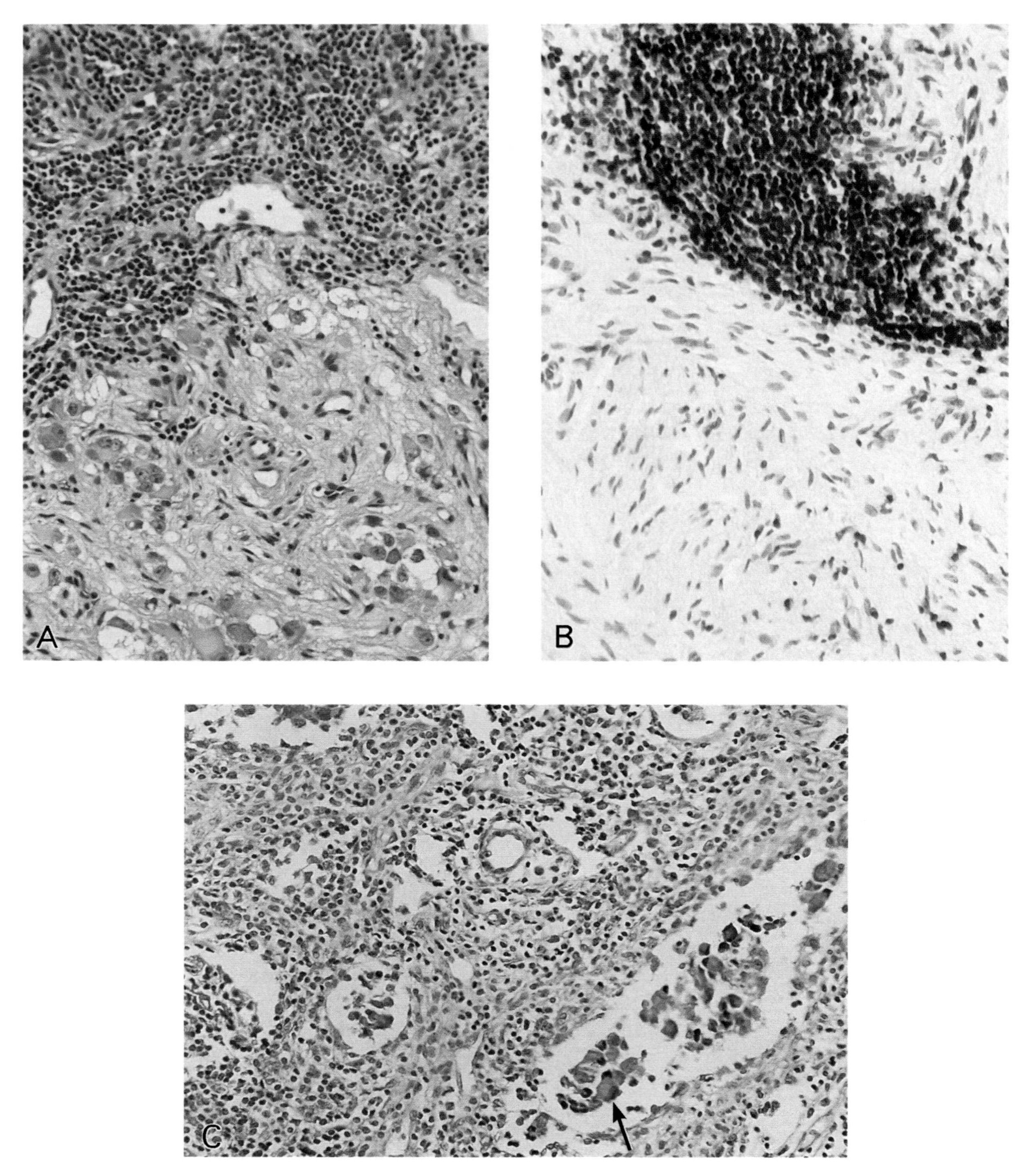

Figure 23-26
GANGLIONEUROBLASTOMA

A: There are perivascular aggregates of small cells with darkly stained nuclei which represent lymphocytes.

B: Immunostain for leukocyte common antigen highlights the aggregates of lymphocytes. (X200, Peroxidase- antiperoxidase stain)

C: Primary adrenal ganglioneuroblastoma had abundant lymphocytes and scattered lymphoid follicles with reactive germinal centers. Areas of tumor had dense infiltrates of lymphocytes with few residual islands of tumor showing some ganglion cell differentiation (arrow).

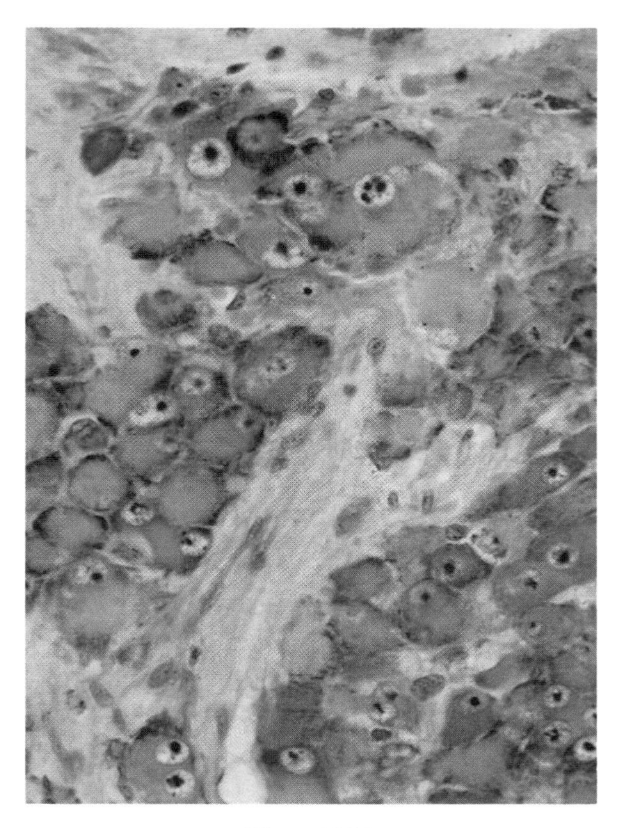

Figure 23-27
GANGLIONEUROBLASTOMA
There is a high level of ganglion cell differentiation. Note the coarsely granular material near the cell borders (Nissl substance) which has a similar tinctorial staining as the prominent nucleoli. (X200, Toluidine blue eosin stain)

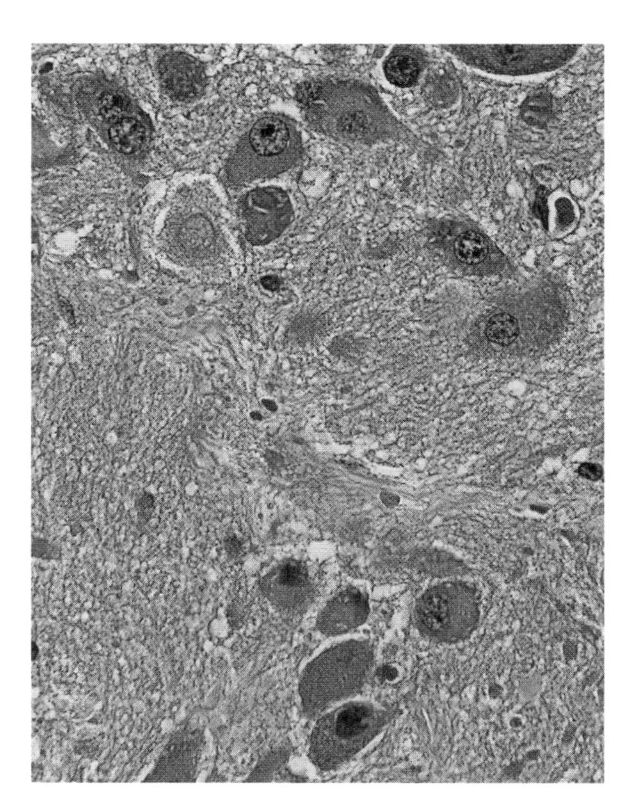

Figure 23-28
GANGLIONEUROBLASTOMA
Ganglioneuroblastoma, stroma-poor by the Shimada classification, in a 4-year-old child with watery diarrhea and elevated level of serum vasoactive intestinal peptide (VIP). There was a low mitosis-karyorrhexis index (MKI) and a high proportion of differentiating elements, placing the tumor in a favorable subgroup.

Cytomorphologic evidence of ganglion cell differentiation includes nuclear enlargement along with increasing amounts of eosinophilic cytoplasm and distinct cell borders. Nuclei may be eccentric in location with prominent nucleoli. Granular amphophilic material in the peripheral cytoplasm corresponds to Nissl substance, which represents rough endoplasmic reticulum; metachromatic stains may accentuate this material (fig. 23-27) (99). A GNB may be composed almost purely of fibrillar matrix and scattered ganglion cells (fig. 23-28), but this is an uncommon feature. Occasionally there is prominent brown, finely granular pigment, which is probably neuromelanin (90,91,93,101). Interestingly, the phenotype of NB cells in vitro may be schwannian and even melanocytic, replete with pigmented cells containing melanosomes (105).

Alterations in Stroma. Hemorrhage or necrosis may be a conspicuous feature in these tumors, and not infrequently there is dystrophic calcification which appears as fine, dust-like basophilic stippling or coarse, plaque-like areas (fig. 23-29). Intensely hemorrhagic NB may mimic a hematoma (fig. 23-30), with wide separation of nests of neuroblasts (fig. 23-31, left); rarely, an angiomatoid pattern is seen (fig. 23-31, right). An angiomatoid NB with intracytoplasmic glycogen has been reported (95). Some NBs undergo marked cystic alteration and simulate an adrenal cyst (fig. 23-32) or hematoma. A recent review of cystic NBs indicated a favorable prognosis (96). A focal sclerosing pattern has also been reported (94).

Ultrastructural Findings. Cytoplasmic organelles are generally sparse in NBs, with few mitochondria, small amounts of rough endoplasmic

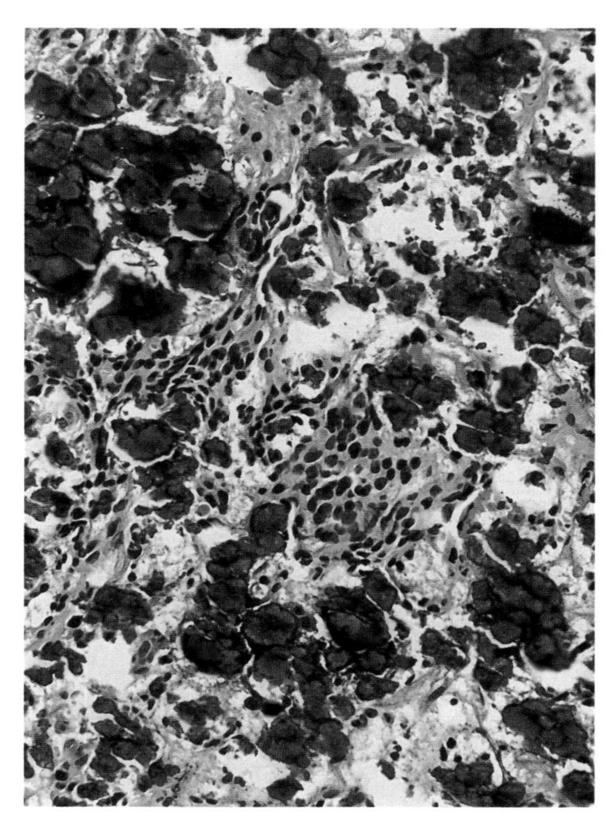

Figure 23-29
NEUROBLASTOMA
Neuroblastoma with irregular foci of dystrophic calcification. Prominent mineralization may give the tumor a faintly gritty consistency on sectioning.

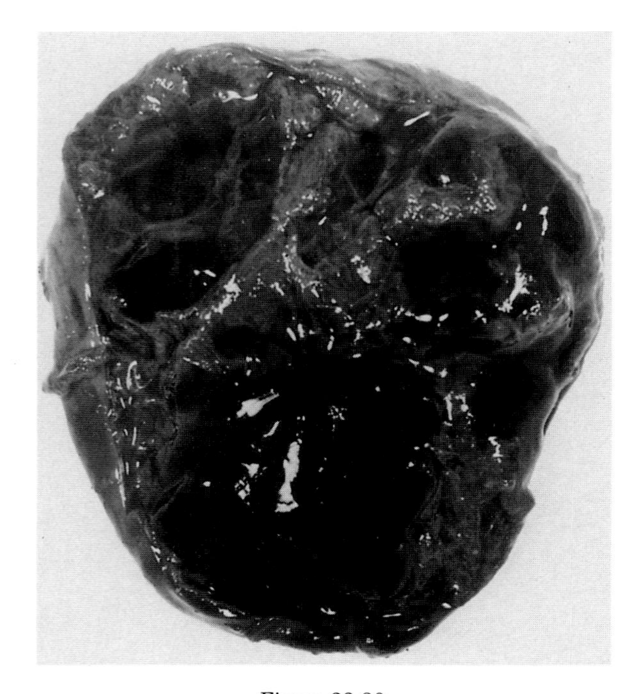

Figure 23-30
HEMORRHAGIC CYSTIC NEUROBLASTOMA
Congenital cystic neuroblastoma from an 11-day-old female. On cross section the tumor is markedly congested and hemorrhagic.

reticulum, and free ribosomes (fig. 23-33). The neuritic extensions of cell cytoplasm can be impressive in some tumors, with a prominent fibrillary matrix at the light microscopic level, and where there is matted neuropil-like matrix, a complicated, seemingly haphazard intertwining of cell processes may be seen ultrastructurally (fig. 23-34). Nuclei are often rounded with a regular contour, finely dispersed nuclear chromatin, and some margination at the periphery; occasionally, the nuclear membrane is slightly irregular or indented and one or more small nucleoli may be seen. A characteristic morphologic feature of NB and GNB is the presence of small, dense-core neurosecretory granules, usually within neuritic cell processes, but they may be sparse and difficult to distinguish from primary lysosomes (109,115,116). Neurosecretory granules can occasionally be recognized in the perinuclear cytoplasm or perikaryon. The granules are usually small and uniform, and are about one third to half the size of dense-core neurosecretory granules in pheochromocytomas (113). The average size of granules in one study was 100 nm (112). The diagnostic features include the presence of dense-core neurosecretory granules along with neuritic cell processes with fine neurofilaments 8 to 12 nm wide and neurotubules 24 to 26 nm in diameter (108,112–116). A positive correlation has been shown between the number of neurosecretory-type granules in undifferentiated NBs and prognostically favorable histochemical excretory patterns (112).

With advancing levels of cellular differentiation in GNB, some cells may acquire structural features resembling ganglionic cells in a fully mature ganglioneuroma. The nucleus has an eccentric location with a prominent nucleolus and frequent margination of heterochromatin against the nuclear membrane (fig. 23-35). There may be small, disorderly profiles of rough endoplasmic reticulum, particularly in the peripheral cytoplasm, and only rarely are there

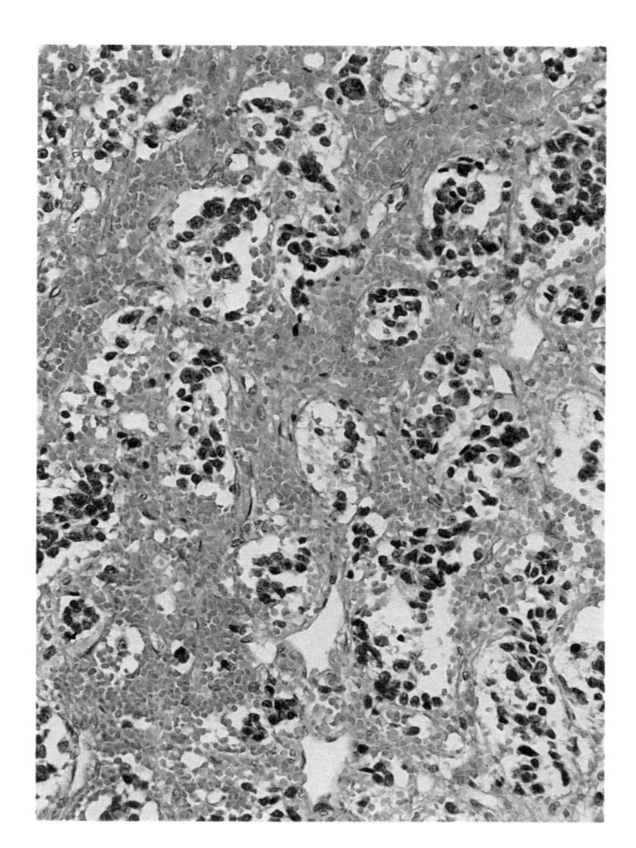
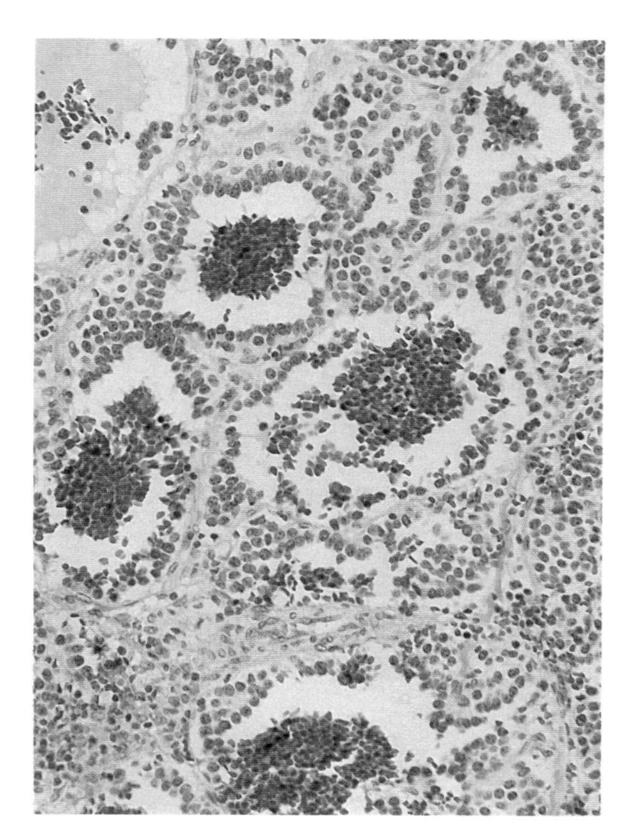

Figure 23-31
NEUROBLASTOMA
Left: Neuroblastoma with marked hemorrhage separating small irregular nests of tumor cells.
Right: Neuroblastoma with an angiomatoid pattern.

orderly stacks or lamellar profiles, which may be found in a fully mature ganglion cell (Nissl substance) (109). Thin cytoplasmic processes can partially envelop cells with ganglionic differentiation consistent with satellite cells. It is uncommon to obtain a ganglion cell with an attached neuritic or neuronal extension in the same plane of section. The terms "neuritic" or "neuronal" are appropriately noncommittal for these cytoplasmic extensions since it is not possible to be specific as to whether the process is a classic axon or dendrite (109). In GNBs with a spindle cell, schwannian matrix, there are Schwann cells with a well-developed myelin sheath enclosing neuritic cell processes (fig. 23-36). Glycogen has been noted within some NBs (110, 117,118), but is uncommon. In a large study of nearly 100 NBs, intracytoplasmic glycogen was noted in less than 5 percent (110); if abundant intracellular glycogen is noted, prompt consideration should be given to other neoplasms in the differential diagnosis (109). Primitive intercellular junctions have been described (110).

Immunohistochemical Findings. Sometimes the primitive cytomorphology of undifferentiated NB has muted or equivocal immunophenotypic "signals" of diagnostic value, and careful correlation with other findings such as ultrastructure may be indicated (137). Immunostaining for NSE is usually readily apparent in NB and GNB (158), with highlighting of neuritic extensions in the form of rosettes, matted neuropil, or sparse internuclear fibrillar matrix (fig. 23-37). Cells with neuronal or ganglionic differentiation may also be immunoreactive. The wide range of structures stained with NSE may mandate correlation with routine morphology and other features to ensure specificity. Virtually all

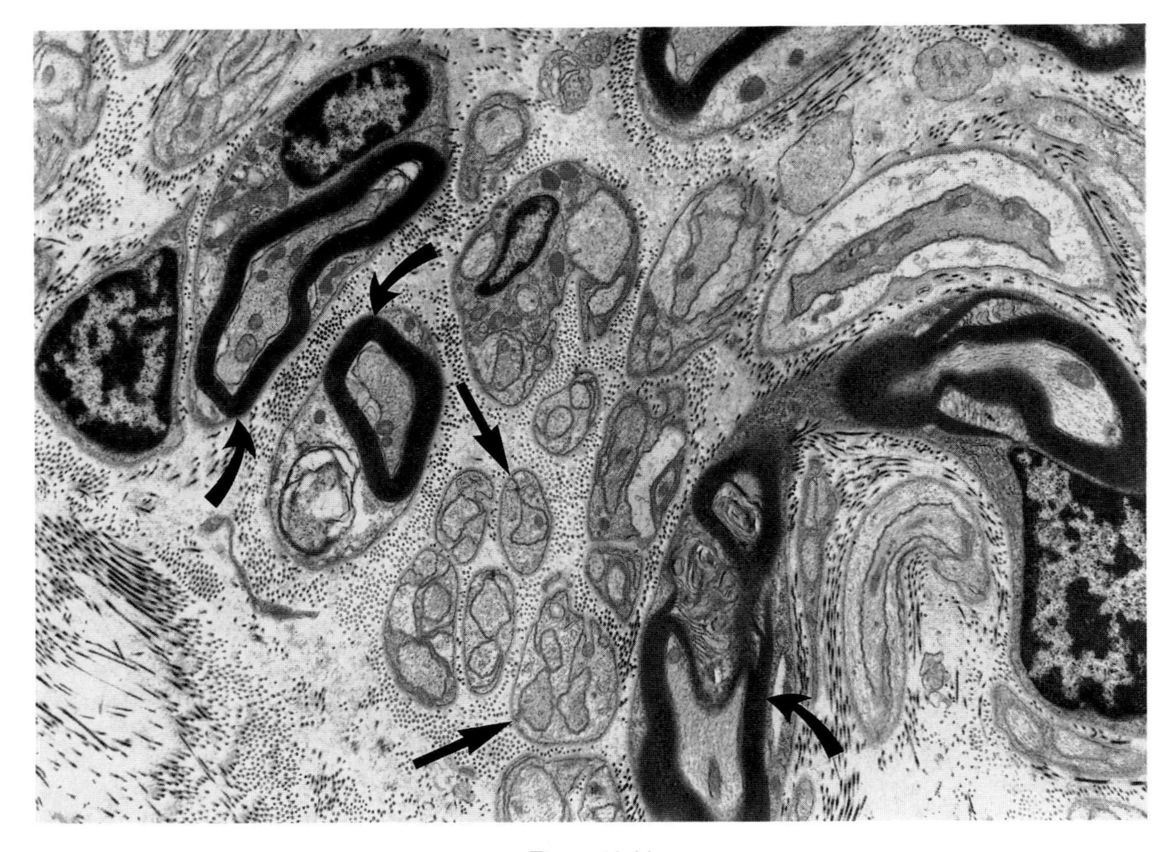

Figure 23-36
NEUROBLASTOMA, STROMA-RICH, INTERMIXED IN THE SHIMADA CLASSIFICATION
The spindle cell, schwannian matrix is composed of numerous neuritic processes ensheathed by Schwann cells forming mesaxons (straight arrows). A well-developed myelin sheath (curved arrows) is seen. (X6,000)

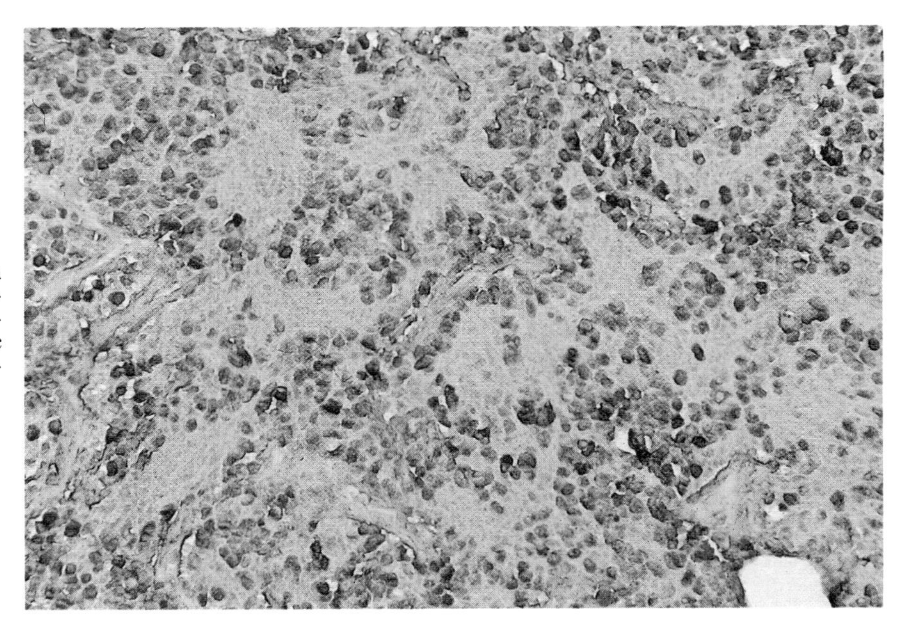

Figure 23-37
HEMORRHAGIC NEUROBLASTOMA
Hemorrhagic neuroblastoma stained for neuron-specific enolase. The tumor cells are separated by edema and hemorrhagic stroma. (X100, Peroxidase-antiperoxidase stain)

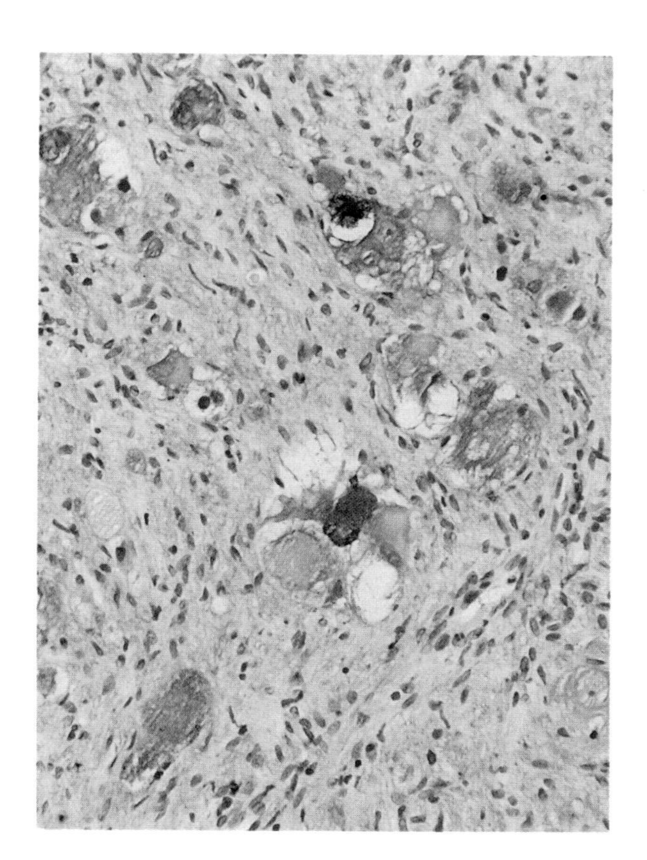

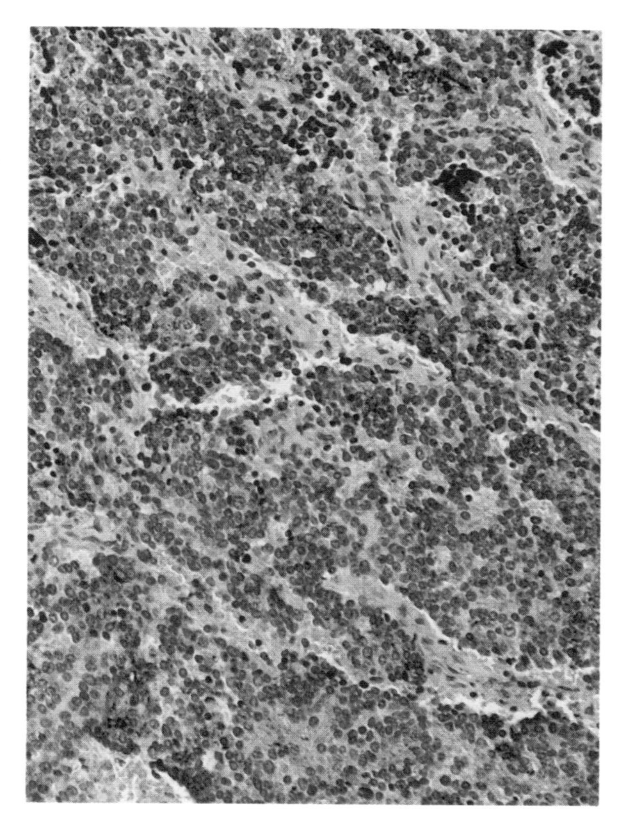

Figure 23-38
STROMA-RICH INTERMIXED NEUROBLASTOMA AND STROMA-POOR NEUROBLASTOMA

Left: Immunoreactivity for chromogranin A is most evident in scattered ganglionic cells, but could also be seen in pale fibrillar areas with overlapping, intertwining neuritic processes. (X200, Peroxidase-antiperoxidase stain)

Right: Tumor stains for chromogranin A, particularly in the Homer Wright rosettes where there is intertwining and overlapping of neuritic processes. (X200, Peroxidase-antiperoxidase stain)

staining for norepinephrine might be related to neuronal uptake of this catecholamine (138). Detection of intracytoplasmic catecholamines is possible by fluorescence methods using formaldehyde (128,130) or glyoxylic acid (154), but because of technical problems and availability of other diagnostic tests, this is seldom necessary.

Human NB cells in vitro have been shown to have a diverse morphologic phenotype including: 1) neuronal cells with neuritic processes and neurosecretory granules; 2) cells resembling Schwann cells; and 3) melanocytic cells replete with melanosomes (160). Interconversion (or transdifferentiation) of nonadrenergic cells and melanocytic cells has been demonstrated as well as an intermediate cell type, possibly representing a multipotential precursor (126). In normal adrenal neuroblasts the sequential expression of genes coding for tyrosine hydroxylase, chromogranin A, pG2, and beta$_2$-microglobulin marks successive stages in maturation of the chromaffin cell lineage, while cells of NB are "arrested" in this sequence, thus raising the possibility that malignant transformation of cells at different stages of maturation may account for some of the phenotypic diversity that characterizes these tumors (127).

Immunostaining for chromogranin A has been demonstrated in NBs, GNBs (fig. 23-38, left) (127, 131–134,138,142,146,153), and GNs (132,134, 142,163); positive results are expected where the concentration of neurosecretory granules is greatest, such as ganglionic cells with active synthesis or areas with overlapping or intertwining of numerous neuritic processes (e.g., Homer Wright rosettes) (fig. 23-38, right) or matted

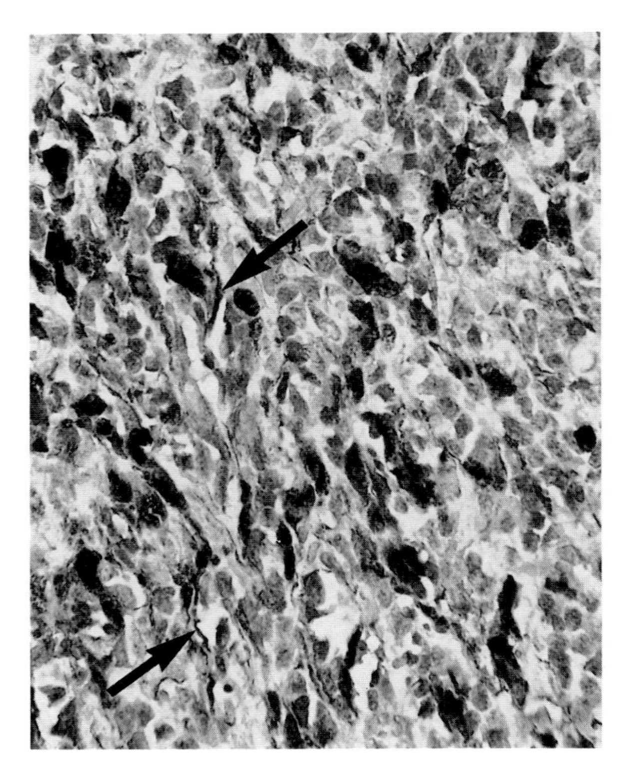

Figure 23-39
GANGLIONEUROBLASTOMA
Immunostain for neurofilament protein highlights slender to plump neuritic processes (arrows). The cytoplasm of some cell bodies is also intensely positive. (X200, Peroxidase-antiperoxidase stain)

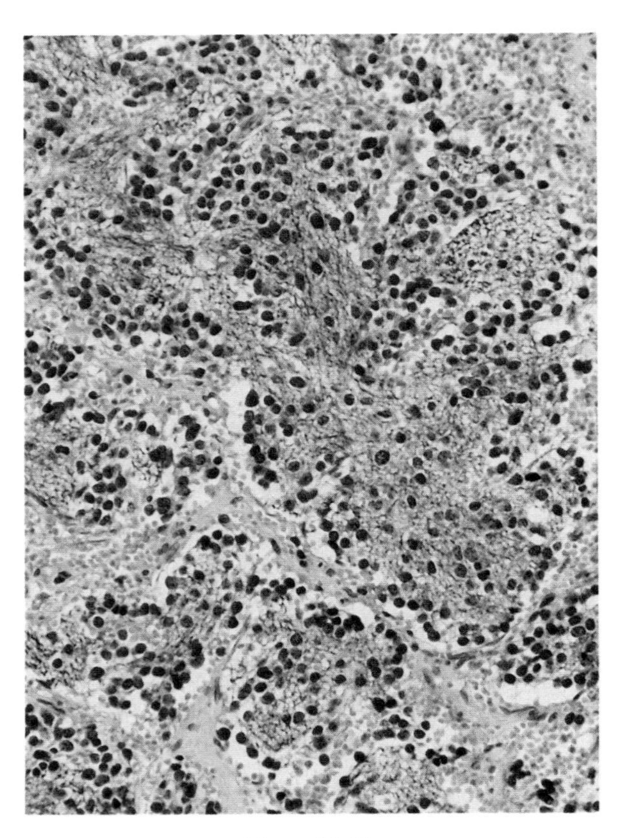

Figure 23-40
NEUROBLASTOMA
Immunostain for MAP-2 highlights abundant neuritic processes. A nearly identical pattern was seen with stain for J-1 tubulin. (X200, Peroxidase-antiperoxidase stain)

neuropil. Immunohistochemical staining has also been demonstrated for other neuroendocrine markers, such as other members of the chromogranin family (146), synaptophysin (131,134, 142), protein gene product (PGP) 9.5 (163), HNK-1 (137), and HISL (163). There may be immunostaining for neurofilament proteins (fig. 23-39), with some variability in staining for the three types (120,133,142,145). Monoclonal antibodies to neuronal microtubule–associated proteins (MAP-1 and MAP-2) may be strongly reactive with neuroblasts (fig. 23-40), ganglion cells, and neurofibrils; staining for alpha- and beta-tubulin may show a similar pattern of reactivity (120,124). Immunostaining has also been reported for peripherin, a type of intermediate filament expressed in the peripheral nervous system (149); it has been regarded as evidence of cell maturation in NB and enhanced expression has been associated with improved prognosis (139).

As already noted, some tumors may be associated with a watery diarrhea syndrome due to the secretion of vasoactive intestinal peptide (VIP); VIP can be demonstrated in cells showing neuronal and ganglionic differentiation (fig. 23-41). The distribution of VIP mRNA is confined to the cytoplasm of cells with ganglionic differentiation and not undifferentiated neuroblastic cells (164). Increased VIP levels in NB have been correlated with cellular differentiation and favorable tumor stage (152), and there is some suggestion that both VIP and somatostatin may function as autocrine growth factors at the cellular level, with perhaps some modulation of differentiation (144,151, 152). P glycoprotein, encoded by the *mdr*-1 gene, has a role in multidrug resistance to chemotherapy through a drug efflux pump at the cellular level which is ATP dependent; it has been expressed

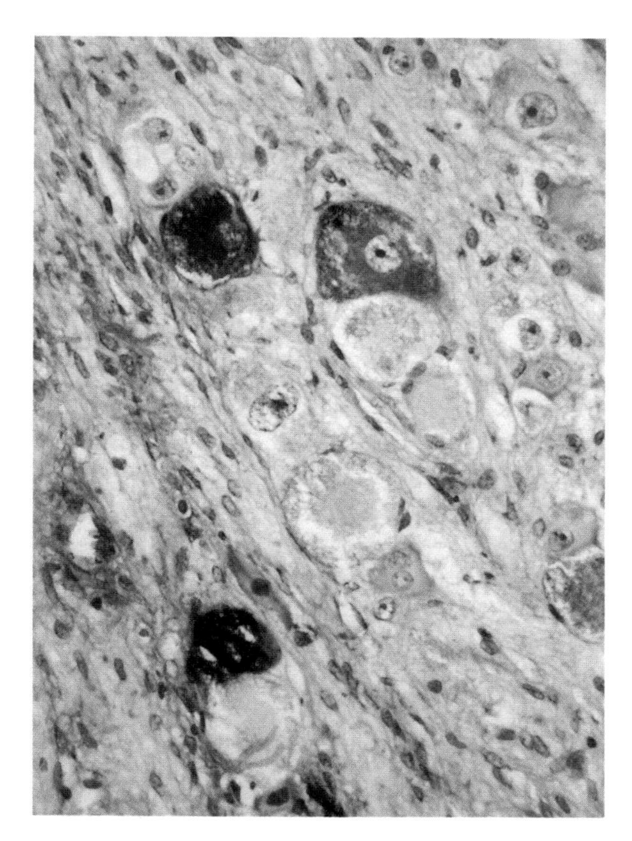

Figure 28-41
NEUROBLASTOMA, STROMA-RICH
Neuroblastoma, stroma-rich, intermixed in the Shimada classification, was associated with watery diarrhea syndrome and elevated serum level of vasoactive intestinal peptide (VIP). Immunostaining demonstrated numerous ganglionic cells positive for VIP. (X300, Peroxidase-antiperoxidase stain)

immunohistochemically in stage IV NB, but was not detected in a recent study of stage IV-S NBs (125). Expression of *mdr*-1/p-glycoprotein is reported to be increased in differentiating cells such as mature ganglion cells (121). The protein encoded by the N-*myc* oncogene (136,159) or N-*myc* RNA expression (159) can also be detected, and quantitation of this protein may be correlated with prognosis (129,136). A significant proportion of aggressive NBs lack genomic amplification of N-*myc*, yet some tumors can express N-*myc* RNA and protein (162).

Immunostaining for S-100 protein may demonstrate small to elongate dendritic-shaped cells in NB and GNB, particularly in fibrovascular septa separating nests of tumor cells (fig. 23-42, left); these have been regarded as Schwann cells or precursor cells, suggesting an avenue of differentiation within the tumor (141). These S-100 positive cells are also situated in the same area in which sustentacular cells are found in paragangliomas. Some cells in close proximity to neuronal or ganglion cells are consistent with satellite cells, and may also be immunoreactive for S-100 protein (fig. 23-42, right). Immunoreactivity for S-100 protein has been used to evaluate differentiation of NB cells into Schwann cells, and may provide some information regarding prognosis (119,123,141,155), even though it is not entirely specific for Schwann cells (135,161). Immunoreactivity for S-100 protein has been correlated with other prognostic factors such as age and mitosis-karyorrhexis index (MKI) (155) and favorable and unfavorable stroma-rich categories in the Shimada classification (119). An inverse relationship has been reported between immunopositivity for S-100 protein and ferritin with an increased number of ferritin-positive cells (stromal septa and NB cells) being associated with unfavorable outcome (119).

Differentiating neuronal or ganglionic cells of NB are strongly positive for transforming growth factors beta-1 and beta-3, a group of regulatory proteins with a variable effect on cell growth and differentiation (140). Expression of other molecular markers such as TRK-A (122) and lack of high-affinity nerve growth factor receptors (157) may have some influence on prognosis. Hopefully, future studies will provide further information on the molecular aspects of these tumors and lead to major advances in treatment (137).

Cytology and Fine-Needle Aspiration Biopsy. Fine-needle aspiration (FNA)/biopsy or exfoliative cytology of NB and GNB typically shows a cellular specimen with small primitive cells which have a high nuclear/cytoplasmic ratio (fig. 23-43); amorphous fibrillar material may be seen in the background or attached directly to the cells. There may be one or two small nucleoli or small aggregates of chromatin that form chromocenters. Smear/imprint preparations of surgically resected specimens may provide valuable cytologic information (fig. 23-44). It is relatively uncommon to see Homer Wright rosettes in the aspirate (165, 168), and when found, may be intact or poorly formed (169). Ancillary diagnostic techniques such as electron microscopy and immunohistochemistry may be necessary to ensure

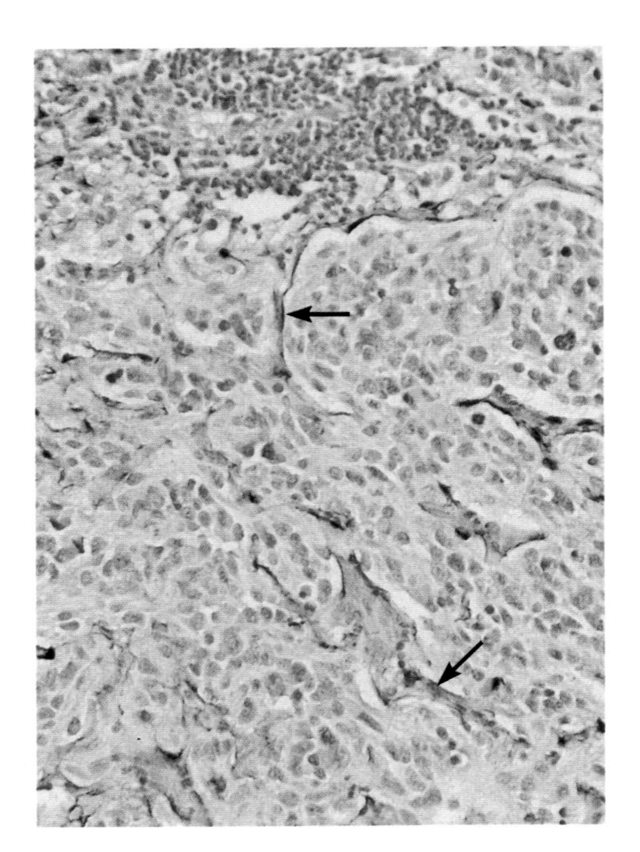
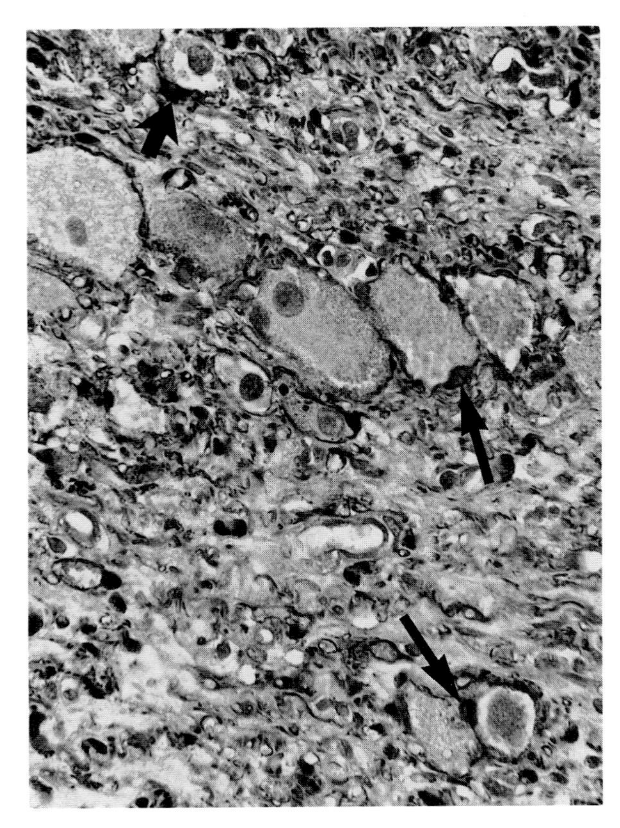

Figure 23-42
NEUROBLASTOMA AND GANGLIONEUROBLASTOMA

Left: In this neuroblastoma, stellate to dendritic cells immunoreactive for S-100 protein are adjacent to vascular septa (arrows). Cells are consistent with Schwann (or sustentacular) cells. (X120, Peroxidase-antiperoxidase stain)

Right: In this ganglioneuroblastoma, cells in intimate contact with ganglion cells (arrows) show intense staining for S-100 protein and are in the typical location of satellite cells. (X200, Peroxidase-antiperoxidase stain)

accuracy of interpretation in difficult cases, and of course close clinical correlation is always indicated. Small tissue fragments attained during FNA may provide valuable morphologic information, and in this context cell block preparations may yield diagnostic material and enable immunohistochemical study. In one series of exfoliative cytology specimens of malignant tumors in children, over half of the specimens positive for NB were from cerebrospinal fluid (fig. 23-43), followed by peritoneal fluid and two positive urine cytologies (166). GN has also been diagnosed by FNA (fig. 23-45) (167), but one must be aware of some of the stroma-rich tumors in which definitive resection may overturn a benign cytologic interpretation (167). Some tumors are accessible by disposable trucut needle biopsy as seen in figure 23-46.

Quantitation of DNA and Nucleolar Organizer Regions. Quantitative analysis of DNA has been shown to have prognostic value in patients with NB (170,173–181), with the most favorable group of tumors having hyperdiploid or aneuploid DNA histograms. Abnormal DNA content has also been reported in GNs when a significant number of ganglion cell nuclei are recovered (180). A favorable clinical outcome has been associated with an aneuploid stemline and low percentage of cells in the S, G2, and M phases of the cell cycle (173). In some studies favorable stage and DNA aneuploidy have been found to be independent prognostic indicators (180). Evaluation of DNA ploidy along with N-*myc* gene amplification may be complementary and together provide useful information regarding prognosis (176). A significant correlation has

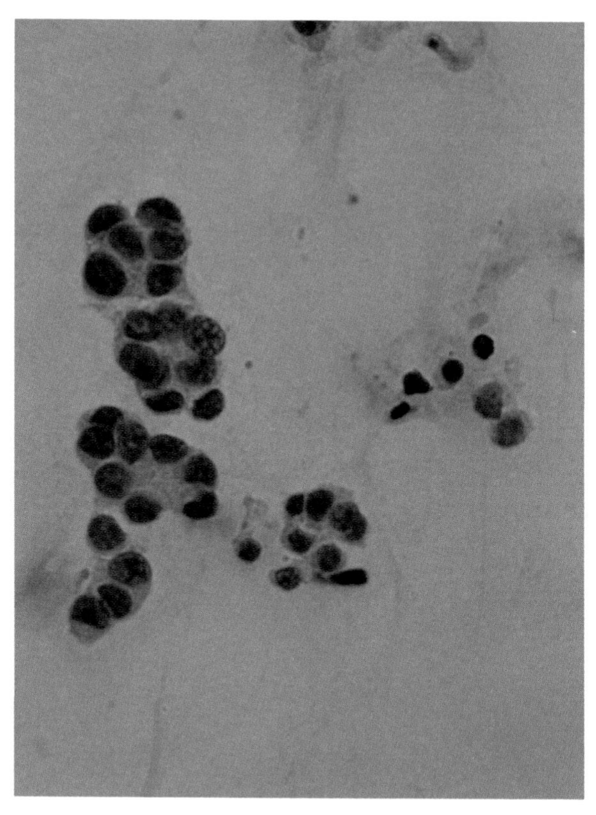

Figure 23-43
NEUROBLASTOMA
Neuroblastoma cells are evident in an exfoliative cytology preparation of cerebrospinal fluid. (Courtesy of Dr. Steven I. Hajdu, New York, NY.)

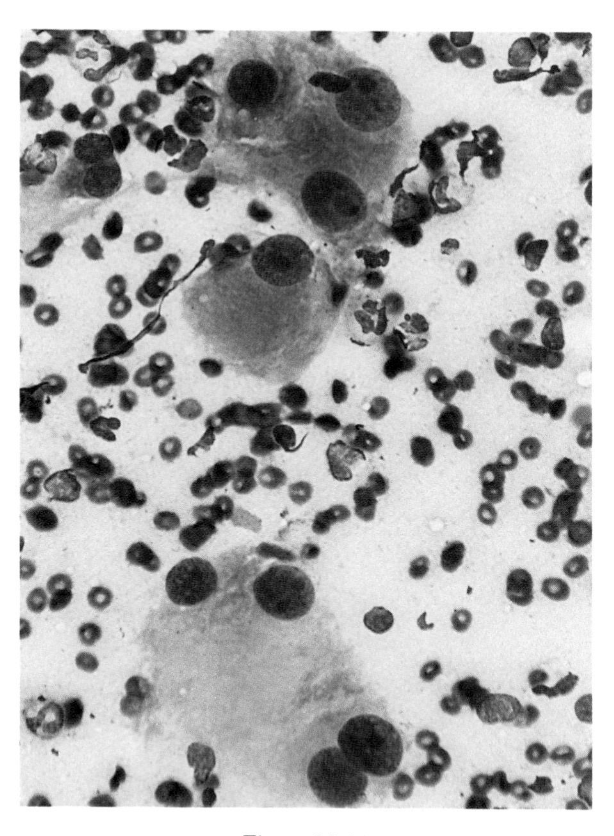

Figure 23-44
SMEAR/IMPRINT OF A GANGLIONEUROBLASTOMA
Cells with ganglionic differentiation show ample cytoplasm, eccentric nuclei, and a single prominent nucleolus. (X400, Diff-Quik stain)

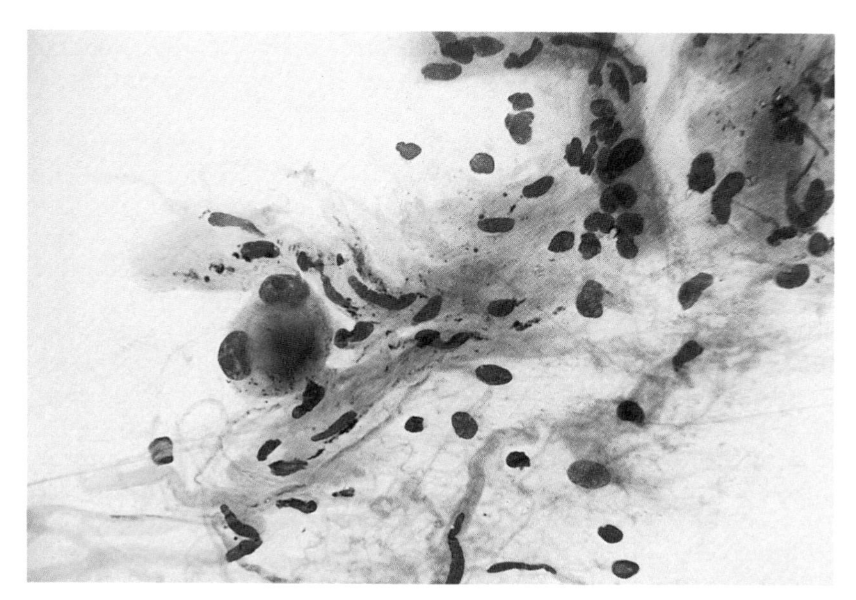

Figure 23-45
GANGLIONEUROMA
Fine-needle aspiration of a paravertebral mass in an adult shows ganglion cells and a spindle cell component representing Schwann cells. The tumor was diagnosed as a ganglioneuroma which was subsequently confirmed on pathologic examination of the resected tumor. (X400, Papanicolaou stain)

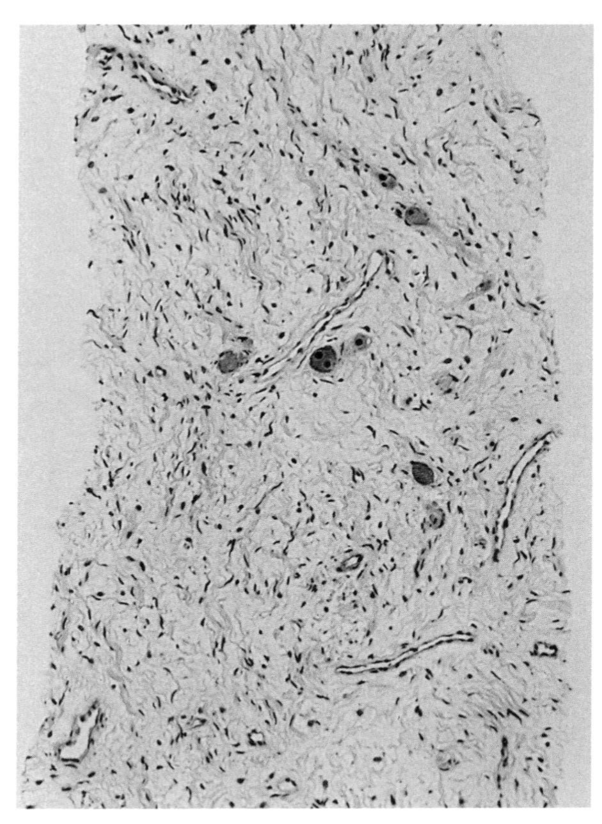

Figure 23-46
GANGLIONEUROMA
Transrectal trucut needle biopsy of a presacral ganglioneuroma in a 28-year-old woman.

been noted between the mean numbers of nucleolar organizer regions (AgNORs) with differentiation and the MKI in stroma-poor tumors, while stroma-rich tumors had the lowest average number of AgNORs (172). Increased numbers of AgNORs correlate with poor survival (171,172,179): it is lowest in the primary tumor, intermediate in regional lymph node metastases, and highest in distant metastases (179).

Grading and Other Prognostic Factors. Various grading schemes have been proposed over the last several decades for NB and GNB (183,196,203); some studies have combined biochemical and histologic determinants in an attempt to predict prognosis (194). The proportion of fibrillar (neuropil-like) matrix has been incorporated as a factor in prognosis (194,203–205, 209) as well as the number of neurosecretory granules with urinary excretion pattern of catecholamines in "undifferentiated" NB (208). Survival has also been correlated with stage, level of serum ferritin, and favorable versus unfavorable histology in the Shimada age-linked classification (191). Dehner (190) has suggested that recent cytogenetic and molecular biologic findings may render purely histopathologic classifications obsolete, but combining morphologic parameters with clinical (e.g., age) or other factors may be valuable, particularly with respect to prognosis. A recent study (although small with regard to number of patients) suggested that when assessing prognosis, N-*myc* oncogene amplification offered no significant advantage over the Shimada classification if the tumor was sampled thoroughly (210).

An age-linked classification of NB and GNB was introduced in 1984 by Shimada et al. (213) and involves subcategorization into stroma-rich and stroma-poor tumors; stroma-rich tumors have an extensive growth of schwannian, spindle cell stroma, but the precise amount is not specified (fig. 23-47). Three subgroups of tumors are recognized in the stroma-rich group: well-differentiated, intermixed, and nodular. The well-differentiated and intermixed stroma-rich tumors can grossly resemble a ganglioneuroma (GN) (fig. 23-48). The well-differentiated stroma-rich tumors have only a few randomly distributed aggregates of immature neuroblastic cells (see fig. 23-20), while the intermixed group has ganglioneuromatous tissue interspersed with scattered nests of variably differentiated neuroblastic cells which are sharply defined, making a "space" in the stroma (fig. 23-49). Nodular stroma-rich tumors have grossly identifiable components of mature and immature tumor, either one within the other in the primary tumor (fig. 23-50), or one in the primary tumor and one in the metastasis (189,213); this subgroup largely corresponds to the composite tumors reviewed by Stout in 1947 (214). Favorable and unfavorable prognosis groups are indicated along with survival data in figure 23-47.

Stroma-poor tumors (fig. 23-51) are divided into two prognostic subgroups based upon age at diagnosis, degree of cytologic differentiation (i.e., maturation into ganglion cells), and the mitosis-karyorrhexis index (MKI) (Table 23-4) (213). Since it is often difficult to distinguish mitotic figures from karyorrhexis these are counted together as mitosis-karyorrhexis and quantified as

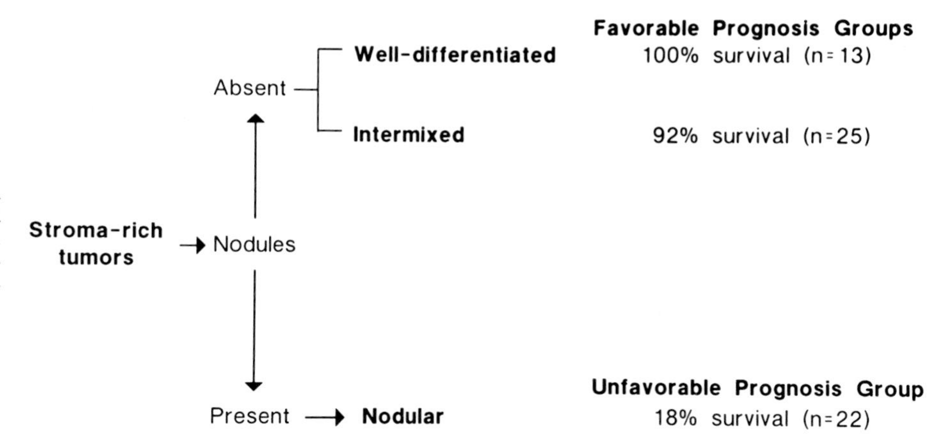

Figure 23-47
SUBGROUPING OF STROMA-RICH TUMORS

Subgrouping of stroma-rich tumors using the age-linked classification of Shimada et al. (213). Survival data in favorable and unfavorable prognosis groups are indicated.

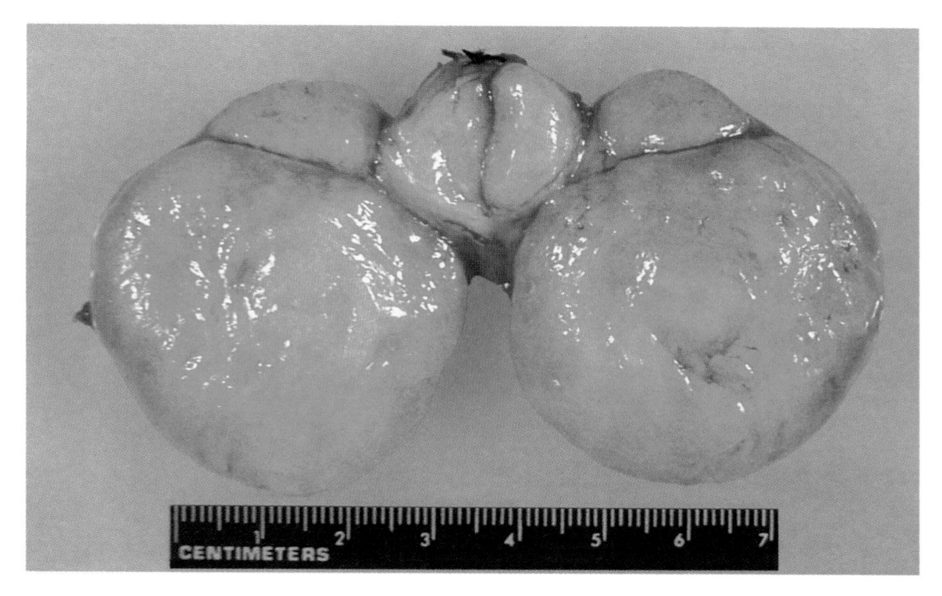

Figure 23-48
GANGLIO-NEUROBLASTOMA

Paravertebral intra-abdominal ganglioneuroblastoma from a 3-year-old girl was stroma-rich, intermixed in the Shimada classification. Tumor grossly resembles a ganglioneuroma.

an index (i.e., counting of 5,000 cells in randomly selected fields). The MKI was introduced to decrease the interobserver and intraobserver variability in identifying and counting mitotic figures (213), but a less rigorous method for counting may be possible (189). Stroma-poor tumors have more of the typical gross and histologic features of NB and GNB already discussed. Using the Shimada classification, stage IV-S NBs are classified in a favorable prognosis group of stroma-poor tumors (195). Although problems may exist in the Shimada classification, such as determination of histologic details, interobserver discrepancy can be reduced considerably if the tumor is assigned to a particular prognostic subgroup (i.e., favorable versus unfavorable histology), because of age at diagnosis (189). Others agree with this (200).

Another age-linked classification of childhood NB has recently been described (197), along with some modification in terminology and reinstitution of the terms NB and GNB (197,198). The term "neuroblastic tumor" includes all tumors of the sympathetic nervous system of neuroblastic origin (i.e., NBs, GNBs, and GNs). NB is divided into undifferentiated, poorly differentiated, or differentiating on the basis of proportion of differentiating neuroblasts (0 percent, 5 percent or less, and more than 5 percent, respectively).

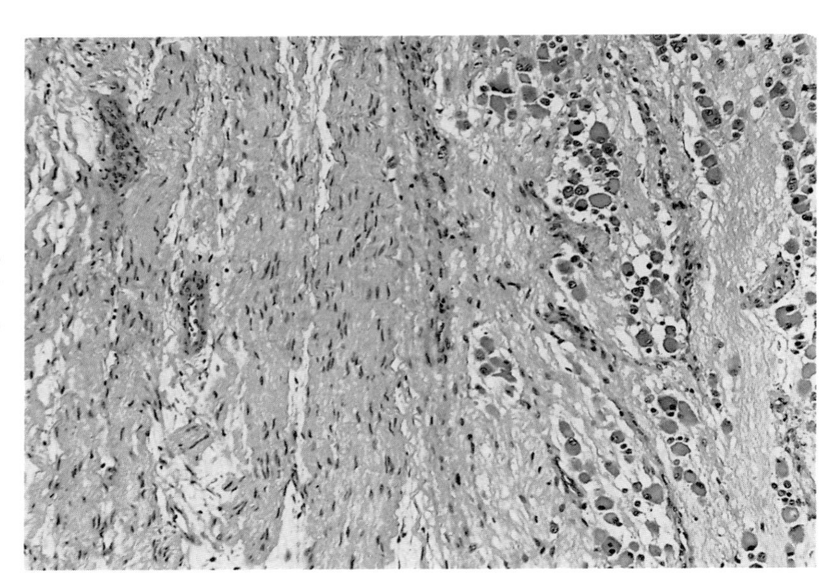

Figure 23-49
GANGLIONEUROBLASTOMA

This ganglioneuroblastoma conforms to the stroma-rich, intermixed subgroup in the Shimada classification. Note the abundant spindle cell (schwannian) stroma in the left half of the field and the fibrillary matrix and immature ganglion cells in the right half.

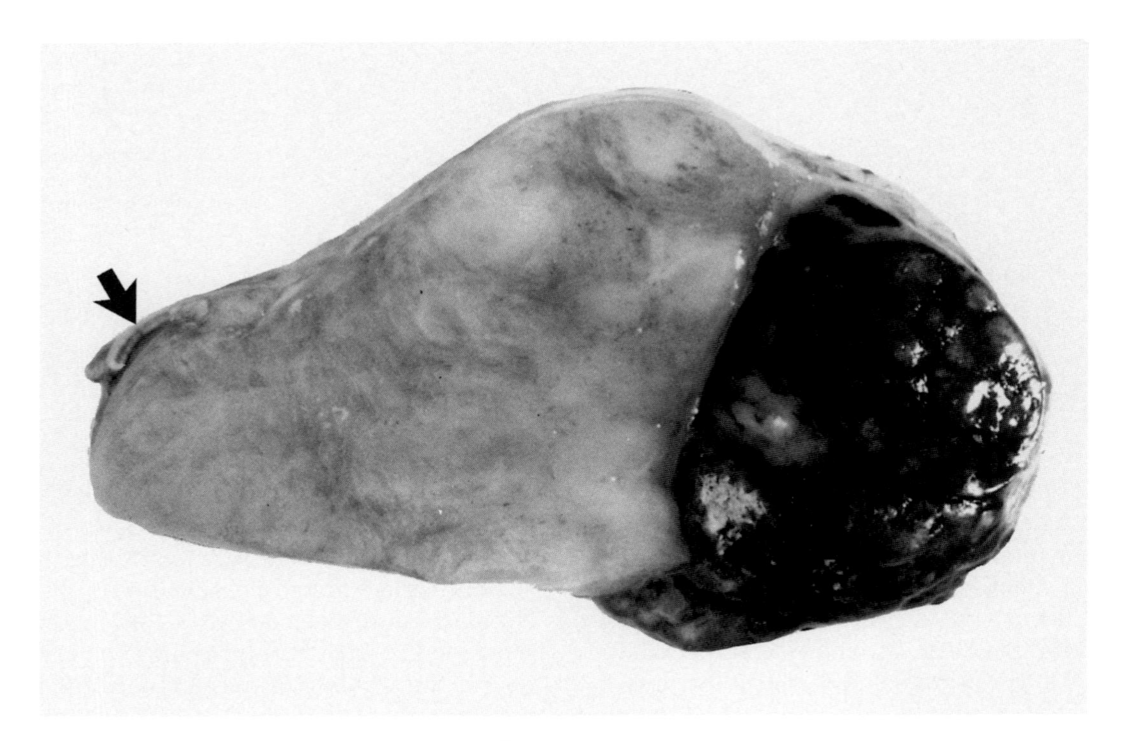

Figure 23-50
COMPOSITE ADRENAL GANGLIONEUROBLASTOMA

Composite adrenal ganglioneuroblastoma or stroma-rich, nodular subtype in the Shimada classification. Note the adrenal remnant (straight arrow). Patient was a 7-year-old girl who died of widespread metastases to liver, lung, spleen, lymph nodes, and bone. The bulging hemorrhagic nodule on the right was typical neuroblastoma while the remainder of the tumor was completely differentiated ganglioneuroma. (Modified from fig. 7-19 from Lack EE, Kozakewich HP. Adrenal neuroblastoma, ganglioneuroblastoma, and related tumors. In: Lack EE, ed. Pathology of the adrenal glands. New York: Churchill Livingstone, 1990:291.)

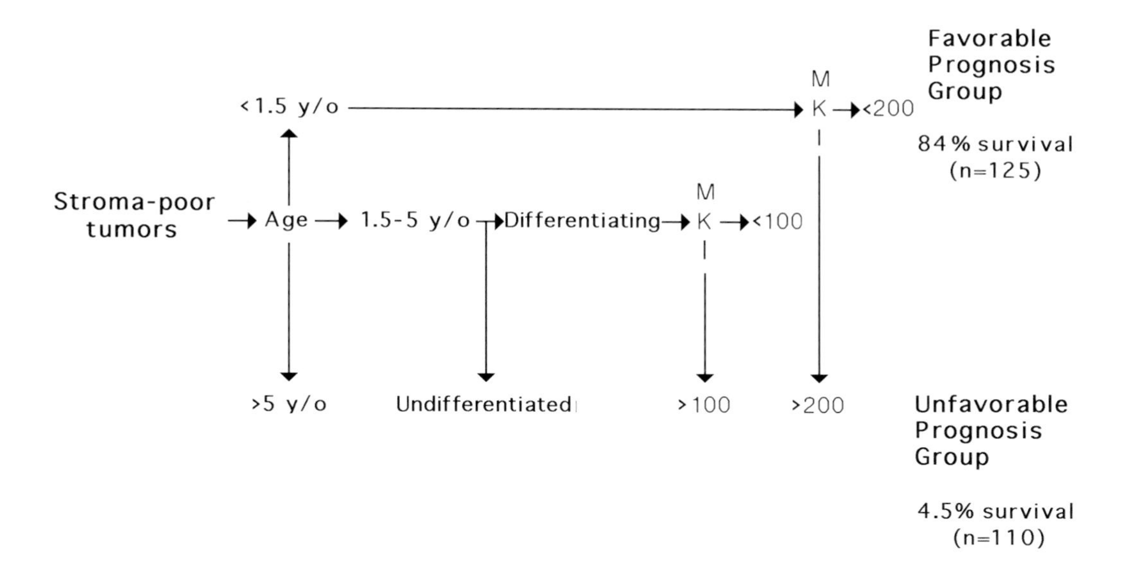

Figure 23-51
PROGNOSIS OF STROMA-POOR TUMORS
Stroma-poor tumors in the Shimada classification classified into favorable and unfavorable prognosis groups based upon age at diagnosis, proportion of differentiating cells, and mitosis-karyorrhexis index (MKI). Survival data are indicated.

Neuroblasts and neuropil constitute the predominant (greater than 50 percent) or exclusive component of the tumor. GNB is divided into nodular, intermixed, or borderline tumors and is composed of a predominantly (greater than 50 percent) ganglioneuromatous component and a small neuroblastomatous component. Low mitotic rate (10 or less mitoses per 10 high-power fields) and the presence of calcification are the most significant prognostic features. Grading of the neoplasms is based upon mitotic rate and presence or absence of calcification, with two risk groups being identified. A correlation between dystrophic calcification and improved survival has been noted in other studies (189,199). Grade 1 tumors have a low mitotic rate (10 or less per 10 high-power fields) with identifiable calcifications; grade 2 tumors also have a low mitotic rate or contain calcifications; and grade 3 tumors have a high mitotic rate (more than 10 per 10 high-power fields) and no calcifications. The low-risk group is defined as grade 1 NB (1 year or less or greater than 1 year of age) or grade 2 NB (1 year or less of age), and the high risk group is grade 2 NB (over 1 year of age) or grade 3 NB (1 year or less or greater than 1 year of age) (197). There is a high degree of interobserver concordance in the low-risk versus high-risk groups, and the favorable and unfavorable histologic subgroups in the Shimada age-linked classification; the survival curves, therefore, are very similar (fig. 23-52). The availability of adequate and representative histologic material from a primary tumor prior to

Table 23-4

HISTOLOGIC FACTORS INVOLVED IN CLASSIFICATION OF STROMA-POOR NEUROBLASTOMAS*

Levels of differentiation
Undifferentiated: less than 5% differentiating elements
Differentiating: 5% or greater differentiating elements
Mitosis-karyorrhexis index (MKI)**
Low: less than 100
Intermediate: less than 200
High: greater than 200

*Data from reference 213.
**Originally based upon 5,000 cell count in random fields.

Tumors of the Adrenal Gland and Extra-Adrenal Paraganglia

N-*myc* is normally found on chromosome 2, but it appears to be translocated to the short arm of chromosome 1 and may become amplified, which helps explain the chromosome 1p abnormalities and poor prognosis compared with patients who have normal chromosome 1p and hyperdiploidy (234). As discussed above, three distinct genetic subsets of NB have been recognized (see Grading and Other Prognostic Factors). The locus of the NB tumor suppressor gene has recently been mapped to 1p36 on the distal arm of chromosome 1 in a constitutional cytogenetic study done on blood lymphocytes (218). Other genetic abnormalities reported in NBs include hyperdiploidy, "double minute" chromosomes (dmin) and "homogeneously staining regions" (hsrs); the dmin and hsrs usually represent amplification of the oncogene N-*myc* (219). Schwann cells in maturing neuroblastomas have been shown to be genetically different from the neuronal cells suggesting that these cells may be a reactive population of normal cells that invade the neuroblastoma (216a).

Identification of the role of N-*myc* oncogene amplification in rapid tumor progression in many patients with NB (230) has been a major step in better understanding molecular biology of this tumor and has been confirmed in a number of other studies (225,231,235,236). About 50 percent of aggressive NBs lack N-*myc* amplification, suggesting that another mechanism may be operative; in some cases, N-*myc* expression is associated with poor clinical outcome even in the absence of gene amplification (237). For the individual patient, therefore, lack of N-*myc* amplification does not exclude a poor prognosis (228). Patients with NB and opsoclonus/myoclonus have been reported to have a good prognosis independent of stage or age at diagnosis, and tumors from several patients have shown no evidence of N-*myc* gene amplification (221). N-*myc* amplification and expression has been noted in localized, stroma-rich GNB suggesting that morphologic differentiation in vivo is not necessarily associated with decreased expression or an adverse prognosis (223). Other cytogenetic alterations have been described involving *ras* proto-oncogenes (217,227), the c-*src* proto-oncogene (222, 226), and the *ret* proto-oncogene (222,232). Newer techniques exist for more rapid and direct methods of determination of N-*myc* amplification, chromosome 1 copy number, presence of 1p deletion, and ploidy using fluorescence in situ hybridization (FISH) on imprints of tumor made directly onto glass slides and on standard bone marrow smears. It is therefore possible to define distinct prognostic groups on the basis of this genetic information and other parameters and thus permit stratification in therapies (233).

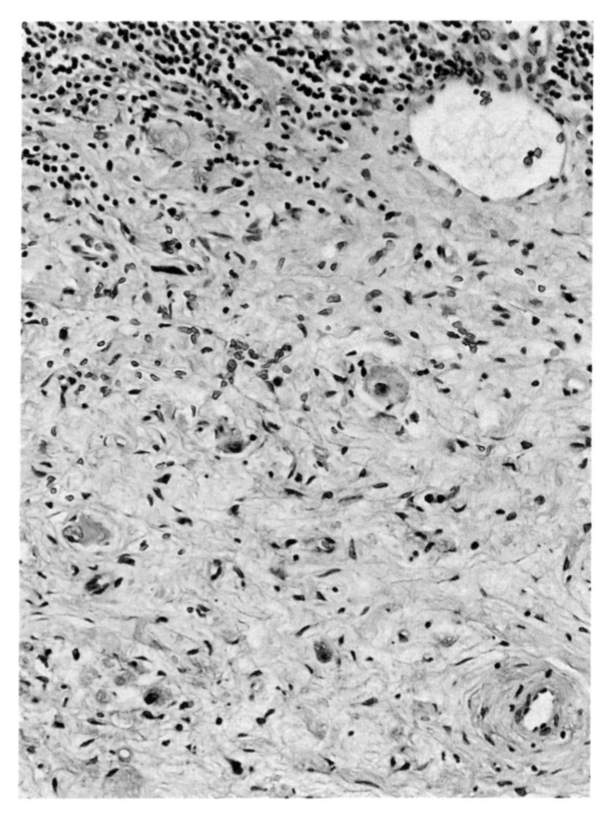

Figure 23-53
CERVICAL LYMPH NODE REPLACED BY GANGLIONEUROMA

Cervical lymph node from young adult partially replaced by fully mature ganglioneuroma. Patient had advanced stage neuroblastoma as a young child.

Spontaneous Regression or Maturation. Childhood NBs are complex neoplasms that occasionally undergo complete regression or mature to ganglioneuroma (fig. 23-53) (242). In a review of the incidence of spontaneous regression of cancer in humans, Everson and Cole (240) indicate that the figures for childhood NB may be variable and cite an overall incidence of 1 to 2 percent. The term "spontaneous" may be a misnomer since therapeutic efforts may have been inadequate (243), or there may well be an

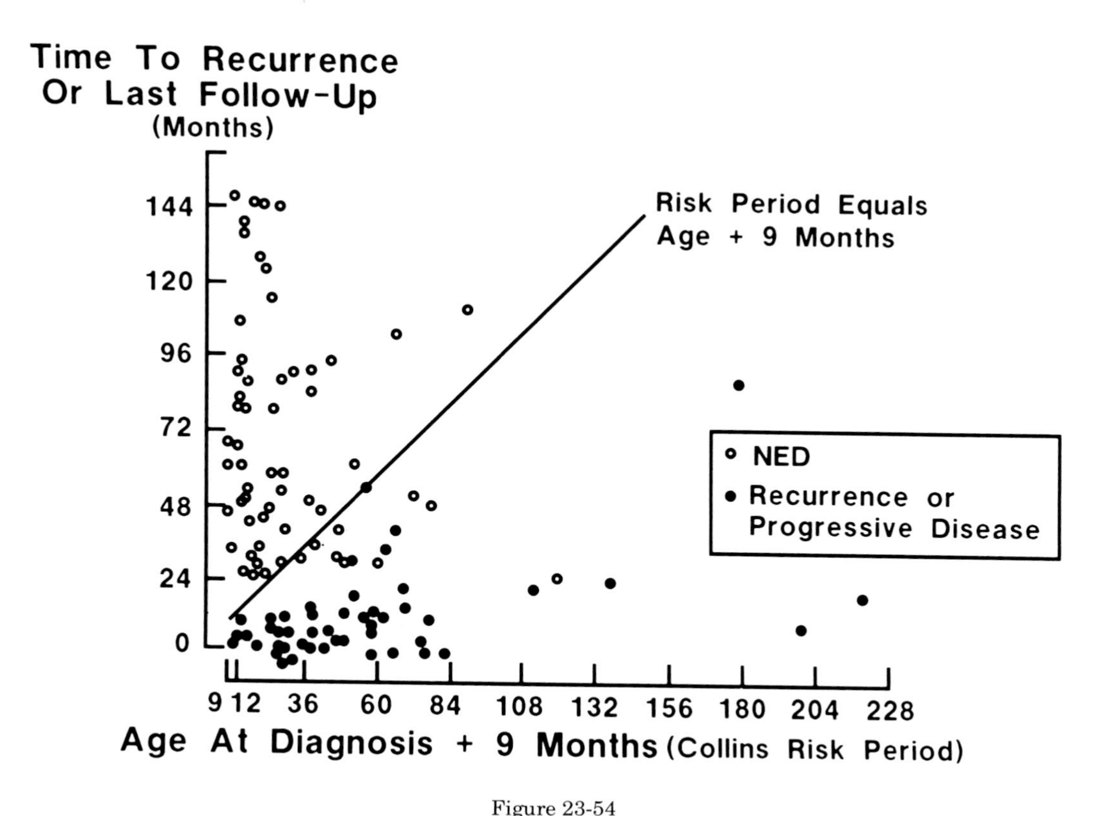

Figure 23-54

GRAPH OF 118 PATIENTS WITH NEUROBLASTOMA BASED UPON COLLINS' RISK PERIOD

Fifty-three patients had recurrent or progressive tumor (closed circles), all within the Collins' risk period of age at diagnosis plus 9 months. (Fig. 2 from Rosen EM, Cassady JR, Frantz CN, Kretschmar C, Levey R, Sallan SE. Neuroblastoma: the Joint Center for Radiation Therapy/Dana-Farber Cancer Institute/Children's Hospital experience. J Clin Oncol 1984;2:719–32.)

underlying biologic explanation which remains undetected (238). The first documented case of tumor maturation was reported by Cushing and Wolbach in 1927 (239) in a child who had cerebellar symptoms with nystagmus. In a follow-up report by Fox et al. (241), the same patient was apparently free of residual or recurrent tumor nearly 46 years later; the other patient in their report had multiple subcutaneous nodules of metastatic NB along with a large adrenal GNB diagnosed at 7 months of age, and biopsy of one of the skin nodules nearly 20 years later showed fully mature ganglioneuroma.

Survival and Patterns of Metastasis. Approximate survival data are indicated in Table 23-6. A more detailed discussion of survival rates and metastatic spread from a historical perspective can be found elsewhere (257). The concept of Collins' law (246) has been used to predict survival for children with NB (fig. 23-54) (264). Based upon a period of risk equal to the patient's age at diagnosis plus 9 months, it predicts that a child who has not been cured will relapse within this time span. Metastases in NBs usually involve bone marrow (78 percent), bone (69 percent; fig. 23-55), lymph nodes (42 percent; figs. 23-56, 23-57), liver (20 percent), skin (2 percent), testis (2 percent), and intracranial structures (7 percent) (245). Ovarian metastases can also occur (272). Bone marrow biopsy (fig. 23-58, left), usually bilateral, has been shown to be more reliable than bone marrow aspiration (fig. 23-58, right) in detecting tumor, but ancillary techniques such as immunohistochemistry may enhance sensitivity (257). Cranial involvement is essentially limited to calvarial bone, leptomeninges, and dura (fig. 23-59) (247,257), while intrinsic involvement of brain parenchyma is uncommon (247,249,255,265). Secondary encroachment on adjacent venous sinuses

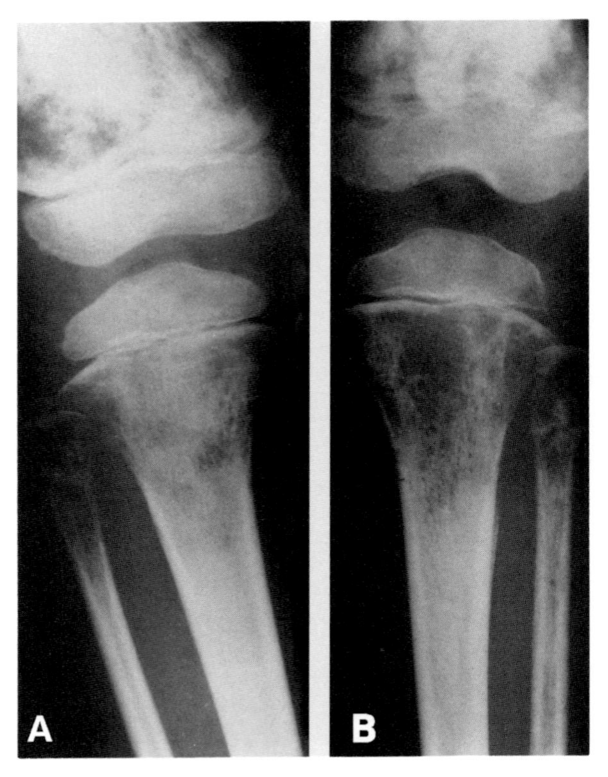

Figure 23-55
WIDELY METASTATIC NEUROBLASTOMA
IN A 4-YEAR-OLD BOY

The bony metastases seen here (A and B) involve predominantly the metaphyses of upper tibia and lower femur on both sides.

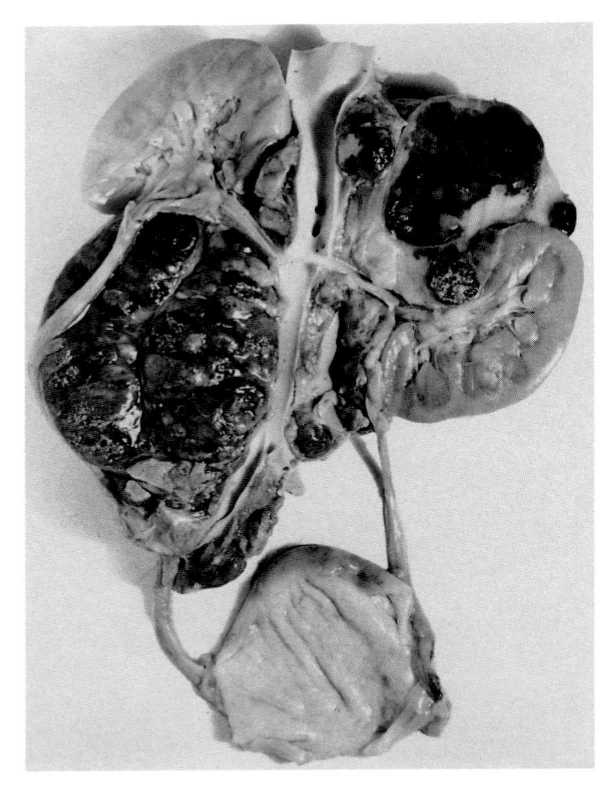

Figure 23-56
METASTATIC NEUROBLASTOMA

Widely metastatic neuroblastoma in a 4-year-old child. Posterior view of viscera shows an adrenal neuroblastoma replacing the right adrenal gland and invading kidney. The tumor extensively involved para-aortic lymph nodes. (Fig. 7-27 from Lack EE, Kozakewich HP. Adrenal neuroblastoma, ganglioneuroblastoma, and related tumors. In: Lack EE, ed. Pathology of the adrenal glands. New York: Churchill Livingstone, 1990:298.)

Figure 23-57
METASTATIC NEUROBLASTOMA

Metastatic neuroblastoma to lymph node shows extensive involvement with areas of lymphatic permeation adjacent to the node (left side of field).

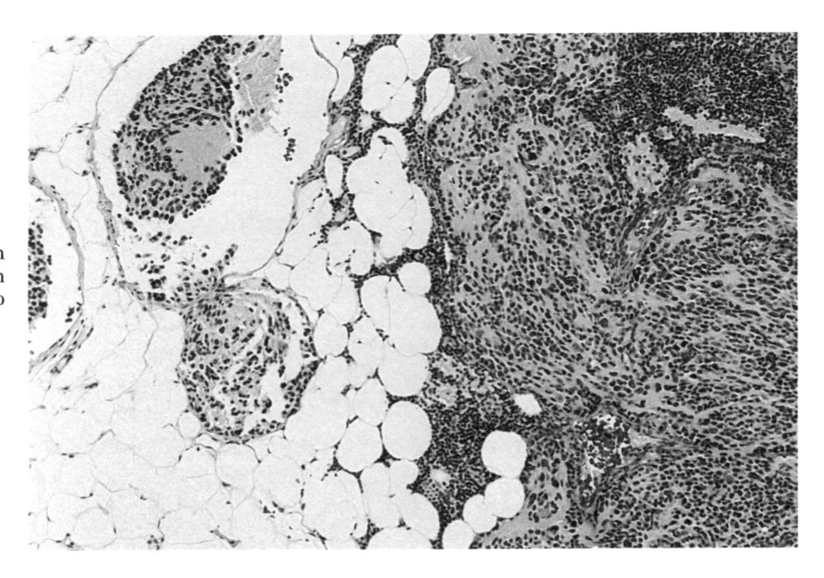

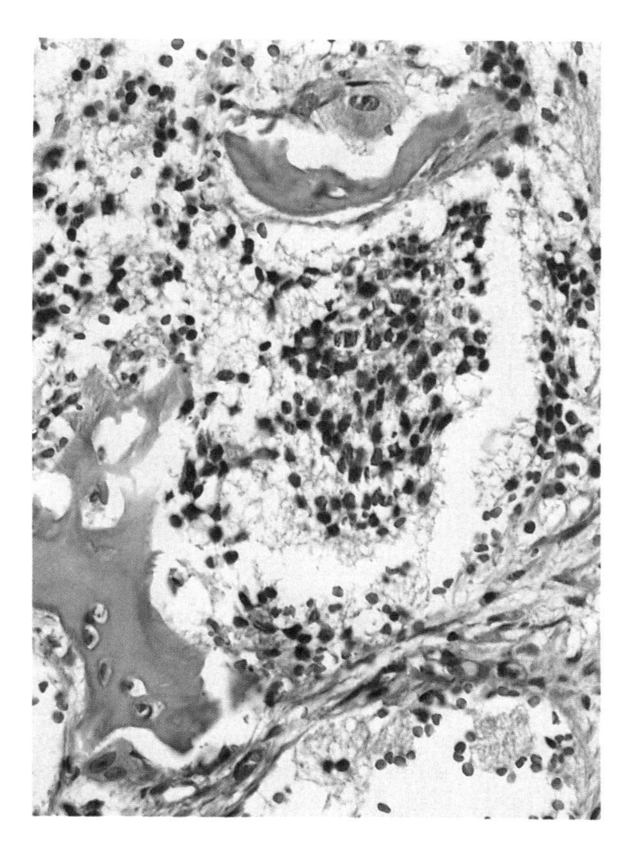

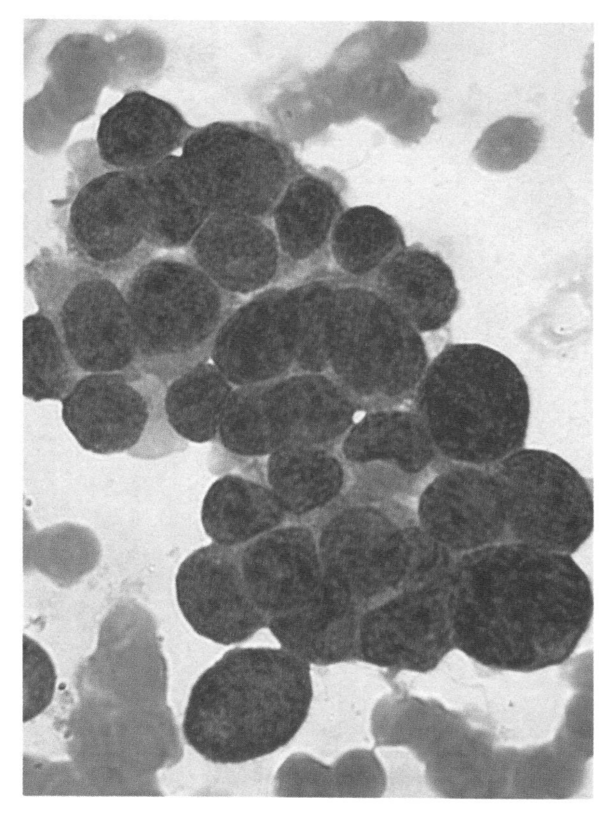

Figure 23-58
METASTATIC NEUROBLASTOMA TO BONE AND BONE MARROW
Left: Tumor cells have small, darkly stained nuclei with the important diagnostic hallmark of reticular neuritic cell processes. Right: Bone marrow aspirate has some clumps of metastatic neuroblastoma cells with finely dispersed nuclear chromatin.

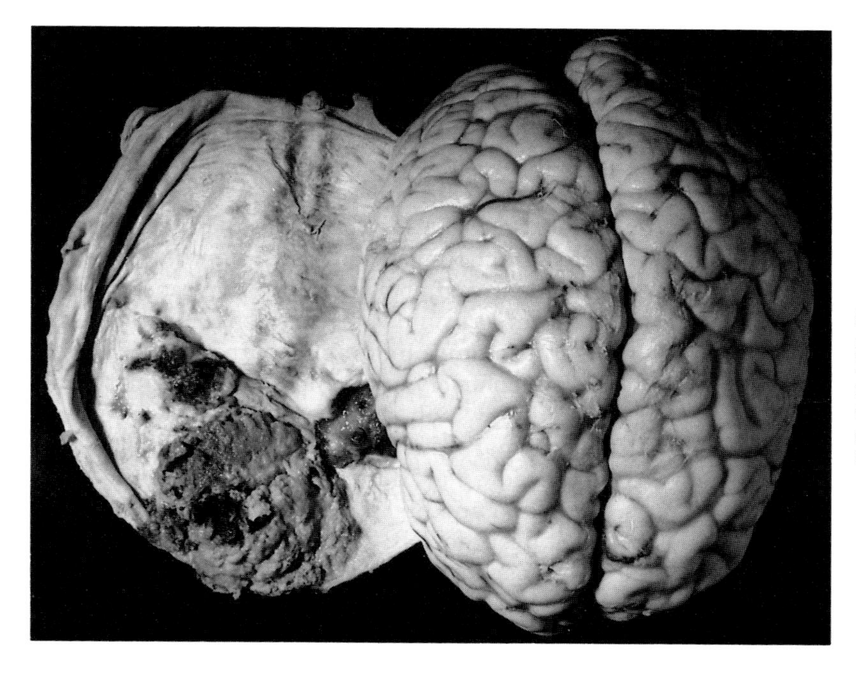

Figure 23-59
METASTATIC NEUROBLASTOMA TO CALVARIAL BONE AND DURA MATER
Leptomeninges over cerebral convexities were free of tumor, and there were no brain metastases. (Fig. 7-30 from Lack EE, Kozakewich HP. Adrenal neuroblastoma, ganglioneuroblastoma, and related tumors. In: Lack EE, ed. Pathology of the adrenal glands. New York: Churchill Livingstone, 1990:300.)

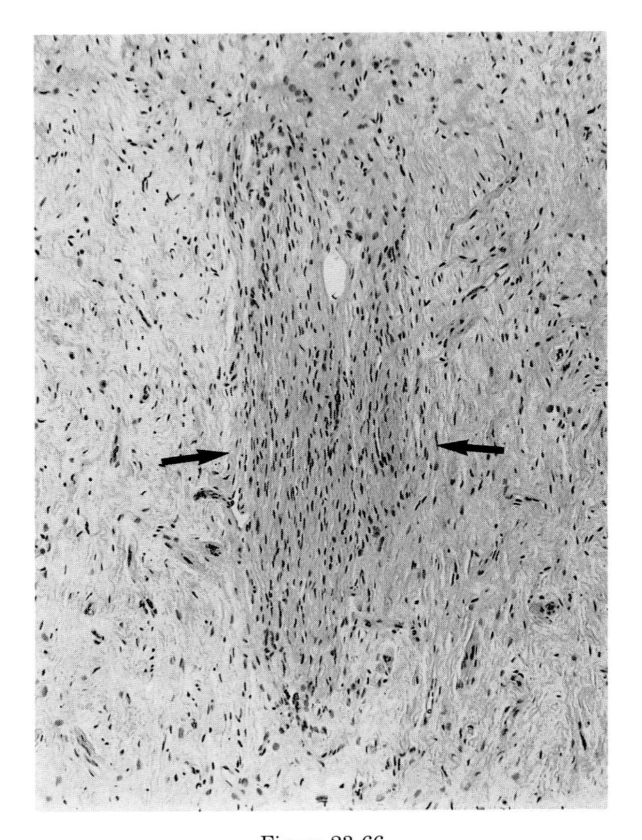

Figure 23-66
GANGLIONEUROMA
Ganglioneuroma had rare foci showing small bundles of myelinated nerve (arrows).

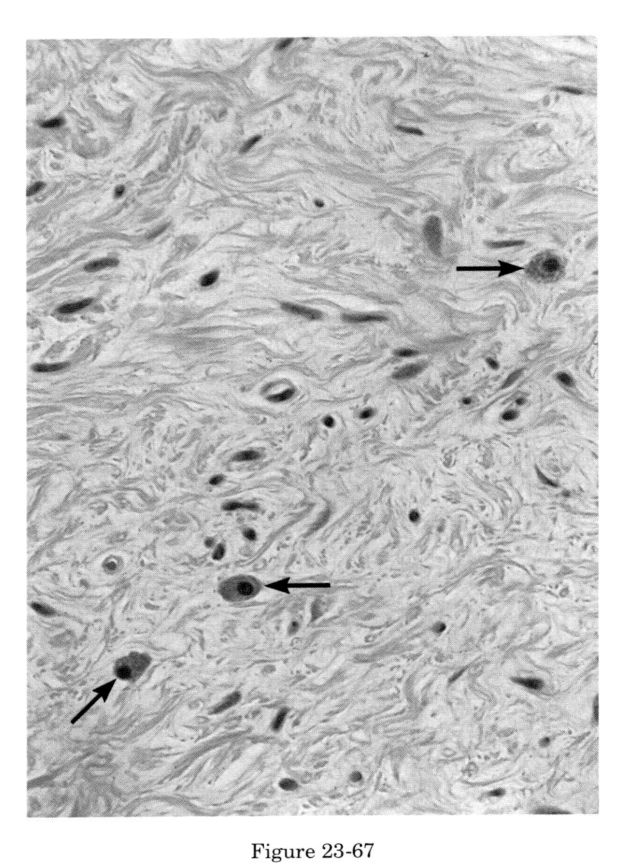

Figure 23-67
GANGLIONEUROMA
A ganglioneuroma contained a few areas with identifiable mast cells (arrows).

Figure 23-68
GANGLIONEUROMA
The ganglion cells of this ganglioneuroma contain abundant granular pigment consistent with neuromelanin. Mature ganglion cells are encircled by cells consistent with satellite cells.

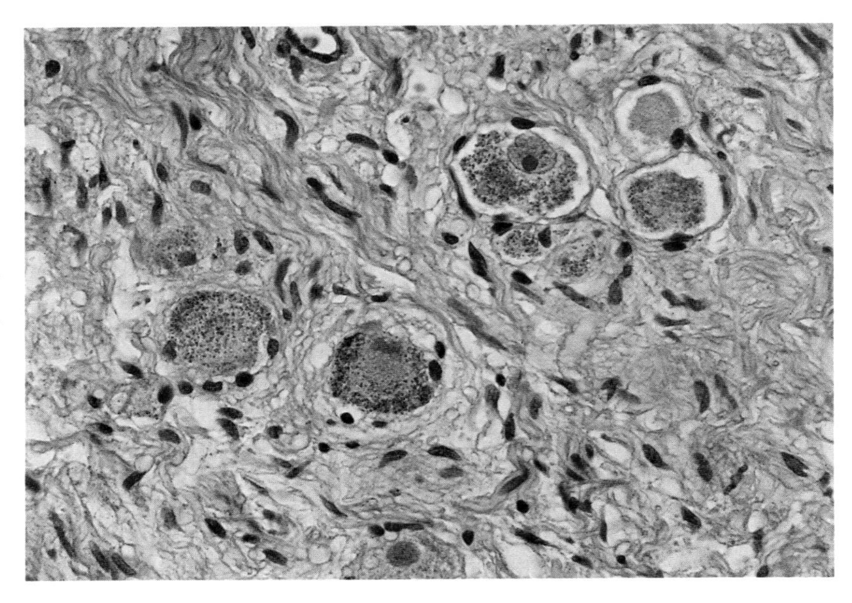

There is still some controversy as to whether GN arises de novo or by maturation or differentiation of a preexisting NB or GNB; the latter has certainly been well-documented (see figure 23-53). Others feel that GN arises de novo given the significant differences in age distribution and location compared with childhood NB (294).

Ultrastructural Findings. Fully mature GN is composed of ganglion cells that may be difficult to recognize in random sampling of tissue submitted for ultrastructural study unless a more directed search is made in multiple pilot sections preparatory to fine structural study. The morphologic features of note are ganglion cells (similar to those in figure 23-35), Schwann cells, and neuritic cell processes (similar to those in figure 23-36), but in most cases examination by electron microscopy is not necessary for diagnosis. The ultrastructure of GN is addressed in several other works (295,302). Rarely, mast cells can be encountered, and the large, nonhomogeneous granules should not be confused with dense-core neurosecretory granules (299).

Malignant Transformation of Ganglioneuroma. There have been rare examples of malignant transformation of GN into malignant peripheral nerve sheath tumor (PNST, malignant schwannoma) either de novo (308,310,311) or following abdominal radiation for NB or GNB (312–314). A case of malignant PNST has also been reported in an adrenal GN in an adult male homosexual (307). Three other cases have been described, but there was no mention of antecedent radiation treatment (309). Figure 23-69 shows a malignant PNST arising in a GN 17 years after abdominal radiation for a large unresectable NB which was initially diagnosed when the patient was 13 months of age (313). The presumed sequence of events in this case is radiation-induced or -associated maturation of NB to GN, and then after a latency of 17 years evolution of a malignant PNST from the Schwann cell component (313).

MASCULINIZING GANGLIONEUROMA

Masculinizing adrenal GNs (fig. 23-70, left) are rare neoplasms in which there is an admixture of ganglioneuroma along with Leydig cells containing pathognomonic crystalloids of Reinke (315), or strands or clusters of cells resembling adrenal cortical cells (316,318). Scully and Cohen (317) reported a case of GN containing cells morphologically identical to hilus (or Leydig) cells in a 50-year-old woman, but there was no evidence of virilization (fig. 23-70, right); the 3.5-cm adrenal tumor was an incidental finding in a patient whose symptoms suggested biliary tract disease. On rare occasion heterotopic hilus cells have been identified within the adrenal gland (see fig. 7-36).

REFERENCES

Epidemiology

1. Bundy S, Evans K. Survivors of neuroblastoma and ganglioneuroma and their families. J Med Genet 1982;19:16–21.
2. Cooney DR, Voorhess ML, Fisher JE, Brecher M, Karp MP, Jewett TC. Vasoactive intestinal peptide producing neuroblastoma. J Ped Surg 1982;17:821–5.
3. Farrelly C, Daneman A, Chan HS, Martin DJ. Occult neuroblastoma presenting with opsomyoclonus: utility of computed tomography. AJR Am J Roentengol 1984;142:807–10.
4. Green M, Cooke RE, Lattanzi W. Occurrence of chronic diarrhea in three patients with ganglioneuromas. Pediatrics 1959;23:951–5.
5. Hansen LP, Lund HT, Fahrenkrug J, Sogaard H. Vasoactive intestinal polypeptide (VIP)-producing ganglioneuroma in a child with chronic diarrhea. Acta Pediatr Scand 1980;69:419–24.
6. Hardy PC, Nesbit ME Jr. Familial neuroblastoma: report of a kindred with a high incidence of infantile tumors. J Pediatr 1972;80:74–7.
7. Iida Y, Nose O, Kai H, et al. Watery diarrhea with vasoactive intestinal peptide-producing ganglioneuroblastoma. Arch Dis Child 1980;55:929–36.
8. Jaffe N, Cassady R, Filler RM. Heterochromia and Horner syndrome associated with cervical and mediastinal neuroblastoma. J Pediatr 1975;87:75–7.
9. Jansen-Goemans A, Engelhardt J. Intractable diarrhea in a boy with vasoactive intestinal peptide-producing ganglioneuroblastoma. Pediatrics 1977;59:710–6.
10. Kimura N, Yamamoto H, Okamoto H, Wakasa H, Nagura H. Multiple-hormone gene expression in ganglioneuroblastoma with watery diarrhea, hypokalemia, and achlorhydria syndrome. Cancer 1993;71:2841–6.
11. Knudson AG Jr, Strong LC. Mutation and cancer: neuroblastoma and pheochromocytoma. Amer J Hum Genet 1972;24:514–32.

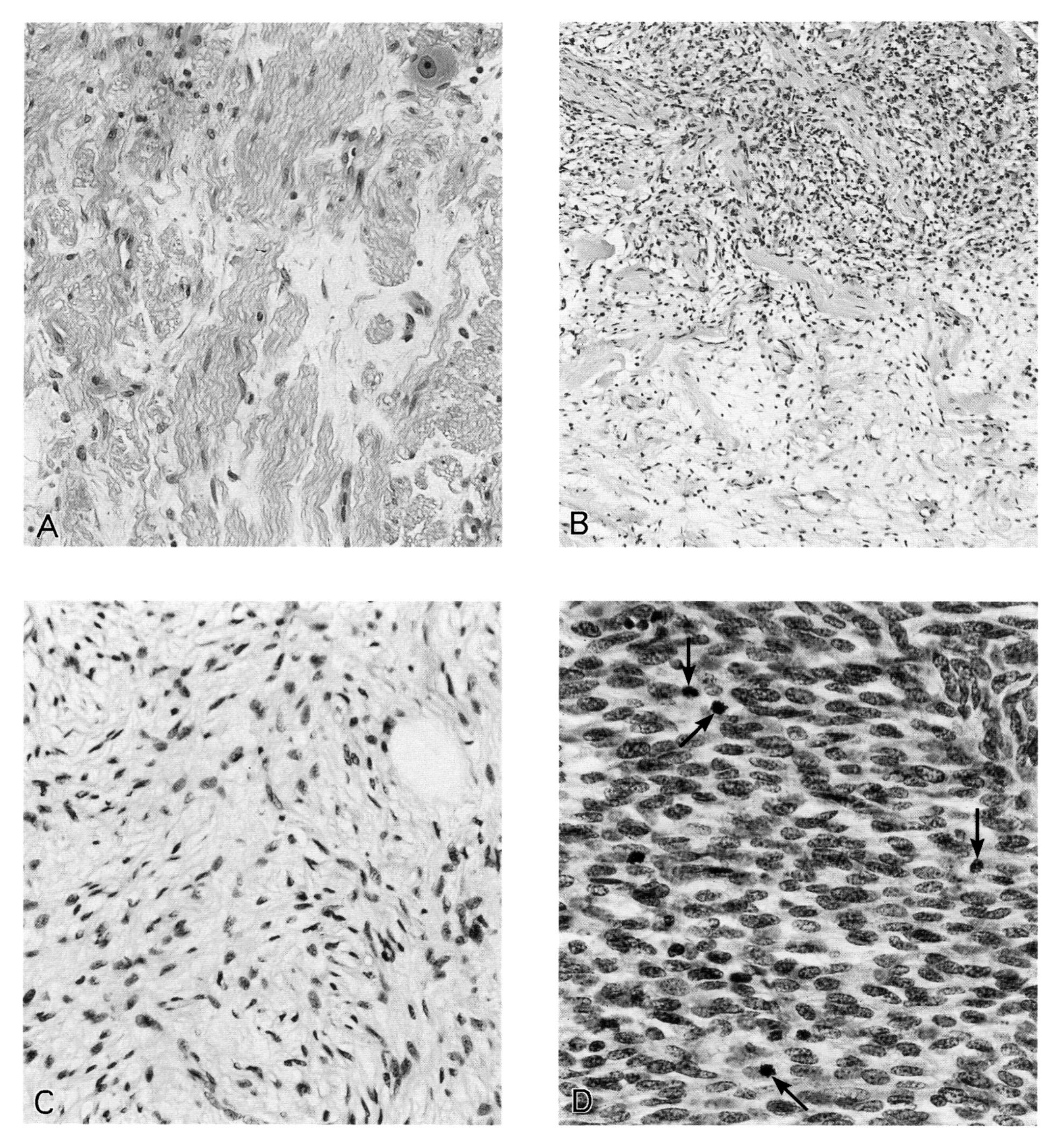

Figure 23-69

MALIGNANT TRANSFORMATION OF A GANGLIONEUROMA

Malignant transformation of a ganglioneuroma 17 years after abdominal megavoltage radiation for unresectable abdominal neuroblastoma at age 13 months. (Figures A–D are from the same case.)

A: Mature ganglioneuroma was seen in much of the tumor resected when the patient was a little over 18 years of age during a "debulking" procedure.

B: Other areas of the same tumor show transition to malignant peripheral nerve sheath tumor.

C: Transition zone of a malignant peripheral nerve sheath tumor.

D: Areas showed pure malignant peripheral nerve sheath tumor with numerous mitotic figures (arrows) while other areas were necrotic. (Courtesy of Dr. M. R. Sper, Cincinnati, OH.)

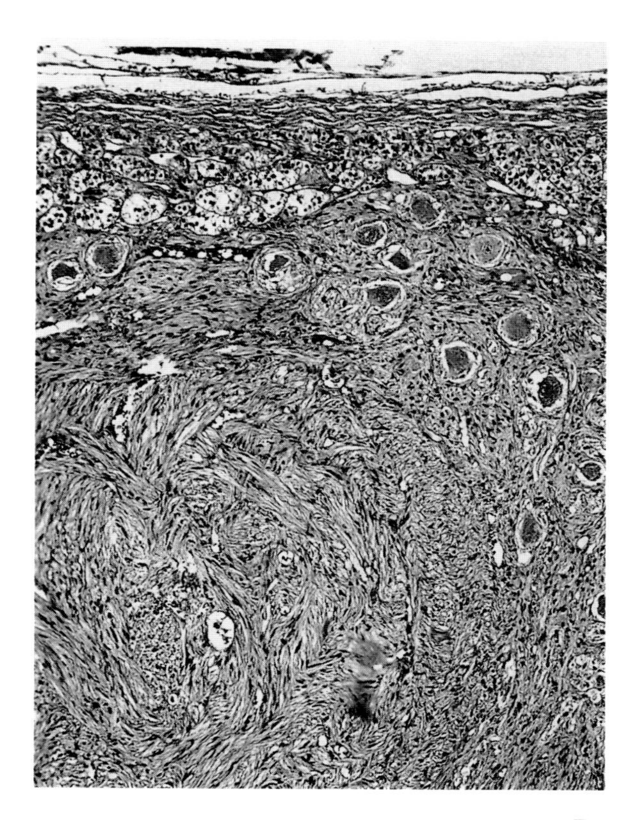

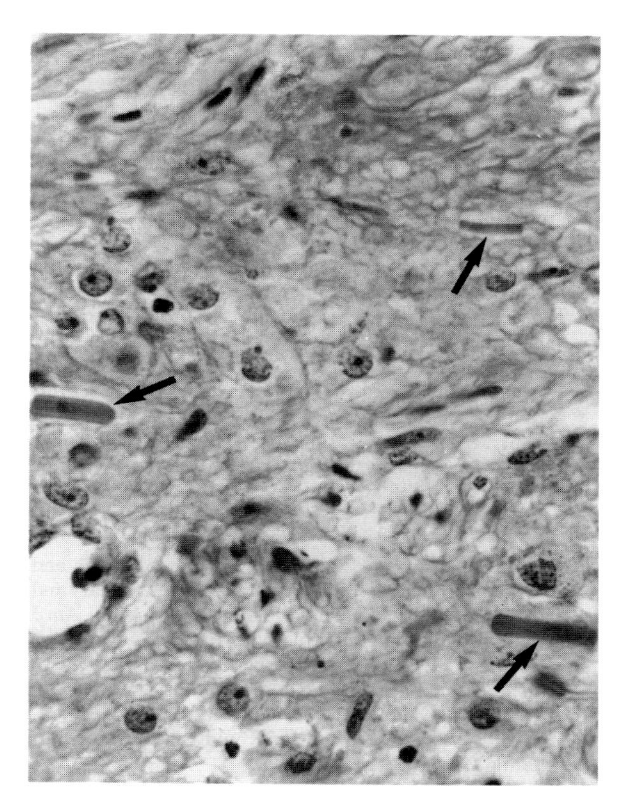

Figure 23-70
ADRENAL GANGLIONEUROMA

Left: This adrenal ganglioneuroma from a 50-year-old woman contains numerous ganglion cells with interspersed fascicles of Schwann cells. Other fields contained Leydig cells. (Fig. 4 from Aguirre P, Scully RE. Testosterone-secreting adrenal ganglioneuromas containing Leydig cells. Am J Surg Pathol 1983;7:699–705.)

Right: Areas of different tumor contained typical hilus cells with crystalloids of Reinke (arrows). The patient had no evidence of virilization. (From Scully RE, Cohen RB. Ganglioneuroma of adrenal medulla containing cells morphologically identical to hilus cells [extraparenchymal Leydig cells]. Cancer 1961;14:421–5.)

12. Kogut MD, Kaplan SA. Systemic manifestation of neurogenic tumors. J Pediatr 1962;60:694–704.
13. Kushner BH, Gilbert F, Helson L. Familial neuroblastoma. Case reports, literature review and etiologic considerations. Cancer 1986;57:1887–93.
14. Lack EE. Pathology of adrenal and extra-adrenal paraganglia. In: Major problems in pathology, Vol 29. Philadelphia: WB Saunders, 1994.
15. Long RG, Bryant MG, Mitchell SJ, Adrian TE, Polak JM, Bloom SR. Clinicopathological study of pancreatic and ganglioneuroblastoma tumours secreting vasoactive intestinal polypeptide (vipomas). Br Med J 1981;282:1767–71.
16. McRae D Jr, Shaw A. Ganglioneuroma, heterochromasia iridis, and Horner's syndrome. J Pediatr Surg 1979; 14:612–4.
17. Mendelsohn G, Eggleston JC, Olson JL. Vasoactive intestinal peptide and its relationship to ganglion cell differentiation in neuroblastic tumors. Lab Invest 1979;41:144–9.
18. Miller RW. Ethnic differences in cancer occurrence: genetic and environmental influences with particular reference to neuroblastoma. In: Mulvihill JJ, Miller RW, Fraumeni JF Jr, eds. Genetics of human cancer. New York: Raven Press, 1977:1–14.
19. Miller RW, Young JL Jr, Novakovic B. Childhood cancer. Cancer 1995;75:395–405.
20. Rosen EM, Cassady JR, Frantz CN, Kretschmar C, Levey R, Sallan SE. Neuroblastoma: the Joint Center for Radiation Therapy/Dana-Farber Cancer Institute/Children's Hospital experience. J Clin Oncol 1984;2:719–32.
21. Sayed AK, Miller BA, Lack EE, Sallan SE, Levey RH. Heterochromia iridis and Horner's syndrome due to paravertebral neurilemoma. J Surg Oncol 1983;22:15–6.
22. Trump DL, Livingstone JN, Baylin SB. Watery diarrhea syndrome in an adult with ganglioneuroma-pheochromocytoma: identification of vasoactive intestinal peptide, calcitonin, and catecholamines and assessment of their biologic activity. Cancer 1977;40:1526–32.
23. Young JL Jr, Miller RW. Incidence of malignant tumors in US children. J Pediatr 1975;86:254–8.
24. Young JL Jr., Ries LG, Silverberg E, Horm JW, Miller RW. Cancer incidence, survival, and mortality for children younger than age 15 years. Cancer 1986;58:598–602.

222. El-Badry OM, Israel MA. Growth regulation of human neuroblastoma. In: Benz CC, Liu ET, eds. Oncogenes and tumor supressor genes in human malignancies. Boston: Kluwer Academic Publishers, 1993:108–18.
223. Fabbretti G, Valenti C, Loda M, et al. N-myc gene amplification/expression in localized stroma-rich neuroblastoma (ganglioneuroblastoma). Hum Pathol 1993;24:294–7.
224. Gilbert F, Feder M, Balaban G, et al. Human neuroblastomas and abnormalities of chromosomes 1 and 17. Cancer Res 1984;44:5444–9.
225. Grady-Leopardi EF, Schwab M, Ablin AR, Rosenau W. Detection of N-myc oncogene expression in human neuroblastoma by in situ hybridization and blot analysis: relationship to clinical outcome. Cancer Res 1986;46:3196–9.
226. Horii Y, Sugimoto T, Sawada T, Imanishi J, Tsuboi K, Hatanaka M. Differential expression of N-myc and c-src proto-oncogenes during neuronal and Schwannian differentiation of human neuroblastoma cells. Int J Cancer 1989;43:305–9.
227. Ireland CM. Activated N-ras oncogenes in human neuroblastoma. Cancer Res 1989;49:5530–3.
228. Oppedal BR, Qien O, Jahnsen T, Brandtzaeg P. N-myc amplification in neuroblastomas: histopathological, DNA ploidy, and clinical variables. J Clin Pathol 1989;42:1148–52.
229. Schneider NR. Cytogenetic evaluation of childhood neoplasms. Arch Pathol Lab Med 1993;117:1220–4.
230. Seeger RC, Brodeur GM, Sather H, et al. Association of multiple copies of the N-myc oncogene with rapid progression of neuroblastomas. N Engl J Med 1985;313:1111–6.
231. Slave I, Ellenbogen R, Jung WH, et al. Myc gene amplification and expression in primary human neuroblastoma. Cancer Res 1990;50:1459–63.
232. Tahira T, Ishizaka Y, Itoh F, Nakayasu M, Sugimura T, Nagao M. Expression of the ret proto-oncogene in human neuroblastoma cell lines and its increase during neuronal differentiation induced by retinoic acid. Oncogene 1991;6:2333–8.
233. Taylor CP, McGuckin AG, Bown NP, et al. Rapid detection of prognostic genetic factors in neuroblastomas using fluorescence in situ hybridization on tumour imprints and bone marrow smears. United Kingdom Children's Cancer Study. Br J Cancer 1994;69:445–51.
234. Triche TJ. Neuroblastoma and other childhood neural tumors: a review. Pediatr Pathol 1990;10:175–93.
235. Tsuda H, Shimosato Y, Upton MP, et al. Retrospective study on amplification of N-myc and c-myc genes in pediatric solid tumors and its association with prognosis and tumor differentiation. Lab Invest 1988;59:321–7.
236. Tsuda T, Obara M, Hirano H, et al. Analysis of N-myc amplification in relation to disease stage and histologic types in human neuroblastomas. Cancer 1987;60:820–6.
237. Wada RK, Seeger RC, Brodeur GM, et al. Human neuroblastoma cell lines that express N-myc without gene amplification. Cancer 1993;72:3346–54.

Spontaneous Regression or Maturation

238. Bolande RP. The spontaneous regression of neuroblastoma. Experimental evidence for a natural host immunity. Pathol Annu 1991;26(pt. 2):187–99.
239. Cushing H, Wolbach SB. The transformation of a malignant paravertebral sympathicoblastoma into a benign ganglioneuroma. Am J Path 1927;3:203–16.
240. Everson TC, Cole WH. Spontaneous regression of cancer. Philadelphia: WB Saunders, 1966:88–163.
241. Fox F, Davidson J, Thomas LB. Maturation of sympathicoblastoma into ganglioneuroma. Report of 2 patients with 20- and 46-year survivals respectively. Cancer 1959;12:108–16.
242. MacMillan RW, Blanc WB, Santulli TV. Maturation of neuroblastoma to ganglioneuroma in lymph nodes. J Ped Surg 1976;11:461–2.
243. Stewart FW. Experiences in spontaneous regression of neoplastic disease in man. Texas Rep Biol Med 1951;10:239–53.

Survival and Patterns of Metastasis

244. Anderson HJ, Hariri J. Congenital neuroblastoma in a fetus with multiple malformations. Metastasis in the umbilical cord as a cause of indrauterine death. Virchows Arch [A] 1983;400:219–22.
245. Berthold F. Overview: biology of neuroblastoma. In: Pochedly C, ed. Neuroblastoma: tumor biology and therapy, Boca Raton: CRC Press, 1990:1–27.
246. Collins VP. Wilms' tumor: its behavior and prognosis. J La State Med Soc 1955;107:474–80.
247. de la Monte SM, Moore GW, Hutchins GM. Nonrandom distribution of metastases in neuroblastic tumors. Cancer 1983;52:915–25.
248. Erttmann R, Heller M, Veelken N, Landbeck G. Intracranial metastatic neuroblastoma. Z Kinderchir 1983;38:333–5.
249. Feldges AJ, Stanisic M, Morger R, Waidelich E. Neuroblastoma with meningeal involvement causing increased intracranial pressure and coma in two children. Am J Pediatr Hematol Oncol 1986;8:355–7.
250. Glorieux P, Bouffet E, Philip I, et al. Metastatic interstitial pneumonitis after autologous bone marrow transplantation. A consequence of reinjection of malignant cells? Cancer 1986;58:2136–9.
251. Graeve JL, de Alarcon PA, Sato Y, Pringle K, Helson L. Miliary pulmonary neuroblastoma. A risk of autologous bone marrow transplantation? Cancer 1988;62:2125–7.
252. Hawthorne HC Jr, Nelson JS, Witzleben CL, Giangiacomo J. Blanching subcutaneous nodules in neonatal neuroblastoma. J Pediatr 1970;77:297–300.
253. Hutchison R. On suprarenal sarcoma in children with metastases in skull. Q J Med 1907;1:33–8.
254. Kellie SJ, Hayes FA, Bowman L, et al. Primary extracranial neuroblastoma with central nervous system metastases: characterization by clinicopathologic findings and neuroimaging. Cancer 1991;68:1999–2006.
255. Koizumi JH, Dal Canto MC. Retroperitoneal neuroblastoma metastatic to brain. Report of a case and review of the literature. Child's Brain 1980;7:267–79.
256. Kushner BH, Gulati SC, Kwon JH, O'Reilly RJ, Exelby PR, Cheung NK. High-dose melphalan with 6-hydroxydopamine-purged autologous bone marrow transplantation for poor-risk neuroblastoma. Cancer 1991;68:242–7.

257. Lack EE. Pathology of adrenal and extra-adrenal paraganglia. Major problems in pathology, Vol 29. Philadelphia: WB Saunders, 1994.
258. Lucky AW, McGuire J, Komp DM. Infantile neuroblastoma presenting with cutaneous blanching nodules. J Am Acad Dermatol 1982;6:389–91.
259. Moss TJ, Sanders DG. Detection of neuroblastoma cells in blood. J Clin Oncol 1990;8:736–40.
260. Musarella MA, Chan HS, DeBoer G, Gallie BL. Ocular involvement in neuroblastoma: prognostic implications. Ophthalmology 1984;91:936–40.
261. Pereira F, Crist W, McKaig S. Neuroblastoma leukemia a rarity? Report of a case. Clin Pediatr 1978;17:701–4.
262. Phillips R. Neuroblastoma. Ann Roy Med Coll Surg Engl 1953;12:29–48.
263. Raney RB Jr, Lyon GM Jr, Porter FS. Neuroblastoma simulating acute leukemia. J Pediatr 1976;89:433–5.
264. Rosen EM, Cassady JR, Frantz CN, Kretschmar C, Levey R, Sallan SE. Neuroblastoma: the Joint Center for Radiation Therapy/Dana-Farber Cancer Institute/Children's Hospital experience. J Clin Oncol 1984;2:719–32.
265. Shaw PJ, Eden T. Neuroblastoma with intracranial involvement: an ENSG study. Med Pediatr Oncol 1992;20:149–55.
266. Shown TE, Durfee MF. Blueberry muffin baby: neonatal neuroblastoma with subcutaneous metastases. J Urol 1970;104:193–5.
267. Smith CR, Chan HS, deSa DJ. Placental involvement in congenital neuroblastoma. J Clin Pathol 1981;34:785–9.
268. Strauss L, Driscoll SG. Congenital neuroblastoma involving the placenta. Reports of two cases. Pediatrics 1964;34:23–31.
269. Towbin R, Gruppo RA. Pulmonary metastases in neuroblastoma. AJR Am J Roentgenol 1982;138:75–8.
270. van der Slikke JW, Balk AG. Hydramnios with hydrops fetalis and disseminated fetal neuroblastoma. Obstet Gynecol 1980;55:250–3.
271. Willis RA. The spread of tumours in the human body, 3rd ed. London: Butterworth, 1973:102–5.
272. Young RH, Kozakewich HP, Scully RE. Metastatic ovarian tumors in children: a report of 14 cases and review of the literature. Int J Gynecol Pathol 1993;12:8–19.

Differential Diagnosis of Neuroblastoma

273. Angervall L, Enzinger FM. Extraskeletal neoplasm resembling Ewing's sarcoma. Cancer 1975;36:240–51.
274. Burger PC, Scheithauer BW. Tumors of the central nervous system. Atlas of Tumor Pathology, 3rd Series, Fascicle 10. Washington, D.C.: Armed Forces Institue of Pathology, 1994.
275. Dehner LP. Peripheral and central primitive neuroectodermal tumors. A nosologic concept seeking a consensus. Arch Pathol Lab Med 1986;110:997–1005.
276. Dehner LP. Primitive neuroectodermal tumor and Ewing's sarcoma. Am J Surg Pathol 1993;17:1–13.
277. Gerald WL, Miller HK, Battifora H, Miettinen M, Silva EG, Rosai J. Intra-abdominal desmoplastic small round-cell tumor. Report of 19 cases of a distinctive type of high-grade polyphenotypic malignancy affecting young individuals. Am J Surg Pathol 1991;15:499–513.
278. Goldblum JR, Beals TF, Weiss SW. Neuroblastoma-like neurilemoma. Am J Surg Pathol 1994;18:266–73.
279. Hartman KR, Triche TJ, Kinsella TJ, Miser JS. Prognostic value of histopathology in Ewing's sarcoma. Long-term follow-up of distal extremity primary tumors. Cancer 1991;67:163–71.
280. Isayama T, Iwasaki H, Kikuchi M, Yoh S, Takagishi N. Neuroectodermal tumor of bone. Evidence for neural differentiation in a cultured cell line. Cancer 1990;65:1771–81.
281. Kushner BH, Hajdu SI, Gulati SC, et al. Extracranial primitive neuroectodermal tumors. The Memorial Sloan-Kettering Cancer Center experience. Cancer 1991;67:1825–9.
282. Lack EE. Pathology of adrenal and extra-adrenal paraganglia. Major problems in pathology, Vol 29. Philadelphia: WB Saunders, 1994.
283. Ladanyi M, Gerald W. Fusion of the EWS and WT1 genes in the desmoplastic small round cell tumor. Cancer Res 1994;54:2837–40.
284. Marina NM, Etcubanas E, Parham DM, Bowman LC, Green A. Peripheral primitive neuroectodermal tumor (peripheral neuroepithelioma) in children. A review of the St. Jude experience and controversies in diagnosis and management. Cancer 1989;64:1952–60.
285. Ordóñez NG, El-Naggar AK, Ro JY, Silva EG, Mackay B. Intra-abdominal desmoplastic small cell tumor: a light microscopic, ultrastructural, and flow cytometric study. Hum Pathol 1993;24:850–65.
286. Parham DM, Weeks DA, Beckwith JB. The clinicopathologic spectrum of putative extrarenal rhabdoid tumors. An analysis of 42 cases studied with immunohistochemistry or electron microscopy. Am J Surg Pathol 1994;18:1010–29.
287. Shimada H, Newton WA Jr, Soule EH, Qualman SJ, Aoyama C, Maurer HM. Pathologic features of extraosseous Ewing's sarcoma: a report from the Intergroup Rhabdomyosarcoma Study. Hum Pathol 1988;19:442–53.
288. Weeks DA, Beckwith JB, Mierau GW, Luckey DW. Rhabdoid tumor of kidney. A report of 111 cases from the National Wilms' Tumor Study Pathology Center. Am J Surg Pathol 1989;13:439–58.
289. Whang-Peng J, Freter CE, Knutsen T, Nanfro JJ, Gazdar A. Translocation t(11;22) in esthesioneuroblastoma. Cancer Genet Cytogenet 1987;29:155–7.

Ganglioneuroma

290. Abell MR, Hart WR, Olson JR. Tumors of the peripheral nervous system. Hum Pathol 1970;1:503–51.
291. Ackerman LV, Taylor FH. Neurogenous tumors within the thorax. A clinicopathologic evaluation of 48 cases. Cancer 1951;4:669–91.
292. Bove KE, McAdams AJ. Composite ganglioneuroblastoma. An assessment of the significance of histological maturation in neuroblastoma diagnosed beyond infancy. Arch Pathol Lab Med 1981;105:325–30.
293. Carpenter WB, Kernohan JW. Retroperitoneal ganglioneuromas and neurofibromas. A clinicopathological study. Cancer 1963;16:788–97.
294. Enzinger FM, Weiss SW. Soft tissue tumors. St Louis: CV Mosby, 1988:828–31.

295. Erlandson RA. Diagnostic transmission electron microscopy of tumors: with clinicopathological, immunohistochemical, and cytogenetic correlations. New York: Raven Press, 1994.
296. Hamilton JP, Koop CE. Ganglioneuromas in children. Surg Gynec Obstet 1965;121:803–12.
297. Harkin JC, Reed RJ. Tumors of the peripheral nervous system. Atlas of Tumor Pathology, 2nd Series, Fascicle 3. Washington, D.C.: Armed Forces Institute of Pathology, 1969.
298. Hazarika D, Naresh KN, Rao CR, Gowda BM. Parapharyngeal ganglioneuroma. Report of a case diagnosed by fine needle aspiration. Acta Cytol 1993;37:552–4.
299. Lack EE. Pathology of adrenal and extra-adrenal paraganglia. Major problems in pathology, Vol 29. Philadelphia: WB Saunders, 1994.
300. Nassiri M, Ghazi C, Stivers JR, Nadji M. Ganglioneuroma of the prostate. A novel finding in neurofibromatosis. Arch Pathol Lab Med 1994;118:938–9.
301. Pachter MR, Lattes R. Neurogenous tumors of the mediastinum: a clinicopathologic study based on 50 cases. Dis Chest 1963;44:79–87.
302. Ricci A Jr, Callihan T, Parham DM, Green A, Woodruff JM, Erlandson RA. Malignant peripheral nerve sheath tumors arising from ganglioneuromas. Am J Surg Pathol 1984;8:19–29.
303. Shekitka KM, Sobin LH. Ganglioneuromas of the gastrointestinal tract. Relation to von Reckinghausen disease and other multiple tumor syndromes. Am J Surg Pathol 1994;18:250–7.
304. Stout AP. Ganglioneuroma of the sympathetic nervous system. Surg Gynecol Obstet 1947;84:101–10.
305. Wyman HE, Chappell BS, Jones WR Jr. Ganglioneuroma of bladder: report of a case. J Urol 1950;63:526–32.
306. Zarabi M, LaBach JP. Ganglioneuroma causing acute appendicitis. Hum Pathol 1982;13:1143–6.

Malignant Transformation of Ganglioneuroma

307. Chandrasoma P, Shibata D, Radin R, Brown LP, Koss M. Malignant peripheral nerve sheath tumor arising in an adrenal ganglioneuroma in an adult male homosexual. Cancer 1986;57:2022–5.
308. Banks E, Yum M, Brodhecker C, Goheen M. A malignant peripheral nerve sheath tumor in association with a paratesticular ganglioneuroma. Cancer 1989;64:1738–42.
309. Enzinger FM, Weiss SW. Soft tissue tumors. St. Louis: CV Mosby, 1988:828–31.
310. Fletcher CD, Fernando IN, Braimbridge MV, McKee PH, Lyall JR. Malignant nerve sheath tumor arising in a ganglioneuroma. Histopathology 1988;12:445–8.
311. Ghali VS, Gold JE, Vincent RA, Cosgrove JM. Malignant peripheral nerve sheath tumor arising spontaneously from retroperitoneal ganglioneuroma: a case report, review of the literature, and immunohistochemical study. Hum Pathol 1992;23:72–5.
312. Keller SM, Papazoglou S, McKeever P, Baker A, Roth JA. Late occurrence of malignancy in a ganglioneuroma 19 years following radiation therapy to a neuroblastoma. J Surg Oncol 1984;25:227–31.
313. Lack EE. Pathology of adrenal and extra-adrenal paraganglia. Major problems in pathology, Vol 29. Philadelphia: WB Saunders, 1994.
314. Ricci A Jr, Callihan T, Parham DM, Green A, Woodruff JM, Erlandson RA. Malignant peripheral nerve sheath tumors arising from ganglioneuromas. Am J Surg Pathol 1984;8:19–29.

Masculinizing Ganglioneuroma

315. Aguirre P, Scully RE. Testosterone-secreting adrenal ganglioneuromas containing Leydig cells. Am J Surg Pathol 1983;7:699–705.
316. Mack E, Sarto GE, Crummy AB, Carlson IH, Curet LB, Ulu J. Virilizing adrenal ganglioneuroma. JAMA 1978;239:2273–4.
317. Scully RE, Cohen RB. Ganglioneuroma of adrenal medulla containing cells morphologically identical to hilus cells (extraparenchymal Leydig cells). Cancer 1961;14:421–5.
318. Takahashi H, Yoshizaki K, Kato H, et al. A gonadotrophin-responsive virilizing adrenal tumour identified as a mixed ganglioneuroma and adreno-cortical adenoma. Acta Endocrinol 1978;89:701–9.

✧✧✧

Index

*Numbers in boldface indicate table and figure pages.